WITHDRAWN
WRIGHT STATE UNIVERSITY LIBRARIES

H. Franklin Bunn, M.D.
Professor of Medicine
Director of Hematology Research
Harvard Medical School
Brigham and Women's Hospital
Boston, Massachusetts

Bernard G. Forget, M.D.
Professor of Medicine
Chief of Hematology Section
Yale University School of Medicine
New Haven, Connecticut

Hemoglobin: Molecular, Genetic and Clinical Aspects

1986
W. B. Saunders Company

Philadelphia   London   Toronto   Mexico City   Rio de Janeiro   Sydney   Tokyo   Hong Kong

W. B. Saunders Company: West Washington Square
Philadelphia, PA 19105

Library of Congress Cataloging in Publication Data

Bunn, H. Franklin (Howard Franklin), 1935—

Hemoglobin—molecular, genetic, and clinical aspects.
1. Hemoglobinopathy. 2. Hemoglobin. I. Forget, Bernard G. II. Title. [DNLM: 1. Hemoglobins.
2. Hemoglobinopathies. WH 190 B942h]
RC641.7.H35B858 1986   616.1'5   83–14480
ISBN 0–7216–2181–3

Editor: John Dyson
Production Manager: Laura Tarves
Manuscript Editor: Karen McFadden
Illustration Coordinator: Walt Verbitski
Indexer: Susan Thomas

Hemoglobin: Molecular, Genetic and Clinical Aspects   ISBN 0-7216-2181-3

© 1986 by W. B. Saunders Company. Copyright under the Uniform Copyright Convention. Simultaneously published in Canada. All rights reserved. This book is protected by copyright. No part of it may be reproduced, stored in a retrieval system, or transmitted in any form or by any means, electronic, mechanical, photocopying, recording, or otherwise, without written permission from the publisher. Made in the United States of America. Press of W. B. Saunders Company. Library of Congress catalog card number 83-14480.

Last digit is the print number: 9   8   7   6   5   4   3   2   1

PREFACE

Hemoglobin is a beguiling molecule. Its accessibility and obvious biological importance continue to make it a subject of intense scrutiny. In their infancy, protein chemistry and molecular biology cut their teeth on hemoglobin. Indeed, a student can become reasonably well grounded in these disciplines by focusing solely on this protein. Hemoglobin has equal appeal for the clinician. Knowledge of its chemistry, physiology, and genetics provides insights into a broad array of disorders.

Nine years have elapsed since we wrote *Human Hemoglobins* in collaboration with Dr. Helen Ranney. In the interval, considerable progress has been made in understanding the hemoglobin molecule in its various guises. The recent explosion of information in molecular genetics began with a detailed exploration of the structure and expression of globin genes. This book includes a comprehensive discussion of the human globin genes and abnormalities in their expression, the thalassemias. In an effort to broaden the scope of this book, we have added a chapter on animal hemoglobins and their molecular evolution. The coverage of sickle hemoglobin has been expanded and split in two chapters, molecular and clinical. Finally, we have added new chapters on four other topics: the history of hemoglobin, the minor (but important) hemoglobin components, methemoglobin, and carboxyhemoglobin.

The book contains other features that we hope will aid in the digestion and assimilation of a diverse and sometimes bewildering bill of fare. The presentation of the structure-function relationships in human and animal hemoglobins has been embellished by the addition of a number of stereoscopic diagrams and models that allow the reader to gain a better grasp of important stereochemical interactions. The reader is urged to obtain a pair of stereo glasses in order to take advantage of this dividend.* A center section of color plates has been added that covers three diverse topics: molecular structure, blood morphology, and clinical features. Finally, we have attempted to "humanize" our book by including brief biographical sketches of some contemporary investigators who have made major contributions.

Thus, *Hemoglobin: Molecular, Genetic and Clinical Aspects* is an extension and expansion of *Human Hemoglobins*. We fully admit that a bigger book may not be a better one. It is likely that the current understanding of hemoglobin is approaching an apogee. Therefore, we believe that this book is timely and hope that it will be useful for both broad-based biologists as well as clinicians.

In preparing this book, we received an enormous amount of help. Karen McFadden has been a first-rate copy editor. She responded to all of our entreaties with enthusiasm and effective action. Maria Isikli provided superb secretarial assistance. Her common sense, good will, and verbal skills greatly facilitated the preparation of this book. Linda Boynton also provided excellent secretarial assistance.

---

*A compact stereo viewer (Stereopticon-707) can be purchased for $3.00 from Taylor Merchant Corporation, 212 West 35th Street, New York, New York 10001.

Richard Feldman and the Computer Graphics Division of the National Institutes of Health constructed many of the stereodiagrams that appear in this book.

The following colleagues provided valuable advice, information and/or graphic material: Gary Ackers, Jay Berzofsky, Thomas Bradley, Robert Broyles, Maurizio Brunori, Margaret Clark, Francis Collins, Carol Crowley, William Daniels, Virgil Fairbanks, Stuart Edelstein, Franklin Epstein, Morris Goodman, Eric Henry, Chien Ho, Ernst Jaffé, Lee Jampol, Danny Jue, Irving Klotz, Dominique Labie, Lawrence Lessin, Irving London, Paul Milner, Winston Moo-Penn, Ronald Nagel, Arthur Nienhuis, Constance Noguchi, Thalia Papayannopoulou, Jack Peisach, Max Perutz, Eliezer Rachmilevitz, Austen Riggs, Griffin Rodgers, Jean Rosa, Zelda Rose, Rose Schneider, Graham Serjeant, Boas Shaanon, Steven Shohet, Lawrence Solomon, L. W. Statius van Eps, Robert Terwilliger, David Todd, Ernst van Bruggen, Carola van Kapff, David Weatherall, Roy Weber, James White, and Ruth Wrightstone.

We are indebted to the following colleagues for thorough and incisive reviews of individual chapters:

Arthur Arnone	Donald Hultquist
Joseph Bonaventura	Martin Karplus
Robert Bookchin	Melisenda McDonald
Samuel Charache	Masako Nagai
Ronald Coburn	Orah Platt
John Edsall	Wendell Rosse
Robert Garlick	

Alan Schechter and Robin Carrell each read several chapters and provided a wealth of ideas and suggestions.

Two colleagues served as primary reviewers for the entire book. Each chapter was read with ruthless attention to detail and returned to us with reasoned and imaginative suggestions. Dave Ginsburg provided the response of the intelligent but uninitiated reader. He had an unflagging eye for errors and inconsistencies as well as deviations from clarity. Bill Eaton furnished expert commentary on nearly all aspects of this book. Many aspects of its organization and focus, as well as numerous details, are a direct reflection of his intellect, zest, and generosity.

Finally, we thank our families, who tolerated us during the past 3 years. To them we dedicate this book.

H. FRANKLIN BUNN AND BERNARD G. FORGET

CONTENTS

1
HISTORICAL BACKGROUND 1
   Determination of Hemoglobin Structure 4
   Hemoglobin Function 8

2
HEMOGLOBIN STRUCTURE 13
   Primary Structure 13
   Secondary Structure 18
   Tertiary and Quaternary Structure 19

3
HEMOGLOBIN FUNCTION 37
   The Bohr Effect 39
   Carbamino Formation 42
   Interaction with Inorganic Anions 44
   Interaction with Organic Phosphates 45
   Other Properties of Hemoglobin 47
   Properties of Isolated Chains 48
   Cooperativity 48
   How Does Hemoglobin Work? 51

4
HEMOGLOBINS A_2, F, AND A_{Ic} AND OTHER HUMAN HEMOGLOBIN COMPONENTS 61
   Hemoglobin A_2 61
   Embryonic Hemoglobins 67
   Hb F (Fetal Hemoglobin) 68
   Glycated Hemoglobins 75
   Other Post-Translational Modifications 82

5
OXYGEN AND CARBON DIOXIDE TRANSPORT IN HEALTH AND DISEASE 91
   Oxygen Transport 91
   Determinants of Blood Oxygen Affinity 95
   Metabolic Control of Red Cell 2,3-DPG 98
   Alterations of Oxygen Affinity in Various Clinical States 105
   Overall Significance of Erythrocyte Oxygen Affinity 115

6
ANIMAL HEMOGLOBINS ... 126
- Invertebrates ... 127
- Vertebrates ... 140

7
MOLECULAR GENETICS AND BIOSYNTHESIS OF HEMOGLOBIN ... 169
- General Processes Involved in Gene Expression and Protein Synthesis ... 169
- Normal Human Globin Gene Structure and Organization ... 172
- Process of Normal Globin Gene Expression ... 190
- Evolutionary Considerations ... 201

8
THE THALASSEMIAS: MOLECULAR PATHOGENESIS ... 223
- Studies of Globin-Chain Synthesis in Intact Thalassemic Erythroid Cells ... 225
- Early Molecular Biology Studies ... 228
- Functional Studies of Thalassemic Globin mRNA in Cell-Free Protein Synthesizing Systems ... 231
- Quantitative Studies of Globin mRNA and Gene DNA in Thalassemia by Molecular Hybridization and Other Assays ... 234
- Gene Mapping Using Restriction Endonuclease Digestion of Total Cellular DNA ... 246
- Characterization of Thalassemic Globin Genes by Gene Cloning, Nucleotide Sequence Analysis, and Expression Studies in Gene Transfer Systems ... 267
- Implications for Prenatal Diagnosis of Thalassemia ... 291
- Applications of Population Surveys and Analysis of Genetic Mechanisms ... 295
- Thalassemia-Like Disorders Associated with Structurally Abnormal Globin Chains ... 297
- Animal Models of Thalassemia ... 302
- Conclusions and Future Prospects for Gene Therapy ... 303

9
THE THALASSEMIAS—CLINICAL MANIFESTATIONS ... 322
- Historical Background ... 322
- Incidence and Population Genetics ... 323
- Pathophysiology of the Anemia in Thalassemia ... 324
- Classification of the Thalassemia Syndromes ... 327
- The Alpha-Thalassemia Syndromes ... 328
- The Beta Thalassemias ... 333
- $\gamma\delta\beta$ and γ Thalassemia ... 344
- δ Thalassemia ... 345
- Hereditary Persistence of Fetal Hemoglobin (HPFH) and Related Disorders ... 345
- Management of the Thalassemia Syndromes ... 350

10
HUMAN HEMOGLOBIN VARIANTS ... 381
- Detection of Hemoglobin Variants ... 382
- Clinical Classification ... 402
- Genetic Basis of the Hemoglobin Variants ... 403
- Assembly of Hemoglobin Variants ... 417
- Common Hemoglobin Variants ... 421

11
SICKLE CELL DISEASE—MOLECULAR AND CELLULAR PATHOGENESIS ... 453
- Historical Background ... 453
- Overview ... 455
- Structure of the Sickle Hemoglobin Fiber ... 455
- Polymerization of Sickle Hemoglobin ... 464

Polymerization in Intact Sickle Cells 474
The Membrane of Sickle Red Cells 484
Inhibition of Polymerization 490

12
SICKLE CELL DISEASE—CLINICAL AND EPIDEMIOLOGICAL ASPECTS 502
Historical Background 502
Epidemiology of the Sickle Gene 502
Sickle Cell Trait 508
Sickle Cell Disease 510
Sickling Disorders Other Than SS Disease 533
Prognosis 538
Treatment of Sickle Cell Disease 541
Prevention 550

13
UNSTABLE HEMOGLOBIN VARIANTS—CONGENITAL HEINZ BODY HEMOLYTIC ANEMIA 565
Introduction 565
Pathogenesis 566
Clinical Manifestations 579
Laboratory Diagnosis of CHBA 581
Treatment 586

14
HEMOGLOBINOPATHY DUE TO ABNORMAL OXYGEN BINDING 595
Molecular Pathogenesis 599
Properties of High-Affinity Variants 603
Physiological Aspects 609
Clinical Manifestations 611
Variants with Low Oxygen Affinity 614

15
M HEMOGLOBINS 623
Structure-Function Relationships 624

16
HEMOGLOBIN OXIDATION: METHEMOGLOBIN, METHEMOGLOBINEMIA, AND SULFHEMOGLOBINEMIA 634
Properties of Methemoglobin 635
The Oxidation of Hemoglobin 638
The Reduction of Methemoglobin 644
Pathophysiologic Considerations 649
Congenital Methemoglobinemia: Cytochrome b_5 Reductase Deficiency ... 650
Toxic Methemoglobinemia 653
Sulfhemoglobinemia 654

17
CARBOXYHEMOGLOBIN AND CARBOXYHEMOGLOBINEMIA 663
Sources of Carbon Monoxide 664
Carboxyhemoglobin: Structure and Function 665
Carboxyhemoglobinemia 668
Toxicity of CO 669

INDEX 677

HISTORICAL BACKGROUND*

1

In 1533, the Spanish theologian and divine Michael Servetus described how blood changes color as it passes through the lungs. Servetus was the first in Western Christendom to challenge Galen's ancient dogma that blood passed directly from the right ventricle of the heart to the left through invisible pores in the septum. Despite the crowning achievements recounted in "De Motu Cordis" (1628), William Harvey remained puzzled as to why blood is obliged to circulate through the lungs. He guessed that the lungs provided either a cooling or a nutritive function. A few years later, Marcello Malpighi, Professor of Theoretical Medicine at Pisa, proposed an alternative explanation: "I . . . believe that the lungs are made by nature for mixing the mass of blood."[4]

The relationship between air and blood awaited the dawn of a new science, chemistry, at the end of the Enlightenment. The great English experimentalist Robert Boyle (1627–1691) (Fig. 1–1) established the relationship between the volume and pressure of a confined gas. He demonstrated that an animal placed in an airtight chamber could not survive. He concluded that "there is in the air . . . a vital quintessence,"[5] necessary not only for life on earth but also in the sea: "Air lurks in water . . . and of it fishes may make some use when they strain the water through their gills."[5] A distinguished contemporary of Boyle, Richard Lower (Fig. 1–2), established beyond doubt that the function of the pulmonary circulation is the aeration of venous blood:

On this account it is extremely probable that the blood takes in air in its course through the lungs, and owes its bright colour entirely to the admixture of air. Moreover, after the air has in large measure left the blood again within the body and the parenchyma of the viscera, and has transpired through the pores of the body, it is equally consistent with

---

*The preparation of this chapter was greatly facilitated by three superb historical reviews, one by André Cournand[1] and two by John Edsall.[2,3]

1

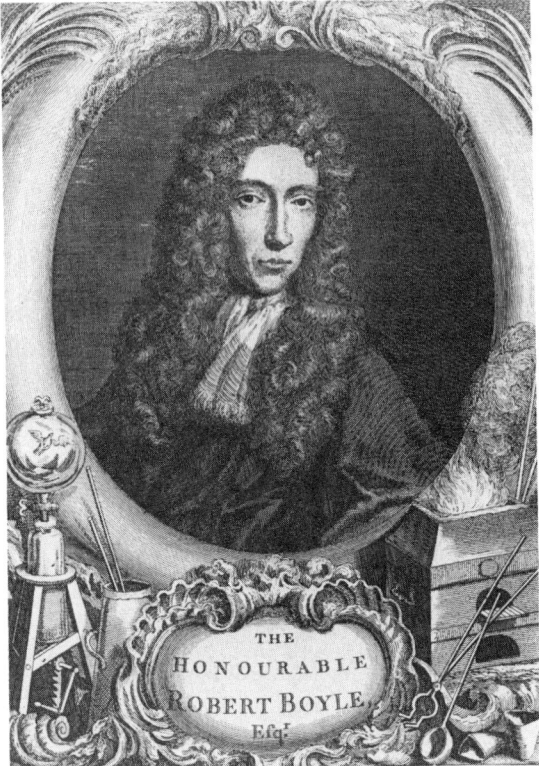

Figure 1–1. Robert Boyle. This portrait hangs in the Royal Society, London.

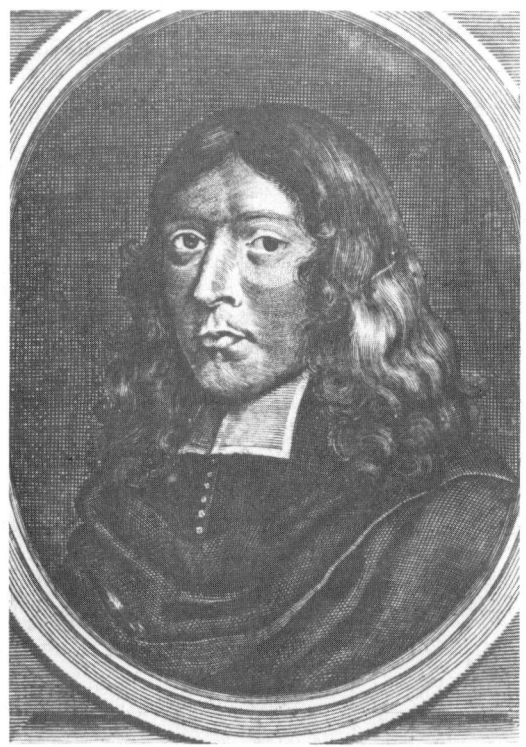

Figure 1–2. Richard Lower.

reason that the venous blood, which has lost its air, should forthwith appear darker and blacker.

From this it is easy to imagine the great advantage accruing to the blood from the admixture of air, and the great importance attaching to the air taken in being always healthy and pure; one can see, too, how greatly in error are those who altogether deny this intercourse of air and blood. Without such intercourse, any one would be able to live in as good health in the stench of a prison as among the most pleasant vegetation. Wherever, in a word, a fire can burn sufficiently well, there we can equally well breathe.[6]

Although the discovery of oxygen is credited to Priestly and Scheele, Antoine Laurent Lavoisier (Fig. 1–3) gained the first foothold on understanding its chemistry. He drew a logical analogy between the respiration of living animals and the combustion of inert substances: Oxygen is utilized, and carbon dioxide and water are produced.

Eminently respirable air that enters the lung, leaves it in the form of chalky aeriform acid [CO_2] . . . in almost equal volume. . . .

Respiration only acts on the portion of pure air that is eminently respirable . . . the excess, that is, its mephitic portion [nitrogen], is a purely passive medium which enters and leaves the lung . . . without change or alteration.

The respirable portion of air has the property to combine with blood and its combination results in its red color. . . .[7]

On the basis of what we know, and in limiting ourselves to simple ideas, that anyone can easily understand, we shall generally state that respiration is a slow combustion of carbon analogous to that operating in a lamp or in a lighted candle, and from this point of view animals which breathe are really combustible substances burning and consuming themselves.[8]

In 1799, Sir Humphrey Davy showed that blood contained more oxygen and carbon dioxide than could be explained by simple solution in a pure liquid. Thirty-seven years later, Gustav Magnus[9] demonstrated that arterial blood contained more oxygen and less carbon dioxide than venous blood.

The nature of the binding of oxygen to blood became a topic of considerable interest during the remainder of the nineteenth century. The central role of the red pigment of blood for binding oxygen was established by crude spectroscopic measurements. In 1862, Felix Hoppe (later known as Hoppe-Seyler) (Fig. 1–4) first used the term "hemoglobin" to describe this pigment. He observed the characteristic optical absorption of oxyhemoglobin.[10] Hoppe's work attracted the interest of George G. Stokes (Fig. 1–5), Luscasian Professor of Mathematics at Cambridge, who is best known for his work

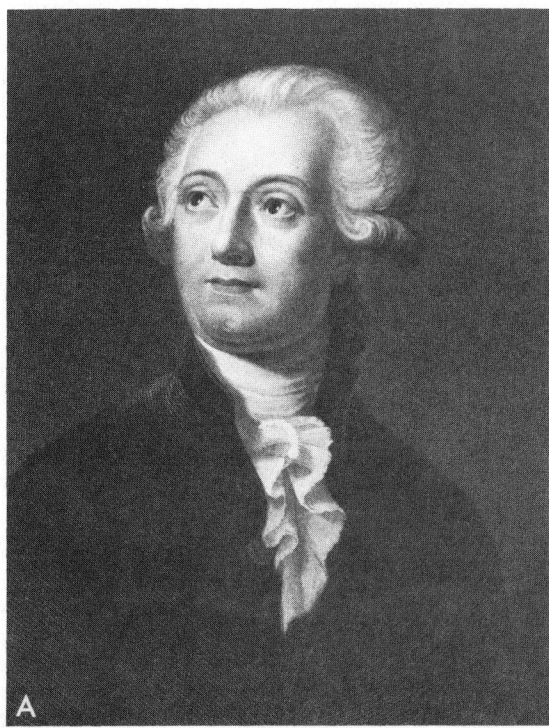
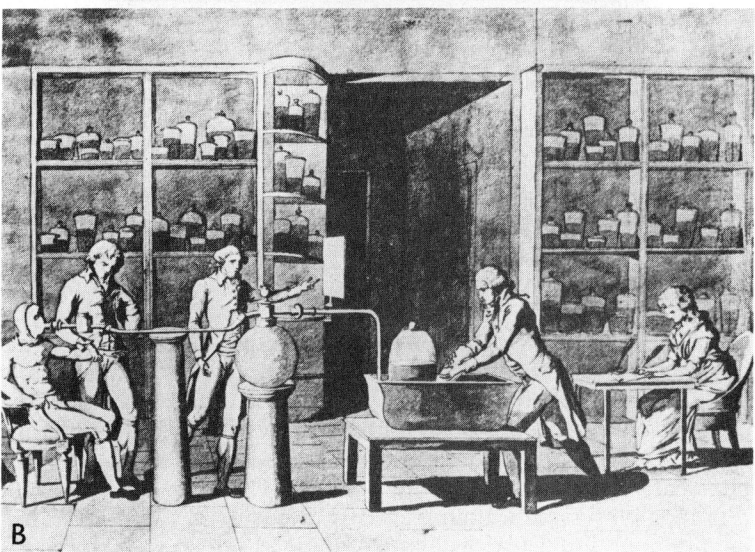

Figure 1–3. *A*, A. L. Lavoisier. *B*, Lavoisier in his laboratory studying the respiration of a human subject. (Drawn by Madame Lavoisier.)

on fluid mechanics. He noted a marked spectral change when oxygen was removed by chemical reduction with ferrous sulfate (Fig. 1–6).[11] The purple solution resumed its red color when re-exposed to oxygen:

I had no sooner looked at the spectrum, than the extreme sharpness and beauty of the absorption-bands of blood excited a lively interest in my mind, and I proceeded to try the effect of various reagents. . . . It seemed to me to be a point of special interest to inquire whether we could imitate the change of colour of arterial into that of venous blood, on the supposition that it arises from reduction. In my experiments I generally employed the blood of sheep or oxen obtained from a butcher; but Hoppe has shown that the blood of animals in general exhibits just the same bands. . . . The two highly characteristic dark bands seen before (oxyhemoglobin) are now replaced by a *single* band, somewhat broader and less sharply defined at its edges than either of the former, and occupying nearly the position of the bright band separating the dark bands of the original solution. . . . If the purple solution be exposed to the air in a shallow vessel, it quickly returns to its original condition, showing the two characteristic bands the same as before; and this change takes place immediately,

HISTORICAL BACKGROUND

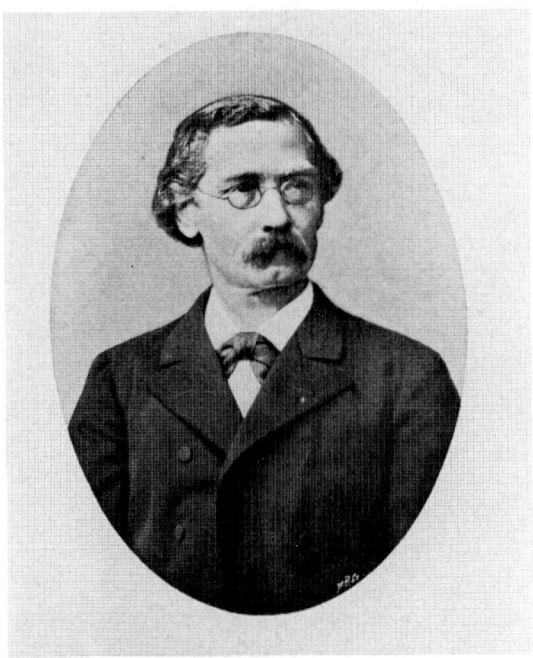

Figure 1–4. Felix Hoppe-Seyler.

provided a small quantity only of the reducing agent was employed, when the solution is shaken up with air. If an additional quantity of the reagent be now added, the same effect is produced as at first, and the solution may thus be made to go through its changes any number of times.

This experiment provided the first demonstration of reversible oxygen binding to hemoglobin.

Ten years earlier, Teichmann had separated heme from globin by treating blood with hot glacial acetic acid. He showed that the reddish-brown crystals, later called hemin, contained iron. A number of chemists independently demonstrated that the iron content of hemoglobin from various animals was about 0.33 per cent, a surprisingly accurate value. Thus, if hemoglobin were a homogeneous molecule, its minimum molecular weight would be about 16,600 daltons, an incredibly large molecule by standards of the late nineteenth century.

For a while, the nature of the interaction of hemoglobin with oxygen was a subject of lively debate. In 1908, Wolfgang Ostwald[12] advanced the hypothesis that the small oxygen molecules became adherent to the surface of the large hemoglobin molecule by some type of electrical attraction. About this time, Peters[13] (later Professor of Biochemistry at Oxford) began to make painstaking measurements of the oxygen and iron content of red cells. According to a method devised by J. S. Haldane (Fig. 1–7), heme iron was oxidized by the addition of an excess of ferricyanide. The oxygen that was quantitatively liberated could then be measured manometrically. A refinement of this technique developed by Van Slyke is still used for the precise measurement of oxygen content in blood. Elemental iron was measured after red cells had been carefully ashed. Peters obtained a mean value of 0.975 mole of O_2 per mole of iron. This stoichiometric relationship indicated that oxygen reacted with hemoglobin at specific sites on that molecule rather than through nonspecific absorption. However, there was still doubt as to whether hemoglobin was uniform in size or structure.

DETERMINATION OF HEMOGLOBIN STRUCTURE

With the explosive emergence of organic chemistry at the turn of the century, the iron-containing prosthetic group of hemoglobin attracted considerable interest. The structure of heme was established by Kuster in 1912.[14] Several years later, heme was synthesized in the laboratory of Hans Fischer.[15] This remarkable achievement permitted a detailed comparison of the natural and synthetic compounds, which were shown to be functionally identical. It soon became apparent that this particular porphyrin was the prosthetic group not only of hemoglobins of a wide variety of species but also of other respiratory proteins such as myoglobins and some of the cytochrome enzymes.

Various forms of hemoglobin were associated with specific absorption bands in the visible spectra. The development of adequate monochromators and photomultiplier tubes for the measurement of small differences in absorbed light permitted the detailed determination of the spectral properties of hemoglobin.[16, 17] The absorption spectra in the visible region were shown to be the most accurate and convenient measure of the binding of oxygen to hemoglobin. There was excellent agreement between spectrophotometric and gasometric measurements of oxygen binding to hemoglobin. The oxidation of hemoglobin to methemoglobin and the interaction of hemoglobin with various other heme ligands such as carbon monoxide and nitric oxide were also shown to result in characteristic alterations in the visible absorption spectra. Some of these are shown in Figure 1–6.

Once the nature of the prosthetic group of hemoglobin was known, a more complete understanding of its interrelationship with the protein globin was possible. Techniques for measuring the size of the hemoglobin molecule

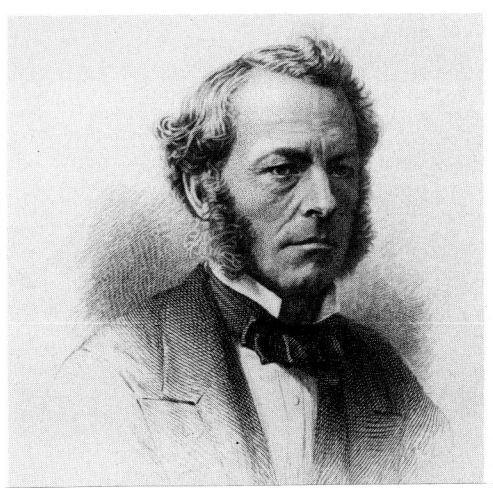

Figure 1–5. George G. Stokes.

did not become available until the 1920's. G. S. Adair (Fig. 1–8) became interested in hemoglobin while a student of Barcroft at Cambridge University. He was one of the first practitioners of a new discipline, biochemistry. Adair was well grounded in thermodynamics. He was one of the few investigators who was familiar with the writings of Willard Gibbs. He set about to determine the molecular weight of hemoglobin by means of osmotic pressure measurements[18, 19] (Fig. 1–8, middle panel). Solving the problem demanded not only a thorough understanding of physical chemistry but also meticulous experimental technique. He developed collodion membranes that were freely permeable to water and salts but not to hemoglobins. The rigor as well as the pace of the best science of that era is epitomized by

Figure 1–6. A, Reproduction of spectra of hemoglobin derivatives obtained by Stokes when viewing solutions with a light source and a prism. This figure is a direct reproduction from Stokes' paper.[11] "Fig. 1" is oxyhemoglobin. D and E represent absorption bands at 576 and 540 nm, respectively, in the spectrum shown below (B). "Fig. 2" is deoxyhemoglobin, showing a single band that corresponds to the 555-nm peak in the spectrum shown below. "Fig. 3" is methemoglobin, with the band between B and D corresponding to the 630-nm peak in the spectrum below. B, Absorption spectra of oxyhemoglobin, deoxyhemoglobin, methemoglobin, and cyanmethemoglobin.

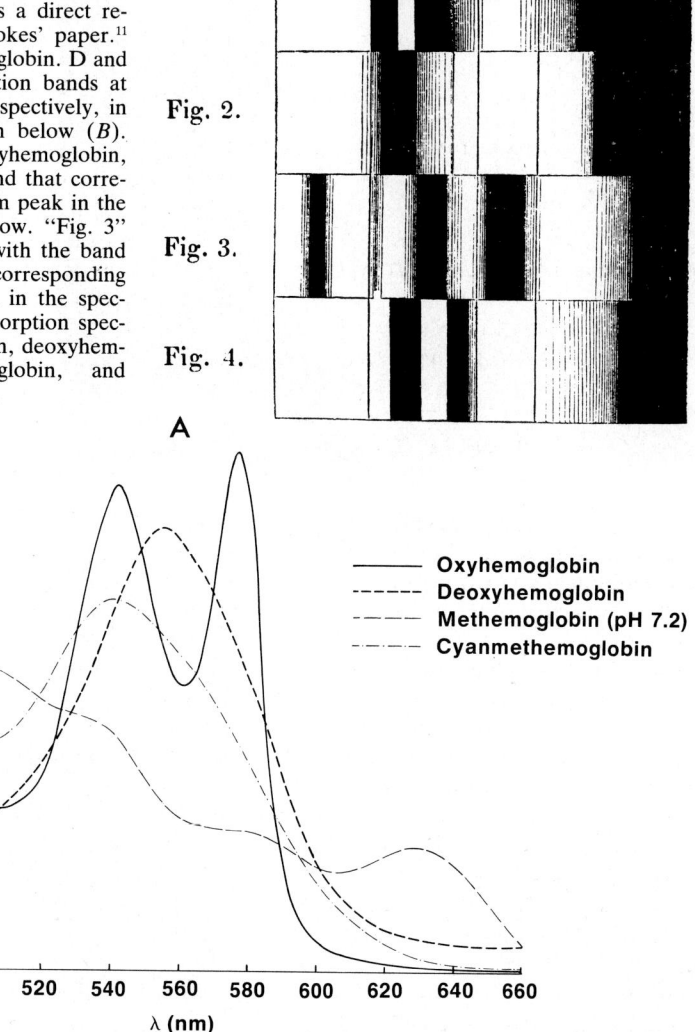

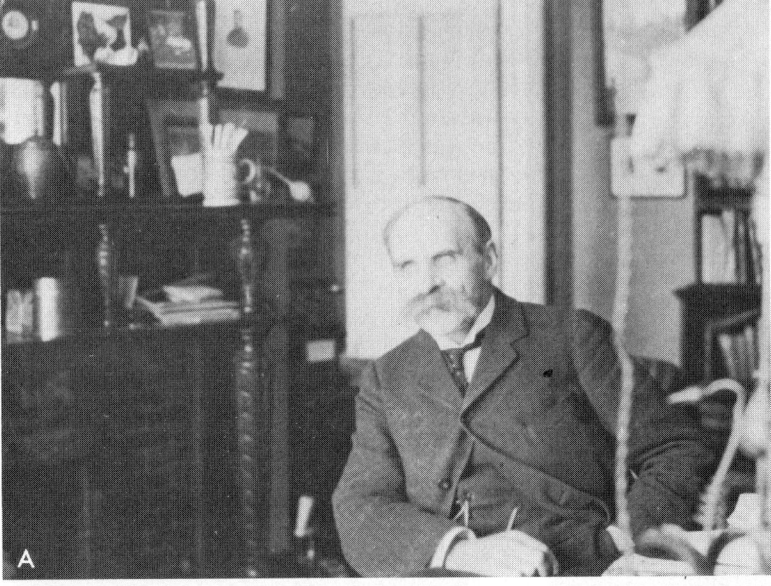
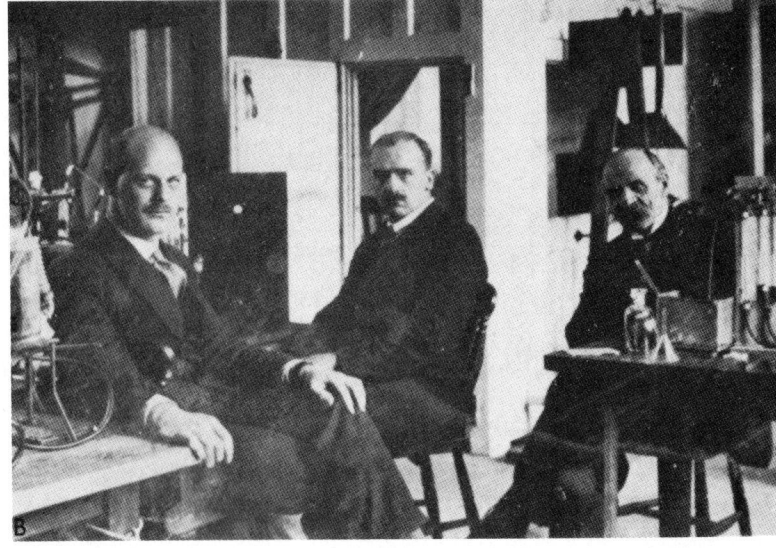

Figure 1–7. A, John Scott Haldane. *B,* John Scott Haldane (right) in his laboratory at Cherwell, North Oxford, with his son J. B. S. Haldane (center) and C. G. Douglas (left).

his statement that "after a few years' practice, the proportion of failures was below ten per cent."[18] Adair's patience reaped great rewards. To his astonishment along with that of his colleagues, his measurements indicated that hemoglobin had the staggering molecular weight of 67,000 daltons. A few years later, The Svedberg (Fig. 1–9) gave hemoglobin the honor of being the first protein to be analyzed by his newly developed technique, analytical centrifugation.[20] All of the vertebrate hemoglobins that he tested had a molecular weight of about 68,000 daltons, which was in complete agreement with the results of Adair. These estimates of molecular size strongly suggested that hemoglobin was likely to be a uniform molecule composed of four heme-containing subunits. As discussed in detail in Chapter 6, Svedberg went on to determine the molecular weights of many of the larger invertebrate hemoglobins. This rigorous and exhaustive body of information provided valuable insights into the nature of the polymeric respiratory proteins.

In contrast to the uniformity of the heme in vertebrate hemoglobins, comparisons of physical and chemical properties pointed to differences in the globin. Although hemoglobins in general were found to have identical absorption spectra in visible light, many differed in functional properties such as oxygen affinity. In 1866, Körber[21] had noted that hemoglobins differed markedly in their rates of denaturation in strong acid and alkali. His observation that

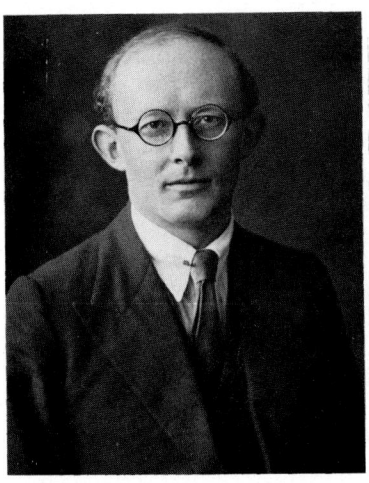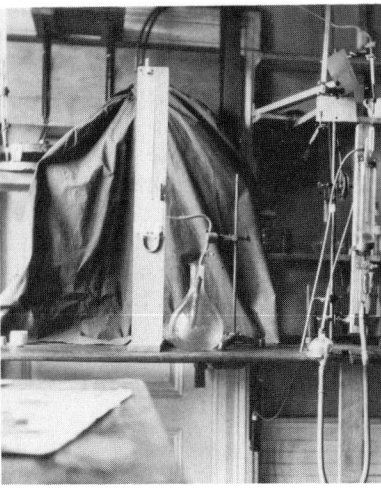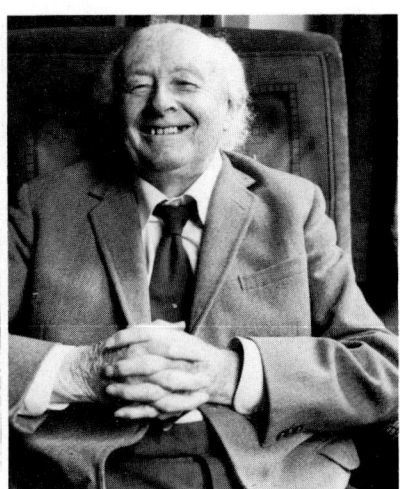

Figure 1–8. *Left,* Gilbert S. Adair at age 30. *Middle,* Photograph of Adair's apparatus for measuring osmotic pressure. *Right,* Adair at age 80.

the hemoglobin of human newborns is remarkably resistant to alkali denaturation provided the basis for the method of estimating fetal hemoglobin that is still widely used in clinical laboratories. Differences in the solubilities[22] and crystalline forms[23] of various mammalian hemoglobins were also noted. Titration of sulfhydryl groups showed that mammalian hemoglobins differed in cysteine content.[24, 25] From these considerations, it was anticipated that a great deal of heterogeneity existed among globins of various species, despite uniformity of size.

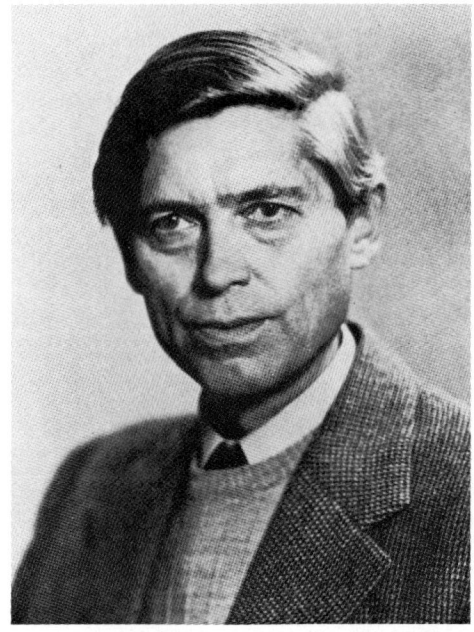

Figure 1–9. The Svedberg.

From the molecular weight of hemoglobin and its amino acid composition, it was apparent that the globin moiety contained approximately 580 residues. The presence of subunits was suspected because of the existence of four heme groups per molecule. A major breakthrough occurred in 1956, when Ingram[26] separated the peptides produced after globin had been hydrolyzed with the proteolytic enzyme trypsin, which cleaves polypeptides only at lysine and arginine residues. Although arginine and lysine account for 60 amino acid residues per mole of hemoglobin, only 30 tryptic peptides were obtained, strongly suggesting that hemoglobin consisted of two identical half molecules. Careful re-examination of N-terminal sequences of human globin by Rhinesmith, Schroeder, and Pauling[27] and by Braunitzer[28] revealed 2 moles of Val-Leu and 2 moles of Val-His-Leu per mole of globin. Taken together, the evidence thus indicated that hemoglobin was a tetramer composed of two pairs of unlike polypeptide chains, which were designated alpha and beta. It seemed reasonable to assume that each globin chain was attached to a heme group.

The advent of new and powerful methods for the determination of protein structure in the early 1960's allowed the structure of hemoglobin to be worked out over a very few years. Rapid progress was made on two fronts. First, techniques became available for the determination of primary amino acid sequences of the subunits of human and animal hemoglobins (see Chapters 2, 4, and 6). Second, Perutz and associates at Cambridge, England, successfully determined the three-dimensional structure of

HISTORICAL BACKGROUND

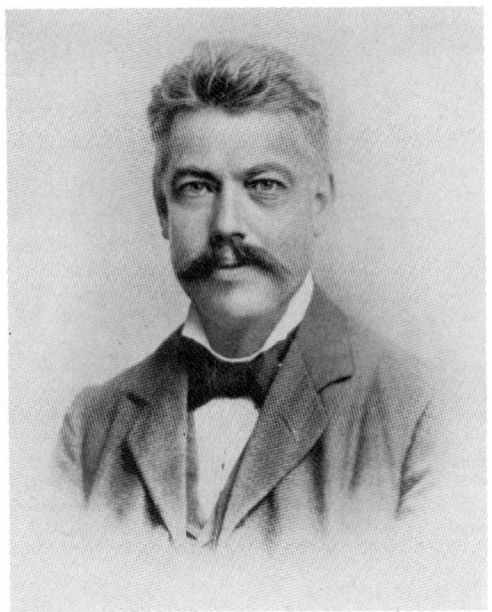

Figure 1–10. Christian Bohr.

oxyhemoglobin and deoxyhemoglobin. Many relevant observations preceded the elegant studies of Perutz. The crystalline forms of a variety of mammalian hemoglobins had been thoroughly catalogued.[23] Furthermore, it was known that the oxy and deoxy forms of horse hemoglobin differed in crystalline structure. Haurowitz[29] observed that when crystals of horse deoxyhemoglobin were exposed to oxygen, extensive disintegration (crazing) took place. These observations provided the first evidence that oxygenation results in a marked change in the conformation of hemoglobin and provided a strong incentive for Perutz to compare the three-dimensional structures of deoxyhemoglobin and oxyhemoglobin. It is not surprising that Perutz and Haurowitz were in close contact with one another because they are cousins-in-law. The solution of the three-dimensional structure of hemoglobin earned Perutz a Nobel Prize in 1962. During the past two decades, his laboratory has continued to define hemoglobin structure in greater detail, as described further in Chapter 2.

HEMOGLOBIN FUNCTION

The gradual accumulation of information on hemoglobin structure permitted increasing insights into its physiologic role in oxygen and carbon dioxide transport as well as its molecular mechanisms of action. This work began at the turn of the century, when the reversible binding of oxygen by hemoglobin was analyzed quantitatively by a group of distinguished physiologists, including Bohr and Krogh in Denmark, Barcroft and the elder Haldane in England, and Henderson in the United States.

In 1904, Christian Bohr (Fig. 1–10) wrote two important papers. In one, he presented the first data demonstrating the sigmoid shape of the oxyhemoglobin dissociation curve.[30] In the other, he showed that the position of the curve was sensitive to changes in carbon dioxide pressure.[31] As explained below, Bohr and associates are credited with establishing the relationship between pH and the oxygen affinity of hemoglobin. In addition, Bohr was the father of Niels Bohr, a pioneer in atomic

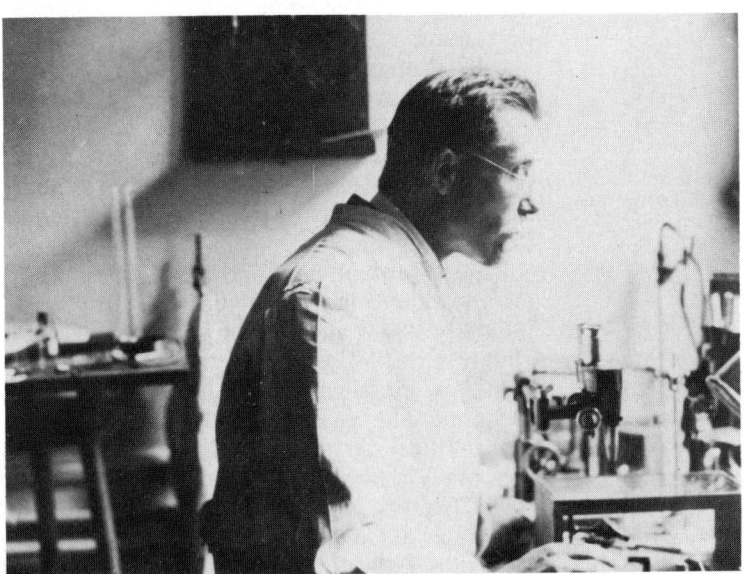

Figure 1–11. August Krogh.

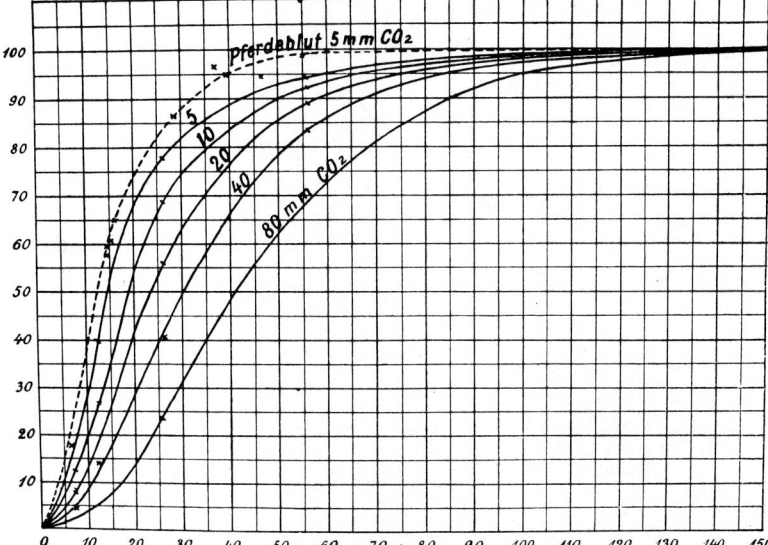

Figure 1–12. Experiment of Bohr, Hasselbalch, and Krogh[31] showing the effect of carbon dioxide tension on the binding of O_2 to hemoglobin. The ordinate scale shows the percentage of saturation of hemoglobin with O_2. The abscissa scale shows oxygen tension in mm Hg. Note that the experimental points demonstrate sigmoid binding. This figure was taken directly from the original paper of Bohr and associates.[31]

physics who first conceived of the planetary atom, and a grandfather of Aage Bohr, a recent Nobel laureate in physics. One wonders which of these achievements constitutes Christian Bohr's most important legacy.

Bohr's demonstration of the sigmoid shape of the oxygen binding curve did not receive unanimous acceptance. Painstaking chemical analyses by Gustav von Hufner[32] had helped to establish the stoichiometry of oxygen binding to the heme iron. Hufner made the reasonable assumption that oxygen reacts with hemoglobin by simple bimolecular combination:

$$Hb + O_2 \rightarrow HbO_2$$

He realized that such a reaction scheme required that the shape of the oxygen binding curve be a rectangular hyperbola. Hufner then obtained experimental data that indeed verified his prediction. His measurements on solutions of hemoglobin revealed hyperbolic O_2 binding with high affinity. Hufner also measured the molecular weight of hemoglobin by osmotic pressure and obtained a value of 16,000 daltons. In retrospect, some of Hufner's experimental results may be regarded as wishful thinking, attempts to make practice fit theory. The issue of the true shape of the oxygen binding curve remained controversial. If Hufner's approach to the problem was theoretical, Bohr's was strictly empirical. He was not beholden to any preconceived model of the oxygenation of hemoglobin. His primary aim was to obtain accurate data. To this end, he derived enormous benefit from the collaboration of his younger colleague, August Krogh (Fig. 1–11),* who designed a microtonometer that equilibrated blood and hemoglobin with various gas mixtures and measured the uptake of O_2 and CO_2. From these data, the sigmoid shape of the oxygen binding curve was clearly apparent (Fig. 1–12). The validity of this observation was not firmly established until Barcroft (Fig. 1–13) amassed a large and unassailable body of oxygen binding data. The

---

*Krogh went on to make important contributions in respiratory and circulatory physiology (see Chapter 5).

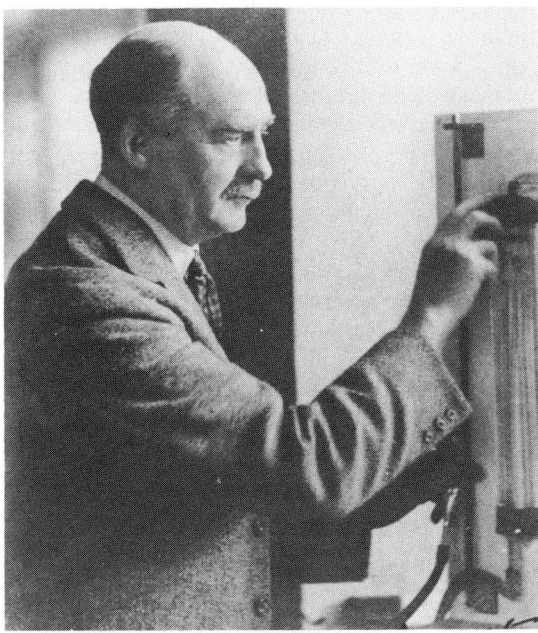

Figure 1–13. Sir Joseph Barcroft with the manometric device he developed for measuring the content of gases in blood.

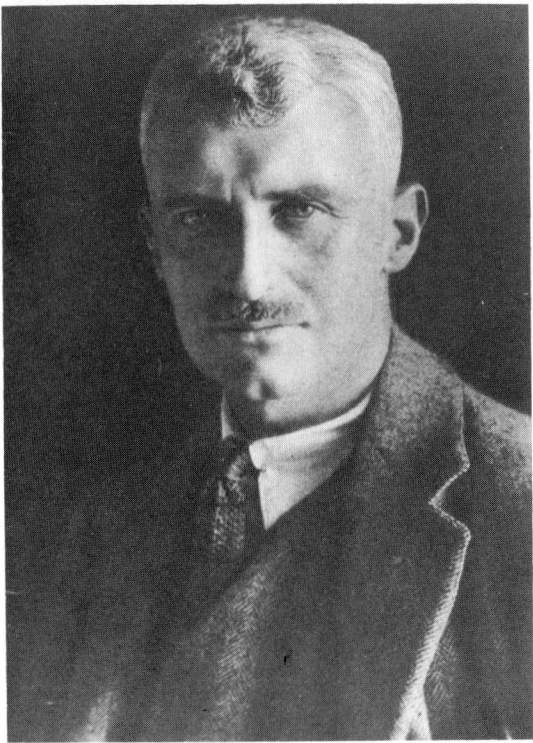

Figure 1–14. Archibald Vivian Hill.

precision of his measurements was greatly abetted by the use of improved gasometric methods for measuring the oxygen content of blood (described earlier). Barcroft and Peters showed unequivocally that not only oxygen but also carbon monoxide bound to hemoglobin in a sigmoid fashion.[33] The physiological significance of this phenomenon was not lost on these investigators. As J. S. Haldane (Fig. 1–7) stated so emphatically, "A man would die on the spot of asphyxia if the oxygen dissociation curve of his blood were suddenly altered so as to assume the form which Hufner supposed it to have in the living body."[34] The physical basis of the sigmoid curve attracted the attention of Archibald Vivian Hill (Fig. 1–14), who had just entered Barcroft's laboratory after completing a mathematics degree at Cambridge. He concluded that the sigmoid curve was best explained by the presence of aggregates of oxygen binding units of hemoglobin and interaction between members of these aggregates.[35] Thus, Hill was the first to envision cooperative behavior in a protein. These assumptions led to the following equation:

$$Y = Kp^n/(1 + Kp^n)*$$

---

*In Chapter 3 (p. 49), the same equation is expressed as $Y/(1 - Y) = Kp^n$.

where Y is the fractional saturation, p is the oxygen pressure, K is a constant, and n is the number of oxygen binding units in the aggregate. The Hill equation is remarkable because it made a prediction about subunit interactions in hemoglobin at a time when its molecular weight was a total mystery. One can imagine Hill's heightened curiosity, when in 1924 (as described previously), another student in Barcroft's laboratory, G. S. Adair, made the first accurate measurement of hemoglobin's molecular weight. The combination of precise structural and functional information allowed Adair to formulate a series of equations that define the binding of four successive ligands to the hemoglobin tetramer.[36] The Adair equations are still widely used in analyses of ligand binding to hemoglobin. The collective contributions of the Barcroft laboratory set the stage for a further half century of inquiry into the cooperative behavior of hemoglobin (see Chapter 3).

These early studies of oxygen binding to hemoglobin employed equilibrium measurements. In the 1930's, F. J. W. Roughton (Fig. 1–15) and H. Hartridge constructed a stopped-flow apparatus to measure the kinetics of oxygen binding[37] and dissociation.[38] In these initial studies, as much as one liter of sheep blood was needed to establish a single data point. These kinetic measurements yielded two important insights. First, Roughton and Hartridge showed that the rates of oxygen binding to and release from hemoglobin were signifi-

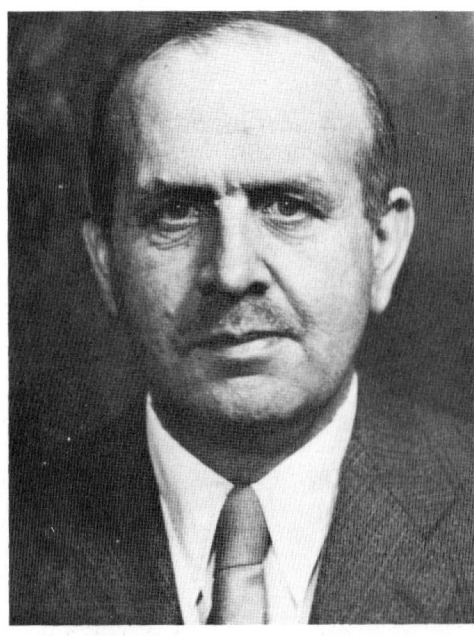

Figure 1–15. F. J. W. Roughton.

cantly faster than the circulation time of red cells through capillaries. Therefore, physiologic interpretations could safely be drawn from equilibrium measurements. Second, as explained in Chapter 3, kinetic measurements, employing both stopped-flow and flash photolysis,[39] provided independent information about the nature of partially liganded hemoglobin and the mechanism of cooperativity.

The growing body of structural and functional information on hemoglobin attracted the interest of Linus Pauling, the leading chemist of the mid-twentieth century. His prediction of the nature of the binding of oxygen to heme iron[40] was subsequently verified by elaborate spectroscopic probes. Moreover, Pauling was the first to view the cooperative behavior of hemoglobin as a chemical problem. He reasoned that the binding of oxygen to one of the heme groups in the tetramer imposed a structural alteration in the protein that makes the remaining hemes more avid for oxygen.[41] This can be considered the first allosteric model of hemoglobin function.

The demonstration by Bohr and colleagues[31] of the effect of carbon dioxide on oxygen binding to hemoglobin not only proved to be a phenomenon of clear-cut and general physiological significance (see Chapter 5) but also provided the first experimental evidence of a linked function in a protein. The growing body of information on the carbon dioxide-bicarbonate system for both buffering and excretion of acid allowed the Bohr-Hasselbalch-Krogh experiment to be interpreted. It became clear that the major effect of CO_2 on the oxygen affinity of hemoglobin was through its alteration in pH. Indeed, the pH dependency of oxygen affinity has become universally recognized as the Bohr effect, although one can make a strong case for giving Krogh an equal share of recognition. The Harvard physiologist L. J. Henderson (Fig. 1-16), along with Bohr's colleague, Hasselbalch, worked out the relationship between carbon dioxide tension and the concentrations of H^+ and HCO_3^-. Henderson was the first to perceive the basic linkage relationship between the interaction of oxygen and carbon dioxide with hemoglobin.[42] According to thermodynamic principles, if CO_2 tension affected oxygen binding to hemoglobin, the extent of oxygenation must have a reciprocal effect on CO_2 binding. Although earlier experiments that tested this relationship were equivocal, a definitive proof of the O_2-CO_2 linkage was provided by Haldane and colleagues.[43] Further experiments in a number of laboratories identified the precise role of

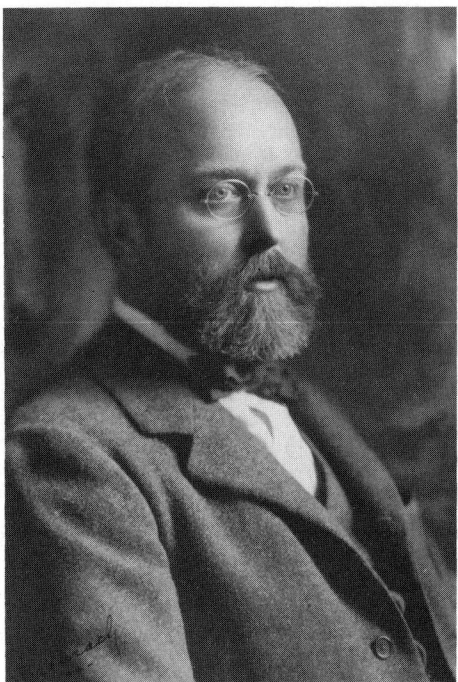

Figure 1–16. L. J. Henderson.

pH in binding O_2 and of oxygenation in binding protons. The direct contribution of CO_2 in the form of a weakly covalent carbamino complex was provided by F. J. W. Roughton and colleagues, who devoted a generation of painstaking effort to this problem. CO_2 and O_2 were shown to bind reciprocally to hemoglobin, just like protons and O_2. Detailed information on the physiological and chemical significance of complexes of protons and CO_2 with hemoglobin is provided in Chapter 3. More recently, intracellular organic phosphates, particularly 2,3-diphosphoglycerate, were also shown to interact with hemoglobin in a similar fashion.[44, 45]

As this brief chapter describes, the cumulative understanding of hemoglobin structure and function emerged spasmodically. The experiments that were so beautifully executed at the beginning of this century provided both immediate and compelling insights into oxygen and carbon dioxide transport and seeds of understanding of allosteric regulation of multisubunit proteins.

References

1. Cournand, A.: Air and blood. *In* Fishman, A. W., and Richards, D. W. (eds.): Circulation of the Blood, Men and Ideas. Oxford, Oxford University Press, 1964, pp. 3–70.
2. Edsall, J. T.: Blood and hemoglobin: The evolution

of knowledge of functional adaptation in a biochemical system. J. Hist. Biol. 5:205, 1972.
3. Edsall, J. T.: Hemoglobin and the origins of the concept of allosterism. Fed. Proc. 39:226, 1980.
4. Malpighi, M.: De Pulmonibus, Observationes Anatomicae. Bologna, 1661.
5. Boyle, R.: A Continuation of New Experiments Physico-Mechanical, Touching the Spring and Weight of the Air, and Their Effects—The Second Part. London, Flesher, 1682.
6. Lower, R.: Tractatus de Corde. Translated by K. J. Franklin. In Gunther, R. T.: Early Science at Oxford, Vol. IX. Oxford, Clarendon Press, 1932.
7. Lavoisier, A. L.: Expériences sur la respiration des animaux et sur les changements qui arrivent à l'air en passant par leur poumon. In Oeuvres, Tome II. Mémoires de chimie et de physique. Paris, Imprimerie Impériale, 1862, p. 174.
8. Lavoisier, A. L., and Seguin, A.: Premier mémoire sur la respiration des animaux. In Oeuvres, Tome II. Mémoires de chimie et de physique. Paris, Imprimerie Impériale, 1862, p. 688.
9. Magnus, G.: Ueber die im Blute enthaltenen Gase, Sauerstoff, Stickstoff and Kohlensaure. Poggendorff's Ann. Phys. Chem. 40:583, 1837.
10. Hoppe, F.: Über das Verhalten des Blutfarbstoffes im Spectrum des Sonnenlichtes. Virchows Arch. Path. Anat. Physiol. 23:446, 1862.
11. Stokes, G. G.: On the reduction and oxidation of the colouring matter of the blood. Proc. R. Soc. Lond. 13:355, 1864.
12. Ostwald, W.: Ueber die Natur der Bindung der Gase im Blut und in seinen Bestandteilen. Kolloidzeitschrift 2:264, 1907–08.
13. Peters, R. A.: Chemical nature of specific oxygen capacity of hemoglobin. J. Physiol. 44:131, 1912.
14. Kuster, W.: Beitrage zur Kenntnis des Bilirubins und Hämins. Hoppe-Seyler's Z. Physiol. Chem. 82:463, 1912.
15. Fischer, H., and Orth, H.: Die Chemie des Pyrrols, Pyrrolfarbstoffe. II. Erste Halfte. Leipzig Akadem. Verlagsgesellschaft, 1937, p. 372.
16. Drabkin, D. L.: Aspects of the oxygenation functions. In Roughton, F. J. W., and Kendrew, J. C. (eds.): Haemoglobin (Barcroft Symposium). New York, Interscience, 1949, p. 35.
17. Heilmeyer, L.: Spectrophotometry in Medicine. Translated by A. Jordan and T. L. Tippell. Glasgow, Maclehose, 1943.
18. Adair, G. S.: A critical study of the direct method of measuring the osmotic pressure of hemoglobin. Proc. R. Soc. 108A:627, 1925.
19. Adair, G. S.: The osmotic pressure of hemoglobin in the absence of salts. Proc. R. Soc. 109A:292, 1925.
20. Svedberg, T., and Nichols, J. B.: The application of the oil turbine type of ultracentrifuge to the study of the stability region of carbon monoxide hemoglobin. J. Am. Chem. Soc. 49:2920, 1927.
21. Körber, E.: Inaugural dissertation: Uber differenzen Blutfarbstoffes. Dorpat, 1866. Cited by Bischoff, H.: Z. Exp. Med. 48:472, 1926.
22. Jope, H. M., and O'Brien, J. R. P.: Crystallization and solubility studies on human adult and foetal haemoglobins. In Roughton, F. J. W., and Kendrew, J. C. (eds.): Haemoglobin (Barcroft Symposium). New York, Interscience, 1949, p. 269.
23. Reichert, E. T., and Brown, A. P.: The Differentiation and Specificity of Corresponding Proteins and Other Vital Substances in Relation to Biological Classification and Organic Evolution: The Crystallography of Hemoglobins. Washington, D.C., Carnegie Institute of Washington, Pub. No. 116, 1909.
24. Ingram, V. M.: Sulfhydryl groups in haemoglobins. Biochem. J. 59:653, 1955.
25. Allison, A. C., and Cecil, R.: The thiol groups of normal adult human haemoglobin. Biochem. J. 69:27, 1958.
26. Ingram, V. M.: A specific chemical difference between the globins of normal human and sickle cell anemia haemoglobin. Nature 178:792, 1956.
27. Rhinesmith, H. S., Schroeder, W. A., and Pauling, L.: A quantitative study of the hydrolysis of human dinitrophenyl (DNP) globin: The number and kind of polypeptide chains in normal adult human hemoglobin. J. Am. Chem. Soc. 79:4682, 1957.
28. Braunitzer, G.: Vergleichende Untersuchungen zur Primarstruktur der Proteinkomptonente einiger Hamoglobine. Z. Physiol. Chem. 312:72, 1958.
29. Haurowitz, F.: Das Gleichgewicht zwischen Hämoglobin und Sauerstoff. Hoppe-Seyler's Z. Physiol. Chem. 254:266, 1938.
30. Bohr, C.: Theoretische Behandlung der quantitativen Verhaltnis bei der Sauerstoffaufnahme des Hamoglobins. Abl. Physiol. 17:682, 1904.
31. Bohr, C., Hasselbalch, L., and Krogh, A.: Ueber einen in biologischer Beziehung wichtigen Einfluss, den die Kohlensäurespannung des Blutes auf dessen Sauerstoffbindung ubt. Skand. Arch. Physiol. 16:402, 1904.
32. Hufner, G.: Ueber das oxyhämoglobin des Pferdes. Hoppe-Seyler's Z. Physiol. Chem. 8:338, 1884.
33. Barcroft, J.: The Respiratory Function of the Blood. Part II. Haemoglobin. Cambridge, Cambridge University Press, 1928.
34. Haldane, J. S.: Respiration. 1st ed. New Haven, Connecticut, Yale University Press, 1922, p. 72.
35. Hill, A. V.: The possible effects of aggregation of the molecules of hemoglobin on its dissociation curve. J. Physiol. 40:4, 1910.
36. Adair, G. S.: The hemoglobin system. VI. The oxygen dissociation curve of hemoglobin. J. Biol. Chem. 63:529, 1925.
37. Hartridge, H., and Roughton, F. J. W.: The kinetics of haemoglobin. III. The velocity with which oxygen combines with reduced hemoglobin. Proc. R. Soc. A. 107:654, 1925.
38. Hartridge, H., and Roughton, F. J. W.: The kinetics of haemoglobin. II. The velocity with which oxygen dissociates from its combination with haemoglobin. Proc. R. Soc. A. 104:395, 1923.
39. Gibson, Q. H.: The photochemical formation of a quickly reacting form of haemoglobin. Biochem. J. 71:293, 1959.
40. Pauling, L., and Coryell, C. D.: The oxygen equilibrium of hemoglobin and its structural interpretation. Proc. Natl. Acad. Sci. USA 22:210, 1936.
41. Pauling, L.: The oxygen equilibrium of hemoglobin and its structural interpretation. Proc. Natl. Acad. Sci. USA 21:186, 1935.
42. Henderson, L. J.: Blood, A Study in General Physiology. New Haven, Yale University Press, 1928.
43. Christiansen, J., Douglas, C. G., and Haldane, J. S.: The absorption and dissociation of carbon dioxide by human blood. J. Physiol. 48:244, 1914.
44. Chanutin, A., and Curnish, R. R.: Effect of organic and inorganic phosphates on the oxygen equilibrium of human erythrocytes. Arch. Biochem. Biophys. 121:96, 1967.
45. Benesch, R. E., and Benesch, R.: The effect of organic phosphates from the human erythrocyte on the allosteric properties of hemoglobin. Biochem. Biophys. Res. Commun. 26:162, 1967.

HEMOGLOBIN STRUCTURE

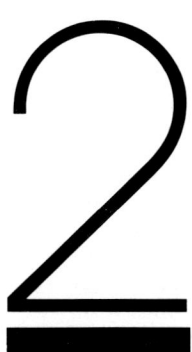

Solving the structure of hemoglobin has been one of the great triumphs of modern molecular biology. The historical events that led to this achievement are reviewed in the preceding chapter. In this chapter, we present detailed information on the primary as well as the three-dimensional structure of hemoglobin. This subject has direct bearing on all other topics that are covered in this book. Chapter 3 will discuss how structural information can be used to better understand hemoglobin's functional properties.

PRIMARY STRUCTURE

The globin of hemoglobin is a protein. Proteins are polymers consisting of amino acids arranged in specific linear sequence and linked by peptide bonds. The general structure of such a polypeptide polymer is

The "R's" represent the side groups of the 20 amino acid residues. These residues are building blocks used in the construction of proteins. There is convincing evidence that the primary amino acid sequence is the important determinant of the folding of the protein in three-dimensional space.[1] Proteins may be linked to carbohydrates (glycoproteins), lipids (lipoproteins), and specific functional prosthetic groups such as heme. The presence of groups such as these has an additional influence in determining the tertiary (and quaternary) structure of the protein and its functional properties.

Determination of Primary Sequence

Human hemoglobin A (Hb A) is generally designated $\alpha_2^A \beta_2^A$. Alpha chains also form stable tetramers with other hemoglobin chains differing in structure from the β chain. Hb F is $\alpha_2 \gamma_2$,

$$^+NH_3-\underset{R}{C}-\underset{\|}{\overset{O}{C}}-NH-\underset{R}{C}-\underset{\|}{\overset{O}{C}}-NH-\underset{R}{C}-\underset{\|}{\overset{O}{C}}---NH-\underset{R}{C}-\underset{\|}{\overset{O}{C}}-NH-\underset{R}{C}-\overset{O}{C}O^-$$

13

MAX PERUTZ

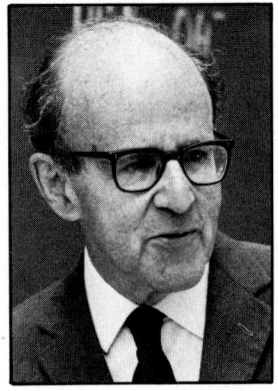

Making a discovery is such a wonderful thing. It's like falling in love and getting to the top of the mountain all in one. When you get to the top after a hard climb, a view of a new landscape opens before you.

If the hemoglobin story has a hero, it is Max Perutz. In 1936, Perutz left his native Austria to pursue a Ph.D. degree at the Cavendish Laboratory in Cambridge. He became a pupil of J. D. Bernal, an Irishman of extraordinary breadth and vision, whose scientific mission was analyzing protein crystals by x-ray diffraction, and later of W. L. Bragg, director of the Cavendish Laboratory and a founding father of x-ray crystallography.

Perutz got the idea of studying hemoglobin from discussions with his cousin-in-law Felix Haurowitz, a biochemist in Prague. Thus began a 20-year quest. Perutz obtained perfect crystals of horse hemoglobin from G. S. Adair (see Fig. 1–8) and soon developed beautiful x-ray diffraction patterns. He attempted to solve the three-dimensional structure by the Patterson method, but this approach proved to be inadequate for such a complex irregular molecule. With the encouragement of Bragg, Perutz pursued the problem doggedly throughout the next decade. He was confounded by the great difficulty of solving the phase problem (see text of this chapter). In 1953, Austen Riggs, then at Harvard, sent Perutz a reprint of a paper showing that hemoglobin, modified by having two atoms of mercury linked to its two reactive sulfhydryl groups, had nearly normal oxygen binding properties. This provided a way of putting an electron-dense atom into the molecule without disturbing its overall conformation. The use of isomorphous replacement not only enabled Perutz to solve the phase problem in hemoglobin but also proved crucial in the subsequent analysis of other proteins. This breakthrough enabled Perutz to determine the three-dimensional structure of methemoglobin in 1959, for which he won the Nobel Prize in Chemistry. Bragg wrote to Bernal, "I've just been over to see the three dimensional map of hemoglobin that Max had calculated. It seems amazing that diffraction effects should reveal the position of atoms in such a maze." Three years later, Perutz solved the structure of deoxyhemoglobin and showed how oxygen binding dramatically alters the conformation of hemoglobin.

Continued refinement of the two hemoglobin structures over the next decade enabled Perutz to explain critical functional properties, including the Bohr effect, interaction with organic phosphates, and cooperative oxygen binding. This structural information also provided insights into the properties of hemoglobin variants that are responsible for various clinical disorders (see Chapters 10 to 15). In recent years, Perutz has employed a number of other biophysical probes to better understand how the binding of oxygen to the heme iron triggers the conformational changes that underlie hemoglobin's cooperative behavior. He continues to spend the bulk of his time at the laboratory bench.

Perutz has given us another legacy of untold importance. He was the founder and, for nearly 20 years, the director of the Medical Research Council (MRC) Laboratory of Molecular Biology in Cambridge. This institute and its forerunner at the Cavendish Laboratory, more than any other, spawned the development of molecular biology. The impetus for its creation was the vision of Bernal, who in the 1930's foresaw that knowledge of the structure of living molecules would lead to an understanding of their function. The MRC laboratory, modest by current-day standards of cost and size, provided an exciting arena where Perutz along with Crick, Watson, Brenner, Ingram, Kendrew, Klug, and a number of other distinguished scientists could work and talk to one another.

Perutz remains the leading apostle of the new biology. His extraordinary energy and involvement lead him to many international meetings in which he participates with full enthusiasm. Priority is given to locations convenient to skiing and mountain climbing. He is a gifted teacher and generous colleague. The contents of this book are in large measure a reflection of his contributions.

and Hb A_2 is $\alpha_2\delta_2$. These hemoglobins are discussed in Chapter 4. Before a detailed analysis of hemoglobin structure could be undertaken, it was necessary to isolate the constituent polypeptide chains. The human α and non-α chains differ widely in their isoelectric points and therefore can be readily separated by methods dependent on differences in the overall surface charge of the protein. For initial structural work, human α and β chains were separated by countercurrent distribution.[2] Subsequently, a much more convenient and effective method of chain separation was developed[3,4] using ion-exchange chromatography in the presence of a high concentration of urea.

Establishment of the primary sequence of normal human globin chains was due in large part to contributions from the laboratories of Braunitzer in Munich, Konigsberg and Hill in New York, and Schroeder in Pasadena. Their basic methodological approach, outlined here, is still employed in the determination of the primary structure of protein subunits. Isolated chains are digested with an enzyme to break them up into smaller peptides. Trypsin, the most generally used of these enzymes, cleaves the polypeptide chain specifically on the carbonyl side of lysine and arginine residues. Thus, the number of peptides obtained is dictated by the number of lysine and arginine residues in the chain. Except for the C-terminal peptide, the other peptides will have one of these two residues at their C terminus.

Ingram[5] analyzed globin peptides by means of *fingerprinting*. The enzyme digest is spotted on filter paper and separated by high-voltage electrophoresis. Then the peptides are further separated from one another by paper chromatography done at a 90-degree angle to the electrophoresis. After appropriate staining, a two-dimensional pattern appears, consisting of a spot for each peptide. This pattern is reproducible for a given globin chain under defined experimental conditions, hence the term "fingerprint." A fingerprint of a tryptic digest of the β chain of human hemoglobin is shown in Figure 2–1. Alternatively, peptides can be separated by ion-exchange column chromatography.[6] Individual peptides are then eluted from the fingerprint (or the column). The total amino acid composition (but not the sequence)

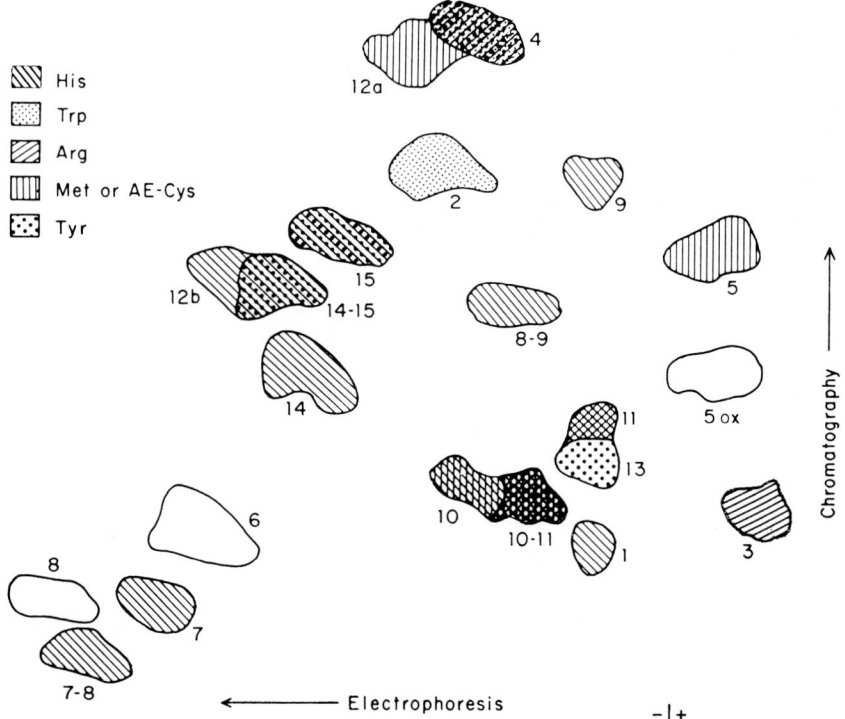

Figure 2–1. Two-dimensional peptide map (fingerprint) of normal human β chain. The purified β chain was digested with trypsin and then applied to a small spot in the lower right hand corner. After the peptides were separated by electrophoresis (horizontal direction), they were separated further by ascending chromatography. The peptides can be identified by a Ninhydrin stain. They are numbered sequentially from the N-terminal peptide (1) to the C-terminal peptide (15). The key shows how special stains can be used to detect peptides containing histidine, tryptophan, arginine, sulfur-containing amino acids, and tyrosine. (From Stamatoyannopoulos, G., et al.: J. Clin. Invest. 52:342, 1973.)

16 HEMOGLOBIN STRUCTURE

is determined following hydrolysis of the peptide bonds in strong acid.

The amino acid sequence of individual peptides can be determined by Edman analysis, which removes residues in order, beginning at the N terminus. This analytical approach has been completely automated and permits sequencing of polypeptide chains up to 60 residues in length. Alternatively, the structure of peptides can be partially or completely established by digestion with carboxypeptidase, which cleaves amino acid residues sequentially at the C terminus.

Finally, the order of the peptides in the

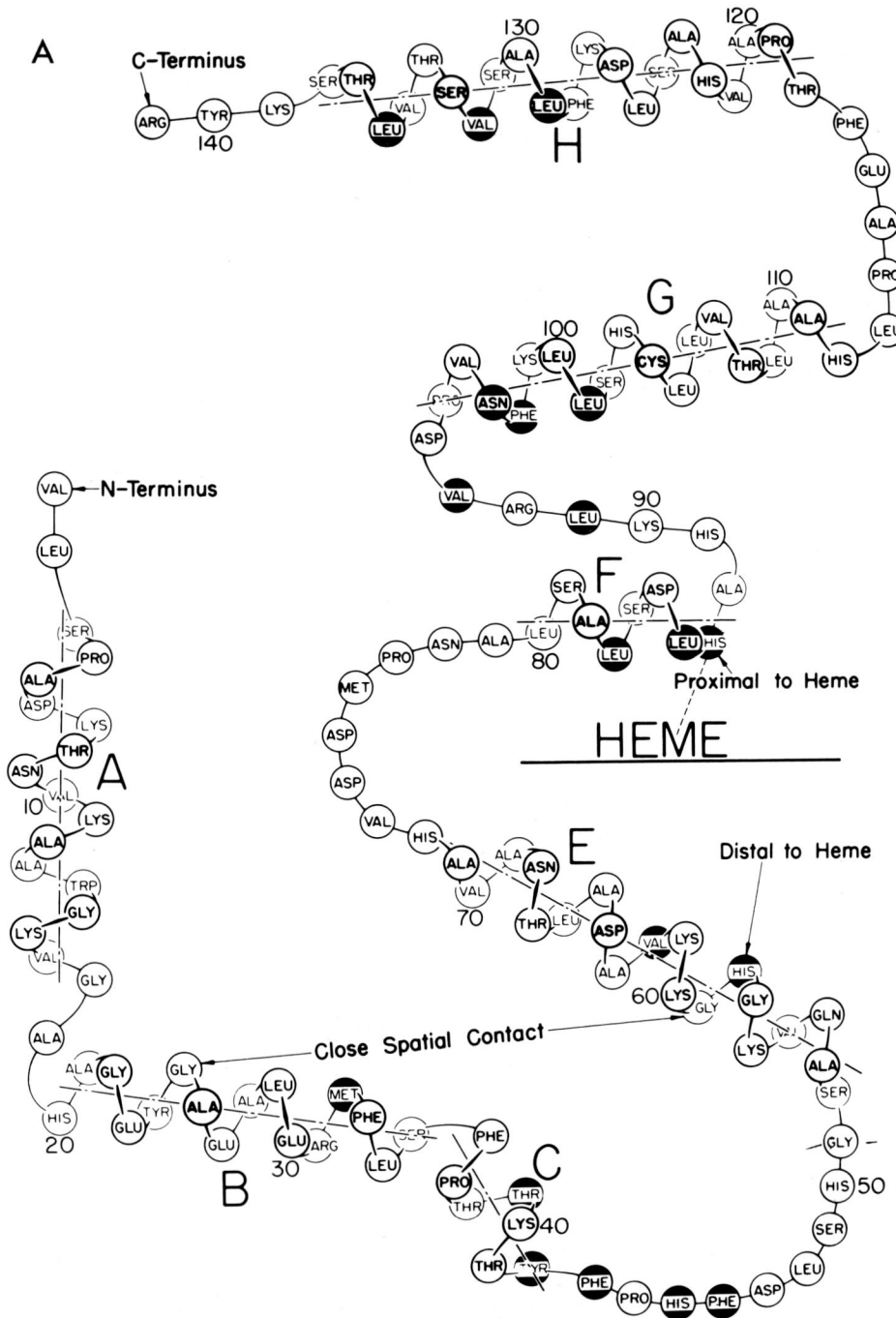

Figure 2–2. A, Primary structure of the α chain. The α-helical segments are shown by large capital letters. The half black circles indicate residues in contact with the heme.

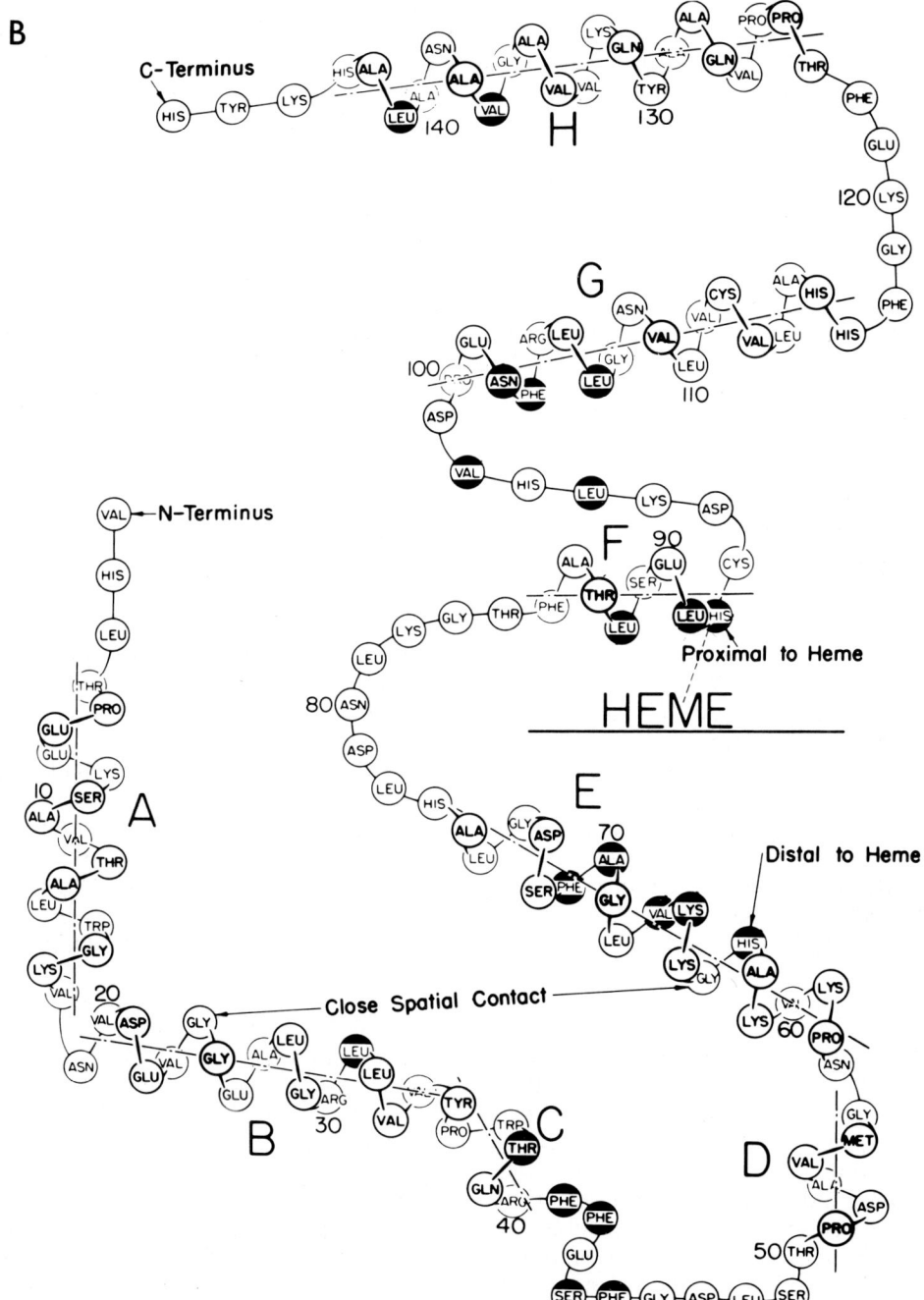

Figure 2-2 *Continued. B,* Primary structure of the β chain. (From Huisman, T. H. J., and Schroeder, W. A.: New Aspects of the Structure, Function, and Synthesis of Hemoglobins. Boca Raton, Florida, CRC Press, 1971.)

chain must be determined. This can be done by structural analyses of peptides formed by other enzymes that attack the protein at alternate sites. For example, the overlapping peptides formed by pepsin and chymotrypsin, as well as trypsin, were analyzed in working out the structure of human α and β chains.

The determination of the primary amino acid sequence of proteins resembles the challenge of solving a complex but ultimately logical jigsaw puzzle. Once the structure of normal human α, β, γ, and δ chains was established, the analysis of hemoglobin variants became much less formidable, because these generally represent single amino acid replacements. Therefore, a fingerprint of the variant subunit usually reveals the displacement of only one of the tryptic peptides, and attention is directed to this peptide.

With the advent of the new technology of molecular genetics, the primary structure of many proteins can now be solved by determining the base sequence of the corresponding mRNA or DNA. This approach is as reliable as classic amino acid sequencing but is less labor-intensive and, therefore, should be useful in determining the primary structures of various animal hemoglobins that have not yet been analyzed. This information will provide valuable insights into phylogenetic relationships and molecular evolution (see Chapters 6 and 7).

Primary Structure of Human Globin Subunits

α Chain

The human α chain consists of 141 amino acids in linear sequence. Its primary structure is shown in Figure 2–2A. As this figure indicates diagrammatically, the heme group is bound covalently by a linkage between the heme iron and the imidazole of a histidine residue at position 87 (counting from the N-terminal end of the polypeptide). This is the so-called proximal histidine. A more detailed treatment of the heme-globin linkage will be presented at the end of this chapter.

β Chain

The β chain is slightly longer than the α chain (146 residues). Its primary structure is shown in Figure 2–2B. Heme binds at β His 92. Unlike many other proteins, such as gamma globulin, ribonuclease, or insulin, there are no disulfide bridges (cystine residues) either within or between hemoglobin subunits. The cysteine residue at position 93 of the β chain is highly reactive and readily undergoes oxidation to form mixed disulfides and other thio ethers. This phenomenon may be involved in hemoglobin catabolism and will be discussed in Chapter 13, Unstable Hemoglobin Variants.

δ, γ, ε, and ζ Chains

The primary sequences of the other human globin chains are shown in Table 4–1. It is clear that there is considerable structural homology between δ, γ, ε, and β chains. Indeed, these are the products of tandem genes located on chromosome 11 (see Chapter 7). In like manner, the ζ chain is homologous with the α chain. They are products of tandem genes on chromosome 16. Chapter 4 contains information on the hemoglobins that are composed of these subunits.

SECONDARY STRUCTURE

The amino acid sequence is the primary determinant of how a protein is arranged in three-dimensional space. Secondary structure refers to the spatial relationship between residues that are close to one another in the linear sequence. Segments of polypeptide chains can be stabilized by folding into one of two regular conformations: the α helix and the β pleated sheet. Some insoluble fibrous proteins such as keratin or myosin are in the form of an α helix, whereas others such as silk fibroin are in the form of a β pleated sheet. Collagen, which is rich in proline and hydroxyproline, cannot form either structure and has its own unique secondary structure. Soluble globular proteins can be divided into four classes:[7] those consisting of only α-helix secondary structure; those formed from only β-sheet secondary structure; those composed of α-helix and β-sheet secondary structures that are spatially segregated; and those having alternating segments of α-helix and β-sheet secondary structure. The subunits of hemoglobin are good examples of an all α-helix folding pattern. The structure of the α helix was elucidated by Pauling and Corey.[8] It consists of a single-stranded helix or coil with 3.6 amino acid residues per turn (Fig. 2–3). The side groups of the residues are oriented externally in a radial fashion. The helix is stabilized by hydrogen bonding between the carbonyl group of each residue and the amino group four residues away.

In its native state, about 75 per cent of the hemoglobin molecule is α-helical. This relatively high helical content in comparison to other globular proteins simplified the solution of the three-dimensional structure of hemoglobin. Upon the removal of heme, the helical content of globin decreases to about 50 per cent.[9] At specific locations in the hemoglobin subunits, the α helix is interrupted by segments that lack a helical configuration. At these sites, the polypeptide chain can turn corners, accounting for the complex convoluted three-dimensional structures of hemoglobin and myoglobin. In some segments of the polypeptide chains, the interruption of the α helix is due to the presence of proline, which is unable

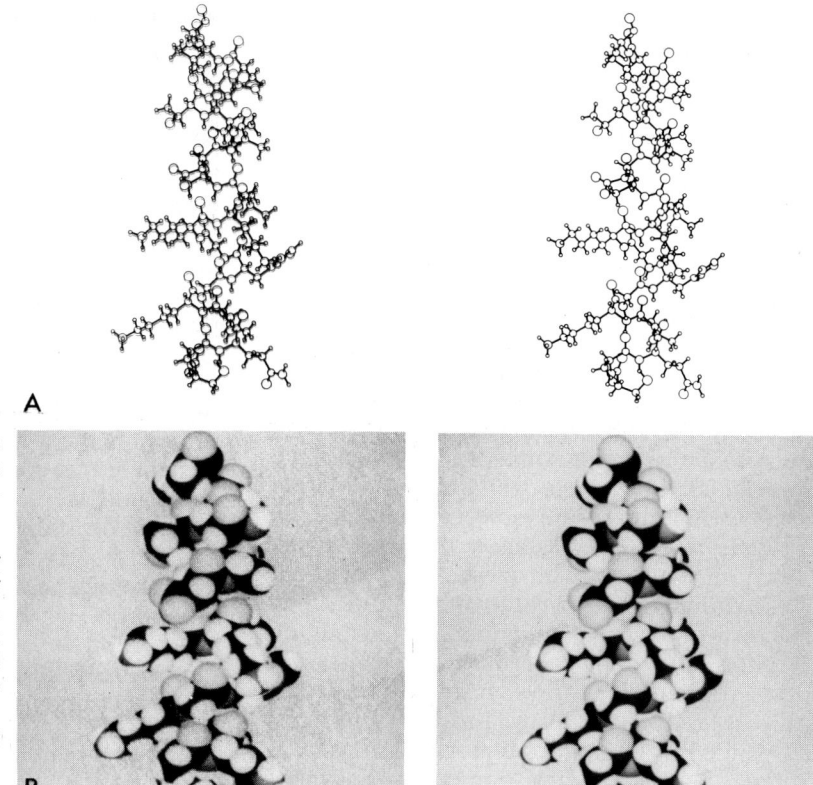

Figure 2–3. *A* and *B*, Stereo views of the E helix of the α chain. The sequence is N-Ser-Ala-Gln-Val-Lys-Gly-His-Gly-Lys-Lys-Val-Ala-Asp-Ala-Leu-Thr-Asn-Ala-C (see Figure 2–2*A*). The N end of the helix begins at the bottom of the figure and spirals upward as a right handed (clockwise) α helix toward the top (C end). *A*, Ball and stick model. The atoms are shown in proportion to their size; O > N > C > H. *B*, Space-filling model of the same structure. (Courtesy of Richard Feldman, National Institutes of Health.)

to participate in this configuration except at the first three residues from the N-terminal end.

During the investigation of the three-dimensional structures of hemoglobin and myoglobin by x-ray crystallography, Perutz and associates realized that the individual subunits of hemoglobin and myoglobin showed striking conformational similarities. They concluded that these protein subunits probably had analogous helical segments. The β subunit was shown to have eight helical segments, lettered A through H. The helical segments of the α chain are closely comparable to those of the β chain, but the residues making up the D helix of the β chain are absent in the α chain. Accordingly, amino acid residues in these subunits can be assigned helical designations. For example, the "proximal" or heme-linked histidine is F8 (see Fig. 2–2). When these chains are aligned according to their helical designations, maximal homology between subunits is apparent (see Table 4–1).

Chapter 6, in which the structure and function of animal hemoglobins are discussed, contains information on the homology between hemoglobin subunits of different species. With few exceptions, residues that are particularly important to hemoglobin function are shared by a diverse group of animals. Each of these invariant residues can be identified by its helical designation.

TERTIARY AND QUATERNARY STRUCTURE

X-Ray Crystallography

The information contained in the primary and secondary structure of the globin subunits provides very little insight into how hemoglobin works. An understanding of a protein's functional properties depends on detailed knowledge of its three-dimensional structure, namely the position of all of its atoms in three-dimensional space. Tertiary structure refers to the steric relationships of amino acid residues that are far apart in the linear sequence. Quaternary structure refers to the way in which the subunits are packed together. The three-dimensional structure of molecules can be determined from the x-ray diffraction patterns of their crystals. At present, the tertiary and quaternary structures of oxyhemoglobin and deoxyhemoglobin have been solved by x-ray crystallography with such a high degree of resolution (2.0 to 2.5 Å) that almost all of the nonhydrogen atoms of this complex molecule can be positioned with an accuracy of 0.5 Å or better. This remarkable achievement can be attributed entirely to Max Perutz and associates at the Medical Research Council Laboratory in Cambridge, England.

Principles of X-Ray Diffraction

The elucidation of the three-dimensional crystal structure of a macromolecule by x-ray diffraction can be viewed as analogous to the reconstruction of an image from microscopic sections. The theoretical resolution limit of a microscope is approximately equal to the wavelength of the electromagnetic radiation used to illuminate the object. Therefore, in order to resolve the distances between atoms, x-rays must be used with a wavelength of about 1 Å. Although, in theory, x-ray crystallography is a form of microscopy, in practice the method is difficult to apply because no one has yet devised a lens for x-rays. Instead, the procedure is as follows: A well-formed crystal is suspended in its mother liquor. The crystal is rotated in a beam consisting of parallel monochromatic x-rays. The rays are diffracted by the crystal in the same way that an optical grating diffracts visible light. The diffracted rays either are collected on a photographic plate, giving a geometric pattern of spots of varying intensities, or are analyzed individually by means of a diffractometer. At certain angles, x-rays penetrating planes of the crystal are mutually reinforced and result in geometrically ordered spots radiating from the x-ray beam. This phenomenon is expressed quantitatively by Bragg's law: $\lambda = 2d \sin \theta$, where θ is the angle of the incident rays, d is the distance between planes, and λ is the wavelength. The amount of scattering of the x-rays depends on the number of electrons encountered by the beam. Accordingly, the relative intensity of the spots is a function of electron density within the unit cell of the crystal. From the amplitudes and phase angles of all diffracted rays, the coordinates of the atoms in the unit cell can be calculated by means of a mathematical operation known as a Fourier summation, the solution of which is greatly facilitated by the use of a computer. The computer is in effect the lens of the "x-ray microscope." The results generated from Fourier summations can be expressed in terms of contour maps that reflect electron density in a given plane. (For an example, see Figure 2–10.)

Application to Hemoglobin

The central problem in solving the structure of complex molecules is the determination of the phase angles of the diffracted x-rays. In their analysis of hemoglobin, Perutz and colleagues solved this problem by the development and application of isomorphous replacement. This method requires that the protein be labeled with an electron-rich ligand, such as a heavy metal, at a specific site (or sites) on the molecule. If the crystalline structure of the chemically modified hemoglobin is isomorphous with that of the protein, its x-ray diffraction pattern can be used to determine the phases of the x-rays scattered from the native (unlabeled) protein. Paramercuribenzoate and silver ions were shown to interact specifically with the β 93 sulfhydryl group of hemoglobin,[10] and these derivatives provided the first test of isomorphous replacement as applied to protein structure. This approach was also used in the x-ray analysis of sperm whale myoglobin in Dr. John Kendrew's laboratory, and by 1960 the three-dimensional structure of myoglobin had been determined at a very high degree of resolution (2.0 Å).[10] During this time, Perutz and colleagues[12] had worked out a 5.5-Å resolution Fourier synthesis of horse methemoglobin.* Their results indicated that the subunits in the hemoglobin tetramer had a tertiary structure very similar to that of myoglobin. Perutz and associates also took advantage of the growing body of information on the amino acid sequences of hemoglobin subunits. Knowledge of the primary structure was very useful in interpreting the computer-generated electron-density maps.

During the past 20 years, Perutz and colleagues at the MRC Laboratory in Cambridge have continued to refine the structure of hemoglobin. Human deoxyhemoglobin has been solved at a resolution of 1.7 Å.[13] This derivative was shown to have a unique quaternary structure, the so-called "deoxy" structure, which differs significantly from that of liganded hemoglobins such as oxy, carboxy, cyanomet, and fluoromet along with methemoglobin, all of which have nearly identical quaternary structure, loosely termed the "oxy" structure.†

---

*Crystals of oxyhemoglobin autoxidized to methemoglobin during the x-ray analysis.
† The "deoxy" structure is commonly designated as the T (or tense) quaternary structure; the "oxy" structure is designated as the R (or relaxed) quaternary structure. The concept of R and T quaternary structures has been very useful in considering the allosteric behavior of hemoglobin (see Chapter 3).

Human carboxyhemoglobin has been analyzed at 2.7Å resolution.[14] The structure of oxyhemoglobin has been elusive. During the initial studies of oxyhemoglobin, the crystals gradually autoxidized to methemoglobin owing to the prolonged period of time required for analysis. The structure of horse methemoglobin has now been solved at high resolution [2.0 Å].[15] The use of an oscillation camera at $-2°C$ has permitted rapid x-ray diffraction analysis of human oxyhemoglobin with minimal autoxidation to methemoglobin.[16] The detailed structure at 2.1Å resolution has recently been published.[16a]

The three-dimensional structure of a protein can be further analyzed by calculations of the potential energy of the molecule.[17] This approach has provided insight into how heme ligation leads to alterations in tertiary structure. In contrast to this static view of the protein, the dynamics of movement of its atoms can be calculated by integrating Newton's equations of motion over a very short period of time.[18] These investigations, which combine structural data with theoretical calculations, should eventually provide a powerful new means of defining the atomic events that underly hemoglobin's cooperative behavior.

Subunit Interactions

The subunits of hemoglobin form a tetrahedron having a twofold (or dyad) axis of symmetry (Fig. 2–4). This means that if any part of the molecule is rotated 180 degrees about this axis, it will superimpose on a seg-

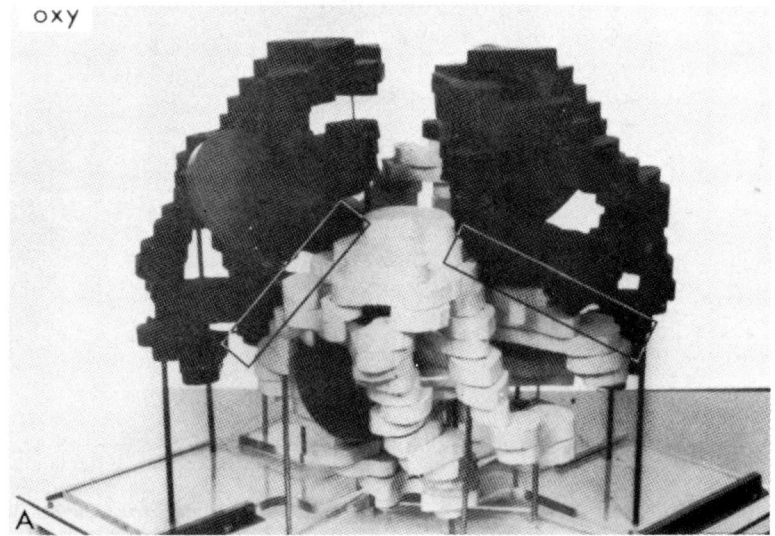
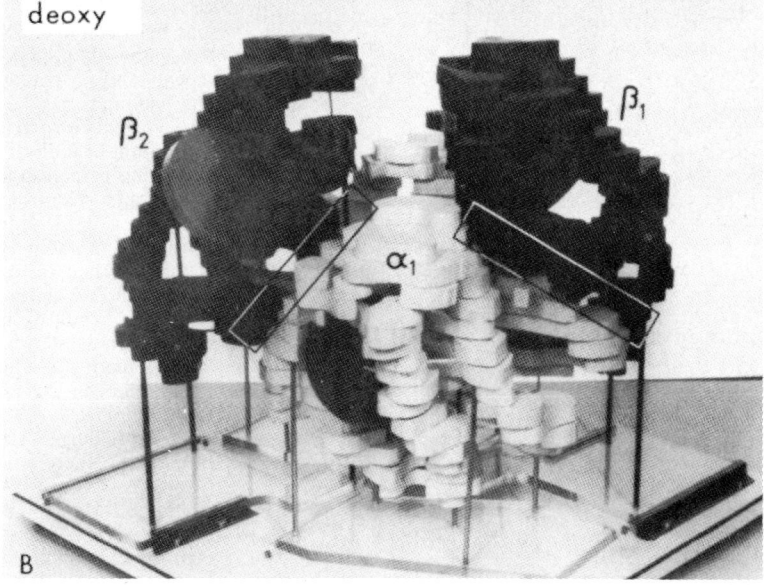

Figure 2–4. A three-dimensional model of hemoglobin, based on early x-ray crystallographic analysis (*A*, oxy; *B*, deoxy). The α chains are shown in white, the β chains in black; the boxed areas are the αβ contact areas. The heme groups are depicted as disks inserted into each subunit. There is an axis of symmetry that is parallel to the plane of the paper. Note the difference in conformation between oxyhemoglobin and deoxyhemoglobin. (From Muirhead, H., et al.: J. Mol. Biol. *28*:117, 1967.)

ment of identical structure. This axis runs down a water-filled cavity in the center of the molecule. One particularly provocative finding of the early x-ray analyses was the marked difference found in the quaternary structures of horse methemoglobin and human deoxyhemoglobin. This oxygenation-dependent conformational isomerization has been confirmed in a comparison of the carboxy and deoxy forms of the same species (human hemoglobin) (Fig. 2–5A). Following deoxygenation, the β chains move apart by about 7 Å, a relatively large distance compared with the overall dimensions of the hemoglobin tetramer (an el-

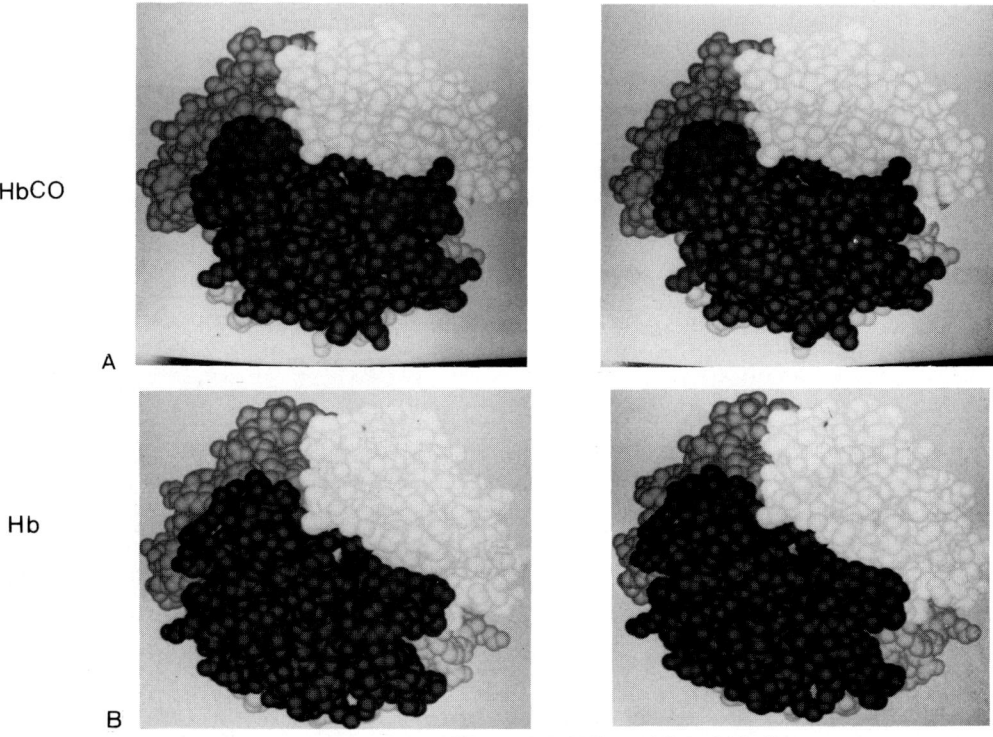

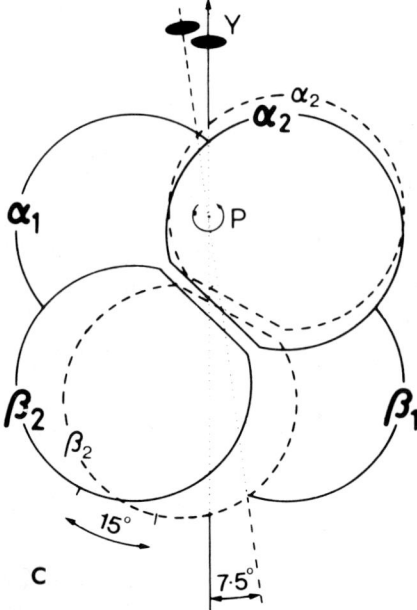

Figure 2–5. Effect of ligand binding on quaternary structure, i.e., the relationship between hemoglobin subunits. *A* and *B,* Space-filling models comparing three-dimensional structures of human carboxyhemoglobin *(A)* and deoxyhemoglobin *(B)* based on coordinates obtained from x-ray crystallography. Heme groups are not shown. The four hemoglobin subunits are shown in different shades. Full views of the α_2 (white) and β_2 (black) subunits are shown. Only a part of the α_1 (dark gray) and β_1 (light gray) subunits can be seen in the background. The $\alpha_1\beta_1$ dimer has been spatially fixed in this figure, whereas the orientation of the $\alpha_2\beta_2$ dimer (foreground) changes markedly when carbon monoxide (or oxygen) binds to deoxyhemoglobin. The orientation of the subunits is the same as that in *C* but is different from that in Figure 2–4. (This figure was prepared by Eric Henry and Richard Feldman at the National Institutes of Health.) *C,* Change in the position of one dimer ($\alpha_2\beta_2$) relevant to its partner dimer ($\alpha_1\beta_1$) as a result of ligation of the heme groups. Deoxyhemoglobin is shown by a solid line and the liganded hemoglobin by an interrupted line. The orientation of the subunits in this diagram is the same as that in *A* and *B*. With reference to $\alpha_1\beta_1$, which is fixed, there is considerable rotation (15 degrees) of the $\alpha_2\beta_2$ dimer upon heme ligation. In addition, there is a 7.5-degree rotation of the twofold (dyad) axis. (From Fermi, G., and Perutz, M.: Haemoglobin and Myoglobin. *In* Phillips, D. C., and Richards, F. M. (eds.): Atlas of Molecular Structures in Biology. Oxford, Clarendon Press, 1981.)

Table 2–1. DISTANCES BETWEEN HEME IRON ATOMS

	Oxy	Deoxy
	(Å)	
α_1–α_2	36.0	34.9
α_1–β_2 (α_2–β_1)	25.0	24.6
α_1–β_1 (α_2–β_2)	35.0	36.9
β_1–β_2	33.4	39.9

lipsoid measuring approximately 64 × 55 × 50 Å). The rotation and translation of the β chain are shown diagrammatically in Figure 2–5B. The heme groups are approximately equidistant from one another. The distances between the iron atoms of the four hemes of oxyhemoglobin and deoxyhemoglobin are shown in Table 2–1. Thus, the "heme-heme interaction" encountered in the cooperative binding of oxygen to hemoglobin could not be explained on the basis of direct contact between heme groups and must depend on interactions between subunits.

The change in quaternary structure upon oxygenation is quite compatible with the large number of physical and chemical differences known to exist between oxyhemoglobin and deoxyhemoglobin (see Table 3–1). This structural alteration involves movement of hemoglobin subunits relative to one another. From inspection of a three-dimensional model of hemoglobin, such as that depicted in Figure 2–4, it is apparent that each α chain impinges upon the two β chains along two different surfaces. Hence, if the subunits are designated α_1, α_2, β_1, and β_2, two interfaces between unlike subunits can be defined as $\alpha_1\beta_1$ and $\alpha_1\beta_2$. From considerations of symmetry, the $\alpha_1\beta_1$ interface is structurally identical to $\alpha_2\beta_2$, and the $\alpha_1\beta_2$ interface is identical to $\alpha_2\beta_1$. These interfaces are depicted in Figure 2–6.

The subunits of hemoglobin interact with one another by means of relatively weak, noncovalent bonds such as Van der Waals forces and hydrogen bonds. In addition, as discussed below, deoxyhemoglobin is stabilized by both intrasubunit and intersubunit salt bonds. The interactions between the amino acid residues at the $\alpha_1\beta_1$ and $\alpha_1\beta_2$ interfaces are shown in Figure 2–7. A much better grasp of these contacts can be obtained by viewing the superb stereodiagrams in the atlas of hemoglobin structure compiled by Fermi and Perutz.[19] In keeping with the fact that the $\alpha_1\beta_1$ interface remains relatively fixed during oxygenation, the contacts between the α_1 and β_1 subunits (and therefore between the α_2 and β_2 subunits) are identical in oxyhemoglobin and deoxyhemoglobin. There are about 40 contacts between residues at this interface, including nine hydrogen bonds.

In contrast, there is considerable movement at the $\alpha_1\beta_2$ interface during oxygenation. The two subunits slip over one another in tongue-and-groove fashion (see Figure 14–2). The primary sites for contact are the FG corner and C helix of one subunit with complementary (C and FG) regions of the other subunit (see Figure 2–6). Thus, there are four major areas of interaction. Good contacts can be made only if the orientation of the C and FG regions is the same in both αβ dimers. This suggests that the quaternary structure must be either oxy (R) or deoxy (T)[20, 21] and provides structural support for the two-state allosteric model discussed in Chapter 3.

Because of the movement along the $\alpha_1\beta_2$ interface, the contacts are entirely different in

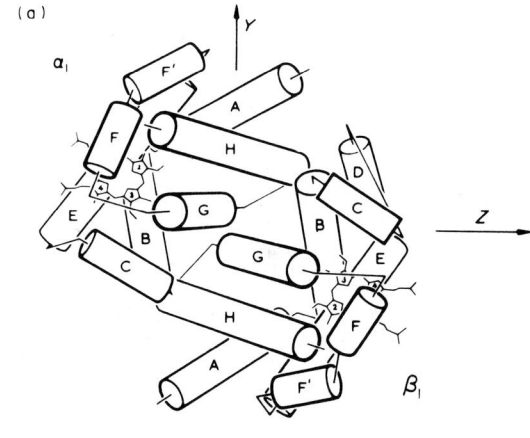

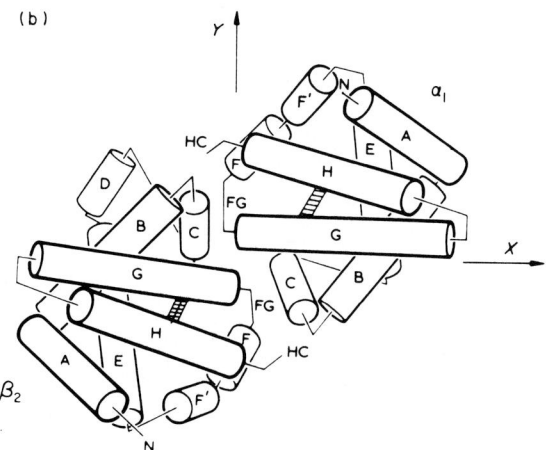

Figure 2–6. Three-dimensional orientation of the subunits in carboxyhemoglobin. The letter on each cylinder designates specific regions of α helix (see Figure 2–2). The top panel (a) shows the $\alpha_1\beta_1$ dimer and the heme groups of the α and β chains. The bottom panel (b) shows the $\alpha_1\beta_2$ interface. (From Baldwin, J. M.: J. Mol. Biol. 136:103, 1980.)

deoxyhemoglobin compared with oxyhemoglobin (Figs. 2–7B and C). In deoxyhemoglobin, there are about 40 contacts, including 19 hydrogen bonds. When hemoglobin is oxygenated, the total number of contacts drops to about 22, including 12 hydrogen bonds. In view of the important role that conformational isomerization plays in hemoglobin function, it is not surprising that residues at the $\alpha_1\beta_2$ interface are "invariant," i.e., highly conserved throughout vertebrate evolution (see Chapter 6). Accordingly, human hemoglobin variants

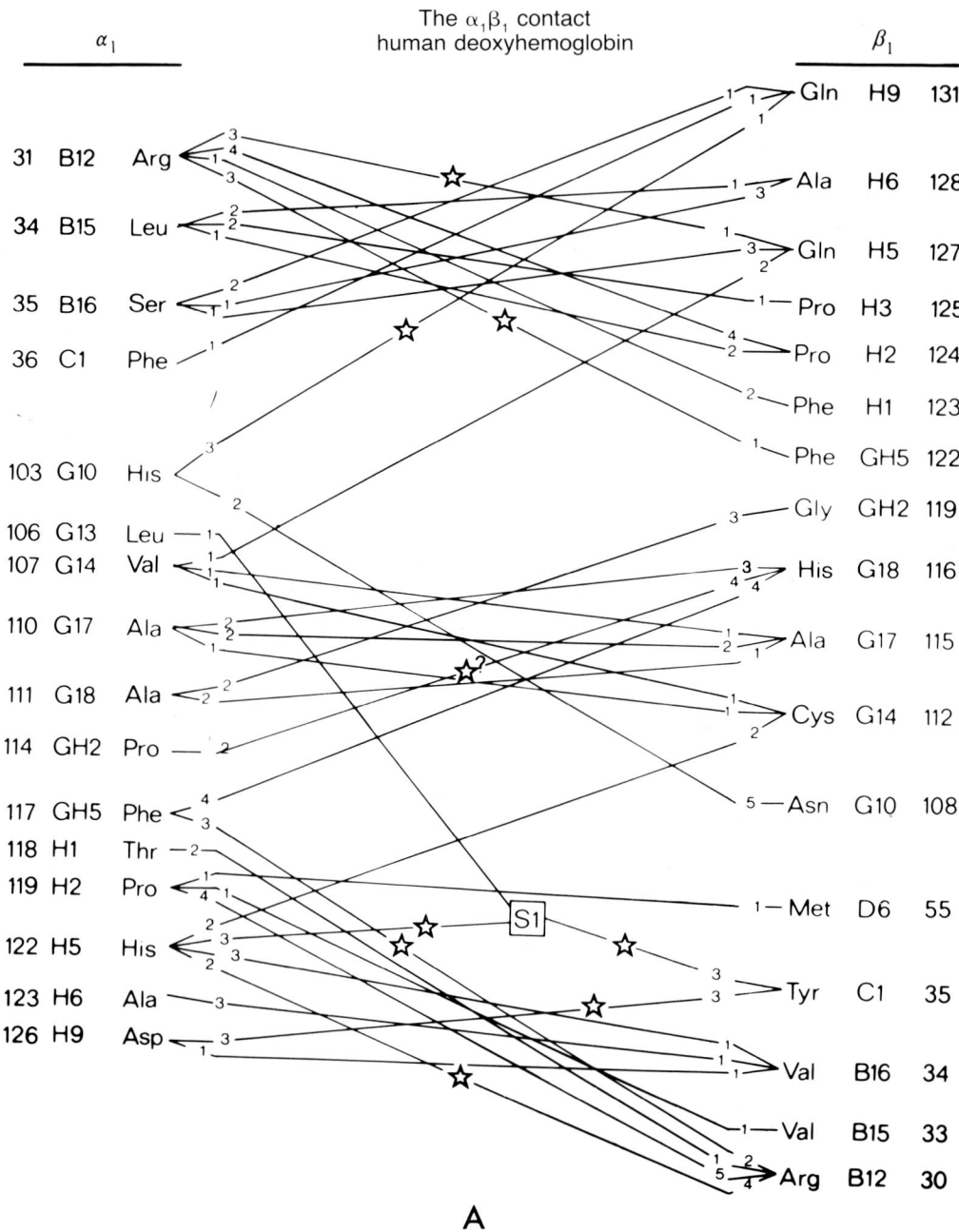

A

Figure 2–7. Contacts between subunits of hemoglobins. The $\alpha_1\beta_1$ contacts for oxyhemoglobin are virtually identical to those for deoxyhemoglobin *(A)*. The $\alpha_1\beta_2$ contacts for human oxyhemoglobin and carboxyhemoglobin are nearly identical to those for horse methemoglobin. Connecting lines indicate distances across subunit interface of less than 4 Å. Lines with star indicate that the contact includes a hydrogen bond. Small numbers along the contact lines indicate the number of contributing atoms. Boxes denote bound solvent molecules. *A*, The human $\alpha_1\beta_1$ contact in human deoxyhemoglobin.
Illustration continued on opposite page

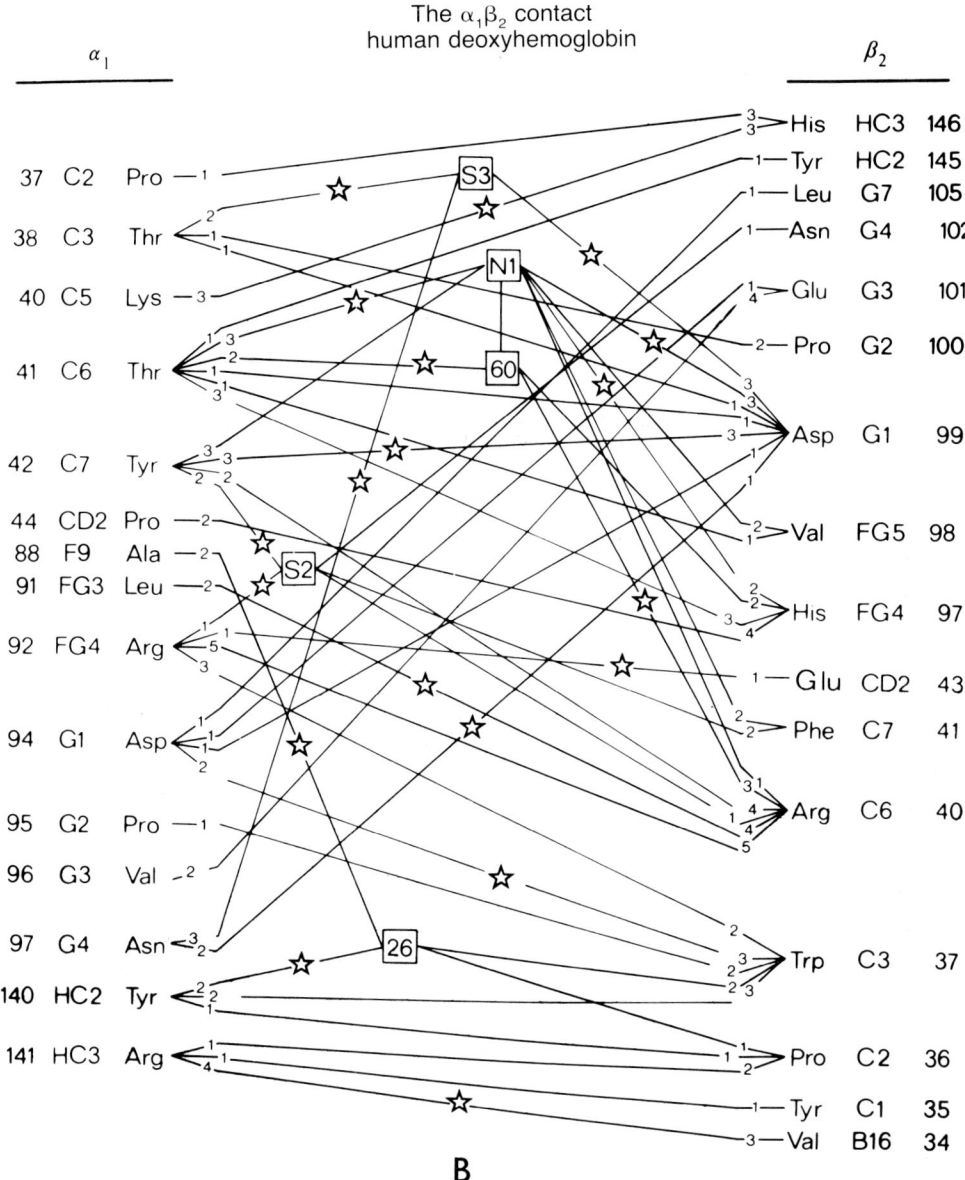

Figure 2–7 *Continued.* B, The $\alpha_1\beta_2$ contact in human deoxyhemoglobin.

Illustration continued on following page

with substitutions at the $\alpha_1\beta_2$ interface usually have drastic alterations in their functional properties (see Chapter 14).

Under physiologic conditions oxyhemoglobin dissociates reversibly into like dimers:

$$\alpha_2\beta_2 \rightleftharpoons 2\,\alpha\beta$$

The reduction in contacts at the $\alpha_1\beta_2$ interface following oxygenation suggests that the dissociation occurs here rather than at the $\alpha_1\beta_1$ interface. Independent evidence for dissociation at the $\alpha_1\beta_2$ interface has been provided.[22] The extent to which hemoglobin dissociates symmetrically into dimers depends markedly on whether it is oxygenated. Subunit dissociation occurs about 10^6 times more readily in oxyhemoglobin than in deoxyhemoglobin. Thus, the binding energy between $\alpha\beta$ dimers must be considerably greater in the deoxygenated form. The molecular basis for this resides primarily in the increased number as well as the different nature[21] of the $\alpha_1\beta_2$ contacts in deoxyhemoglobin compared with those of oxyhemoglobin (see Figures 2–7B and C). In particular, deoxyhemoglobin contains a number of intersubunit salt bonds that are absent or very much weaker in oxyhemoglobin.[23]

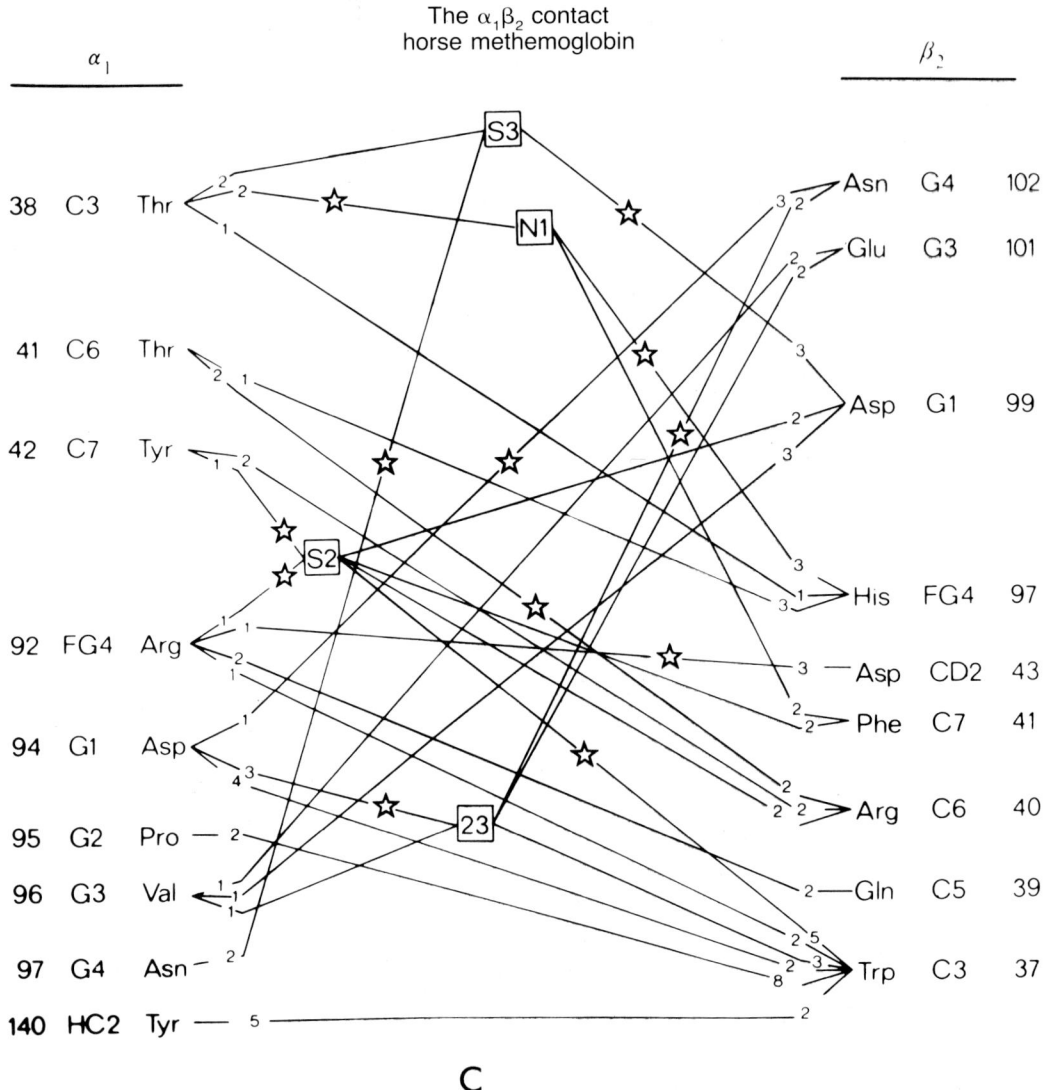

Figure 2–7 Continued. C, The $\alpha_1\beta_2$ contact in horse methemoglobin. (From Fermi, G., and Perutz, M.: Hemoglobin and myoglobin. In Phillips, D. C., and Richards, F. M. (eds.): Atlas of Molecular Structures in Biology. Oxford, Clarendon Press, 1981.)

The salt bridges between $\alpha_1\beta_1$ and $\alpha_2\beta_2$ dimers of deoxyhemoglobin, shown diagrammatically in Figures 2–8 and 2–9, include α_1–α_2 and α_1–β_2 interactions. The carboxyl group of the C-terminal arginine of one α chain interacts with the ε-amino group of 132 (H10) lysine from the other α chain. The guanidinium group of this C-terminal arginine forms an electrostatic bond with the carboxyl group of 131 (H9) aspartic acid of the other α chain. In addition, a chloride ion is thought to form ionic contacts with both the guanidinium group of C-terminal arginine and the NH_2-terminal amino group of the opposite α chain. These $\alpha_1\alpha_2$ salt bridges cannot be formed in oxyhemoglobin because the space between $\alpha_1\beta_1$ and $\alpha_2\beta_2$ dimers is too small.[21] The C-terminal histidine of each β chain of deoxyhemoglobin is involved in two electrostatic interactions (Fig. 2–9). Its positively charged imidazole forms a salt bridge with the FG1 aspartate from the same subunit, and its negatively charged carboxyl group spans the $\alpha_1\beta_2$ interface to form a salt bridge with α 40 (C5) lysine. When hemoglobin is oxygenated, these residues are now too far apart for this interaction to take place, and as a result, the salt bridge is broken.

In deoxyhemoglobin, the penultimate tyrosine residue of each of the four subunits is

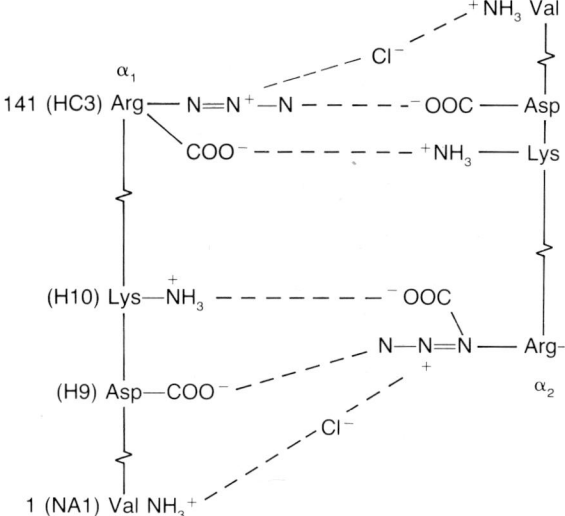

Figure 2–8. Electrostatic interactions between α chains in deoxyhemoglobin. The helical notations for certain amino acids are shown in parentheses.

firmly anchored in a pocket between the F and H helices. This is also illustrated in Figure 2–9. Upon oxygenation, these tyrosines are evicted, freeing the C-terminal portion of each subunit.

Although these interactions are important in stabilizing the deoxy quaternary structure and contribute to the Bohr effect (see Chapter 4), just how large a role they play in the overall energy of subunit cooperativity is a matter of continuing investigation.

Binding of 2,3-DPG

Organic phosphates also enhance the stability of the deoxy conformation. In mammals, 2,3-diphosphoglycerate (2,3-DPG) has been shown to mediate intracellular hemoglobin function. The physiological importance of this cofactor will be discussed in detail in Chapters 3, 5, and 6. X-ray diffraction studies by Arnone[24] indicate that 2,3-DPG binds electrostatically to the β chains of deoxyhemoglobin at a specific site in the entrance to the central cavity along the dyad axis of symmetry. The phosphate groups of 2,3-DPG form salt bonds with the β N-terminal amino groups and the imidazoles of β 2 histidine and β 143 histidine. The carboxyl group of 2,3-DPG is bonded to the ε-amino group of β 82 lysine. Figure 2–10 is an electron-density map showing 2,3-DPG situated at this site. A more diagrammatic representation is shown in Figure 2–11. The plane of these figures is perpendicular to the dyad axis. The x-ray data indicate that the

HEMOGLOBIN STRUCTURE 27

binding of 2,3-DPG results in a small change in the tertiary structure of the β subunits.[24]

The change in quaternary configuration with oxygenation is shown diagrammatically in Figure 2–12. As the four heme groups are successively oxygenated, the inter- and intrasubunit salt bonds are successively broken. The 2,3-DPG molecule, chloride ions, and protons are ejected. Fully oxygenated hemoglobin has fewer constraints, enabling it to dissociate along the $\alpha_1\beta_2$ interface more readily than deoxyhemoglobin. The change in tertiary and quaternary conformation during oxygen binding is the basis for cooperativity, a subject that will be discussed in Chapter 3, Hemoglobin Function.

Heme-Globin Interactions

Heme

The prosthetic group of hemoglobin is ferroprotoporphyrin IX. Its structure is shown in Figure 2–13. Heme is also the prosthetic group of myoglobin, catalase, peroxidase, and cyto-

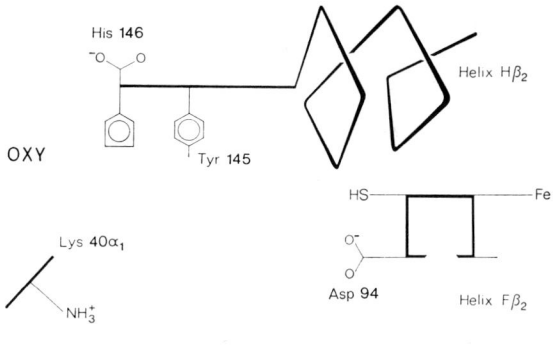

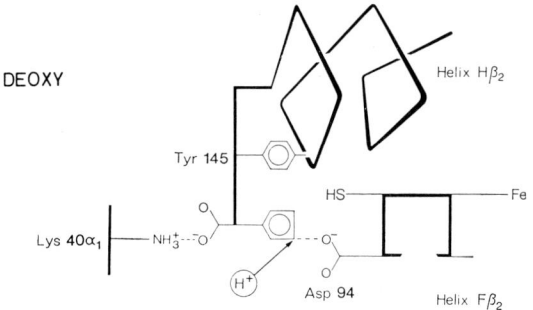

Figure 2–9. Change in conformation of C-terminal residues of β chain. The salt bridges of β 146 His probably break when the quaternary structure changes from T to R or when the β-chain hemes take up oxygen, whichever comes first. (From Perutz, M.: Nature 228:734, 1970.)

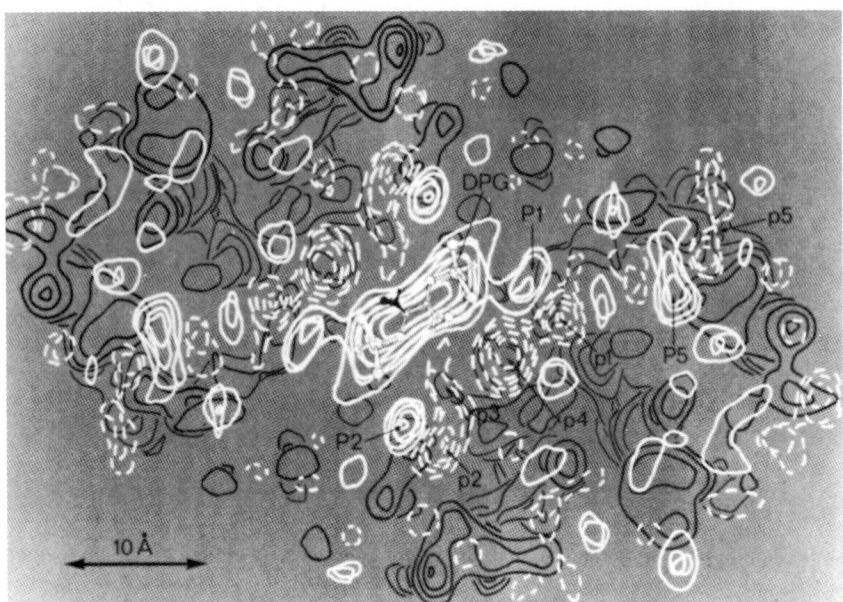

Figure 2–10. Electron-density map of human deoxyhemoglobin, showing the same parts of the molecule sketched in Figure 2–11. Sections are perpendicular to the twofold axis of symmetry. The effect of 2,3-DPG on the tertiary structure of the β chain is shown. White lines show difference electron density map ± 2,3-DPG. Solid contours and upper case letters mark positive difference density; broken contours and lower case letters mark negative difference density. (From Arnone, A.: Nature *237*:146, 1972.)

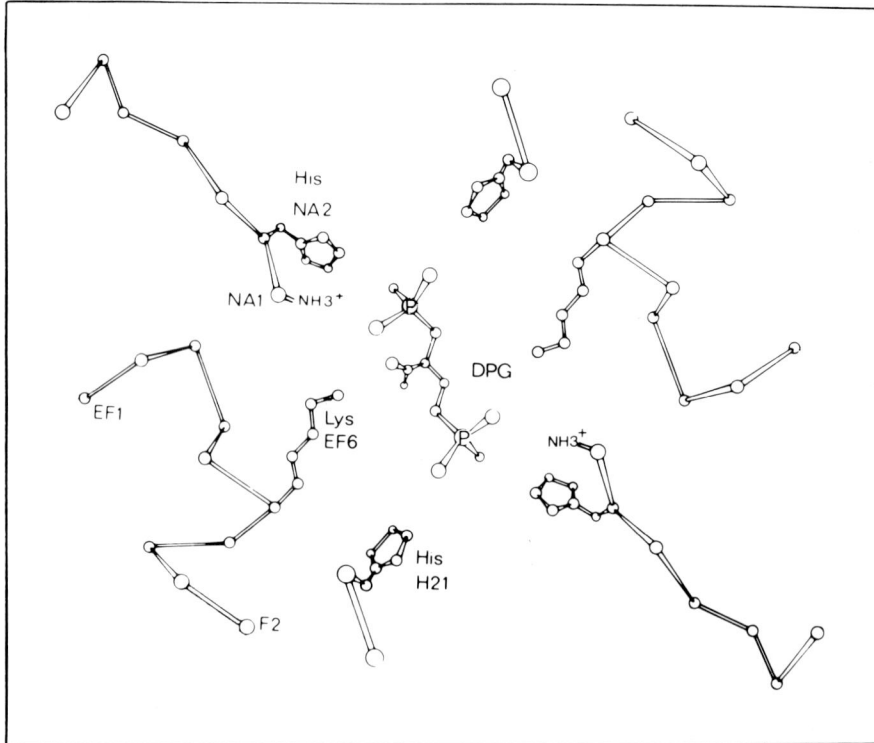

Figure 2–11. The binding of DPG to human deoxyhemoglobin. The stereochemistry of DPG complements the basic residues of the central cavity to form salt bridges with N-terminal valines and histidines 2 and 143 of both β chains and with lysine 82 of one β chain. (From Arnone, A.: Nature *249*:34, 1974.)

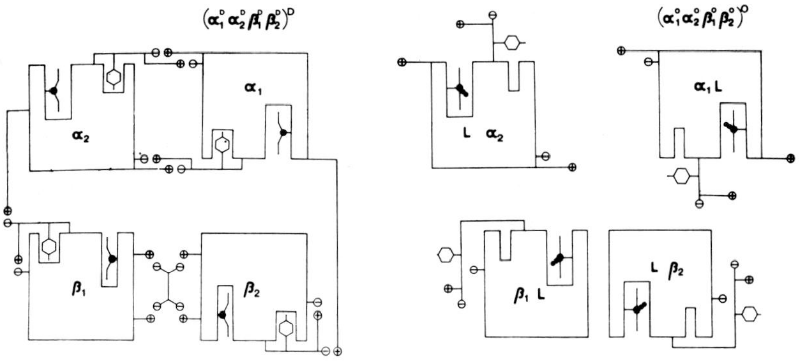

HEMOGLOBIN STRUCTURE

Figure 2–12. Diagrammatic representation of the quaternary configurations of deoxyhemoglobin (left) and oxyhemoglobin (right). Intrasubunit and intersubunit salt bonds are broken upon oxygenation. (From Perutz, M. F.: Nature 228:734, 1970.)

chromes of class *b*. Heme has a molecular weight of 614. The four heme groups therefore account for about 4 per cent of the mass of the hemoglobin molecule (M.W. = 64,400). Heme can be prepared by diluting hemoglobin in cold acid acetone, which precipitates the globin, leaving the heme in solution. During this extraction, the iron is completely oxidized. In alkaline solution, this brown pigment is called hematin; at lower pH, it is called hemin. The biosynthesis of heme is described in Chapter 7. Asymmetry is introduced into the molecule at two steps in the synthesis. Uroporphyrin isomerase enables uroporphyrinogen III to be formed in preference to the symmetrical uroporphyrinogen I. Protoporphyrinogen IX is formed from coproporphyrinogen III by the selective oxidation of two of the four propionic acid groups, located on adjacent pyrroles. It is likely that the final product, ferroprotoporphyrin IX, has been "engineered" during its evolutionary development to provide optimal fit with apoproteins such as globin. Indeed, the interactions of globin with a variety of other synthetic protoporphyrins are less stable.

High-resolution x-ray studies have provided precise information on the details of the heme-globin linkage. The heme is inserted in a cleft between the E and F helices. The iron is linked

Figure 2–13. A, Structure of heme (ferroprotoporphyrin IX). B, Stereo view of heme having the same orientation as in A. The atoms are shown in proportion to their size: Fe >> O > N > C >> H. (Courtesy of Richard Feldman, National Institutes of Health.)

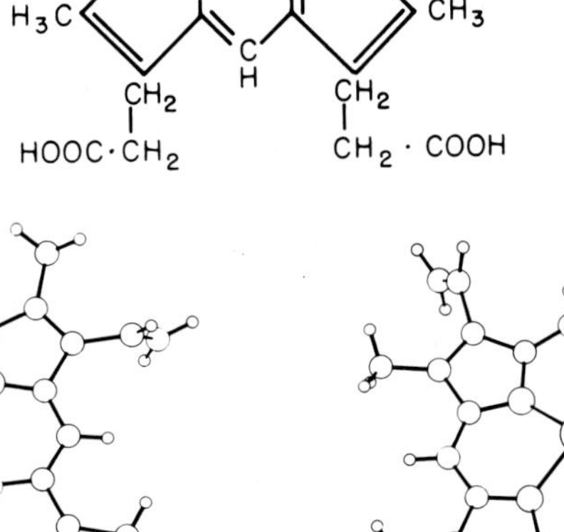

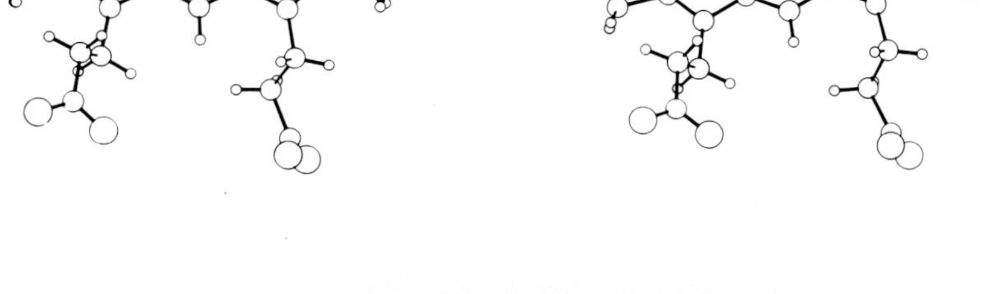

covalently to the imidazole nitrogen of the "proximal" F8 histidine. Residue β E11 valine appears to "guard" the access of oxygen to the heme pocket. This is also an invariant residue that is substituted in three of the unstable hemoglobin variants discussed in Chapter 13. The heme is so oriented that the asymmetrically placed nonpolar vinyl groups are buried deep in the hydrophobic interior of the cleft, while on the other side of the porphyrin, the charged propionic acid groups are oriented toward the hydrophilic surface of the subunit. The heme is stabilized by a large number of interatomic contacts. There is a high degree of complementarity between heme and globin structure (Fig. 2–14).

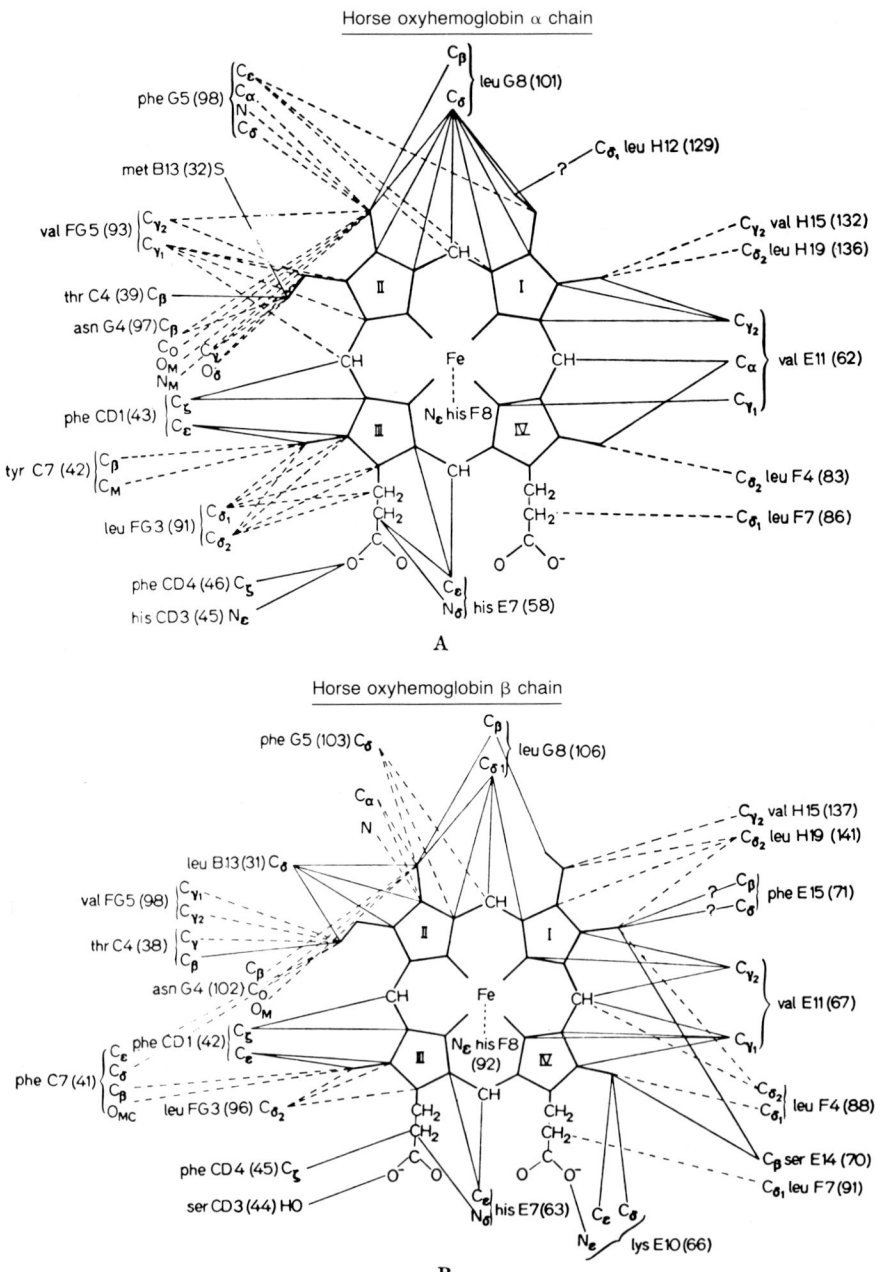

Figure 2–14. Contacts between the heme group and residues of the globin in *(A)* the α chain and *(B)* the β chain. All contacts of approximately 4 Å or less are listed. Plain lines indicate contacts on the side of helix E (distal histidine); broken lines indicate contacts on the side of helix F (proximal histidine). The suffix M means "main chain." (From Perutz, M. F., et al.: Nature 219:131, 1968.)

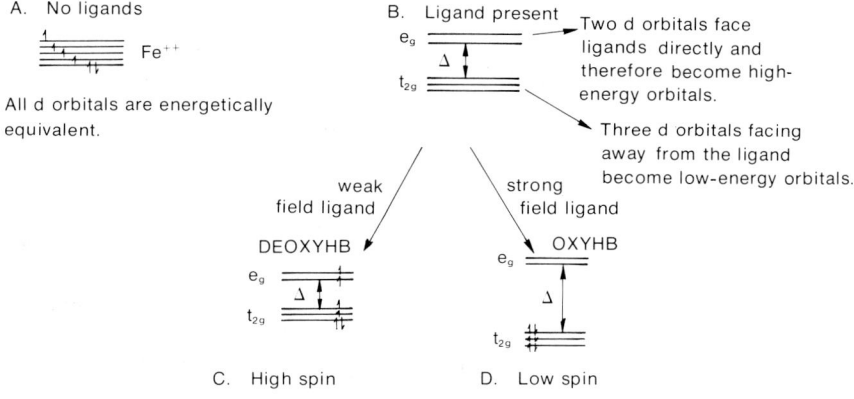

Δ represents the energy difference between e_g and t_{2g} orbitals.

Figure 2–15. State of d orbitals of ferrous iron (Fe^{++}) and the effect of ligand. (Courtesy of V. S. Sharma.)

The Iron Atom

In heme, an iron atom occupies the center of the porphyrin ring. Iron is a transition metal having an atomic number of 26. Its electronic configuration depends on its ionic state:

Elemental iron	$1s^2\ 2s^2\ 2p^6\ 3s^2\ 3p^6\ 3d^6\ 4s^2$
Ferrous iron (Fe^{++})	$1s^2\ 2s^2\ 2p^6\ 3s^2\ 3p^6\ 3d^6$
Ferric iron (Fe^{+++})	$1s^2\ 2s^2\ 2p^6\ 3s^2\ 3p^6\ 3d^5$

In general, the electrons of the outermost 3d orbitals of transition metals are involved in the formation of coordination compounds. The physicochemical properties (such as visible spectra, ionic radii, magnetic moments, and so on) of these compounds depend on the detailed electronic configuration of 3d electrons. In the absence of ligands the five d orbitals are energetically equivalent, and the first five d electrons occupy these orbitals singly (Fig. 2–15A). The last electron, however, has no vacant orbital available to it and therefore is forced to pair with one of the other five electrons. As we can see, in this state there are four unpaired electrons in the d orbitals of the metal ion. However, in the presence of ligands,* the five d orbitals are not equivalent. This is because electrons on the donor atoms of a ligand exert repulsion on d-orbital electrons. Two of the orbitals face ligands directly and therefore experience the repulsive force most. They become high-energy orbitals (Fig. 2–15B), not favored by the electrons. The remaining three d orbitals are at relatively lower energy because they are oriented away from the ligands. If the ligand (or a group of ligands) exerts only a small repulsive force (i.e., weak field ligands), the energy separating t_{2g} and e_g orbitals is small; then, the first five electrons are able to occupy the five d orbitals just as they do in the absence of ligands, and only the sixth electron is forced to pair.

Iron in deoxyhemoglobin is five-coordinated, with the four pyrrole→nitrogens of the porphyrin and the imidazole nitrogen of the proximal histidine (F8). Accordingly, the field due to the ligands is a relatively weak one. The distribution of electrons in deoxyhemoglobin is represented in Figure 2–15C.

In contrast, the iron in oxyhemoglobin is six-coordinated. As an additional ligand, oxygen enhances the overall ligand field strength. This is due in part to the increased number of ligands around the metal ion and in part to the distance between the metal ion and the four porphyrin nitrogen donors. Accordingly, the energy separation between t_{2g} and e_g orbitals is much larger. As electrons prefer to occupy lower-energy orbitals, the first three electrons go in the t_{2g} orbitals. The fourth, fifth, and sixth electrons find the energy difference between t_{2g} and e_g orbitals too great to transfer up into the e_g orbitals and therefore are forced to pair with electrons already in the t_{2g} orbitals (Fig. 2–15D). As a result, there are no unpaired electrons in oxyhemoglobin. As we can see from Figures 2–15C and D, the number of electrons in the orbitals facing the ligands (i.e., e_g orbitals) has also decreased from two to zero.

---

*In the context of this discussion, the term "ligand" refers to any atom that forms a bond with the iron atom.

No doubt the picture given above is oversimplified and inadequate to explain some of the more complex phenomena associated with hemoglobin chemistry. Yet, it is good enough to explain one frequently discussed difference between deoxyhemoglobin and oxyhemoglobin—namely, reduced magnetic moment or spin state of oxyhemoglobin. Upon oxygenation, the electrons become paired, resulting in a low spin state and a reduction of magnetic moment. In like manner, methemoglobin (Fe^{+++}) at neutral or acid pH has a high spin state. Upon the addition of negatively charged ligands such as OH^-, cyanide (CN^-), or azide (N_3^-), the heme iron becomes low spin.

The Iron-Oxygen Linkage

Both x-ray[16] and spectroscopic[25, 26] analyses have provided definitive information on the orientation of the oxygen molecule in the heme pocket. These studies confirm a prediction made by Pauling and Coryell in 1936[27] that oxygen is bound to the iron atom by end-on geometry with a tilt away from the axis perpendicular to the porphyrin plane:

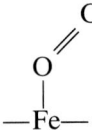

Furthermore, the oxygen atom not bound to the iron atom forms a hydrogen bond with the imidazole nitrogen of the distal (E7) histidine,[16] just as in myoglobin[28] and cobalt hemoglobin.[29] This interaction appears to be stronger in the α subunit, and by causing increased polarization of the oxygen, it might favor dissociation of superoxide anion, thereby explaining the increased tendency of the α subunit to autoxidize (see Chapter 16).

The Trigger

The most fundamental information to be derived from the structural analysis of hemoglobin is how the binding of oxygen can trigger the marked alteration in conformation that is implicit in subunit cooperativity. A closely linked question is how the transition from the T to the R quaternary structure affects the environment of the unliganded hemes in such a way that oxygen affinity is increased. Perutz and colleagues[30, 31] have provided a broad array of experimental evidence supporting the reciprocal relationship between quaternary structure and heme environment. A comparison of the high-resolution structures of deoxyhemoglobin and oxyhemoglobin provides insights into the nature of the trigger. Previous structural analyses of synthetic iron-porphyrin compounds had shown that the length of the bond from the iron atoms to the nitrogen atoms of the porphyrin ring depends on the spin state of the iron.[32] It is 2.06 Å in high spin ferric compounds and 1.99 Å in low spin ferric compounds. In iron-free porphyrin, the distance from the center of the ring to the nitrogen atoms is 2.01 Å. Thus, in low spin iron-porphyrin compounds, the iron atom lies in the plane of the porphyrin ring. Application of the Pythagorean theorem to the interatomic distances in the high spin ferric porphyrins indicates that in these compounds the iron atom is about 0.4 Å outside the plane. It is likely that in *ferrous* porphyrins the same relationship pertains. Thus, in low spin oxyhemoglobin and carboxyhemoglobin, the iron atom should also lie in the plane of the porphyrin ring, whereas in high spin deoxyhemoglobin, the iron atom should be significantly out of the plane.[20, 23] This prediction has proved to be correct. As shown in Figure 2–16, in deoxyhemoglobin, the iron atom is pulled about 0.6 Å out of the plane of the porphyrin ring, toward the proximal histidine,[13] primarily owing to translation and tilt of the F helix away from the heme. Because of the asymmetrical position of the proximal histidine relative to the porphyrin, the C_ϵ carbon atom of the imidazole group is in close contact with one of the pyrrole nitrogens of the heme. Accordingly, steric hindrance would prevent the iron atom from moving into the plane of the porphyrin ring. Thus, in deoxyhemoglobin, the bond between the iron atom and the imidazole nitrogen of the proximal histidine is under increased strain. Resonance Raman measurements indicate that the Fe–N bond is stretched by about 0.03 Å in the α subunits and 0.01 Å in the β subunits of deoxyhemoglobin, compared with oxyhemoglobin.[33, 34] The resultant displacement of the iron atom out of the plane of the porphyrin is associated with decreased oxygen affinity. The switch from the T to the R quaternary structure results in a more symmetrical orientation of the proximal histidine, allowing this group to move closer to the heme group with less steric hindrance and less strain on the bond between the iron atom and the imidazole nitrogen. This structural transition permits the iron atom to sit flush in the plane of the porphyrin, an orientation that permits stronger binding between the heme iron and

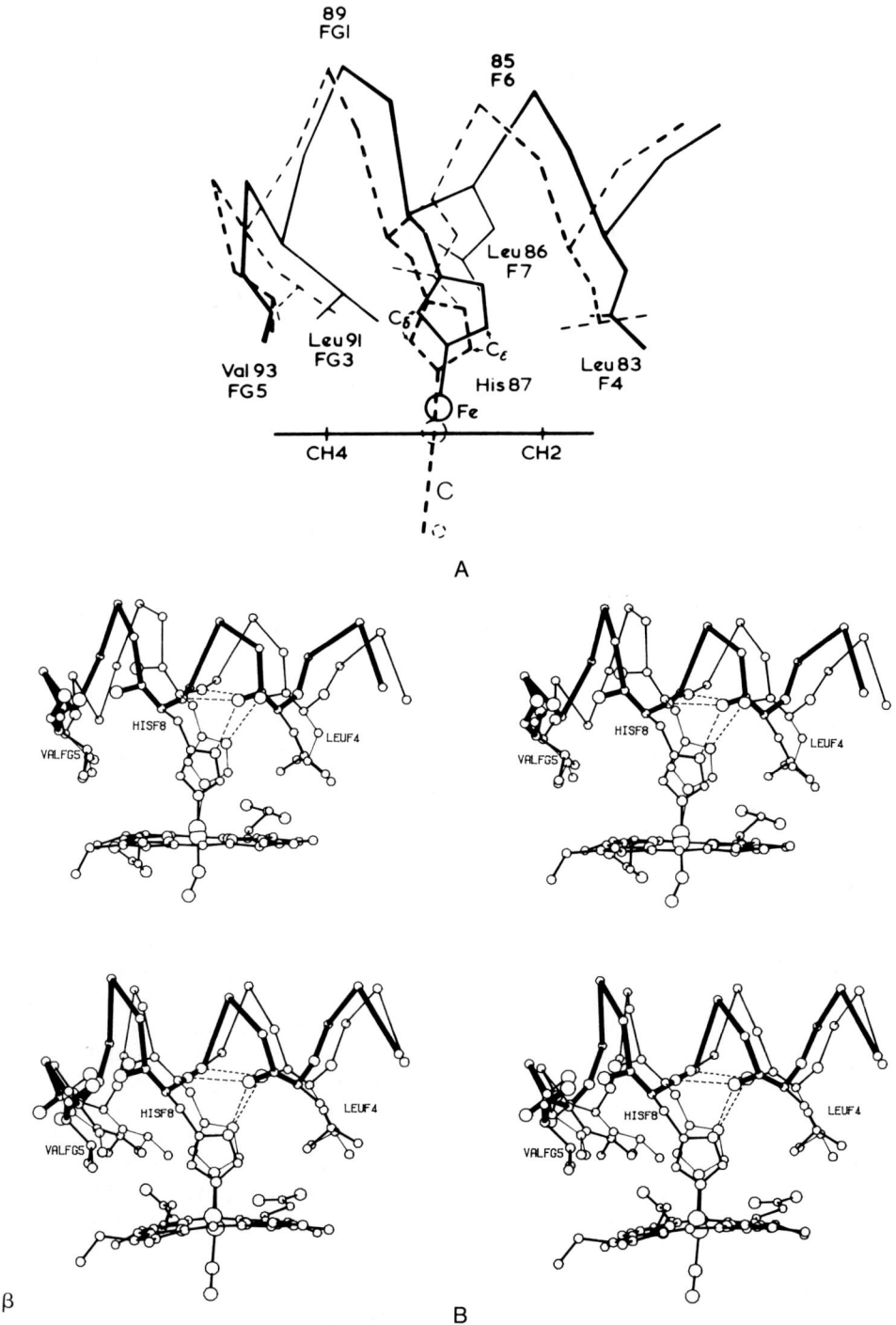

Figure 2–16. *A*, Effect of oxygenation on the orientation of the proximal histidine of the α chain (α His 87) and neighboring residues of the F helix. The hemes of the oxy and deoxy structures have been superimposed, and the plane of the heme (and CH1 to CH3 of the heme) is perpendicular to the plane of the paper. Liganded hemoglobin (oxy and carboxy) is shown by dashed lines, and deoxyhemoglobin is shown by solid lines. Upon oxygenation, the F helix moves across the heme plane and slightly toward it, altering the position of the proximal histidine (87) and the iron atom (Fe) relative to the heme. Similar movement is seen in the β subunit. (From Baldwin, J., and Chothia, C.: J. Mol. Biol. *129*:175, 1979.) *B*, Stereo view of the hemes and the proximal side of the α subunit *(top)* and β subunit *(bottom)*. The orientation of this figure is the same as that of *A*. The plane of the heme group is perpendicular to the plane of the page. Oxyhemoglobin is shown in heavy lines and deoxyhemoglobin in lighter lines. The heme groups of HbO_2 and Hb have been superimposed for clarity. Only the HbO_2 heme is shown. (From Shaanan, B.: J. Mol. Biol. *171*:31, 1983.)

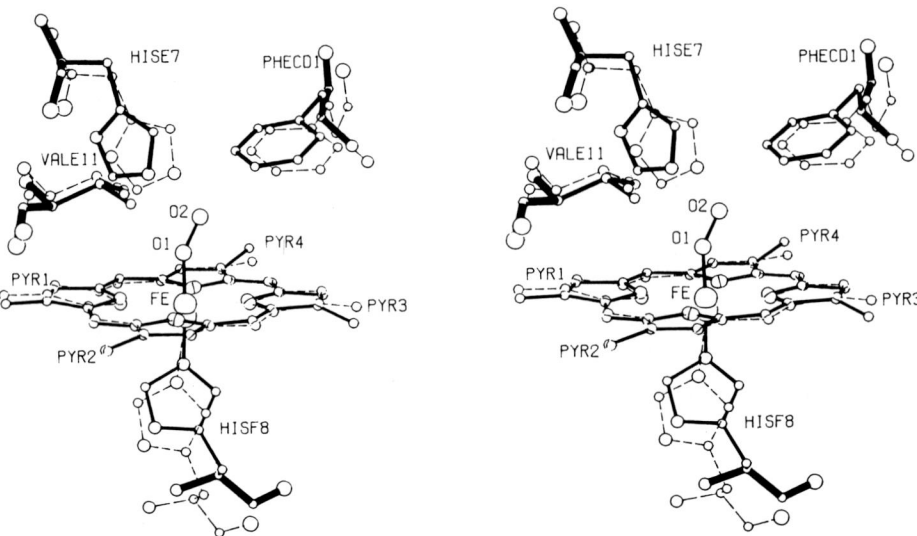

Figure 2–17. Stereo view of the heme group of the α chain of oxyhemoglobin (heavy lines) and deoxyhemoglobin (interrupted lines). The hemes of HbO$_2$ and Hb have been superimposed and the other residues transformed accordingly. Note the movement of the proximal (F8) histidine (shown also in Figure 2–16B) as well as the distal (E7) histidine and CD1 phenylalanine on the O$_2$ binding side of the heme group. Note also the slight alteration in the structure of the heme group. (From Shaanan, B.: J. Mol. Biol. *171*:31, 1983.)

oxygen. The strain on the α-chain Fe–N bond in deoxyhemoglobin amounts to approximately 0.15 KCal, a fraction of the 2.5 KCal involved in subunit cooperativity (see Chapter 3). It is likely that the trigger involves other important structural transitions such as doming or ruffling of the porphyrin (Fig. 2–17).

Gelin and Karplus[17] have proposed a reaction path whereby movement of the heme iron atom is linked to structural perturbations at the subunit interface. From their calculations of conformational energies, they conclude that the strain on the heme groups in deoxyhemoglobin increases markedly upon oxygen binding, as the iron atom moves toward the plane of the porphyrin ring. As a result, the heme group is forced into a slight tilt that leads to small movements in residues at the FG corner and C helix (i.e., the α$_1$β$_2$ interface). Baldwin and Chothia[35] have confirmed this reaction path by detailed examination of high-resolution structures of deoxyhemoglobin and carboxyhemoglobin. They propose that oxygen binding to deoxyhemoglobin leads to strain at the α$_1$β$_2$ interface that can be relieved by a flip to the R quaternary structure. The remaining unliganded heme groups then acquire a substantial increase in oxygen affinity. This structural explanation of subunit cooperativity (or heme-heme interaction) is tentative and undoubtedly oversimplified, but it is basically consistent with a two-state allosteric model. This topic will be discussed in detail in the next chapter.

Conclusion

The x-ray studies on human oxyhemoglobin and deoxyhemoglobin have progressed to the point at which the three-dimensional coordinates of their 4600 nonhydrogen atoms are established with a high degree of certainty. This information—the culmination of 35 years of dedication to this project—permits a deeper understanding of the way in which hemoglobin functions. On a television broadcast, Perutz was asked what he thought was the essence of scientific creativity. He parapharased an admonition of Sir Isaac Newton: "Always keep the problem foremost in your mind."

References

1. Anfinsen, C. B.: Principles that govern the folding of protein chains. Science *181*:223, 1973.
2. Hill, R. J., and Craig, L. C.: Countercurrent distribution studies with adult human hemoglobin. J. Am. Chem. Soc. *81*:2272, 1959.
3. Chernoff, A. I.: The amino acid composition of hemoglobin. I. An improved method for separating the peptide chains of human hemoglobin. J. Chromatogr. *6*:252, 1961.

4. Clegg, J. B., Naughton, M. A., and Weatherall, D. J.: Abnormal human hemoglobins. Separation and characterization of the α and β chains by chromatography, and the determination of two new variants Hb Chesapeake and Hb J (Bangkok). J. Mol. Biol. *19*:91, 1966.
5. Ingram, V. M.: A specific chemical difference between the globins of normal human and sickle cell anaemia haemoglobin. Nature *178*:792, 1956.
6. Jones, R. T.: Structural studies of aminoethylated hemoglobins by automatic peptide chromatography. Cold Spring Harbor Symp. Quant. Biol. *29*:297, 1964.
7. Levitt, M., and Chothia, C.: Structural patterns in globular proteins. Nature *261*:552, 1976.
8. Pauling, L., and Corey, R. B.: Atomic coordinates and structure factors for two helical configurations of polypeptide chains. Proc. Natl. Acad. Sci. USA *37*:235, 1951.
9. Beychok, S., Tyuma, I., Benesch, R. E., and Benesch, R.: Optically active absorption bands of hemoglobin and its subunits. J. Biol. Chem. *242*:2460, 1967.
10. Green, D. W., Ingram, V. M., and Perutz, M. F.: The structure of haemoglobin. IV. Sign determination by the isomorphous replacement method. Proc. R. Soc. Lond. A. *225*:287, 1954.
11. Kendrew, J. C., Dickerson, R. E., Strandberg, B. E., Hart, R. G., Davis, D. R., Phillips, D. C., and Shore, V. C.: Structure of myoglobin. A three-dimensional Fourier synthesis at 2 Å resolution. Nature *185*:422, 1960.
12. Perutz, M. F., Rossman, M. G., Cullis, A. F., Muirhead, H., Will, G., and North, A. C. T.: Structure of haemoglobin. A three-dimensional Fourier synthesis at 5.5 Å resolution, obtained by x-ray analysis. Nature *185*:416, 1960.
13. Fermi, G., Perutz, M. F., Shaanan, B., and Fourme, B.: The crystal structure of human deoxyhemoglobin at 1.7 Å resolution. J. Mol. Biol. *175*:159, 1984.
14. Baldwin, J. M.: The structure of human carbonmonoxyhaemoglobin at 2.7 Å resolution. J. Mol. Biol. *136*:103, 1980.
15. Ladner, R. C., Heidner, E. J., and Perutz, M. F.: The structure of horse methemoglobin at 2 Å resolution. J. Mol. Biol. *114*:385, 1977.
16. Shaanan, B.: The iron-oxygen bond in human oxyhaemoglobin. Nature *296*:683, 1982.
16a. Shaanan, B.: The structure of human oxyhaemoglobin at 2.1 Å resolution. J. Mol. Biol. *171*:31, 1983.
17. Gelin, B. R., and Karplus, M.: Mechanism of tertiary structural change in hemoglobin. Proc. Natl. Acad. Sci. USA *74*:801, 1977.
18. Levitt, M.: Protein conformation dynamics and folding by computer simulation. Ann. Rev. Biophys. Bioeng. *11*:251, 1982.
19. Fermi, G., and Perutz, M.: Haemoglobin and myoglobin. In Phillips, D. C., and Richards, F. M. (eds.): Atlas of Molecular Structures in Biology. Oxford, Clarendon Press, 1981.
20. Perutz, M. F.: Stereochemical mechanism of oxygen transport by haemoglobin. Proc. R. Soc. Lond. B. *208*:135, 1980.
21. Baldwin, J.: Structure and cooperativity of haemoglobin. Trends in Biochemical Sciences *5*:224, 1980.
22. Rosemeyer, M. A., and Huehns, E. R.: On the mechanism of the dissociation of haemoglobin. J. Mol. Biol. *25*:253, 1967.
23. Perutz, M. F.: Stereochemistry of cooperative effects in haemoglobin. Nature *228*:726, 1970.
24. Arnone, A.: X-ray diffraction study of binding of 2,3-diphosphoglycerate to human deoxyhaemoglobin. Nature *237*:146, 1972.
25. Barlow, C. H., Maxwell, J. C., Wallace, W. J., and Caughey, W. S.: Elucidation of the mode of binding of oxygen to iron in oxyhemoglobin by infra-red spectroscopy. Biochem. Biophys. Res. Commun. *55*:91, 1973.
26. Duff, L. L., Appelman, E. H., Shriver, D. F., and Klotz, I. M.: Steric disposition of O_2 in oxyhemoglobin as revealed by its resonance Raman spectrum. Biochem. Biophys. Res. Commun. *90*:1098, 1979.
27. Pauling, L., and Coryell, C. D.: The magnetic properties and structure of hemoglobin, oxyhemoglobin and carbonmonoxyhemoglobin. Proc. Natl. Acad. Sci. USA *22*:210, 1936.
28. Phillips, S. E. V., and Schoenborn, B. P.: Neutron diffraction reveals oxygen histidine bond in oxymyoglobin. Nature *292*:81, 1981.
29. Imai, K., Ikeda-Saito, M., and Yonetani, T.: Studies on cobalt myoglobins and hemoglobins. XIII. A consequence of the occurrence of glutamine at the E7(58) site of α subunits in opossum hemoglobin. J. Mol. Biol. *144*:551, 1980.
30. Perutz, M. F., Ladner, J. E., Simon, S. R., and Ho, C.: Influence of globin structure on the state of the heme. Biochemistry *13*:2163, 1974.
31. Perutz, M. F., Fersht, A. R., Simon, S. R., and Roberts, G. C. K.: Influence of globin structure on the state of the heme. II. Allosteric transitions in methemoglobin. Biochemistry *13*:2174, 1974.
32. Countryman, R., Collins, D. M., and Hoard, J. L.: Stereochemistry of the low spin nonporphyrin, bis (imidazole)-α,β,γ,δ-tetraphenylporphinato iron (III) chloride. J. Am. Chem. Soc. *91*:5166, 1969.
33. Nagai, K., and Kitagawa, T.: Difference in Fe(II)-N (His-F8) stretching frequencies between deoxyhemoglobin in the two alternative quaternary structures. Proc. Natl. Acad. Sci. USA *77*:2033, 1980.
34. Nagai, K., Kitagawa, T., and Morimoto, H.: Quaternary structures and low molecular vibrations of deoxy and oxyhaemoglobin studied by resonance Raman scattering. J. Mol. Biol. *136*:271, 1980.
35. Baldwin, J., and Chothia, C.: Haemoglobin: The structural changes related to ligand binding and its allosteric mechanism. J. Mol. Biol. *129*:175, 1979.

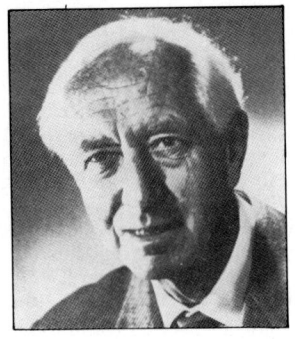

JEFFRIES WYMAN

Jeffries Wyman is one of the undisputed leaders in theoretical biology. He has used hemoglobin as a stepping stone toward understanding how complex macromolecules function.

Wyman harkens back to an earlier era when rigorous classical training was coupled with an insatiable appetite for all aspects of nature. His curiosity extends far beyond protein chemistry. He is well known for his travels, on foot, in far-flung corners of the world. He is a painter, a linguist, and an expert in archeology and classical art, interests that induced him to live major portions of his life in Cairo and Rome.

Wyman's heritage is a significant part of his persona. His grandfather, Jeffries Wyman (1814–1874), was Professor of Anatomy at Harvard and defended Darwin when his views on evolution were challenged by the famous biologist Louis Agassiz. At Harvard Medical School hangs a large group portrait that includes the elder Wyman with Oliver Wendell Holmes.

The younger Wyman read philosophy at Harvard and was awarded a degree *summa cum laude*. He also became strongly grounded in mathematics and biology, a combination that helped to shape his scientific career. He wrote a classic text on protein chemistry with his lifelong friend John Edsall. Since 1936, hemoglobin has been the focal point of Wyman's research. He became concerned with two fundamental problems: the Bohr effect and the basis of cooperativity. He and David Allen made the prescient conclusion that histidine residues were responsible for binding Bohr protons. Furthermore, they were the first to realize that cooperative oxygen binding implied a change in protein conformation.

In 1960, Wyman moved to Rome and began a long and fruitful collaboration with Eraldo Antonini and Maurizio Brunori. They provided him with a large body of experimental results. Wyman placed the functional properties of hemoglobin into a rigorous thermodynamic formalism. He developed the principles of linked functions (see text of this chapter), which provided quantitative insights into how allosteric proteins work and led him, together with Monod and Changeux, to propose the two-state model of allostery. The MWC model was a novel and heuristic way of explaining the functional behavior not only of hemoglobin but also of other multisubunit proteins.

Wyman remains actively engaged in research. Using hemoglobin as a model, he has extended the application of linkage theory to steady-state systems and is currently investigating the role of proteins as transducers of biological energy.

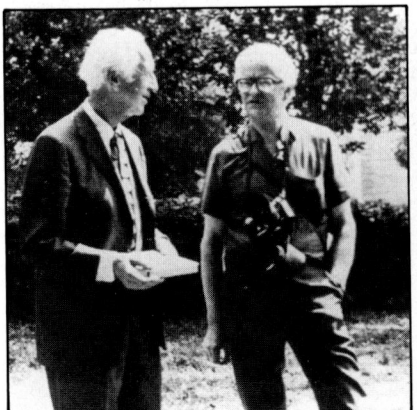

Wyman and Kendrew.

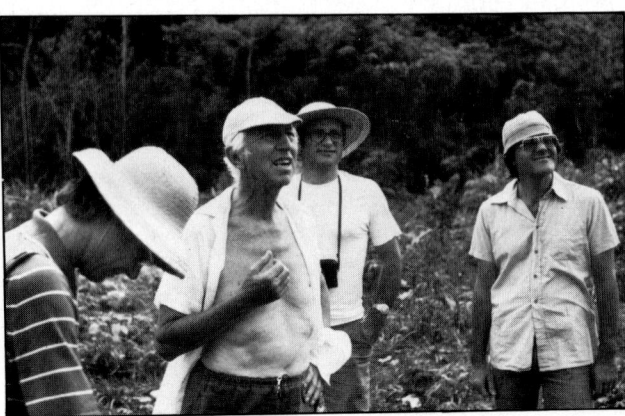

Wyman in the Amazon jungle with (L to R) Joseph Bonaventura, Morris Reichlin, and Maurizio Brunori.

3
HEMOGLOBIN FUNCTION

As discussed in Chapter 1, a number of distinguished physiologists at the turn of the century began to study hemoglobin in order to gain a better understanding of oxygen transport. They developed a sophisticated conception of hemoglobin's function at a time when knowledge of its structure was rather primitive It is difficult to improve on Barcroft's assessment[1] of the important physiological requisites of a respiratory pigment:

1. "Capability of transporting a large quantity of oxygen."
2. "Great solubility."
3. The uptake and release of oxygen at "appropriate pressures."
4. "Power of buffering a bicarbonate solution."

Experiments readily showed that the oxygen-carrying pigment in red blood cells had both high binding capacity and great solubility.

Demonstration of the ability of hemoglobin to load and unload oxygen at physiologic oxygen tensions depended on the development of suitable methods for determining the equilibrium between hemoglobin and oxygen, the so-called oxygen dissociation curve. Initially, there was considerable uncertainty in these measurements. However, by 1930, the classic sigmoid shape of the oxygen dissociation curve was well established for both whole blood and hemoglobin in solution (Fig. 3–1). The physiological significance of this phenomenon was readily appreciated. At the oxygen tension found in the air sacs of the lung, the hemoglobin in red cells becomes 97 per cent saturated with oxygen. Thus, normal blood, having a hemoglobin concentration of 15 g/dl would carry 1.34×15, or 20 ml of O_2 per 100 ml of blood (20 volumes/dl).* Following circulation through capillary beds, the mixed venous oxygen tension is normally about 40 mm Hg. As

---

*1 mole of O_2 at standard pressure and temperature is 22.4 l. Therefore, at 97 per cent saturation:
$$\frac{0.97 \times 1 \times 22,400}{16,100} = 1.34 \text{ ml } O_2/g \text{ Hb}$$

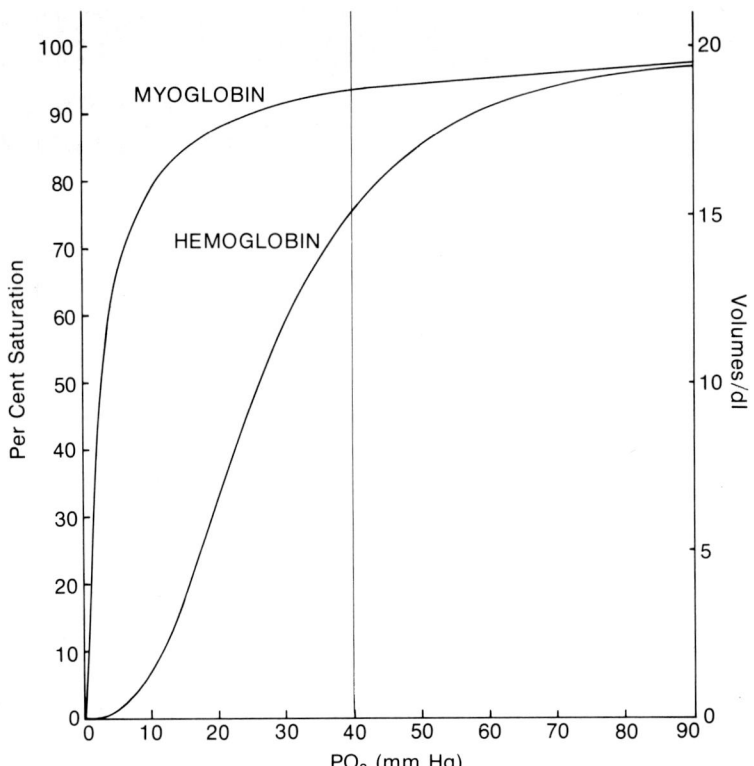

Figure 3–1. Oxygen binding curves of hemoglobin (whole blood) and myoglobin at 37°C and pH 7.4. The ordinate on the right applies to whole blood (15 g Hb/dl).

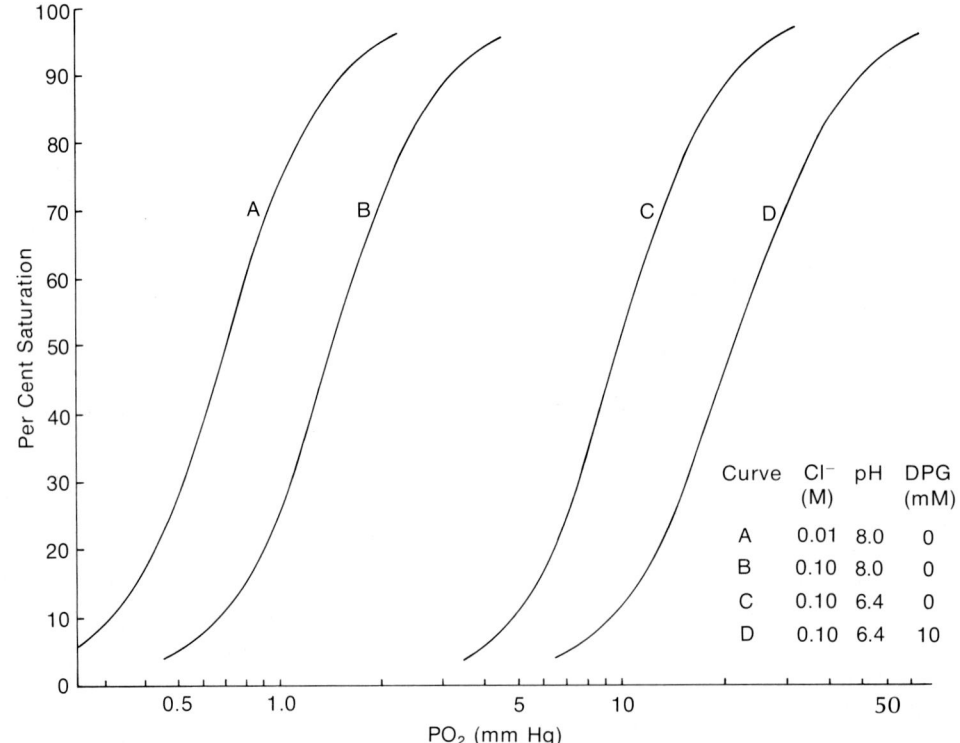

Curve	Cl⁻ (M)	pH	DPG (mM)
A	0.01	8.0	0
B	0.10	8.0	0
C	0.10	6.4	0
D	0.10	6.4	10

Figure 3–2. Effect of ionic strength, pH, and 2,3-DPG on oxygen affinity of human hemoglobin A at 20°C.

shown by the oxygen dissociation curve for whole blood of normal individuals (Fig. 3–1), at a PO_2 of 40 mm Hg, hemoglobin is about 75 per cent saturated with oxygen. Thus, blood normally gives up an average of $1.34 \times 15 \times (0.97-0.75)$, or 4.5 volumes of oxygen per dl, during its circulation through the tissues. Oxygen is released at a high enough PO_2 to maintain an adequate supply for intracellular utilization. Such an efficient mechanism for oxygen transport would not be possible were it not for the sigmoid shape of the oxygen dissociation curve. This sigmoid curve reflects the fact that hemoglobin binds oxygen in a cooperative fashion. If each of the four heme groups of the hemoglobin molecule bound oxygen independently of the others, the oxygen dissociation curve would have a hyperbolic shape, like that of myoglobin. As shown in Figure 3–1, such a curve would be most unsuitable for oxygen transport. In going from an arterial PO_2 of 95 mm Hg to a mixed venous PO_2 of 40 mm Hg, only 0.8 volumes/dl of O_2 would be unloaded. Further release of oxygen would be possible only at considerably lower oxygen tension.

In order for hemoglobin to fulfill its physiological role, it must bind to oxygen with an appropriate affinity. If the hemoglobin-oxygen bond were too weak, blood would not become oxygenated in the pulmonary circulation; if it were too strong, insufficient oxygen would be unloaded to tissues. Evolutionary "engineering" of hemoglobin has produced a molecule that can pick up and discharge oxygen at physiological oxygen pressures. The affinity of oxygen for hemoglobin can be conveniently expressed by the term P_{50}, the oxygen tension at which hemoglobin is half saturated. The higher the affinity of hemoglobin for oxygen, the lower the P_{50} and vice versa. Thus, P_{50} is inversely related to oxygen affinity. The P_{50} for human blood at physiologic pH (7.4) and temperature (37°C) is normally 26 ± 1 mm Hg.

A number of genetic and environmental factors can affect the oxygen affinity of human blood. The oxygen affinity of human red cells is significantly altered in a variety of congenital and acquired disorders (see Chapters 5 and 14). Furthermore, oxygen affinity varies considerably among different animals. This wide range in P_{50} is due in part to intrinsic structural differences between animal hemoglobins and in part to differences in intracellular milieu.[2] (See Chapter 6.) The oxygen affinity of hemoglobin can be markedly influenced by alterations in solvent conditions. Figure 3–2 shows how the P_{50} of normal human hemoglobin can vary over a 100-fold range owing to changes in pH, ionic strength, and, in particular, organic phosphates.

In summary, in order to satisfy the third of Barcroft's criteria, the loading and unloading of oxygen at physiologic oxygen tensions, hemoglobin must have an appropriate affinity for oxygen and must bind oxygen cooperatively. In this chapter, we will first discuss the buffering power of hemoglobin (Barcroft's fourth criterion) as part of a detailed consideration of the Bohr effect. Although Barcroft and the other physiologists of his day knew that PCO_2 and pH both influenced oxygen affinity, they were unaware that intracellular anions, primarily 2,3-DPG and chloride ion, also regulate hemoglobin function. In the next section, the interaction of these cofactors with hemoglobin will be reviewed. We will then return to a discussion of subunit interaction and how hemoglobin works. Chapter 5 will be concerned with the function of intact red cells under normal and pathological circumstances.

THE BOHR EFFECT

As described in Chapter 1, Bohr, Hasselbalch, and Krogh[3] discovered that the oxygen affinity of hemoglobin was reduced by increasing amounts of carbon dioxide. Subsequent studies demonstrated that this effect was due primarily to a reduction in pH.

Physiologists readily grasped the significance of these observations. They realized that an organism binds and unloads oxygen and CO_2 reciprocally: Oxygen is picked up by the lungs as CO_2 is expelled. In the tissues, the reverse process occurs. Because of the Bohr effect, CO_2 exchange *facilitates* oxygen exchange and vice versa. As shown in Figure 3–3A, over a physiologic pH range, P_{50} varies inversely with pH. This is the so-called alkaline Bohr effect. As CO_2 is expelled during circulation through the lungs, there is a corresponding increase in pH and a shift to the left in the oxygen dissociation curve. Thus, the relative increase in oxygen affinity favors the binding of oxygen to hemoglobin. Conversely, as blood circulates through capillaries, CO_2 enters the plasma and red cells. Because of the abundance of carbonic anhydrase in red cells, carbonic acid is readily formed: $CO_2 + H_2O \rightleftharpoons H_2CO_3$. The

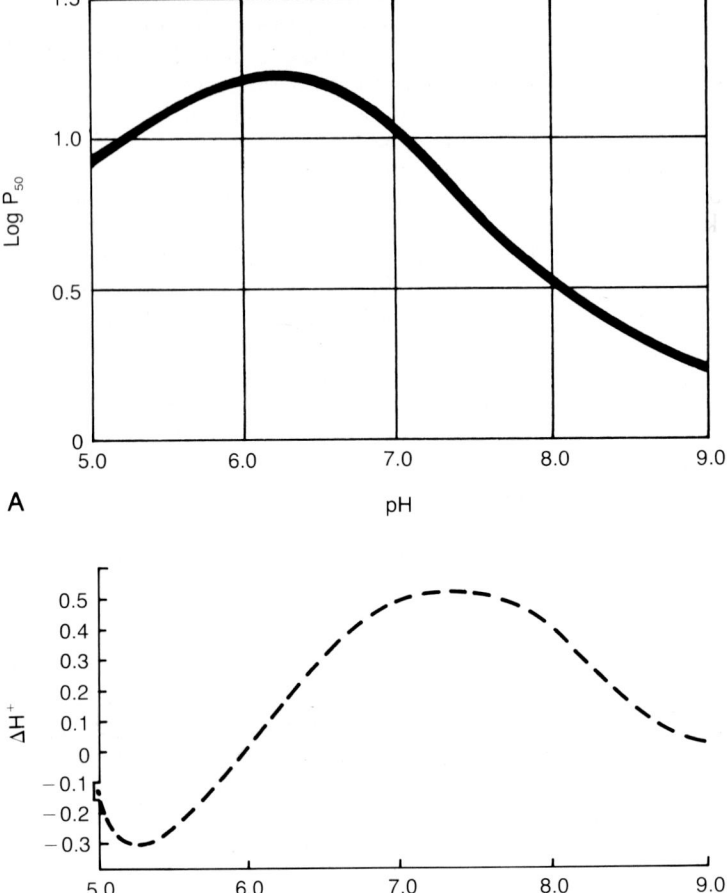

Figure 3–3. A, The effect of pH on oxygen affinity of human hemoglobin. The slope of the curve between pH 6.5 and 7.5 is a measure of the alkaline Bohr effect. B, Bohr protons taken up (pH 5.0 to 6.0) or released (pH > 6.0) upon oxygenation of hemoglobin. The ordinate (ΔH^+) shows the number of protons per heme.

ionization of this weak acid ($H_2CO_3 \rightleftharpoons H^+ + HCO_3^-$) results in a decrease in intracellular pH. Because of the Bohr effect, hemoglobin's oxygen affinity is now relatively decreased, resulting in enhanced unloading of oxygen to the respiring tissues. Thus, the Bohr effect permits a physiologically appropriate cycle for the transport of oxygen and CO_2 by the organism (Fig. 3–4).

As a result of the influx of CO_2 into red cells traversing the capillary circulation, there is an increase in intracellular H^+ and HCO_3^- concentrations. The binding of protons to hemoglobin represents the most important buffer system for maintaining intracellular pH at neutrality. As will be discussed below, this phenomenon is directly dependent on the Bohr effect. The bicarbonate ion diffuses out of the red cell and is replaced by chloride ion, thus preserving electrical neutrality. This anion exchange, the so-called Hamburger effect, is depicted in Figure 3–4. Finally, a minor proportion of the CO_2 that enters the red cell becomes covalently bound to hemoglobin as a carbamino complex. This phenomenon will be covered in the next section of this chapter.

In view of the physiological considerations mentioned above, it is not surprising that direct titrations revealed oxyhemoglobin to be a stronger acid than deoxyhemoglobin (Fig. 3–3B). This phenomenon is a direct corollary of the dependence of oxygen affinity on pH. The Bohr effect is an example of a linked function:

$$\begin{array}{ccc} Hb + 4O_2 & \rightleftharpoons & Hb(O_2)_4 \\ + & & + \\ H^+ & & H^+ \\ \Updownarrow & & \Updownarrow \\ HbH + 4O_2 & \rightleftharpoons & HbH(O_2)_4 \end{array}$$

The equilibria shown horizontally represent the oxygenation of hemoglobin and can readily be demonstrated experimentally by measuring oxygen dissociation curves at different pH's (Fig. 3–3A). The reactions shown vertically represent protonation of deoxyhemoglobin and oxyhemoglobin. These equilibria can be measured directly by following pH during the stepwise addition of alkali (Fig. 3–3B). According to a fundamental thermodynamic principle, the state of a chemical reaction at equilibrium is independent of the path taken. Thus, these two experimental approaches are really measuring the same phenomenon. These relationships were expressed quantitatively by Wyman[4] in terms of linkage equations:

$$\left(\frac{\partial H^+}{\partial Y}\right)_{pH} = \left(\frac{\partial (\log p)}{\partial pH}\right)_{Y}$$

where Y is the fractional saturation of hemoglobin with oxygen and p is oxygen tension. The expression on the right can be measured by oxygen equilibria (Fig. 3–3A), whereas the expression on the left can be determined by titration experiments (Fig. 3–3B). These two methods for measuring the Bohr effect are in excellent agreement. In the physiologic pH range (6.6 to 7.6), $\Delta \log P_{50}/ \Delta pH$ is about -0.6 for normal human hemoglobin. According to the preceding equation, with the binding of 4 moles of O_2 to deoxyhemoglobin, 4×0.6 or 2.4 protons would be released. Thus, the cycle of reactions shown above can be simplified as follows:

$$Hb(H) + 4 O_2 \rightleftharpoons Hb(O_2)_4 + 2.4 H^+$$

The fact that protons bind more readily to deoxyhemoglobin than to oxyhemoglobin must mean that specific groups on the molecule have higher affinity for protons when hemoglobin is in the deoxy or T quaternary structure. Possible candidates include the N termini of the α and β chains and the imidazole groups of histidine residues, because the binding of protons of these groups can change significantly at neutral (i.e., physiologic) pH. A number of experimental approaches have been used to identify the specific sites on the molecule responsible for the physiologic or "alkaline" Bohr effect. Perutz[5] has approached the problem by comparing the three-dimensional structures of T-state (deoxy) and R-state (oxy) hemoglobins and identifying salt bonds that are present in the T structure but are broken in the R structure. Protons are bound more readily when salt bonds are formed than when they are broken:

$$RNH_3 \cdots {}^-OOCR' \rightleftharpoons RNH_2 + R'COO^- + H^+$$

Perutz[5] has made specific assignments of Bohr protons by examining the high-resolution structures of deoxyhemoglobin and oxyhemoglobin and determining sites where salt bridges, such as that shown above, are present in the former but not in the latter. These assignments of Bohr protons can be tested by observation on mutant or chemically modified hemoglobins in which specific sites on the molecule have been altered. This dual approach has enabled the identification of three sites that contribute to the alkaline Bohr effect[6,7]: (1) the imidazole of β 146 histidine (see Figure 2–9); (2) the N-terminal amino

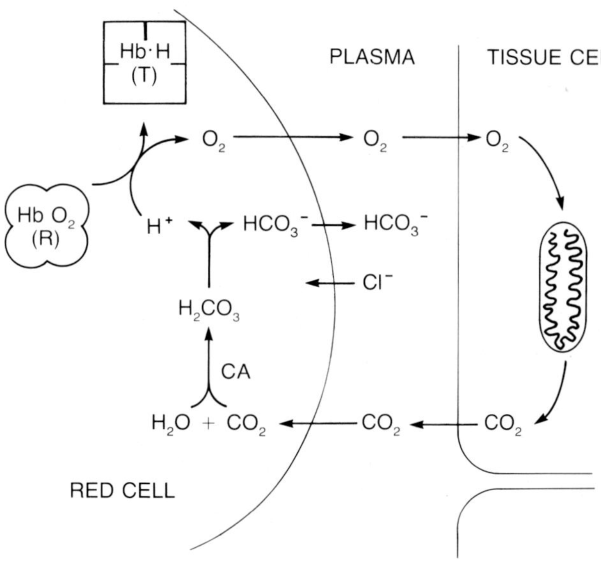

Figure 3–4. The unloading of oxygen and the uptake of protons and CO_2 during the circulation of the red cell through tissues. The formation of carbonic acid (H_2CO_3) from CO_2 and water is catalyzed by carbonic anhydrase (CA). The dissociation of O_2 from hemoglobin and the binding of protons are associated with a change from the R to the T quaternary structure.

group of the α chain; and (3) the imidazole of α 122 histidine.[8] Although it is likely that this conclusion is substantially correct, the precise (quantitative) contribution of each of these as well as other sites is uncertain and, at this time, somewhat controversial. Conclusions drawn from comparisons of normal and modified hemoglobins may be difficult to interpret because the modification sometimes has widespread effects on functional properties. Alternative approaches to identify the sites responsible for the alkaline Bohr effect include physical probes such as nuclear magnetic resonance (NMR) spectroscopy[9, 10] and hydrogen exchange measurements.[10a, 11] A study utilizing deuterium exchange has confirmed that under physiological conditions (0.1 M Cl^-), β 146 His contributes about 50 per cent to the alkaline Bohr effect.[10a] However, contrary results have been obtained from NMR titrations of β 146 His.[9, 10] Although difficult to interpret, Hydrogen exchange measurements suggest that other residues may also be important participants in the Bohr effect.[11] In fact, calculations of electrostatic interactions based on the three-dimensional structure of deoxyhemoglobin and the change in quaternary structure on ligand binding suggest that the Bohr effect may be spread over many sites, including a number of lysine residues.[12, 13] However, these calculations need to be refined by use of coordinates for liganded hemoglobin.

CARBAMINO FORMATION

Early gasometric measurements established the reciprocal relationship between the oxygen and carbon dioxide content of blood. As explained in the previous section, carbon dioxide is transported primarily as bicarbonate, following its hydration and ionization within the red cell. In addition, a portion of carbon dioxide is bound chemically to hemoglobin.[14] Hemoglobin solutions contain more total analyzable CO_2 than a protein-free solution of comparable pH and PCO_2. From a consideration of the structure of carbon dioxide

$$\ddot{\text{O}} :: \text{C} :: \ddot{\text{O}}$$

it can be seen that its electron-poor carbon atom is capable of attack on nucleophiles such as electron-rich amino groups

$$\text{H} : \ddot{\text{N}} : \text{R}$$
$$\text{H}$$

to form a carbamino complex

$$^-:\ddot{\text{O}}:\text{C}:\ddot{\text{N}}:\text{R} + \text{H}^+$$
$$\quad\quad :\ddot{\text{O}}: \quad \text{H}$$

This reaction depends on the existence of free primary amino groups in the protein. If an amino group is protonated (H_3^+NR), the reaction will not occur. In proteins, free (primary) amino groups occur in two forms: the N-terminal amino group of each polypeptide chain and the ε-amino group of lysine residues. The latter amino groups have a pK of about 9. Thus, at neutral (physiologic) pH, they are 99 per cent protonated and unable to bind CO_2. In contrast, the pK of N-terminal amino groups is close to neutrality.[15] On chemical grounds, it seems reasonable that CO_2 can combine nonenzymatically with the N-terminal amino groups of hemoglobin. Experimental verification has been provided by measurement of CO_2 binding to hemoglobins that had been modified by selective blocking of the N termini of the α and β chains.[16, 17] From these considerations, it is not surprising that carbamino formation would vary directly with pH (Fig. 3–5).[18] Moreover, at a given pH, deoxyhemoglobin binds CO_2 more readily than does oxyhemoglobin. Thus, the combination of CO_2 and hemoglobin to form a carbamino complex is an example of an oxygen-linked reaction. Other oxygen-linked functions include the interaction of protons and organic phosphates with hemoglobin. Similar linkage equations can be written for all these interactions.[19] In the case of CO_2, the following equilibrium applies:

$$\text{Hb}(CO_2)_n + 4\,O_2 \rightleftharpoons \text{Hb}(O_2)_4 + n\,CO_2$$

This reaction is identical in form to that shown in the previous section on the Bohr effect, except that the H^+ ion is replaced by CO_2. Analogous to the binding of protons to hemoglobin, the above reaction implies that, at a given pH, carbamino hemoglobin has a lower affinity for oxygen than has hemoglobin in the absence of CO_2. This relationship can be readily demonstrated by measuring the oxygen dissociation curves at various pH's in the presence and absence of CO_2. As Figure 3–6 shows, CO_2 has a minimal effect on P_{50} at a pH of less than 6.8 because the N-terminal amino groups are now predominantly in the

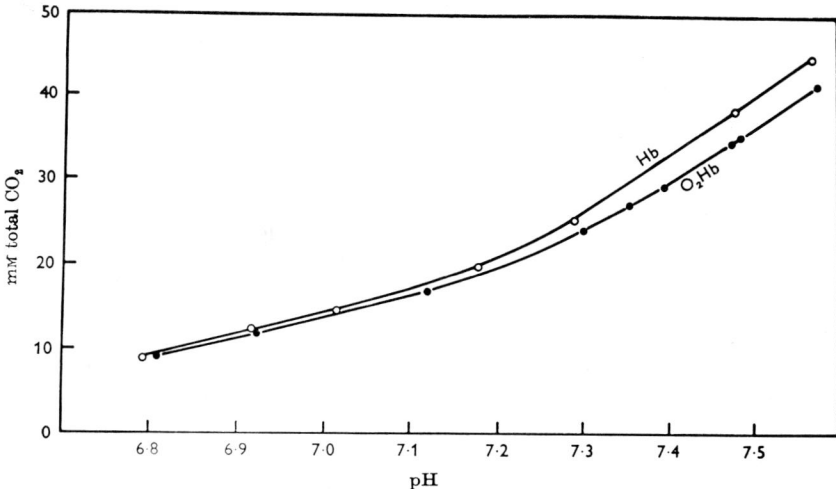

Figure 3–5. The effect of pH and oxygenation on the binding of carbon dioxide to a concentrated solution of hemoglobin at 37°C, $PCO_2 = 42$ mm Hg. (From Kilmartin, J. V., and Rossi-Bernardi, L.: Physiol. Rev. 53:836, 1973.)

protonated form. The stereochemical basis for the interaction of CO_2 and hemoglobin is less well understood than that of the Bohr effect. It seems likely that CO_2, like protons, stabilizes the deoxy conformation. Arnone[20] has completed x-ray diffraction analysis of crystals of human deoxyhemoglobin in the presence and absence of CO_2. He was able to demonstrate the carbamino complex at the N termini of the β chains. No gross perturbation in the tertiary structure of the subunit was observed.

Unexpectedly, no carbamate formation at the N termini of the α chains was demonstrated.

As the x-ray diffraction analysis suggests, α and β chains differ in their interaction with carbon dioxide. In the absence of organic phosphates such as 2,3-DPG, the β chains of deoxyhemoglobin bind CO_2 with an affinity about threefold that of α chains.[21] Upon oxygenation, the β chains release a considerable portion of their bound CO_2, whereas the CO_2 bound to the N termini of α chains is nearly

Figure 3–6. The effect of pH, PCO_2, and organic phosphates on the oxygen affinity of human hemoglobin. A (○) represents phosphate-free Hb, $PCO_2 = 0$; B (◑) represents phosphate-free hemoglobin, $PCO_2 = 40$ mm Hg; C represents hemoglobin containing equimolar ATP (□) or 2,3-DPG (▽), $PCO_2 = 0$; D represents hemoglobin containing equimolar ATP (●) or 2,3-DPG (▲), $PCO_2 = 40$ mm Hg. (From Kilmartin, J. V., and Rossi-Bernardi, L.: Physiol. Rev. 53:836, 1973.)

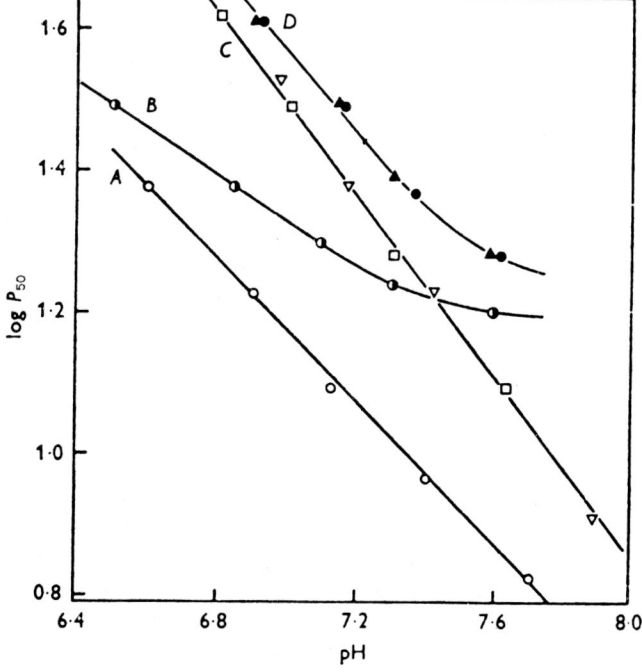

unaffected by oxygenation.[22-25] The addition of organic phosphates such as 2,3-DPG or inositol hexaphosphate (IHP) causes a marked reduction in the binding of CO_2 to the β chains of deoxyhemoglobin. Interestingly, this heterogeneity in the binding of CO_2 is reflected in studies on isolated subunits.[26] Like Hb A ($\alpha_2\beta_2$), the β_4 tetramer binds CO_2 more readily when deoxygenated. It follows that CO_2 causes a reduction in the oxygen affinity of β_4. In contrast, CO_2 has no effect on the oxygen affinity of isolated α chains.[26]

It is difficult to determine how significant a role carbamino formation plays in CO_2 transport. Certainly, the reciprocal binding of CO_2 and O_2 is physiologically appropriate. That is, as oxygen is given up to respiring tissues, direct CO_2 uptake by hemoglobin is enhanced. As mentioned in the section on the Bohr effect (see Figure 3–4), CO_2 is transported primarily as bicarbonate ions and protons bound to hemoglobin. Under physiologic conditions, only about 10 per cent of CO_2 produced by respiring tissues is transported as a carbamino complex with hemoglobin.[27] An earlier estimate by Roughton was too high because it failed to account for the fact that CO_2 and 2,3-DPG compete for the same binding site on the β chain (see the section below and Figure 3–6).

INTERACTION WITH INORGANIC ANIONS

The important role of organic ions, particularly 2,3-DPG, in regulating intracellular hemoglobin function (discussed below) was partially anticipated by earlier studies showing that inorganic ions have a marked effect on the oxygenation of hemoglobin.[1, 28, 29] Oxygen affinity is progressively lowered in the presence of increasing concentrations of inorganic phosphate or chloride ion. Comparable to the interaction of hemoglobin with protons, CO_2, and organic phosphates, linkage considerations dictate that these inorganic anions bind more strongly to deoxyhemoglobin than to oxyhemoglobin. The sites of binding to deoxyhemoglobin have been identified by x-ray analysis.[30, 31] They include the N termini of the β chains as well as specific sites on the α chains. As shown in Figure 3–7, one chloride interacts with the protonated N-terminal amino group of α_2 valine and the hydroxyl group of α_2 131 serine, and another is positioned between the

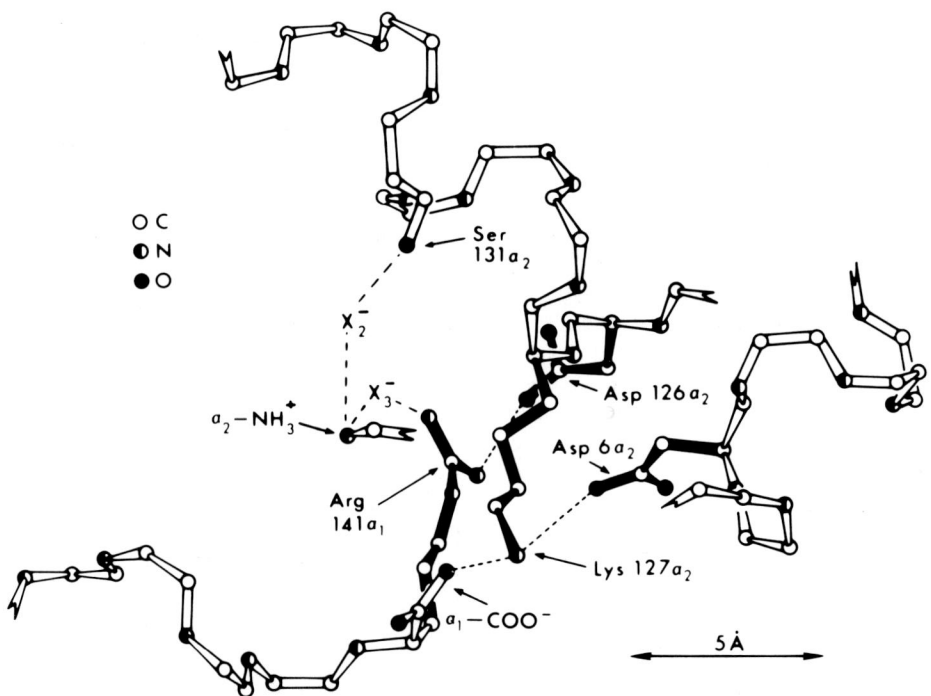

Figure 3–7. Diagram of the N-terminal amino group of the α_2 chain in deoxyhemoglobin A. Anion binding sites are shown as X_2^- and X_3^-. The broken lines indicate salt bonds. For clarity, the peptide backbone between the first and fifth residues of the α_2 chain has been deleted. The black portion represents structure penetrating below the plane of the page. (From O'Donnell, S., et al.: J. Biol. Chem. *254*:12204, 1979.)

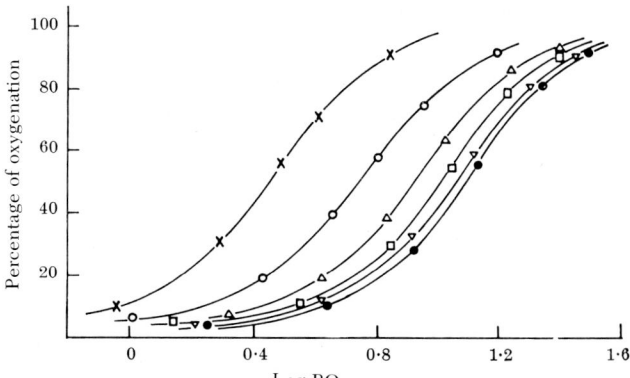

Figure 3–8. The effect of 2,3-DPG on the oxygenation of phosphate-free hemoglobin (X = no 2,3-DPG; ○ = 0.2 mM 2,3-DPG; △ = 0.4 mM 2,3-DPG; □ = 0.6 mM 2,3-DPG; ▽ = 0.8 mM 2,3-DPG; ● = 1.0 mM 2,3-DPG). (From Benesch, R., and Benesch, R. E.: Nature 221:618, 1969.)

α_2 valine N-terminal amino group and the guanidinium group of α_1 141 arginine (i.e., on the other α chain). In addition, there are the two corresponding symmetry-related binding sites not shown in Figure 3–7. There are several other sites on hemoglobin that bind chloride, but because the interactions are weaker and not oxygen-linked, they are much less significant.

The binding of chloride ion to hemoglobin has been studied directly by ^{35}Cl nuclear magnetic resonance[32, 33] and indirectly by oxygen equilibria and acid-base titrations on normal, chemically modified, and mutant hemoglobins.[31, 34, 35] There are two classes of binding sites. Only the high-affinity sites are oxygen-linked,[32] i.e., stronger binding to deoxyhemoglobin than to oxyhemoglobin. In the absence of organic phosphates, there appear to be two sites on deoxyhemoglobin that have relatively high affinity for chloride (K_D = 0.01 M): the α amino group of the α chain and the ε-amino group of β 82 (EF6) lysine.[34] The former site agrees with the structural analysis mentioned above. Because the latter is an important 2,3-DPG binding site, it probably does not bind significant amounts of chloride under physiologic conditions. In contrast, the interaction of chloride at the N terminus of the α chain appears to be an important determinant of hemoglobin function. Chloride binding at this site stabilizes the protonation of this amino group, thereby raising its pKa. Upon oxygenation, both the chloride ion and the proton are released:

$$\alpha\text{-NH}_3^+\text{Cl}^- \rightleftharpoons \alpha\text{-NH}_2 + \text{H}^+ + \text{Cl}^-$$

Deoxy   Oxy

Thus, part of the pH dependency of oxygenation (the Bohr effect) is linked to chloride binding. In fact, the alkaline Bohr effect decreases by about half if the chloride ion concentration is reduced from physiologic (0.1 M) to zero.[36]

INTERACTION WITH ORGANIC PHOSPHATES

In view of the known effect of inorganic anions on oxygen affinity (discussed in the preceding section), it is difficult to understand why the specific anions that exist in the red cell were not explored until 1967. The erythrocyte of humans and most other mammals has a very high concentration of the glycolytic intermediate 2,3-DPG. Although it is the most abundant organic phosphate of the red cell, it is present only in trace amounts in other tissues. Its concentration within the red cell is normally about 5 mM per liter of packed cells, roughly equivalent to the concentration of hemoglobin tetramer and about fourfold that of ATP. All other organic phosphates are present in much lower concentrations. In 1967, Chanutin and Curnish[37] and Benesch and Benesch[38] independently demonstrated that 2,3-DPG is a potent modifier of hemoglobin function. Hemoglobin that had been carefully "stripped" of all red cell organic phosphates had an unexpectedly high oxygen affinity, although heme-heme interaction[39] and the Bohr effect[40] remained intact. As shown in Figure 3–8, the addition of a low concentration of 2,3-DPG (0.2 to 1.0 mM) results in a progressive decrease in oxygen affinity. ATP is almost as effective as 2,3-DPG. The relative potency of other organic phosphates in lowering the oxygen affinity of hemoglobin is roughly proportional to their anionic strength.

The structure of 2,3-DPG is shown in Figure 3–9. It has five titratable acid groups. As the

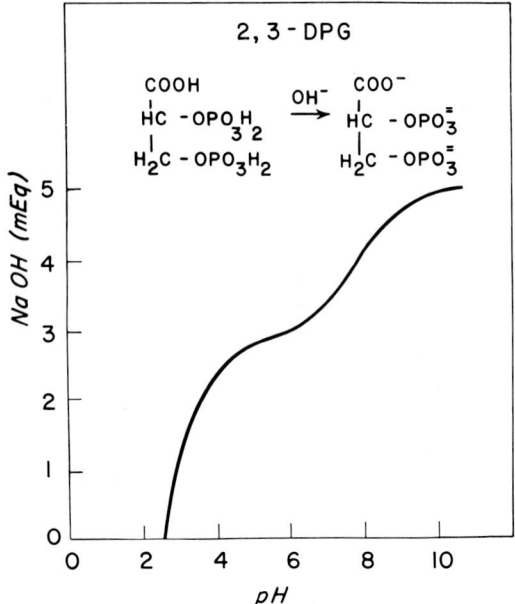

Figure 3–9. Structure of 2,3-DPG and titration curve showing five titratable protons.

titration curve shows, at physiologic pH, 2,3-DPG has about 3.5 negative charges. Thus, it qualifies as a potent polyanion. On this basis, the Beneschs considered it likely that 2,3-DPG interacted electrostatically with positively charged groups on the hemoglobin molecule. They measured the binding of 2,3-DPG to hemoglobin at physiologic pH and ionic strength by means of a modified form of equilibrium dialysis.[41] As shown in Figure 3–10, 2,3-DPG bound to deoxyhemoglobin in a 1:1 molar ratio.* From this diagram, it can be seen that half of the hemoglobin was bound when

---

*One mole of 2,3-DPG per mole of deoxyhemoglobin tetramer.

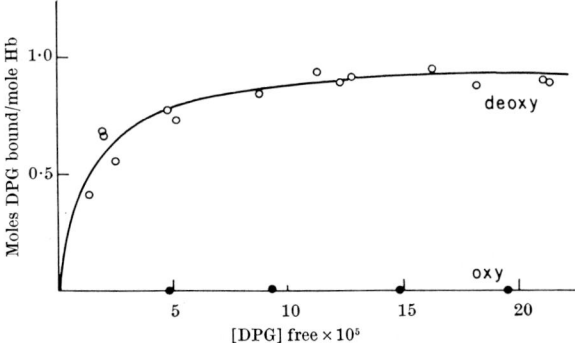

Figure 3–10. The binding of 2,3-DPG to oxyhemoglobin and deoxyhemoglobin. (From Benesch, R., and Benesch, R. E.: Nature 221:618, 1969.)

the concentration of free 2,3-DPG was 2.5×10^{-5} M. Thus, the equilibrium dissociation constant (K_D) for the binding of 2,3-DPG to deoxyhemoglobin can be expressed as follows:

$$\frac{[Hb][DPG]}{[HbDPG]} = K_D = 2.5 \times 10^{-5} \text{ M}$$

In contrast, under the same experimental conditions, 2,3-DPG binds much less strongly to oxyhemoglobin (Fig. 3–10) and other liganded forms of hemoglobin such as carboxyhemoglobin and cyanomethemoglobin.[41] ATP binds to hemoglobin competitively with 2,3-DPG and, like 2,3-DPG, in a 1:1 molar ratio.[42] At low pH and low ionic strength, 2,3-DPG and other polyanions bind nonspecifically to both deoxyhemoglobin and oxyhemoglobin.[43] For this reason, some studies on the binding of 2,3-DPG to hemoglobin are difficult to interpret.[44,45] More recently, the binding of organic phosphates to hemoglobin has been defined more precisely under physiologic conditions, by a variety of techniques, including membrane dialysis,[46] oxygen equilibria,[47,48] measurement of associated proton binding,[49] and phosphorus NMR.[50,51] These studies indicate that the K_D for 2,3-DPG and deoxyhemoglobin is about 3×10^{-5} M, whereas that for oxyhemoglobin is about 3×10^{-3} M. These equilibrium constants indicate that 2,3-DPG binds much more strongly to hemoglobin than does chloride ion (see section above).

In addition to protons, CO_2, and Cl^-, 2,3-DPG is another cofactor that binds to hemoglobin reciprocally with oxygen. Accordingly, linkage equations can be written,[19] similar to those for the Bohr effect and carbamino formation. The following net reaction pertains:

$$HbDPG + 4 O_2 \rightleftharpoons Hb(O_2)_4 + DPG$$

This equilibrium is identical in form to those shown previously for H^+ and CO_2 interaction. The equilibrium constant that the Beneschs obtained from direct measurement of the binding of 2,3-DPG to deoxyhemoglobin was in good agreement with the constant derived indirectly from the measurement of oxygen affinity in the absence and presence of 2,3-DPG. This is entirely analogous to the two experimental approaches for measuring the Bohr effect (see above).

In view of its potent effect on the oxygen dissociation curve, 2,3-DPG must act as an allosteric modifier of hemoglobin function. It was therefore of prime importance to determine the precise site on the hemoglobin molecule at which 2,3-DPG binds. Considerable evidence indicated that the N-terminal amino groups of the β chain were involved. Human hemoglobins A_{Ic} and F_I, which are blocked at the N terminus of their non-α chains, have markedly impaired reactivity to 2,3-DPG.[52] Furthermore, 2,3-DPG and CO_2 were shown to be competitors in their binding to hemoglobin.[53-55] The long recognized high oxygen affinity of blood of the fetus and neonate can be explained by the impaired reactivity of human Hb F (F_{II}) with 2,3-DPG.[56,57] Among the differences in primary sequence between the β and γ chains is position 143 (H21): histidine in the β chain and uncharged serine in the γ chain. Fitting 2,3-DPG to a high-resolution (2.5 Å) model of deoxyhemoglobin, Perutz[58] concluded that the organic polyanion could form salt bonds with the β N-terminal amino groups, the imidazoles of β 143 histidine, and the amino groups of β 82 (EF6) lysine. By contrast, in oxyhemoglobin, the β H helices are too close together and the β N termini are too far apart to permit a satisfactory fit. Subsequently, Arnone[59] analyzed crystals of deoxyhemoglobin bound to 2,3-DPG by x-ray diffraction and established this as the correct binding site. A diagram of the 2,3-DPG binding site is shown in Chapter 2 (see Figure 2–11). Phosphorus NMR studies indicate that 2,3-DPG binds to the same residues in oxyhemoglobin.[51]

In summary, 2,3-DPG binds firmly to a specific site on deoxyhemoglobin, whereas the conformational change induced by oxygenation results in much weaker binding to oxyhemoglobin. One can then ask how well does 2,3-DPG bind to partially oxygenated forms of hemoglobin, and at what point in oxygenation is the cofactor ejected? In general, it is difficult to design appropriate experiments that provide information on the properties of the partially liganded intermediates. One can prepare hemoglobin derivatives, such as $\alpha_2^{CNMet}\beta_2$ and $\alpha_2\beta_2^{CNMet}$, in which the α or β chains are frozen in the r tertiary structure. These analogues of partially oxygenated hemoglobin bind 2,3-DPG, although more weakly than native deoxyhemoglobin.[60,61] The two-state allosteric model (see below) predicts that 2,3-DPG binds firmly to partially oxygenated hemoglobins that still possess the T quaternary conformation. When the tetramer flips into the R conformation, 2,3-DPG would be ejected. Thus, interaction with organic phosphates could be considered a probe of quaternary structure. Experimental results utilizing spin-labeled analogues of 2,3-DPG are in accord with this model.[62,63] There are both kinetic[64] and equilibrium[65] studies that indicate that 2,3-DPG is released following the binding of the third oxygen to the tetramer.

OTHER PROPERTIES OF HEMOGLOBIN

There is a large body of information on the various physical and chemical properties of hemoglobin. In general, it is striking how many of these are dependent on the quaternary structure, that is, whether hemoglobin is in the T (deoxy) or R (oxy) conformation. A broad comparison is shown in Table 3–1. Many of the differences in the chemical properties of

Table 3–1. PHYSICAL AND CHEMICAL DIFFERENCES BETWEEN OXYHEMOGLOBIN AND DEOXYHEMOGLOBIN

	Oxyhemoglobin	Deoxyhemoglobin	References
Physical Properties			
Visible spectrum: absorbance peak(s)	576,540 nm	555 nm	
Soret spectrum: absorbance peak	415 nm	430 nm	
Magnetic susceptibility	Low (diamagnetic)	High (paramagnetic)	
Chemical Properties			
Solubility	High	Lower	
Dissociation into αβ dimers	Fast	Slow	113
Binding to haptoglobin	Fast	Slow	114
Digestion by carboxypeptidase	Fast	Slow	115
Reactivity of β 93-cysteine SH	Fast	Slow	68–70
Reactivity to bromothymol blue	Slow	Fast	116
Reactivity to cyanate	Slow	Slower	117, 118
Functional Properties			
Affinity for heme ligands	High	Low	
Affinity for protons	Low	High	
Relative affinity for CO_2	Low	High	
Affinity for organic phosphates	Low	High	

oxyhemoglobin and deoxyhemoglobin can be interpreted and even predicted in terms of the three-dimensional structures established by Perutz and associates.

As shown in Table 3–1, deoxyhemoglobin dissociates into dimers much less readily than oxyhemoglobin:

$$\text{Deoxyhemoglobin} \quad \alpha_2\beta_2 \rightleftharpoons 2\alpha\beta$$

$$\text{Oxyhemoglobin} \quad \alpha_2\beta_2 \rightleftharpoons 2\alpha\beta$$

This difference is due primarily to the intersubunit salt bonds, including 2,3-DPG, which stabilize the deoxy structure (see Chapter 2). The dissociation of hemoglobin into dimers appears to be necessary for its binding to haptoglobin[66] and for the filtration of hemoglobin through renal glomeruli.[67]

The sulfhydryl groups have proved to be useful probes of hemoglobin conformation. As shown in Table 3–1, the sulfhydryl group of the cysteine residue at β 93 is 70-fold less reactive with hemoglobins in the deoxy or T structure than when it is liganded.[68–70] The structural explanation for this finding is that when hemoglobin is deoxygenated, this group is partially hidden and therefore less accessible to attack by sulfhydryl reagents. This cysteine (β F9) is adjacent to the proximal (F8) histidine. Both are invariant residues, present in all mammalian hemoglobins of known structure. The functional significance of F9 cysteine is not understood. It is worth noting that animal hemoglobins having serine at this site have a markedly exaggerated Bohr effect (see Chapter 6). The other two cysteine residues in hemoglobins, α 104 (G11) and β 112 (G14), are located at the $\alpha_1\beta_1$ interface. The study of the vibrational transitions of these sulfhydryl groups by infrared spectroscopy has proved to be a useful probe of perturbations at the $\alpha_1\beta_1$ interface.[71, 72]

PROPERTIES OF ISOLATED CHAINS

Because the behavior of hemoglobin is strongly dependent on interactions between the α and β globin subunits, it is no surprise that the functional properties of isolated chains are markedly different from those of the intact tetramer.

Alpha and beta chains can be prepared from human hemoglobin by treating a hemolysate with p-chloromercuribenzoate, which forms a complex with the globin sulfhydryl groups.[73] Following isolation of the subunit and chemical removal of the mercury compound, these preparations closely resemble native hemoglobin subunits. Naturally occurring, free β chains can be found in hemolysates of some individuals with α thalassemia. The functional properties of so-called hemoglobin H are identical to those of β chains prepared from normal hemoglobin A.

Like myoglobin, isolated α chains are monomers (16,000 M.W.).[74] These heme proteins share the following properties[75, 76]:

1. High oxygen affinity.
2. Absence of subunit cooperativity (Hill n = 1.0). The oxygen binding curve is in the form of a rectangular hyperbola (see Figure 3–1).
3. Absent Bohr effect.
4. No effect of organic phosphates or CO_2 on oxygenation.

In contrast, β chains aggregate to form a β_4 tetramer (Hb H). Subunit dissociation of β_4 differs from that of $\alpha_2\beta_2$. Unlike Hb A, oxy β_4 dissociates less readily than deoxy β_4.[77] The oxygen affinity of β_4 is even higher than that of β monomers, and subunit cooperativity is not detectable.[75, 76] In dilute solutions, in which β monomers appear, oxygen affinity decreases,[78] as dictated by thermodynamic linkage considerations. Unlike α chains, the oxygenation of β_4 is affected by allosteric modifiers such as protons,[79, 80] organic phosphates,[81] and CO_2[26] although to a much lesser extent than Hb A.

Isolated α chains and β_4 behave like mutant and chemically modified $\alpha_2\beta_2$ tetramers that have high oxygen affinity and lack subunit cooperativity. The deoxy forms of these hemoglobins have a characteristic absorption spectrum in the 400 to 450 nm range. Furthermore, a similar spectrum appears transiently upon rapid removal of oxygen or carbon monoxide from normal hemoglobin by means of flash photolysis (see below). In all cases, the hemoglobin appears to be in an "oxy" conformation even when fully deoxygenated.

COOPERATIVITY

The sigmoid shape of the oxygen-hemoglobin binding curve indicates the presence of cooperativity. As discussed in Chapter 1, A. V. Hill,[82] a student in Bancroft's laboratory, devised an empirical expression for the equilibrium of hemoglobin with oxygen. This equation was derived before it was established that one molecule of hemoglobin binds four molecules of oxygen. Therefore, it is without apparent physical basis. Nevertheless, the Hill equation has proved useful in expressing oxygen binding data. If hemoglobin binds oxygen according to the reaction

$$Hb + nO_2 \rightleftharpoons Hb(O_2)_n,$$

the dissociation equilibrium constant is

$$K_D = \frac{[Hb][PO_2]^n}{[Hb(O_2)_n]},$$

and the fractional saturation of hemoglobin with oxygen is

$$Y = \frac{[Hb(O_2)_n]}{[Hb] + [Hb(O_2)_n]}.$$

Therefore,

$$\frac{Y}{1-Y} = \frac{[PO_2]^n}{K_D}.$$

At $Y = 0.5$,

$$PO_2 = P_{50}$$
$$K_D = (P_{50})^n.$$

Thus,

$$\log \frac{Y}{1-Y} = n \log \left(\frac{PO_2}{P_{50}}\right) \quad \text{(Hill equation)}.$$

If measurements of oxygen equilibria are plotted according to the Hill equation with $\log Y/1-Y$ on the ordinate and $\log PO_2$ on the abscissa, a linear plot would be expected. As shown in Figure 3–11, a Hill plot of oxygen binding data is generally linear for values of Y between 0.1 and 0.9 (10 to 90 per cent saturation). The x intercept of this line at $Y = 0.5$ gives the P_{50} value. The slope of this line, n, is a measure of subunit cooperativity. The Hill plots of normal human hemoglobin (and those of most other mammalian hemoglobins) reveal n values of 2.8 to 3.0. This number is without direct physical meaning. Heme proteins that have a single subunit, such as isolated α chains or myoglobin, have n values of 1.0. Thus, their oxygen binding curves have the form of a rectangular hyperbola. Likewise, tetrameric hemoglobins that fail to change conformation on oxygenation have an absence of subunit cooperativity and Hill plots in which $n = 1.0$. Examples include hemoglobin H ($β_4$),[75, 76] certain high-affinity variants such as hemoglobins Bethesda and Kempsey (see Chapter 14), and certain chemically modified hemoglobins.[83-85] In contrast, if the oxygenation of one subunit of hemoglobin resulted in an infinite increase in the affinity of the other three hemes for oxygen, the partially oxygenated intermediate would not exist and the slope of the Hill plot would be 4.0. Thus, the Hill plots of normal (native) hemoglobins indicate that there is a strong but not infinite degree of cooperativity between subunits.

In the initial stages of oxygen binding (Y <

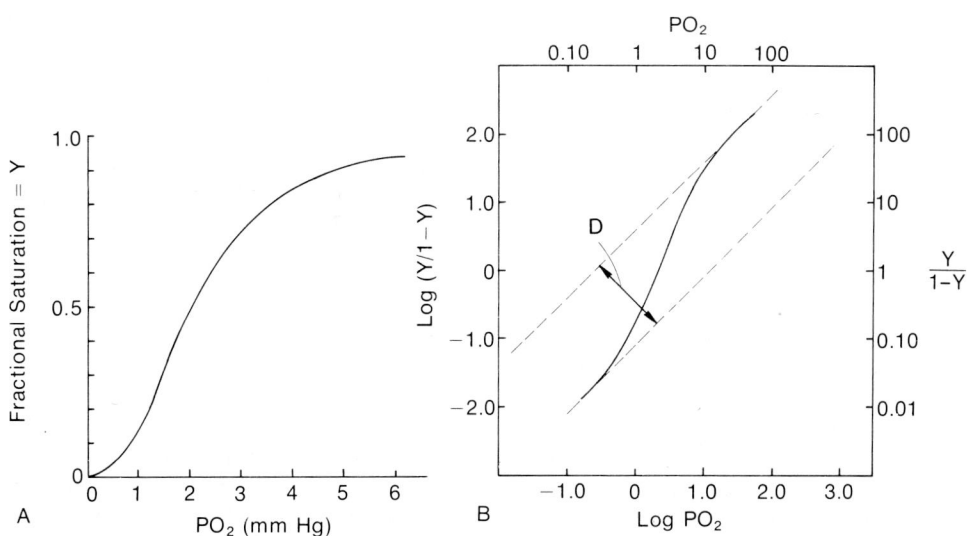

Figure 3–11. Oxygen binding curve of human hemoglobin A at 25°C and pH 7.4. *A,* Arithmetic plot. *B,* Hill plot. (This figure was constructed from data of Tyuma, I., Shimizu, K., and Imai, K.: Biochem. Biophys. Res. Commun. 43:423, 1971.)

0.1) there is no subunit cooperativity, as documented by the fact that the slope of the Hill plot approaches 1.0 (Fig. 3–11). It is likely that during this initial binding of ligand to heme, the hemoglobin remains in the "deoxy" quaternary structure (designated the T or tense structure in the terminology of allosteric models discussed below). The affinity of deoxyhemoglobin for oxygen is markedly affected by solvent conditions. Protons and organic phosphates that stabilize the deoxy structure (see Chapter 2) cause a significant shift to the right of this asymptote (i.e., reduction in O_2 affinity). When all hemoglobin molecules are at least 75 per cent saturated (Y > 0.9), the slope of the Hill plot again approaches 1.0, and the hemoglobin again becomes noncooperative. The hemoglobin is now in the "oxy" quaternary structure (designated R or relaxed in allosteric terminology). Compared with T-state hemoglobin, the oxygen affinity of this R-state hemoglobin is much less responsive to solvent conditions. It resembles the behavior of isolated subunits and certain mutant and chemically modified hemoglobins mentioned previously. These noncooperative hemoglobins appear to be locked in an "oxy" or R structure throughout the whole range of oxygen saturation.

Wyman[4] has shown that the free energy of cooperativity of normal hemoglobin can be determined from the distance (D) between the asymptotes of the Hill plot, that is, the difference in binding affinities of the first and last ligand, K_1 and K_4. The minimum interaction energy (cal/mole heme) is equal to 2.3 D RT $\sqrt{2}$.* Thus, in Figure 3–11, precise measurements of oxygen equilibrium of human hemoglobin indicate that the free energy change in going from deoxy (T) to oxy (R) conformation is about 9 to 12 Cal/mole of tetramer.

Early measurements of the oxygenation of hemoglobin both in red cells and in dilute solution established that oxygen affinity varies inversely with temperature. Precise determinations of the oxygen binding curve at different temperatures permit the calculation of the thermodynamic parameters enthalpy (ΔH) and entropy (ΔS) involved in the binding of ligands to hemoglobins. A reaction associated with a decrease in enthalpy ($-\Delta H$) is exothermic. Examples include the binding of oxygen and of 2,3-DPG to deoxyhemoglobin. Any structural interpretation of enthalpies of reactions involving a macromolecule is tenuous. Each of the separate components of the system must be considered, including the heat of solution of oxygen, the heat of water binding, Bohr proton binding, anion binding, and so on. A chemical reaction having a decrease in entropy involves in its totality increased ordering or less "randomness." Again, this measurement is very difficult to interpret in structural terms.

In his early analyses of the thermodynamics of oxygen binding to hemoglobin, Wyman[4] found that the general shape of the sigmoid curve (and the corresponding Hill plot) was not affected by change in temperature and therefore concluded that the free energy of cooperativity was primarily entropic. Subsequently, the development of instrumentation for accurate determination of the extremes of the binding curve enabled Imai[86, 87] to demonstrate that the shape of the oxygen dissociation curve is in fact significantly altered by temperature. Both entropy and enthalpy contribute to the free energy of cooperativity. As hemoglobin is successively oxygenated, the enthalpy fluctuates but is compensated by a corresponding change in entropy, so that the free energy of the first three steps in oxygenation are approximately equal ($K_1 = K_2 = K_3$).

In order to obtain a complete understanding of the thermodynamics of oxygenation of hemoglobin, the following variables should be systematically controlled: oxygen tension, temperature, pH, PCO_2, organic phosphate, inorganic anion, and subunit dissociation. Thus, a full definition of the hemoglobin system requires that all but one of these variables be fixed in a particular equilibrium measurement. The importance of these independent factors was not adequately appreciated until recently. For example, before 1970, many experiments employed hemoglobin containing unknown amounts of 2,3-diphosphoglycerate. Furthermore, the interpretation of oxygen equilibria in most earlier experiments has been confounded by the fact that dilute hemoglobin solutions were utilized, which therefore contained a significant proportion of $\alpha\beta$ dimer.[88]

Ackers and colleagues[88–92] have been making a sustained effort to obtain comprehensive thermodynamic measurements of the hemoglobin system. Obviously, this is a formidable task. For example, if data were collected at five different values for each variable listed above, a full set of oxygen equilibria would require 5^7 or 78,125 separate measurements! During the past five years, these investigators have compiled a highly rigorous and self-consistent set of measurements on the dissociation of hemoglobin tetramer to dimer as a function

---

*R = the molar gas constant, and T = absolute temperature.

of oxygenation and pH. The rationale for these extensive studies is that the $\alpha_1\beta_2$ contact, where tetramer dissociation takes place, is the major site of structural perturbations that accompany oxygenation (see Chapter 2). The thermodynamic parameters for the oxygenation of hemoglobin dimers and tetramers as well as for the assembly of deoxy, half-oxygenated, and fully oxygenated dimers into tetramers were measured at different pH values. The contributions of enthalpy and entropy to the free energy of tetramer formation indicate that deoxyhemoglobin is stabilized predominantly by hydrogen bond formation.[92] This conclusion is consistent with structural studies that have demonstrated the importance of intrasubunit and extrasubunit salt bonds (see Chapter 2). In addition, these thermodynamic analyses suggest that hydrophobic interactions are not important in stabilizing deoxyhemoglobin at the $\alpha_1\beta_2$ interface. These investigators conclude that the release of Bohr protons is an important source of the free energy of cooperativity. As mentioned previously, it is uncertain whether these interactions are localized to a few specific sites or distributed over a number of residues.

HOW DOES HEMOGLOBIN WORK?

Understanding the mechanism underlying the cooperative behavior of hemoglobin remains a major challenge. The solution to this intricate and beguiling puzzle will depend on assembling a detailed model that is not only compatible with the high-resolution structural information that continues to emerge (see Chapter 2) but that also satisfies experimental observations on hemoglobin's functional properties. Thermodynamic measurements discussed in the preceding section are highly respected because they are based on immutable scientific laws and are not dependent on a particular model or mechanism. However, the latter characteristic is also a limitation of thermodynamics, because it provides no information about the pathway or the steps involved in going from one state to another. In the case of hemoglobin, other means must be used to understand the nature and properties of the partially liganded tetramer.

This section begins with a consideration of hemoglobin as an allosteric protein and models that attempt to explain its cooperative behavior. The chapter will end with a discussion of experiments designed to test which model best explains hemoglobin's cooperative behavior.

Allosteric Models

Hemoglobin can be considered a prototype of an allosteric protein in which binding of ligand is cooperative. Generally, allosteric proteins undergo an alteration in conformation upon successive binding of ligand. Many enzymes have multiple subunits, and in some, cooperativity has been demonstrated. Enzymes that qualify as allosteric proteins[93] include aspartate transcarbamylase, phosphorylase, glutamate dehydrogenase, isocitrate dehydrogenase, phosphofructokinase, and cyclic AMP–dependent protein kinase. Allosteric enzymes cannot be analyzed by simple Michaelis-Menten kinetics. As with hemoglobin, the affinity of the multisubunit enzyme for substrate depends on its fractional saturation with substrate. This is known as homotropic interaction. In this way, the reaction rate can be closely regulated by small changes in substrate concentration. In addition, allosteric enzymes may be controlled by the participation of modulators, either activators or inhibitors, which bind at sites different from the substrate binding site. This is known as heterotropic interaction. In the case of hemoglobin, the binding of oxygen increases the affinity of the remaining hemes for oxygen (homotropic interaction) and lowers the affinity of various effectors (modulators) such as protons, 2,3-DPG, and CO_2 at other sites on the hemoglobin molecule (heterotropic interactions).

Two models have been proposed to explain the molecular basis of allosteric control. In an early and provocative analysis of the oxygenation of hemoglobin, Pauling[94] proposed a simple model consisting of a single heme-oxygen binding constant and an interaction constant that depended on the geometry of the four subunits. Subsequent determination of the three-dimensional structure of hemoglobin ruled out direct chemical interaction between heme groups. However, more recently, Koshland, Nemethy, and Filmer[95] presented a more general form of Pauling's sequential model in which the binding of ligand to each subunit of the molecule results in a change in the tertiary structure of that subunit. This conformational alteration affects the affinity of neighboring subunits for ligands. This "induced fit," illustrated by the diagonal in Figure 3–12, results in several intermediate conformational species, depending on the number of ligand binding sites in the molecule.

Monod, Wyman, and Changeux (MWC)[96] proposed an alternative model based on a

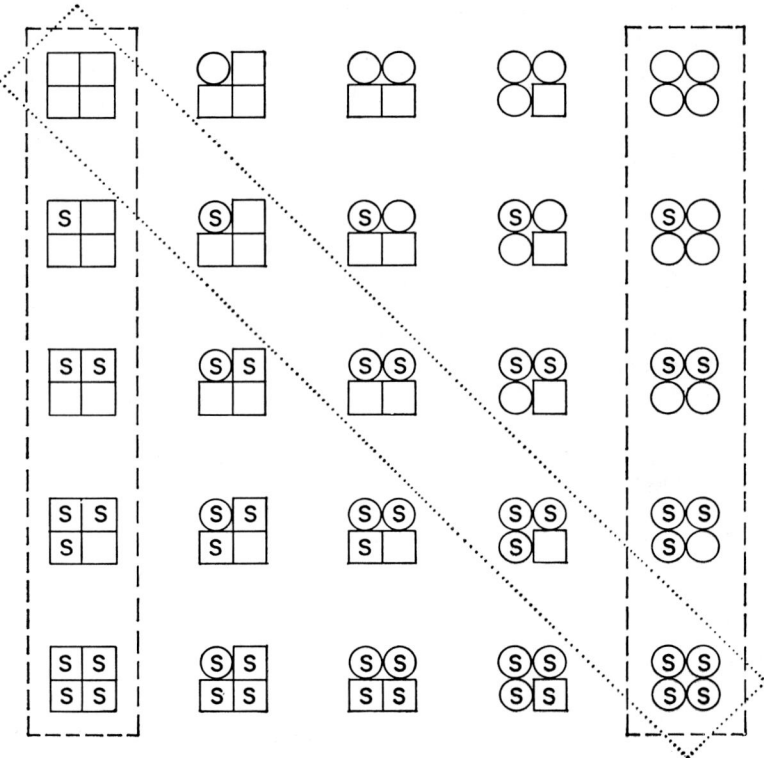

Figure 3–12. A general allosteric model for the binding of substrate (S) to a four-subunit enzyme. In the case of hemoglobin, S = O$_2$. The squares represent the t conformation and the circles the r conformation. The model proposed by Monod and associates is shown by the dashed lines, and that proposed by Koshland and coworkers is shown by the dotted lines. (From Hammes, G. G., and Wu, C.: Science *172*:1205, 1971.)

novel and heuristic concept. They suggested that an allosteric protein exists in an equilibrium between two conformers designated the R (or relaxed) and T (or tense) structures, which differ in affinity for ligand or substrate. The binding of ligand to the subunits of the protein results in a concerted change in conformation, so that the affinity of the unreacted subunits for ligand changes abruptly. Thus, the equilibrium between the two conformers is markedly altered by the binding of ligand. Effectors have a different affinity for the R and T states and thus will also alter the conformational equilibrium. The simplest form of the two-state MWC model is shown diagrammatically in the two vertical rectangles in Figure 3–12.

According to this version of the MWC model, the system can be defined by two independent variables: L and c. L is an indicator of the relative stabilities of the R and T conformers when the heme groups are completely unsaturated:

$$L = [T]/[R]$$

Under physiologic conditions, in which deoxyhemoglobin is almost entirely in the T structure, $L \cong 10,000$. The second variable, c, is the ratio of heme ligand affinities for the two states:

$$c = K_R/K_T$$

K_R and K_T are dissociation equilibrium constants:

$$K = \frac{[Hb][O_2]}{[HbO_2]}$$

As mentioned above and depicted in Figure 3–3, when the oxygen binding curve for normal cooperative hemoglobin is plotted according to the Hill equation, the extremes of the curve approach a slope of 1.0. These asymptotes represent the oxygenation of T-state hemoglobin (at low saturation) and R-state hemoglobin (at high saturation) and, when extrapolated to 50 per cent saturation (log $[Y/1-Y] = 0$), give values for K_T and K_R, respectively. The ratio of the oxygen affinity of the hemoglobin over that of R-state hemoglobin is designated as $\alpha_{1/2}$:

$$\alpha_{1/2} = P_{50}/K_R$$

These variables are sufficient to describe the cooperative behavior of hemoglobin. Experimental oxygen equilibrium data can be fitted quite readily to this scheme. Hill's n at intermediate degrees of oxygenation ($Y > 0.1, < 0.9$) can be expressed as follows:

$$n = 1 + 3\left[\frac{(1 - c\alpha_{1/2})(\alpha_{1/2} - 1)}{(1 + c\alpha_{1/2})(\alpha_{1/2} + 1)}\right]$$

This model in its simplest form assumes that under all solvent conditions K_R and K_T are invariant and therefore hemoglobin's cooperative behavior is based on changes in the equilibrium between the R and T conformers during ligand binding.

Experiments That Test Allosteric Models

A variety of investigational tools have been employed to investigate the stereochemical basis of hemoglobin cooperativity. The large and detailed body of structural information gleaned from x-ray crystallography has been summarized in Chapter 2. However, the x-ray data provide information only on the two extreme states of hemoglobin: fully deoxy and fully liganded. In order to understand subunit cooperativity, it is necessary to have information on the intermediate states of heme ligation. Independent information on partially saturated hemoglobin can be obtained by kinetic measurements as well as by studies on various modified hemoglobins such as mutants, valence hybrids, and heme-substituted hemoglobins. Although a detailed review of these topics is beyond the scope of this book, this section will summarize how some of these approaches can be useful in providing new insights into the mechanism of hemoglobin function.

Kinetics. Beginning with the pioneering work of Gibson and Roughton, a large body of information has been collected on the rates of reaction of hemoglobin with heme ligands as well as with allosteric effectors (such as 2,3-DPG and IHP). Furthermore, the kinetics of subunit assembly has been thoroughly investigated. This section presents a brief discussion of hemoglobin kinetics. More detailed information may be obtained from recent reviews.[97-99]

The binding of oxygen to hemoglobin as well as its dissociation from hemoglobin is sufficiently fast relative to the circulation of red cells that the oxygenation of red cells in the pulmonary and systemic capillary beds is in equilibrium with plasma oxygen tension (see Chapter 5). Thus, kinetic measurements provide little or no physiologic insights beyond what is given by much simpler equilibrium measurements. However, kinetic measurements do provide important insights into how hemoglobin works.

Most kinetic experiments have employed a stopped-flow apparatus in which reactants are placed in separate syringes: for example, deoxyhemoglobin in one and carbon monoxide in the other. A pneumatic device forces a small quantity from each syringe into a mixing chamber that serves as a cuvette, with a monochromatic light source on one side and a photomultiplier tube on the opposite side. The change in light transmission can be followed on an oscilloscope. The stopped-flow apparatus has been widely used for the following kinetic measurements:

1. The combination of carbon monoxide with deoxyhemoglobin:

$$Hb + 4CO \xrightarrow{l'} Hb(CO)_4.*$$

In cooperative hemoglobin, this reaction is autoaccelerating: CO combines slowly with deoxy (T-state) hemoglobin but rapidly after the hemoglobin has been partially saturated with CO (Fig. 3–13). In noncooperative hemoglobins that are frozen in the R quaternary structure, CO combination is much more rapid.

2. The dissociation of oxygen from oxyhemoglobin:

$$Hb(O_2)_4 \xrightarrow{k} Hb + 4O_2.$$

Figure 3–14 shows the dissociation of oxygen from fully and partially oxygenated hemoglobin A. Initially, oxygen is more tightly bound while hemoglobin is fully saturated. As the average oxygen saturation decreases, the rate of dissociation increases.

3. The replacement of oxygen in oxyhemoglobin with carbon monoxide:

$$Hb(O_2)_4 \xrightarrow{k_4} Hb(O_2)_3 + O_2$$

$$Hb(O_2)_3 + CO \xrightarrow{l'_4} Hb(O_2)_3CO$$

---

*By convention, equilibrium constants employ capital letters, whereas kinetic constants use lower case letters. K and k refer to oxygen; L and l refer to carbon monoxide. The superscript ' refers to an "on" reaction. A numerical subscript denotes the heme ligand number. For example, k_4 denotes the dissociation of one oxygen molecule from fully saturated oxyhemoglobin (Hb(O$_2$)$_4$); l'_1 denotes the combination of the first molecule of carbon monoxide with deoxyhemoglobin.

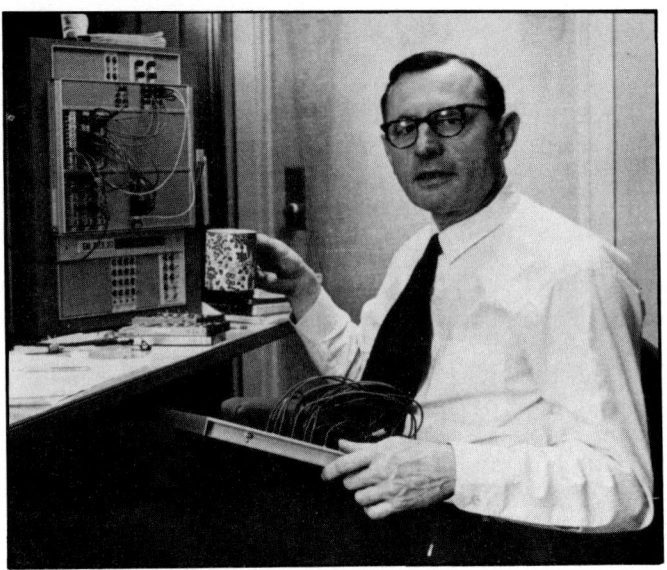

QUENTIN GIBSON

Quentin Gibson is the doyen and leading practitioner of heme-protein kinetics. His career path has been somewhat tortuous. He was born in Scotland but spent his youth in Northern Ireland, during a relatively tranquil period. He completed his medical degree at the University of Belfast and was bent upon a career in midwifery. During his training, he encountered a rural practitioner who believed ascorbic acid to be of value in treating congestive heart failure. While making rounds in a remote Irish village, they came upon two brothers who were deeply cyanotic. Both brothers had normal hearts: one belonged to a field hockey team. The athletic brother was treated with ascorbic acid, and the other served as a control. The resulting contrast in appearance was gratifying to the practitioner but mystifying to Gibson. So began one of the most productive careers in hemoglobin research.

Gibson assumed a research position at the University of Belfast under Henry Barcroft, son of Sir Joseph Barcroft (see Fig. 1–13). The doctoral candidate soon completed a brilliant series of investigations elucidating the enzymatic basis for methemoglobin reduction and the pathogenesis of congenital methemoglobinemia (see Chapter 16). The bulk of current understanding of this disorder is contained within Gibson's original papers.

Methemoglobinemia piqued Gibson's interest in the functional behavior of hemoglobin. He went to his workshop and constructed one of the first apparatus for measuring rapid reactions in biologic molecules. Stopped flow kinetics has become an essential tool for investigating a wide range of metabolic processes. Armed with his new apparatus, Gibson began a highly fruitful collaboration with F. J. W. Roughton (see Fig. 1–15), one of the pioneer investigators of hemoglobin physiology. Roughton was a stern taskmaster. He once returned the fourth draft of a manuscript with the exhortation, "Come, Gibson. Remember, we are writing a classic." In part from Roughton's training but mainly by natural inclination, Gibson has remained a master of experimental design and execution. His experiments on photodissociation of carbon monoxide from hemoglobin provided the first solid evidence that hemoglobin has two conformational states of widely different ligand affinity. As explained in this chapter, his systematic investigation of ligand binding kinetics of various types of hemoglobin has provided information on the intermediate states of heme ligation that is crucial to understanding the cooperativity problem.

Gibson has been in the Biochemistry Department at Cornell University since 1965. During this tenure, he has trained a sizable proportion of investigators currently working on rapid kinetics of biochemical reactions. He is the prototype of the genial and courtly British professor, documented in the photograph above that shows him relaxing in front of a bank of electronic gear, holding his English tea cup. Indeed, Gibson's mania for hands-on research is such that it has been alleged that the primary function of his technician is making tea. The extraordinary scope and validity of Gibson's research on hemoglobin and cytochromes along with his accessibility and enthusiasm have made him a one-man clearing house of information.

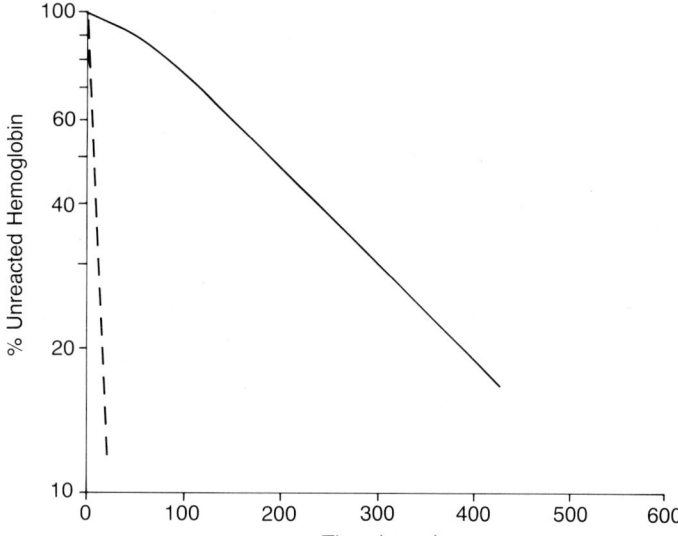

Figure 3–13. Time course for the binding of carbon monoxide with normal hemoglobin (—) and a hemoglobin such as β_4 (Hb H) or Hb Kempsey (see Chapter 14) that is frozen in the R quaternary structure (– – –). Note that the reaction for normal cooperative hemoglobin is much slower and autoaccelerating. (0.05 M bis-TRIS, pH 6.0, 20°C.) (Courtesy of Melisenda J. McDonald.)

The first reaction (k_4) is rate-limiting. Because this reaction involves only fully liganded hemoglobin, it is generally a property of "oxy-like" or R-state hemoglobin.

Important kinetic information can also be obtained from flash photolysis. When carboxyhemoglobin or oxyhemoglobin is subjected to a strong light source, the heme ligand will dissociate and eventually depart from the heme pocket. Subsequently, it will recombine with the deoxy heme group. Gibson[100] showed that when carbon monoxide is rapidly removed from CO-hemoglobin by flash photolysis, the initial recombination with CO was rapid. Subsequently, the hemoglobin became slow-reacting, just like normal deoxyhemoglobin:

$$Hb(CO)_4 \rightarrow Hb^* + 4CO$$

$$Hb^* + CO \rightarrow HbCO \text{ (fast)}$$

$$Hb^* \rightarrow Hb$$

$$Hb + CO \rightarrow HbCO \text{ (slow)}$$

The absorbance spectrum of the fast-reacting species (Hb*) differed from that of normal

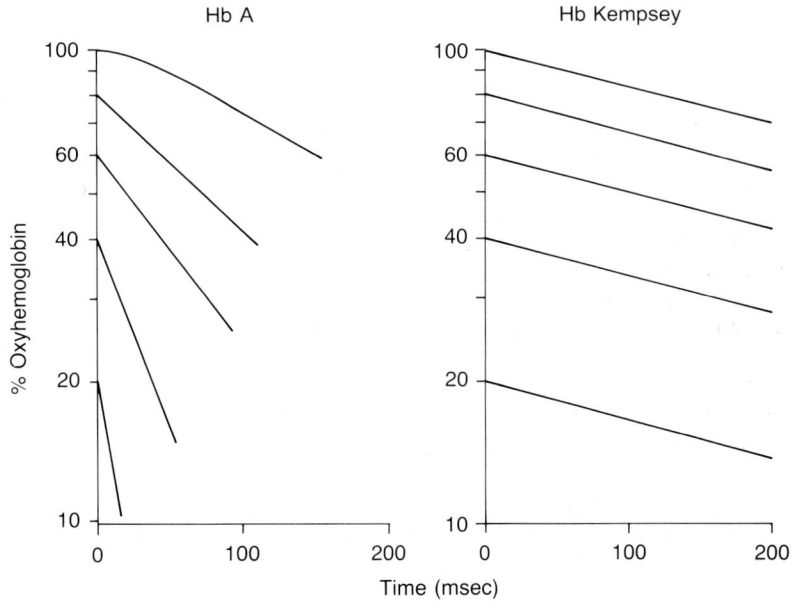

Figure 3–14. Time course for the dissociation of oxygen from hemoglobin of varying degrees of saturation. Oxygen dissociates slowly from hemoglobins such as Hb Kempsey that are frozen in the R quaternary structure (right panel). As shown in the left panel, oxygen dissociates slowly from fully oxygenated Hb A that is in the R state but much more rapidly from partially oxygenated Hb A that has undergone transition to the T structure. (Courtesy of Melisenda J. McDonald.)

deoxyhemoglobin tetramer and resembled that of isolated α and β chains (see section above on isolated chains). These experiments could be explained by different quaternary structures. Upon photolysis, the deoxyhemoglobin remains transiently in the "oxy-like" or R structure but then rapidly relaxes into the "deoxy" or T structure.

All of the kinetic experiments described above can be readily interpreted in terms of a two-state allosteric model. The autoacceleration noted when CO binds to deoxyhemoglobin can be explained by the switch from T to R quaternary structure upon partial heme ligation. Likewise, the kinetics of dissociation of oxygen (k) is compatible with a switch of partially oxygenated hemoglobin from R to T quaternary structure. Finally, as mentioned above, the flash photolysis experiments are readily explained by a rapid change in quaternary structure from R to T structure when CO is rapidly removed from carboxyhemoglobin.

Most of the kinetic experiments described above have taken place in the millisecond time scale. In the past few years, monochromatic laser pulses have been used for photolysis experiments. Thanks to advances in optics and solid-state circuiting, high-resolution spectra can be generated within nanoseconds or even picoseconds after photolysis.[101] Resonance Raman spectroscopy has also proved to be useful in monitoring these ultrafast processes. These experiments will permit a deeper understanding of the sequential alterations in and around the heme pocket resulting from ligand binding and conformational transitions.

What has been learned from these kinetic measurements? Kinetics has sometimes provided special and unique insights into the existence and properties of intermediate species. For example, a combination of flash photolysis and stopped flow has provided information on the stage in heme ligation at which the transition in quaternary structure takes place.[102] Kinetic measurements have also been useful in demonstrating asymmetry between globin subunits. Perhaps the most fundamental use of kinetic data has been to gain a partial understanding of the transition states involved in heme ligation.[101] It has been long appreciated that heme ligands differ markedly from one another not only in their affinity for hemoglobin but also in the relative contribution of the "on" and "off" reaction rates. Furthermore, the kinetic basis of subunit cooperativity is ligand-dependent. For oxygen, the "off" rate changes markedly with partial ligand binding ($k_1/k_4 = 150$). The "on" reaction changes much less ($k'_4/k'_1 = 6$). In contrast, for carbon monoxide, most of the subunit cooperativity resides in the "on" rates ($1'_4/1'_1 = 40$). The "off" rates change much less ($1_1/1_4 = 10$). Szabo[103] has explained these puzzling results in terms of ligand-dependent differences in the transition state between unbound and bound heme.

Study of Partially Oxygenated Intermediates. A full understanding of subunit cooperativity depends on having firm information on the partially liganded intermediates. Many questions come to mind: What is the sequence of oxygen binding to α and β subunits? How much alteration in tertiary structure accompanies the oxygenation of a subunit? How many quaternary structures exist in normal hemoglobin and at what stages(s) in heme ligation does quaternary structure change? At what stages do the Bohr protons and 2,3-DPG dissociate? As mentioned above, kinetic studies have provided answers to some of these questions. Other physical-chemical probes have also been valuable in providing independent information. For example, the sequence of oxygen binding has been investigated by both proton nuclear magnetic resonance[104, 105] and by the use of a spin label attached to either α or β heme groups.[106] Both studies indicate that the α and β chains of purified human hemoglobin bind oxygen with equal affinity. However, upon addition of 2,3-DPG, the affinity of the β chain is selectively reduced. The transition in quaternary structure from T to R probably occurs abruptly, as a result of (1) successive rupture of the salt bonds that stabilize the deoxy structure and (2) constraints imposed at the interface between $α_1$ and $β_2$ subunits.[107] There is some experimental evidence that this "click" in quaternary structure occurs after the third O_2 has been bound.[102] In keeping with this conclusion, 2,3-DPG is probably released after the third oxygen is bound to hemoglobin (see earlier section on 2,3-DPG binding). Despite these experimental observations, it is more generally correct to say that the point in ligation at which the transition occurs is dependent on the solvent conditions that affect the relative stability of the R and T structures.

From these studies on hemoglobin, and many others not included here, a great deal of experimental evidence has been marshaled in support of one or both of the two allosteric models described above. A model involving sequential change in structure predicts a linear relationship between fractional ligand concentration and parameters sensitive to hemoglobin structure (e.g., release of Bohr protons and change in EPR sectra). In contrast, the MWC two-state model predicts a significant departure from linearity. A number of independent studies have indicated that conformational changes do in fact take place in a concerted fashion, in keeping with a two-state model. A thorough review of the literature through 1975 by Shulman and colleagues[108] indicates that the bulk of the experimental evidence on normal hemoglobin, mutants, and chemically modified hemoglobins is consistent with the MWC model. The original stereochemical model proposed by Perutz[5] and subsequent analyses of higher-resolution x-ray data[107] emphasize the tongue-and-groove "click" between the "deoxy" and "oxy" structures at the $\alpha_1\beta_2$ interface, a consideration that also provides strong support for the existence of only two quaternary structures, i.e., a two-state model. Szabo and Karplus[109–111] have applied a statistical thermodynamic analysis to Perutz's structural model and have determined a series of parameters that agree very well with experimental data on normal hemoglobin as well as mutant and chemically modified hemoglobins. Their analysis, which provides a pivotal link between structural and functional data, is also compatible with a modified two-state model.

A large amount of experimental evidence poses a significant challenge to the simplest form of the MWC model presented above. For example, there is rather convincing proof that both the affinity parameters, K_R and K_T, vary somewhat with solvent conditions. In addition, under certain circumstances, hemoglobin exhibits considerable chain heterogeneity, which confounds the simplest form of the MWC model. Finally, NMR studies suggest that oxygenation of the α chain can impose a perturbation in tertiary structure of the β chain without any change in quaternary structure.[112] Nevertheless, in most cases, these experimental observations can be reconciled with a modified version of the two-state model.

Although many details await clarification, recent advances in structural analyses as well as modern biophysical probes have provided considerable insights into the mechanism whereby heme ligation effects changes in tertiary and quaternary structure and vice versa. The solution of this problem may permit a better understanding of how other, more complex allosteric proteins work.

References

1. Barcroft, J.: The Respiratory Function of the Blood. Part II. Haemoglobin. London, Cambridge University Press, 1928.
2. Bunn, H. F.: Differences in the interaction of 2,3-diphosphoglycerate with certain mammalian hemoglobins. Science *172*:1049, 1971.
3. Bohr, C., Hasselbalch, K., and Krogh, A.: Ueber einen in biologischer Beziehung wichtigen Einfluss, den die Kohlensaurespannung des Blutes auf dessen Sauerstoffbindung ubt. Skand. Arch. Physiol. *16*:402, 1904.
4. Wyman, J.: Linked functions and reciprocal effects in hemoglobin: A second look. Adv. Protein Chem. *19*:223, 1964.
5. Perutz, M. F.: Stereochemistry of cooperative effects in haemoglobin. Nature *228*:726, 1970.
6. Perutz, M. F., Kilmartin, J. V., Nishikura, K., Fogg, J. H., Butler, P. J. G., and Rollema, H. S.: Identification of residues contributing to the Bohr effect of human haemoglobin. J. Mol. Biol. *138*:649, 1980.
7. Kilmartin, J. V., Fogg, J. H., and Perutz, M. F.: Role of C-terminal histidine in the alkaline Bohr effect of human hemoglobin. Biochemistry *19*:3189, 1980.
8. Nishikura, K.: Identification of histidine-122 α in human haemoglobin as one of the unknown alkaline Bohr groups by hydrogen-tritium exchange. Biochem. J. *173*:671, 1978.
9. Ho, C., and Russu, I. M.: Proton nuclear magnetic resonance studies of sickle cell hemoglobin. *In* Caughey, W. S. (ed.): Biochemical and Clinical Aspects of Hemoglobin Abnormalities. New York, Academic Press, 1978, pp. 179–194.
10. Russu, I. M., Ho, N. T., and Ho, C.: Role of the β146 histidyl residue in the alkaline Bohr effect of hemoglobin. Biochemistry *19*:1043, 1980.
10a. Matsukawa, S., Itatani, Y., Mawatari, K., Shimokawa, Y., and Yoneyama, Y.: Quantitative evaluation for the role of beta 146 His and beta 143 His residues in the Bohr effect of human hemoglobin in the presence of 0.1 M chloride ion. J. Biol. Chem. *259*:479, 1984.
11. Ohe, M., and Kajita, A.: Change in pK_a values of individual histidine residues of human hemoglobin upon reaction with carbon monoxide. Biochemistry *19*:4443, 1980.
12. Matthew, J. B., Hanania, G. I. H., and Gurd, F. R. N.: Electrostatic effects in hemoglobin: Hydrogen ion equilibria in human deoxy- and oxyhemoglobin A. Biochemistry *10*:1919, 1979.
13. Matthew, J. B., Hanania, G. I. H., and Gurd, F. R. N.: Electrostatic effects in hemoglobin: Bohr effect and ionic strength dependence of individual groups. Biochemistry *10*:1928, 1979.
14. Ferguson, J. K. W., and Roughton, F. J. W.: The chemical relationships with physiological importance of carbamino compounds of CO_2 with haemoglobin. J. Physiol. (Lond.) *83*:87, 1934.
15. Garner, M. H., Bogardt, R. A., and Gurd, F. R. N.: Determination of the pK values of the α amino groups of human hemoglobin. J. Biol. Chem. *250*:4398, 1975.
16. Kilmartin, J. V., and Rossi-Bernardi, L.: Inhibition of CO_2 combination and reduction of the Bohr

effect in haemoglobin chemically modified at its α-amino groups. Nature 222:1243, 1969.
17. Kilmartin, J. V., and Rossi-Bernardi, L.: The binding of carbon dioxide by horse haemoglobin. Biochem. J. *124*:31, 1971.
18. Rossi-Bernardi, L., and Roughton, F. J. W.: The specific influence of carbon dioxide and carbamate compounds on the buffer power and Bohr effect in human haemoglobin solutions. J. Physiol. (Lond.) *189*:1, 1967.
19. Garby, L., Robert, M., and Zaar, B.: Proton and carbamino linked oxygen affinity of normal human blood. Acta Physiol. Scand. *84*:482, 1972.
20. Arnone, A.: X-ray studies of the interaction of CO_2 with human deoxyhaemoglobin. Nature *247*:143, 1974.
21. Perrella, M., Bresciani, D., and Rossi-Bernardi, L.: The binding of CO_2 to human hemoglobin. J. Biol. Chem. *250*:5413, 1975.
22. Perrella, M., Kilmartin, J. V., Fogg, J., and Rossi-Bernardi, L.: Identification of the high and low affinity CO_2-binding sites of human haemoglobin. Nature *256*:759, 1975.
23. Bauer, C., Baumann, R., Engels, U., and Pacyna, B.: The carbon dioxide affinity of various human hemoglobins. J. Biol. Chem. *250*:2173, 1975.
24. Morrow, J. S., Matthew, J. B., Wittebort, R. J., and Gurd, F. R. N.: Carbon 13 resonances of $^{13}CO_2$ carbamino adducts of α and β chains in human adult hemoglobin. J. Biol. Chem. *251*:477, 1976.
25. Matthew, J. B., Morrow, J. S., Wittebort, R. J., and Gurd, F. R. N.: Quantitative determination of carbamino adducts of α and β chains in human adult hemoglobin in presence and absence of carbon monoxide and 2,3-diphosphoglycerate. J. Biol. Chem. *252*:2234, 1977.
26. Bauer, C., and Kurtz, A.: Oxygen-linked CO_2 binding to isolated β subunits of human hemoglobin. J. Biol. Chem. *252*:2952, 1977.
27. Bauer, C., and Schroeder, E.: Carbamino compounds of haemoglobin in human adult and foetal blood. J. Physiol. (Lond.) *227*:457, 1972.
28. Rossi-Fanelli, A., Antonini, E., and Caputo, A.: Studies on the relations between molecular and functional properties of hemoglobin. II. The effect of salts on the oxygen equilibrium of human hemoglobin. J. Biol. Chem. *236*:397, 1961.
29. Rossi-Fanelli, A., Antonini, E., and Caputo, A.: Studies on the relations between molecular and functional properties of hemoglobin. I. The effect of salts on the molecular weight of human hemoglobin. J. Biol. Chem. *236*:391, 1961.
30. Arnone, A., and Williams, D. L.: Crystallographic evidence for anion binding sites at the NH_2-termini of the α subunits of human deoxyhemoglobin. In Labie, D., Pogart, C., Rosa, J. (eds.): Interactions Moléculaires de l'Hémoglobines. Paris, INSERM, 1977, p. 15.
31. O'Donnell, S., Mandaro, R., Schuster, T. M., and Arnone, A.: X-ray diffraction and solution studies of specifically carbamylated human hemoglobin A. J. Biol. Chem. *254*:12204, 1979.
32. Chiancone, E., Norne, J. E., Forsen, S., Antonini, E., and Wyman, J.: Nuclear magnetic resonance quadripole relaxation studies of chloride binding to human oxy- and deoxyhaemoglobin. J. Mol. Biol. *70*:675, 1972.
33. Chiancone, E., Norne, J. E., Forsen, S., Bonaventura, J., Brunori, M., Antonini, E., and Wyman, J.: Identification of chloride-binding sites in hemoglobin by nuclear magnetic resonance quadripole-relaxation studies of hemoglobin digests. Eur. J. Biochem. *55*:385, 1975.
34. Nigen, A. M., Manning, J. M., and Alben, J. O.: Oxygen-linked binding sites for inorganic anions to hemoglobin. J. Biol. Chem. *255*:5525, 1980.
35. Van Beek, G. G. M., and deBruin, S. H.: Identification of the residues involved in the oxygen linked chloride ion binding sites in human deoxyhemoglobin and oxyhemoglobin. Eur. J. Biochem. *105*:353, 1980.
36. Rollema, H. S., deBruin, S. H., Janssen, L. H. M., and vanOs, G. A. J.: The effect of potassium chloride on the Bohr effect of human hemoglobin. J. Biol. Chem. *250*:1333, 1975.
37. Chanutin, A., and Curnish, R. R.: Effect of organic and inorganic phosphates on the oxygen equilibrium of human erythrocytes. Arch. Biochem. Biophys. *121*:96, 1967.
38. Benesch, R., and Benesch, R. E.: The effect of organic phosphates from the human erythrocyte on the allosteric properties of hemoglobin. Biochem. Biophys. Res. Commun. *26*:162, 1967.
39. Benesch, R., Benesch, R. E., and Enoki, Y.: The interaction of hemoglobin and its subunits with 2,3-diphosphoglycerate. Proc. Natl. Acad. Sci. USA *61*:1102, 1968.
40. Benesch, R. E., Benesch, R., and Yu, C. I.: The oxygenation of hemoglobin in the presence of diphosphoglycerate. Effect of temperature, pH, ionic strength and hemoglobin concentration. Biochemistry *8*:2567, 1969.
41. Benesch, R., Benesch, R. E., and Yu, C. I.: Reciprocal binding of oxygen and diphosphoglycerate by human hemoglobin. Proc. Natl. Acad. Sci. USA *59*:526, 1968.
42. Lo, H. H., and Schimmel, P. R.: Interaction of human hemoglobin with adenine nucleotides. J. Biol. Chem. *244*:5084, 1969.
43. Berman, M., Benesch, R., and Benesch, R. E.: The removal of organic phosphates from hemoglobin. Arch. Biochem. Biophys. *145*:236, 1971.
44. Chanutin, A., and Hermann, E.: The interaction of organic and inorganic phosphates with hemoglobin. Arch. Biochem. Biophys. *131*:180, 1969.
45. Luque, J., Diederich, D., and Grisolia, S.: Binding of 2,3-diphosphoglycerate to oxyhemoglobin. Biochem. Biophys. Res. Commun. *36*:1019, 1969.
46. Hamasaki, N., and Rose, Z. B.: The binding of phosphorylated red cell metabolites to human hemoglobin A. J. Biol. Chem. *249*:7896, 1974.
47. Goodford, P. J., St.-Louis, J., and Wootton, R.: A quantitative analysis of the effects of 2,3-diphosphoglycerate, adenosine triphosphate and inositol hexaphosphate on the oxygen dissociation curve of human hemoglobin. J. Physiol. *283*:397, 1978.
48. Imaizumi, K., Imai, K., and Tyuma, I.: The linkage between the four-step binding of oxygen and the binding of heterotropic anionic ligands in hemoglobin. J. Biochem. *86*:1829, 1979.
49. Van Beek, G. M., and deBruin, S. H.: The pH dependence of the binding of d-glycerate 2,3-biphosphate to deoxyhemoglobin and oxyhemoglobin. Eur. J. Biochem. *100*:497, 1979.
50. Gupta, R. K., Benovic, J. L., and Rose, Z. B.: Magnetic resonance studies of the binding of ATP and cations to human hemoglobin. J. Biol. Chem. *253*:6165, 1978.
51. Gupta, R. K., Benovic, J. L., and Rose, Z. B.: Location of the allosteric site for 2,3-bisphospho-

51. glycerate on human oxy- and deoxyhemoglobin as observed by magnetic resonance spectroscopy. J. Biol. Chem. 254:8250, 1979.
52. Bunn, H. F., and Briehl, R. W.: The interaction of 2,3-diphosphoglycerate with various human hemoglobins. J. Clin. Invest. 49:1088, 1970.
53. Bauer, C.: Antagonistic influence of CO_2 and 2,3-diphosphoglycerate on the Bohr effect of human hemoglobin. Life Sci. 8:1041, 1969.
54. Rossi-Bernardi, L., Roughton, F. J. W., et al.: The effect of organic phosphates on the binding of CO_2 to human hemoglobin and CO_2 transport in the circulating blood. In Rorth, M., and Astrup, P. (eds.): Oxygen Affinity of Hemoglobin and Red Cell Acid-Base Status. Copenhagen, Munksgaard, 1972, p. 225.
55. Tomita, S., and Riggs, A.: Studies of the interaction of 2,3-diphosphoglycerate and carbon dioxide with hemoglobins from mouse, man, and elephant. J. Biol. Chem. 246:547, 1971.
56. Bauer, C., Ludwig, I., and Ludwig, M.: Different effects of 2,3-diphosphoglycerate and adenosine triphosphate on the oxygen affinity of adult and foetal human hemoglobin. Life Sci. 7:1339, 1968.
57. Tyuma, I., and Shimizu, K.: Different response to organic phosphates of human fetal and adult hemoglobins. Arch. Biochem. Biophys. 129:404, 1969.
58. Perutz, M. F.: The Bohr effect and combination with organic phosphates. Nature 228:734, 1970.
59. Arnone, A.: X-ray diffraction study of binding of 2,3-diphosphoglycerate to human deoxyhaemoglobin. Nature 237:146, 1972.
60. Bauer, C., Henry, Y., and Banerjee, R.: Binding of 2,3-diphosphoglycerate to haemoglobin valency hybrids. Nature [New Biol.] 242:208, 1973.
61. Haber, J. E., and Koshland, D. E.: The effect of 2,3-diphosphoglyceric acid on the changes in $\beta\beta$ interactions in hemoglobin during oxygenation. J. Biol. Chem. 246:7790, 1971.
62. Ogata, R., and McConnell, H. M.: The binding of a spin-labeled triphosphate to hemoglobin. Cold Spring Harbor Symp. Quant. Biol. 36:325, 1971.
63. Ogata, R., and McConnell, H. M.: Mechanism of cooperative oxygen binding to hemoglobin. Proc. Natl. Acad. Sci. USA 69:334, 1972.
64. Salhany, J. M., Mathers, D. H., and Eliot, R. S.: The deoxygenation kinetics of hemoglobin partially saturated with carbon monoxide. J. Biol. Chem. 247:6985, 1972.
65. Caldwell, P. R. B., Nagel, R. L., and Jaffe, E. R.: The effect of oxygen, carbon dioxide, pH and cyanate on the binding of 2,3-diphosphoglycerate to human hemoglobin. Biochem. Biophys. Res. Commun. 44:1504, 1971.
66. Nagel, R. L., and Gibson, Q. H.: The binding of hemoglobin to haptoglobin in its relation to subunit dissociation of hemoglobin. J. Biol. Chem. 246:69, 1971.
67. Bunn, H. F., Esham, W. T., and Bull, R. W.: The renal handling of hemoglobin. I. Glomerular filtration. J. Exp. Med. 129:909, 1969.
68. Riggs, A.: The binding of N-ethylmaleimide by human hemoglobin and its effect upon the oxygen equilibrium. J. Biol. Chem. 236:1948, 1961.
69. Benesch, R. E., and Benesch, R.: The influence of oxygenation on the reactivity of the -SH groups of hemoglobin. Biochemistry 1:735, 1962.
70. Geraci, G., and Parkhurst, L. J.: Effects of hemoglobin and chain-chain interactions on the conformation of human hemoglobins. A kinetic study. Biochemistry 12:3414, 1973.
71. Alben, J. O., Bare, G. H., and Bromberg, P. A.: Sulphydryl groups as a new molecular probe at the $\alpha_1\beta_1$ interface in haemoglobin using Fourier transform infrared spectroscopy. Nature 252:736, 1974.
72. Alben, J. O., and Bare, G. H.: Ligand dependent heme protein interactions in human hemoglobin studied by Fourier transform infrared spectroscopy. J. Biol. Chem. 255:3892, 1980.
73. Bucci, E., and Fronticelli, C.: A new method for the preparation of α and β subunits of human hemoglobin. J. Biol. Chem. 240:PC551, 1964.
74. Ranney, H. M., Briehl, R. W., and Jacobs, A. S.: Oxygen equilibrium of hemoglobin α A and of hemoglobin reconstituted from hemoglobins α A and H. J. Biol. Chem. 240:2442, 1965.
75. Brunori, M., Noble, R. W., Antonini, E., and Wyman, J.: The reactions of the isolated α and β chains of human hemoglobin with oxygen and carbon monoxide. J. Biol. Chem. 241:5238, 1966.
76. Tyuma, I., Benesch, R. E., and Benesch, R.: The preparation and properties of the isolated alpha and beta subunits of hemoglobin A. Biochemistry 5:2957, 1966.
77. Valdes, R., and Ackers, G. K.: Self-association of hemoglobin β^{SH} chains is linked to oxygenation. Proc. Natl. Acad. Sci. USA 75:311, 1978.
78. Kurtz, A., and Bauer, C.: The oxygen affinity of hemoglobin β^{SH} chains is concentration dependent. Biochem. Biophys. Res. Commun. 84:852, 1978.
79. McDonald, M. J., and Noble, R. W.: The effect of pH on the rates of ligand replacement reactions of human adult and fetal hemoglobins and their subunits. J. Biol. Chem. 247:4282, 1972.
80. Rollema, H. S., deBruin, S. H., and vanOs, G. A. J.: The Bohr effect of isolated α and β chains of human hemoglobin. FEBS Lett. 61:148, 1976.
81. Bonaventura, J., Bonaventura, C., Amiconi, G., Tentori, L., Brunori, M., and Antonini, E.: Allosteric interactions in non-α chains isolated from normal human hemoglobin, fetal hemoglobin, and hemoglobin Abruzzo (β143(H21)His$\rightarrow$Arg). J. Biol. Chem. 250:6278, 1975.
82. Hill, A. V.: The possible effects of the aggregation of the molecules of haemoglobin on its dissociation curve. J. Physiol. 40:iv, 1910.
83. Simon, S. R., and Konigsberg, W. H.: Chemical modification of hemoglobins: A study of conformation restraint by internal bridging. Proc. Natl. Acad. Sci. USA 56:749, 1966.
84. Antonini, E., Wyman, J., Zito, R., Rossi-Fanelli, A., and Caputo, A.: Studies on carboxypeptidase digests of human hemoglobin. J. Biol. Chem. 236:PC60, 1961.
85. Neer, E. J., and Konigsberg, W.: The characterization of modified human hemoglobin. II. Reaction with 1-fluoro-2,4-dinitrobenzene. J. Biol. Chem. 243:1966, 1968.
86. Imai, K., and Yonetani, T.: Thermodynamical studies of oxygen equilibrium of hemoglobin. J. Biol. Chem. 250:7093, 1975.
87. Imai, K.: Thermodynamic aspects of the cooperativity in four-step oxygenation equilibria of haemoglobin. J. Mol. Biol. 133:233, 1979.
88. Mills, F. C., Johnson, M. L., and Ackers, G. K.: Oxygen-linked subunit interactions in human hemoglobin: Experimental studies on the concentration dependence of oxygenation curves. Biochemistry 15:5350, 1976.

89. Ip, S. H. C., and Ackers, G. K.: Thermodynamic studies on subunit assembly in human hemoglobin. J. Biol. Chem. 252:82, 1977.
90. Mills, F. C., and Ackers, G. K.: Quaternary enhancement in binding of oxygen by human hemoglobin. Proc. Natl. Acad. Sci. USA 76:273, 1979.
91. Chu, A. H., and Ackers, G. K.: Mutual effects of protons, NaCl, and oxygen on the dimer-tetramer assembly of human hemoglobin. J. Biol. Chem. 256:1199, 1981.
92. Ackers, G. K.: Energetics of subunit assembly and ligand binding in human hemoglobin. Biophys. J. 32:331, 1980.
93. Hammes, G. G., and Wu, C. W.: Regulation of enzyme activity. Science 172:1205, 1971.
94. Pauling, L.: The oxygen equilibrium of hemoglobin and its structural interpretation. Proc. Natl. Acad. Sci. USA 21:186, 1935.
95. Koshland, D. E., Jr., Nemethy, G., and Filmer, D.: Comparison of experimental binding data and theoretical models in proteins containing subunits. Biochemistry 5:365, 1966.
96. Monod, J., Wyman, J., and Changeux, J. P.: On the nature of allosteric transitions: A plausible model. J. Mol. Biol. 12:88, 1965.
97. Parkhurst, L. J.: Hemoglobin and myoglobin ligand kinetics. Ann. Rev. Phys. Chem. 30:503, 1979.
98. Olsen, J. S.: Stopped-flow, rapid mixing measurements of ligand binding to hemoglobin and red cells. In Antonini, E., Rossi-Bernardi, L., and Chiancone, E. (eds.): Methods in Enzymology, Vol. 76. New York, Academic Press, 1981, p. 631.
99. Brunori, M., Coletta, M., and Ilgenfritz, G.: Temperature jump of hemoglobin. In Antonini, E., Rossi-Bernardi, L., and Chiancone, E. (eds.): Methods in Enzymology, Vol. 76. New York, Academic Press, 1981, p. 681.
100. Gibson, Q. H.: The photochemical formation of a quickly reacting form of haemoglobin. Biochem. J. 71:293, 1959.
101. Hofrichter, J., Sommer, J. H., Henry, E. R., and Eaton, W. A.: Nanosecond absorption spectroscopy of hemoglobin: Elementary processes in kinetic cooperativity. Proc. Natl. Acad. Sci. USA 80:2235, 1983.
102. Gibson, Q. H., and Parkhurst, L. J.: Kinetic evidence for a tetrameric functional unit in hemoglobin. J. Biol. Chem. 243:5521, 1968.
103. Szabo, A.: Kinetics of hemoglobin and transition state theory. Proc. Natl. Acad. Sci. USA 75:2108, 1978.
104. Viggiano, G., Ho, N. T., and Ho, C.: Proton nuclear magnetic resonance and biochemical studies of oxygenation of human adult hemoglobin in deuterium oxide. Biochemistry 18:5238, 1979.
105. Viggiano, G., and Ho, C.: Proton nuclear magnetic resonance investigation of structural changes associated with cooperative oxygenation of human adult hemoglobin. Proc. Natl. Acad. Sci. USA 76:3673, 1979.
106. Asakura, T., and Lau, P-W.: Sequence of oxygen binding by hemoglobin. Proc. Natl. Acad. Sci. USA 75:5462, 1978.
107. Baldwin, J., and Chothia, C.: Hemoglobin: The structural changes related to ligand binding and its allosteric mechanism. J. Mol. Biol. 129:175, 1979.
108. Shulman, R. G., Hopfield, J. J., and Ogawa, S.: Allosteric interpretation of hemoglobin properties. Q. Rev. Biophys. 8:325, 1975.
109. Szabo, A., and Karplus, M.: A mathematical model of structure-function relationships in hemoglobin. J. Mol. Biol. 72:163, 1972.
110. Szabo, A., and Karplus, M.: Analysis of cooperativity in hemoglobin. Valence hybrids, oxidation and methemoglobin replacement reactions. Biochemistry 14:931, 1975.
111. Szabo, A., and Karplus, M.: Analyses of the interaction of organic phosphates with hemoglobin. Biochemistry 15:2869, 1976.
112. Miura, S., and Ho, C.: Preparation and proton nuclear magnetic resonance investigation of cross-linked mixed valency hybrid hemoglobins: Models for partially oxygenated species. Biochemistry 21:6280, 1982.
113. Benesch, R. E., Benesch, R., and Williamson, M. E.: The influence of reversible oxygen binding on the interaction between hemoglobin subunits. Proc. Natl. Acad. Sci. USA 48:2071, 1962.
114. Nagel, R. L., Rothman, M. C., Bradley, T. B., and Ranney, H. M.: Comparative haptoglobin binding properties of oxyhemoglobin and deoxyhemoglobin. J. Biol. Chem. 240:PC4543, 1965.
115. Zito, R., Antonini, E., and Wyman, J.: The effect of oxygenation on the rate of digestion of human hemoglobins by carboxypeptidases. J. Biol. Chem. 239:1804, 1964.
116. Antonini, E., Wyman, J., Moretti, R., and Rossi-Fanelli, A.: The interaction of bromothymol blue with hemoglobin and its effect on oxygen equilibrium. Biochim. Biophys. Acta 71:124, 1963.
117. Lee, C. K., and Manning, J. M.: Kinetics of carbamylation of the amino groups of sickle cell hemoglobin by cyanate. J. Biol. Chem. 248:5861, 1973.
118. Jensen, M., Nathan, D., and Bunn, H. F.: The reaction of cyanate with the α and β subunits of hemoglobin: Effects of oxygenation, phosphates and carbon dioxide. J. Biol. Chem. 248:8057, 1973.

HEMOGLOBINS A₂, F, AND A_Ic AND OTHER HUMAN HEMOGLOBIN COMPONENTS

4

In normal human erythrocytes, Hb A ($\alpha_2\beta_2$) composes about 90 per cent of the total hemoglobin. Its structure has been presented in detail in Chapter 2, and its functional properties have been discussed in Chapter 3. Besides Hb A, human red cells contain other hemoglobin components that are of considerable interest (Table 4–1). Some of these, such as Hbs A_2 and F, are products of additional globin-chain genes, and others such as Hb A_{Ic} are post-translational modifications of Hb A. Information on these hemoglobin components is useful not only for a better understanding of globin-gene expression but also in the diagnosis of a variety of disorders. Moreover, minor hemoglobin components may serve as "reporter molecules," reflecting accumulation of various metabolites or toxins.

HEMOGLOBIN A_2

When Kunkel and Wallenius[1] analyzed human hemolysates by starch gel electrophoresis, they found a minor component that had less negative charge than Hb A and composed about 2.5 per cent of the total. This component was designated Hb A_2 (Fig. 4–1). Subsequently, these investigators demonstrated increased amounts of Hb A_2 in individuals with β thalassemia.[2] Structural analysis of the globin of Hb A_2 revealed normal α chains combined with chains whose structure differed significantly from that of normal β chains. These non-α subunits were designated δ chains.[3]

Structure. The primary sequence of the human δ chain is shown in Table 4–2. There is marked structural homology between the δ and β globin chains. In fact, the primary sequence of the δ chain differs from that of the β chain in only 10 out of 146 residues.[3] More recent structural analyses of δ-chain protein[4,5] and the corresponding gene DNA[6] have verified the primary sequence of the human δ chain.

In addition to man, apes and New World monkeys have a minor component similar to Hb A_2[2,7] that composes 0.6 to 6.0 per cent of the total hemoglobin.[7] This component is lack-

Table 4-1. HUMAN HEMOGLOBINS

Hemoglobin	Structure	% of Normal Adult Hemolysate	Increased In	Decreased In
A	$\alpha_2\beta_2$	92		
A_2	$\alpha_2\delta_2$	2.5	β thalassemia (Table 4-3)	Iron deficiency, α thalassemia (Table 4-3)
A_{Ia}	Not known	<1		
A_{Ib}	" "	<2	Diabetes mellitus	Hemolytic anemia
A_{Ic}	$\alpha_2(\beta\text{-N-glucose})_2$	3		
F	$\alpha_2\gamma_2$	<1	Fetal red cells, β thalassemia, HPFH, Marrow "stress", Sickle cell anemia, pernicious anemia, etc. (Table 4-4)	
F_I	$\alpha_2(\gamma\text{-N-acetyl})_2$	<1		
Gower-1	$\zeta_2\epsilon_2$	0		
Gower-2	$\alpha_2\epsilon_2$	0	Early embryo	
Portland	$\zeta_2\gamma_2$	0		
H	β_4	0	α thalassemias (Chapter 9)	
Bart's	γ_4	0		

ing in Old World monkeys and other mammals. Primates that lack detectable Hb A_2 have δ-chain genes that are functionally silent because of various mutations. This will be discussed further in Chapter 8.

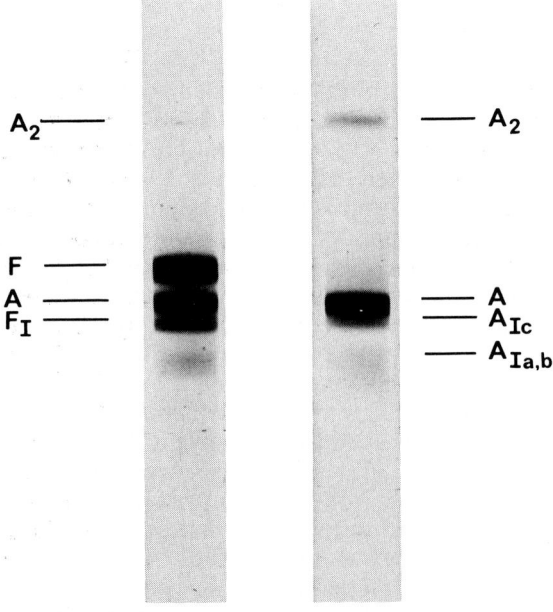

Figure 4-1. Analysis of human umbilical cord and adult blood hemolysates by gel electrofocusing. The gels have been overloaded in order to demonstrate Hb A_2.

It is likely that the δ chain arose by a recent duplication of the β-chain gene (~40 million years ago), although there is some controversy on this point (see Chapter 7). The impaired expression of the δ-chain gene is primarily due to reduced transcription[8-10] in erythroid cells causing a relatively low level of δ-chain mRNA. Lower levels of δ-gene transcription may be due to known differences in the base sequence flanking the 5' end of the β and δ genes.[6] The synthesis of δ chains declines further during erythroid maturation,[11, 12] probably owing to instability of δ-chain mRNA.[13] There is virtually no detectable δ-chain production in reticulocytes. Unlike Hb F, Hb A_2 appears to be evenly distributed among red cells.[14, 15]

Functional Properties. In view of its low amount in red cells, Hb A_2 is unlikely to have any physiological role in oxygen transport. Moreover, it is unlikely that this gene product serves any other useful function. Its oxygen binding properties resemble those of Hb A: The two hemoglobins have similar oxygen affinity,[16-19] subunit cooperativity, Bohr effect,[16, 18] and response to 2,3-DPG.[17-19] Hb A_2 is more resistant to thermal denaturation than Hb A[20] is. This can be explained by an additional contact at the $\alpha_1\delta_1$ interface (δ 116 Arg⋯α 114 Pro), which confers enhanced stability to the αδ dimer.[21] The apparent lack of a physiological role for Hb A_2 is compatible with greater differences in primary structure among the δ chains of primates compared with

Table 4–2. PRIMARY STRUCTURE OF HUMAN GLOBIN SUBUNITS

Helix*	α	ζ	Helix*	β	δ	γ	ε
NA1	1 Val	Ser	NA1	1 Val	Val	Gly	Val
			NA2	2 His	His	His	His
NA2	2 Leu	Leu	NA3	3 Leu	Leu	Phe	Phe
A1	3 Ser	Thr	A1	4 Thr	Thr	Thr	Thr
A2	4 Pro	Lys	A2	5 Pro	Pro	Glu	Ala
A3	5 Ala	Thr	A3	6 Glu	Glu	Glu	Glu
A4	6 Asp	Glu	A4	7 Glu	Glu	Asp	Glu
A5	7 Lys	Arg	A5	8 Lys	Lys	Lys	Lys
A6	8 Thr	Thr	A6	9 Ser	Thr	Ala	Ala
A7	9 Asn	Ile	A7	10 Ala	Ala	Thr	Ala
A8	10 Val	Ile	A8	11 Val	Val	Ile	Val
A9	11 Lys	Val	A9	12 Thr	Asn	Thr	Thr
A10	12 Ala	Ser	A10	13 Ala	Ala	Ser	Ser
A11	13 Ala	Met	A11	14 Leu	Leu	Leu	Leu
A12	14 Trp	Trp	A12	15 Trp	Trp	Trp	Trp
A13	15 Gly	Ala	A13	16 Gly	Gly	Gly	Ser
A14	16 Lys	Lys	A14	17 Lys	Lys	Lys	Lys
A15	17 Val	Ile	A15	18 Val	Val	Val	Met
A16	18 Gly	Ser					
AB1	19 Ala	Thr					
B1	20 His	Gln	B1	19 Asn	Asn	Asn	Asn
B2	21 Ala	Ala	B2	20 Val	Val	Val	Val
B3	22 Gly	Asp	B3	21 Asp	Asp	Glu	Glu
B4	23 Glu	Thr	B4	22 Glu	Ala	Asp	Glu
B5	24 Tyr	Ile	B5	23 Val	Val	Ala	Ala
B6	25 Gly	Gly	B6	24 Gly	Gly	Gly	Gly
B7	26 Ala	Thr	B7	25 Gly	Gly	Gly	Gly
B8	27 Glu	Glu	B8	26 Glu	Glu	Glu	Glu
B9	28 Ala	Thr	B9	27 Ala	Ala	Thr	Ala
B10	29 Leu	Leu	B10	28 Leu	Leu	Leu	Leu
B11	30 Glu	Glu	B11	29 Gly	Gly	Gly	Gly
B12	31 Arg	Arg	B12	30 Arg	Arg	Arg	Arg
B13	32 Met	Leu	B13	31 Leu	Leu	Leu	Leu
B14	33 Phe	Phe	B14	32 Leu	Leu	Leu	Leu
B15	34 Leu	Leu	B15	33 Val	Val	Val	Val
B16	35 Ser	Ser	B16	34 Val	Val	Val	Val
C1	36 Phe	His	C1	35 Tyr	Tyr	Tyr	Tyr
C2	37 Pro	Pro	C2	36 Pro	Pro	Pro	Pro
C3	38 Thr	Gln	C3	37 Trp	Trp	Trp	Trp
C4	39 Thr	Thr	C4	38 Thr	Thr	Thr	Thr
C5	40 Lys	Lys	C5	39 Gln	Gln	Gln	Gln
C6	41 Thr	Thr	C6	40 Arg	Arg	Arg	Arg
C7	42 Tyr	Tyr	C7	41 Phe	Phe	Phe	Phe
CE1	43 Phe	Phe	CD1	42 Phe	Phe	Phe	Phe
CE2	44 Pro	Pro	CD2	43 Glu	Glu	Asp	Asp
CE3	45 His	His	CD3	44 Ser	Ser	Ser	Ser
CE4	46 Phe	Phe	CD4	45 Phe	Phe	Phe	Phe
			CD5	46 Gly	Gly	Gly	Gly
CE5	47 Asp	Asp	CD6	47 Asp	Asp	Asn	Asn
CE6	48 Leu	Leu	CD7	48 Leu	Leu	Leu	Leu
CE7	49 Ser	His	CD8	49 Ser	Ser	Ser	Ser
CE8	50 His	Pro	D1	50 Thr	Ser	Ser	Ser
			D2	51 Pro	Pro	Ala	Pro
			D3	52 Asp	Asp	Ser	Ser
			D4	53 Ala	Ala	Ala	Ala
			D5	54 Val	Val	Ile	Ile
			D6	55 Met	Met	Met	Leu
CE9	51 Gly	Gly	D7	56 Gly	Gly	Gly	Gly
E1	52 Ser	Ser	E1	57 Asn	Asn	Asn	Asn
E2	53 Ala	Ala	E2	58 Pro	Pro	Pro	Pro
E3	54 Gln	Gln	E3	59 Lys	Lys	Lys	Lys
E4	55 Val	Leu	E4	60 Val	Val	Val	Val
E5	56 Lys	Arg	E5	61 Lys	Lys	Lys	Lys
E6	57 Gly	Ala	E6	62 Ala	Ala	Ala	Ala
E7	58 His	His	E7	63 His	His	His	His
E8	59 Gly	Gly	E8	64 Gly	Gly	Gly	Gly

Table continued on following page

Table 4–2. PRIMARY STRUCTURE OF HUMAN GLOBIN SUBUNITS (Continued)

Helix*	α	ζ	Helix*	β	δ	γ	ε
E9	60 Lys	Ser	E9	65 Lys	Lys	Lys	Lys
E10	61 Lys	Lys	E10	66 Lys	Lys	Lys	Lys
E11	62 Val	Val	E11	67 Val	Val	Val	Val
E12	63 Ala	Val	E12	68 Leu	Leu	Leu	Leu
E13	64 Asp	Ala	E13	69 Gly	Gly	Thr	Thr
E14	65 Ala	Ala	E14	70 Ala	Ala	Ser	Ser
E15	66 Leu	Val	E15	71 Phe	Phe	Leu	Phe
E16	67 Thr	Gly	E16	72 Ser	Ser	Gly	Gly
E17	68 Asn	Asp	E17	73 Asp	Asp	Asp	Asp
E18	69 Ala	Ala	E18	74 Gly	Gly	Ala	Ala
E19	70 Val	Val	E19	75 Leu	Leu	Ile, Thr	Ile
E20	71 Ala	Lys	E20	76 Ala	Ala	Lys	Lys
EF1	72 His	Ser	EF1	77 His	His	His	Asn
EF2	73 Val	Ile	EF2	78 Leu	Leu	Leu	Met
EF3	74 Asp	Asp	EF3	79 Asp	Asp	Asp	Asp
EF4	75 Asp	Asp	EF4	80 Asn	Asn	Asn	Asn
EF5	76 Met	Ile	EF5	81 Leu	Leu	Leu	Leu
EF6	77 Pro	Gly	EF6	82 Lys	Lys	Lys	Lys
EF7	78 Asn	Gly	EF7	83 Gly	Gly	Gly	Pro
EF8	79 Ala	Ala	EF8	84 Thr	Thr	Thr	Ala
F1	80 Leu	Leu	F1	85 Phe	Phe	Phe	Phe
F2	81 Ser	Ser	F2	86 Ala	Ser	Ala	Ala
F3	82 Ala	Lys	F3	87 Thr	Gln	Gln	Lys
F4	83 Leu	Leu	F4	88 Leu	Leu	Leu	Leu
F5	84 Ser	Ser	F5	89 Ser	Ser	Ser	Ser
F6	85 Asp	Glu	F6	90 Glu	Glu	Glu	Glu
F7	86 Leu	Leu	F7	91 Leu	Leu	Leu	Leu
F8	87 His	His	F8	92 His	His	His	His
F9	88 Ala	Ala	F9	93 Cys	Cys	Cys	Cys
FG1	89 His	Tyr	FG1	94 Asp	Asp	Asp	Asp
FG2	90 Lys	Ile	FG2	95 Lys	Lys	Lys	Lys
FG3	91 Leu	Leu	FG3	96 Leu	Leu	Leu	Leu
FG4	92 Arg	Arg	FG4	97 His	His	His	His
FG5	93 Val	Val	FG5	98 Val	Val	Val	Val
G1	94 Asp	Asp	G1	99 Asp	Asp	Asp	Asp
G2	95 Pro	Pro	G2	100 Pro	Pro	Pro	Pro
G3	96 Val	Val	G3	101 Glu	Glu	Glu	Glu
G4	97 Asn	Asn	G4	102 Asn	Asn	Asn	Asn
G5	98 Phe	Phe	G5	103 Phe	Phe	Phe	Phe
G6	99 Lys	Lys	G6	104 Arg	Arg	Lys	Lys
G7	100 Leu	Leu	G7	105 Leu	Leu	Leu	Leu
G8	101 Leu	Leu	G8	106 Leu	Leu	Leu	Leu

Table continued on opposite page

β chains.[7, 22] Thus, certain mutations that significantly alter hemoglobin function or stability could be tolerated in Hb A_2 but not in the major component responsible for O_2 transport.

Fourteen δ-chain variants have been discovered thus far (see Table 10–2C). This subject has been reviewed by Vella.[23] It is likely that hundreds of δ-chain variants exist, comparable to the 200-odd known β-chain variants, but because of their small quantity, they are less likely to be detected. Because δ-gene mutations are more apt to be adaptively neutral than β-gene mutations, it would be of interest to compare the functional properties of human δ-chain variants as well as the various A_2 hemoglobins among the apes and New World primates. It is likely that many of these hemoglobins have significant functional abnormalities. Indeed, one human δ-chain variant has very high oxygen affinity.[24]

Measurement of Hb A_2. Most methods for assaying Hb A_2 take advantage of the large difference in surface charge between Hb A_2 (pI = 7.40) and Hb A (pI = 6.95). Thus, the two components are easily separated by zone electrophoresis and can be quantitated by densitometric scanning.[25] Alternatively, small disposable columns may provide more reliable results.[26, 27] Because of similarity in overall surface charge, Hb A_2 is difficult to separate from Hbs C and E. This problem is obviated when Hb A_2 is assayed by immunological techniques.[28] Further information on methods for measuring Hb A_2 is provided elsewhere.[29, 30]

Hb A_2 in Congenital Disorders. Hb A_2 is elevated about twofold in individuals with β thalassemia minor (see Chapter 9) and sickle/β thalassemia (see Chapter 12). Exceptionally high levels of Hb A_2 (8 to 15 per cent) have been encountered in two families with β thal-

Table 4-2. PRIMARY STRUCTURE OF HUMAN GLOBIN SUBUNITS (Continued)

Helix*	α	ζ	Helix*	β	δ	γ	ε
G9	102 Ser	Ser	G9	107 Gly	Gly	Gly	Gly
G10	103 His	His	G10	108 Asn	Asn	Asn	Asn
G11	104 Cys	Cys	G11	109 Val	Val	Val	Val
G12	105 Leu	Leu	G12	110 Leu	Leu	Leu	Met
G13	106 Leu	Leu	G13	111 Val	Val	Val	Val
G14	107 Val	Val	G14	112 Cys	Cys	Thr	Ile
G15	108 Thr	Thr	G15	113 Val	Val	Val	Ile
G16	109 Leu	Leu	G16	114 Leu	Leu	Leu	Leu
G17	110 Ala	Ala	G17	115 Ala	Ala	Ala	Ala
G18	111 Ala	Ala	G18	116 His	Arg	Ile	Thr
G19	112 His	Arg	G19	117 His	Asn	His	His
GH1	113 Leu	Phe	GH1	118 Phe	Phe	Phe	Phe
GH2	114 Pro	Pro	GH2	119 Gly	Gly	Gly	Gly
GH3	115 Ala	Ala	GH3	120 Lys	Lys	Lys	Lys
GH4	116 Glu	Asp	GH4	121 Glu	Glu	Glu	Glu
GH5	117 Phe	Phe	GH5	122 Phe	Phe	Phe	Phe
H1	118 Thr	Thr	H1	123 Thr	Thr	Thr	Thr
H2	119 Pro	Ala	H2	124 Pro	Pro	Pro	Pro
H3	120 Ala	Glu	H3	125 Pro	Gln	Glu	Glu
H4	121 Val	Ala	H4	126 Val	Met	Val	Val
H5	122 His	His	H5	127 Gln	Gln	Gln	Gln
H6	123 Ala	Ala	H6	128 Ala	Ala	Ala	Ala
H7	124 Ser	Ala	H7	129 Ala	Ala	Ser	Ala
H8	125 Leu	Trp	H8	130 Tyr	Tyr	Trp	Trp
H9	126 Asp	Asp	H9	131 Gln	Gln	Gln	Gln
H10	127 Lys	Lys	H10	132 Lys	Lys	Lys	Lys
H11	128 Phe	Phe	H11	133 Val	Val	Met	Leu
H12	129 Leu	Leu	H12	134 Val	Val	Val	Val
H13	130 Ala	Ser	H13	135 Ala	Ala	Thr	Ser
H14	131 Ser	Val	H14	136 Gly	Gly	Gly, Ala	Ala
H15	132 Val	Val	H15	137 Val	Val	Val	Val
H16	133 Ser	Ser	H16	138 Ala	Ala	Ala	Ala
H17	134 Thr	Ser	H17	139 Asn	Asn	Ser	Ile
H18	135 Val	Val	H18	140 Ala	Ala	Ala	Ala
H19	136 Leu	Leu	H19	141 Leu	Leu	Leu	Leu
H20	137 Thr	Thr	H20	142 Ala	Ala	Ser	Ala
H21	138 Ser	Glu	H21	143 His	His	Ser	His
HC1	139 Lys	Lys	HC1	144 Lys	Lys	Arg	Lys
HC2	140 Tyr	Tyr	HC2	145 Tyr	Tyr	Tyr	Tyr
HC3	141 Arg	Arg	HC3	146 His	His	His	His

*The residues have been aligned to demonstrate homology between subunits.

assemia.[31,32] Theoretically, this could be due to crossover between the δ and β genes at sites where the full δ-chain sequence is preserved. In one of these families, restriction endonuclease mapping ruled out this possibility.[32] Individuals who are heterozygous for both β thalassemia and a δ-chain variant have equivalent levels of the normal and variant A_2 hemoglobins with a total that is twice the normal level.[24,33] Thus, the increased Hb A_2 in β thalassemia is derived from the δ chains both in *cis* and in *trans* to the β-thalassemia gene. Red cells of individuals with β thalassemia minor contain about 70 per cent as much hemoglobin as normal red cells. Because the proportion of Hb A_2 is increased about twofold, there is an absolute increase in Hb A_2 in these cells. However, as discussed below, this need not imply an absolute increase in δ-chain synthesis. As shown in Table 4-3, Hb A_2 is significantly elevated in individuals with sickle trait[34,34a] as well as in many individuals with an unstable hemoglobin variant (see Chapter 13). Patients with homozygous sickle cell anemia have normal levels of Hb A_2 (mean = 2.7 per cent)[35] However those SS patients with

Table 4-3. ALTERATIONS IN Hb A_2 IN VARIOUS DISORDERS

	Elevated	Reduced
Congenital	β-thalassemia trait Unstable hemoglobin variants Sickle trait (AS) SS with α thalassemia	α thalassemia δβ thalassemia δ thalassemia HPFH
Acquired	Megaloblastic anemias Hyperthyroidism	Iron deficiency Sideroblastic anemias

coexisting α thalassemia have significantly higher levels: αα/α- = 3.1 per cent; α-/α- = 3.8 per cent.[35]

The situation is complex in β-thalassemia homozygotes. Although the range is very wide, the mean proportion of Hb A_2 is 2.3 to 3.0 per cent.[30] However, because of marked microcytosis, the absolute amount of Hb A_2 per red cell may be *less* than normal. The Hb A_2 is particularly low in those cells containing increased Hb F.[30] Nevertheless, in bone marrow cells from β-thalassemia homozygotes, the rate of δ-gene transcription exceeds that of normal cells.[36] Thus, the relatively low level of Hb A_2 in circulating red cells of homozygotes can be explained by the preferential survival of the Hb F–containing cells.

In contrast to values in individuals with β thalassemia, levels of Hb A_2 are decreased in individuals with α thalassemia[37, 38] (Fig. 4–2). There is not yet adequate information on how well the level of Hb A_2 correlates with the number of α-chain genes that have been deleted. Markedly reduced levels of Hb A_2 have been encountered in Hb H disease.[39, 40] Hb A_2 is also decreased in δβ thalassemia and in δ thalassemia (see Chapter 9).

Hb A_2 in Acquired Disorders. In patients with iron deficiency, Hb A_2 is decreased to about 60 per cent of normal values[38, 40–42] (Table 4–3). Levels return to normal within six weeks after iron therapy. The fact that this rate of response is considerably shorter than the red cell life span suggests that the new red cells produced after iron treatment contain supernormal amounts of Hb A_2.[43] Decreased Hb A_2 in iron deficiency has been attributed to preferential synthesis of Hb A in the late erythroid precursors.[41] However, as discussed below, an alternative explanation seems equally plausible. Decreased Hb A_2 is also encountered in sideroblastic anemia,[44, 45] another acquired disorder that impairs heme synthesis. Finally, low levels of Hb A_2 have been reported in occasional patients with erythroleukemia,[46] although most patients with this disorder have normal Hb A_2.[40]

Elevated levels of Hb A_2 have been encountered in several unrelated acquired disorders. Patients with megaloblastic anemia due to a deficiency of either vitamin B_{12} or folic acid often have elevated Hb A_2[40, 47, 48, 48a] (Table 4–3), particularly if their anemia is severe.[40] Hb A_2 levels will return to normal after appropriate replacement therapy.[40] Because DNA replication and therefore cell division are impaired in megaloblastic anemias, it is likely that compared with normal, a relatively larger proportion of hemoglobin synthesis occurs in less mature erythroid precursors. The relative synthesis of δ chains should be correspondingly greater in the less mature erythroid cells.[11, 12]

Patients with hyperthyroidism also have significantly elevated levels of Hb A_2 (Table 4–3).[49, 50, 50a] Following treatment with thyroid hormone, the levels of Hb A_2 return to normal. It is worth noting that while patients are hyperthyroid, they have slight microcytosis.[50a]

Initial reports from two widely distant parts of the world[51, 52] suggested that Hb A_2 was also elevated in patients with malaria. However, this finding has not been confirmed in a large number of follow-up studies (reference 53 and references therein).

A unifying hypothesis that explains the alterations in Hb A_2 in various conditions is presented in Chapter 10. The basic premise is that α chains combine more readily with β chains than with δ chains. The competition between β and δ chains for α chains is relaxed in β thalassemia (owing to a relative excess of α chains) and exaggerated in α thalassemia, in which α chains are decreased. Accordingly, Hb A_2 should increase in β thalassemia and decrease in α thalassemia. The low levels of Hb A_2 in iron deficiency and sideroblastic anemias (and perhaps in some cases of erythroleukemia) are compatible with this hypothesis because relative deficiency of α-chain production has been documented in all three disorders (see Chapter 7). Moreover, the increased level of Hb A_2 in sickle trait red cells may reflect the fact that α chains bind less readily to $β^S$ chains than to $β^A$ chains and are therefore more available to combine with δ chains.

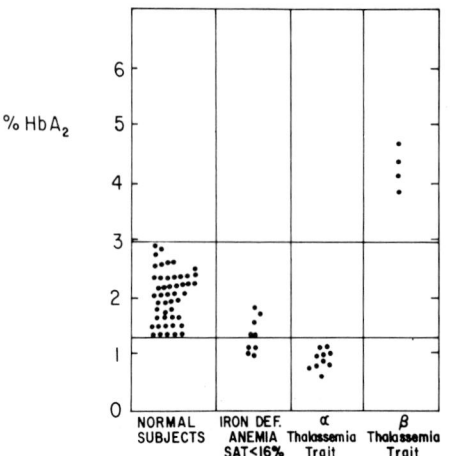

Figure 4–2. Levels of Hb A_2 in normal individuals and in those with various hematologic disorders. (From McCormack, M. K.: Clin. Chim. Acta *105*:387, 1980.)

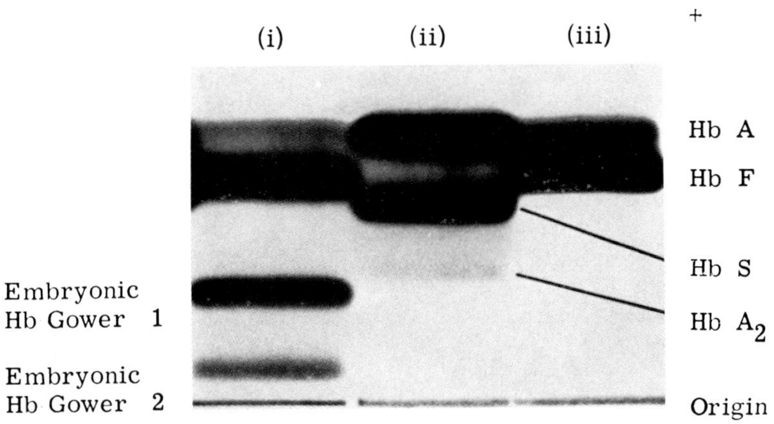

Figure 4-3. Starch gel electrophoresis (pH 8.6) of (i) hemolysate from a 3.5-cm (crown–rump) human embryo; (ii) mixture of Hbs S + A; and (iii) hemolysate from a normal newborn (umbilical cord blood). (From Huehns, E. R., and Shooter, E. M.: J. Med. Genet. 2:48, 1965.)

EMBRYONIC HEMOGLOBINS

In 1961, Huehns and colleagues[54] discovered two hemoglobin components in the blood of human embryos that differed from Hb A and fetal hemoglobin (Hb F). These components migrated more slowly than Hb A_2 when analyzed by starch gel electrophoresis (pH 8.6) (Fig. 4–3). They were designated Hb Gower-1 and Hb Gower-2 in honor of the street in London where University College Hospital is located. Hb Gower-2 was shown to be a tetramer composed of two α chains and two novel subunits, designated ε chains. The primary sequence of ε chains is shown in Table 4–2. The ε chains are encoded by a gene in the β globin gene complex on chromosome 11. The ε gene is located on the 5′-side of the $^G\gamma$ gene. The molecular genetics of the embryonic globin subunits are discussed in Chapter 7.

A third human embryonic hemoglobin was found to have the electrophoretic mobility of Hb A at pH 8.6 but could be separated from Hb A at lower pH.[55, 56] This hemoglobin, designated Hb Portland, was shown to be a tetramer composed of two γ chains and two novel subunits, designated ζ chains.[57] The ζ chain was found to bear strong structural homology to the α chain.[58] Subsequently, the ζ gene was identified at a site 5′ to the α-chain genes on chromosome 16 (see Chapter 7).

Structural analyses have shown Hb Gower-1 to be a tetramer composed entirely of embryonic subunits: $\zeta_2\epsilon_2$. Earlier reports stated incorrectly that Hb Gower-1 was a tetramer of ε chains (ϵ_4).

These three embryonic hemoglobins, $\alpha_2\epsilon_2$, $\zeta_2\epsilon_2$ and $\zeta_2\gamma_2$, serve as physiologic oxygen carriers. Red cells from early embryos in which these three hemoglobins predominate have an affinity for oxygen similar to that of cord blood cells and a sigmoid oxygen dissociation curve indicative of subunit cooperativity.[59] Furthermore, the alkaline Bohr effect in embryonic red cells was similar to that of fetal red cells. Oxygen equilibria have also been determined on purified Hb Portland ($\zeta_2\gamma_2$).[60] This hemoglobin has a significantly higher oxygen affinity than Hb A, lower subunit cooperativity (Hill's $n = 2.0$) than Hb A, and an alkaline Bohr effect about half that of Hb A.

The embryonic hemoglobins are produced in the yolk sac during the third through eighth weeks of gestation. From about the eighth to the twenty-eighth week, the liver becomes the major site of erythropoiesis. During the last half of gestation, red cell production gradually shifts from the liver and spleen to the bone marrow. As shown in Figure 4–4, when the embryo reaches a crown-rump length of 35 mm (at about seven weeks' gestation) Hb F composes about 50 per cent of the total hemoglobin, and when the embryo exceeds a crown-rump length of 50 mm (about nine weeks' gestation), about 90 per cent of the total is Hb F.[61, 62] Thereafter, the embryonic hemoglobins are no longer detectable,* and Hb F is the predominant hemoglobin in fetal red cells. However, β-chain synthesis begins early in fetal development. At the sixth week of gestation, Hb A composes about 7 per cent of the total hemoglobin and increases slowly until about the thirtieth week,[66, 67] when there is a much more concerted "switch" from γ-chain to β-chain production. The biosynthesis of the

---

*Two interesting exceptions have been noted. Moderate amounts (10 to 25 per cent) of Hb Portland ($\zeta_2\gamma_2$) can be detected in babies born with homozygous α thalassemia-1 (hydrops fetalis).[63, 64] Furthermore, the adult human leukemia cell line K562 synthesizes Hbs Gower-1 and Portland in response to stimulation by certain inducing agents.[65]

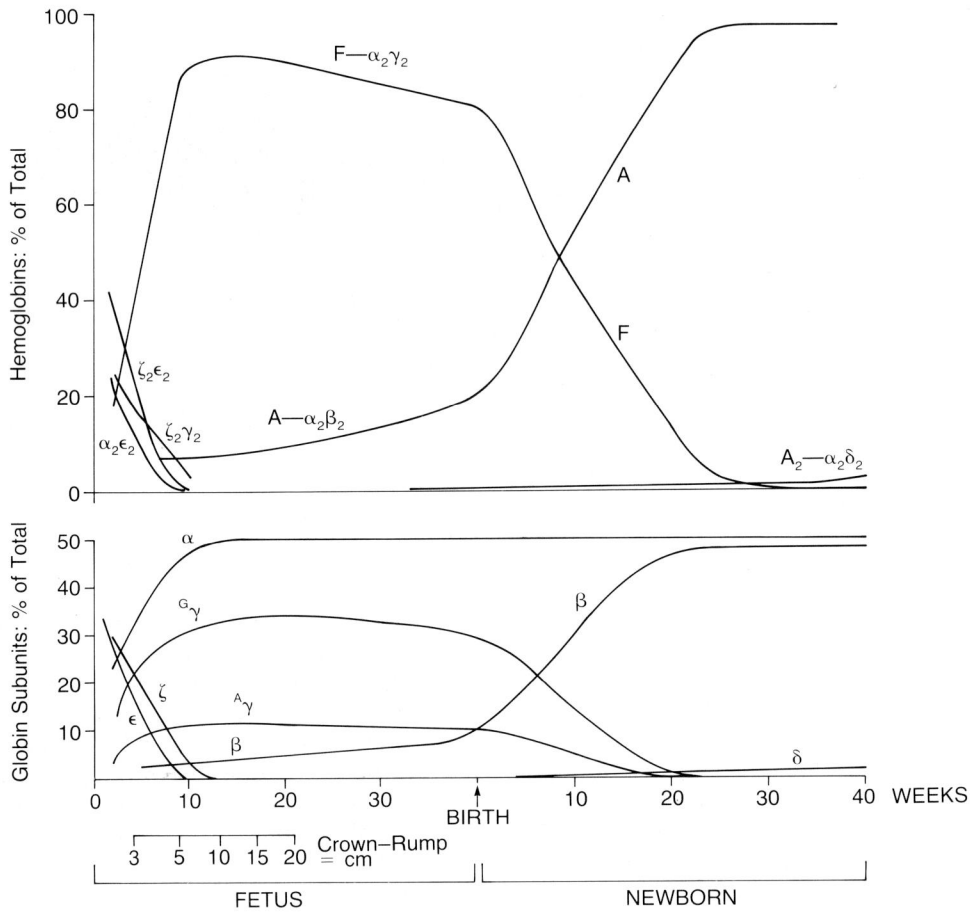

Figure 4–4. Changes in hemoglobin tetramers (top panel) and in globin subunits (bottom panel) during human development from embryo to early infancy.

embryonic and fetal hemoglobins as well as the switch will be discussed in considerably more detail in Chapter 7.

Hb F (FETAL HEMOGLOBIN)

The discovery by Körber in 1866[68] that hemolysates of newborn red cells were resistant to alkaline denaturation suggested that these cells contained a structurally distinct hemoglobin. This conclusion was strengthened by the demonstration that the hemoglobin from a newborn had increased absorbance in the ultraviolet spectrum,[69] a finding now known to be due to an additional tryptophan residue in the γ chain (γ 130 Trp). Subsequently, N-terminal amino acid analysis showed that the alkali-resistant hemoglobin of the newborn did indeed differ from normal adult hemoglobin.[70] The development of chromatographic[71,72] and electrophoretic techniques enabled the isolation and characterization of human fetal hemoglobin (designated Hb F) (see Figure 4–1). More precise N-terminal analyses of purified Hb F suggested that it was a tetramer with two identical subunits in common with Hb A (α chains). However, the two other subunits had a common structure different from either of the subunits of Hb A.[73]

Structure. The primary structure of the human γ chain was determined by Walter Schroeder and colleagues.[74] As shown in Table 4–2, the amino acid sequence of the γ chain is strongly analogous to that of the β chain. The sequences of the two proteins differ in 39 of 146 residues. Twenty-two of these residues are on the external surface of the molecule and are therefore unlikely to have a significant effect on the properties of Hb F other than surface charge. The internal substitutions are "conservative," involving amino acids of similar polarity. Four substitutions occur at the $\alpha_1\beta_1$ ($\alpha_1\gamma_1$) interface and probably account for the increased stability of Hb F and its decreased dissociation into monomers (see below). In contrast, no substitution occurs at the $\alpha_1\beta_2$ ($\alpha_1\gamma_2$) interface that is so important for subunit cooperativity. Thus, the structural differences between γ and β chains would not be expected to cause any gross functional perturbations. However, the differences in primary structure of γ and β chains can satisfactorily explain several of the unique properties of Hb F discussed in the section below.

Hb F has two types of structural heterogeneity: genetic and post-translational. As shown in the electrophoretic analysis of cord blood hemolysate (see Figure 4–1), two fetal hemoglobin components can be resolved. The major component, Hb F (also designated Hb F_o or Hb F_{II}), is unmodified $\alpha_2\gamma_2$ and composes the majority of the total hemoglobin. A less abundant fetal hemoglobin component (Hb F_I) with a lower isoelectric point (more negative charge) differs from Hb F only by having acetyl groups linked at the N termini of the γ chains. Additional minor fetal hemoglobin components are formed by nonenzymatic glycosylation. These post-translational modifications of Hb F will be discussed at the end of this chapter.

A second and more important kind of structural heterogeneity of Hb F arises from different γ-chain genes. Five years after establishing the primary structure of the γ chain, Schroeder and colleagues,[75] discovered totally unexpected heterogeneity in the γ-chain sequence by conventional chromatographic and electrophoretic analyses of Hb F chains and peptides. They found that in Hb F isolated from red cells of newborns, about 75 per cent of the γ chains had glycine at position 136, and 25 per cent had alanine at this site. The former has been designated $^G\gamma$, and the latter is called $^A\gamma$ (Fig. 4–5). The proportion of $^G\gamma$ to $^A\gamma$ is constant throughout fetal development.[76, 77] In contrast, the small amount of Hb F in adult red cells contains about 40 per cent $^G\gamma$ and 60 per cent $^A\gamma$. The transition from the fetal $^G\gamma/^A\gamma$ ratio to the "adult" ratio takes place during the first 10 months of life.[78, 78a]

Initial determinations of the relative proportions of $^G\gamma$ and $^A\gamma$ chains in Hb F required isolation of an appropriate γ-chain peptide, followed by precise amino acid analysis. However, this determination has been greatly simplified by the discovery that $^G\gamma$ and $^A\gamma$ chains can be readily separated by electrophoresis in a buffer containing urea and an acidic buffer as well as a detergent such as Triton[79, 80] or by gel electrofocusing.[80a, 81] These subunits can also be cleanly separated by high-performance liquid chromatography.[82, 83] Schroeder and his colleague Titus H. J. Huisman have completed definitive studies of the γ 136 heterogeneity in a large number of populations as well as in individuals with various hemoglobin disorders. This cumulative information (reviewed concisely in reference 84 and more extensively in reference 85) has provided important insights into the expression of globin genes. The interpretation of these data was facilitated by structural analyses of the β-globin gene complex, which revealed that $^G\gamma$ and $^A\gamma$ chains are encoded by adjacent (tandem) genes on the 5′-side of the δ-chain gene (see Chapter 7). It follows that γ-chain variants will have either glycine or alanine at position 136 (see Table 10–2D). In certain disorders such as sickle cell disease and most forms of β thalassemia, both $^G\gamma$ and $^A\gamma$ genes are synthesized. However, in certain forms of δβ thalassemia and HPFH, only one of the two γ chains is predominantly synthesized. This topic is thoroughly discussed in Chapters 8 and 9.

More recently, another important γ-chain heterogeneity has been documented.[86] In the Hb F of about 30 per cent of white newborns and 20 per cent of black newborns, a minority of γ chains (about 18 per cent) have threonine rather than isoleucine at position 75.[86–89] In a much smaller number of homozygotes, this γ subunit composes about 30 per cent of the newborn Hb F. There is convincing evidence that this substitution resides exclusively on the $^A\gamma$ chain.[88, 89] Thus, this subunit has been designated $^A\gamma^T$ (Fig. 4–5). Before the high frequency of the $^A\gamma^T$ subunit was realized, it was recognized as a γ-chain variant: Hb F-Sardinia ($\alpha_2\gamma_2$ 75 Ile→Thr).[90] Thus, $^A\gamma^T$ can be viewed as an extremely common γ-chain variant (i.e., polymorphism). In individuals with β thalassemias and δβ thalassemias, the proportion of the $^A\gamma^T$ subunit in Hb F is often significantly increased.[87, 88]

Hb F-Sardinia ($\alpha_2^A\gamma^T_2$) can be separated and measured by isoelectric focusing on polyacrylamide slabs.[81] Moreover, $^A\gamma^T$ can be separated from $^A\gamma^I$ and $^G\gamma$ by means of high-performance liquid chromatography.[83] Thirty-four other γ-chain variants have been discovered to date. They are tabulated and discussed in Chapter 10. In 18 of these variants, the residue at position 136 has also been identified: 50 per

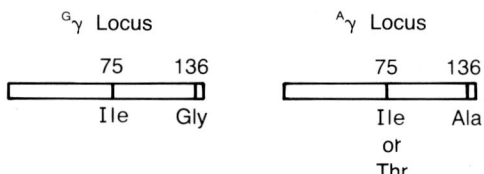

Figure 4–5. Structural heterogeneity of human γ-globin subunits.

cent are mutations of the $^G\gamma$ gene, and the remainder are mutations of the $^A\gamma$ gene. The $^G\gamma$ variants tend to compose 15 to 25 per cent of the total hemoglobin in newborn red cells, whereas the $^A\gamma$ variants compose about 5 to 15 per cent. This difference is consistent with the 3:1 ratio of $^G\gamma$ to $^A\gamma$ in the Hb F of newborns.

Three-Dimensional Structure. Crystals of deoxyhemoglobin F have been analyzed by x-ray diffraction.[91] The three-dimensional structure has been solved at a resolution of 2.5 Å. Difference Fourier electron-density maps of deoxy Hb F versus deoxy Hb A are largely featureless, except where primary sequences of the γ and β subunits differ. The only detectable difference in the tertiary structure of the γ and β subunits is at the N-terminal segments. The impaired binding of 2,3-DPG to Hb F (compared with Hb A) may be due in part to increased distance between the phosphate groups and γ 2 His. However, as explained in Chapter 2, the substitution β 143 His→γ 143 Ser is probably the more important contributor to the diminished interaction of Hb F with 2,3-DPG.

The solubility of deoxy Hb F is significantly higher than that of deoxy Hb A. This appears to be due to a weakening of one electrostatic contact between neighboring molecules in the Hb F crystal. This contact may contribute to the marked inhibition of polymerization of sickle hemoglobin by Hb F.[91] (This subject is discussed in more detail in Chaper 11.)

The increased resistance of Hb F to alkali denaturation compared with Hb A can also be explained by structural differences at the interface between subunits in the $\alpha\gamma$ versus the $\alpha\beta$ dimer. There are two residues buried within the β chain of hemoglobin A (112 Cys and 130 Tyr) that may become ionized by alkali and hydrated, favoring the formation of readily denatured hemoglobin monomers.[92] In contrast, on the γ chain, threonine is at position 112 and tryptophan is at position 130. These residues are not altered in the presence of alkali and therefore do not contribute to the denaturation of Hb F.[92]

Information on the three-dimensional structure of Hb F is relevant to consideration of its stability and assembly. As mentioned above, the resistance of Hb F to alkali denaturation appears to be based on structural features at the interface between subunits of the $\alpha\gamma$ dimer. It is likely that the intersubunit bonding is stronger in the $\alpha\gamma$ dimer than in the $\alpha\beta$ dimer. This may explain earlier recombination experiments in which incubation of mixtures of Hb F and Hb H (β_4^A) failed to produce any Hb A, whereas comparable incubations of Hb C and β_4^A did produce appreciable amounts of Hb A.[93] The dissociation of the $\alpha\gamma$ dimer into monomers is probably slower than the dissociation of the $\alpha\beta$ dimer.

Oxygen Binding. Red cells from the fetus and the newborn have higher oxygen affinity than adult red cells. In contrast, when hemolysates of newborn and adult red cells are dialyzed against buffered saline (300 mOsm/l), they have nearly identical oxygen binding.[94] These observations suggest that some type of dialyzable factor is responsible for the difference in the oxygen affinity of fetal and adult red cells.[94] The level of 2,3-DPG is at least as high in fetal and newborn red cells as it is in adult red cells. However, 2,3-DPG has a much smaller effect on the oxygen affinity of Hb F than on that of Hb A[95, 96] (Fig. 4–6). The stereochemical basis of this impaired interaction is explained above. In Hb F_I the N-terminal amino groups of the γ chains are blocked, thereby further impairing binding of 2,3-DPG. As shown in Figure 4–6, the oxygen affinity of this hemoglobin is totally unresponsive to the addition of 2,3-DPG.[17]

Hb F also has impaired interaction with other allosteric modifiers. The effect of chloride ion on the oxygen affinities of purified Hb F and Hb A is shown in Figure 4–7. At low concentrations of chloride (0.005 to 0.05 M), Hb F has significantly lower oxygen affinity than Hb A.[97] It is likely that the deoxy or T quaternary structure of stripped Hb F is more stable than that of stripped Hb A because Hb F has fewer repelling positive charges in its central cavity.[97, 98] In contrast, at physiologic concentrations of chloride, Hbs F and A have identical oxygen affinities. This result is consistent with the aforementioned observations on dialyzed hemolysates from fetal and maternal red cells. As mentioned in Chapter 3, the oxygen-linked binding of chloride ion to Hb A takes place at the "DPG binding site." Thus, it is not surprising that chloride ion has less effect on the oxygenation of Hb F than on that of Hb A.[97] A third important allosteric modifier, CO_2, also has less effect on Hb F than on Hb A.[99, 100] At any given PCO_2, Hb F forms less protein-linked carbamate than Hb A, owing to the fact that the N-terminal group of the γ chain has a pKa of 8.1, substantially higher than that of β chain of the Hb A (pKa = 6.6). Thus, at physiologic pH, about 90 per cent of the N-terminal amino groups of the γ chains are protonated and unable to bind CO_2.

Observations of both fetal red cells and

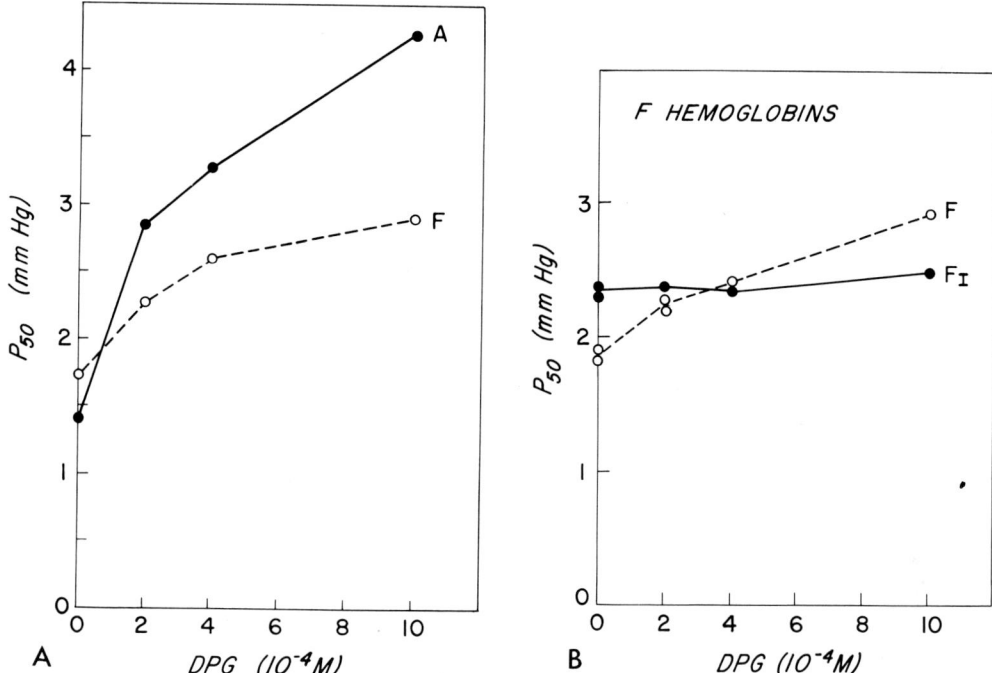

Figure 4–6. The effect of 2,3-DPG on the oxygen affinity of Hbs A and F *(A)* and the purified components, Hbs F_I and F *(B)*. Oxygen equilibria were performed in 0.05 M bis-TRIS, pH 7.2, 0.1 M Cl$^-$, 4°C. (Constructed from data of Bunn, H. F., and Briehl, R.: J. Clin. Invest. *49*:1088, 1970.)

purified Hb F have revealed an enhanced physiologic (alkaline) Bohr effect. This pertains even in the absence of 2,3-DPG and CO_2. The alkaline Bohr effect of Hb F (pH 6.5 to 8.5), like that of Hb A, is markedly dependent on chloride ion.[97] As shown in Figure 4–8, at low chloride ion concentration (0.005 M), the two hemoglobins have identical Bohr effects. However, at physiologic chloride ion concentration, the Bohr effect of Hb F is about 20 per cent higher than that of Hb A. It is likely that the lower Bohr effect in Hb A is due to β 143 His, which at low pH is protonated and binds chloride ion while in the oxy or R structure. This enhancement of the stability of the R structure by chloride and proton contributes to the acid Bohr effect of Hb A (pH 5.0 to 6.5). The absence of this interaction in Hb F would lower its acid Bohr effect and thereby increase its alkaline Bohr effect.

Figure 4–7. The effect of chloride ion on the oxygen affinity of Hbs F and A. Oxygen equilibria were performed in 0.02–0.05 M bis-TRIS, pH 7.0, 25°C. (From Poyart, C., et al.: Pfluegers Arch. *376*:169, 1978.)

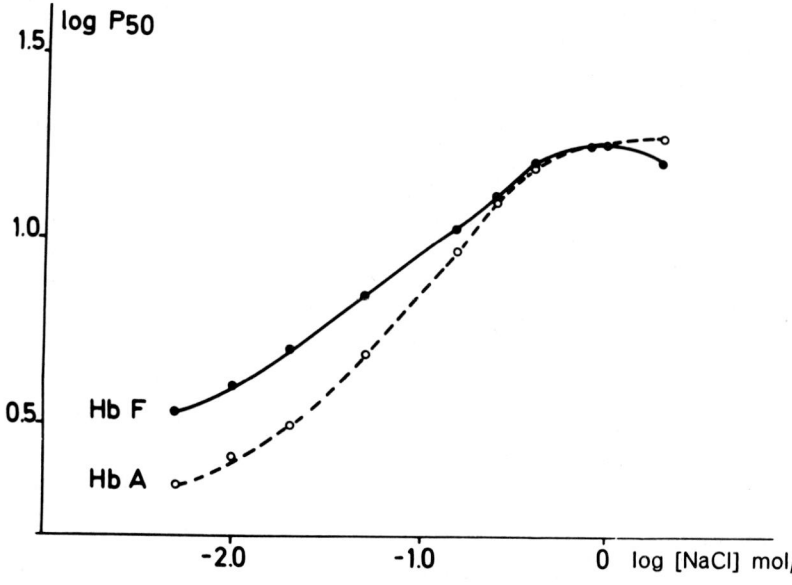

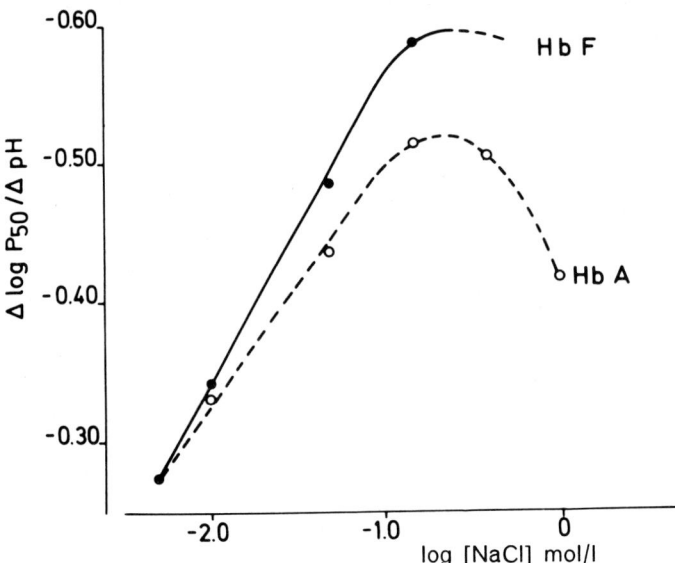

Figure 4–8. The effect of chloride ion on the Bohr effect ($\Delta \log P_{50}/\Delta$ pH) of Hbs F and A. Conditions as in Figure 4–7. (From Poyart, C., et al.: Pfluegers Arch. *376*:169, 1978.)

The enhanced alkaline Bohr effect of fetal red cells is probably of considerable physiologic importance. It operates in concert with the maternal Bohr effect to maximize oxygen transport to the fetus. Thus, the fall in pH of maternal blood as it passes through the placenta facilitates oxygen unloading. In contrast, the pH of fetal blood increases as it circulates through the placenta owing to release of CO_2. The uptake of O_2 by the fetal red cells is facilitated by their large Bohr effect. This difference in Bohr effect accounts for about 40 per cent of the total O_2 transfer between the mother and the fetus. Furthermore, the large Bohr effect of fetal red cells contributes about half of the oxygen delivery to fetal tissues.[97]

More information on physiological and pathological aspects of oxygen transport in the fetus and newborn is presented in Chapter 5.

Detection and Measurement. Hb F is unevenly distributed in red cells of normal individuals of all ages as well as in red cells of most patients with various congenital and acquired disorders. The increased resistance of Hb F to acid denaturation has been exploited for the detection of Hb F–containing cells.[101] As shown in Figure 4–9A, Hb F in newborn blood is localized in about 80 per cent of red cells. In the remaining 20 per cent, Hb A has been eluted, leaving pale, empty cells. In red cells of a patient with δβ thalassemia, Hb F is localized to about 50 per cent of red cells (Fig. 4–9C). In contrast, Hb F is more evenly distributed in an individual heterozygous for pancellular hereditary persistence of Hb F (HPFH) (Fig. 4–9B).

The detection and quantification of Hb F in individual red cells have been greatly improved by the use of monospecific anti-Hb F antibodies.[102, 103] These antibodies permit not only the identification of red cells containing Hb F (see Color Plate III*C* and *F*) but also the quantitation of the amount of Hb F per cell. The significance of "F cells" in peripheral blood as well as in erythroid cell culture is discussed in Chapter 7.

The percentage of Hb F in a hemolysate can be determined by chromatographic,[104, 105] electrophoretic, and immunologic[106, 107] methods as well as by the classic measurement by alkali denaturation[108–111] In general, an immunologic assay is recommended for samples containing less than 2 per cent Hb F; alkali denaturation is suggested for samples containing 2 to 40 per cent Hb F; and chromatography is recommended if the amount of Hb F exceeds 40 per cent.[112] For methodologic details, see the monograph of Schroeder and Huisman.[29]

The measurement of $^G\gamma$, $^A\gamma^T$, and $^A\gamma^I$ chains has been discussed in the preceding section on the structure of Hb F.

Levels of Hb F in Health and Disease. Red cells of newborns contain 80 ± 10 per cent Hb F, of which about 15 per cent is Hb F_1 ($\alpha_2[\gamma\text{-N-acetyl}]_2$). As shown in Figure 4–4, the amount of Hb F drops continuously during the first six months of life,[61] owing to a progressive decrease in the synthesis of Hb F.[113, 114] The rate of decline of Hb F is slower in babies born prematurely as well as in infants of diabetic mothers[114a] and in those with D_1 trisomy.[115, 116] In contrast, infants with Down's syndrome[117] and with C/D translocation[118] have precocious synthesis of Hb A and therefore a more rapid decline in the amount of Hb F. (See Chapter 7.)

During early childhood, there is a further decrease in Hb F.[62] As shown in Figure 4–10,

HEMOGLOBINS A_2, F, AND A_{Ic} AND OTHER HUMAN HEMOGLOBIN COMPONENTS

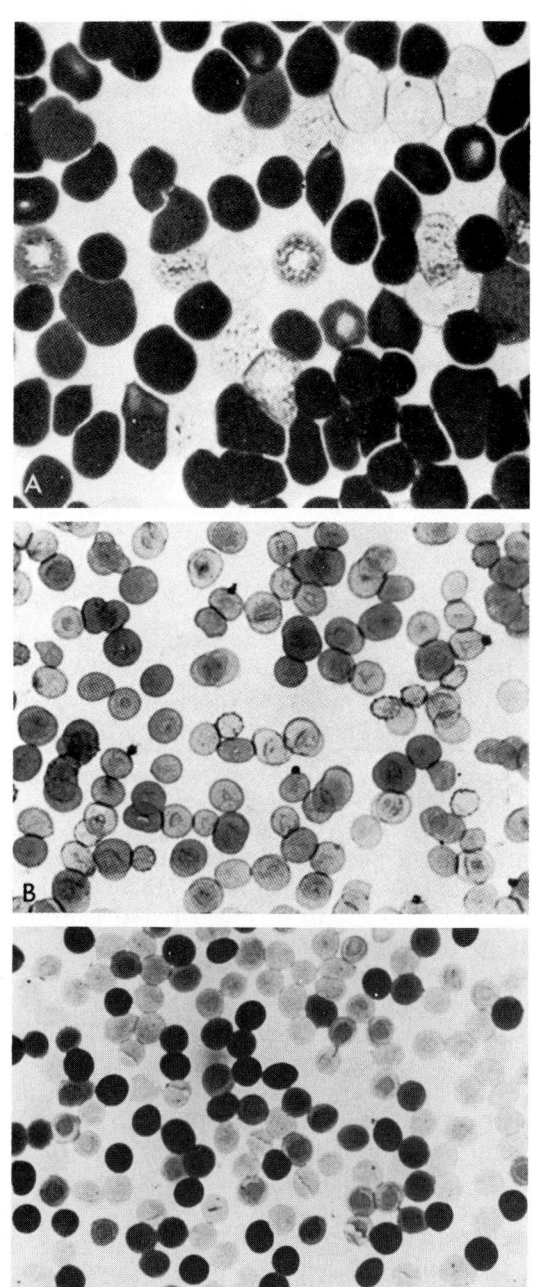

Figure 4–9. Acid elution preparations of umbilical cord blood (A), blood from a black heterozygous for hereditary persistence of Hb F (HPFH) (B), and from a black with $\delta\beta$ thalassemia (C). (From Weatherall, D. J., et al.: Clin. Haematol. 3:467, 1974.)

hemolysates[120, 121] and the proportion of "F cells"[120] in a population of normal adults is skewed toward higher values. Each F cell contains about 20 per cent Hb F. The levels of Hb F among normal adults is under genetic control.[120, 122] It is likely that individuals who are at the high end of this distribution would develop much more marked elevation of Hb F if they were subjected to erythropoietic stress (see below).

There is a modest but significant increase in the proportion of Hb F during normal midpregnancy.[123] This elevation is caused primarily by increased production of maternal F cells[124] rather than by fetal red cells that have entered the maternal circulation through small breaks in the placental barrier. A more marked increase in Hb F is encountered in women with hydatidiform moles.[125, 143] Thus, F cell production is partially responsive to chorionic gonadotrophin and perhaps other hormones related to pregnancy.

Hb F may be elevated in a variety of congenital disorders. The various forms of hereditary persistence of Hb F will be discussed in detail in Chapters 8 and 9. The levels of Hb F

about 80 per cent of children six months to two years of age have greater than 1 per cent Hb F, whereas only 4 per cent of normal adults have greater than 1 per cent Hb F.[119]

The small amount of hemoglobin F present in adult red cells is restricted to between 0.1 per cent and 7 per cent of the total red cells[103, 119] (see Color Plate IIIF). However, the distribution of both the percentage of Hb F in

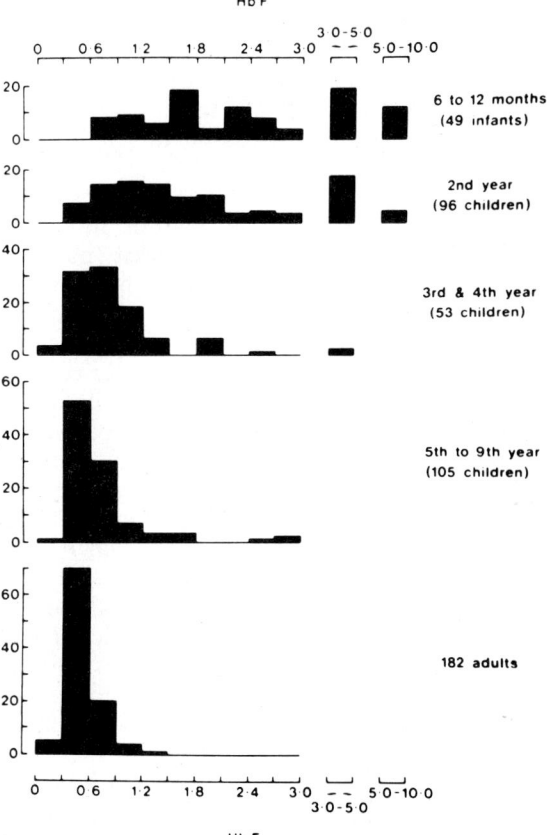

Figure 4–10. Levels of Hb F of normal individuals ranging from infants (top) to adults (bottom). (From Weatherall, D. J., et al.: Clin. Haematol. 3:467, 1974.)

Table 4–4. ACQUIRED DISORDERS ASSOCIATED WITH ELEVATED Hb F*

Condition	Approximate Frequency of ↑ Hb F	Approximate Range of % Hb F	References†
Juvenile chronic myeloid leukemia	Invariable	Up to 70%	62, 133–135
Fanconi's anemia	,,	2–85%	
Erythroleukemia	Common	Up to 60%	136
Erythroleukemia induced by chronic chemotherapy	,,	,,	137
Paroxysmal nocturnal hemoglobinuria	,,	2–20%	
Refractory anemias—pre-leukemia	,,	,,	
Aplastic anemia—following marrow engraftment	,,	,,	139
Hydatidiform mole	,,	1–10%	125, 143
Kala-azar	,,	1–8%	144
Aplastic anemia	Less common	1–10%	
Adult chronic myeloid leukemia	,,	1–12%	131
Acute leukemias	,,	1–10%	130, 131
Polycythemia vera	,,	1–10%	141
Myelofibrosis	,,	1–8%	
Choriocarcinoma	,,	1–5%	
Osteopetrosis	,,	Up to 20%	142
Testicular malignancies	,,	2–15%	130, 132
Bronchogenic carcinoma	,,	Up to 38%	
Hepatoma	,,	Up to 22%	
Thyrotoxicosis	,,	2–20%	

*Modified from Weatherall, D. J., et al.: Clin. Haematol. 3:467, 1974.
†For additional references see Weatherall, D. J., et al.: Clin. Haematol. 3:467, 1974.

in the β thalassemias is highly variable, ranging from normal (< 1 per cent) in many individuals with β-thalassemia trait to nearly 100 per cent in homozygous β^0 or δβ thalassemia. (The thalassemias will be discussed in Chapters 8 and 9.)

Individuals with most types of congenital hemolytic anemia have normal or modestly elevated levels of Hb F. In contrast, patients with sickle cell anemia generally have much higher levels of Hb F. In a large group of SS homozygotes, the mean Hb F was 5.8 per cent, with a range of 0.4 per cent to 18.8 per cent.[126] Higher amounts are encountered in homozygotes from Saudi Arabia in association with a mild form of the disease. Two factors contribute to the elevation of Hb F in sickle cell disease: First, the overall production of F cells and the amount of Hb F in individual F cells are both increased.[127] Second, there is preferential survival of Hb F–containing cells owing to the marked inhibition of Hb F on sickling.[128] The relevance of Hb F to the genetics, molecular and cellular pathogenesis, and prognosis of sickle cell disease will be discussed in Chapters 11 and 12.

Elevations of Hb F have also been noted in a variety of acquired disorders, primarily those involving impaired erythropoiesis.[62, 129] Among malignancies, leukemias and other myeloproliferative disorders often have increased Hb F[130, 131] (Table 4–4). Occasional patients with solid tumors, particularly testicular malignancies,[132, 132a] also have increased Hb F. In all of these conditions, Hb F is distributed unevenly among red cells.

The frequency with which elevations of Hb F are encountered varies widely among these disorders. A marked elevation of Hb F (up to 70 per cent) invariably accompanies juvenile chronic myelocytic leukemia.[62, 133] As a rule, other proteins in these red cells also revert to a fetal pattern.[134, 135] Patients with erythroleukemia (DiGuglielmo's disease) sometimes have marked increases in Hb F, whereas lower levels (< 10 per cent) are seen in other types of leukemia. In some of these patients, red cells may also display other fetal markers.[136, 137]

Increased levels of Hb F are found in a wide variety of other primary bone marrow disorders, as shown in Table 4–4. The broad association of increased production of F cells with disorders of erythropoiesis may reflect defects in terminal maturation.[138]

The percentage of F cells, and therefore of Hb F, often goes up considerably when the bone marrow recovers from severe depression of erythropoiesis, such as following (a) bone marrow transplantation[139] or androgen therapy for aplastic anemia, (b) chemotherapy for acute leukemia, or (c) transient erythroblastopenia of childhood.[138, 140] Less marked increases in F cell production have been observed within a week following treatment of iron deficiency anemia.[138, 140]

GLYCATED HEMOGLOBINS

Glycosylation of proteins may be enzymatic or nonenzymatic. The linkage of sugars to certain residues such as serine, asparagine, and hydroxylysine is under strict enzymatic control. Enzymatic glycosylation serves a wide variety of functions, such as facilitating secretion of a protein from its cell of origin, enhancing a protein's survival in the circulation, providing a protective coat or barrier, or forming specific receptors for hormones and other humoral substances.

In contrast, proteins can also condense nonenzymatically with sugars to form a variety of adducts. This phenomenon, sometimes called the "browning reaction," has been well known in the food industry for 50 years. It was generally assumed that nonenzymatic glycation† depended on the presence of a high concentration of the free sugar and required nonphysiological incubation conditions of temperature, pH, or state of hydration. Browning reactions tend to be heterogeneous, but the most common type involves condensation of aldehydes, ketones, and reducing sugars with amino groups on proteins,[145] peptides,[146] and amino acids.[147] The carbonyl group on sugars forms a Schiff base with the amino group, followed by an Amadori rearrangement.[148]

During the last few years, it has become increasingly apparent that nonenzymatic glycation can occur under physiological conditions. This phenomenon accounts for the formation of several minor hemoglobin components in normal red cells. Furthermore, nonenzymatic glycation takes place in other tissues and may play a role in the pathogenesis of the complications of diabetes.

†The term "glycation" is preferable to "glycosylation" for designating ketoamine-linked glucose-protein adducts.

When human hemolysate is analyzed by cation-exchange chromatography, several negatively charged minor hemoglobin components can be isolated.[71, 149] They have been designated Hbs A_{Ia}, A_{Ib}, and A_{Ic} according to their order of elution. Hb A_{Ia} actually contains two distinct hemoglobin components, called Hb A_{Ia1} and Hb A_{Ia2}.[150] Hb A_{Ic} is the most abundant minor hemoglobin component in human red cells, composing about 4 per cent of the total. Interest in Hb A_{Ic} has been stimulated by the discovery that this hemoglobin is glycated and is elevated twofold to threefold in patients with diabetes.[151-154]

Structural Studies

Hb A_{Ic} is identical to the major component Hb A except for a blocking group attached to the N terminus of the β chain by a borohydride-reducible linkage.[155] Mass spectroscopic analysis by Bookchin and Gallop[156] revealed that the blocking group was a hexose. The identity of the hexose and the nature of the protein linkage was established by Bunn and colleagues.[157] Acid hydrolysis of Hb A_{Ic} produced a 25 per cent yield of reducing sugar, consisting of glucose and mannose in a 3:1 ratio.[157] Following reduction of Hb A_{Ic} with [³H]-borohydride and oxidation with periodate, labeled formic acid was obtained, but no labeled formaldehyde. The latter product would be formed if the sugar were attached by a Schiff base. These results provide direct evidence that the sugar in Hb A_{Ic} is glucose and that the attachment is via a Schiff base that undergoes an Amadori rearrangement to the more stable ketoamine linkage:[157]*

*Both forms react readily with the reducing agent sodium borohydride to give stable products, N-1-deoxysorbitol and N-1-deoxymannitol. The use of [³H]-borohydride is an effective way of fixing a radioactive label to the sugar adduct.

$$\beta-NH_2 + \begin{array}{c} HC=O \\ | \\ HCOH \\ | \\ HOCH \\ | \\ HCOH \\ | \\ HCOH \\ | \\ CH_2OH \end{array} \underset{k_{-1}}{\overset{k_1}{\rightleftharpoons}} \begin{array}{c} HC=N-\beta A \\ | \\ HCOH \\ | \\ HOCH \\ | \\ HCOH \\ | \\ HCOH \\ | \\ CH_2OH \end{array} \xrightarrow[k_2]{Amadori} \begin{array}{c} CH_2-N^+H_2-\beta A \\ | \\ C=O \\ | \\ HOCH \\ | \\ HCOH \\ | \\ HCOH \\ | \\ CH_2OH \end{array}$$

glucose   aldimine   Ketoamine
(Schiff base)

$$Hb\ A \underset{}{\overset{rapid}{\rightleftharpoons}} pre\text{-}A_{Ic} \xrightarrow{slow} Hb\ A_{Ic}$$

Hydrolysis of the ketoamine yields both glucose and its C2 epimer, mannose.

Several lines of evidence support this structure. Following hydrolysis of Hb A_{Ic}, 5-hydroxymethylfurfural (5-HMF) can be recovered.[158] This dehydrated sugar could be formed only from a glucose adduct that had undergone the Amadori rearrangement. Furthermore, when synthetic Hb A_{Ic} was prepared with glucose tritiated at the second carbon atom, the loss of the tritium label provided a direct demonstration of the rearrangement.[158] Finally, synthetic 1-deoxysorbitol-N-valylhistidine and 1-deoxymannitol-N-valylhistidine had the same proton nuclear magnetic resonance spectra and elution pattern on gas chromatography as the borohydride-reduced β-chain N-terminal dipeptide prepared from Hb A_{Ic}.[159] These studies provide rigorous proof of the attachment of glucose to the β N terminus by a ketoamine linkage. It is likely that Hb A_{Ic} as well as other ketoamine-linked glucose adducts are primarily in a ring structure:

$$
\begin{array}{c}
CH_2-NH-\beta A \\
| \\
C=O \\
| \\
HOCH \\
| \\
HCOH \\
| \\
HCOH \\
| \\
CH_2OH
\end{array}
\quad \overset{H^+}{\rightleftharpoons} \quad
\begin{array}{c}
CH_2-N^+H_2-\beta A \\
| \\
C=O \\
| \\
HOCH \\
| \\
HCOH \\
| \\
HCOH \\
| \\
CH_2OH
\end{array}
$$

Ketoamine

$$
\begin{array}{c}
H_2C-NH-\beta A \\
| \\
COH \\
| \\
HOCH \\
| \\
HCOH \\
| \\
HC \\
| \\
CH_2OH
\end{array}
\quad \overset{H^+}{\rightleftharpoons} \quad
\begin{array}{c}
H_2C-N^+H_2-\beta A \\
| \\
COH \\
| \\
HOCH \\
| \\
HCOH \\
| \\
HC \\
| \\
CH_2OH
\end{array}
$$

β-N-valyl-
1-deoxyfructose

rather than the open ketone form.[160]

The separation of Hb A_{Ic} as a discrete chromatographic peak appears to be somewhat fortuitous, depending on a sufficient reduction in the pKa of the β N terminus at a pH that is optimal for its resolution. Furthermore, the most commonly used chromatographic resin, BioRex 70, may be particularly sensitive to hemoglobin modified at the 2,3-DPG binding site. Glucose also forms ketoamine linkages with the N-terminal amino group of the α chain as well as the ε-amino group of several lysine residues in both the α and β chains[161, 162] (Fig. 4–11). Among the 25 lysine residues in the αβ dimer, only a few are selectively modified. In order of relative abundance they are β 66, α 61, β 17, α 40, and β 8.[162] It is of considerable interest that β 66 and α 61 are residues on the carboxyl side of Lys-Lys primary sequences. Furthermore, the identical situation pertains in human serum albumin, in which the primary site of glycation is Lys 525.[163] It appears as if the pKa of the residue on the carboxyl side of Lys-Lys sequences is sufficiently decreased to make it a reactive site. In contrast to Hb A_{Ic}, hemoglobin glycation at these sites cannot be separated by ordinary chromatographic or electrophoretic means, probably because the positive charge on the ε-amino group is not significantly altered by glycation. However, all of these glycated hemoglobins can be readily isolated by means of boronate-affinity chromatography.[162, 164] The combination of ion-exchange and boronate-affinity chromatography along with structural analyses has enabled a precise determination of the distribution of ketoamine-linked glucose at the N-terminal amino groups of the α and β chain as well as the selected lysine residues listed above.[164] This information is summarized in Table 4–5. Note that in diabetic red cells, hemoglobin glycated at these sites is increased in close proportion to the increase in Hb A_{Ic}.[165]

The formation of adducts of Hb A with glucose raises the question of whether other sugars within the red cell may also interact with hemoglobin. The red cell contains a group of sugar phosphates that are involved in glycolytic metabolism, but their concentrations are at least 100-fold less than that of glucose. Nevertheless, in comparison with glucose, hexoses containing an aldehyde at C1 (or a ketone group at C2) and a negatively charged group such as phosphate (or a carboxyl) at C6 react much more rapidly with hemoglobin and with a greater degree of specificity.[166, 167] The phosphate group serves as an affinity label, interacting with positively charged groups at the 2,3-DPG binding site and permitting the aldehyde (or ketone) function to form a Schiff base with the N-terminal amino group.

Hbs A_{Ia1}, A_{Ia2}, and A_{Ib}, like Hb A_{Ic}, all have blocking groups covalently linked to the N terminus of the β chain (see Figure 4–11).

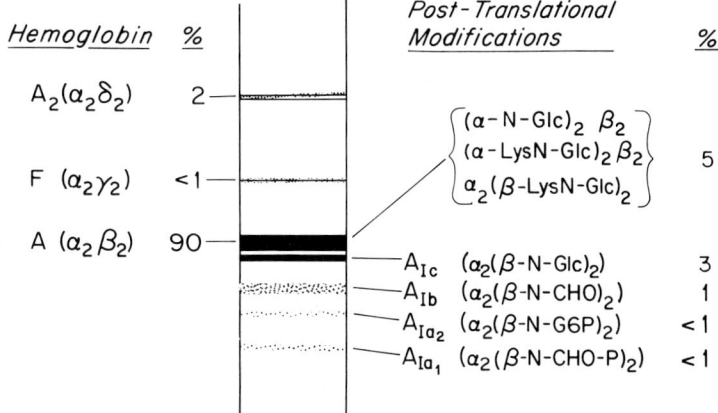

Figure 4–11. Separation of hemoglobin components in a normal hemolysate by means of gel electrofocusing. Glycated hemoglobins are shown on the right, along with the percentage of components in normal individuals.

Furthermore, the fact that Hbs A_{Ia2} and A_{Ib} incorporate tritium from [^{3}H]-borohydride at this site suggests that these adducts also involve a ketoamine or aldimine linkage. Hb A_{Ia1} contains about 2 moles of phosphate per β chain, whereas Hb A_{Ia2} has 1 mole and Hb A_{Ib} and Hb A_{Ic} have none. Hb A_{Ia2} is probably an adduct of hemoglobin with glucose-6-phosphate. The phosphate content of Hb A_{Ia1} indicates that it may be an adduct with sugar diphosphates or triphosphates, such as fructose-1,6-diphosphate, ADP, or ATP. The structure of the β-N-terminal blocking group in Hb A_{Ib} is unknown. Biosynthetic data in the monkey indicate that Hb A_{Ib} may be formed from Hb A_{Ic}.[168]

Biosynthesis

Knowledge of the structure of these minor hemoglobin components raises obvious questions about their mode of synthesis: Is the glycation of hemoglobin under enzymatic control? At what stage in red cell development does the conversion take place? When human reticulocytes and bone marrow were incubated with ^{59}Fe- or ^{14}C-labeled amino acids, significantly less radioactivity was incorporated into the glycated minor hemoglobins in comparison with the major component Hb A_o.[169] These *in vitro* studies were consistent with Hbs A_{Ia}, A_{Ib}, and A_{Ic} being post-translational modifications of Hb A_o. Much better definition of the biosynthesis of the glycated hemoglobins was achieved by *in vivo* studies. As shown in Figure 4–12, a normal human volunteer was given an intravenous injection of ^{59}Fe bound to transferrin. The specific radioactivity of major and minor hemoglobin components was determined over the next three months. As expected, the specific activity of Hb A_o reached a maximum within 10 days following the injection of the iron pulse label and fell very slowly thereafter during the life span of this cohort of labeled red cells. In contrast, the specific activity of Hbs A_{Ia}, A_{Ib}, and A_{Ic} increased in a nearly linear fashion, crossing that of Hb A_o by day 60, half the life-span of the red cell. These data indicate that glycation of hemoglobin takes place slowly and continuously throughout the 120-day life span of the red cell. In support of this conclusion are the facts that old red cells have significantly higher levels of Hb A_{Ic} than young red cells[170] and that Hb A_{Ic} is decreased in red cells of patients with hemolytic anemia.[169, 171]

Glycation of animal hemoglobins occurs in a similar way.[172] The data on mouse hemoglobin are less well defined, because labeled red cells were transferred from one animal into another and their survival was unexpectedly curtailed. Biosynthetic data in the rhesus monkey parallel the results obtained in man.[168]

Table 4–5. **GLYCOSYLATED HEMOGLOBIN IN HEMOLYSATES***

	Normals (15)	Diabetics (15)
Total glycosylated Hb[1]	7.5 ± 0.5	16.8 ± 4.5
% Glycosylated Hb A_o[2]	5.2 ± 0.5	10.5 ± 2.6
% Hb A_{Ic} (BioRex)[3]	4.4 ± 0.6	9.1 ± 2.1
% Hb A_{Ic} (corrected)[4]	2.9 ± 0.4	6.7 ± 1.7

*From Garlick, R. L., et al.: J. Clin. Invest. 71:1062, 1983. The values shown in this table are means ± 1 S.D.
[1]Percent of hemoglobin in hemolysate that adhered to boronate-affinity resin.
[2]Percent of Hb A_o (purified on BioRex 70 chromatography) that adhered to boronate-affinity resin. Hb A_o is the major hemoglobin component isolated by column chromatography.
[3]Percent of hemolysate that elutes in the Hb A_{Ic} peak on BioRex 70 chromatography.
[4]Correction of BioRex A_{Ic} peak for that portion (70 ± 4%) that adhered to boronate-affinity resin.

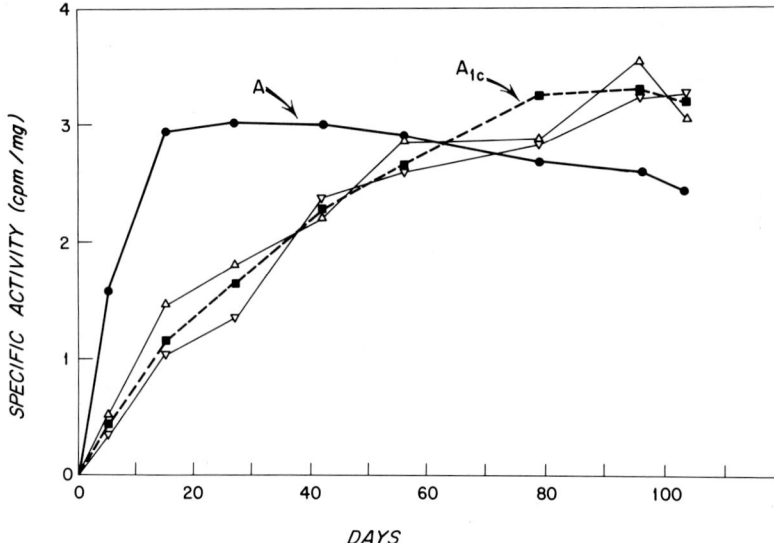

Figure 4–12. The biosynthesis of glycated hemoglobins *in vivo*. A normal human volunteer was given an intravenous injection of ^{59}Fe-transferrin on day 0. Blood samples were withdrawn over the ensuing 100 days, and the hemoglobin components were separated by chromatography on BioRex-70 cation-exchange resin. The specific radioactivities of Hbs A_{Ia} (△), A_{Ib} (▽), A_{Ic} (■), and A_o (●) are shown on the ordinate. (From Bunn, H. F., et al.: J. Clin. Invest. 57:1652, 1976.)

The slow conversion of Hb A to A_{Ic} indicates that the process is a nonenzymatic condensation of two abundant reactants within the red cell: glucose and hemoglobin. In fact, Hb A_{Ic} can be synthesized *in vitro* by incubating column-purified Hb A with glucose.[158, 161] The product has the chromatographic behavior, structure, and functional properties of authentic Hb A_{Ic}.[158, 173] The rate of formation of Hb A_{Ic} in these incubations agrees quite well with the rate calculated from the *in vivo* kinetic data.[174]

These biosynthetic results indicate that the proportion of Hb A_{Ic} in red cells is a function of the mean blood-glucose concentration and the red cell life span. It follows that measurements of Hb A_{Ic} should provide an assessment of diabetic control (see below).

Because glycation of hemoglobin is nonenzymatic, a variety of monosaccharides are potential candidates to form adducts with hemoglobin similar to Hb A_{Ic}. In general, aldoses are more reactive than ketoses such as fructose. The rate at which various aldoses condense with hemoglobin is determined primarily by the equilibrium between the open and the ring form of the sugar[175]; the former (open) structure is required for the aldimine (Schiff base) linkage. One of the main reasons the reaction is so slow is that the ring structure is heavily favored in most aldoses. The fact that galactose and mannose condense with hemoglobin even more readily than glucose[176, 177] is in keeping with their having a higher fraction of molecules in the open form.[178] Because the condensation of the aldehyde function with proteins involves nonprotonated amino groups, the rate of glycation of hemoglobin increases directly with pH over a physiological range.[158, 175]

Functional Properties

Because these minor hemoglobins are modified by specific sugars at specific sites, their functional properties are of special interest. In the absence of organic phosphates, Hb A_{Ic} has oxygen affinity very similar to that of Hb A.[179, 180] However, Hb A_{Ic} has decreased reactivity to 2,3-DPG[179, 180] (Fig. 4–13) and inositol hexaphosphate.[173] This observation provided initial evidence that the N terminus of the β chain is one of the sites involved in the binding of 2,3-DPG.[179] Hb A_{Ia1} and Hb A_{Ia2} have much lower oxygen affinities than Hb A, in keeping with the covalent linkage of sugar phosphate to the 2,3-DPG binding site.[173] Hbs A_{Ia1} and A_{Ia2} are even less responsive to the addition of organic phosphate than Hbs A_{Ib} and A_{Ic}. Kinetic parameters such as the rate of binding of carbon monoxide to deoxyhemoglobin are entirely consistent with the oxygen equilibria. Thus, the functional properties of the glycated fit well with what is known about their structure. Because of the alterations in oxygen affinity induced by the minor glycated hemoglobins, functional studies on unseparated human hemolysate may be subject to error, particularly measurements at the extremes of the oxygen binding curve.

Despite the pronounced effects of glycation on hemoglobin function, the oxygenation of intact red cells is probably not significantly affected by elevations in Hb A_{Ic} and the other minor components. Several groups[181-183] have examined the whole blood oxygen dissociation curves of a large number of diabetics and found that the mean oxygen affinity of diabetic blood was identical to that of normal blood. When compared with nondiabetic blood having comparable levels of 2,3-DPG, diabetic blood had a very slight increase of oxygen affinity (~2 mm Hg), which can probably be attributed to increased levels of Hb A_{Ic}.[182] (Fig. 4–13). It is most unlikely that this trivial alteration in intracellular hemoglobin function has any clinical significance. In diabetic patients, perturbations in acid-base balance are much more likely to affect oxygen transport because of the Bohr effect as well as secondary effects on red cell 2,3-DPG.[183]

Relevance to Diabetes

In 1968, Rahbar[153] screened a group of 1200 patients in Iran for hemoglobin abnormalities and found two with an apparently abnormal minor component. Both these patients had diabetes mellitus. Furthermore, he found this abnormality in 47 other diabetics. Subsequent studies proved that this electrophoretic abnormality was due to a twofold to threefold increase in Hb A_{Ic}.[184] These findings in diabetics were readily confirmed in several other studies. Furthermore, observations on twins indicated that this phenomenon could not be explained by genetic linkage and was more likely a reflection of the metabolic state of the diabetic patient.[185] From the structural and biosynthetic studies presented above, it is clear that Hb A_{Ic} is formed slowly and irreversibly by the condensation of two very abundant reactants within the red cell: glucose and hemoglobin. Accordingly, the percentage of Hb A_{Ic} in red cells should be an integrated measurement of mean plasma glucose concentration. Determination of Hb A_{Ic} in diabetics has proved to be a useful index of metabolic control during the preceding two to three months.[186-188] Such information is valuable to the clinician because blood glucose determinations are subject to rather marked fluctuations owing not only to the severity of the diabetes but also to other variables such as exercise, prior ingestion of food, or the administration of insulin or other hypoglycemic agents. Determination of Hb A_{Ic} may prove useful in screening large patient populations for the presence of unsuspected diabetes. The test should have a diagnostic accuracy comparable to that of fasting blood sugar determinations and superior to testing for urine glucose. Furthermore, the validity of the hemoglobin test does not require the patient's cooperation and is not dependent on the variables mentioned above. The standard oral glucose tolerance test (OGTT) appears to be a more sensitive test for detecting subclinical diabetes than measurement of Hb A_I (see reference 189 and references therein). About half of patients judged to have borderline diabetes by OGTT have normal Hb A_{Ic}. Nevertheless, Hb A_{Ic} may still provide useful

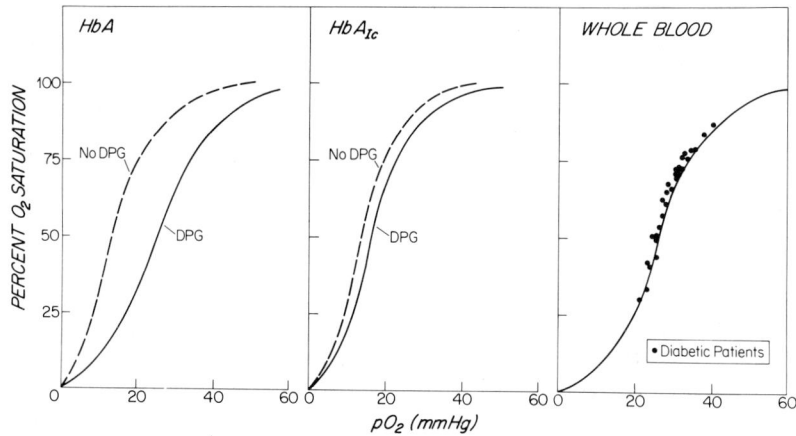

Figure 4–13. Effect of 2,3-DPG on the oxygenation of purified Hb A (left panel) and Hb A_{Ic} (middle panel) (pH 7.4, 37°C). The right panel shows oxygenation of whole blood of various diabetic patients (●) having elevated Hb A_{Ic} compared with normal blood (solid line) at standard pH (7.4), temperature (37°C), and red cell 2,3-DPG (5 mM). (The whole blood data were obtained from Arturson, G., et al.: Scand. J. Clin. Lab. Invest. *34*:19, 1974.) (From Bunn, H. F. and Cahill, G. F.: *In* Isselbacher, K. J., Adams, R. O., Braunwald, E., Petersdorf, R. G., and Wilson, J. D., (eds.): Updates: Harrison's Principles of Internal Medicine. New York, McGraw Hill, 1981, p. 33.)

independent information in screening patients for diabetes. When diabetic women become pregnant, there is a significant decrease in Hb A_I by the third trimester.[190, 191] This finding may reflect better diabetic control. Alternatively, the decrease in Hb A_{Ic} may be due to an influx of young red cells (low in glycated hemoglobin) because of the expansion in red cell mass that accompanies pregnancy. In accord with the latter explanation, a significant decrease in Hb A_{Ic} has been noted when nondiabetic women become pregnant.[192]

Measurement and Interpretation

A variety of methods are available to measure glycated hemoglobins.* This section contains a summary of the commonly used methods and their relative merits and drawbacks (Table 4–6).

Ion-Exchange Chromatography. Chromatography on BioRex 70 cation-exchange resin[154] has been the method most often employed and is therefore the standard with which other assays should be compared. Most clinical applications of this technique detect not only Hb A_{Ic} but also the other glycated hemoglobin components Hb A_{Ia1}, Hb A_{Ia2}, and Hb A_{Ib}. In addition, the rapid assays also include pre-A_{Ic}. The combination of these minor components is often called Hb A_I or "fast hemoglobin." Chromatographic methods are necessarily cumbersome and time-consuming, but these concerns are minimized by the availability of simple and inexpensive disposable columns.[193, 194] The reproducibility of these analyses depends on maintenance of reasonably uniform temperatures ($\pm$ 1°C).[195] Laboratories that have a large demand for Hb A_I measurements should consider a high-performance liquid chromatography system that can be completely automated and provides highly reliable data with a turn-around time of approximately 20 minutes.[196, 197] Interpretation of chromatographic data is thwarted by increased levels (> 0.5 per cent) of Hb F, which co-chromatographs with Hb A_{Ic}, and by hemoglobin variants such as Hbs S, C, D, G, and so on.[198, 199] In addition, falsely high values for Hb A_I are obtained in patients with uremia,[200, 201] possibly in alcoholics,[202, 203, 203a] and in patients with lead poisoning.[204] Lactescent plasma will also cause falsely high values if whole blood is analyzed by a rapid chromatographic assay.[205]

---

*This topic has been thoroughly reviewed by Goldstein and associates.[192a]

Affinity Chromatography. Boronic acid forms a weak covalent linkage with vicinal hydroxyl groups of sugars:

$$\begin{array}{c} | \\ C-O \\ | \\ C-O \\ | \end{array} \diagdown B \diagup \begin{array}{c} OH \\ OH \end{array}$$

Accordingly, resins linked to phenylboronic acid have proved to be useful in separating glycosylated from nonglycosylated proteins.[161, 164, 206, 207] An analysis of a diabetic hemolysate on boronate-affinity resin is shown in Figure 4–14. Nonglycated hemoglobin fails to adhere to the resin and is eluted in the void volume. The adherent glycated hemoglobin can then be eluted by the application of a competing sugar, sorbitol. This component contains not only Hb A_{Ic}, but also the adducts of glucose to other sites on hemoglobin (glycated Hb A_o). This measurement of total glycated hemoglobins is as reliable as the measurement of the single component Hb A_{Ic}. Table 4–5 shows a comparison between total glycated hemoglobin, Hb A_{Ic} and glycated Hb A_o in normals and diabetics. Note that the actual level of Hb A_{Ic} is lower than previous estimates. Hb A_{Ic} composes about 40 per cent of the total glycated hemoglobin in both normal and diabetic specimens.

This method offers many advantages over others currently in use. It is precise, simple to perform, and, unlike all but the colorimetric TBA test, is specific for glycated hemoglobin.

Electrophoretic Techniques. Two electrophoretic methods have been adapted for measuring Hb A_{Ic}. Isoelectric focusing on thin (1-mm) slabs (but not cylinders) of polyacrylamide gel provides a clean separation of Hb A_{Ic} from Hb A_o,[177, 208] but the method requires a moderate level of technical skill and a high-quality densitometer for quantitation. Electrophoresis on agar gel at pH 6.5[209, 210] provides a much wider separation than that obtained by gel electrofocusing, and quantitation is easier.

Colorimetric Methods. Fluckiger and Winterhalter[180] have devised a colorimetric test that takes advantage of the fact that when A_{Ic} is subjected to mild acid hydrolysis, 5-hydroxymethylfurfural (5-HMF) is released and can combine with thiobarbituric acid (TBA) to form a colored product. This method has been adapted for routine use[211–213] and generally gives reliable results. The TBA test has several advantages over chromatographic and electrophoretic methods. Because it is specific for ketoamine-linked glucose, it is unaffected by

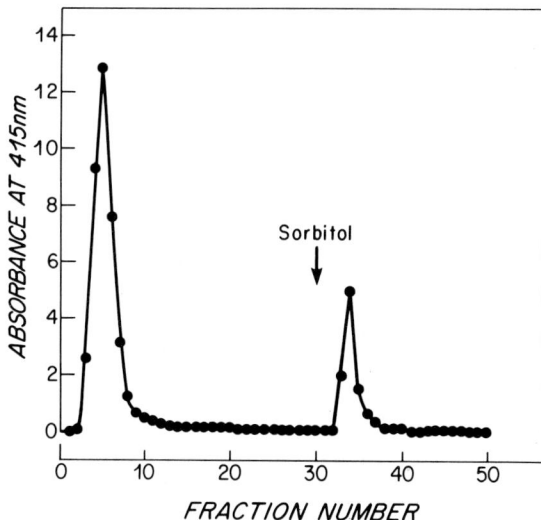

Figure 4–14. Separation of glycated hemoglobins of a diabetic hemolysate by chromatography on a phenylboronate affinity resin. The nonglycated hemoglobin eluted in the void volume (left-hand peak). The glycated hemoglobins adhered to the resin and were discharged by the addition of a competing sugar, sorbitol (right-hand peak). (From Garlick, R. L., et al.: J. Clin. Invest. 71:1062, 1983.)

the presence of Hb F, hemoglobin variants, and other post-translational modifications of hemoglobin. The test requires only a simple colorimeter and inexpensive stable reagents. However, the TBA test is difficult to standardize because the yield of 5-HMF from Hb A_{Ic} is only about 30 per cent and is considerably less for glycated Hb A_o.[162, 164] Falsely high values may result because of the de novo formation of 5-HMF as a result of condensation of free glucose (in high concentration) with hemoglobin.[214] Furthermore, the precision of the TBA test is limited by a variable degree of background color absorbance from nonglycated hemoglobin.

Other colorimetric tests have been devised for measurement of glycated hemoglobin. One involves the fluorometric detection of formaldehyde that is released following oxidation of glycated hemoglobin by periodate.[215] This is a well-designed assay that is currently undergoing evaluation in a number of laboratories. Another less sensitive colorimetric test involves the detection of hydrolyzed sugars by means of the well-known phenol sulfuric acid test.[216]

Immunologic Assays. Radioimmune[217] and nephelometric[218] assays have been developed utilizing antisera raised against Hb A_{Ic}. The precision and reliability of these assays are limited by the fact that the antibodies show cross-reactivity to Hb A. Thus far, there has been little utilization of immunologic methods for clinical studies.

Interpretation. The results of measurements of glycated hemoglobin must be considered in terms of factors listed in Table 4–6 that give falsely high results. In addition, the inclusion of the Schiff base (aldimine) precursor (pre-A_{Ic}) also detracts from the reliability and utility of the test because this adduct fluctuates rapidly in proportion to blood glucose levels. This precursor component normally composes 10 per cent of the total Hb A_{Ic} but can be substantially higher if recent blood glucose levels have increased over the average for the preceding two to three months. Pre-A_{Ic} can be abolished by thorough dialysis of the sample[219]

Table 4–6. COMPARISON OF COMMONLY USED METHODS TO MEASURE GLYCATED HEMOGLOBIN

Method	Precision	False Increase Due to	False Decrease Due to
Ion-exchange chromatography		Pre-A_{Ic}, A_{Ia1}, A_{Ia2}, A_{Ib} Hb F, Hb G, and other negatively charged hemoglobins	
Disposable columns	Good	Uremia; ? alcoholism; ? high-dose aspirin; ? lead poisoning	Hb S, Hb C, Hb E, and other positively charged variants
HPLC	Excellent	Lactescent plasma Storage of hemolysate	
Boronate-affinity chromatography	Good	None	None
Electrophoresis			
Gel electrofocusing	Good	Pre-A_{Ic}	
Agar gel electrophoresis	Good	Pre-A_{Ic}	
Colorimetry (TBA test)	Good	Baseline color absorbance De novo formation of 5-HMF in sample containing high level of glucose	

or by incubating the washed red cells in saline solution prior to preparing the hemolysate.[220]

Significance of Nonenzymatic Glycation

Several centers are now conducting prospective studies that will relate the level of glycated hemoglobin with other clinical parameters in an attempt to ascertain whether the degree of control of hyperglycemia is related to the development of complications. The establishment of a correlation does not imply causality. For example, a number of investigators have examined the association between glycated hemoglobin and various clinical manifestations such as retinopathy, nerve conduction velocity, weight of babies born to diabetic mothers, coagulation parameters, and serum lipid profiles. Positive correlations do not mean that hyperglycemia was directly responsible for the observed clinical abnormality. Some studies are attempting to determine whether the observed abnormality is reversible following the establishment of tight control.

Perhaps the most important issue concerning nonenzymatic glycation of proteins is whether this phenomenon contributes to the long-term complications of diabetes. Those tissues that bear the brunt of diabetic complications do not require insulin for entry of glucose into cells.[221] Thus, basement membrane proteins, lens crystallin, and nerve myelin protein are exposed to high levels of glucose in diabetics. All of these proteins normally undergo nonenzymatic glycation, and they do so to an increased extent when diabetes is present. It is not yet clear whether nonenzymatic glycation affects the function of these proteins.

OTHER POST-TRANSLATIONAL MODIFICATIONS

Although glucose adducts are by far the most common and abundant type of post-translation modification of hemoglobin, other small molecules are also capable of forming covalent linkages with hemoglobin and may reflect significant metabolic perturbations.

Carbamylated Hemoglobin

Urea is normally present in the plasma in a concentration of about 2.5 mM. However, patients with renal failure may have plasma levels as high as 40 mM. Urea is in equilibrium with ammonium and cyanate ions:

$$H_2N\overset{O}{\overset{\|}{C}}NH_2 \rightleftharpoons NH_4^+ + CNO^-$$

Cyanate can combine with amino groups on proteins to form irreversible covalent adducts:

$$HbNH_2 + CNO^- + H^+ \longrightarrow HbNH\overset{O}{\overset{\|}{C}}NH_2$$

When hemoglobin is incubated with cyanate *in vitro*, the primary sites of modification are the N-terminal amino groups of the α and β chains.[222] Because carbamylation of hemoglobin S greatly reduces its tendency to polymerize, cyanate has been used in the treatment of sickle cell disease[223] (see Chapters 11 and 12).

The presumed presence of increased levels of cyanate in the plasma of uremic patients raises the possibility that their hemoglobin becomes carbamylated *in vivo*. Increased amounts of "Hb A_I" have been observed in uremics, despite normal levels of glycated hemoglobin.[201, 224] Amino acid analyses demonstrated that this additional negatively charged hemoglobin was carbamylated at the N-terminal amino group of the α and β chains. Patients on hemodialysis had about 1 to 2 per cent carbamylated hemoglobin, whereas those who had not received dialysis had levels as high as 4 per cent. This minor degree of modification would have no significant effect on hemoglobin function. However, other proteins may become carbamylated in uremia and perhaps contribute to the clinical manifestations of the uremic syndrome.

Acetaldehyde-Hemoglobin Adducts

When ethanol is metabolized *in vivo* it is oxidized to acetaldehyde. This highly reactive compound forms Schiff base linkages with amino groups on proteins:

$$RNH_2 + CH_3\overset{O}{\overset{\|}{C}}H \rightleftharpoons RN=CCH_3$$

When hemoglobin is incubated with acetaldehyde, negatively charged minor components that have the chromatographic behavior of Hbs $A_{Ia} + A_{Ib}$ are formed.[202, 225] Alcoholics have increased levels of negatively charged hemoglobin that does not appear to be glycated.[202, 203, 203a] It is uncertain whether this hemoglobin component is composed of acetaldehyde adducts. A thorough structural analysis of these minor components has not yet been performed. Because acetaldehyde-protein adducts are readily reversible, it is unlikely that this modification causes any long-term impairment of protein function.

Acetylated Hemoglobin

A wide variety of proteins are acetylated at the NH_2 terminus.[226, 227] The acetylation event is catalyzed by an acetyltransferase enzyme using acetyl-CoA as substrate[228] and occurs early in the life of a protein molecule, perhaps during growth of the nascent polypeptide chain.[229, 230] The NH_2-terminal acetylation of proteins appears to depend in part on primary structure. Proteins having alanine or serine at the NH_2 terminus are readily acetylated, whereas those having glycine at the NH_2 terminus are acetylated somewhat less readily. Proteins having other residues at the NH_2 terminus generally escape acetylation.

Hemoglobins are acetylated much less readily than most other proteins. Among mammalian hemoglobins, only three are known to be acetylated: human and primate hemoglobin F_I,[231, 232] hemoglobin Raleigh,[233] and cat hemoglobin.[234] In each case, the NH_2-terminal residue is one that favors acetylation. The hemoglobin variant Hb Raleigh involves the replacement β 1 Val $\rightarrow$ Ala. The NH_2-terminal residue of the β chain of cat hemoglobin B is serine. Acetylation of these hemoglobins appears to be complete; the NH_2-terminus of the β chain is totally blocked. In contrast, only about 10 to 15 per cent of the NH_2-terminal glycine of γ chains of human Hb F are acetylated. Thus, the extent of acetylation of these hemoglobins is consistent with their NH_2-terminal residues. It is likely that during molecular evolution, hemoglobins have been selected that have N-terminal sequences resistant to acetylation because these regions of the molecule are important sites for anion binding (see Chapters 2, 3, and 6).

Hb F_I. As shown in Figure 4-1, hemolysates from newborns contain a negatively charged component, designated Hb F_I, that composes about 10 per cent of the total hemoglobin. Structural analyses show that the majority of this component is identical to Hb F except that the N-terminal amino groups of the γ chains are acetylated.[231, 235] In addition, a small amount of glycated Hb F has the same chromatographic and electrophoretic behavior.[236, 237] Despite this ambiguity, we will reserve the term Hb F_I for the acetylated species. Hb F_I is encountered in all stages of fetal development[238] as well as in patients with various disorders associated with elevated levels of Hb F.[239] In all cases, the ratio of Hb F_I to Hb F is about 1:6 to 1:10. The acetylation of $^G\gamma$ and $^A\gamma$ chains is comparable.[75, 240]

It is likely that the synthesis of Hb F_I, like that of other acetylated proteins, depends on enzymatic transfer from acetyl-coenzyme A. Cord blood hemolysate can support the acetylation of Hb F *in vitro*.[228] The modification can also take place nonenzymatically but at a much slower rate.[241] For most proteins, including cat Hb B,[242] N-terminal acetylation takes place on the nascent polypeptide during translation. The acetylation of human γ chains seems to be less efficient because only a minority of subunits are modified. It is likely that only the nascent chain or the completed free subunit are substrates for acetylation. A markedly enhanced rate of formation of Hb F_I occurs in reticulocytes,[239, 240] probably owing to increased availability of free γ subunits in these cells, with sluggish protein synthesis and a declining pool of free α chains.

When hemoglobin or red cells are incubated with acetylsalicylic acid (aspirin), a significant amount of acetylated hemoglobin is formed.[243, 244] However, unlike Hb F_I, the acetyl groups are located at several lysine residues on the α and β chains.[244, 245] Patients who are receiving high doses of aspirin appear to have a slight increase in negatively charged hemoglobin,[244, 246] but this finding needs to be documented with structural analyses.

Hemoglobin as a Reporter Molecule

It is likely that under various circumstances other reactive compounds in the plasma can modify hemoglobin. For example, vitamins, drugs, or toxins may form adducts with hemoglobin. One component of the most negatively charged hemoglobins in normal hemolysate (Hb A_{Ia}) may be an adduct with pyridoxal phosphate.[247] Penicillin can form covalent linkages with hemoglobin.[248] Individuals addicted to high doses of opiates may also have negatively charged minor hemoglobin components.[249] Some patients with lead poisoning have a negatively charged hemoglobin component[204] that may arise because some of the heme groups have been substituted by zinc protoporphyrin.[250]

In conclusion, the latter half of this chapter has been concerned with structural modifications of hemoglobin due to the presence of variable amounts of reactive compounds that are capable of forming covalent adducts. These modified hemoglobins can be viewed as reporter molecules because they provide clues not only to the diagnosis of such diverse diseases as diabetes, uremia, and alcoholism but also to the extent of the metabolic derangement. More importantly, these well-defined chemical modifications on the hemoglobin molecule may serve as prototypes of similar modifications on other proteins that contribute to the pathogenesis of disease.

References

1. Kunkel, H. G., and Wallenius, G.: New hemoglobins in normal adult blood. Science *122*:288, 1955.
2. Kunkel, H. G., Ceppellini, R., Muller-Eberhard, U., and Wolf, J.: Observations on the minor basic hemoglobin components in the blood of normal individuals and patients with thalassemia. J. Clin. Invest. *36*:1615, 1957.
3. Ingram, V. M., and Stretton, A. O. W.: Human hemoglobin A_2: Chemistry, genetics and evolution. Nature *190*:1079, 1961.
4. Lehmann, H., and Casey, R.: Residues 124 and 125 (H2 and H3) of the human haemoglobin δ-chain. Acta Haematol. *56*:84, 1976.
5. Braunitzer, G., Schrank, B., Stangl, A., and Grillemeier, M.: Notiz zur Sequenz der δ-Ketten der menschlichen Hamoglobine (Hb A_2 = $\alpha_2\delta_2$). Hoppe-Seyler's Z. Physiol. Chem. *359*:777, 1978.
6. Spritz, R. A., DeRiel, J. K., Forget, B. G., and Weissman, S. M.: Complete nucleotide sequence of human δ gene. Cell *22*:639, 1980.
7. Boyer, S. H., Crosby, E. F., Thurmon, T. F., Noyes, A. N., Fuller, G. F., Leslie, S. E., and Shepard, M. K.: Hemoglobins A and A_2 in New World primates: Comparative variation and its evolutionary implications. Science *166*:1428, 1969.
8. Benz, E. J., Jr., Scarpa, A. L., Tonkonow, B. L., Pierson, H. A., and Ritchey, A. K.: Posttranscriptional defects in β-globin messenger RNA metabolism in β-thalassemia. J. Clin. Invest. *68*:1529, 1981.
9. Kantor, J. A., Turner, P. H., and Nienhuis, A. W.: Beta thalassemia: Mutations which affect processing of the β-globin mRNA precursor. Cell *21*:149, 1980.
10. Humphries, R. K., Ley, T., Turner, P., Moulton, A. D., and Nienhuis, A. W.: Differences in human α-, β-, and δ-globin gene expression in monkey kidney cells. Cell *30*:173, 1982.
11. Rieder, R. F., and Weatherall, D. J.: Studies on hemoglobin biosynthesis: Asynchronous synthesis of hemoglobin A and hemoglobin A_2 by erythrocyte precursors. J. Clin. Invest. *44*:42, 1965.
12. Roberts, A. V., Weatherall, D. J., and Clegg, J. B.: The synthesis of human hemoglobin A_2 during erythroid maturation. Biochem. Biophys. Res. Commun. *47*:81, 1972.
13. Wood, W. G., Old, J. M., Roberts, A. V. S., Clegg, J. B., Weatherall, D. J., and Quattrin, N.: Human globin gene expression: Control of β, δ and γ chain production. Cell *15*:437, 1978.
14. Matioli, G. T., and Niewisch, H. B.: Electrophoresis of hemoglobin in single erythrocytes. Science *150*:1824, 1965.
15. Heller, P., and Yakulis, V.: The distribution of hemoglobin A_2. Ann. N.Y. Acad. Sci. *165*:54, 1969.
16. Eddison, G. G., Briehl, R. W., and Ranney, H. M.: Oxygen equilibria of hemoglobin A_2 and hemoglobin Lepore. J. Clin. Invest. *43*:2323, 1964.
17. Bunn, H. F., and Briehl, R. W.: The interaction of 2,3-diphosphoglycerate with various human hemoglobins. J. Clin. Invest. *49*:1088, 1970.
18. deBruin, S. H., and Janssen, L. H. M.: Comparison of the oxygen and proton binding behavior of human hemoglobin A and A_2. Biochim. Biophys. Acta *295*:490, 1973.
19. Adachi, K., Asakura, T., Gill, F. M., and Schwartz, E.: Comparative studies of Hb Lepore Boston, Hb A_2, and Hb A. J. Biol. Chem. *253*:382, 1978.
20. Kinderlerer, J., Lehmann, H., and Tipton, K. F.: Thermal denaturation of human hemoglobin. Biochem. J. *119*:66P, 1970.
21. Perutz, M. F., and Raidt, H.: Stereochemical basis of heat stability in bacterial ferredoxins and in haemoglobin A_2. Nature *255*:256, 1975.
22. Day, T. H.: Is hemoglobin A_2 important? Biochem. Genet. *8*:403, 1973.
23. Vella, F.: Variation in hemoglobin A_2. Hemoglobin *1*:619, 1977.
24. Salkie, M. L., Gordon, P. A., Rigal, W. M., Lam, H., Wilson, J. B., Headlee, M. E., and Huisman, T. H. J.: Hb A_2-Canada or $\alpha_2\delta_2$ 99 (G1) Asp → Asn, a newly discovered delta chain variant with increased oxygen affinity occurring *in cis* to β-thalassemia. Hemoglobin *6*:223, 1982.
25. Gottfried, E. L., Wall, B., and Robertson, N. A.: Reliable estimation of hemoglobin A_2 concentration by electrophoresis with densitometry. Am. J. Clin. Pathol. *72*:415, 1979.
26. Huisman, T. H. J., Schroeder, W. A., Brodie, A. N., Mayson, S. M., and Jakway, J.: Microchromatography of hemoglobins. III. A simplified procedure for the determination of hemoglobin A_2. J. Lab. Clin. Med. *86*:700, 1975.
27. Moors, A., Melis-Liekens, J., DeVlieger-Bensel, M., DeGroof-Cornelis, E., and VanRos, G.: Evaluation of a simplified microchromatographic technique for hemoglobin A_2 determination. Acta Haematol. *61*:15, 1979.
28. Chudwin, D. S., and Rucknagel, D. L.: Immunologic quantification of hemoglobin F and A_2. Clin. Chim. Acta *50*:413, 1974.
29. Schroeder, W. A., and Huisman, T. H. J.: The Chromatography of Hemoglobin. New York, Marcel Dekker, Inc., 1980.
30. Weatherall, D. J., and Clegg, J. B.: The Thalassemia Syndromes. 3rd ed. Oxford, Blackwell Scientific Publications, 1981.
31. Schroeder, W. A., Huisman, T. H. J., Hyman, C., Shelton, J. R., and Apell, G.: An individual with "Miyada"-like hemoglobin indistinguishable from hemoglobin A_2. Biochem. Genet. *10*:135, 1975.
32. Steinberg, M. H., Coleman, M. B., and Adams, J. G., III: Beta-thalassemia with exceptionally high hemoglobin A_2. J. Lab. Clin. Med. *100*:548, 1982.
33. Huisman, T. H. J., Punt, K., and Schaad, J. D. G.: Thalassemia minor associated with hemoglobin B_2 heterozygosity, a family report. Blood *17*:747, 1961.
34. Whitten, W. J., and Rucknagel, D. L.: The proportion of Hb A_2 is higher in sickle cell trait than in normal homozygotes. Hemoglobin *5*:371, 1981.
34a. Francina, A., Dorléac, E., Baudonnet, C., Jaccoud, P., and Delaunay, J.: Microchromatofocusing of hemoglobins. Increased hemoglobin A_2 percentage in sickle cell trait. Clin. Chim. Acta *121*:261, 1982.
35. Higgs, D. R., Aldridge, B. E., Lamb, J., Clegg, J. B., Weatherall, D. J., Hayes, R. J., Grandison,

Y., Lowrie, Y., Mason, K. P., Serjeant, B. E., and Serjeant, G. R.: The interaction of alpha-thalassemia and homozygous sickle-cell disease. N. Engl. J. Med. 306:1441, 1982.
36. Ley, T. J., Anagnou, N. P., Pepe, G., and Nienhuis, A. W.: RNA processing errors in patients with β-thalassemia. Proc. Natl. Acad. Sci. USA 79:4775, 1982.
37. Matuonto, V., Cappellini, M. D., and Fiorelli, G.: Comparison between electrophoresis and DEAE-microchromatography for the quantitation of haemoglobin A_2. J. Chromatogr. 92:174, 1974.
38. McCormack, M. K.: Quantitation of hemoglobin A_2 in alpha thalassemia trait by microcolumn chromatography. Clin. Chim. Acta 105:387, 1980.
39. Wasi, P., Na-Nakorn, S., Pootrakul, S., Sookanek, M., Disthasongchan, P., Pornpatkul, M., and Panick, V.: Alpha- and beta-thalassemia in Thailand. Ann. N.Y. Acad. Sci. 165:60, 1969.
40. Alperin, J. B., Dow, P. A., and Petteway, M. B.: Hemoglobin A_2 levels in health and various hematologic disorders. Am. J. Clin. Pathol. 67:219, 1977.
41. Kuczynski, A.: The relationship between the serum iron concentration and erythrocytic haemoglobin A_2 level. J. Med. 2:136, 1971.
42. Kurlekar, N., and Mehta, B. C.: Hemoglobin A_2 levels in iron-deficiency anemia. Isr. J. Med. Res. 73:77, 1981.
43. Bannerman, R. M., and Lehmann, H.: Hemoglobin A_2—What is it for? J. Med. 1:129, 1970.
44. Reed, L. J., and Mollin, D. W.: Synthesis of hemoglobin A_2 in sideroblastic and megaloblastic anemias. In Abstracts of the XIIth Congress of the International Society of Hematology. New York, The International Society of Hematology, 1968, p. 63.
45. White, J. M., Brain, M. D., and Ali, M.: Globin synthesis in sideroblastic anaemia, I. Alpha and beta peptide chain synthesis. Br. J. Haematol. 20:263, 1971.
46. Aksoy, M., and Erdem, S.: Decrease in the concentration of Hb A_2 during erythroleukemia. Nature 213:522, 1967.
47. Josephson, A. M., Masri, M. S., Singer, L., Dworkin, D., and Singer, K.: Starch block electrophoretic studies of human hemoglobin solutions. II. Results in cord blood, thalassemia and other hematologic disorders: Comparison with Tiselius electrophoresis. Blood 13:543, 1958.
48. Henshaw, L. A., Tizzard, J. L., Booth, K., and Beard, M. E. J.: Haemoglobin A_2 levels in vitamin B_{12} and folate deficiency. J. Clin. Pathol. 31:960, 1978.
48a. Mehta, B. C., and Agarwal, M. B.: Hemoglobin A_2 in nutritional megaloblastic anemia. Indian J. Med. Res. 77:478, 1983.
49. Kendall, A. G., and Bastomsky, C. H.: Hemoglobin A_2 in hyperthyroidism. Hemoglobin 5:571, 1981.
50. Krishnamoorthy, R., Elion, J., Kuhn, J. M., Lagrange, J. L., Rochette, J., Luton, J. P., Bricaire, H., and Labie, D.: Haemoglobin A_2 is elevated in hyperthyroid patients. Nouv. Rev. Fr. Hematol. 24:39, 1982.
50a. Kuhn, J.-M., Rieu, M., Rochette, J., Krishnamoorthy, R., Labie, D., Elion, J., Luton, J.-P., and Bricaire, H.: Influence of thyroid status on hemoglobin A_2 expression. J. Clin. Endocrinol. Metab. 57:344, 1983.
51. Arends, T.: High concentrations of hemoglobin A_2 in malaria patients. Nature 215:1517, 1967.
52. LieInjo, L. E., Lopex, C. G., and Lopex, M.: Hemoglobin A_2 in malaria patients. Trans. R. Soc. Trop. Med. Hyg. 65:480, 1971.
53. VanRos, G., Moors, A., DeVlieger, M., and DeGroof, E.: Hemoglobin A_2 levels in malaria patients. Am. J. Trop. Med. Hyg. 27:659, 1978.
54. Huehns, E. R., Flynn, F. V., Butler, E. A., and Beaven, G. H.: Two new haemoglobin variants in the very young human embryo. Nature 189:496, 1961.
55. Kaltsoya, A., Fessas, P., and Stavropoulos, A.: Hemoglobins of early human embryonic development. Science 153:1417, 1966.
56. Capp, G. L., Rigas, D. A., and Jones, R. T.: Hemoglobin Portland 1: A new human hemoglobin unique in structure. Science 157:65, 1967.
57. Capp, G. L., Rigas, D. A., and Jones, R. T.: Evidence for a new haemoglobin chain (ζ-chain). Nature 228:278, 1970.
58. Kamuzora, H., Jones, R. T., and Lehmann, H.: The ζ-chain, an α-like chain of human embryonic haemoglobin. FEBS Lett. 46:195, 1974.
59. Huehns, E. R., and Farooqui, A. M.: Oxygen dissociation properties of human embryonic red cells. Nature 254:335, 1975.
60. Tuchinda, S., Nagai, K., and Lehmann, H.: Oxygen dissociation curve of haemoglobin Portland. FEBS Lett. 49:390, 1975.
61. Huehns, E. R., and Beaven, G. H.: Developmental changes in human hemoglobins. Clin. Dev. Med. 37:175, 1971.
62. Weatherall, D. J., Pembrey, M. E., and Pritchard, J.: Fetal haemoglobin. Clin. Hematol. 3:467, 1974.
63. Wood, W. G., Whittaker, J. H., Clegg, J. B., and Weatherall, D. J.: Haemoglobin synthesis in human bone marrow culture. Biochim. Biophys. Acta 277:413, 1972.
64. Todd, D., Lai, M. C. S., Beaven, G. H., and Huehns, E. R.: The abnormal haemoglobins in homozygous alpha-thalassemia. Br. J. Haematol. 19:27, 1970.
65. Rutherford, T. R., Clegg, J. B., and Weatherall, D. J.: K562 human leukaemic cells synthesize embryonic haemoglobin in response to haemin. Nature 280:164, 1979.
66. Kazazian, H. H., and Woodhead, A. P.: Hemoglobin A synthesis in the developing fetus. N. Engl. J. Med. 289:58, 1973.
67. Wood, W. G., and Weatherall, D. J.: Haemoglobin synthesis during human foetal development. Nature 244:162, 1973.
68. Körber, E.: Inaugural dissertation: "Über differenzen Blutfarbstoffes." Dorpat, 1866. Cited by Bischoff, H.: Z. Exp. Med. 48:472, 1926.
69. Jope, E. M.: The ultra-violet spectral absorption of haemoglobin inside and outside the red blood cell. In Roughton, F. J. W., and Kendrew, J. C. (eds.): Haemoglobin. London, Butterworth, 1949, p. 205.
70. Porter, R. R., and Sanger, F.: The free amino groups of hemoglobins. Biochem. J. 42:287, 1948.
71. Allen, D. W., Schroeder, W. A., and Balog, J.: Observations on the chromatographic heterogeneity of normal adult and fetal human hemoglobin. J. Am. Chem. Soc. 80:1628, 1958.
72. Huisman, T. H. J., and Prins, H. K.: Chromatographic estimation of four different human hemoglobins. J. Lab. Clin. Med. 46:255, 1955.
73. Rhinesmith, H. S., Schroeder, W. A., and Pauling, L.: A quantitative study of the hydrolysis of human dinitrophenyl (DNP) globin: The number and kind of polypeptide chains in normal adult human hemoglobin. J. Am. Chem. Soc. 79:4682, 1957.
74. Schroeder, W. A., Shelton, J. R., Shelton, J. B.,

Cormack, J., and Jones, R. T.: The amino acid sequence of the γ-chain of human fetal hemoglobin. Biochemistry 2:992, 1963.
75. Schroeder, W. A., Huisman, T. H. J., Shelton, J. R., Shelton, J. B., Kleinhauer, E. F., Dozy, A. M., and Robberson, B.: Evidence for multiple structural genes for γ chain of human fetal hemoglobin. Proc. Natl. Acad. Sci. USA 60:537, 1968.
76. Nute, P. E., Pataryas, H. A., and Stamatoyannopoulos, G.: The $^G\gamma$ and $^A\gamma$ hemoglobin chains during human fetal development. Am. J. Hum. Genet. 25:271, 1973.
77. Alter, B. P.: The $^G\gamma{:}^A\gamma$ composition of fetal hemoglobin in fetuses and newborns. Blood 54:1158, 1979.
78. Schroeder, W. A., Huisman, T. H. J., Brown, A. K., Uy, R., Bouver, N. G., Lerch, P. O., Shelton, J. R., Shelton, J. B., and Apell, G.: Postnatal changes in the chemical heterogeneity of human fetal hemoglobin. Pediatr. Res. 5:493, 1971.
78a. Jensen, M., Attenberger, H., Schneider, C. H., and Walther, J.-U.: The developmental change in the $^G\gamma$ and $^A\gamma$ globin proportions in hemoglobin F. Eur. J. Pediatr. 138:311, 1982.
79. Rovera, G., Magarian, C., and Borun, T. W.: Resolution of hemoglobin subunits by electrophoresis in acid urea polyacrylamide gels containing Triton X-100. Ann. Biochem. 85:506, 1978.
80. Alter, B. P., Goff, S. C., Efremov, G. D., Gravely, M. E., and Huisman, T. H. J.: Globin chain electrophoresis: A new approach to the determination of $^G\gamma/^A\gamma$ ratio in fetal hemoglobin and to studies of globin synthesis. Br. J. Haematol. 44:527, 1980.
80a. Comi, P., Giglioni, B., Ottolenghi, S., Gianni, A. M., Ricco, G., Mazza, U., Saglio, G., Camaschella, C., Pich, P. G., Gianazza, E., and Righetti, P.-G.: $^G\gamma$ and $^A\gamma$ globin chain separation and quantitation by isoelectric focusing. Biochem. Biophys. Res. Commun. 87:1, 1979.
81. Chen-Marotel, J., Beuzard, Y., Trung, B. K., Braconnier, F., Rosa, J., Guerrasio, A., Saglio, G., Camaschella, C., and Ricco, G.: Polymorphism of human fetal haemoglobin studied by isoelectric focusing. FEBS Lett. 115:68, 1980.
82. Congote, L. F., Bennett, H. P. J., and Solomon, S.: Rapid separation of the α, β, $^G\gamma$ and $^A\gamma$ human globin chains by reversed-phase high pressure liquid chromatography. Biochem. Biophys. Res. Commun. 89:851, 1979.
83. Huisman, T. H. J., Altay, C., Webber, B., Reese, A. L., Gravely, M. E., Okonjo, K., and Wilson, J. B.: Quantitation of three types of gamma chain of Hb F by high pressure liquid chromatography; application of this method to the Hb F of patients with sickle cell anemia or the S-HPFH condition. Blood 57:75, 1981.
84. Schroeder, W. A.: The synthesis and chemical heterogeneity of human fetal hemoglobin. Hemoglobin 4:431, 1980.
85. Huisman, T. H. J.: The human fetal hemoglobins. Tex. Rep. Biol. Med. 40:29, 1981.
86. Ricco, G., Mazza, V., Turi, R. M., Pich, P. G., Camaschella, G., Saglio, G., and Bernini, L. F.: Significance of a new type of human fetal hemoglobin carrying a replacement isoleucine-threonine at position 75 (E19) of the γ chain. Hum. Genet. 32:305, 1976.
87. Huisman, T. H. J., Schroeder, W. A., Reese, A., Wilson, J. B., Lam, H., Roger, J., Shelton, J. B., Shelton, J. R., and Baker, S.: The $^T\gamma$ chain of human fetal hemoglobin at birth and in several abnormal hematologic conditions. Pediatr. Res. 11:1102, 1977.
88. Schroeder, W. A., Huisman, T. H. J., Efremov, G. D., Shelton, J. R., Shelton, J. B., Phillips, R., Reese, A., Gravely, M., Harrison, J. M., and Lam, H.: Further studies on the frequency and significance of the $^T\gamma$-chain of human fetal hemoglobin. J. Clin. Invest. 63:268, 1979.
89. Saglio, G., Ricco, G., Mazza, U., Camaschella, C., Pich, P. G., Gianni, A. M., Gianazza, E., Righetti, P. G., Giglioni, B., Comi, P., Gusmeroli, M., and Ottolenghi, S.: Human $^T\gamma$ globin chain is a variant of $^A\gamma$ chain ($^A\gamma$ Sardinia). Proc. Natl. Acad. Sci. USA 76:3420, 1979.
90. Grifoni, V., Kamuzora, H., Lehmann, H., and Charlesworth, D.: A new Hb variant: F Sardinia γ75(E19) Isoleucine → Threonine found in a family with Hb G-Philadelphia, β-chain deficiency and a Lepore-like hemoglobin indistinguishable from Hb A_2. Acta Haematol. 53:347, 1975.
91. Frier, J. A., and Perutz, M. F.: Structure of human foetal deoxyhaemoglobin. J. Mol. Biol. 112:97, 1977.
92. Perutz, M. F.: Mechanism of denaturation of haemoglobin by alkali. Nature 247:341, 1974.
93. Huehns, E. R., Beaven, G. H., and Stevens, B. L.: Recombination studies on haemoglobins at neutral pH. Biochem. J. 92:440, 1964.
94. Allen, D. W., Wyman, J., and Smith, C. A.: The oxygen equilibrium of foetal and adult human hemoglobin. J. Biol. Chem. 203:81, 1953.
95. Bauer, C., Ludwig, I., and Ludwig, M.: Different effects of 2,3-diphosphoglycerate and adenosine triphosphate on the oxygen affinity of adult and foetal human hemoglobin. Life Sci. 7:1339, 1968.
96. Tyuma, I., and Shimizu, K.: Different response to organic phosphates of human fetal and adult hemoglobins. Arch. Biochem. Biophys. 129:404, 1969.
97. Poyart, C., Bursaux, E., Guesnon, P., and Teisseire, B.: Chloride binding and the Bohr effect of human fetal erythrocytes and Hb F_{II} solutions. Pfluegers Arch. 37:169, 1978.
98. Bonaventura, J., Bonaventura, C., Sullivan, B., Ferruzzi, G., McCurdy, P. R., Fox, J., and Moo-Penn, W. F.: Hemoglobin Providence. Functional consequences of two alterations of the 2,3-diphosphoglycerate binding site at position beta 82. J. Biol. Chem. 251:7563, 1976.
99. Gros, G., and Bauer, C.: High pK value of the N-terminal amino group of the γ-chain causes low CO_2 binding of human fetal hemoglobin. Biochem. Biophys. Res. Commun. 80:56, 1978.
100. Bursaux, E., Poyart, C., Guesnon, P., and Teisseire, B.: Comparative effects of CO_2 on the affinity for O_2 of fetal and adult erythrocytes. Pfluegers Arch. 378:197, 1979.
101. Kleihauer, E., Braun, H., and Betke, K.: Demonstration von fetalem Hamoglobin in den Erythrozyten eines Blutausstrichs. Klin. Wochenschr. 35:637, 1957.
102. Katsura, S.: A new serological method for the detection of fetal hemoglobin in the single erythrocyte. Yokohama Med. Bull. 15:117, 1964.
103. Boyer, S. H., Belding, T. K., Margolet, L., and Noyes, A. N.: Fetal hemoglobin restriction to a few erythrocytes (F cells) in normal human adults. Science 188:361, 1975.
104. Abraham, E. C., Reese, A., Stallings, M., Garver, F. A., and Huisman, T. H. J.: An improved chromatographic procedure for quantitation of human fetal hemoglobin. Hemoglobin 1:547, 1977.
105. Huisman, T. H. J., Henson, J. B., and Wilson, J.

B.: A new high performance liquid chromatographic procedure to quantitate hemoglobin A_{Ic} and other minor hemoglobins in blood of normal, diabetic and alcoholic individuals. J. Lab. Clin. Med. 102:163, 1983.
106. Garver, F. A., Jones, S. C., Baker, M. M., Gultekin, A., Barton, B. P., Gravely, M., and Huisman, T. H. J.: Specific radioimmunochemical identification and quantitation of hemoglobins A_2 and F. Am. J. Hematol. 1:459, 1976.
107. Makler, M. T., and Pesce, A. J.: ELISA assay for measurement of human hemoglobin A and hemoglobin F. Am. J. Clin. Pathol. 74:673, 1980.
108. Singer, K., Chernoff, A. I., and Singer, L.: Studies on abnormal hemoglobins. I. Their demonstration in sickle cell anemia and other hematologic disorders by means of alkali denaturation. Blood 6:413, 1951.
109. Jonxis, J. H. P., and Huisman, T. H. J.: The detection and estimation of fetal hemoglobin by means of alkali denaturation test. Blood 11:1009, 1956.
110. Betke, K., Marti, H. R., and Schlicht, I.: Estimation of small percentages of foetal hemoglobin. Nature 184:1877, 1959.
111. Molden, D. P., Alexander, N. M., and Neeley, W. E.: Fetal hemoglobin: Optimum conditions for its estimation by alkali denaturation. Am. J. Clin. Pathol. 77:568, 1982.
112. International Committee for Standardization in Haematology: Recommendations for fetal haemoglobin reference preparations and fetal haemoglobin determination by the alkali denaturation method. Br. J. Haematol. 42:133, 1979.
113. Bard, H.: The postnatal decline of hemoglobin F synthesis in normal full-term infants. J. Clin. Invest. 55:395, 1975.
114. Dover, G. J., Boyer, S. H., and Bell, W. R.: Microscopic method for assaying F cell production: Illustrative changes during infancy and in aplastic anemia. Blood 52:664, 1978.
114a. Perrine, S. P., Greene, M. F., Kan, Y. W., and Faller, D. V.: Absence of the fetal globin switch in infants of diabetic mothers. (Abstract.) Blood, in press.
115. Huehns, E. R., Hecht, F., Keil, J. V., and Motulsky, A. G.: Developmental hemoglobin anomalies in a chromosomal triplication: D_1 trisomy syndrome. Proc. Natl. Acad. Sci. USA 51:89, 1964.
116. Bard, H.: Postnatal fetal and adult hemoglobin synthesis in D_1 trisomy syndrome. Blood 40:523, 1972.
117. Wilson, M. G., Schroeder, W. A., and Graves, D. A.: Postnatal change of hemoglobins F and A_2 in infants with Down's syndrome (G trisomy). Pediatrics 42:349, 1968.
118. Weller, S. D. V., Apley, J., and Raper, A. B.: Malformations associated with precocious synthesis of adult hemoglobin. Lancet 1:777, 1966.
119. Wood, W. G., Stamatoyannopoulos, G., Lim, G., and Nute, P. E.: F-cells in the adult: Normal values and levels in individuals with hereditary and acquired elevations of Hb F. Blood 46:671, 1975.
120. Zago, M. A., Wood, W. G., Clegg, J. B., Weatherall, D. J., O'Sullivan, M., and Gunson, H.: Genetic control of F cells in human adults. Blood 53:977, 1979.
121. Vgenopoulos, T., and Marti, H. R.: Hamoglobin F bei erworbenen Anamien. Klin. Wochenschr. 52:1011, 1974.
122. Dover, G. J., Boyer, S. H., and Pembrey, M. E.: F cell production in sickle cell anemia; regulation by genes linked to β-hemoglobin locus. Science 211:1441, 1981.
123. Pembrey, M. E., Weatherall, D. J., and Clegg, J. B.: Maternal synthesis of haemoglobin F in pregnancy. Lancet 16:1351, 1973.
124. Boyer, S. H., Belding, T. K., Margolet, L., Noyes, A. N., Burke, P. J., and Bell, W. R.: Variations in the frequency of fetal hemoglobin-bearing erythrocytes (F-cells) in well adults, pregnant women, and adult leukemics. Johns Hopkins Med. J. 137:105, 1975.
125. Bromberg, Y. M., Salzberger, M., and Abrahamov, A.: Alkali type of hemoglobin in women with molar pregnancy. Blood 12:1122, 1957.
126. Serjeant, G. R.: Irreversibly sickled cells and splenomegaly in sickle cell anemia. Br. J. Haematol. 19:635, 1970.
127. Dover, G. J., Boyer, S. H., Charache, S., and Heintzelman, K.: Individual variation in the production and survival of F-cells in sickle cell disease. N. Engl. J. Med. 299:1428, 1978.
128. Bertles, J. F., and Milner, P. F.: Irreversibly sickled erythrocytes: A consequence of the heterogeneous distribution of hemoglobin types in sickle cell anemia. J. Clin. Invest. 47:1731, 1968.
129. Newman, D. R., Pierre, R. V., and Linman, J. W.: Studies on the diagnostic significance of hemoglobin F levels. Mayo Clin. Proc. 48:199, 1973.
130. Chudwin, D. S., Rucknagel, D. L., Scholnik, A. P., Waldmann, T. A., and McIntire, K. R.: Fetal hemoglobin and α-fetoprotein in various malignancies. Acta Haematol. 58:288, 1977.
131. Dasgupta, A., Pavri, R. S., and Advani, S. H.: Hemoglobin abnormalities in hematological malignancies. Isr. J. Med. Res. 73:82, 1981.
132. Dainiak, N., and Hoffman, R.: Hemoglobin-F production in testicular malignancy. Cancer 45:2177, 1980.
132a. Müderrisoğlu, C., Kansu, E., Akdas, A., Lateli, Y., and Firat, D.: Haemoglobin F levels in urogenital cancers. Br. J. Urol. 55:264, 1983.
133. Hardisty, R. M., Speed, D. E., and Till, M.: Granulocytic leukaemia in childhood. Br. J. Haematol. 10:551, 1964.
134. Weatherall, D. J., and Brown, M. J.: Juvenile chronic myeloid leukaemia. Lancet 1:526, 1970.
135. Maurer, H. S., Vida, L. N., and Honig, G. R.: Similarities of the erythrocytes in juvenile chronic myelogenous leukemia to fetal erythrocytes. Blood 39:778, 1972.
136. Pagnier, J., Lopez, M., Mathiot, C., Habibi, B., Zamet, P., Varet, B., and Labie, D.: An unusual case of leukemia with high fetal hemoglobin: Demonstration of abnormal hemoglobin synthesis localized in red cell clone. Blood 50:249, 1977.
137. Krauss, J. S., Rodriguez, A. R., and Milner, P. F.: Erythroleukemia with high fetal hemoglobin after therapy for ovarian carcinoma. Am. J. Clin. Pathol. 76:721, 1981.
138. Papayannopoulou, T., Vichinsky, E., and Stamatoyannopoulos, G.: Foetal Hb production during acute erythroid expansion. Br. J. Haematol. 44:535, 1980.
139. Alter, B. P., Rappeport, J. M., Huisman, T. H. J., Schroeder, W. A., and Nathan, D. G.: Fetal erythropoiesis following bone marrow transplantation. Blood 48:843, 1976.
140. Dover, G. J., Boyer, S. H., and Zinkham, W. H.: Production of erythrocytes that contain fetal hemoglobin in anemia. J. Clin. Invest. 63:173, 1979.
141. Hoffman, R., Papayannopoulou, T., Landaw, S., Wasserman, L. R., DeMarsh, Q. B., Chen, P., and Stamatoyannopoulos, G.: Fetal hemoglobin in polycythemia vera: Cellular distribution in 50 unselected patients. Blood 53:1148, 1979.

142. Schiliro, G., Musumeci, S., Pizzarelli, G., Russo, A., Marinucci, M., Tentori, L., and Russo, G.: Fetal haemoglobin in early malignant osteopetrosis. Br. J. Haematol. 38:339, 1978.
143. Lee, J. C., Hayashi, R. H., and Shepard, M. K.: Fetal hemoglobin in women with normal and with hydatidiform molar pregnancy. Am. J. Hematol. 13:131, 1982.
144. Schiliro, G., Musumeci, S., Russo, A., Marino, S., Sciotto, A., and Russo, G.: Transient increase of fetal haemoglobin in kala-azar. Br. J. Haematol. 46:207, 1980.
145. Clark, A. V., and Tannenbaum, S. R.: Isolation and characterization of pigments from protein-carbamyl browning systems: Models for two insulin-glucose pigments. J. Agric. Food Chem. 22:1089, 1974.
146. Dixon, H. B. F.: A reaction of glucose with peptides. Biochem. J. 129:203, 1972.
147. Adhikari, H. R., and Tappe, A. L.: Fluorescent products in a glucose-glycine browning reaction. J. Food Sci. 38:486, 1973.
148. Hodge, J. E.: The Amadori rearrangement. Adv. Carbohydr. Chem. 10:169, 1955.
149. Huisman, T. H. J., and Meyering, C. A.: Studies on the heterogeneity of hemoglobin. I. The heterogeneity of different hemoglobin types in carboxymethyl cellulose and in Amberlite IRC-50 chromatography: Qualitative aspects. Clin. Chim. Acta 5:103, 1960.
150. McDonald, M. J., Shapiro, R., Bleichman, M., Solway, J., and Bunn, H. F.: Glycosylated minor components of human adult hemoglobin. J. Biol. Chem. 253:2327, 1978.
151. Shibata, S., Miyaji, T., Ueda, S., and Takeda, I.: An abnormal hemoglobin component discovered in the blood of diabetic patients. Acta Haematol. Jpn. 25:327, 1962.
152. Huisman, T. H. J., and Dozy, A. M.: Studies on the heterogeneity of hemoglobin V binding of hemoglobin with oxidized glutathione. J. Lab. Clin. Med. 60:302, 1962.
153. Rahbar, S.: An abnormal hemoglobin in red cells of diabetics. Clin. Chim. Acta 22:296, 1968.
154. Trivelli, L. A., Ranney, H. M., and Lai, H.: Hemoblobin components in patients with diabetes mellitus. N. Engl. J. Med. 284:353, 1971.
155. Holmquist, W. R., and Schroeder, W. A.: A new N-terminal blocking group involving a Schiff base in hemoglobin A_{Ic}. Biochemistry 5:2489, 1966.
156. Bookchin, R. M., and Gallop, P. M.: Structure of hemoglobin A_{Ic}: Nature of the N-terminal chain blocking group. Biochem. Biophys. Res. Commun. 32:86, 1968.
157. Bunn, H. F., Haney, D. N., Gabbay, K. H., and Gallop, P. M.: Further identification of the nature and linkage of the carbohydrate in hemoglobin A_{Ic}. Biochem. Biophys. Res. Commun. 67:103, 1975.
158. Fluckiger, R., and Winterhalter, K. H.: In vitro synthesis of hemoglobin A_{Ic}. FEBS Lett. 71:356, 1976.
159. Koenig, R. J., Blobstein, S. H., and Cerami, A.: The structure of carbohydrate of hemoglobin A_{Ic}. J. Biol. Chem. 252:2992, 1977.
160. Fischer, R. W., and Winterhalter, K. H.: The carbohydrate moiety in hemoglobin A_{Ic} is present in the ring form. FEBS Lett. 135:145, 1981.
161. Bunn, H. F., Shapiro, R., McManus, M., Garrick, L., McDonald, M. J., Gallop, P. M., and Gabbay, K. H.: Structural heterogeneity of human hemoglobin A due to non-enzymatic glycosylation. J. Biol. Chem. 254:3892, 1979.
162. Shapiro, R., McManus, M. J., Zalut, C., and Bunn, H. F.: Sites of non-enzymatic glycosylation of human hemoglobin A. J. Biol. Chem. 255:3120, 1980.
163. Garlick, R. L., and Mazer, J. S.: The principal site of nonenzymatic glycosylation of human serum albumin in vivo. J. Biol. Chem. 258:6142, 1983.
164. Garlick, R. L., Mazer, J. S., Higgins, P., and Bunn, H. F.: Characterization of glycosylated hemoglobins: Relevance to monitoring of diabetic control and analysis of other proteins. J. Clin. Invest. 71:1062, 1983.
165. Gabbay, K. H., Sosenko, J. M., Banuchi, G. A., Minninsohn, M. J., and Fluckiger, R.: Glycosylated hemoglobins: Increased glycosylation of hemoglobin A in diabetic patients. Diabetes 28:337, 1979.
166. Haney, D. N., and Bunn, H. F.: Glycosylation of hemoglobin in vitro: Affinity labeling of hemoglobin by glucose-6-phosphate. Proc. Natl. Acad. Sci. USA 73:3534, 1976.
167. Stevens, V. J., Vlassara, H., Abati, A., and Cerami, A.: Non-enzymatic glycosylation of hemoglobin. J. Biol. Chem. 252:2998, 1977.
168. Solway, J., McDonald, M. J., and Bunn, H. F.: Biosynthesis of glycosylated hemoglobins in the monkey. J. Lab. Clin. Med. 93:962, 1979.
169. Bunn, H. F., Haney, D. N., Kamin, S., Gabbay, K. H., and Gallop, P. M.: The biosynthesis of human hemoglobin A_{Ic}; slow glycosylation of hemoglobin in vivo. J. Clin. Invest. 57:1652, 1976.
170. Fitzgibbons, J. F., Koler, R. D., and Jones R. T.: Red cell age related changes of hemoglobins A_{Ia+b} and A_{Ic} in normal and diabetic subjects. J. Clin. Invest. 58:820, 1976.
171. Horton, B. F., and Huisman, T. H. J.: Studies on the heterogeneity of haemoglobin. VII. Minor haemoglobin components in haematological disease. Br. J. Haematol. 11:296, 1965.
172. Koenig, R. J., and Cerami, A.: Synthesis of hemoglobin A_{Ic} in normal and diabetic mice: Potential model of basement membrane thickening. Proc. Natl. Acad. Sci. USA 72:3687, 1975.
173. McDonald, M. J., Bleichman, M., Bunn, H. F., and Noble, R.: Functional properties of the glycosylated minor components of human adult hemoglobin. J. Biol. Chem. 254:702, 1979.
174. Higgins, P. J., and Bunn, H. F.: Kinetic analysis of the non-enzymatic glycosylation of hemoglobin. J. Biol. Chem. 256:5204, 1981.
175. Bunn, H. F., and Higgins, P. J.: Reaction of monosaccharides with proteins: Possible evolutionary significance. Science 213:222, 1981.
176. Dolhofer, R., and Wieland, O. H.: In vitro glycosylation of hemoglobins by different sugars and sugar phosphates. FEBS Lett. 85:86, 1978.
177. Spicer, K. M., Allen, R. C., Hallett, D., and Buse, M. G.: Synthesis of hemoglobin A_{Ic} and related minor hemoglobins by erythrocytes. J. Clin. Invest. 64:40, 1979.
178. Hayward, L. D., and Angyal, S. J.: A symmetry role for the circular dichroism of reducing sugars, and the proportion of carbonyl forms in aqueous solutions thereof. Carbohydr. Res. 53:13, 1977.
179. Bunn, H. F., and Briehl, R. W.: The interaction of 2,3-diphosphoglycerate with various human hemoglobins. J. Clin. Invest. 49:1008, 1970.
180. Fluckiger, R., and Winterhalter, K. H.: Glycosylated hemoglobins. In Labie, D., Poyart, C., and Rosa,

181. Rorth, M., Parving, H.-H., and Munkgaard, S.: Red cell oxygen affinity and 2,3-diphosphoglycerate in diabetes. Lancet *1*:1179, 1972.
182. Arturson, G., Garby, L., Robert, M., and Zaar, B.: Oxygen affinity of whole blood *in vivo* and under standard conditions in subjects with diabetes mellitus. Scand. J. Clin. Lab. Invest. *34*:19, 1974.
183. Ditzel, J., and Standl, E.: The problem of tissue oxygenation in diabetes mellitus. Acta Med. Scand. Suppl. *578*:59, 1975.
184. Rahbar, S., Blumenfeld, O., and Ranney, H. M.: Studies of an unusual hemoglobin in patients with diabetes mellitus. Biochem. Biophys. Res. Commun. *36*:838, 1969.
185. Tattersall, R. B., Pyke, D. A., Ranney, H. M., and Bruckheimer, S. M.: Hemoglobin components in diabetes mellitus. Studies in identical twins. N. Engl. J. Med. *293*:1171, 1975.
186. Koenig, R. J., Peterson, C. M., Jones R. L., Saudek, C., Lehrman, M., and Cerami, A.: Correlation of glucose regulation and hemoglobin A_{Ic} in diabetes mellitus. N. Engl. J. Med. *295*:417, 1976.
187. Gabbay, K. H., Hasty, K., Breslow, J. L., Ellison, R. C., Bunn, H. F., and Gallop, P. M.: Glycosylated hemoglobins and long-term blood glucose control in diabetes mellitus. J. Clin. Endocrinol. Metab. *44*:859, 1977.
188. Gonen, B., Rubenstein, A. H., Rochman, H., Tanega, S. P., and Horwitz, D. L.: Haemoglobin A_1: An indication of the metabolic control of diabetic patients. Lancet *2*:734, 1977.
189. Dunn, P. J., Cole, R. A., Soeldner, J. S., and Gleason, R. E.: Reproducibility of hemoglobin A_{Ic} and sensitivity to various degrees of glucose intolerance. Ann. Intern. Med. *91*:390, 1979.
190. Schwartz, H. C., King, K. C., Schwartz, A. L., Edmunds, D., and Schwartz, R.: Effects of pregnancy on hemoglobin A_{Ic} in normal, gestational diabetic and diabetic women. Diabetes *25*:1118, 1976.
191. Leslie, R. D. G., John, P. N., Pyke, D. A., and White, T. M.: Haemoglobin A_1 in diabetic pregnancy. Lancet *2*:958, 1978.
192. Lind, T., and Cheyne, G. A.: Effect of normal pregnancy upon the glycosylated hemoglobins. Br. J. Obstet. Gynaecol. *86*:210, 1979.
192a. Goldstein, D. E., Little, R. R., Wiedmeyer, H. M., England, J. D., and Parker, K. M.: Recent advances in glycosylated hemoglobin measurement. CRC Crit. Rev. Clin. Lab. Sci. *21*:187, 1984.
193. Kynoch, P. A. M., and Lehmann, H.: Rapid estimation (2½ hours) of glycosylated haemoglobin for routine purposes. Lancet *2*:16, 1977.
194. Jones, M. B., Koler, R. D., and Jones, R. T.: Microcolumn method for the determination of hemoglobin minor fractions A_{Ia+b} and A_{Ic}. Hemoglobin *2*:53, 1978.
195. Rosenthal, M. A.: The effect of temperature on the fast hemoglobin test system. Hemoglobin *3*:215, 1979.
196. Cole, R. A., Soeldner, J. S., Dunn, P. H., and Bunn, H. F.: A rapid method for the determination of glycosylated hemoglobins using high pressure liquid chromatography. Metabolism *27*:289, 1978.
197. Davis, J. E., McDonald, J. M., and Jarrett, L.: A high performance liquid chromatography method for hemoglobin A_{Ic}. Diabetes *27*:102, 1978.
198. Abraham, E. C., Stallings, M., Cameron, B. F., and Huisman, T. H. J.: Minor hemoglobins in sickle cell heterozygotes with and without diabetes. Biochim. Biophys. Acta *625*:109, 1980.
199. Sosenko, J. M., Fluckiger, R., Platt, O. S., and Gabbay, K. H.: Glycosylation of variant hemoglobins in normal and diabetic subjects. Diabetes Care *3*:590, 1980.
200. deBoer, M.-J., Miedema, K., and Casparie, A. F.: Glycosylated hemoglobin in renal failure. Diabetologia *18*:437, 1980.
201. Fluckiger, R., Harmon, W., Meier, W., Loo, S., and Gabbay, K. H.: Hemoglobin carbamylation in uremia. N. Engl. J. Med. *304*:823, 1981.
202. Stevens, V. J., Fantl, W. J., Newman, C. B., Sims, R. V., Cerami, A., and Peterson, C. M.: Acetaldehyde adducts with hemoglobin. J. Clin. Invest. *67*:361, 1981.
203. Hoberman, H. D., and Chiodo, S. M.: Elevation of the hemoglobin A_I fraction in alcoholism. Alcoholism: Clin. Exp. Res. *6*:260, 1982.
203a. Hoberman, H. D.: Post-translational modification of hemoglobin in alcoholism. Biochem. Biophys. Res. Commun. *113*:1004, 1983.
204. Charache, S., and Weatherall, D. J.: Fast hemoglobin in lead poisoning. Blood *28*:377, 1966.
205. Dix, D., Cohen, P., Kingsley, S., Lea, M. J., Senkbeil, J., and Sexton, K.: Interference by lactescence in the glycohemoglobin analysis. Clin. Chem. *25*:494, 1979.
206. Mallia, A. K., Hermanson, G. T., Krohn, R. I., Fujimoto, E. K., and Smith, P. K.: Preparation and use of a boronic acid affinity support for separation and quantitation of glycosylated hemoglobins. Anal. Lett. *14*:649, 1981.
207. Yue, D. K., McLennan, S., Church, D. B., and Turtle, J. R.: The measurement of glycosylated hemoglobin in man and animals by aminophenylboronic acid affinity chromatography. Diabetes *31*:701, 1982.
208. Basset, P., Beuzard, Y., Garel, M. C., and Rosa, J.: Isoelectric focusing of human hemoglobin: Its application to screening, to the characterization of 70 variants, and to the study of modified fractions of normal hemoglobins. Blood *51*:971, 1978.
209. Allen, R. C., Stastny, M., Hallett, D., and Simmons, M. A.: A comparison of isoelectric focusing and electrochromatography for the separation and quantification of hemoglobin A_{Ic}. *In* Radola, B. J. (ed.): Electrophoresis, 1979. Berlin, de Gruyter, 1980, p. 663.
210. Menard, L., Dempsey, M. E., Blankstein, L. A., Aleyassine, H., Wacks, M., and Soeldner, J. S.: Quantitative determination of glycosylated hemoglobin A_I by agar gel electrophoresis. Clin. Chem. *26*:1598, 1980.
211. Pecoraro, R. E., Graf, R. J., Beiler, H., and Porte, D.: Comparison of a colorimetric assay for glycosylated hemoglobin with ion exchange chromatography. Diabetes *28*:1120, 1979.
212. Fischer, R. W., DeJong, C., Voigt, E., Berger, W., and Winterhalter, K. H.: The colorimetric determination of Hb A_{Ic} in normal and diabetic subjects. Clin. Lab. Haematol. *2*:129, 1980.
213. Yue, D. K., Morris, McLennan, S., and Turtle, J. R.: Glycosylation of plasma protein and its relation to glycosylated hemoglobin in diabetes. Diabetes *29*:296, 1980.
214. Kennedy, A. L., Mehl, T. D., and Merimee, T. J.: Non-enzymatically glycosylated serum protein: Spurious elevation due to free glucose in serum. Diabetes *29*:413, 1980.

215. Gallop, P. M., Fluckiger, R., Hanneken, A., Mininsohn, M. M., and Gabbay, K. H.: Chemical quantitation of hemoglobin glycosylation: Fluorometric detection of formaldehyde released upon periodate oxidation of glycoglobin. Anal. Biochem. *117*:427, 1981.
216. Nayak, S. S., and Pattabiraman, T. N.: A new colorimetric method for the estimation of glycosylated hemoglobin. Clin. Chim. Acta *109*:267, 1981.
217. Javid, J., Pettis, P. K., Koenig, R. J., and Cerami, A.: Immunologic characterization and quantification of haemoglobin A_{Ic}. Br. J. Haematol. *38*:329, 1978.
218. Chou, P. P., Kerkay, J., and Gupta, M. K.: Development of a laser nephelometric method for the quantitation of human glycohemoglobins. Anal. Lett. *14*(B13):1071, 1981.
219. Svendsen, P. A., Christiansen, J. S., Soegaard, U., Welinder, B. S., and Nerup, J.: Rapid changes in chromatographically determined haemoglobin A_{Ic} induced by short term changes in glucose concentration. Diabetologia *19*:130, 1980.
220. Goldstein, D. B., Path, S. B., England, J. D., Hess, R. L., and DaCosta, J.: Effects of acute changes in blood glucose on Hb A_{Ic}. Diabetes *29*:623, 1980.
221. Spiro, R. G.: Search for a biochemical basis of diabetic microangiopathy. Diabetologia *12*:1, 1976.
222. Kilmartin, J. V., and Rossi-Bernardi, L.: Inhibition of CO_2 combination and reduction of the Bohr effect in haemoglobin chemically modified at its α-amino groups. Nature *222*:1243, 1969.
223. Cerami, A., and Manning, J. M.: Potassium cyanate as an inhibitor of the sickling of erythrocytes *in vitro*. Proc. Natl. Acad. Sci. USA *68*:1180, 1971.
224. Oimomi, M., Ishikawa, K., Kawasaki, T., Kubota, S., Yoshimura, Y., and Baba, S.: Glycosylated haemoglobin in renal failure. Diabetologia *21*:163, 1981.
225. Tsuboi, K. K., Thompson, D. J., Rush, E. M., and Schwartz, H. C.: Acetaldehyde-dependent changes in hemoglobin and oxygen affinity of human erythrocytes. Hemoglobin *5*:241, 1981.
226. Jörnvall, H.: Acetylation of protein N-terminal amino groups. Structural observations on alpha-amino acetylated proteins. J. Theor. Biol. *55*:1, 1975.
227. Bloemendal, H.: The vertebrate eye lens. Science *197*:127, 1977.
228. Marchis-Mouren, G., and Lippman, F.: On the mechanism of acetylation of fetal and chicken hemoglobins. Proc. Natl. Acad. Sci. USA *53*:1147, 1965.
229. Granger, M., Tesser, G. I., DeJong, W. W., and Bloemendal, H.: Model studies of enzymatic NH_2-terminal acetylation of proteins with des-$N^{\alpha 1}$-acetyl-α-melanotropin as a substrate. Proc. Natl. Acad. Sci. USA *73*:3010, 1976.
230. Palmiter, R. D., Gagnon, J., and Walsh, K. A.: Ovalbumin: A secreted protein without a transient hydrophobic leader sequence. Proc. Natl. Acad. Sci. USA *75*:94, 1978.
231. Schroeder, W. A., Cua, J. T., Matsuda, G., and Fenninger, W. D.: Hemoglobin F_I, an acetyl-containing hemoglobin. Biochim. Biophys. Acta *63*:532, 1962.
232. Mahoney, W. C., and Nute, P. E.: Fetal hemoglobin of the Rhesus monkey, *Macaca mulatta*: Complete primary structure of the γ-chain. Biochemistry *19*:4436, 1980.
233. Moo-Penn, W. F., Bechtel, K. C., Schmidt, R. M., Johnson, M. H., Jue, D. L., Schmidt, D. E., Dunlap, W. M., Opella, S. J., Bonaventura, J., and Bonaventura, C.: Hemoglobin Raleigh (β1 Valine→Acetylalanine): Structural and functional characterization. Biochemistry *16*:4872, 1977.
234. Taketa, F., Attermeir, M. H., and Mauk, A. G.: Acetylated hemoglobins in feline blood. J. Biol. Chem. *247*:33, 1972.
235. Huehns, E. R., and Shooter, E. M.: The properties and reactions of hemoglobin F and their bearing on the dissociation equilibrium of hemoglobin. Biochem. J. *101*:852, 1966.
236. Abraham, E. C., Cope, N. D., Braziel, N. N., and Huisman, T. H. J.: On the chromatographic heterogeneity of human fetal hemoglobin. Biochim. Biophys. Acta *577*:159, 1979.
237. Abraham, E. C.: Glycosylated minor components of human fetal hemoglobin. Chromatographic separation, identification, and functional characterization. Biochim. Biophys. Acta *667*:168, 1981.
238. Matsuda, G., Schroeder, W. A., Jones, R. T., and Weliky, N.: Is there an "embryonic" or "primitive" human hemoglobin? Blood *16*:984, 1960.
239. Garlick, R. L., Shaeffer, J. R., Chapman, P. B., Kingston, R. E., Mazer, J. S., and Bunn, H. F.: Synthesis of acetylated human fetal hemoglobin. J. Biol. Chem. *256*:1727, 1981.
240. Garlick, R. L., Mazer, J. S., Himmelstein, A., Stamatoyannopoulos, G., and Shaeffer, J. R.: Enhanced synthesis of acetylated human fetal hemoglobin in senescent reticulocytes. Biochim. Biophys. Acta *799*:29, 1984.
241. Garbutt, G. J., and Abraham, E. C.: Non-enzymatic acetylation of human hemoglobins. Biochim. Biophys. Acta *670*:190, 1981.
242. Kasten-Jolly, J., and Taketa, F.: Biosynthesis and amino terminal acetylation of cat hemoglobin B. Arch. Biochem. Biophys. *214*:829, 1982.
243. Klotz, I. M., and Tam, J. W. D.: Acetylation of sickle cell hemoglobin by aspirin. Proc. Natl. Acad. Sci. USA *70*:1313, 1973.
244. Bridges, K. R., Schmidt, G. J., Jensen, M., Cerami, A., and Bunn, H. F.: The acetylation of hemoglobin by aspirin: *in vitro* and *in vivo*. J. Clin. Invest. *56*:201, 1975.
245. Shamsuddin, M., Mason, R. G., Ritchey, J. M., Honig, G. R., and Klotz, I. M.: Sites of acetylation of sickle cell hemoglobin by aspirin. Proc. Natl. Acad. Sci. USA *71*:4693, 1974.
246. Nathan, D. M., Francis, T. B., and Palmer, J. L.: Effect of aspirin on determination of glycosylated hemoglobin. Clin. Chem. *29*:466, 1983.
247. Srivastava, S. K., VanLoon, C., and Beutler, E.: Characterization of a previously unidentified hemoglobin fraction. Biochim. Biophys. Acta *278*:617, 1972.
248. Winterhalter, K. H.: Personal communication, 1983.
249. Ceriello, A., Giugliano, P., Dello Russo, P., Sgambato, S., and D'Onofrio, F.: Increased glycosylated haemoglobin A_I in opiate addicts: Evidence for a hyperglycemic effect of morphine. Diabetologia *22*:379, 1982.
250. Lamola, A. A., Piomelli, S., Poh-Fitzpatrick, M. B., Yamane, T., and Harber, L. C.: Erythropoietic protoporphyria and lead intoxication: The molecular basis for difference in cutaneous photosensitivity. II. Different binding of erythrocyte protoporphyrin to hemoglobin. J. Clin. Invest. *56*:1528, 1975.

OXYGEN AND CARBON DIOXIDE TRANSPORT IN HEALTH AND DISEASE

5

Chapter 3 presented a review of the chemistry of hemoglobin with particular emphasis on its interaction with gaseous ligands such as oxygen and carbon monoxide and with various allosteric effectors: hydrogen ion, carbon dioxide, and organic phosphates. Most of this information was developed from experiments done on dilute solutions of hemoglobin under artificially controlled conditions of temperature, pH, and ionic strength. It is no surprise that the properties of hemoglobin are significantly affected by conditions peculiar to the living red cell. In order to understand hemoglobin's physiologic function, it is necessary to study whole blood under *in vivo* conditions. In this chapter, we will first consider the physiology of oxygen transport and especially the uptake and release of oxygen by the circulating red cell. In subsequent sections, we will discuss the metabolic control of red cell 2,3-DPG and its perturbation in various pathological states. From this information, we can draw some conclusions about the role of red cell oxygen affinity under both physiologic and pathological conditions.

OXYGEN TRANSPORT

At sea level, the air we breathe contains 20.95 per cent oxygen. The ambient oxygen tension (PO_2) is approximately 0.21×760 or 160 mm Hg. As air is drawn into the upper air passage, it becomes fully saturated with water. Within the airways and lungs, the inspired air mixes with both dead space gas and alveolar gas that is continuously altered by uptake of O_2 and release of CO_2 from blood passing through the lung capillaries. Accordingly, the PO_2 in the alveolar air drops to about 95 mm Hg.

The amount of oxygen transported across the alveolar capillary membrane per unit time is a product of the diffusing capacity of the membrane per unit time and the PO_2 difference between alveolar gas and pulmonary cap-

RUTH AND REINHOLD BENESCH

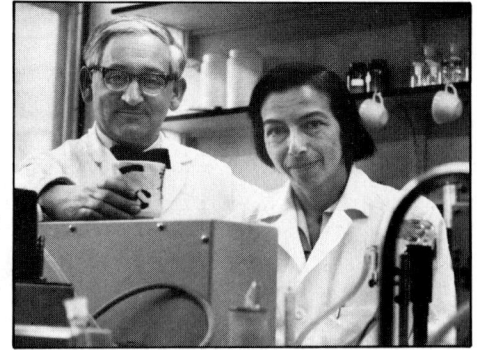

Synergism is a highly valued property in science and perhaps even more in scientific collaborations. The most eminent partnership in hemoglobin research is that of Ruth and Reinhold Benesch. Each brings a special flavor that makes the blend so distinctive. Reinhold is imaginative, unorthodox, and iconoclastic; like many creative scientists, he is a bit clumsy in the laboratory. Ruth is rigorous and thoroughly disciplined in both thought and execution; her facility at the laboratory bench is reminiscent of the grace and economy of a great pianist.

The Benesches fled from Central Europe to England just before the outbreak of World War II. Like most scientists in England during the war, Reinhold Benesch worked on a project of military relevance. His assignment was to develop a way of making eggs soft so that they could be packed closely into cubical containers and shipped to the troops without breaking. He solved the problem by feeding hens an inhibitor of carbonic anhydrase that prevented the deposition of calcium carbonate in the eggshell. Benesch's ingenious egg experiment was commemorated 40 years later (1983) at the New York Academy of Sciences' Symposium on Carbonic Anhydrase.

Throughout his career, Reinhold Benesch's flair for broad comedy has been a personal trademark, greatly appreciated by professional and lay colleagues. Once he was asked to give a learned discourse on the scientific principles underlying the preparation of fine beer. His lecture provoked such hilarity that the brewmasters in attendance thought he was an unemployed Broadway actor posing as a scientist.

The Benesches married in London in 1946 and emigrated to the United States a year later. Their infatuation with the hemoglobin molecule began in 1960. Their measurements of sulfhydryl reactivity and subunit dissociation provided compelling evidence for the alterations in hemoglobin conformation imposed by ligand binding. The fact that purified α and β subunits lacked these oxygen-linked properties established the importance of interaction between unlike subunits in the hemoglobin tetramer. These ideas were summarized in a review article entitled "Homos and heteros among the hemos" that the Benesches wrote for *Science*.

In 1967, the Benesches took note of a fact known to a few hematologists and physiologists: normal human red cells contain the metabolic intermediate 2,3-diphosphoglycerate (2,3-DPG) at a concentration of 5 mM, equivalent to that of hemoglobin tetramer and a 1000-fold higher than that in other cells. They wondered whether this abundant organic phosphate could interact stoichiometrically with hemoglobin. As discussed in Chapter 3, they designed elegant experiments showing that 2,3-DPG causes a marked reduction in oxygen affinity by virtue of its preferential binding to deoxyhemoglobin. The Benesches were quick to recognize the physiologic significance of 2,3-DPG as a modulator of intracellular oxygen binding. During the next decade, research on red cell 2,3-DPG became a growth industry, and a considerable amount was learned about oxygen transport in health and disease (see text of this chapter).

During the past decade, the Benesches' research has focused on sickle hemoglobin. By measuring the gelation and solubility of hybrid hemoglobins containing β^s and mutant α chains, they have been able to determine some of the sites in the α chain that make contacts in the sickle polymer. In addition, the Benesches have coupled their expertise in protein chemistry with their knowledge of hemoglobin structure to prepare stereospecific compounds that inhibit polymerization of sickle hemoglobin.

The Benesches' work is characterized by a combination of authenticity and originality, with an unfailing eye for relevance. They are spirited critics of their own work as well as that of their colleagues. After hearing Austen Riggs present his clever experiments on hybrids prepared from hemoglobins of diverse animals, Reinhold Benesch rose from the audience and offered the following benediction:

> The bullephant and elefrog
> Entangled in genetic smog,
> Enjoy their promiscuity,
> Despite some incongruity.

illary blood. This membrane is about 0.2 micron thick, consisting of surfactant, alveolar epithelium, basement membrane, interstitial tissue, basement membrane, and capillary endothelium.[1] Oxygen is transported passively across the alveolar capillary membrane. In normal lung tissue, the resistance to gas movement across this membrane is negligible. In order for there to be a measurable difference between alveolar and end-capillary oxygen tension, the membrane thickness would have to be many fold greater.[2] One factor that contributes slightly to an alveolar-capillary oxygen gradient is lung tissue, including metabolically active macrophages that take oxygen directly from alveolar gas. As mentioned in Chapter 3, expulsion of CO_2 in the pulmonary circulation results in an increase in intracellular pH. Because of the Bohr effect, the oxygen affinity of the hemoglobin increases, facilitating transport of oxygen into the red cell.

Blood from pulmonary capillaries becomes mixed with blood from bronchial, pleural, and thebesian veins. Normally, this shunt amounts to about 1 to 2 per cent of the pulmonary circulation and results in a further drop in PO_2 in the pulmonary vein to about 90 mm Hg. This partial pressure of oxygen is maintained until the blood reaches the arterioles.

The diffusion of oxygen into and out of red cells is impaired by the high intracellular concentration of hemoglobin. The red cell membrane does not pose an additional barrier, but a stagnant water layer surrounding the cell further retards the rate of oxygen uptake[3] and egress. Altogether, the rates of oxygenation and deoxygenation of red cell suspensions are roughly 10 times slower than an equimolar solution of hemoglobin. Nevertheless, the transit times in pulmonary and peripheral capillaries are about fivefold the half times for oxygenation and deoxygenation. In an individual at rest, the red cell spends about 0.75 second in transit through pulmonary capillaries. It has been estimated that equilibration with alveolar gas is complete within 0.35 second.[4] Thus, under normal circumstances, there is probably no kinetic limitation to oxygen uptake and release from red cells. Accordingly, equilibrium measurements have direct physiologic relevance.

Why Red Cells?

This chapter will focus on the various factors that determine the oxygen binding properties of human blood under physiologic conditions. It is reasonable to ask why hemoglobin of man, and indeed of all other vertebrates, is so neatly packaged in corpuscles. If hemoglobin were circulating free in plasma at a concentration of 15 g per 100 ml, the oncotic pressure would be prohibitively high. One of the primary functions of the red cell membrane is to extrude intracellular cation and water in order to prevent osmotic lysis. For hemoglobin to function in free solution, it would have to be in the form of large polymers such as the macrohemoglobins of worms and the hemocyanins of arthropods and molluscs (see Chapter 6). It has often been stated that hemoglobin in solution would have a significantly higher viscosity compared with blood having the same oxygen-carrying capacity. This has been shown to be untrue for human hemoglobin.[5] However, the viscosity of a comparable concentration of a high–molecular-weight polymeric hemoglobin would be prohibitively high. The viscosity of whole blood varies with the hematocrit in such a way that maximal oxygen transport occurs when the packed cell volume is in the normal range.[6]

The design of the red cell appears optimal. Its overall contour allows efficient diffusion of gas throughout the cell interior. The excess of surface area relative to volume enables the cell to distort its shape in such a way that it can readily traverse small-bore capillaries. Such distensibility would be impossible if the erythrocyte were spherical. Thus, the packaging of hemoglobin into pliable, biconcave discs appears to solve a number of problems in the transport of oxygen and carbon dioxide.

Unloading of Oxygen to Tissues

The transport of oxygen to tissues is governed by three independent variables that can be expressed quantitatively in the Fick equation:

$$VO_2 = 0.139 \cdot Q \cdot Hb \cdot (S_AO_2 - S_{\bar{V}}O_2)$$

where VO_2 is the amount of oxygen released (l/min), 1.39 is the amount (in milliliters) of O_2 bound by 1 gram of fully saturated hemoglobin, Q is blood flow (l/min), and S_AO_2 and $S_{\bar{V}}O_2$ are arterial and mixed venous oxygen saturations (%). Here the small amount of O_2 that is physically dissolved in blood is disregarded.

The *hemoglobin concentration* of the blood is the resultant of the balance between erythropoiesis and red cell destruction (or loss). As discussed in detail below, increased red cell mass, as mediated by erythropoietin, represents an important adaptation to hypoxia.

The *blood flow* to a given tissue or organ is controlled by a complex interplay of local, neural, and hormonal factors. Alteration in blood flow to a given organ is generally appropriate to its metabolic demands. For example, during vigorous muscular exercise, increased cardiac output accompanies enhanced blood flow through exercising muscle. Unused capillaries are recruited in order to maximize oxygen delivery and clearance of metabolic wastes. Considerable alterations in the distribution of blood flow often occur without any significant change in the cardiac output. Familiar examples include the increased blood flow to the intestine following meals and the marked effect of ambient temperature on circulation to the skin. Because of the body's wisdom in tailoring regional circulation to local and temporal demands, the determinants of blood flow at the tissue level are very complex. Thus, it is very difficult to obtain a good estimate of blood flow through a given capillary bed.

The third factor in the Fick equation ($S_AO_2 - S_{\bar{V}}O_2$) is a quantitative expression of the *fractional unloading of oxygen from hemoglobin* during the flow of blood from artery to vein. This parameter is dependent on the blood's oxyhemoglobin dissociation curve, which determines the amount of oxygen the blood can release for a given decrement in PO_2. Under physiologic conditions, the dissociation curve is poised so that blood becomes nearly fully saturated with oxygen during the circulation through the lungs. During flow through systemic capillaries, a steeper portion of the curve is encompassed, permitting a relatively large amount of oxygen to be unloaded over a relatively small drop in PO_2. This allows oxygen to be released into the plasma at sufficiently high concentration to provide an adequate gradient into the interior of cells.

In addition to the three important determinants expressed by the Fick equation, a number of other variables at the tissue level influence oxygen delivery. In capillaries, the plasma oxygen tension is estimated to be about 1 mm Hg less than that inside red cells.[7] The PO_2 gradient between the plasma and the interior of tissue cells depends on a number of independent factors, including the pattern and density of capillaries as well as their relative flow rates. Furthermore, this gradient is affected by differences in oxygen diffusion among various

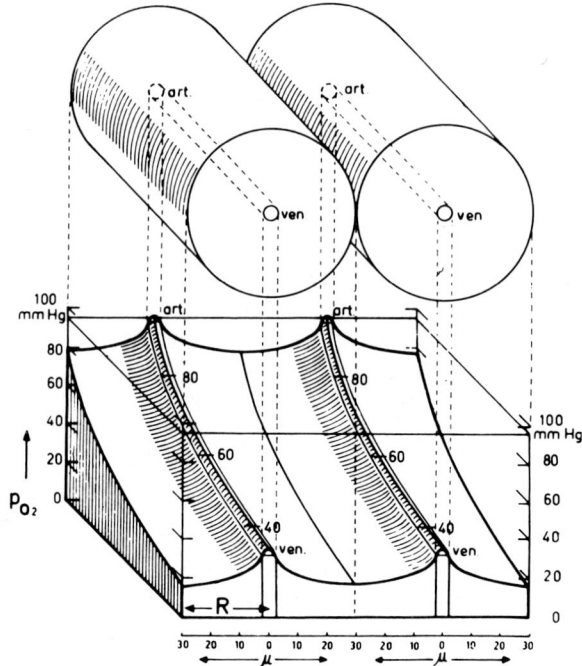

Figure 5–1. Model of adjacent tissue cylinders supplied by parallel capillaries. Blood is flowing from back to front. PO_2 is shown as a function of flow from artery to vein and as a function of distance from the capillary. (From Theus, G.: *In* Schade, J. P., and McMenemy, W. H. (eds.): Selective vulnerability of the brain in hypoxemia. Oxford, Blackwell Scientific Publications, 1963, pp. 27–35.)

tissues and the oxygen affinity of oxygen-utilizing enzymes.[8] Each capillary supplies a cylinder of tissue,[9] as depicted diagrammatically in Figure 5–1. There is a progressive fall in intravascular oxygen tension as red cells flow through the capillary as well as a progressive decrease in tissue oxygen tension with increasing distance from the capillary. This cylindrical model of Krogh[9] is a considerable oversimplification. It fails to account for gas exchange in larger-bore blood vessels and shunting from arterioles to venules, as well as variations in flow and geometry of capillaries and in local oxygen consumption.

In most tissues, the transport of oxygen into the cell is diffusion-limited. The transfer of O_2 through tissue protoplasm may be faster than through an equivalent thickness of water.[10] Skeletal and cardiac muscles have high concentrations of myoglobin within the cell cytoplasm. Because of its high O_2 affinity, this heme protein scavenges and stores oxygen. Myoglobin also facilitates the transport of oxygen into the cell.[11]

The PO_2 within the muscle cells of the myocardium has been estimated to be 5 mm

Hg.[12] A PO_2 of about 0.5 mm Hg is required for normal respiration of isolated mitochondria.[13] If O_2 tension falls below 0.1 mm Hg, tissue respiration ceases and cell death occurs. Thus, oxygen is generally present in excess at the mitochondrial level. Under normal circumstances, cellular respiration is thought to be limited by ADP levels rather than by availability of oxygen, substrate, or respiratory chain enzymes.

DETERMINANTS OF BLOOD OXYGEN AFFINITY

The oxygen affinity of hemoglobin is generally measured as P_{50}, the partial pressure of O_2 at which hemoglobin is half oxygenated (and half deoxygenated). Measurement of P_{50} takes no account of the shape of the O_2 dissociation curve (heme-heme interaction) but designates the position of the mid-portion of the curve. As O_2 affinity increases, P_{50} decreases and vice versa. Under physiologic conditions (T = 37°C, PCO_2 = 40 mm Hg, pH = 7.4), blood from normal males has a P_{50} of about 26 mm Hg. When measurements are made in the same laboratory, the standard error of the mean is relatively low (~ 0.4), indicating only a small amount of variation of P_{50} values in normals.[14]

Females tend to have somewhat higher P_{50} levels.[15] These values depend somewhat on the method used to measure whole blood oxygen affinity. As we will discuss in detail below, P_{50} values vary considerably in a number of clinical disorders. Widely varying oxygen affinities have been noted in the blood of different mammals (see Chapter 6).

The three primary determinants of oxygen affinity of whole blood are depicted in Figure 5–2:
1. Temperature
2. pH
3. Red cell 2,3-DPG

Temperature

The effects of temperature on the oxygen affinity of dilute solutions of purified hemoglobin A are discussed in detail in Chapter 3. The P_{50} of whole blood has a similar temperature dependence. For example, an increase in temperature from 20°C to 30°C increases the P_{50} of normal human blood 88 per cent[16, 16a] and that of phosphate-free hemoglobin A (pH 7.2) 93 per cent.[17] The relationship between temperature and oxygen affinity appears to be physiologically appropriate. Thus, under conditions of relative hypothermia, metabolic de-

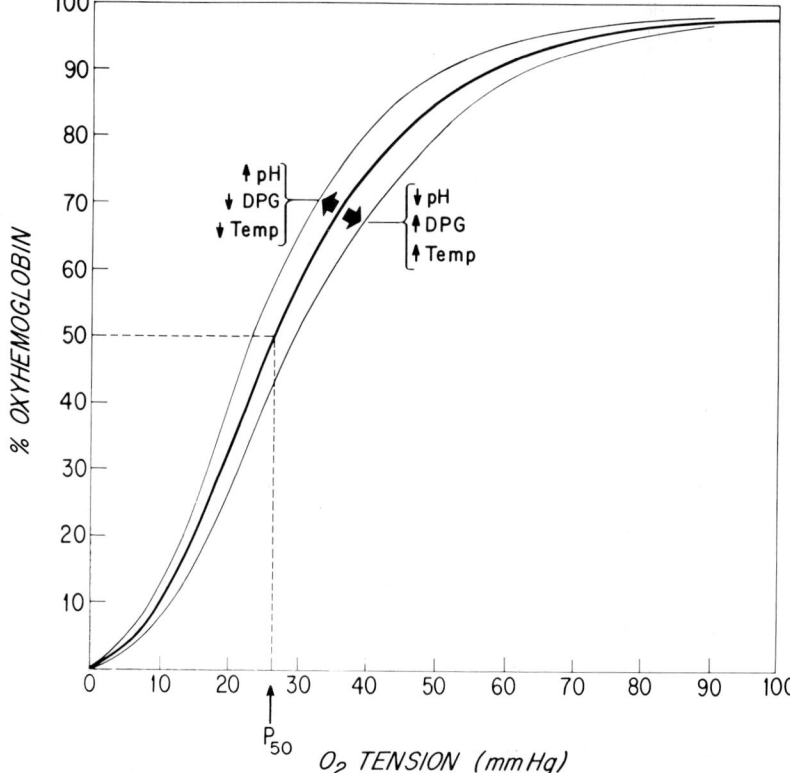

Figure 5–2. The principal factors that influence the position of the oxyhemoglobin dissociation curve.

mands are comparatively low. Because of the left shift in the oxygen dissociation curve, less oxygen is released to tissues. Conversely, if temperature is increased above normal, the right-shifted curve should result in increased oxygen unloading, helping to meet the higher requirement that fever is known to engender. In homeotherms such as man and other mammals, only a slight variation in body temperature is possible. In order for this phenomenon ($\Delta P_{50}/\Delta T$) to be physiologically significant, it must be pronounced. This is the case for human hemoglobin where a 10-degree increase in temperature results in nearly a twofold increase in P_{50}.

pH and the Bohr Effect

The Bohr effect can be readily demonstrated in whole blood by measurement of P_{50} at various values of pH. For normal human blood at 37°C, PCO_2 = 40 mm Hg, $\Delta \log P_{50}/\Delta pH \cong -0.5$.[16] This value happens to be quite close to that determined for dilute solutions of phosphate-free hemoglobin.[17] The stereochemical basis and the physiological significance of the Bohr effect have also been covered in Chapter 3. Because of the direct binding of CO_2 in the formation of carbamino complexes, the PCO_2 of whole blood can alter its oxygen affinity independent of its effect on pH (see below). Changes in red cell 2,3-DPG[17–20] and PCO_2[19, 20] can result in significant alteration in the Bohr effect.

2,3-DPG

The red cell's concentration of 2,3-DPG is the third important determinant of the oxygen affinity of whole blood. The level of 2,3-DPG in normal adult red cells is about 15 ± 1.5 µmoles per gram of hemoglobin or 5 mmoles per liter of packed red cells. There is some variability in red cell 2,3-DPG values depending on the methods employed. Females may have a slightly higher level than males. Young children (< 5 years old) tend to have a slightly higher red cell 2,3-DPG concentration than adults.[21] Conversely, red cell 2,3-DPG declines significantly in elderly individuals.[22]

Because whole blood oxygen binding curves are customarily determined under standard physiologic conditions (37°C, pH = 7.4, PCO_2 = 40 mm Hg), variations in P_{50} are due primarily to alterations in red cell 2,3-DPG.* This has been documented for blood specimens from patients with a variety of disorders associated with a wide range of values for O_2 affinity.[23] As expected from the measurements of oxygen equilibria of dilute hemoglobin solutions (see Chapter 3), the P_{50} of whole blood increases directly with 2,3-DPG (Fig. 5–3). However, this increase is significantly modified by the conditions that pertain in the intact red cell. The binding affinity of 2,3-DPG to deoxyhemoglobin may decrease significantly at hemoglobin concentrations approaching those of the red cell,[24, 25] although contrary results have been reported.[26] Furthermore, there is significant binding of 2,3-DPG to oxyhemoglobin under these circumstances.[27]

Two,3-DPG has an important effect on intracellular oxygen affinity that is independent of its preferential binding to deoxyhemoglobin. The fact that 2,3-DPG is a highly charged

---

*Unless otherwise stated, P_{50} values in this chapter have been corrected to standard conditions.

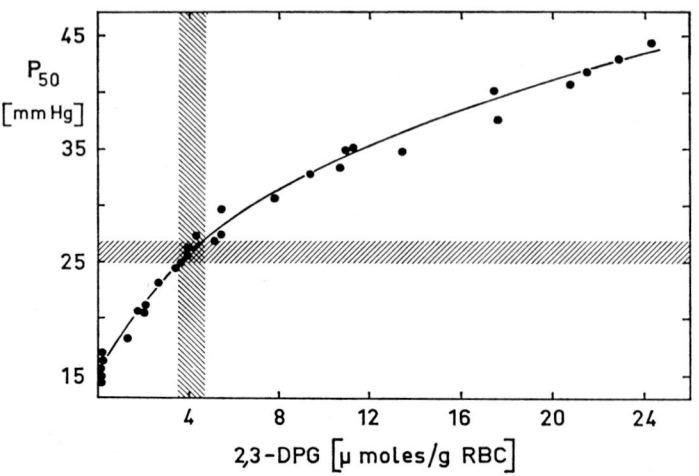

Figure 5–3. The relationship between red cell 2,3-DPG and oxygen affinity. Shaded area indicates normal range. (From Duhm, J.: Pfluegers Arch. 326:341, 1971.)

impermeant anion makes it strongly affect the difference in pH between the inside and outside of the cell.[28, 29] Indeed, 2,3-DPG and hemoglobin itself are the two principal impermeant anions of the erythrocyte. The distribution of permeant ions between these two compartments obeys the Gibbs-Donnan law, as expressed in the following equation:

$$\frac{H_e^+}{H_i^+} = \frac{OH_i^-}{OH_e^-} = 0.92 \frac{Cl_i^-}{Cl_e^-} = 0.93 \frac{(HCO_3^-)_i}{(HCO_3^-)_e}$$

where e = extracellular concentration and i = intracellular concentration. This relationship follows from a consideration of the chemical activities of the permeant ions at equilibrium and the requirement for electrical neutrality inside and outside the cell. The factors 0.92 and 0.93 are due to small differences between the activities and concentrations of the anions. Because of the presence of hemoglobin and 2,3-DPG inside the red cell, the ratio of intracellular to extracellular chloride ion is approximately 0.7. From the equation above, one can calculate that the pH_i should be about 0.20 unit lower than pH_e. This is in good agreement with direct measurements showing that at a plasma pH of 7.4 (37°C), the intracellular pH is about 7.20 to 7.25.[30]

Because of the Bohr effect, the oxygen affinity of whole blood is dependent not only on the plasma pH but also on the difference between intracellular and extracellular pH. This ΔpH increases in direct proportion to red cell 2,3-DPG.[31, 32] Red cells having a sixfold increase in 2,3-DPG have an intracellular pH of 6.85 when extracellular pH is 7.40. Thus, 2,3-DPG has a dual effect in lowering oxygen affinity: It interacts directly with hemoglobin, and it lowers intracellular pH relative to extracellular pH. As shown in Figure 5–3, at levels greater than 5 mmoles per liter of packed red cells, 2,3-DPG has a smaller effect on oxygen affinity that is due almost entirely to a progressive lowering of intracellular pH. These considerations explain why the relationship between red cell 2,3-DPG and P_{50} shown in Figure 5–3 is biphasic.

Other Determinants of Red Cell Oxygen Affinity

In comparison with temperature, pH, and red cell 2,3-DPG, other factors are much less important determinants of red cell oxygen affinity.

1. *Carbon dioxide* affects red cell oxygen

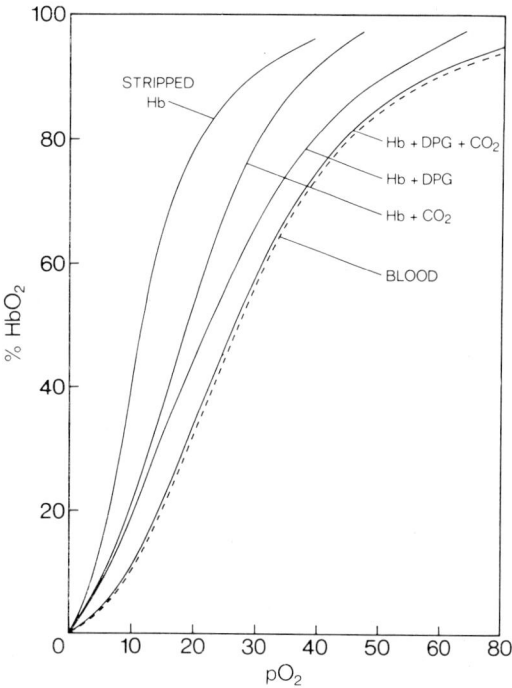

Figure 5–4. The effect of 2,3-DPG and CO_2 on the oxygen binding of phosphate-free human hemoglobin (37°C, pH 7.2). At physiologic concentrations of 2,3-DPG and PCO_2, the oxygen affinity of the hemoglobin solution is very close to that of the intact red cell. (From Kilmartin, J. V., and Rossi-Bernardi, L.: Physiol. Rev. 53:836, 1973.)

affinity independent of its contribution to intracellular pH. The interaction between CO_2 and hemoglobin to form the carbamino complex is discussed in Chapter 3. Under physiologic conditions, the PCO_2 of 40 mm Hg contributes significantly to the P_{50} of normal blood. As shown in Figure 5–4, the P_{50} of a concentrated solution of stripped (phosphate-free) hemoglobin, at pH 7.2, increases from 10 mm Hg to 20 mm Hg with the addition of 2,3-DPG (1.2 moles per hemoglobin tetramer).[33] If the PCO_2 of this solution is then increased from 0 to 40 mm Hg and the pH is kept at 7.2, the P_{50} of the solution rises to 25 mm Hg. This is very close to the value obtained for normal human blood (26 mm Hg). From these results, it is apparent that wide deviations of PCO_2 from normal would be required to affect significantly the oxygen affinity of red cells directly through the formation of carbamino complexes. The relatively narrow range of PCO_2 values encountered in various clinical states would have little direct influence on whole blood oxygen affinity. The indirect effect of PCO_2 on pH is much more significant.

2. *ATP* is the second most abundant organic phosphate in human red cells. Normally, its

concentration is about one-fourth that of 2,3-DPG. ATP per se is almost as strong a modifier of hemoglobin as 2,3-DPG.[34-36] However, because ATP has a much higher affinity for divalent cations than has 2,3-DPG, the bulk of red cell ATP is bound to magnesium ion.[27, 36, 37] The MgATP complex has no significant effect on the oxygenation of hemoglobin.[36] Thus, red cell ATP probably has no effect on the oxygen affinity of whole blood. In contrast to human red cells, ATP is the prime mediator of oxygen affinity of fishes and most amphibians (see Chapter 6).

3. *MCHC* (the mean corpuscular hemoglobin concentration) probably has a small effect on the oxygen affinity of red cells. The oxygen affinity of phosphate-free hemoglobin decreases slightly with increasing hemoglobin concentration.[17] Although a significant positive correlation between MCHC and P_{50} has been reported,[38] its functional significance is uncertain. When normal red cells were artificially swollen and contracted by suspension in hypotonic and hypertonic media, no significant change in P_{50} was observed when corrections were made for changes in intracellular pH.[39, 40] These results indicate that the oxygen affinity of red cells is not significantly affected by changes in the intracellular concentration of hemoglobin.

4. *Carboxyhemoglobin.* Normal red cells contain about 0.5 per cent carboxyhemoglobin, owing to the endogenous production of carbon monoxide. Smokers and individuals exposed to high levels of carbon monoxide in the air will have much higher levels of carboxyhemoglobin (2 to 10 per cent). As explained in Chapter 17, carboxyhemoglobin causes a significant increase in oxygen affinity.

From these considerations, one would conclude that the P_{50} of normal human red cells is determined within rather narrow limits by temperature, plasma pH, PCO_2, and red cell 2,3-DPG. Because all but the last are fixed experimentally or corrected for in the measurement of oxygen binding to whole blood, it follows that variations in P_{50} are dependent primarily on red cell 2,3-DPG. In general, this appears to be true in a wide variety of clinical settings. Nevertheless, some interesting exceptions have been noted. Red cells from the fetus and the newborn have increased oxygen affinity because of impaired interaction between 2,3-DPG and hemoglobin F (see Chapters 3 and 4). The red cells of patients with diabetes mellitus have a slightly lower P_{50} than one would predict from red cell 2,3-DPG levels,[41] probably related to the presence of increased concentration of hemoglobin A_{Ic}.[42, 43] Hemoglobin A_{Ic} also fails to interact normally with 2,3-DPG[44] (see Chapter 4). Erythrocytes of patients with hereditary spherocytosis (HS) have somewhat higher P_{50} values than one would expect from red cell 2,3-DPG levels.[45] If the human red cell contains structurally abnormal hemoglobin, its oxygen binding properties may be significantly altered. This includes many of the hemoglobin variants (see Chapters 13 to 15) as well as acquired abnormalities in hemoglobin structure.

Red cell oxygen affinity also may be altered in the presence of certain *exogenous agents*. Several of these influence the oxygenation of the red cell by affecting intracellular pH. For example, the P_{50} of red cells is promptly and significantly increased by the addition of small amounts of propranolol (1 to 5×10^{-4} M),[46, 47] which has no effect on the oxygen affinity of hemoglobin solutions. Propranolol appears to lower red cell oxygen affinity by causing a leakage of potassium ions, thus lowering the pH inside the cell because of an alteration in the Donnan equilibrium.[48] The decrease in oxygen affinity observed after the addition of hypertonic solutions of neutral salts[49, 50] can also be explained by a relative decrease in intracellular pH.[40] High concentrations of iodinated dyes, used as contrast media in radiology, *increase* blood oxygen affinity.[51] These agents are relatively impermeant anions that decrease the pH gradient between the inside and outside of the red cell, an effect opposite to that of propranolol.[52, 53]

A number of exogenous agents are known to increase the oxygen affinity of intact red cells. Cyanate increases oxygen affinity by carbamylating the N-terminal amino groups of α and β chains, sites that are crucial to the molecule's function.[54, 55] Small concentrations (1.5 mM) of zinc chloride increase the oxygen affinity of both intact red cells and hemoglobin solutions.[56] Red cell oxygen affinity is also increased in a hyperbaric environment (50 Atm).[57] The mechanisms for these last two observations have not yet been worked out.

METABOLIC CONTROL OF RED CELL 2,3-DPG

Because the level of 2,3-DPG within the red cell is a prime determinant of whole blood oxygen affinity, it is appropriate to examine the factors involved in the regulation of this glycolytic intermediate. This information is necessary for an understanding of how the concentration of red cell 2,3-DPG changes in response to environmental perturbations.

Red Cell Metabolism

The red cell's sole *raison d'être* is the efficient transport of oxygen from lung to tissues and CO_2 in the reverse direction. As emphasized in the preceding section, the red cell is especially well engineered for this purpose. It has differentiated to the extent that only essential metabolic pathways are in operation. Thus, the adult erythrocyte has a relatively simple organization: a metabolically active membrane enclosing a homogeneous cytoplasm that contains by weight 34 per cent hemoglobin and about 2 per cent nonheme proteins, primarily carbonic anhydrase and glycolytic enzymes. The red cell has very limited metabolic obligations: (a) maintenance of the sodium-potassium pump in order to prevent colloid osmotic lysis (see above); (b) maintenance of hemoglobin in the reduced (ferrous) state, because the oxidized form, methemoglobin (ferrihemoglobin), is unable to bind oxygen; (c) repair of the membrane by acylation of phospholipids[58]; and (d) protection of the cell membrane and interior against oxidant stress. These functions can be accomplished with a relatively low expenditure of ATP (the metabolic currency of the cell) and reducing equivalents, NADH and NADPH.

During its maturation in the bone marrow, the red cell loses it organelles and, with them, the capability for mitochondrial respiration and fatty acid and protein synthesis. Only two metabolic pathways remain intact in the mature erythrocyte: anaerobic glycolysis (the Embden-Meyerhof pathway) and the pentose phosphate pathway (hexose monophosphate shunt). These metabolic processes are diagrammed in Figure 5–5. Under physiologic conditions, glucose is the only important substrate for red cell metabolism. It enters the cell by facilitated diffusion. Once phosphorylated, the glycolytic intermediates are locked within the cell until they are metabolized to pyruvate and lactate. These two non-phosphorylated products are free to diffuse out of the red cell and constitute the prime source of plasma pyruvate and lactate under resting conditions.

In the red cell, 2,3-DPG is by far the most abundant organic phosphate. In this respect, the red cell differs dramatically from other tissues in which 2,3-DPG is present only in the minute concentration that is required for it to serve as a cofactor in the monophosphoglycerate mutase reaction (see Figure 5–6).

Regulation of Red Cell 2,3-DPG

During red cell glycolysis, the intermediate 1,3-diphosphoglycerate is at a crossroad. As depicted in Figure 5–5, it can be converted to 3-phosphoglycerate (3-PG) with the concomitant conversion of ADP to ATP, or it can be isomerized to 2,3-DPG. The latter reaction is energetically wasteful, involving the loss of a high-energy phosphate bond. By hydrolysis, 2,3-DPG is catabolized to 3-phosphoglycerate and inorganic phosphate. These two reactions constitute the Rapoport-Luebering shunt[59] (Fig. 5–6).

In essence, the level of red cell 2,3-DPG is determined by three factors: (1) the rate of formation of substrate 1,3-DPG; (2) the relative amount of 1,3-DPG going into the Rapoport-Luebering shunt versus that undergoing conventional glycolysis; and (3) the rate at which 2,3-DPG is hydrolyzed. It is apparent that the concentration of 2,3-DPG is the resultant of a complex array of independent and interdependent factors, a number of which are altered by environmental stimuli. We shall consider these in order.

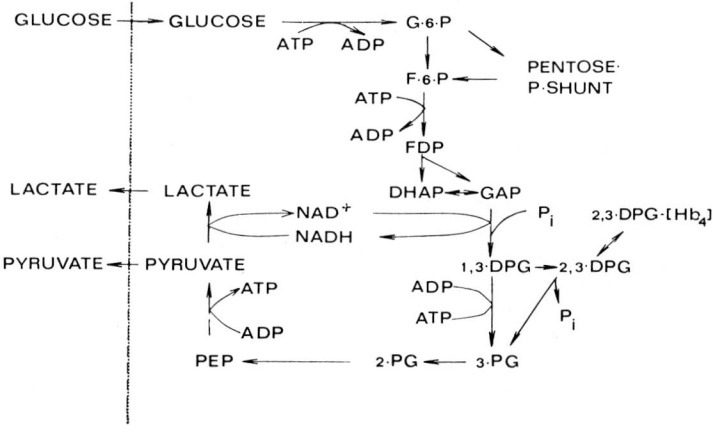

Figure 5–5. Glycolytic pathway within red cells. Glucose enters the red cell and is metabolized to lactate and pyruvate, which escape from the cell. (From Rörth, M.: Ser. Haematol. 5:1, 1972.)

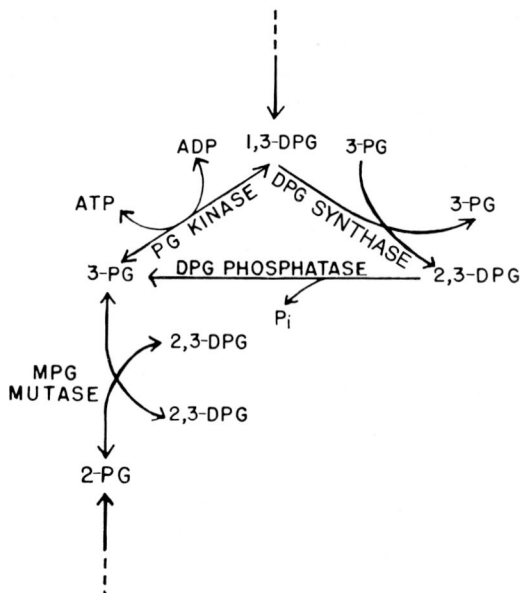

Figure 5–6. The Rapoport-Luebering cycle. 1,3-Diphosphoglycerate (1,3-DPG) can be isomerized to 2,3-DPG or, alternatively, can be converted directly to 3-phosphoglycerate (3-PG) with the formation of one equivalent of ATP. (Modified from Keitt, A. S.: Am. J. Med. *41*:762, 1966.)

Glycolysis

The synthesis of 2,3-DPG in the red cell is directly dependent on the rate of glycolysis—i.e., the rate at which glucose is converted to lactate. From measurements of various glycolytic intermediates before and after a given change in incubation conditions, one can demonstrate which enzymatic steps of the glycolytic sequence remain in equilibrium and which are perturbed by the change. The latter, called crossover points, indicate those enzymes that are subject to metabolic control.[60] In the red cell, phosphofructokinase (PFK) is a particularly sensitive step. The positive and negative effectors that regulate the activity of this enzyme are shown by the following reaction:

$$\text{Fructose-6-PO}_4 + \text{MgATP} \xrightarrow[-:\text{ATP, H}^+]{+:\text{ADP, P}_i}$$

$$\text{Fructose-1,6-diphosphate} + \text{MgADP}$$

This reaction is unusual in that it is activated by product (ADP) and inhibited by substrate (ATP). In addition, PFK is activated by inorganic phosphate and inhibited by hydrogen ions. Thus, the rate of red cell glycolysis varies directly with pH and with inorganic phosphate. Both *in vivo* (in appropriate clinical states discussed below) and *in vitro*, corresponding changes in red cell 2,3-DPG have been observed.[61, 62]

The ratio of NAD to NADH is an important determinant of the rate of synthesis of 1,3-DPG (see Figure 5–5). Thus, the incubation of red cells with appropriate oxidants such as pyruvate[23, 31] or methylene blue[63] will increase this ratio and, by enhancing levels of 1,3-DPG, will promote synthesis of red cell 2,3-DPG. This observation has been exploited in the design of a suitable medium for preservation of red cells (see below).

Which of the two reaction pathways 1,3-DPG takes is determined in part by the ratio of ADP to ATP. A relative increase in ADP will favor the conversion of 1,3-DPG to 3-phosphoglycerate. Conversely, if ADP is relatively decreased, the synthesis of 2,3-DPG will be favored. This probably explains why levels of red cell 2,3-DPG and ATP are often reciprocal. The ADP/ATP ratio depends on a complex interaction between the glycolytic rate and the metabolic demands of the cell.

Enzymology of 2,3-DPG Synthesis and Degradation*

The level of 2,3-DPG also depends on the rates of its synthesis and breakdown according to the following overall reactions:

$$1,3\text{-DPG} \xrightarrow{\text{DPG synthase}\dagger} 2,3\text{-DPG}$$

$$2,3\text{-DPG} + \text{H}_2\text{O} \xrightarrow{\text{``DPG phosphatase''}} 3\text{-PG} + \text{P}_i$$

There is convincing evidence that a single enzyme is responsible for both the synthesis (synthase†) and hydrolysis ("phosphatase") of 2,3-DPG.[64, 65] This enzyme is called bisphosphoglycerate synthase (or bisphosphoglycerate synthase-phosphatase[65]). In addition, this enzyme is capable of catalyzing, albeit weakly, the conversion of 3-phosphoglycerate to 2-phosphoglycerate:

$$3\text{-PG} \xrightarrow{\text{``PG mutase''}} 2\text{-PG}$$

The red cell contains another enzyme protein called phosphoglycerate mutase[66] (or

---

*The enzymology of 2,3-DPG is discussed in considerably more detail in reviews by Chiba and Sasaki[65] and by Z. B. Rose.[66]

†This enzyme was formerly designated diphosphoglycerate mutase.

Table 5–1. COMPARISON OF RATES OF THE THREE REACTIONS CATALYZED BY DIPHOSPHOGLYCERATE SYNTHASE (DPGS) AND MONOPHOSPHOGLYCERATE MUTASE (MPGM)*

Reaction			Name	k_{cat}^a (sec^{-1})	
				MPGM[b]	DPGS[c]
3-PG	$\xrightarrow{2,3-DPG}$	2-PG	Mutase	1333	1.7
1,3-DPG	$\longrightarrow$	2,3-DPG	Synthase	0.4	12.5
2,3-DPG	$\longrightarrow$	PG + P$_i$	Phosphatase	2.78[d]	2.57[d]

*From Rose, Z. B.: Adv. Enzymol. 51:211, 1980.
[a]k_{cat} values are for subunits of about 30,000 daltons. Rates were determined at pH 7.5, 25°C.
[b]Chicken muscle enzyme.
[c]Horse red blood cell enzyme.
[d]Activated by glycolate-2-P.

monophosphoglycerate mutase) that is primarily responsible for the conversion of 3-PG to 2-PG. This protein is also capable of catalyzing the other two reactions listed above. Thus, the red cell contains two distinct enzyme proteins, each of which is trifunctional for all three reactions. The relative activities of the two enzymes for these three reactions are shown in Table 5–1. It is apparent that bisphosphoglycerate synthase is the enzyme responsible for the conversion of 1,3-DPG to 2,3-DPG. The phosphatase activities of the two enzymes are similar and are enhanced by a variety of anions,[67, 68] particularly glycolate-2-phosphate.[69] Because the number of molecules of bisphosphoglycerate synthase in normal red cells greatly exceeds that of monophosphoglycerate mutase, the former enzyme is primarily responsible for the hydrolysis of 2,3-DPG. The phosphatase activity of bisphosphoglycerate synthase is greatly stimulated by certain sulfur-containing anions, particularly bisulfite and dithionite.[68] The addition of these anions to a red cell suspension results in rapid depletion of red cell 2,3-DPG.[70]

The two enzymes have striking similarities. Each is a dysmutase. The substrate becomes cofactor, while another molecule of the cofactor becomes product:

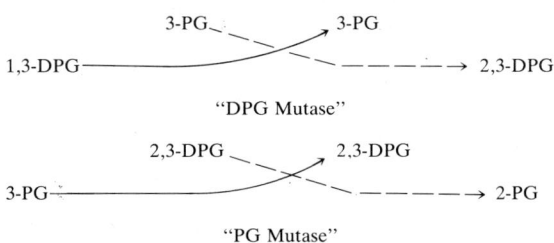

Both enzymes can become phosphorylated by transfer of a phosphate group from either 1,3-DPG or 2,3-DPG.[66, 71] As shown in the scheme in Figure 5–7, the fate of the phosphorylated complex depends on the availability of acceptors.[66] PG will incorporate the phosphate from the phospho-enzyme to form 2,3-DPG. On the other hand, glycolate-2-phosphate and other anions will allow hydrolysis of the protein-bound phosphate, resulting in "phosphatase" activity.

These two enzymes share significant structural features. There is striking homology in the primary amino acid sequence of the phosphorylated peptides of the two proteins.[71] In phosphoglycerate mutase, the catalytic site involves a rosette of positively charged residues, reminiscent of the 2,3-DPG binding site of deoxyhemoglobin. As shown in Figure 5–8, a specific histidine residue becomes phosphorylated. It is likely that the other protein, bisphosphoglycerate synthase, has a similar active site.

DPG Synthase Activity

The level of 2,3-DPG in red cells is determined in part by the activity of the synthase. This activity is markedly diminished in red cells of cats and ruminants, which contain very low amounts of 2,3-DPG (< 0.5 mmoles/liter

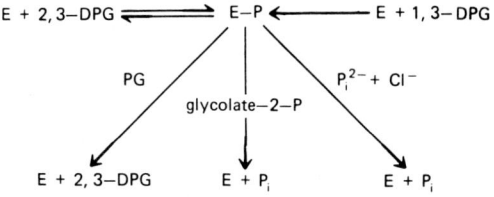

Figure 5–7. Generalized scheme for the mechanism of the two trifunctional enzymes, bisphosphoglycerate synthase and phosphoglycerate mutase. The enzyme becomes phosphorylated by phosphoryl groups from either 2,3-DPG or 1,3-DPG (glycerate-1,3-P$_2$). In the presence of 3-PG, the phosphorylated enzyme transfers its phosphate to form 2,3-DPG (synthase activity). Alternatively, in the presence of glycolate-2-P or other anions, the phosphate-enzyme bond is hydrolyzed, resulting in net "phosphatase activity." (From Rose, Z. B.: Adv. Enzymol. 51:211, 1980.)

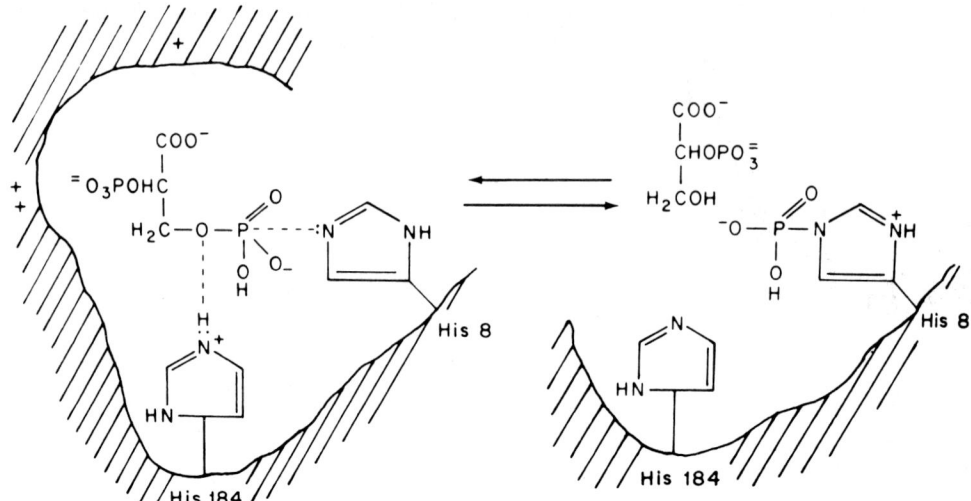

Figure 5–8. Diagram of active site of phosphoglycerate mutase in which a phosphoenzyme intermediate serves as a precursor to phosphorylation (←——) or as a product of hydrolysis (——→) ("phosphatase activity"). (From Rose, Z. B.: Adv. Enzymol. *51*:211, 1980.)

of red blood cells)[72] (see Chapter 6). Indeed, analysis of the enzyme in red cells of various mammals by means of a monospecific precipitating antibody failed to reveal any detectable enzyme protein in the adult goat.[73] Deficiency of "DPG mutase" activity of human red cells has been encountered in several kindred. There is considerable variability in the hematological status of affected individuals. Surprisingly, in families in which there is a partial deficiency of enzyme, affected individuals tend to have varying degrees of hemolysis.[74–75a] In contrast, in two individuals with absent enzyme activity, there was erythrocytosis (due to very low red cell 2,3-DPG and therefore increased oxygen affinity) but no detectable hemolysis.[73, 76] More information on variant enzymes is needed in order to determine factors affecting red cell life span.

DPG synthase activity is induced during erythroid differentiation.[76a] The levels of both the enzyme activity and 2,3-DPG increase in parallel during maturation of erythroid precursor cells from rabbit bone marrow.[77] Both enzyme and product are also increased when murine (Friend)[78] or human (K562)[78a] leukemia cell lines are induced toward erythroid differentiation.

Studies on purified DPG synthase are in reasonably good agreement with observations on intact red cells. The maximum velocity of the enzyme for 2,3-DPG synthesis is 240 μmoles/hr/ml of packed red cells.[79] In comparison, the estimated rate in normal human red cells under physiologic conditions is 0.17 μmole/hr/ml, which is about 7 per cent of the glycolytic rate. This estimate is in reasonable agreement with careful measurements of metabolic intermediates in human red cells that indicate that 10 to 20 per cent of glycolysis passes through the Rapoport-Luebering cycle.[80, 81] The primary reason why the synthesis of 2,3-DPG falls so far short of the maximal velocity of DPG synthase is that the enzyme is markedly inhibited by its product, 2,3-DPG.[82] The activity of the synthase increases directly with pH up to pH 9.75.[82, 83] The increase in red cell 2,3-DPG induced by alkalosis is probably due in part to this pH effect on the synthase as well as the stimulation to glycolysis discussed above.

As mentioned above, a number of anions stimulate the "phosphatase" activity of DPG synthase.[67, 69] In the normal intact cell, inorganic phosphate and chloride contribute to about 20 per cent of the activation of the phosphatase.[69] Part of the remaining 80 per cent of the activation appears to be due to small concentrations (2 to 5 μM) of glycolate-2-phosphate. This compound appears to be formed by phosphorylation of glycolate via pyruvate kinase. Thus, the increased amount of 2,3-DPG in the red cells of patients with pyruvate kinase deficiency can be explained in part by decreased activation of 2,3-DPG phosphatase. Glycolate-2-phosphate is hydrolyzed by a specific phosphatase, phosphoglycolate phosphatase.[84] Theoretically, the level of glycolate-2-phosphate could be an important independent regulator of red cell 2,3-DPG.[79]

However, the lack of correlation between phosphoglycolate phosphatase activity and levels of 2,3-DPG in anemic patients and experimental animals[84a] argues against this possibility.

Metabolic "Functions" of 2,3-DPG

It is apparent that 2,3-DPG fulfills a number of physiologic and metabolic functions in the erythrocyte.

Regulation of Oxygen Affinity. By far the most important function, of course, is the reduction of oxygen affinity by direct binding to a specific site on hemoglobin. Because it is a highly charged impermeant anion, 2,3-DPG effectively lowers intracellular pH and thereby causes a further reduction in oxygen affinity. These two phenomena are discussed in detail above.

Effects on Red Cell Metabolism. Because 2,3-DPG is present in such high concentrations in the red cell, it may serve as an energy source under certain circumstances such as during storage of bank blood (see below). In addition, 2,3-DPG affects the activity of a number of other red cell enzymes. Among the glycolytic enzymes, it inhibits hexokinase[85-88] (cf. reference 89), phosphofructokinase[87, 88] (cf. reference 90), aldolase,[87] glyceraldehyde-3-phosphate dehydrogenase,[87] and phosphoglucomutase.[87] The first four of these are proximal to 2,3-DPG synthesis. Thus, the inhibition of these enzymes may serve as a form of negative feedback, controlling 2,3-DPG formation.[87] In addition, other red cell enzymes are inhibited by 2,3-DPG, including AMP deaminase,[91, 92] phosphoribosyl pyrophosphate synthetase,[93, 94] and IMP:pyrophosphate phosphoribosyl transferase.[94] By inhibiting the catabolism of AMP, 2,3-DPG helps to preserve the red cell pool of adenine nucleotides.

Because 2,3-DPG can chelate with divalent cations, it may play a role in determining the concentration of free and bound magnesium ion within the red cell. Hemoglobin and Mg^{++} can be considered as competitors for binding to the two main organic phosphates, 2,3-DPG and ATP. From a knowledge of the stability constants for the various complexes under physiologic conditions, the distribution of the various species in the oxygenated and deoxygenated red cell can be estimated[36, 95, 96] (Fig. 5–9). The inhibition by 2,3-DPG of phosphofructokinase may be due to its ability to chelate magnesium and thus reduce the concentration of the substrate MgATP. The increase in free magnesium with deoxygenation may increase the activity of reactions involving MgADP, such as pyruvate kinase.

Other Effects. The initiation of protein synthesis in erythroid cells may be influenced by 2,3-DPG.[97] Physiologic levels of 2,3-DPG inhibit the phosphorylation of the β subunits of initiation factor 2 (eIF-2) by casein kinase II. The importance of the phosphorylation state of βeIF-2 is not yet established.

Finally, the stability of the red cell membrane appears to be influenced by the circulation of 2,3-DPG. The interaction of intrinsic membrane proteins such as the anion channel (Band 3) and glycophorin with the cytoskeleton is weakened by polyanions such as inositol triphosphate and 2,3-DPG.[98] The lateral mobility of the intrinsic proteins is significantly enhanced by these organic phosphates.

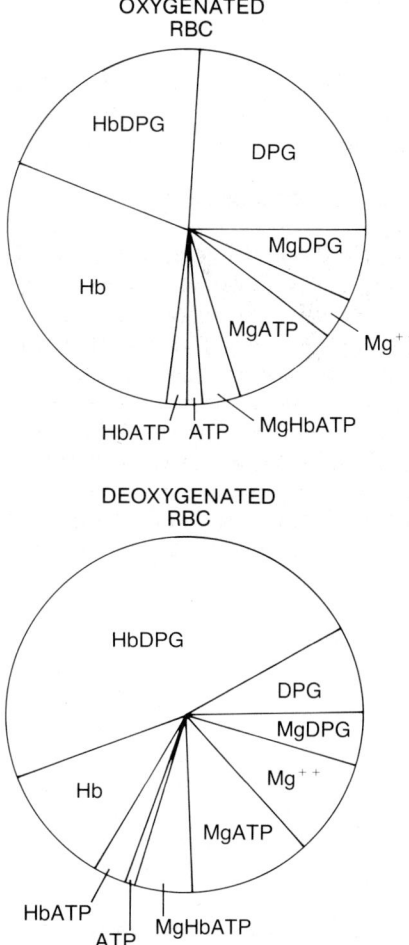

Figure 5–9. Distribution of hemoglobin, 2,3-DPG, ATP, magnesium ion, and their respective complexes in human erythrocytes. (These results are the mean values calculated from the data of Berger, H., et al.: Eur. J. Biochem. 38:553, 1973, and Gupta, R. K., et al.: J. Biol. Chem. 253:6172, 1978.)

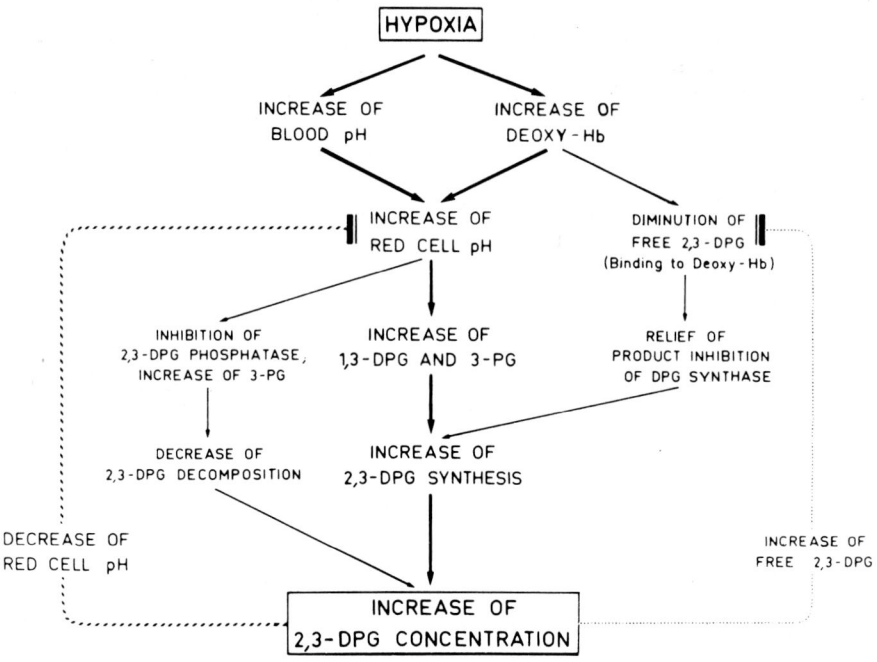

Figure 5–10. Probable mechanisms for increased red cell 2,3-DPG induced by hypoxia. (Courtesy of Dr. J. Dühm.)

2,3-DPG and Hypoxia

One of the most intriguing features of the metabolic control of red cell 2,3-DPG is the fact that this organic phosphate becomes elevated in various pathological and experimental states of hypoxia. Moreover, this change is often physiologically appropriate, because the resultant shift to the right in the oxygen dissociation curve may increase oxygen delivery to tissues. Two mechanisms have been proposed for this adaptation (Fig. 5–10). Hypoxia is generally accompanied by a respiratory alkalosis. In addition, enhanced extraction of oxygen during capillary circulation results in a further increase in red cell pH because of proton binding by deoxyhemoglobin. As discussed above, red cell 2,3-DPG increases primarily because alkalosis stimulates glycolysis but also because of a direct effect of pH on diphosphoglycerate synthase. It has been shown both in man[99] and in experimental animals[100] that acute hypoxia will not induce an increase in red cell 2,3-DPG if alkalosis is prevented.

In addition, the increase in deoxyhemoglobin in hypoxic states decreases the level of free 2,3-DPG in the red cell (Fig. 5–10). This affords partial relief of the strong inhibition that 2,3-DPG exerts on its own synthesis. Applying the Michaelis-Menten equation for competitive inhibition to the diphosphoglycerate synthase reaction,*

$$v = \frac{V_{max}}{1 + \dfrac{K_m}{(1,3\text{-DPG})}\left(1 + \dfrac{2,3\text{-DPG}}{K_i}\right)},$$

it can be calculated that the velocity of the enzyme would be enhanced about 130 per cent going from the oxygenated to the completely deoxygenated state. Even in severe hypoxemia, oxygen extraction is seldom greater than 50 per cent (except in the coronary circulation). Thus, the increase in 2,3-DPG synthesis induced by deoxygenation *in vivo* would be correspondingly less. Oski and colleagues[101] have shown that under conditions in which pH has been carefully controlled, deoxygenation of hemoglobin A favors the synthesis of 2,3-DPG. In a parallel experiment, this augmentation was not observed with hemoglobin F, presumably because it fails to bind strongly to 2,3-DPG. These observations are difficult to

---

*K_m (1,3-DPG) = 3.1 µM; K_i (2,3-DPG) = 20 µM[83]; concentration of 1,3-DPG = 0.7 µM[104]; and 2,3-DPG = 3190 µM in oxygenated red cells and 1190 µM in deoxygenated red cells.[96] The rate equation is an approximation in which the term including 3-PG has been omitted; that term would be insignificant because 3-PG is always saturating.

reconcile with the *in vivo* experiments cited above[99, 100] or the *in vitro* data cited below.[100]

It is likely that the former mechanism (pH increase) is the more important means by which hypoxia increases red cell 2,3-DPG. Duhm and Gerlach[100] found that in red cells containing low levels of 2,3-DPG but high levels of the triose phosphate precursors, deoxygenation made no difference in the rate of 2,3-DPG formation.

Another approach to this question is to examine 2,3-DPG levels in individuals who are hypoxic and yet do not have increased oxygen extraction. For example, there are families in which polycythemia accompanies the presence of a hemoglobin variant with increased oxygen affinity (see Chapter 14). Red cell 2,3-DPG levels have been measured in about six of these and have been consistently normal.[102] In like manner, carbon monoxide can cause a significant shift to the left in the oxygen dissociation curve. Animals chronically exposed to carbon monoxide were found to have increased red cell 2,3-DPG.[103] A patient with congenital methemoglobinemia due to diaphorase I deficiency had a 70 per cent increase in 2,3-DPG, which approached normal on treatment with methylene blue.[105] These diverse observations are difficult to reconcile and therefore do not provide firm evidence concerning the mechanism by which hypoxia induces increased red cell 2,3-DPG. Red cells with increased O_2 affinity lack both the pH increment contributed by the Bohr effect and the enhanced binding of 2,3-DPG by deoxyhemoglobin.

Even though chronic hypoxemia results in marked changes in red cell 2,3-DPG, it is unlikely that the transient oxygenation and deoxygenation of blood circulating through the lungs and tissues have any significant bearing on red cell metabolism. The turnover of most enzymatic reactions is too slow to be influenced by any such oscillations in pH, free 2,3-DPG, and so on. Reports showing significantly lower 2,3-DPG in arterial red cells compared with venous red cells[106, 107] have not been confirmed in another laboratory.[108] This discrepancy could be due to slight changes in red cell 2,3-DPG that may occur between drawing the blood and preparing the protein-free extract.

In Vivo Red Cell Aging

During the red cell's 120-day life span, oxygen affinity increases considerably.[109] Red cells become more dense as they age *in vivo*. Accordingly, "young" and "old" red cells can be separated by centrifugation. Young (top layer) red cells have a P_{50} of 33.5 mm Hg compared with a P_{50} of 27 mm Hg for old (bottom layer) cells.[109] By developing a special microspectrophotometric technique for measuring the oxygen affinity of individual red cells, Waldeck[110] obtained a distribution of P_{50} values that approximate this range. After hemolysates of young and old cells are dialyzed against a salt solution, there is no longer any difference in oxygen affinity.[111] The dialyzable substance that accounts for the difference in P_{50} is 2,3-DPG.[112] Several studies have shown significantly higher levels of 2,3-DPG in young cells compared with old red cells[113–115] (cf. reference 116). These differences adequately explain the observed change in P_{50} with red cell aging. The fact that 2,3-DPG of normal whole blood specimens does not correlate with an age-related enzyme (erythrocyte glutamic-oxaloacetic transaminase)[117] cannot be considered as evidence to the contrary.

ALTERATIONS OF OXYGEN AFFINITY IN VARIOUS CLINICAL STATES

Over the past few decades, whole blood oxygen affinity has been measured in a wide variety of clinical disorders. One conclusion that emerges from these studies is that oxygen affinity is decreased in patients with various types of hypoxia. In all instances, the "shift to the right" has been found to be due to increased red cell 2,3-DPG. As discussed in the previous section, the mechanism by which this phenomenon occurs is not fully understood. Yet, as shown in Figure 5–11, it may serve as an adaptation to hypoxia. In certain clinical situations (described below), the decreased oxygen affinity of the blood enables an increased amount of oxygen to be unloaded to tissues. In this section, we will consider a number of adaptational and clinical situations in which displacement of the oxygen dissociation curve has been reported.

Hypoxic States

Anemia

From the relationship $VO_2 = 0.139 \cdot Q \cdot Hb \cdot (S_AO_2 - S_{\bar{V}}O_2)$, it is apparent that if there is a primary deficit in red cell mass (Hb), oxygen delivery to an organ or tissue (VO_2) can be maintained by an increase in blood flow or in

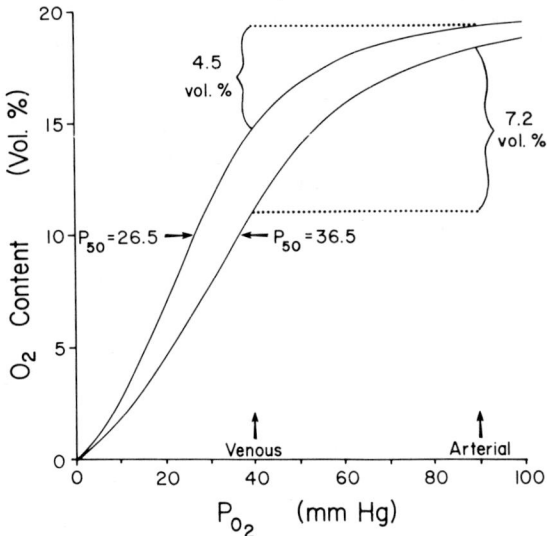

Figure 5–11. Enhancement of oxygen unloading due to a decrease in red cell oxygen affinity. Normal oxygen binding curve: P_{50} = 26.5 mm Hg; right-shifted curve: P_{50} = 36.5 mm Hg. (From Klocke, R. A.: Chest 62(Suppl):79S, 1972.)

oxygen unloading. Patients with mild or moderate anemia maintain a normal cardiac output. If the packed cell volume falls below 25 per cent, cardiac output increases in proportion to the severity of the anemia. However, even with lesser degrees of anemia, alterations in the distribution of blood flow occur so that circulation to vital organs is enhanced. The second mode of compensation, increased oxygen extraction, is made possible by a decrease in whole blood oxygen affinity. Unlike individuals at altitude and those with chronic lung disease or cyanotic heart defects (discussed below), anemic patients have normal arterial oxygen saturation. Therefore, a "shift to the right" permits a steeper portion of the oxygen dissociation curve to be encompassed. It is apparent from the oxygen dissociation curves shown in Figure 5–12 that in the anemic patient the "shift to the right" compensates in part for the decrease in red cell mass. The patient shown in this figure has a hemoglobin level that is half normal. However, because of this compensation, the amount of oxygen unloaded at a given venous PO_2 is 73 per cent normal.

In patients with anemias of differing etiology and severity, red cell 2,3-DPG varies inversely with hemoglobin concentration.[116, 118–120] Indeed, this correlation has even been established in normal subjects.[120, 121] Thus, the product of hemoglobin concentration and oxygen extraction is fixed within rather narrow limits. Card and Brain[21] have postulated that the hemoglobin and red cell mass in children are set at a slightly decreased level because oxygen unloading is increased owing to a modest reduction in oxygen affinity.

Red cell age probably has a bearing on the level of 2,3-DPG in anemic patients. Because 2,3-DPG decreases as cells age (see above), patients with hemolysis should have higher levels than those with anemia of similar severity due to failure of red cell production. Clinical surveys indicate that this is true[122, 123] (Table 5–2). Nevertheless, patients with aplastic anemia and presumably a near-normal mean red cell age have elevated 2,3-DPG. This is observed even in patients who are dependent on transfusions of 2,3-DPG–depleted red cells.[124]

Anemic patients often have a slight respiratory alkalosis that may offset the effect of elevated 2,3-DPG on red cell oxygen affinity.[125] Thus, such individuals generally have a normal *in vivo* oxygen dissociation curve. However, it does not follow that 2,3-DPG is an unimportant mode of compensation in these anemic patients. After all, if red cell 2,3-DPG remained fixed, these patients would have left-shifted oxygen dissociation curves and, consequently, impaired oxygen release.

In most types of anemia, the level of red cell 2,3-DPG depends on the deficit in red cell mass[118] as well as on red cell age. However, there are interesting exceptions. In congenital

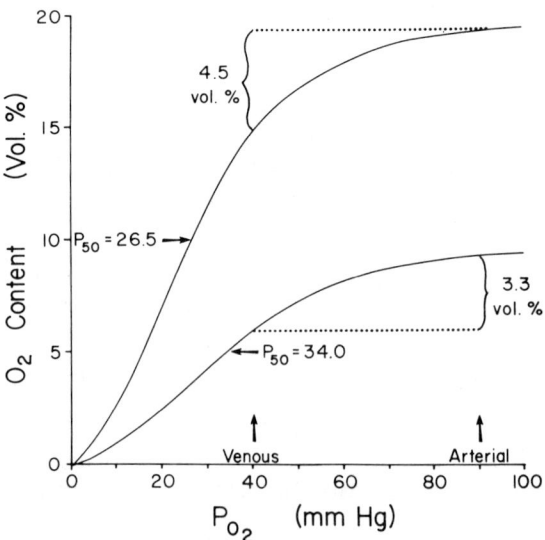

Figure 5–12. Enhancement of oxygen unloading by decreased red cell oxygen affinity in a patient with anemia. An anemic patient with a 50 per cent reduction in hemoglobin concentration has only a 27 per cent reduction in oxygen unloading. (From Klocke, R. A.: Chest 62(Suppl):79S, 1972.)

Table 5–2. LEVELS OF RED CELL 2,3-DPG IN VARIOUS TYPES OF ANEMIA*

Group	Diagnosis	Number of Patients	Hb (g/100 ml)	Arterial pH	2,3-DPG μmol/g Hb	2,3-DPG mmol/l RBC
1	Iron Deficiency	9	8.2	7.39	27.9	7.15
2	Hepatic Cirrhosis	8	8.7	7.43	22.4	6.15
3	Hemolytic Anemia	7	7.5	7.38	24.0	7.66
4	Leukemia	22	8.3	7.42	18.5	5.68
5	Aplastic Anemia	11	8.0	7.41	19.9	6.11
6	Uremia	16	6.9	7.32	15.6	4.95
NORMALS		50	15.8	7.38	13.2	4.10

*From Humpeler, E., et al.: Blut 29:382, 1974.

nonspherocytic hemolytic anemia due to a deficiency in one of the glycolytic enzymes, red cell 2,3-DPG may be determined by the primary metabolic abnormality. Patients with pyruvate kinase deficiency have unusually high red cell 2,3-DPG, whereas those with hexokinase deficiency have subnormal 2,3-DPG.[61] Reduced red cell 2,3-DPG due to deficiency in DPG synthase activity is discussed in the preceding section on enzymology. In hereditary spherocytosis, the 2,3-DPG is unexpectedly low, perhaps because red cells are sequestered in the unfriendly environment of the spleen.[126] Following splenectomy, red cell 2,3-DPG rises to normal.[45, 126] Red cell 2,3-DPG may also be reduced in red cell membrane disorders in which increased cation fluxes result in enhanced consumption of ATP.[127] The increased ADP:ATP ratio favors the conversion of 1,3-DPG to 3-PG, bypassing 2,3-DPG synthesis (see the preceding section entitled "Regulation of Red Cell 2,3-DPG").

Polycythemia*

There are widely conflicting reports on red cell 2,3-DPG levels in patients with polycythemia vera, ranging from 55 per cent[128] to 145 per cent of normal.[120, 129] There is no apparent explanation for this discrepancy. As mentioned below, patients with polycythemia related to pulmonary disease or a cardiac right-to-left shunt have increased 2,3-DPG, whereas those with functionally abnormal hemoglobin variants have normal levels.

Adaptation to High Altitude

Individuals exposed to low ambient oxygen tension adapt to this environmental stress in several ways. Pulmonary ventilation increases, and polycythemia develops. The overall cardiac output is unchanged, although there may be redistribution of blood flow to vital organs. The acclimatized individual is able to maintain normal oxygen consumption and exercise tolerance even at an altitude of 5000 meters (arterial PO_2 = 40 mm Hg). This subject has been reviewed.[130]

It has long been known that individuals living at high altitudes have decreased whole blood oxygen affinity. The mechanism for this "shift to the right" was worked out by Lenfant and associates.[131] A group of normal volunteers were taken from sea level to an altitude of 4530 meters. As shown in Figure 5–13, the whole blood P_{50} increased rapidly, reaching a maximum of about 31 mm Hg* by 36 hours. This change in oxygen affinity was accompanied by a parallel rise in red cell 2,3-DPG. This study was the first to demonstrate that 2,3-DPG mediates a decrease in oxygen affinity following a hypoxic stimulus. Despite the increase in 2,3-DPG, the in vivo P_{50} of individuals at high altitude is normal or even low, owing to concomitant respiratory alkalosis.[131a] This increase in 2,3-DPG can be abolished if volunteers are given acetazolamide, which effectively prevents the development of respiratory alkalosis[99] (see preceding section entitled "2,3-DPG and Hypoxia"). In a large number of individuals living at 3300 meters (Leadville, Colorado), 2,3-DPG was found to be somewhat elevated.[132] Those who had excessive polycythemia had a more impressive increase in red cell 2,3-DPG. Exposure to high altitude does not affect the concentration of other organic phosphates in the red cell.[133]

After a thorough analysis of the various factors determining oxygen delivery to individuals acclimatized at high altitudes, Lenfant and

---

*Although polycythemia is not necessarily associated with hypoxia, it is logical to discuss it after the section on anemia.

*Corrected to pH 7.4.

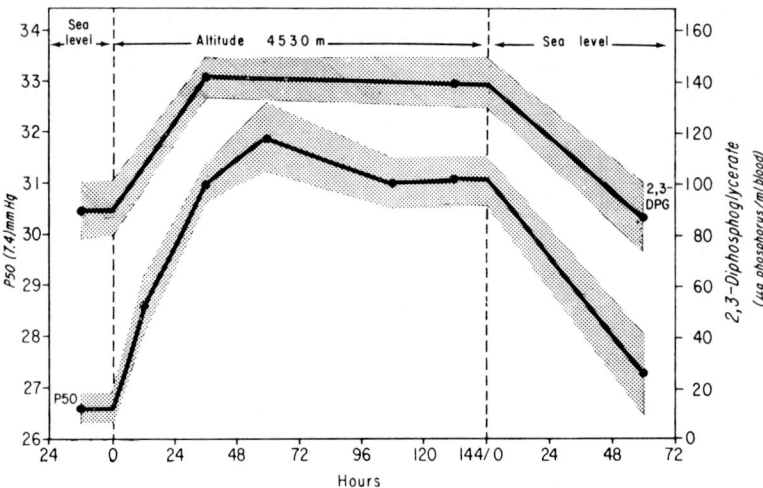

Figure 5–13. The effect of exposure to altitude on red cell 2,3-DPG and oxygen affinity. (From Lenfant, C., et al.: J. Clin. Invest. 47:2652, 1968.)

Sullivan[130] concluded that the "shift to the right" of the oxygen dissociation curve is of very little adaptive value. As shown in Figure 5–14, the portion of the oxygen dissociation curve that is encompassed between a low arterial PO_2 (43 mm Hg) and a mixed venous PO_2 of 30 mm Hg is equally steep at whole blood P_{50}'s of 26 mm Hg and 36 mm Hg. At low alveolar oxygen tension, the arterial saturation is significantly reduced in red cells having an increased P_{50}. This decrease in oxygen-carrying capacity offsets any enhancement of oxygen unloading in the capillaries. Thus, the A-V oxygen content may be minimally affected by the increase in P_{50}. The extent to which this is true varies from one organ to another[134] (see Figure 5–16). Polycythemia is a much more significant adaptation to altitude, because it enhances oxygen-carrying capacity. The fact that those Leadville citizens with the highest levels of 2,3-DPG had the most severe polycythemia[132] suggests that the right-shifted curve in individuals at high altitude is of little benefit and, under certain circumstances, may even impair the delivery of oxygen to tissues.[135] The physiologic significance of red cell oxygen affinity in hypoxic states is discussed in more detail in the last section of this chapter.

Pulmonary Disease

In one of the first surveys of red cell 2,3-DPG in various clinical disorders, Oski and associates[136] showed that patients with chronic obstructive pulmonary disease had significantly elevated levels (5.2 mmoles/l of red blood cells versus normal of 4.1 mmoles/l of red blood cells). This undoubtedly accounts for the "shift to the right" that has been observed in some of these patients. Carefully measured oxygen binding curves have shown that the decreased oxygen affinity in some of these patients can enhance oxygen unloading.[137] In general, this advantage cannot be great in patients with arterial hypoxemia for reasons cited in the section above. (See also reference 138.) There is a wide variation of P_{50} and 2,3-DPG values in patients with chronic pulmonary disease.[138, 139] Those patients with secondary polycythemia tended to have increased P_{50} values, whereas those with normal hematocrits had decreased P_{50} values. This is a complex group of patients to analyze, because they vary greatly in acid-base status and 2,3-DPG is very sensitive to alterations in plasma and red cell

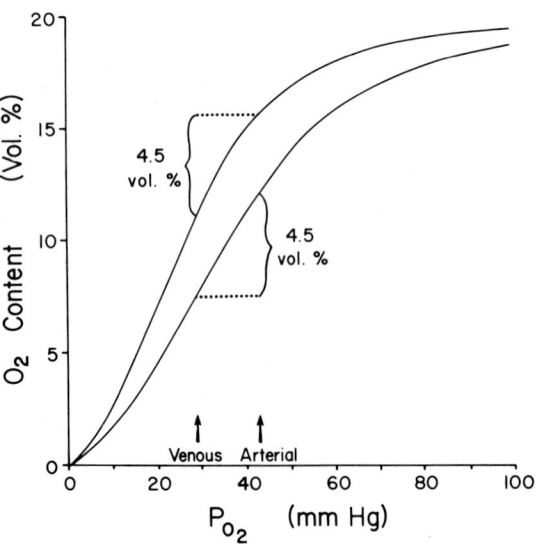

Figure 5–14. Failure of right-shifted oxygen binding curve to enhance oxygen unloading in patients with arterial hypoxemia. (From Klocke, R. A.: Chest 62(Suppl.):79S, 1972.)

pH. For these reasons, it is not surprising that in these groups of patients, red cell 2,3-DPG does not closely parallel the degree of hypoxia. Acute changes in red cell 2,3-DPG, observed after the administration or withdrawal of oxygen therapy, correlate closely with changes in arterial pH.[139] In contrast to patients with chronic lung disease, acute asthmatics have normal red cell 2,3-DPG but slightly increased hemoglobin levels.[140]

Cardiac Disorders

Cardiac function is obviously of critical importance in maintaining oxygen homeostasis. Hypoxia can be seen in a variety of cardiac disorders. Patients with *cyanotic congenital heart disease* shunt blood from the right heart to the left, bypassing the pulmonary circulation. Accordingly, arterial oxygen tension is reduced. Five such patients having a mean arterial oxygen saturation of 72 per cent had a 74 per cent increase in red cell 2,3-DPG.[136] Similar elevations in 2,3-DPG have also been reported in another series of patients[108] and also in dogs with a surgically created right-to-left shunt.[141] It is doubtful whether the resultant decrease in oxygen affinity is of significant advantage, for reasons analogous to those discussed in the previous sections concerning hypoxemia secondary to high altitude or pulmonary disease. Following surgical correction of cyanotic heart defects, red cell 2,3-DPG falls promptly to normal.[108] This may be due in part to reversal of the hypoxia but also to the transfusion of stored blood (see below) and perhaps alterations in red cell metabolism following surgery.[142]

The development of congestive heart failure is accompanied by decreasing cardiac output and impaired perfusion of tissues. Woodson and associates[143] have measured cardiac and hemoglobin function in 39 cardiac patients and found that P_{50} was significantly increased in those whose cardiac index fell below 2.3 liters/min/m². When patients' hemoglobin levels were considered, an inverse linear relationship between "hemoglobin flow" (Hb × cardiac output) and P_{50} was found. Cardiac patients with a functional classification of III or IV had significant elevations in red cell 2,3-DPG and P_{50}. As previously discussed, oxygenation is related to a product of blood flow × hemoglobin × ($S_AO_2 - S_{\bar{V}}O_2$). For patients with cardiac failure in whom blood flow is compromised, enhanced oxygen extraction serves as a compensation.

Decreased oxygen affinity (as measured by P_{50} under standard conditions) has also been noted in patients who have sustained an *acute myocardial infarction*. The degree of the increase in P_{50} correlated with the size of the infarct.[144] However, the "shift to the right" in these patients could not be explained by increased red cell 2,3-DPG. In a thorough hemodynamic study of 23 patients following acute myocardial infarction, increased extraction of oxygen was found to be inversely proportional to "hemoglobin flow" (Hb × cardiac output).[145] About a third of the enhanced oxygen extraction could be explained by a slight decrease in whole blood oxygen affinity.

In contrast to patients with congestive heart failure, those with circulatory collapse due to *cardiogenic* and *septic shock* may have decreased red cell 2,3-DPG[146, 147] and, consequently, decreased P_{50} values.[146] These abnormalities appear to be related to the presence of acidosis.[147] Those patients with low red cell 2,3-DPG had a more precarious clinical status and prognosis.[146, 147] The impairment of oxygen extraction in septic shock is probably secondary to increased oxygen affinity rather than to peripheral arteriovenous shunting.[146] However, the *in vivo* P_{50} of these patients is often close to normal, because the direct effect of acidosis on P_{50} counterbalances the increased O_2 affinity.[148]

It is worth examining the relationship between altered oxygen affinity and the coronary circulation, because the myocardium normally extracts more oxygen than any other tissue. A primary "shift to the left" does not appear to be deleterious to cardiac function. Those individuals having familial polycythemia due to high-affinity hemoglobin variants (see Chapter 14) have no apparent increase in angina pectoris or other cardiac manifestations. However, increased oxygen affinity may be deleterious to patients with pre-existing coronary artery disease. A group of dogs with experimental coronary artery obstruction developed electrocardiographic evidence of ischemia when given blood depleted of 2,3-DPG.[149] Eliot and associates[150, 151] have studied a group of patients with angina pectoris but normal coronary arteries and found that their dialyzed hemolysates had significantly *decreased* oxygen affinity. However, more recently, whole blood P_{50}'s in similar groups of patients were found to be within normal limits.[152, 153] A significant increase in P_{50} has been noted during atrial pacing in coronary sinus blood of some patients with angina pectoris.[154, 155] However, red cell 2,3-DPG was normal.[154] It would be of considerable interest if oxygen affinity were regulated at a local level by some type of feedback control.

Whole blood oxygen affinity may be affected by agents used in the treatment of angina pectoris. The effect of propranolol on red cell oxygenation has been discussed in an earlier section of this chapter (Determinants of Blood Oxygen Affinity). Nitroglycerin may affect oxygen affinity in the coronary circulation. Following the intracoronary perfusion of the drug in dogs, a significant increase in the P_{50} of blood from the coronary sinus has been noted.[156] The mechanism of this effect is unclear.

Metabolic Disorders

Acid-Base Balance

In their survey of cell metabolites in various clinical conditions, Guest and Rapoport[28] showed that 2,3-DPG was increased in patients with alkalosis and decreased in those with acidosis. Forty years later, their observation has been amply confirmed.[38, 157, 158] The importance of pH in the regulation of 2,3-DPG has been stressed in a previous section. Astrup and associates[159, 160] have presented a convincing argument that it is the prime determinant of red cell 2,3-DPG in various clinical disorders. It is apparent that the pH-induced changes in red cell 2,3-DPG influence oxygen affinity in a direction opposite to the direct influence of pH (Bohr effect) (Table 5–3). The net result is that in most chronic acid-base disorders, *in vivo* P_{50} is normal. Thus, 2,3-DPG serves as a buffer to maintain uniform oxygen release irrespective of the patient's plasma pH. However, when this delicate balance is upset by acute changes in a patient's acid-base status, significant and perhaps deleterious changes in *in vivo* oxygen affinity can occur.[38, 157] For example, if metabolic acidosis is rapidly corrected by the infusion of bicarbonate or lactate, the prompt rise in plasma pH is reflected in a corresponding increase in oxygen affinity as dictated by the Bohr effect.[38, 157] There is a lag of several hours before the increase in pH results in higher levels of red cell 2,3-DPG. Meanwhile, the *in vivo* P_{50} is decreased and may compromise oxygen release, particularly in patients who lack other compensatory mechanisms for insuring optimal tissue oxygenation.

The regulation of erythropoiesis may depend in part on the acid-base status of the organism. It has been a puzzle why levels of erythropoietin rise sharply immediately following exposure to a hypoxic environment but then fall toward baseline within 12 to 18 hours. Humans exposed to a simulated altitude of 4500 meters developed alkalosis, accompanied by a temporary drop in P_{50} of about 2 mm Hg until 2,3-DPG increased and normalized the *in vivo* oxygen affinity.[146] The acute rise in serum erythropoietin was blunted when alkalosis was prevented by the administration of acetazolamide. These results suggest the interesting possibility that the initial high levels of erythropoietin could be due in part to the transient "shift to the left." However, it is difficult to understand how this modest increase in oxygen affinity could contribute significantly to the individual's degree of hypoxia in view of the discussion in an earlier section on oxygen affinity in hypoxemic states (see Figure 5–14). The aforementioned experiments do not rule out the possibility that pH or acetazolamide itself has a direct effect on erythropoietin production.

Hypophosphatemia and Hyperphosphatemia

Inorganic phosphate (P_i) plays an important role in red cell metabolism. P_i stimulates glycolysis by activating the important regulatory enzyme phosphofructokinase. In addition, phosphate is a substrate in the synthesis of 1,3-diphosphoglycerate. For these reasons, red cell 2,3-DPG synthesis is enhanced by inorganic phosphate. Red cells incubated in the presence of glucose and inorganic phosphate maintain higher 2,3-DPG levels than those incubated with glucose alone.[61] Patients with hypophosphatemia have low levels of red cell 2,3-DPG and ATP.[28] Decreased 2,3-DPG and a concomitant increase in oxygen affinity have been seen in patients with hypophosphatemia secondary to diarrhea,[161, 162] hyperparathyroidism,[163] and inadequate phosphate supplements during hyperalimentation.[163, 164] In addition, hemolysis may be encountered in association with rigid, ATP-depleted red cells.[161]

Elevations in red cell ATP and 2,3-DPG have been observed in patients with hyperphosphatemia. Those in whom increased serum phosphate is due to chronic renal failure may fail to show these changes because of coexistent acidosis (see below). Children up to the age of 12 have plasma phosphate levels

Table 5–3. EFFECT OF BLOOD pH ON OXYGEN AFFINITY

Clinical State	Red Cell 2,3-DPG	DPG Effect on P_{50}	Direct pH Effect on P_{50}	"In Vivo" P_{50}
Acidosis	↓	↓	↑	Normal
Alkalosis	↑	↑	↓	Normal

that are 50 per cent higher than those of adults. The resulting increase in red cell ATP and more modest elevation in 2,3-DPG account for the slight (1.6 mm Hg) right shift in their oxygen dissociation curve.[21] The physiologic "anemia" of childhood may be attributed to enhanced oxygen unloading secondary to this decrease in oxygen affinity.[21]

Renal Failure

Patients with uremia have a complex array of physiological and metabolic abnormalities. They have varying degrees of anemia, metabolic acidosis, and hyperphosphatemia. All these factors affect the concentration of red cell 2,3-DPG. As a group, uremic patients have decreased oxygen affinity,[119, 165] which is due to increased levels of 2,3-DPG.[119, 162, 166] Uremic patients have about the same[119] or somewhat lower elevations[123, 125, 162, 167] of red cell 2,3-DPG compared with patients with other types of anemia of similar severity. As might be expected, those uremic patients with acidosis tend to have relatively low values, whereas the values are relatively high in those with hyperphosphatemia.[160, 162] Patients with renal failure have about a twofold elevation in red cell ATP.[162] Furthermore, following incubation of uremic plasma with normal red cells, ATP increased about 50 per cent.[162] This was shown to be due to increased P_i in uremic plasma. As we stated in the introduction to this chapter, ATP probably has no significant influence on the P_{50} of normal red cells. Moreover, the elevated levels of ATP in uremic patients do not appear to influence oxygen affinity.[167]

Hemodialysis of uremic patients may result in a significant reduction in serum phosphate and in red cell 2,3-DPG.[168] This occurred despite a concomitant increase in plasma pH. In other studies, the changes induced by dialysis have been less marked.[167, 169] Decreased 2,3-DPG has also been found in patients whose hyperphosphatemia has been corrected by aluminum hydroxide gels.

Hepatic Cirrhosis

Patients with advanced cirrhosis of the liver have decreased whole blood oxygen affinity[170–172] in association with increased red cell 2,3-DPG.[173] The increase in 2,3-DPG in these patients is roughly proportional to the degree of anemia.[174] At a given hemoglobin level, 2,3-DPG is significantly higher in cirrhotic patients than in those without liver disease. The primary basis for increased red cell 2,3-DPG in these patients is hyperventilation, whereby increased red cell pH stimulates synthesis of 2,3-DPG (see above).[175] In addition, patients with advanced hepatic decompensation have decreased arterial oxygen saturation that cannot be explained by moderately decreased oxygen affinity. Perhaps pulmonary arterial-venous shunting contributes to the elevated 2,3-DPG in these patients.

Hyperlipemia

Individuals with familial (Type 1) hyperlipoproteinemia have a marked increase in whole blood oxygen affinity (P_{50} = 18 to 22 mm Hg).[176] This phenomenon cannot be explained by an abnormality in red cell 2,3-DPG or MCHC and appears to depend on a plasma factor. The P_{50} of these red cells approaches normal when they are placed into normal plasma. Conversely, the P_{50} of normal red cells decreases after suspension in lactescent plasma. The red cells of patients with Type 1 hyperlipoproteinemia have a significant reduction in cholesterol and phospholipid. Perhaps distortion of the red cell membrane in some way causes increased intracellular oxygen affinity. In contrast to the striking increase in the oxygen affinity of red cells in these patients, marked hypercholesterolemia has no effect on oxygen binding of rabbit red cells.[177]

Endocrine Disorders

Patients with thyrotoxicosis have an increased rate of metabolism and therefore may have hypoxia at the subcellular level. Accordingly, decreased oxygen affinity would serve as an appropriate compensation. Moderate increases in P_{50} (2 to 3 mm Hg) have been observed in patients with Graves' disease[178] as well as in euthyroid human volunteers[178, 179] and rats[179, 180] who were given triiodothyronine (T_3). Furthermore, following the incubation of rat blood with supraphysiologic amounts of T_3, a significant increase in P_{50} was observed.[180] Increased red cell 2,3-DPG has been observed in patients with hyperthyroidism[178, 181, 182] as well as in normal volunteers given thyroid hormone.[178, 183] However, others have found that red cell 2,3-DPG was normal in both hyperthyroid[184, 185] and hypothyroid[185] patients. Moreover, rats given T_3 in doses known to increase P_{50}[180] showed no significant change in red cell 2,3-DPG[186] (cf. reference 187).

Snyder and Reddy[188] found that in a cell-free system containing a partially purified enzyme preparation, the conversion of 1,3-DPG to 2,3-DPG was enhanced by the addition of thyroxine (10^{-12} M) or T_3 (10^{-14} M). These results indicate that thyroid hormone stimulates diphosphoglycerate synthase activity. However, others have not been able to reproduce these results.[83, 189–191] Thus, the role of thyroid hormone in regulating 2,3-DPG is uncertain.

Thyroid hormone may affect red cell 2,3-DPG levels in the neonatal period. During the first four days of life, red cell 2,3-DPG increases 25 per cent, while total thyroxine and free thyroxine increase 70 per cent and 100 per cent, respectively.[192, 193] However, this association may well be fortuitous.

Patients with panhypopituitarism have anemia accompanied by inappropriately low levels of red cell 2,3-DPG.[194] This has also been observed in a patient with isolated growth hormone deficiency.[194] Administration of thyroxine and human growth hormone acted synergistically to increase red cell 2,3-DPG to normal levels. Investigators in the same laboratory have reported a marked rise in 2,3-DPG of uremic patients given testosterone.[195] This increase was far in excess of that attributable to an influx of young red cells. Androgens will induce an increase in red cell 2,3-DPG in animals,[196, 197] independent of erythropoietin.[197] Furthermore, a significant rise in red cell 2,3-DPG has been observed after in vitro incubation with various androgens.[198]

There is not much information on the effect of adrenal hormones on intracellular hemoglobin function. Rabbits treated with aldosterone had a 2.7 mm Hg increase in P_{50}.[199] A somewhat smaller shift to the right was observed following administration of cortisol. No change in the concentrations of red cell cation was observed. In this study, 2,3-DPG was not measured. In contrast, oxygen affinity was not affected by in vitro incubation with these hormones. High doses of prednisone have resulted in significant increases in 2,3-DPG in patients with leukemia and the nephrotic syndrome.[200] Adrenalin has been reported to increase the level of 2,3-DPG in rats.[187]

During pregnancy, maternal red cell 2,3-DPG rises 25 per cent.[201] It is uncertain whether this increase is mediated by either ovarian or placental hormones. As Rörth[201] has pointed out, this coincides with the development of respiratory alkalosis secondary to hyperventilation. The low maternal PCO_2 may facilitate the efflux of CO_2 from the fetus. It is likely that the combination of increased maternal red cell 2,3-DPG and mild alkalosis results in a normal oxygen affinity in vivo.

Patients with Parkinson's disease have elevated red cell 2,3-DPG for reasons that are unclear.[202]

Exercise

The effect of exercise on red cell oxygen affinity has been of considerable interest to physiologists. Acute exercise induces a complex series of metabolic events, including local lactic acidosis, hyperventilation (with accompanying decreased PCO_2), hyperphosphatemia, and, in some cases, enhanced destruction of red blood cells. In view of the complex interplay of these factors, it is not surprising that there have been conflicting reports on the effect of exercise on red cell 2,3-DPG and oxygen transport.

Immediately following acute spurts of exercise, red cell 2,3-DPG decreases slightly,[203] probably because of lactic acidosis. Thereafter, red cell 2,3-DPG rises slowly and reaches a plateau at about 10 per cent above pre-exercise levels.[203, 204] During more sustained exercise, 2,3-DPG increases steadily with no initial lag period.[203] This elevation in 2,3-DPG may reflect enhanced synthesis due to increased deoxygenation of blood in exercising muscle,[101] perhaps abetted by accompanying hyperphosphatemia. In general, alkalosis cannot be invoked as a contributing factor, because in most study subjects, there has not been a significant rise in mixed venous or arterial pH, despite extreme hyperventilation. Although red cell 2,3-DPG increases slightly following exercise, the corrected P_{50} (pH 7.4, 37°C) is generally unchanged,[205, 206] perhaps owing to a concomitant decrease in mean corpuscular hemoglobin concentration.[205] The in vivo P_{50} during exercise is markedly increased, primarily because of increased blood temperature.[206]

Red cell 2,3-DPG increases about 10 per cent following a prolonged period of intensive physical training,[207–209] and there appears to be a corresponding rise in P_{50}. The increase in 2,3-DPG may be due in part to a younger population of red cells (see earlier section on in vivo aging of red cells).

Oxygen Affinity in the Fetus and Newborn*

The oxygen dissociation curve of blood from the human fetus and newborn is shifted to the left of that of maternal blood. This difference

---

*Oski[213] has written a concise review of this subject. For more detailed information, see the recent monograph by Wimberly.[214]

Table 5–4. POSTNATAL CHANGES IN P_{50}, RED BLOOD CELL 2,3-DPG, AND FETAL HEMOGLOBIN IN TERM INFANTS*

Age of Infant	P_{50} (mm Hg)	2,3-DPG (μmol/ml of RBC)	Fetal Hb (%)
1 day	19.4 ± 1.8	5.4 ± 1.00	77.0 ± 7.3
5 days	20.6 ± 1.7	6.6 ± 0.99	76.8 ± 5.8
3 weeks	22.7 ± 1.0	5.4 ± 0.73	70.0 ± 7.3
6 to 9 weeks	24.4 ± 1.4	5.6 ± 0.75	52.1 ± 11.0
3 to 4 months	26.5 ± 2.0	5.8 ± 1.20	23.2 ± 16.0
6 months	27.8 ± 1.0	5.1 ± 1.60	4.7 ± 2.2
8 to 11 months	30.3 ± 0.7	7.4 ± 0.49	1.6 ± 1.0
Normal adult	27.0 ± 1.1	5.1 ± 0.42	<2.0%

*From Oski, F. A., and Gottlieb, A. J.: Prog. Hematol. 7:33, 1971.

in oxygen affinity has also been observed in a variety of other mammals (see Chapter 6). The only exception reported to date is the cat.[211] The higher oxygen affinity of fetal blood has been considered to be physiologically advantageous in facilitating oxygen transport across the placenta. However, this phenomenon may be of limited significance in man. There have now been several instances reported in which mothers having a markedly left-shifted oxygen binding curve due to the presence of a hemoglobin variant have borne entirely normal offspring who did not inherit the variant.[212] Here, the maternal blood presumably had a higher oxygen affinity than the fetal blood.

The mechanism underlying the increased oxygen affinity of fetal red cells is interesting. The red cells of the newborn contain about 80 per cent hemoglobin F ($\alpha_2\gamma_2$). This hemoglobin, when purified and studied in a phosphate-free buffer, has a slightly *lower* oxygen affinity than hemoglobin A. However, 2,3-DPG binds less strongly to deoxyhemoglobin F.[215] Consequently, a given concentration of 2,3-DPG is less effective in lowering oxygen affinity.[216, 217] The diminished interaction between 2,3-DPG and hemoglobin F is primarily due to the fact that at position β H21, an important binding site, the γ chain has uncharged serine rather than a positively charged histidine residue. Neonatal red cells have normal to slightly increased levels of 2,3-DPG. However, this cofactor is not pulling its weight in newborn erythrocytes, and as a consequence oxygen affinity is significantly higher than "normal."

Following birth, the oxygen affinity of the baby's blood decreases rapidly[218] (Table 5–4). During the first week of life, red cell 2,3-DPG increases about 20 per cent. The postnatal rise in 2,3-DPG is even more marked in healthy premature infants. At one to four weeks of age, their P_{50} values are close to those of normal adults.[214] Although this increment in 2,3-DPG would not have much direct interaction with the fetal hemoglobin, it should lower intracellular pH and thereby decrease oxygen affinity. This rapid change in P_{50} seems appropriate for the increased metabolic demands following birth. A rapid rise in red cell 2,3-DPG during the neonatal period has been observed in several other species (see Chapter 6). During the first six months of life, hemoglobin F decreases from 77 per cent to about 5 per cent of the total. This results in a further increase in P_{50} (see Table 5–4).

In contrast, premature infants with respiratory problems have a marked decrease in red cell 2,3-DPG following birth,[214] owing to the marked effect of pH on 2,3-DPG synthesis. Theoretically, such a left-shifted curve could be an advantage to the newborn who has concurrent hypoxemia and low cardiac output[214] (see section below entitled "Overall Significance of Erythrocyte Oxygen Affinity"). Nevertheless, under most circumstances, the increased oxygen affinity of newborn red cells would result in impaired oxygen delivery to tissues. Oski and associates[219, 220] have found that the mortality of premature newborns with severe respiratory distress syndrome is reduced if these infants are given an exchange transfusion of fresh adult blood having near-normal oxygen affinity. However, one cannot conclude that the enhanced survival was due to a reduction in oxygen affinity. It is possible that the exchange transfusions improved either pulmonary ventilation or pulmonary perfusion.

Transfusion of Stored Blood*

During the first week of storage of blood in acid citrate dextrose (ACD) solution, red cells become depleted of 2,3-DPG and, as a result, have increased oxygen affinity.[49, 114, 222, 223]

---

*This subject has been thoroughly reviewed by Sohmer and Dawson.[221]

Thus, patients who are transfused with large amounts of such blood will have a "left-shifted" oxyhemoglobin dissociation curve.[49] Furthermore, the rates at which red cells take on and release oxygen are reduced by storage.[224] The clinical significance of this alteration in oxygen binding and transport has not been established. At the least, it is safe to say that the recipient does not derive the full physiologic benefit from blood depleted in 2,3-DPG. Following infusion of such donor cells into normal volunteers, their content of 2,3-DPG returns to normal within 6 to 24 hours.[225, 226] However, the reconstitution of red cell 2,3-DPG may be much less rapid following transfusion into critically ill patients. When a patient requires a large amount of blood and his compensatory mechanisms are compromised, the administration of functionally normal red cells is advisable.

Considerable attention has been directed toward ways of modifying storage media in order to preserve red cell 2,3-DPG and normal hemoglobin function. It has been shown that 2,3-DPG and P_{50} are better maintained in citrate phosphate dextrose (CPD) solution[227] because of the higher pH of this medium.[228] In 1971, 10 per cent of the blood banks in the United States used CPD as a preservative, while 90 per cent continued to use ACD. By 1975, the reverse was true; CPD was employed by 90 per cent of American blood banks. Although the shelf life is the same for the two preservatives (21 days), CPD enables red cells to function more physiologically during the first week of storage and therefore is a superior preservative. Since 1978, the standard preservative in the United States has been CPD-adenine. The addition of adenine has extended the shelf life of stored blood to 28 days.

Several laboratories have investigated the inclusion of various substrates to blood storage media that allow the maintenance of physiologic levels of 2,3-DPG and ATP for longer periods. The addition of inosine to the storage medium provides ribose-1-phosphate, a substrate that feeds directly into the glycolytic pathway (Fig. 5–15). The resulting increase in 2,3-DPG is potentiated by the addition of pyruvate,[31, 229] methylene blue,[230] or fructose,[231] all of which undergo reduction, coupled with oxidation of NADH to NAD, thereby providing cofactor for the glyceraldehyde-3-phosphate dehydrogenase reaction. The transfusion of large amounts of blood stored in inosine incurs the risk of hyperuricemia resulting from the catabolism of this purine. Dihydroxyace-

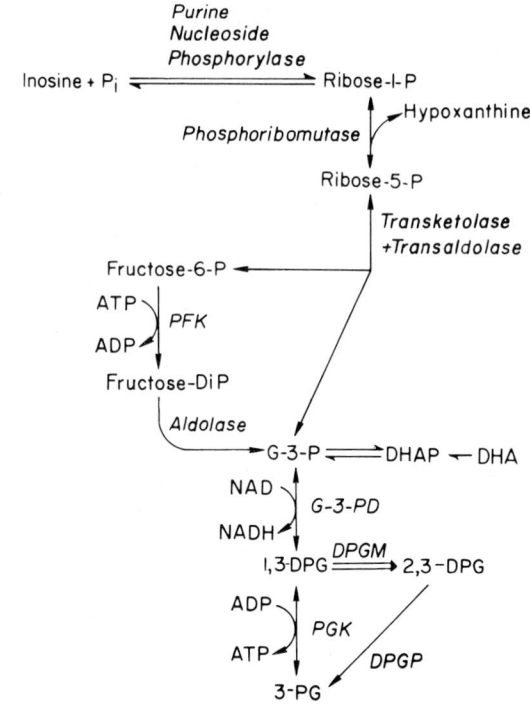

Figure 5–15. The pathway of red cell inosine metabolism to 2,3-DPG. Also shown in this figure is the Rapoport-Luebering cycle, which 1,3-DPG can be converted to 3-PG either directly or via 2,3-DPG. The conversion of dihydroxyacetone (DHA) to dihydroxyacetone phosphate (DHAP) is also shown. (PFK = phosphofructokinase; G-3-PD = glyceraldehyde-3-phosphate dehydrogenase; PGK = phosphoglycerate kinase; DPGM = diphosphoglycerate mutase (synthase); DPGP = diphosphoglycerate phosphatase; P_i = inorganic phosphate; G-3-P = glyceraldehyde-3-phosphate; 3-PG = 3-phosphoglycerate.) (Modified from Oski, F. A., et al.: Blood 37:52, 1971. By permission of Grune & Stratton.)

tone has been proposed as an additive.[232] Red cells contain a kinase that permits this compound to be phosphorylated to dihydroxyacetone phosphate (DHAP). As shown in Figure 5–5, DHAP is a normal intermediate in glycolysis and serves as an effective substrate for the synthesis of 2,3-DPG. Dihydroxyacetone is useful in preserving 2,3-DPG in stored red cells.[232, 233] One great advantage of this preservative is that it would not engender hyperuricemia.

The efficiency of conventional blood banking is severely limited by the finite shelf life of the stored units. Discarding of blood after 28 days' storage is a major waste of a precious resource. The levels of 2,3-DPG and ATP in outdated blood can be restored to normal by incubation with appropriate substrates such as inosine, dihydroxyacetone, pyruvate, or methylene blue. If such rejuvenated blood is frozen in glycerol, the levels of 2,3-DPG and

ATP are well maintained.[234] Upon thawing, the added substrates and waste products are removed along with the glycerol. This "recycling" extends the effective shelf life of stored red cells indefinitely without compromise of either erythrocyte survival or function. The impaired oxygen transport of stored red blood cells can also be restored by incubation with pyridoxal 5'-phosphate.[235]

Measures that increase 2,3-DPG levels in stored blood may also be effective *in vivo*. Monkeys infused with either dihydroxyacetone, or inosine combined with pyruvate and phosphate had a 36 to 50 per cent increase in red cell 2,3-DPG and a 10 per cent increase in P_{50}.[236]

A dramatic reduction in red cell oxygen affinity can be achieved by incubating red cells with lipid vesicles containing the potent allosteric modifier inositol hexaphosphate.[237, 238] These modified cells appear to be stable and retain the incorporated phosphate. However, the practical significance of this innovation is uncertain in view of the success in maintaining or regenerating 2,3-DPG by appropriate storage media.

OVERALL SIGNIFICANCE OF ERYTHROCYTE OXYGEN AFFINITY

This chapter has been concerned with shifts in oxygen affinity that can occur in various physiologic and pathologic states. Before deciding whether these alterations have adaptive or clinical significance, we must take a critical view of the overall importance of whole blood oxygen affinity as a determinant of tissue oxygenation. This question defies an easy answer. It is very difficult to measure the oxygen supply and demand of a given organ or tissue under conditions in which oxygen affinity, hemoglobin concentration, and blood flow can be adequately controlled. In this section, we will review some experimental and clinical studies that address this problem. Interpretation and integration of these studies are complicated by the fact that a variety of species and organ systems have been tested and different means have been used to manipulate oxygen affinity.[239] Nevertheless, some general conclusions can be drawn.

Critical Intracellular PO_2

There is a large gradient in oxygen tension between the capillary, where oxygen is released from red cells, and the intracellular organelles, which utilize oxygen. Assuming that blood flow and oxygen utilization remain unchanged, an increase in oxygen affinity should result in a predictable decrease in capillary PO_2. Would a drop in capillary PO_2 from, for example, 40 mm Hg to 30 mm Hg result in a critical reduction in intracellular PO_2? A consideration of electrical power provides a crude analogy. If the voltage of the high-tension wires from a hydroelectric plant is decreased from 400,000 V to 300,000 V, this drop in power would be reflected proportionately by a decrease in house voltage from 120 V to 90 V. Thus, a significant drop in capillary PO_2 would necessarily reduce the flow of oxygen into cells (see Figure 5-1). At what point is such a reduction metabolically significant? It is estimated that the PO_2 within canine myocardial cells is about 5 mm Hg.[240] Direct measurements of PO_2 in guinea pig brain have revealed a frequency distribution with a range of 5 to 95 mm Hg and a mode of 18 mm Hg.[241] In general, most estimates of intracellular oxygen tensions are much greater than the apparent Km values for oxygen of cytochromes in isolated mitochondria (~ 0.1 mm Hg)[13] and have led to the conclusions that small drops in tissue PO_2 should not affect mitochondrial function. However, the oxygen affinity of cytochromes may be considerably lower *in vivo*.[242] In fact, cytochrome aa_3 is probably not fully saturated.[243] In addition, the affinities of other oxygen-requiring enzymes may be sufficiently low that they would be affected by small changes in intracellular PO_2.[8] Thus, decreased cellular oxygen tension due to increased oxygen affinity could compromise tissue metabolism.

Compensatory Mechanisms

Various modes of compensation are available to offset the impairment in oxygen delivery due to a "shift to the left" in the oxyhemoglobin dissociation curve. As implied in the Fick equation, blood flow may increase, and enhanced erythropoiesis may augment the oxygen-carrying capacity of the blood. Furthermore, in some cases, improved ventilation would increase the oxygenation of arterial blood. In addition, compensation can take place at the tissue level: Unused capillaries may become patent, and with time, new capillaries may form, thereby increasing capillary density. There may also be an enhancement of mitochondrial density or of the activity of the respiratory enzymes. The extent to which an increase in oxygen affinity impairs oxygen delivery depends in large part on how effectively these compensatory adjustments can be called into play. The experimental assessment of the physiologic importance of oxygen affinity has generally depended on either measurements of the aforementioned modes of compensation or determination of abnormalities of organ function.[8]

Hypoxemia

Alterations of blood oxygen affinity may be of considerable importance to man and animals with decreased arterial oxygen saturation (hypoxemia). This problem has been analyzed theoretically[244, 244a] as well as experimentally.[135, 245, 246] As shown in a theoretical plot (Fig. 5–16), the amount of oxygen released to tissues (difference between arterial and venous oxygen saturation) depends on both the oxygen affinity of the blood and the degree of hypoxemia (arterial PO_2). If the hypoxemia is mild or moderate, a right-shifted curve may enable enhanced oxygen unloading. This prediction agrees with experimental measurements on rats[245] as well as on patients with pulmonary disease[137] and is consistent with a clinical evaluation of individuals taken to moderate altitude.[247] On the other hand, if hypoxemia is severe, a right-shifted curve would be detrimental and a left-shifted curve would be beneficial, particularly in tissues in which oxygen extraction is high and therefore venous PO_2 is low (Fig. 5–16). This conclusion is again supported by experimental and clinical observations. Rats whose P_{50} was lowered by the administration of oral sodium cyanate had significantly improved survival when subjected to low ambient oxygen tension. The group with high oxygen affinity had lower heart rates than the control rats subjected to an identical hypoxic stress.[135, 245] Similar conclusions were drawn from investigation of "human llamas."[246] These individuals, who have a hemoglobin variant with high oxygen affinity, showed improved early adaptation to altitude compared with normal siblings. However, interpretation of these observations is obscured by the fact that the "human llamas" also had an elevated red cell mass, which would be expected to give them an added advantage at high altitude.

The bulk of experimental observations indicate that a left-shifted curve is a handicap when arterial blood is well saturated with oxygen (see below) but is beneficial to severely hypoxemic man and animals. Observations of nature provide further support for this conclusion. As discussed in Chapter 6, nearly all animals that have adapted to very high altitude have increased blood oxygen affinity.

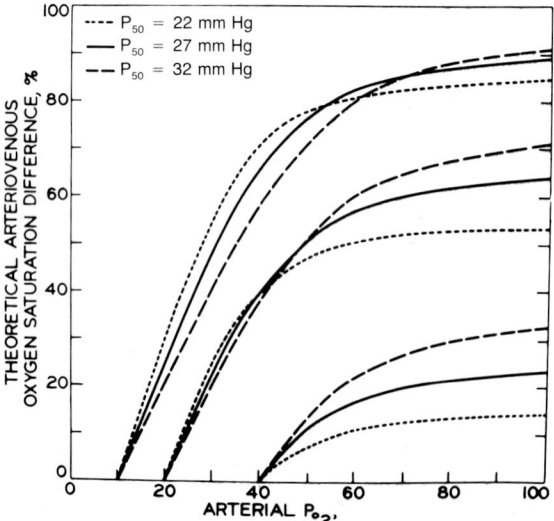

Figure 5–16. Effect of arterial PO_2 on the theoretical difference between arterial and venous oxygen saturation. This figure shows calculations for three different P_{50} values (22, 27, and 32 mm Hg) and three different values of venous PO_2 (10, 20, and 40 mm Hg). (From Woodson, R. D.: Crit. Care Med. 7:368, 1979.)

Normal Arterial PO_2

When the arterial oxygen tension is normal, increased oxygen affinity has the potential to significantly compromise oxygen delivery to tissues. Most studies indicate that rather marked increases in oxygen affinity have little or no effect on the overall circulation and metabolism of individuals or experimental animals who are otherwise normal. When monkeys were given exchange transfusions with blood that had been depleted of 2,3-DPG, the mean P_{50} dropped from 33.9 ± 1.1 (S.D.) mm Hg to 27.2 ± 5.9 mm Hg.[248] However, there was no change in red cell mass, cardiac output, oxygen consumption, or base deficit. Therefore, despite the lowering of venous oxygen tension, the shift to the left did not seem to affect overall oxygen or acid-base homeostasis. In rats, the oxygen tension in skin bubbles fell significantly following exchange transfusion with blood having increased oxygen affinity.[249] However, oxygen tension to more vital tissues may well have been preserved. In rabbits, metabolites in brain tissue were not affected by marked increases in oxygen affinity induced by the administration of cyanate.[250] These studies suggest that animals with increased oxygen affinity have sufficient compensatory mechanisms to maintain oxygenation to vital organs.

Reduction in Red Cell Mass

In view of the modes of compensation described above, it is not surprising that anemic animals are less able to tolerate an increase in red cell oxygen affinity. Woodson and associates[251] have examined the effect of reduction in P_{50} on the work performance of normal and anemic rats. They devised a treadmill that gave an accurate and reproducible end point of muscle exhaustion. All measurements were made on animals breathing room air. The duration of maximal exercise was shown to be linearly related to an animal's red cell mass. Rats with significantly increased oxygen affinity showed a lower exercise tolerance. The authors concluded that a 12 mm Hg (34 per cent) decrease in P_{50} was equivalent to a 10 per cent decrease in red cell mass. Thus, severe impairment of tissue oxygenation was seen in animals having a combination of increased oxygen affinity and reduced red cell mass. The obvious clinical inference that might be drawn is that a significant "shift to the left" is deleterious to those patients who cannot compensate by developing circulatory adjustments and/or secondary erythrocytosis.

As we have mentioned, patients with increased oxygen affinity due to a hemoglobin variant have no apparent clinical manifestations other than secondary erythrocytosis. They maintain normal oxygen consumption and a normal[252] or slightly increased[253] resting cardiac output (see Chapter 14). However, if robbed of their primary mode of compensation by phlebotomy to a normal red cell mass, these individuals have impaired exercise tolerance and a more pronounced increase in cardiac output.

Oski and associates[254] had the unique opportunity of comparing two adolescents with different types of congenital nonspherocytic hemolytic anemia associated with striking differences in red cell 2,3-DPG. The patient with red cell pyruvate kinase (PK) deficiency had a markedly "right-shifted" oxygen binding curve ($P_{50} = 38$ mm Hg) due to the greatly increased red cell 2,3-DPG that almost always accompanies this disorder. In contrast, the patient with hexokinase (HK) deficiency had a left-

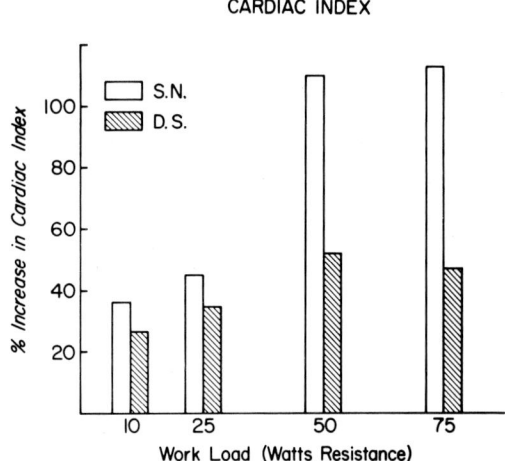

Figure 5–17. The effect of graded exercise on cardiac output in two patients: S. N., with hexokinase deficiency and increased red cell oxygen affinity, and D. S., with pyruvate kinase deficiency and decreased red cell oxygen affinity. (Courtesy of F. A. Oski.)

shifted curve ($P_{50} = 19$ mm Hg) due to a decrease in red cell 2,3-DPG. Otherwise, the two patients were reasonably well matched for age and severity of anemia (9.8 to 10 g/100 ml of hemoglobin). Deficiencies of these two enzymes appear to be restricted to the red cell. During graded exercise, the patient with HK deficiency developed much lower mixed venous oxygen tension and higher cardiac output (Fig. 5–17) than the patient with PK deficiency. These hemodynamic differences were reflected in the performance status of the two patients. The one with HK deficiency was a semi-invalid, whereas the PK-deficient individual played on his junior high school soccer team.

Reduction in Blood Flow

A number of studies indicate that increased oxygen affinity, when combined with reduced blood flow, will result in organ damage. Bakker and colleagues[255] demonstrated how this combination can cause significant impairment of hepatic function. When infused with blood having high oxygen affinity, animals are less able to tolerate hypovolemic shock[256] and have increased mortality.[256, 257] These studies are relevant to the infusion of large amounts of stored blood into patients with hemorrhagic shock.

CONCLUSION

Evolution has endowed man and other animals with a number of independent mechanisms to insure adequate delivery of oxygen to tissues. Under most circumstances, wide shifts in red cell oxygen affinity are well tolerated, owing to adjustments in ventilation, blood flow, and red cell mass. However, the oxygen dissociation curve assumes considerable importance when the organism is robbed of significant modes of compensation.

References

1. Waltemath, C. L.: Oxygen uptake, transport and tissue utilization. Anesth. Analg. 49:184, 1970.
2. Comroe, J. H., Jr.: Physiology of Respiration. Chicago, Year Book Medical Publishers, 1965.
3. Coin, J. T., and Olson, J. S.: The rate of oxygen uptake by human red blood cells. J. Biol. Chem. 254:1178, 1979.
4. Comroe, J. H., Jr., Forster, R. E., Dubois, A. B., Briscoe, W. A., and Carlsen, E.: The Lung. Clinical Physiology and Pulmonary Function Tests. 2nd ed. Chicago, Year Book Medical Publishers, 1962.
5. Schmidt-Nielsen, K., and Taylor, C. R.: Red blood cells: Why or why not? Science 162:274, 1968.
6. Castle, W. B., and Jandl, J. H.: Blood viscosity and blood volumes: Opposing influences upon oxygen transport in polycythemia. Semin. Hematol. 3:193, 1966.
7. Lawson, W. H., Jr., and Forster, R. E.: Oxygen tension gradients in peripheral capillary blood. J. Appl. Physiol. 22:970, 1967.
8. Woodson, R. D.: Physiological significance of oxygen dissociation curve shifts. Crit. Care Med. 7:368, 1979.
9. Krogh, A.: The number and distribution of capillaries in muscles with calculation of the oxygen pressure head necessary for supplying the tissue. J. Physiol. (Lond.) 52:409, 1919.
10. Longmuir, I. S., and Bourke, A.: The measurement of the diffusion of oxygen through respiring tissue. Biochem. J. 76:225, 1960.
11. Wittenberg, J. B.: Myoglobin-facilitated diffusion of oxygen. J. Gen. Physiol. 49(Part 2):57 1965.
12. Coburn, R. F., Ploegmakers, F., Gondrie, P., and Abboud, R.: Myocardial myoglobin oxygen tension. Am. J. Physiol. 224:870, 1973.
13. Chance, B., Cohen, P., and Jobsis, F.: Intracellular oxidation reduction states in vivo. Science 137:499, 1962.
14. Bartels, H., Betke, K., Hilpert, P., Niemeyer, G., and Riegel, K.: Die sogenannte Standard-O_2-dissoziations-kurve des gesunden erwachsenen Menschen. Pfluegers Arch. 272:372, 1961.
15. Humpeler, E., and Amor, H.: Sex differences in the oxygen affinity of hemoglobin. Pfluegers Arch. 343:151, 1973.
16. Astrup, P., Engel, K., Severinghaus, J. W., and Munson, E.: The influence of temperature and pH on the dissociation curve of oxyhemoglobin of human blood. Scand. J. Clin. Lab. Invest. 17:515, 1965.
16a. Reeves, R. B.: The effect of temperature on the oxygen equilibrium curve of human blood. Respir. Physiol. 42:317, 1980.
17. Benesch, R. E., Benesch, R., and Yu, C. I.: The oxygenation of hemoglobin in the presence of diphosphoglycerate. Effect of temperature, pH, ionic strength and hemoglobin concentration. Biochemistry 8:2567, 1969.
18. Riggs, A.: Mechanism of the enhancement of the Bohr effect in mammalian hemoglobins by diphosphoglycerate. Proc. Natl. Acad. Sci. USA 68:2062, 1971.
19. Wranne, B., Woodson, R. D., and Detter, J. C.: Bohr effect: Interaction between H^+, CO_2 and 2,3-DPG in fresh and stored blood. J. Appl. Physiol. 32:749, 1972.
20. Arturson, G., Garby, L., Wranne, B., and Zaar, B.: Effect of 2,3-diphosphoglycerate on the oxygen affinity and on the proton- and carbamino-linked oxygen affinity of hemoglobin in human whole blood. Acta Physiol. Scand. 92:332, 1974.
21. Card, R., and Brain, M.: The "anemia" of childhood. N. Engl. J. Med. 288:388, 1973.
22. Purcell, Y., and Brozovic, B.: Red cell 2,3-diphosphoglycerate concentration in man decreases with age. Nature 251:511, 1974.
23. Oski, F. A., and Gottlieb, A. J.: The interrelationships between red blood cell metabolites, hemoglobin and the oxygen-equilibrium curve. Prog. Hematol. 7:33, 1971.
24. Garby, L., and deVerdier, C. H.: Affinity of human hemoglobin A to 2,3-diphosphoglycerate. Effect of hemoglobin concentration and of pH. Scand. J. Clin. Lab. Invest. 27:345, 1971.
25. Hedlund, B. E., and Lovrien, R.: Thermodynamics of 2,3-diphosphoglycerate association with human oxy- and deoxyhemoglobin. Biochem. Biophys. Res. Commun. 61:859, 1974.
26. Hamasaki, N., and Rose, Z. B.: The binding of phosphorylated red cell metabolites to human hemoglobin A. J. Biol. Chem. 249:7896, 1974.
27. Berger, H., Janig, G.-R., Gerber, G., Ruckpaul, K., and Rapoport, S. M.: Interaction of haemoglobin with ions. Interactions among magnesium, adenosine 5'-triphosphate, 2,3-disphosphoglycerate and oxygenated and deoxygenated human haemoglobin under simulated intracellular conditions. Eur. J. Biochem. 38:553, 1973.
28. Guest, G. M., and Rapoport, S.: Role of acid soluble phosphorus compounds in red blood cells in experimental rickets, renal insufficiency, pyloric obstruction, gastroenteritis, ammonium chloride acidosis and diabetes acidosis. Am. J. Dis. Child. 58:1072, 1939.
29. Battaglia, F. C., McGaughey, H., Makowski, E. L., and Meschia, G.: Postnatal changes in oxygen affinity of sheep red cells: A dual role of 2,3-diphosphoglyceric acid. Am. J. Physiol. 219:217, 1970.
30. Waddell, W. J., and Bates, R. G.: Intracellular pH. Physiol. Rev. 49:285, 1969.
31. Duhm, J.: Effects of 2,3-diphosphoglycerate and other organic phosphate compounds on oxygen affinity and intracellular pH of human erythrocytes. Pfluegers Arch. 326:341, 1971.
32. Salhany, J. M., Keitt, A. S., and Eliot, R. S.: The rate of deoxygenation of red blood cells. Effect of intracellular 2,3-diphosphoglycerate and pH. FEBS Lett. 16:257, 1971.
33. Kilmartin, J. V., and Rossi-Bernardi, L.: Interaction of hemoglobin with hydrogen ions, carbon dioxide,

and organic phosphates. Physiol. Rev. *53*:836, 1973.
34. Benesch, R., and Benesch, R. E.: The effect of organic phosphates from the human erythrocyte on the allosteric properties of hemoglobin. Biochem. Biophys. Res. Commun. *26*:162, 1967.
35. Chanutin, A., and Curnish, R. R.: Effect of organic and inorganic phosphates on the oxygen equilibrium of human erythrocytes. Arch. Biochem. Biophys. *121*:96, 1967.
36. Bunn, H. F., Ransil, B. J., and Chao, A.: The interaction between erythrocyte organic phosphates, magnesium ion and hemoglobin. J. Biol. Chem. *246*:5273, 1971.
37. Rose, I. A.: The state of magnesium in cells as estimated from the adenylate kinase equilibrium. Proc. Natl. Acad. Sci. USA *61*:1079, 1968.
38. Bellingham, A. J., Detter, J. C., and Lenfant, C.: Regulatory mechanisms of hemoglobin oxygen affinity in acidosis and alkalosis. J. Clin. Invest. *50*:700, 1971.
39. May, A., and Huehns, E. R.: The mechanism of the low oxygen affinity of red cells in sickle cell disease. Haematol. Bluttransfus. *10*:279, 1972.
40. Murphy, J. R., Wengerd, M., and Kellermeyer, R. W.: Erythrocyte O_2 affinity: Influence of cell density and *in vitro* changes in hemoglobin concentration. J. Lab. Clin. Med. *84*:218, 1974.
41. Arturson, G., Garby, L., Robert, M., and Zaar, B.: Oxygen affinity of whole blood *in vivo* and under standard conditions in subjects with diabetes mellitus. Scand. J. Clin. Lab. Invest. *34*:19, 1974.
42. Rahbar, S.: An abnormal hemoglobin in red cells of diabetics. Clin. Chim. Acta *22*:296, 1968.
43. Trivelli, L. A., Ranney, H. M., and Lai, H.: Hemoglobin components in patients with diabetes mellitus. N. Engl. J. Med. *284*:353, 1971.
44. Bunn, H. F., and Briehl, R. W.: The interaction of 2,3-diphosphoglycerate with various human hemoglobins. J. Clin. Invest. *49*:1088, 1970.
45. Fernandez, L. A., and Erslev, A. J.: Oxygen affinity and compensated hemolysis in hereditary spherocytosis. J. Lab. Clin. Med. *80*:780, 1972.
46. Oski, F. A., Miller, L. D., Delivoria-Papadopoulos, M., Manchester, J. H., and Shelburne, J. C.: Oxygen affinity in red cells: Changes induced *in vivo* by propranolol. Science *175*:1372, 1972.
47. Pendleton, R. G., Newman, D. J., Sherman, S. S., Brann, E. G., and Maya, W. E.: Effect of propranolol upon the hemoglobin-oxygen dissociation curve. J. Pharmacol. Exp. Ther. *180*:647, 1972.
48. Agostoni, A., Berfasconi, C., Gerli, G. C., Luzzna, M., and Rossi-Bernardi, L.: Oxygen affinity and electrolyte distribution of human blood: Changes induced by propranolol. Science *182*:300, 1973.
49. Valtis, D. J., and Kennedy, A. C.: Defective gas-transport function of stored red blood cells. Lancet *1*:119, 1954.
50. Dawson, R. B.: Hemoglobin function: Effects of salts and glutathione. Vox Sang. *22*:26, 1972.
51. Rosenthal, A., Litwin, S. B., and Laver, M. B.: Effect of contrast media used in angiocardiography on hemoglobin-oxygen equilibrium. Invest. Radiol. *8*:191, 1973.
52. Lichtman, M. A., Whitbeck, A. A., and Murphy, M.: Fictitious changes in binding of oxygen to hemoglobin when based on extracellular pH in the presence of certain blood additives like radiographic contrast media. Invest. Radiol. *10*:225, 1975.
53. Rosenthal, A., and Mesrobian, A.: The relationship between angiography, intraerythrocytic pH and hemoglobin oxygen equilibrium. Invest. Radiol. *10*:140, 1975.
54. Kilmartin, J. V., and Rossi-Bernardi, L.: Inhibition of CO_2 combination and reduction of the Bohr effect in haemoglobin chemically modified at its α-amino groups. Nature *222*:1243, 1969.
55. DeFuria, F. G., Miller, D. R., Cerami, A., and Manning, J. M.: The effects of cyanate *in vitro* on red blood cell metabolism and function in sickle cell anemia. J. Clin. Invest. *51*:566, 1972.
56. Oelshlegel, F. J., Brewer, G. J., Prasad, A. S., Kurtsen, C., and Schoomaker, E. B.: Effect of zinc on increasing oxygen affinity of sickle and normal red blood cells. Biochem. Biophys. Res. Commun. *53*:560, 1973.
57. Kiesow, L. A., Bless, J. W., and Shelton, J. B.: Oxygen dissociation in human erythrocytes: Its response to hyperbaric environments. Science *179*:1236, 1973.
58. Shohet, S. B., Nathan, D. G., and Karnovsky, M. L.: Stages in the incorporation of fatty acids into red blood cells. J. Clin. Invest. *47*:1096, 1968.
59. Rapoport, S., and Luebering, J.: Glycerate-2,3-diphosphatase. J. Biol. Chem. *189*:683, 1951.
60. Williamson, J. R.: General features of metabolic control as applied to the erythrocyte. *In* Brewer, G. J. (ed.): Red Cell Metabolism and Function. New York, Plenum Press, 1970, p. 117.
61. Keitt, A. S.: Pyruvate kinase deficiency and related disorders of red cell glycolysis. Am. J. Med. *41*:762, 1966.
62. Minikami, S.: Effect of oxygen tension on glycolysis in erythrocytes. Forsvarsmedicin *5*:181, 1969.
63. Dawson, R. B., and Kocholaty, W. F.: Hemoglobin function during blood storage. XV. Effects of metabolic additives inosine and methylene blue on P_{50} and 2,3-DPG. *In* Brewer, G. J. (ed.): Hemoglobin and Red Cell Structure and Function. New York, Plenum Press, 1972, p. 495.
64. Rosa, R., Audit, I., and Rosa, J.: Evidence for three enzymatic activities in one electrophoretic band of 3-phosphoglycerate mutase from red cells. Biochimie *57*:1059, 1975.
65. Chiba, H., and Sasaki, R.: Functions of 2,3-bisphosphoglycerate and its metabolism. Curr. Top. Cell Regul. *14*:75, 1978.
66. Rose, Z. B.: The enzymology of 2,3-bisphosphoglycerate. Adv. Enzymol. *51*:211, 1980.
67. Mányai, S., and Várady, Zs.: Elektive Spallung der 2,3-Diphosphoglyzerinsäure in Erythrozyten. Biochim. Biophys. Acta *20*:594, 1956.
68. Harkness, D. R., and Roth, S.: Purification and properties of 2,3-diphosphoglyceric acid phosphatase from human erythrocytes. Biochem. Biophys. Res. Commun. *34*:849, 1969.
69. Rose, Z. B., and Liebowtiz, J.: 2,3-Diphosphoglycerate phosphatase from human erythrocytes. J. Biol. Chem. *245*:3232, 1970.
70. Parker, J. C.: Influence of 2,3-diphosphoglycerate metabolism on sodium-potassium permeability in human red blood cells: Studies with bisulfite and other redox reagents. J. Clin. Invest. *48*:117, 1969.
71. Han, C.-H., and Rose, Z. B.: Active site phosphohistidine peptides from red cell bisphosphoglycerate synthase and yeast phosphoglycerate mutase. J. Biol. Chem. *254*:8836, 1979.
72. Harkness, D. R., Ponce, J., and Grayson, V.: A comparative study on the phosphoglyceric acid

cycle in mammalian erythrocytes. Comp. Biochem. Physiol. 28:129, 1969.
73. Peterson, L. L.: Red cell diphosphoglycerate mutase. Immunochemical studies in vertebrate red cells, including a human variant lacking 2,3-DPG. Blood 52:953, 1978.
74. Alagille, D., Fleury, J., and Odievre, M.: Déficit congénital en 2,3-diphosphoglyceromutase. Soc. Méd. Hôp. Paris 115:493, 1964.
74a. Schroter, W.: Kongenitale nichtspharocytare hamolytische Anamie bei 2,3-Diphosphoglyceratmutase-Mangel der Erythrocyten im fruhen Sauglingsalter. Klin. Wochenschr. 43:1147, 1965.
75. Cartier, P., Labie, D., Leroux, J. P., Najman, A., and Demaugre, F.: Déficit familial en diphosphoglycerate mutase: Étude hématologique et biochimique. Nouv. Rev. Fr. Hematol. 12:269, 1972.
75a. Travis, S. F., Martinez, J., Garvin, J., Jr., Atwater, J., and Gillmer, P.: Study of a kindred with partial deficiency of red cell 2,3-diphosphoglycerate mutase (2,3-DPGM) and compensated hemolysis. Blood 51:1107, 1978.
76. Rosa, R., Prehu, M.-O., Beuzard, Y., and Rosa, J.: The first case of a complete deficiency of diphosphoglycerate mutase in human erythrocytes. J. Clin. Invest. 62:907, 1978.
76a. Sasaki, R., and Chiba, H.: Role and induction of 2,3-bisphosphoglycerate synthase. Mol. Cell. Biochem. 53/54:247, 1983.
77. Narita, H., Ikura, K., Yanagawa, S., Sasaki, R., Chiba, H., Saimyoji, H., and Kumagai, N.: 2,3-bisphosphoglycerate in developing rabbit erythroid cells. J. Biol. Chem. 255:5230, 1980.
78. Narita, H., Yanagawa, S., Sasaki, R., and Chiba, H.: Induction of 2,3-bisphosphoglycerate synthase in Friend leukemia cells. Biochem. Biophys. Res. Commun. 103:90, 1981.
78a. Wu, Y., Dean, A., and Schechter, A. N.: The relationship between 2,3-DPG levels and hemoglobin in K562 cells. Blood 60:59a, 1982.
79. Rose, Z. B., and Salon, J.: The identification of glycolate-2-P as a constituent of normal red blood cells. Biochem. Biophys. Res. Commun. 87:869, 1979.
80. Momsen, G., and Vestergaard-Bogind, B.: Human erythrocyte 2,3-diphosphoglycerate metabolism. Influence of 1,3-diphosphoglycerate and P_i. Arch. Biochem. Biophys. 190:67, 1978.
81. Rapoport, I., Berger, Elsner, R., and Rapoport, S.: pH-dependent changes of 2,3-bisphosphoglycerate in human red cells during transitional and steady states in vitro. Eur. J. Biochem. 73:421, 1977.
82. Rose, Z. B.: The purification and properties of diphosphoglycerate mutase from human erythrocytes. J. Biol. Chem. 243:4810, 1968.
83. Rose, Z. B.: Effects of salts and pH on the rate of erythrocyte diphosphoglycerate mutase. Arch. Biochem. Biophys. 158:903, 1973.
84. Badwey, J. A.: Phosphoglycolate phosphatase in human erythrocytes. J. Biol. Chem. 252:2441, 1977.
84a. Somoza, R., and Beutler, E.: Phosphoglycolate phosphatase and 2,3-diphosphoglycerate in red cells of normal and anemic subjects. Blood 62:750, 1983.
85. Dische, Z.: The pentose phosphate metabolism in red cells. In Bishop, C., and Surgenor, D. M. (eds.): The Red Blood Cell: A Comprehensive Treatise. New York, Academic Press, 1964, p. 189.

86. Brewer, G. J.: Erythrocyte metabolism and function: Hexokinase inhibition by 2,3-diphosphoglycerate and interaction with ATP and Mg^{2+}. Biochim. Biophys. Acta 192:157, 1969.
87. Beutler, E.: 2,3-Diphosphoglycerate affects enzymes of glucose metabolism in red blood cells. Nature [New Biol.] 232:20, 1971.
88. Harkness, D. R., Ponce, J., and Roth, S.: Kinetic studies of the inhibition of glycolytic kinases of human erythrocytes by 2,3-diphosphoglyceric acid. Biochim. Biophys. Acta 250:63, 1971.
89. deVerdier, C. H., and Garby, L.: Glucose metabolism in normal erythrocytes: II. Factors influencing the hexokinase step. Scand. J. Haematol. 2:305, 1965.
90. Staal, G. E., and Koster, J. F.: Influence of 2,3-diphosphoglycerate on phosphofructokinase of human erythrocytes? FEBS Lett. 23:29, 1972.
91. Askari, A., and Rao, S. N.: Regulation of AMP deaminase by 2,3-diphosphoglyceric acid: A possible mechanism for the control of adenine nucleotide metabolism in human erythrocytes. Biochim. Biophys. Acta 151:198, 1968.
92. Lian, C.-Y., and Harkness, D. R.: The kinetic properties of adenylate deaminase from human erythrocytes. Biochim. Biophys. Acta 341:27, 1974.
93. Hershko, A., Razin, A., and Mager, J.: Regulation of the synthesis of 5-phosphoribosyl-1-pyrophosphate in intact red blood cell and in cell free preparations. Biochim. Biophys. Acta 184:64, 1969.
94. Yip, L. C., and Balis, M. E.: Inhibitory effects of 2,3-DPG on enzymes of purine nucleotide metabolism. Biochem. Biophys. Res. Commun. 63:722, 1975.
95. Gerber, G., Berger, H., Janig, G.-R., and Rapoport, S.: Interaction of haemoglobin with ions. Quantitative description of the state of magnesium adenosine 5′-triphosphate, 2,3-diphosphoglycerate and human hemoglobin under simulated intracellular conditions. Eur. J. Biochem. 38:563, 1973.
96. Gupta, R. K., Benovic, J. L., and Rose, Z. B.: The determination of free magnesium level in the human red cell by ^{31}P-NMR. J. Biol. Chem. 253:6172, 1978.
97. Gonzatti-Haces, M. I., and Traugh, J. A.: Kinetics of phosphorylation of eIF-2 by the hemin-controlled repressor and casein kinase II. J. Biol. Chem. 257:6642, 1982.
98. Sheetz, M.: Personal communication, 1983.
99. Lenfant, C., Torrance, J. D., and Reynafarje, C.: Shift of the O_2-Hb dissociation curve at altitude: Mechanism and effect. J. Appl. Physiol. 30:625, 1971.
100. Duhm, J., and Gerlach, E.: On the mechanisms of the hypoxia-induced increase of 2,3-diphosphoglycerate in erythrocytes. Pfluegers Arch. 326:254, 1971.
101. Oski, F. A., Gottlieb, A. J., Miller, W. W., and Delivoria-Papadopoulos, M.: The effects of deoxygenation of adult and fetal hemoglobin on the synthesis of red cell 2,3-diphosphoglycerate and its in vivo consequences. J. Clin. Invest. 49:400, 1970.
102. Lokich, J. J., Maloney, W. C., Bunn, H. F., Bruckheimer, S. M., and Ranney, H. M.: Hemoglobin Brigham ($\alpha_2^A \beta_2^{100\ Pro \rightarrow Leu}$), hemoglobin variant associated with familial erythrocytosis. J. Clin. Invest. 52:2060, 1973.
103. Dinman, B. D., Eaton, J. W., and Brewer, G. J.:

Effects of carbon monoxide on DPG concentrations in the erythrocyte. Ann. N.Y. Acad. Sci. *174*:246, 1970.
104. Rose, I. A., and Warms, J. V. B.: Control of red cell glycolysis: The cause of triose phosphate accumulation. J. Biol. Chem. *245*:4009, 1970.
105. Versmold, H., Kohne, E., Kleihauer, E., and Riegel, K.: Die Sauerstofftransport funktion des Blutis bei hereditar Methamoglobinamie Die Rolle des 2,3-diphosphoglycerates. Monatsschr. Kinderheilkd. *121*:397, 1973.
106. Hamasaki, N., Minakami, S., and Aono, K.: 2,3-Diphosphoglycerate content of human arterial and venous blood. Nature [New Biol] *229*:215, 1971.
107. DeLaMorena, E.: Biochemical differences with respect to the determination of 2,3-diphosphoglycerate in arterial and venous blood of normal individuals. Biochem. Med. *20*:382, 1978.
108. Ravin, M. B., Drury, W. L., Keitt, A. S., and Daicoff, G.: Red cell 2,3-diphosphoglycerate in surgical correction of cyanotic congenital heart disease. Anesth. Analg. *52*:599, 1973.
109. Edwards, M. J., Koler, R. D., Rigas, D. A., and Pitcairn, D. M.: The effect of *in vivo* aging of normal human erythrocytes and erythrocyte macromolecules upon oxyhemoglobin dissociation. J. Clin. Invest. *40*:636, 1961.
110. Waldeck, F.: Ein mikrophotometrisches Verfahren zur Aufnahme der Sauerstoffbindungskurve von einzelnen Erythrocyten. Pfluegers Arch. *295*:1, 1967.
111. Edwards, M. J., and Rigas, D. A.: Electrolyte labile increase of oxygen affinity during *in vivo* aging of hemoglobin. J. Clin. Invest. *46*:1579, 1967.
112. Murphy, J. R., Wengerd, M., and Kellermeyer, R. W.: Erythrocyte O_2 affinity: Influence of cell density and *in vitro* changes in hemoglobin concentration. J. Lab. Clin. Med. *84*:218, 1974.
113. Bernstein, R. E.: Alterations in metabolic energetics and cation transport during aging of red cells. J. Clin. Invest. *38*:1572, 1959.
114. Bunn, H. F., May, M. H., Kocholaty, W., and Shields, C. E.: Hemoglobin function in stored blood. J. Clin. Invest. *48*:311, 1969.
115. Haidas, S., Labie, D., and Kaplan, J. C.: 2,3-Diphosphoglycerate content and oxygen affinity as a function of red cell age in normal individuals. Blood *38*:463, 1971.
116. Hjelm, M.: The content of 2,3-diphosphoglycerate and some other phosphocompounds in human erythrocytes from healthy adults and subjects with different types of anaemia. Forsvarsmedicin *5*:219, 1969.
117. Edwards, M. J., Cannon, B., Albertson, J., and Bigley, R. H.: Mean red cell age, a determinant of blood oxygen affinity. Nature *230*:583, 1971.
118. Valeri, C. R., and Fortier, N. L.: Red-cell 2,3-diphosphoglycerate and creatine levels in patients with red-cell mass deficits or with cardiopulmonary insufficiency. N. Engl. J. Med. *281*:1452, 1969.
119. Torrance, J. D., Jacobs, P., Restrepo, A., Eschbach, J., Lenfant, C., and Finch, C. A.: Intraerythrocytic adaptation to anemia. N. Engl. J. Med. *283*:165, 1970.
120. Koch, H.-H., and Schroter, W.: Kompensatorische Veranderungen der erythrocytaren 2,3-diphosphoglycerat Konzentration bei Anamien und Polyglobulien. Monatsschr. Kinderheilkd. *121*:392, 1973.
121. Eaton, J. W., and Brewer, G. J.: The relationship between red cell 2,3-diphosphoglycerate and levels of hemoglobin in the human. Proc. Natl. Acad. Sci. USA *61*:756, 1968.
122. Opalinski, A., and Beutler, E.: Creatine, 2,3-diphosphoglycerate and anemia. N. Engl. J. Med. *285*:283, 1971.
123. Humpeler, E., Amor, H., and Braunsteiner, H.: Unterschedliche Sauerstoffaffinität des Hämoglobins bei Anamien verschiedener Atiologie. Blut *29*:382, 1974.
124. Dickerman, J. D., Ostrea, E. M., and Zinkham, W. H.: *In vivo* aging of transfused erythrocytes and 2,3-diphosphoglycerate levels. Blood *42*:9, 1973.
125. Lichtman, M. A., Murphy, M. S., Whitbeck, A. A., and Kearney, E. A.: Oxygen binding to hemoglobin in subjects with hypoproliferative anaemia, with and without chronic renal disease: Role of pH. Br. J. Haematol. *27*:439, 1974.
126. Palek, J., Mircevova, A., and Brabec, V.: 2,3-Diphosphoglycerate metabolism in hereditary spherocytosis. Br. J. Haematol. *17*:59, 1969.
127. Albala, M. M., Fortier, N. L., and Glader, B. E.: Physiologic features of hemolysis associated with altered cation and 2,3-diphosphoglycerate content. Blood *52*:135, 1978.
128. Hakim, J., Boucherot, J., Troube, H., and Boivin, P.: Red cell 2,3-diphosphoglycerate and adenosine triphosphate levels in patients with polycythemia vera. Rev. Eur. Étud. Clin. Biol. *17*:99, 1972.
129. Hjelm, M., and Wadman, B.: Eyrthrocyte-DPG and creatine in polycythemia. N. Engl. J. Med. *287*:45, 1972.
130. Lenfant, C., and Sullivan, K.: Adaptation to high altitude. N. Engl. J. Med. *284*:1298, 1971.
131. Lenfant, C., Torrance, J., English, E., Finch, C. A., Reynafarje, C., Ramos, J., and Faura, J.: Effect of altitude on oxygen binding by hemoglobin and on organic phosphate levels. J. Clin. Invest. *47*:2652, 1968.
131a. Winslow, R. M., Samaja, M., and West, J. B.: Red-cell function at extreme altitude on Mount Everest. J. Appl. Physiol. *56*:109, 1984.
132. Eaton, J. W., Brewer, G. J., and Grover, R. F.: Role of red cell 2,3-diphosphoglycerate in the adaptation of man to altitude. J. Lab. Clin. Med. *73*:603, 1969.
133. Torrance, J. D., and Bartlett, G. R.: Altitude hypoxia and erythrocyte phosphates. Biochim. Biophys. Acta *215*:409, 1970.
134. Klocke, R. A.: Oxygen transport and 2,3-diphosphoglycerate. Chest *62*(Suppl.):79S, 1972.
135. Eaton, J. W., Skelton, T. D., and Berger, E.: Survival at extreme altitude: Protective effect of increased hemoglobin-oxygen affinity. Science *183*:743, 1974.
136. Oski, F. A., Gottlieb, A. J., Deliveria-Papadopoulos, M., and Miller, W. W.: Red-cell 2,3-diphosphoglycerate levels in subjects with chronic hypoxemia. N. Engl. J. Med. *280*:1165, 1969.
137. Edwards, M. J., Novy, M. J., Walters, C.-L., and Metcalfe, J.: Improved oxygen release: An adaptation of mature red cells to hypoxia. J. Clin. Invest. *47*:1851, 1968.
138. Flenley, D. C., Fairweather, L. J., Cooke, N. J., and Kerby, B. J.: Changes in haemoglobin binding curve and oxygen transport in chronic hypoxia lung disease. Br. Med. J. *1*:602, 1975.
139. Keitt, A. S., Hinkes, C., and Block, A. J.: Compar-

ison of factors regulating red cell 2,3-diphosphoglycerate (2,3-DPG) in acute and chronic hypoxemia. J. Lab. Clin. Med. *84*:275, 1974.
140. Gallagher, P. J.: 2,3-Diphosphoglycerate in acute asthma. J. Clin. Pathol. *24*:518, 1971.
141. Litwin, S. B., Rosenthal, A., Skogen, W. F., and Laver, M. B.: Long-term studies of hemoglobin-oxygen affinity in hypoxemic dogs with a right-to-left cardiac shunt. J. Surg. Res. *28*:118, 1980.
142. Young, J. A., Lichtman, M. A., and Cohen, J.: Reduced red cell 2,3-diphosphoglycerate and adenosine triphosphate, hypophosphatemia and increased hemoglobin-oxygen affinity after cardiac surgery. Circulation *47*:1313, 1973.
143. Woodson, R. D., Torrance, J. D., Shappell, S. D., and Lenfant, C.: The effect of cardiac disease on hemoglobin-oxygen binding. J. Clin. Invest. *49*:1349, 1970.
144. Kostuk, W. J., Suwa, K., Berstein, E. F., and Sobel, B. E.: Altered hemoglobin oxygen affinity in patients with acute myocardial infarction. Am. J. Cardiol. *31*:295, 1973.
145. Lichtman, M. A., Cohen, J., Young, J. A., Whitbeck, A. A., and Murphy, M.: The relationships between arterial oxygen flow rate, oxygen binding by hemoglobin and oxygen utilization after myocardial infarction. J. Clin. Invest. *54*:501, 1974.
146. Miller, L. D., Oski, F. A., Diaco, J. F., Sugarman, H. J., Gottlieb, A. J., Davidson, D., and Delivoria-Papadopoulos, M.: The affinity of hemoglobin for oxygen: Its control and *in vivo* significance. Surgery *68*:187, 1970.
147. Chillar, R. K., Slawsky, P., and Desforges, J. F.: Red cell 2,3-diphosphoglycerate and adenosine triphosphate in patients with shock. Br. J. Haematol. *21*:183, 1971.
148. Agostoni, A., Lotto, A., Stabilini, R., Bernasconi, C., Gerli, G., Gattinoni, L., Iapichino, G., and Salvede, P.: Hemoglobin oxygen affinity in patients with low-output heart failure and cardiogenic shock after acute myocardial infarction. Eur. J. Cardiol. *3*:53, 1975.
149. Holsinger, J. W., Salhany, J. M., and Eliot, R. S.: Physiologic observations on the effect of impaired blood oxygen release on the myocardium. Adv. Cardiol. *9*:81, 1973.
150. Eliot, R. S., and Bratt, G.: The paradox of myocardial ischemia and necrosis in young women with normal coronary angiograms. Am. J. Cardiol. *23*:633, 1969.
151. Eliot, R. S., Salhany, J., and Mizukami, H.: Angina and infarction occurring with patent coronary arteries and decreased rate of oxygen release. Adv. Cardiol. *5*:106, 1970.
152. Vokonas, P. S., Cohn, P. F., Klein, M. D., Laver, M. B., and Gorlin, R.: Hemoglobin affinity for oxygen in the anginal syndrome with normal coronary arteriograms. J. Clin. Invest. *54*:409, 1974.
153. Verdier, F., Fay, M., and Korobaeff, M.: Mésure de l'affinité de l'hémoglobine pour l'oxygène. Application aux malades atteints d'angine de poitrine avec coronarographie normale étude de dix cas. Nouv. Presse Méd. *4*:1550, 1975.
154. Shappell, S. D., Murray, J. A., Nasser, M. G., Wills, R. E., Torrance, J. D., and Lenfant, C. J. M.: Acute change in hemoglobin affinity for oxygen during angina pectoris. N. Engl. J. Med. *282*:1219, 1970.
155. Colvard, M. C., and Longmuir, I. S.: The effects of pacing on oxygen hemoglobin dissociation and oxygen carrying capacity in patients suspected of coronary artery disease. Am. Heart J., *85*:662, 1973.
156. Gross, G. J., and Hardman, H. F.: Alteration in oxyhemoglobin equilibrium (P-50) and myocardial oxygen consumption (mVO$_2$) by nitroglycerin. J. Pharmacol. Exp. Ther. *193*:346, 1975.
157. Bellingham, A. J., Detter, J. C., and Lenfant, C.: The role of hemoglobin affinity for oxygen and red-cell 2,3-diphosphoglycerate in the management of diabetic ketoacidosis. Trans. Assoc. Am. Phys. *83*:113, 1970.
158. Alberti, K. G. M., Emerson, P. M., Darley, J. H., and Hockaday, T. D. R.: 2,3-Diphosphoglycerate and tissue oxygenation in uncontrolled diabetes mellitus. Lancet *2*:391, 1972.
159. Astrup, P.: Red cell pH and oxygen affinity of hemoglobin. N. Engl. J. Med. *283*:202, 1970.
160. Astrup, P., Rörth, M., and Thorshauge, C.: Dependency on acid-base status of oxyhemoglobin dissociation and 2,3-diphosphoglycerate level in human erythrocytes. II. *In vivo* studies. Scand. J. Clin. Lab. Invest. *26*:47, 1970.
161. Jacob, H. S., and Amsden, T.: Acute hemolytic anemia with rigid red cells in hypophosphatemia. N. Engl. J. Med. *285*:1446, 1971.
162. Lichtman, M. A., Miller, D. R., Cohen, J., and Waterhouse, C.: Reduced red cell glycolysis, 2,3-diphosphoglycerate and adenosine triphosphate concentration and increased hemoglobin-oxygen affinity caused by hypophosphatemia. Ann. Intern. Med. *74*:562, 1971.
163. Sheldon, G. F., Plazak, L. F., Watkins, G. M., and Moore, F. D.: Inorganic phosphate and the oxyhemoglobin dissociation curve. Surg. Forum *22*:81, 1971.
164. Travis, S. F., Sugarman, H. J., Ruberg, R. L., Dudrick, S. J., Deliveria-Papadopoulos, M., Miller, L. D., and Oski, F. A.: Alterations of red-cell glycolytic intermediates and oxygen transport as a consequence of hypophosphatemia in patients receiving intravenous hyperalimentation. N. Engl. J. Med. *285*:763, 1971.
165. Mitchell, T. R., and Pegrum, G. D.: The oxygen affinity in chronic renal failure. Br. J. Haematol. *21*:463, 1971.
166. Hurt, G. A., and Chanutin, A.: Organic phosphate compounds of erythrocytes from individuals with uremia. J. Lab. Clin. Med. *64*:675, 1964.
167. Lichtman, M. A., Murphy, M. S., Byer, B. J., and Freeman, R. B.: Hemoglobin affinity for oxygen in chronic renal disease. The effect of hemodialysis. Blood *43*:417, 1974.
168. Raich, P. C., Rodriguez, J. M., Desai, J. N., and Shahidi, N. T.: Effect of hemodialysis on erythrocyte 2,3-diphosphoglycerate in patients with uremia. Am. J. Med. Sci. *265*:147, 1973.
169. Bursaux, E., Broyer, M., Poyart, C., Bohn, B., and Jean, G.: Oxygen transport in children on maintenance haemodialysis. Clin. Sci. Mol. Med. *54*:85, 1978.
170. Keys, A., and Snell, A. M.: Respiratory properties of the arterial blood in normal man and in patients with disease of the liver: Position of the oxygen dissociation curve. J. Clin. Invest. *17*:59, 1938.
171. Caldwell, P. R. B., Fritts, H. W., and Cournand, A.: Oxyhemoglobin dissociation curve in liver disease. J. Appl. Physiol. *20*:316, 1965.
172. Mulhausen, R., Astrup, P., and Kjeldsen, K.: Oxygen affinity of hemoglobin in patients with cardiovascular diseases, anemia, and cirrhosis of the liver. Scand. J. Clin. Lab. Invest. *19*:291, 1967.

173. Hurt, G. A., and Chanutin, A.: Organic phosphate compounds of erythrocytes from individuals with cirrhosis of the liver. Proc. Soc. Exp. Biol. Med. 118:167, 1965.
174. Astrup, P., and Rörth, ML: Oxygen affinity of hemoglobin and red cell 2,3-diphosphoglycerate in hepatic cirrhosis. Scand J. Clin. Lab. Invest. 31:311, 1973.
175. Farber, M. O., Carlone, S., Serra, P., Capocaccia, L., Rossi-Fannelli, F., Antonini, E., and Manfredi, F.: The oxygen affinity of hemoglobin in hepatic encephalopathy. J. Lab. Clin. Med. 98:135, 1981.
176. Ditzel, J., and Dyerberg, J.: The oxyhemoglobin dissociation curve in patients with familial hyperchylomicronemia. J. Lab. Clin. Med. 89:573, 1977.
177. Cooksey, J., and Reilly, P.: Effect of hypercholesterolemia on the hemoglobin-oxygen dissociation curve of the rabbit. J. Surg. Res. 22:23, 1977.
178. Miller, W. W., Delivoria-Papadopoulos, M., Miller, L., and Oski, F. A.: Oxygen releasing factor in hyperthyroidism. J.A.M.A. 211:1824, 1970.
179. Gahlenbeck, H., and Bartels, H.: Veranderung der Sauerstoffbindungskurven des Blutes bei Hyperthyreosen und nach Gabe von Trijodthyronin bei Gesunden und bei Ratten. Klin. Wochenschr. 46:547, 1968.
180. Gahlenbeck, H., Rathschlag-Schaefer, A-M., and Bartels, H.: Triiodothyronine induced changes of oxygen affinity of blood. Respir. Physiol. 6:16, 1968.
181. Snyder, L. M., and Reddy, W. J.: The effect of 3,5,3-triiodothyronine on red cell 2,3-diphosphoglyceric acid. Clin. Res. 18:416, 1970.
182. Alvares-Sala, J. L., Urbán M. A., Sicilia, J. J., Diaz Fdez, A. J., Mendieta, F. F., and Espinos, D.: Red-cell 2,3-diphosphoglycerate in patients with hyperthyroidism. Acta Endocrinol. 93:424, 1980.
183. Mills, G. C., Bowman, A. B., and Johnson, J. E.: Effects of triiodothyronine on glutathione and phosphate esters of human erythrocytes. Tex. Rep. Biol. Med. 24:629, 1966.
184. Monti, M.: Red cell, 2,3-diphosphoglycerate in patients with hyperthyroidism before and after treatment. Acta Med. Scand. 196:263, 1974.
185. Zaroulis, C. G., Kourides, I. A., and Valeri, C. R.: Red cell 2,3-diphosphoglycerate and oxygen affinity of hemoglobin in patients with thyroid disorders. Blood 52:181, 1978.
186. Duhm, J., Deuticke, B., and Gerlach, E.: Beeinflusst Trijodthyronin den 2,3-Diphosphoglycerat-Gehalt von Eyrhrocyten? Naturwissenschaften 56:329, 1969.
187. Brewer, G. J., Oelschlegel, F. J., Jr., and Eaton, J. A.: Biochemical, physiological and genetic factors in the regulation of mammalian erythrocyte metabolism and DPG levels. In Rörth, M., and Astrup, P. (eds.): Oxygen Affinity of Hemoglobin and Red Cell Acid-Base Status. New York, Academic Press, 1972, p. 539.
188. Snyder, L. M., and Reddy, W. J.: Mechanism of action of thyroid hormones on erythrocyte 2,3-diphosphoglyceric acid synthesis. J. Clin. Invest. 49:1993, 1970.
189. Czernik, A. J., Psychoyos, S., and Cash, W. D.: Failure of thyroid hormones to enhance the activity of diphosphoglycerate mutase. Endocrinology 96:508, 1974.
190. Torrance, J. D.: Diphosphoglycerate mutase assay: The effect of pyruvate, lactate dehydrogenase and thyroid hormone on the assay. Clin. Chim. Acta 50:103, 1974.
191. Lappin, T. R. J., and Elmore, D. T.: The effect of thyroid hormones and other kinetic modifiers on bisphosphoglyceromutase from human erythrocytes. Biochem. Pharmacol. 29:517, 1980.
192. Riegel, K., Versmold, H., Windhorst, H., and Horn, K.: Thyroxine and red cell 2,3-diphosphoglycerate in the newborn period. Klin. Wochenschr. 51:138, 1973.
193. Versmold, H., Horn, K., Windhorst, H., and Riegel, K. P.: The rapid postnatal increase of red cell 2,3-diphosphoglycerate: Its relation to plasma thyroxine. Respir. Physiol. 18:26, 1973.
194. Rodriguez, J. M., and Shahidi, N. T.: Erythrocyte 2,3-diphosphoglycerate in adaptive red-cell-volume deficiency. N. Engl. J. Med. 285:479, 1971.
195. Parker, J. P., Beirne, G. J., Desai, J. N., Raich, P. C., and Shahidi, N. T.: Androgen-induced increase in red-cell 2,3-diphosphoglycerate. N. Engl. J. Med. 287:381, 1972.
196. Gorshein, D., Oski, F. A., and Delivoria-Papadopoulos, M.: Effect of androgens on the red cell 2,3-diphosphoglycerate hemoglobin oxygen affinity and red cell mass in mammals. Proc. Soc. Exp. Biol. Med. 147:616. 1974.
197. Smolin, M. F., Zanjani, E. D., Hoffman, R., and Wasserman, L. R.: Mechanism of androgen action on erythropoiesis. Clin. Res. 23:583A, 1975.
198. Molinari, P. F., Chung, S. K., and Snyder, L. M.: Variations of erythrocyte glycolysis following androgens. J. Lab. Clin. Med. 81:443, 1973.
199. Bauer, C., and Rathschlag-Schaefer, A-M.: The influence of aldosterone and cortisol on oxygen affinity and cation concentration of the blood. Respir. Physiol. 5:360, 1968.
200. Silken, A. B.: Pharmacologic manipulation of human erythrocyte 2,3-diphosphoglycerate levels by prednisone administration. Pediatr. Res. 9:61, 1975.
201. Rörth, M.: Hemoglobin interactions and red cell metabolism. Ser. Haematol. 5:82, 1972.
202. Alevizos, B., and Stefanis, C.: 2,3-Diphosphoglycerate in Parkinson's disease. J. Neruol. Neurosurg. Psychiatry 39:952, 1976.
203. Meen, H. D., Holter, P. H., and Refsum, H. E.: Changes in 2,3-diphosphoglycerate (2,3-DPG) after exercise. Eur. J. Appl. Physiol. 46:177, 1981.
204. Eaton, J. W., Faulkner, J. A., and Brewer, G. J.: Response of the human red cell to muscular activity. Proc. Soc. Exp. Biol. Med. 132:886, 1969.
205. Shappell, S. D., Murray, J. A., Bellingham, A. J., Woodson, R. D., Detter, J. G., and Lenfant, C.: Adaptation to exercise: Role of hemoglobin affinity for oxygen and 2,3-diphosphoglycerate. J. Appl. Physiol. 30:827, 1971.
206. Thomson, J. M., Dempsey, J. A., Chosy, L. W., Shahidi, N. T., and Reddan, W. G.: Oxygen transport and oxyhemoglobin dissociation during prolonged muscular work. J. Appl. Physiol. 37:658, 1974.
207. Braumann, K. M., Boning, D., and Trost, F.: Oxygen dissociation curves in trained and untrained subjects. Eur. J. Appl. Physiol. 42:51, 1979.
208. Remes, K., Vuopio, P., and Harkonen, M.: Effect of long-term training and acute physical exercise on red cell 2,3-diphosphoglycerate. Eur. J. Appl. Physiol. 42:199, 1979.
209. Boswart, J., Kuta, I., Lisy, Z., and Kostiuk, P.: 2,3-Diphosphoglycerate during exercise. Eur. J. Appl. Physiol. 43:193, 1980.

210. Rand, P. W., Norton, J. M., Barker, N., and Lovell, M.: Influence of athletic training on hemoglobin-oxygen affinity. Am. J. Physiol. 224:1334, 1973.
211. Novy, M. J., and Parer, J. T.: Absence of high blood oxygen affinity in the fetal cat. Respir. Physiol. 6:144, 1969.
212. Charache, S., Jacobson, R., Brimhall, B., Murphy, E. A. Hathaway, P., Winslow, R., Jones, R., Rath, C., and Simkovich, J.: Hb Potomac (101 Glu→Asp): Speculations on placental oxygen transport in carriers of high affinity hemoglobins. Blood 51:331, 1978.
213. Oski, F. A.: Clinical implications of the oxyhemoglobin dossociation curve in the neonatal period. Crit. Care Med. 7:412, 1979.
214. Wimberley, P. D.: Fetal hemoglobin, 2,3-diphosphoglycerate and oxygen transport in the newborn premature infant. Scand. J. Clin. Lab. Invest. 42(Suppl. 160):1, 1982.
215. deVerdier, C. H., and Garby, L.: Low binding of 2,3-diphosphoglycerate to haemoglobin F: A contribution to the knowledge of the binding site and an explanation for the high oxygen affinity of foetal blood. Scand. J. Clin. Lab. Invest. 23:149, 1969.
216. Bauer, C., Ludwig, I., and Ludwig, M.: Different effects of 2,3-diphosphoglycerate and adenosine triphosphate on the oxygen affinity of adult and foetal human haemoglobin. Life Sci. 7:1339, 1968.
217. Tyuma, I., and Shimizu, K.: Different response to organic phosphates of human fetal and adult hemoglobins. Arch. Biochem. Biophys. 129:404, 1969.
218. Delivoria-Papadopoulos, M., Roncevic, N. P., and Oski, F. A.: Postnatal changes in oxygen transport of term, premature and sick infants. The role of red cell 2,3-diphosphoglycerate and adult hemoglobin. Pediatr. Res. 5:235, 1971.
219. Delivoria-Papadopoulos, M., Miller, L., Forster, R., and Oski, F. A.: The role of exchange transfusion in the management of low-birth-weight infants with and without severe respiratory distress syndrome. I. Initial observations. J. Pediatr. 89:273, 1976.
220. Gottuso, M., Williams, M., and Oski, F.: Exchange transfusion in low-birth-weight infants. II. Further observations. J. Pediatr. 89:279, 1976.
221. Sohmer, P. R., and Dawson, R. B.: Significance of 2,3-DPG in red blood-cell transfusions. CRC Crit. Rev. Clin. Lab. Sci. 11:107, 1979.
222. Gullbring, B., and Strom, G.: Changes in oxygen carrying function of human hemoglobin during storage in cold acid-citrate-dextrose solution. Acta Med. Scand. 155:413, 1956.
223. Akerblöm, O., deVerdier, C. H., Garby, L., and Högman, C.: Restoration of defective oxygen-transport function of stored red blood cells by addition of inosine. Scand. J. Clin. Lab. Invest. 21:245, 1968.
224. Sirs, J. A.: Effects of storage on the respiratory function and flexibility of red blood cells. Blood Cells 3:409, 1977.
225. Beutler, E., and Wood, L. A.: The in vivo regeneration of red cell 2,3-diphosphoglyceric acid after transfusion of stored blood. J. Lab. Clin. Med. 74:300, 1969.
226. Valeri, C. R., and Hirsch, N. M.: Restoration in vivo of erythrocyte adenosine triphosphate, 2,3-diphosphoglycerate, potassium ion and sodium ion concentrations following the transfusion of acid-citrate-dextrose–stored human red blood cells. J. Lab. Clin. Med. 73:722, 1969.
227. Huisman, T. H. J., Boyd, E. M., Kitchens, J., Mayson, S., and Shepeard, W. L.: Oxygen equilibria and biochemical changes of whole blood stored in different preservation media. Transfusion 9:180, 1969.
228. Dawson, R. B., and Ellis, T. J.: The hemoglobin function of blood stored at 4°C in ACD and CPD with adenine and inosine. Transfusion 10:113, 1970.
229. Oski, F. A., Travis, S. F., Miller, L. D., Delivoria-Papadopoulos, M., and Cannon, E.: The in vitro restoration of red cell 2,3-diphosphoglycerate levels in banked blood. Blood 37:52, 1971.
230. Dawson, R. B., and Kocholaty, W. F.: Hemoglobin function during blood storage. XV. Effects of metabolic additives inosine and methylene blue on P_{50} and 2,3-DPG. In Brewer, G. J. (ed.): Hemoglobin and Red Cell Structure and Function. New York, Plenum Press, 1972, p. 495.
231. Torrance, J. D.: The role of fructose in restoration of organic phosphate compounds in outdated bank blood. J. Lab. Clin. Med. 82:489, 1973.
232. Wood, L., and Beutler, E.: The effect of ascorbate and dihydroxyacetone on the 2,3-diphosphoglycerate and ATP levels of stored human red cells. Transfusion 14:272, 1974.
233. Dawson, R. B.: Blood preservation using metabolic regulators and nutrients: XXI. Further studies on pyruvate and DHA (dihydroxyacetone). Transfusion 16:446, 1976.
234. Valeri, C. R., Zaroulis, C. G., Vecchione, J. J., Valeri, D. A., Anastasi, J., Pivacek, L. E., and Emerson, C. P.: Therapeutic effectiveness and safety of outdated human red blood cells rejuvenated to restore oxygen transport function to normal, frozen for 3 to 4 years at −80°C, washed, and stored at 4°C for 24 hours prior to rapid infusion. Transfusion 20:159, 1980.
235. Maeda, N., Kon, K., Sekiya, M., and Shiga, T.: Restoration of the poor oxygen transport function of ACD-stored blood by pyridoxal 5′-phosphate. Experientia 35:1245, 1979.
236. Pollock, T. W., Rosato, E. F., Delivoria-Papadopoulos, M., and Miller, L. D.: In vivo manipulation of oxygen-hemoglobin affinity. J. Surg. Res. 22:449, 1977.
237. Nicolau, C., and Gersonde, K.: Incorporation of inositol hexaphosphate into intact red blood cells. I. Fusion of effector-containing lipid vesicles with erythrocytes. Naturwissenschaften 66:563, 1979.
238. Gersonde, K., and Nicolau, C.: Incorporation of inositol hexaphosphate into intact red blood cells. II. Enhancement of gas transport in inositol hexaphosphate–loaded red blood cells. Naturwissenschaften 66:567, 1979.
239. Ross, B. K., and Hlastala, M. P.: Increased hemoglobin oxygen affinity does not decrease skeletal muscle oxygen consumption. J. Appl. Physiol. 51:864, 1981.
240. Coburn, R. F., Ploegmakers, F., Gondrie, P., and Abboud, R.: Myocardial myoglobin oxygen tension. Am. J. Physiol. 224:870, 1973.
241. Lubbers, D. W.: Local tissue PO_2: Its measurement and meaning. In Kessler, M., Bruley, D. F., Clark, L. C., Jr., Lubbers, D. W., Silver, I. A., and Strauss, J. (eds.): Oxygen Supply. Baltimore, University Park Press, 1971, p. 151.
242. Rosenthal, M., LaManna, J. C., Jobsis, F. F., Levasseur, J. E., Kontos, H. A., and Patterson, J. L.: Effects of respiratory gases on cytochrome a in intact cerebral cortex. Is there a critical PO_2? Brain Res. 108:143, 1976.
243. Hempel, F. G., Jobsis, F. F., LaManna, J. L.,

Rosenthal, M. R., and Saltzman, H. A.: Oxidation of cerebral cytochrome aa$_3$ by oxygen plus carbon dioxide at hyperbaric pressures. J. Appl. Physiol. 43:873, 1977.
244. Turek, Z., Kreuzer, F., and Hoofd, L. J. C.: Advantage or disadvantage of a decrease of blood oxygen affinity for tissue oxygen supply at hypoxia. Pfluegers Arch. 342:185, 1973.
244a. Willford, D. C., Hill, E. P., and Moores, W. Y.: Theoretical analysis of optimal P$_{50}$. J. Appl. Physiol. 52:1043, 1982.
245. Turek, Z., Kreuzer, F., and Ringnalda, B. E. M.: Blood gases at several levels of oxygenation in rats with a left-shifted blood oxygen dissociation curve. Pfluegers Arch. 376:7, 1978.
246. Hebbel, R. P., Eaton, J. W., Kronenberg, R. S., Zanjani, E. D., Moore, G., and Berger, E. M.: Human llamas: Adaptation to altitude in subjects with high hemoglobin oxygen affinity. J. Clin. Invest. 62:593, 1978.
247. Moore, L. G., and Brewer, G. J.: Beneficial effect of rightward hemoglobin-oxygen dissociation curve shift for short-term high-altitude adaptation. J. Lab. Clin. Med. 98:145, 1981.
248. Riggs, T. E., Shafer, A. W., and Guenter, C. A.: Acute changes in oxyhemoglobin affinity; effects on oxygen transport and utilization. J. Clin. Invest. 52:2660, 1973.
249. Guy, J. T., Bromberg, P. A., Metz, E. N., Ringle, R., and Balcerzak, S. P.: Oxygen delivery following transfusion of stored blood. I. Normal rats. J. Appl. Physiol. 37:60, 1974.
250. Cassel, J., Kogure, K., Busto, R., Kim, C. Y., and Harkness, D. R.: The effect on cerebral energy metabolites of the cyanate produced shift of the oxygen saturation curve. In Bicher, H. I., and Bruley, D. F. (eds.): Oxygen Transport To Tissue. New York, Plenum Press, 1973, p. 319.
251. Woodson, R. D., Wranne, B., and Detter, J. C.: Effect of increased blood oxygen affinity on work performance of rats. J. Clin. Invest. 52:2717, 1973.
252. Novy, M. F., Edwards, M. J., and Metcalfe, J.: Hemoglobin Yakima. II. High blood oxygen affinity associated with compensatory erythrocytosis and normal hemodynamics. J. Clin. Invest. 46:1848, 1967.
253. White, J. M., Szur, L., Gillies, I. D. S., Lorkin, P. A., and Lehmann, H.: Familial polycythaemia caused by a new haemoglobin variant: Hb Heathrow, beta 103 (G5) phenylalanine–leucine. Br. Med. J. 3:665, 1973.
254. Oski, F. A., Marshall, B. E., Cohen, P. F., Sugarman, H. J., and Miller, L. D.: Exercise with anemia: The role of the left-shifted or right-shifted oxygen-hemoglobin equilibrium curve. Ann. Intern. Med. 74:44, 1971.
255. Bakker, J. C., Gortmaker, G. C., and Offerijns, F. G. J.: The influence of the position of the oxygen dissociation curve on oxygen-dependent functions of the isolated perfused rat liver. Pfluegers Arch. 366:45, 1976.
256. Malmberg, P. O., Hlastala, M. P., and Woodson, R. D.: Effect of increased blood oxygen affinity on oxygen transport in hemorrhagic shock. J. Appl. Physiol. 47:889, 1979.
257. Collins, J. A., and Stechenberg, L.: The effects of the concentration and function of hemoglobin on the survival of rats after hemorrhage. Surgery 85:412, 1979.

ANIMAL HEMOGLOBINS

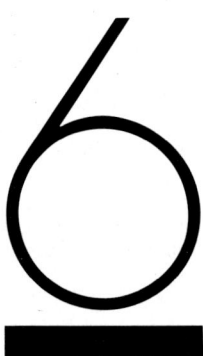

The extraordinary range of morphology and adaptation among members of the animal kingdom is reflected in the diversity in structure and function of their oxygen-carrying proteins. Even though hemoglobins of man have received the lion's share of attention both in this book and elsewhere, a full understanding of the biochemistry, physiology, and molecular genetics of hemoglobins depends on comparative studies. Investigation of a wide span of animal hemoglobins provides a compelling glimpse of molecular evolution. A richly detailed body of information on the animal hemoglobins continues to accumulate. The scope of this book does not permit more than a broad survey of this information. In this chapter, we will try to present a systematic overview of the structural and functional features of oxygen-carrying proteins from various animals and to speculate on ways in which adaptational needs are met.

Those working and thinking in the general framework of human biology are accustomed to tissues and organs operating within very narrow limits of control. Man and his close relatives cannot tolerate much variation in body temperature, pH, osmolarity, or availability of oxygen. The imagination must be stretched to contemplate the enormous vicissitudes in environmental conditions to which other animals may be subjected. Metabolic processes are often at the mercy of wide swings in temperature, pH, salinity, and oxygen tension. Pond-dwelling creatures may enjoy a surfeit of oxygen during the day, when the warm sun allows surrounding flora to engage in photosynthesis. But when the dark of night comes, the pond dwellers may rapidly go into oxygen debt. The importance of oxygen-carrying proteins varies enormously with environmental conditions and with the developmental stage of the animal. Moreover, these molecules may be asked to fulfill additional roles such as oxygen storage or maintenance of buoyancy.

When surveying the properties of respiratory proteins under various experimental conditions, biologists can sometimes to make plausible associations between functional behavior and environmental adaptation. More often, however, the adaptational significance of a particular property is far from obvious. Indeed, this disclaimer will be a recurring theme of this chapter. Invertebrates are especially prone to wide perturbations in environmental conditions. In many cases, there is insufficient information about *in vivo* changes in temperature, pH, PO_2, or ionic strength of the body fluids of the animal in its various habitats to make coherent predictions or explanations about oxygen transport. Although speculations on adaptational significance are entertaining and heuristic, they are usually neither testable nor conclusive and therefore should be taken with a grain of salt.

In this chapter, vertebrates will receive more attention than invertebrates and mammals more than other vertebrates, again an indication of the anthropocentric tenor of this book. Although some might question the "relevance" of some of this information, no one can deny either the intellectual entertainment or the intrinsic beauty of the animal hemoglobins. Moreover, much of the information in this chapter has direct bearing on topics covered elsewhere in this book, including structure-function relationships, regulation of oxygen transport, and control of gene expression. This chapter is lengthy. In the interest of time, some readers may wish to skip the section on invertebrate oxygen-carrying proteins. The remainder of the chapter provides an effective link between the previous sections on structure, function, and physiology and the following sections on hemoglobin synthesis and clinical disorders.

INVERTEBRATES*

The animal kingdom is divided into 31 phyla. Vertebrates compose only a subgroup of one phylum, Chordata. In view of the enormous diversity of invertebrates, it is not surprising that their respiratory proteins are also highly varied and serve a wide range of physiologic functions. In contrast to their universal presence in vertebrates, oxygen-carrying proteins occur sporadically among invertebrates† (Figure 6–1). They appear to be absent in about half of the animal phyla. When present, their concentration in cells or in body fluids is enormously variable and may change drastically with environmental perturbations. Bona fide hemoglobins can be found in relatively simple unicellular organisms such as *Paramecium*.[11] The different types of invertebrate respiratory proteins are distributed over a number of taxonomic groups. Although certain general rules and relationships are apparent, exceptions abound. Moreover, despite growing interest in this topic, there are large information gaps.

The structures of invertebrate oxygen-carrying proteins are complex but elegant. As shown in Table 6–1, they can be divided into four types according to their oxygen binding prosthetic group: hemerythrin, hemocyanin, chlorocruorin, and hemoglobin. These oxygen-carrying proteins display marked variability in size. In general, the high–molecular-weight (polymeric) respiratory proteins range in size from 10^5 to 10^7 daltons and are freely dissolved in tissue fluids such as hemolymph or coelom, whereas the smaller proteins (less than 100,000 daltons) are encased in red cells within the vascular system, coelomic cavity, or certain other tissues. The polymers contribute much less colloid osmotic pressure than a comparable amount of low–molecular-weight protein and therefore prevent excess transit of water from cells into intravascular spaces. The function of these polymeric proteins varies considerably. Some bind oxygen cooperatively, but many do not. Some appear to be affected by small molecules such as protons as well as calcium and chloride ions. These giant molecules are particularly useful model systems for understanding the assembly and functional properties of extended biological structures.

Hemerythrins

Hemerythrin is an intracellular respiratory protein that has a unique design totally different from that of hemoglobin and hemocyanin. This protein is found in certain marine invertebrates from four different phyla‡ (Fig. 6–1).

---

*This section has fewer citations than the rest of the book. Much of the information in this section was obtained from excellent reviews: Klippenstein[1] (hemerythrin); the Bonaventuras,[2,3] Van Holde and Miller,[4] Mangum,[5] and van Bruggen[6] (hemocyanin); Terwilliger,[7] Garlick,[8] and Weber[9] (hemoglobins); and Antonini and Chiancone[10] (hemocyanin and polymeric hemoglobins).

†Hemoglobins have also been encountered in a few species of bacteria and yeast and in the root nodules of leguminous plants (leghemoglobin).

‡Hemerythrin is found in sipunculid worms (phylum Sipunculoidea), priapulids (phylum Priapulida) and in some brachiopods (phylum Brachiopoda) and polychete worms (phylum Annelida).

128 ANIMAL HEMOGLOBINS

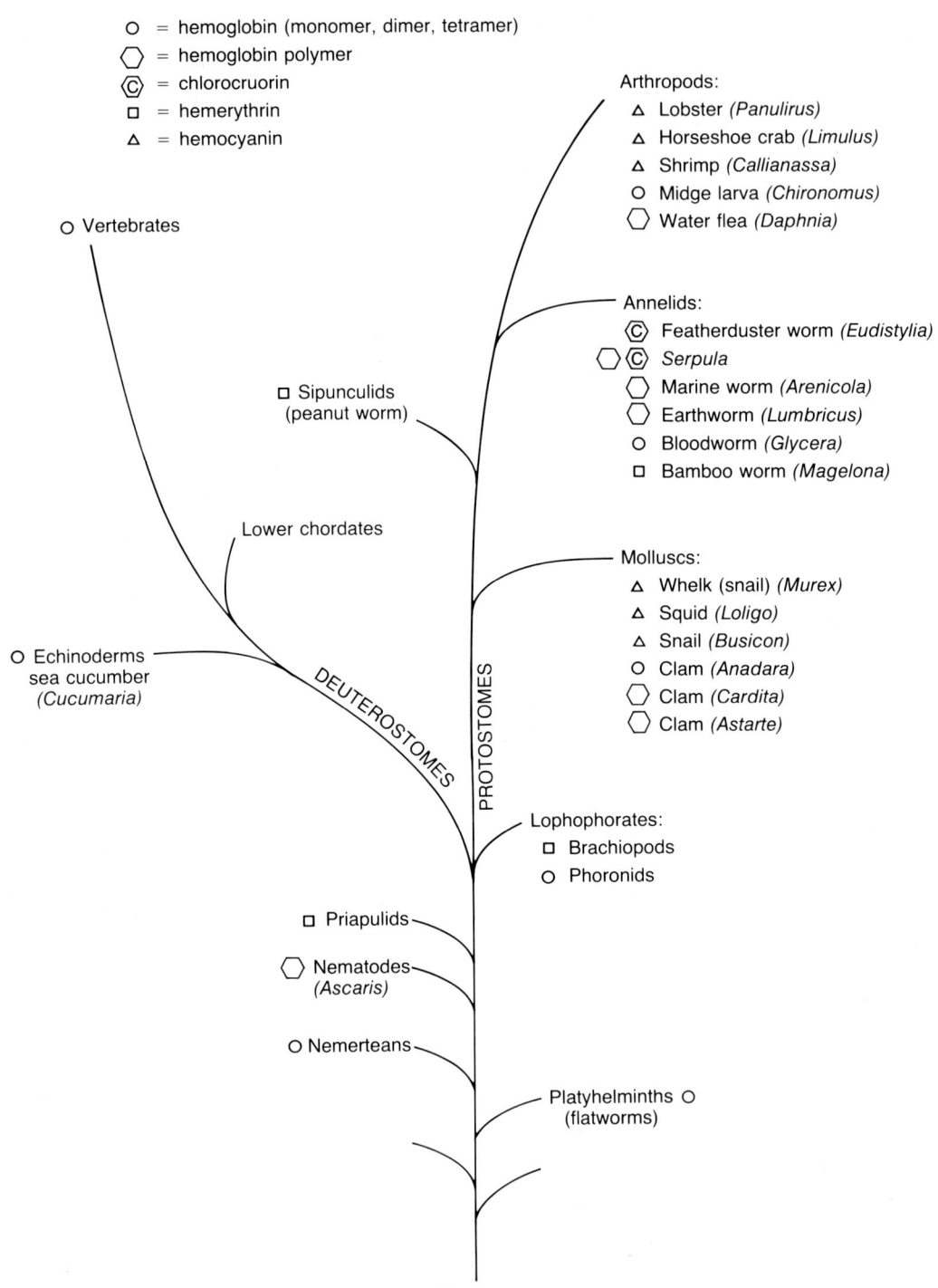

Figure 6–1. Distribution of hemoglobin and other oxygen-transporting proteins (hemerythrin and hemocyanin) in the animal kingdom. Most of the examples discussed in the section on invertebrates are shown here. Both the common name and the genus are included. This figure does not include myoglobin or other oxygen-storing proteins. (Adapted from Terwilliger, R. C.: Am. Zool. *20*:53, 1980, with assistance by Dr. Robert Garlick.)

Table 6–1. COMPARISON OF INVERTEBRATE OXYGEN-TRANSPORT PROTEINS*

	Vertebrate Hemoglobins	Invertebrate Hemoglobins	Chlorocruorin	Hemerythrin	Hemocyanin
Molecular weight (daltons)	65,000	16,000–4 × 10^6	~ 3 × 10^6	40,000–110,000	400,000–9,000,000
Number of subunits	4	1–200	~ 180	3, 4, 8	6–48
Metal:O$_2$	Fe:O$_2$	Fe:O$_2$	Fe:O$_2$	2Fe:O$_2$	2CU:O$_2$
Metal coordination	Protoporphyrin	Protoporphyrin	Formylporphyrin	Protein side chains	Protein side chains
Color					
Oxygenated	Red	Red	Red—concentrated Green—dilute	Violet	Blue
Deoxygenated	Purple	Purple	Red—concentrated Green—dilute	Colorless	Colorless

*Adapted from Klippenstein, G. L.: Am. Zool. 20:39, 1980.

This 110,000-dalton polymer contains eight subunits of identical size (13,600 daltons), each of which binds one molecule of oxygen.* Several structurally distinct subunits often coexist within a given species and probably within the octomer.[1] Hemerythrin subunits from several species have undergone primary sequence analysis. There appears to be a repetition of an internal sequence of about 30 residues that corresponds to symmetrical domains in the tertiary structure of the protein.[12] X-ray analyses have demonstrated that the eight subunits are arranged in two layers of four subunits oriented in an end-to-side manner (Fig. 6–2).[13, 14] This gives the molecule the overall shape of a square doughnut. The quaternary structure is stabilized by a number of electrostatic interactions and hydrogen bonds. In myohemerythrin, these interactions are markedly diminished, and as a result, the protein is monomeric.

The unique oxygen binding site in hemerythrin involves two iron atoms, which are coordinated to a group of specific residues, including five histidines, shown in Figure 6–3.[15, 15a] Understandably, these residues are invariant among hemerythrin subunits whose primary structure has been determined. The two iron atoms are in sufficiently close apposition to bind one atom of O$_2$. Upon binding, the Fe^{2+} iron atoms each transfer an electron to the oxygen, so that the iron atoms now become Fe^{3+} and the oxygen becomes peroxide (O$_2^{2-}$).

*Some sipunculids (Phascolosoma) have trimeric hemerythrin, and in one species it is tetrameric.

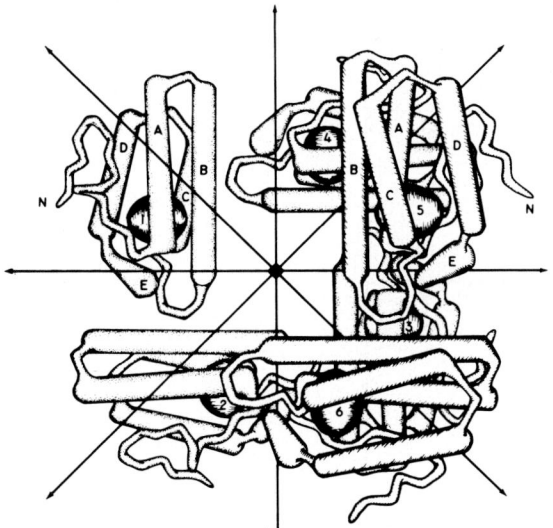
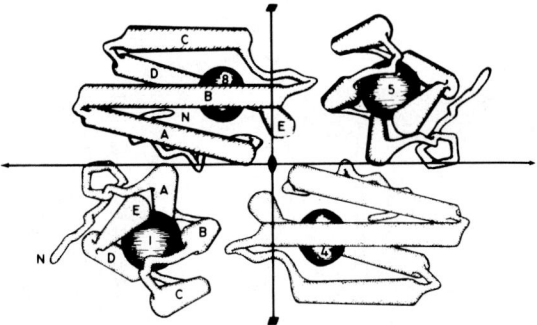

Figure 6–2. The quaternary structure of an octomeric hemerythrin. Left, View of the octomer from above. Two of the four subunits have been removed from the top layer. The oxygen binding regions are shown as darkly shaded spheres. Right, Side view of the octomer. (The letters A to E refer to helical segments. The N terminus is designated by N.) (From Ward, K. B., et al.: Nature 257:818, 1975.)

130 ANIMAL HEMOGLOBINS

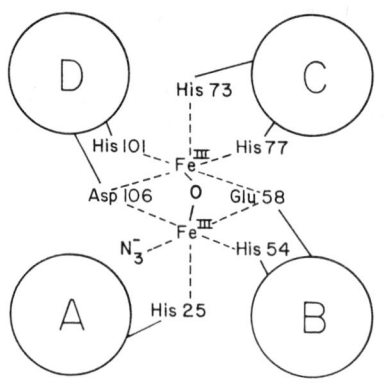

Figure 6–3. Bonding of iron atoms at functional site of hemerythrin, to each other, and to their respective helices (A, B, C, D). The structure of the N_3^- complex of hemerythrin is shown. (From Klotz, I. M., and Kurtz, D. M.: Accounts of Chemical Research. *17*:16, 1984.)

Oxygenated hemerythrin is violet, whereas deoxygenated (apo)hemerythrin is colorless. Despite its multisubunit structure, hemerythrin has minimal subunit cooperativity ($n = 1.0$ to 1.8) and no Bohr effect.[12] Furthermore, it does not appear to be regulated by other intracellular cofactors.

Hemerythrins found in coelomic cells and in muscle are structurally and functionally distinct from the vascular protein. As mentioned previously, myohemerythrin is a monomer with a molecular weight of 13,900 daltons that has a substantially higher oxygen affinity than the octomer found in blood cells. Coelomic hemerythrin is an octomer with intermediate oxygen affinity. The functional differences between these proteins probably facilitate the extraction of oxygen from the surrounding water and its transport from the respiratory surface to metabolizing cells.

Hemocyanins

Hemocyanins are large, extracellular, copper-containing proteins that circulate in the hemolymph of some arthropods and molluscs (Fig. 6–1). These proteins have attracted the interest of biologists for more than a century. The appeal of hemocyanins rests in part on their rich blue color (Fig. 6–4) as well as on the ability of their subunits to assemble into elegant higher-order structures.

The subunit composition and quaternary structure of arthropod and mollusc hemocyanins differ so radically from one another that the question of convergent evolution arises.[2, 10] Arthropod hemocyanin is composed of subunits of 70,000 to 80,000 daltons, each of which binds one molecule of oxygen. Six of these subunits aggregate to form hexamers, which can be readily visualized by electron microscopy. In the lobster *Panulirus interruptus,* the six monomers are arranged into two triangles that lie in parallel planes rotated about 25 degrees around a threefold axis of symmetry.[10] These hexamers are building blocks of higher-order polymers of up to 48 monomers (3.4×10^6 daltons) (Fig. 6–5E). The subunit compo-

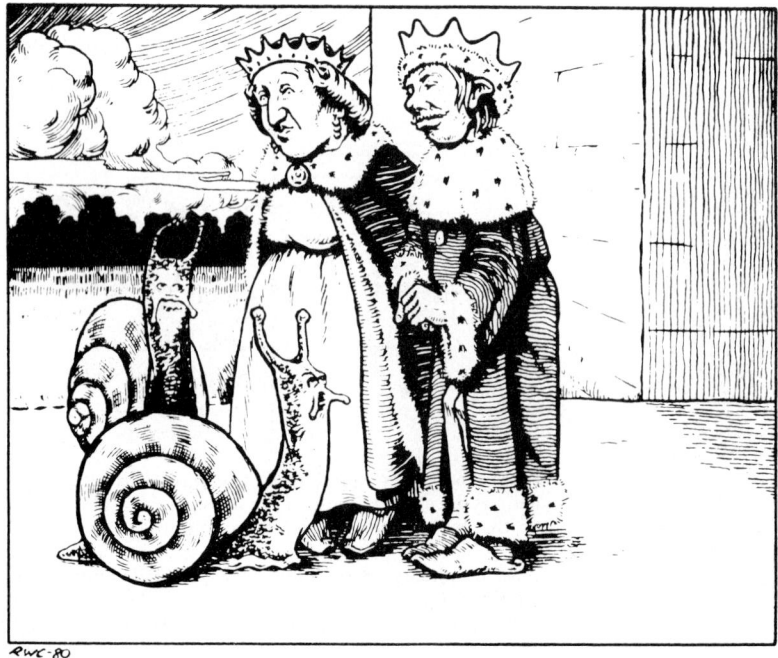

Figure 6–4. "Blue blood indeed! As usual they don't know what they're talking about." (From van Bruggen, E. F. J.: Trends in Biochemical Science 7:185, 1980.)

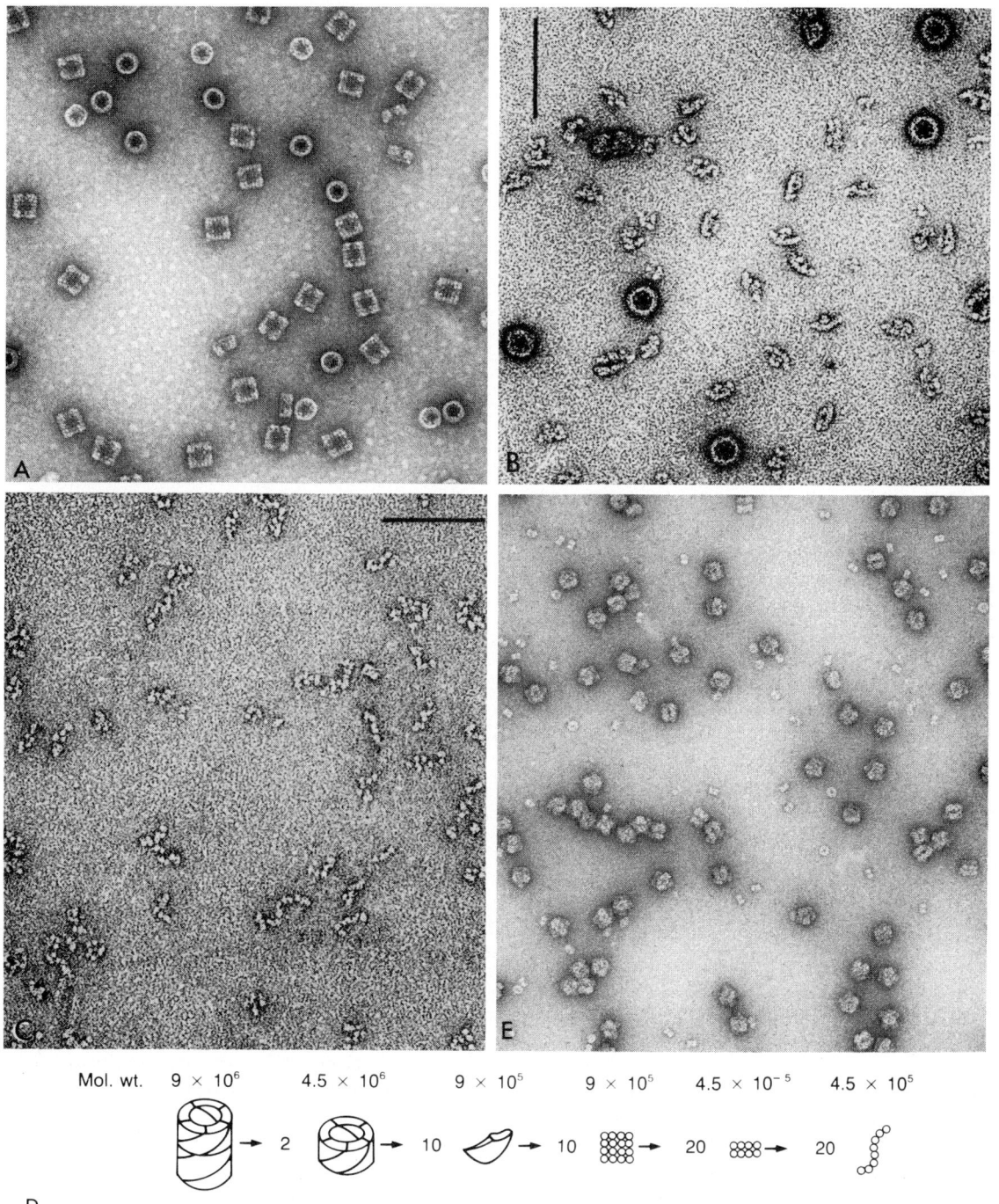

Figure 6–5. A, Electron micrograph of molluscan hemocyanin (from the snail *Helix pomatia*) ($\times$ 218,000). The fully assembled, barrel-shaped macromolecule has a molecular weight of 9×10^6 daltons. Half molecules of 4.5×10^6 daltons are also shown in this figure. *B,* Electron micrograph of *Helix pomatia* hemocyanin that has dissociated into 9×10^5–dalton submultiples. *C,* Further dissociation into 4.5×10^5–dalton subunits, resembling "beads on a string." ($\times$ 218,000). (Courtesy of Ernst van Bruggen.) *D,* Diagram of the assembly of molluscan hemocyanin. The 4.5×10^6 dalton subunit contains about eight oxygen binding domains. This subunit forms a dimer, which then aggregates with four other dimers to form a hollow cylinder of 4.5×10^6 daltons. (From Antonini, E., and Chiancone, E.: Ann. Rev. Biophys. Bioeng. 6:239, 1977.) *E,* Electron micrograph of arthropod hemocyanin from the horsehoe crab *Limulus polyphemus* ($\times$ 218,000). The fully assembled molecule is a 3×10^6–dalton polymer composed of 48 subunits. As shown in this figure, a macromolecule can dissociate into 4×10^5–dalton submultiples. Each of these is composed of six 70,000-dalton subunits. (Courtesy of Ernst van Bruggen.)

sition of these polymers is heterogeneous. Hemocyanin from the horseshoe crab *Limulus* contains five chromatographically distinct polypeptides that differ considerably from one another in oxygen affinity.[2] The aggregation of these proteins into higher-order polymers (dodecamer—48-mer) requires the presence of unlike subunits.[2] In contrast, hemocyanins that do not aggregate beyond hexamers tend to have uniform subunit composition.

Hemocyanins of molluscs are giant molecules composed of large (450,000-dalton) subunits, each of which contains about eight oxygen binding sites. High-resolution electron microscopy of hemocyanin prepared under dissociating conditions reveals a linear array of about seven to eight "beads on a string," which probably correspond to oxygen binding domains.[10] In fact, oxygen binding peptides of about 50,000 daltons can be obtained following limited proteolytic cleavage, but these fragments do not aggregate into polymers. The three-dimensional structure of gastropod hemocyanin has been analyzed by optical diffraction of images obtained by electron microscopy.[16] As shown in Figure 6–5, about 20 of the native subunits assemble into a hollow cylinder that is 380 Å long and 350 Å in diameter and has a molecular weight of about 9×10^6 daltons. At the end of the cylinder is a collar, which is attached to the inner wall. This protein may limit the growth of the cylinder. It is likely that as in arthropod hemocyanin, unlike subunits are required for the assembly of mollusc hemocyanin. Hemocyanin from the whelk *Murex* is composed of equal amounts of two chromatographically distinct subunits and can be represented as an oligomer with the formula $A_{10}B_{10}$.[17] It is likely that other molluscan hemocyanins have similar compositions.

Because the primary sequences of hemocyanin subunits have not been fully determined, the structure of the oxygen binding unit remains poorly understood. The sequence of the putative oxygen binding site of *Limulus* hemocyanin has recently been determined.[17a] The copper atoms are covalently linked to imidazoles of histidine residues, similar to the iron atoms in hemerythrin and, indeed, hemoglobin. Analogous to hemerythrin, one molecule of oxygen binds to two metal atoms. In deoxyhemocyanin, the copper atoms are reduced (Cu^+), but when bound to oxygen, electrons are transferred from the copper atoms to oxygen: Cu^{2+}—O_2^{2-}—Cu^{2+}. Like deoxygenated hemerythrin, deoxyhemocyanin is colorless. In contrast, oxygenated hemocyanin has a deep

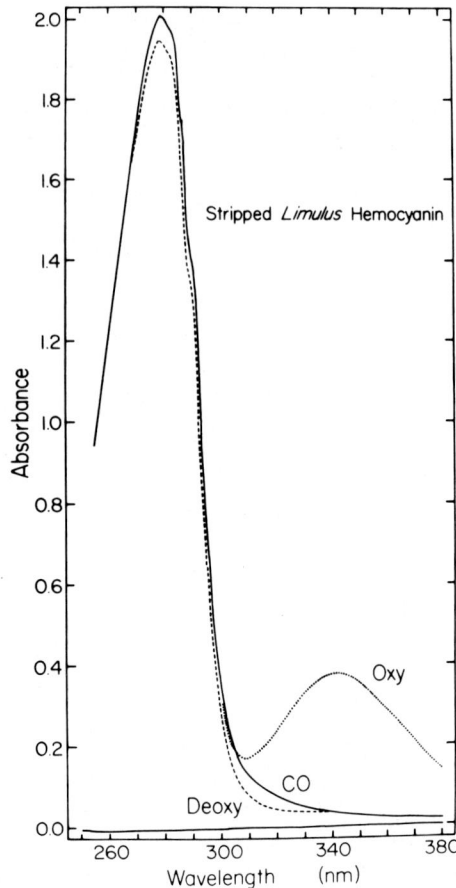

Figure 6–6. Absorption spectra of oxy (. . .), deoxy (– – –), and carboxy (—) forms of *Limulus* hemocyanin. Note that only the oxy form has significant absorbance at 320 to 380 nm. (From Bonaventura, C., et al.: Biochemistry *13*:4784, 1974.)

blue color. The absorption spectrum shows a band at 340 nm (Fig. 6–6). This spectral change is not observed when carbon monoxide binds to hemocyanin. The latter ligand fails to form a bridge between the two copper atoms. Unlike vertebrate hemoglobins, hemocyanins bind carbon monoxide noncooperatively. Furthermore, carbon monoxide binding is not influenced by allosteric effectors (Fig. 6–7).[18]

The oxygen transport function of hemocyanins has been thoroughly investigated not only by physiologists but also by biochemists interested in the behavior of multisubunit proteins. In contrast to hemerythrins, hemocyanins often display significant subunit cooperativity and are responsive to allosteric effectors. The intrinsic oxygen affinity of hemocyanins is generally lower than that of other invertebrate oxygen-carrying proteins.[5] For example, the P_{50} of the hemocyanin from the squid *Loligo* is about 160 mm Hg at 37°C and pH 7.4, and that of the spider *Cupennius salei* is almost as high. The low oxygen affinity raises some doubt as to whether the hemocyanins are adequately saturated *in vivo*. However, most marine animals exist at relatively low temperatures, in which two factors tend to raise oxygen binding. Like most hemoglobins, the oxygen affinity of hemocyanins increases substantially as temperature is lowered. Furthermore, many hemocyanins have a "normal" alkaline Bohr effect ($\Delta \log P_{50}/\Delta pH < 0$). Because the pH of the blood of these animals rises as temperature is lowered, there is an additional increment in oxygen affinity at low temperature. Some animals, particularly marine gastropods and the horseshoe crab *Limulus*, have a reverse Bohr effect ($\Delta \log P_{50}/\Delta pH > 0$). In some cases, this phenomenon appears to be adaptive. For example, in the snail *Busycon*, the circulatory beds are arranged in a series. The blood pH drops progressively as blood passes into the distal circulation. If there were no reverse Bohr effect, the distal tissue would become very hypoxic. The animal might be able to crawl but probably would not be able to make urine in the nephridium.[19]

One of the most thoroughly studied of all the hemocyanins is that of *Limulus*. These 3×10^6–dalton polymers have about 48 oxygen binding sites. In this native state, *Limulus* hemocyanin has a relatively low oxygen affinity, considerable subunit cooperativity, and a substantial reverse Bohr effect[3] (Fig. 6–7). When it is stripped of small molecule effectors, oxygen affinity is markedly increased, with loss of subunit cooperativity and the Bohr effect. These phenomena, measured under carefully controlled laboratory conditions, appear to have adaptive significance.[5] In the spring and early summer, horseshoe crabs enter estuaries to breed. Burrowing and copulation greatly restrict ventilation through their book gills. Under these conditions, both the PO_2 and the pH drop in the postbranchial blood; therefore, the reverse Bohr effect helps maintain adequate oxygenation. Unlike crustacean hemocyanins, *Limulus* hemocyanin has higher oxygen affinity when salinity is decreased. This may reflect an accompanying reduction in allosteric effectors, as demonstrated by the oxygen equilibria shown in Figure 6–7. Marine (salty) waters tend to be well agitated and therefore relatively well saturated with oxygen. In contrast, fresh water in estuaries is often relatively unstirred and stratified and therefore less well oxygenated. Accordingly, the increase in oxygen affinity that accompanies the decrease in salinity probably helps the horseshoe crab maintain adequate oxygenation.

The hemocyanin of the shrimp *Callianassa californiensis* has also been thoroughly investigated.[4] Like many hemocyanins, its function is very sensitive to the presence of divalent cations. In the absence of cations, the protein is noncooperative and has a very low oxygen affinity. Upon addition of Mg^{2+} or Ca^{2+}, the oxygen affinity increases markedly and the binding curve becomes sigmoidal, signifying

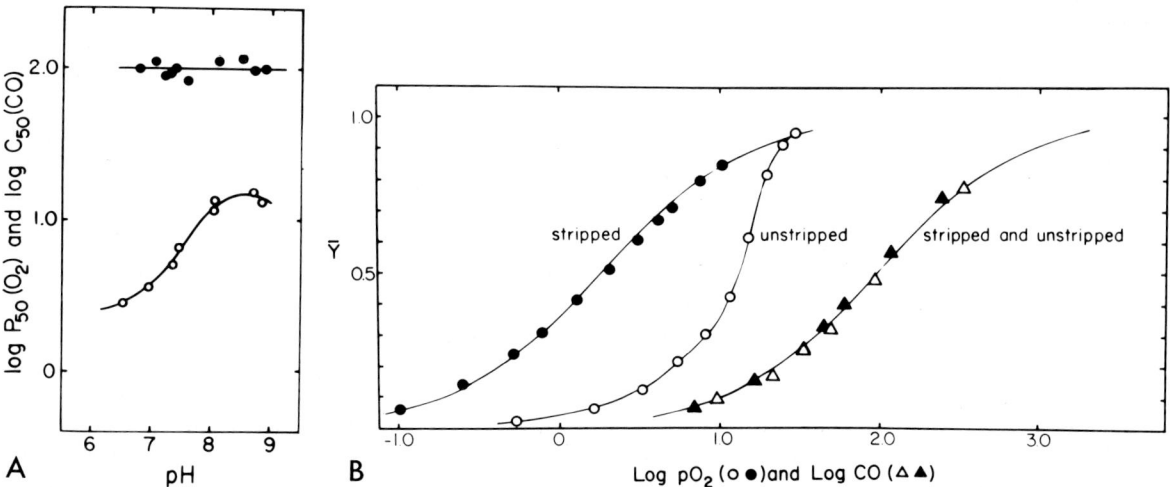

Figure 6–7. A, Effect of pH on the affinity of *Limulus* hemocyanin for oxygen (○) and carbon monoxide (●). Oxygen binding measurements reveal a marked reverse Bohr effect, whereas CO binding is uninfluenced by pH. B, Oxygen (○, ●) and carbon monoxide (△, ▲) binding curves for stripped (closed symbols) and unstripped (open symbols) *Limulus* hemocyanin. The removal ("stripping") of divalent cations results in the dissociation of the polymer and loss of subunit cooperativity. In contrast, CO binding is noncooperative whether or not the hemocyanin has been stripped. (From Bonaventura C., et al.: Biochemistry 13:4784, 1974.)

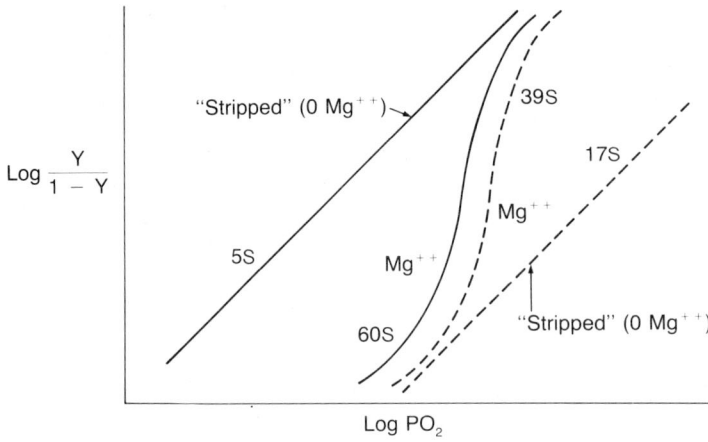

Figure 6–8. Idealized Hill plots comparing the oxygenation of *Limulus* (———) and *Callianassa* (– – –) hemocyanins. Sedimentation coefficients (5S, 60S, and so on) indicate the state of aggregation.

subunit cooperativity. The behavior of this hemocyanin can be explained by a two-state allosteric model.[4] The 17S hexamer has a low affinity for oxygen and for divalent cations. The 39S polymer containing 24 subunits has a high affinity for both oxygen and divalent cations. Thus, in the presence of Mg^{2+} or Ca^{2+}, oxygenation of the hemocyanin will lead to aggregation.

The *Limulus* and *Callianassa* hemocyanins offer an interesting contrast in the behavior of multisubunit proteins. As shown by the Hill plots in Figure 6–8, the cooperative behavior of each of these two proteins depends on subunit aggregation. The stripped proteins, free of divalent cations, have noncooperative oxygen binding curves ($n = 1$). The low–molecular-weight species of *Limulus* hemocyanin appears to be in the R conformation with a high affinity for oxygen and a low affinity for heterotropic effectors. In this way, it resembles lamprey hemoglobin (see below). In the presence of cations, the deoxygenated protein polymerizes and assumes the T conformation. Upon oxygenation, the molecule is converted to R: the polymer partially disaggregates and divalent cations are released.

In summary, the hemocyanins of *Limulus* and *Callianassa* both show strong linkage between oxygenation, cation binding, and subunit aggregation. In *Limulus*, the low–molecular-weight noncooperative species of hemocyanin is in the R structure, whereas in *Callianassa*, it is in the T conformation. In both cases, divalent cations cause aggregation of subunits and induce subunit cooperativity.

Hemoglobins (Erythrocruorins)

In the broadest biological context, hemoglobin may be defined as a protein containing heme (ferroprotoporphyrin IX [see Fig. 2–13]) that binds oxygen at a respiratory surface such as skin, gills, trachea, or lung and transports the oxygen to inner tissues, where it is utilized for metabolism. A wide range of invertebrates have one or more respiratory proteins that fit this general definition (Fig. 6–1). However, the hemoglobins are distributed rather capriciously among taxonomic groups. For example, Lankester,[20] who in 1861 first described red and green pigments in invertebrates, noted that one of two congeneric species of both bivalve clams and polychete worms contained hemoglobin, whereas the other did not. Moreover, the invertebrate hemoglobins show striking variability in size, structure, and function. As mentioned at the beginning of this chapter, low–molecular-weight hemoglobins (16,000 to 120,000 daltons) tend to be encased within circulating red cells. In contrast, the large polymeric hemoglobins (0.25×10^6 to 3.8×10^6 daltons) circulate freely in the blood or hemolymph.[7]* The special term erythrocruorin has traditionally been reserved for all invertebrate heme proteins. However, they cannot be distinguished from vertebrate hemoglobins on the basis of absorption spectra or functional properties.[21] Moreover, because they generally contain heme subunits comparable in size to those of vertebrates[22] and because structural data indicate primary sequence homology with vertebrate hemoglobins[23–25] as well as the presence of a myoglobin fold[26, 27] (Fig. 6–9), characteristic of vertebrate myoglobins and hemoglobins, these invertebrate polymers can rightfully be considered full-fledged members of the hemoglobin family. As Lankester[20] noted, some annelids have a green respiratory protein in which oxygen binds to chloroheme

---

*The bivalve clam *Barbatia reeveana* is a noteworthy exception. Its intracellular hemoglobin is polymeric.[20a]

rather than heme. The chlorocruorins will be discussed at the end of this section.

Lower Phyla. Hemoglobins have been encountered in a single-cell organism, *Paramecium* (phylum Protozoa),[11] as well as in two classes of flatworms (phylum Platyhelminthes) and in nemertine worms (phylum Nemertina)[17] (Fig. 6–1). These proteins have the characteristic size of globin monomers (about 17,000 daltons) and therefore cannot bind oxygen cooperatively. Primary sequence data on hemoglobin from a fluke (phylum Platyhelminthes) show significant homology with vertebrate hemoglobins.[28] In the phylum Nematoda, the parasitic roundworm *Ascaris* has a particularly interesting hemoglobin. Its extracellular hemoglobin appears to be an octomer containing 40,000-dalton subunits. Its myoglobin appears to be a monomer equal in size to the hemoglobin subunit but differing in structure. These heme proteins are striking exceptions to the rule, first suggested by the ultracentrifugation studies of Svedberg,[22] that the great bulk of animal hemoglobins are composed of multiples of subunits of approximately 17,000 daltons. Moreover, perienteric *Ascaris* hemoglobin has an extraordinarily high oxygen affinity[29] (Fig. 6–10). At 20°C, its P_{50} is 0.001 to 0.004 mm Hg. Oxygen dissociates from this hemoglobin extremely slowly (t_{50} = 600 to 750 seconds). These properties make it very unlikely that this hemoglobin is useful for either oxygen transport or storage. Perhaps it functions as a peroxidase or as a storehouse for heme groups.[9]

Annelid Hemoglobins. The respiratory proteins of the segmented worms have aroused considerable interest. As mentioned earlier, intracellular hemerythrin has been noted in some polychetes. In addition, many annelids have low–molecular-weight hemoglobin within coelomic cells. The most thoroughly studied of these is the monomeric hemoglobin of *Glycera dibranchiata*. Its primary sequence shows significant homology with those of vertebrate hemoglobins.[24] Moreover, x-ray diffraction analysis shows that its tertiary structure has the myoglobin fold typical of vertebrate hemoglobins[26] (Fig. 6–9). Because this hemoglobin is monomeric, it is unable to bind oxygen cooperatively (Fig. 6–10).

The predominant oxygen-carrying protein in the annelids is extracellular polymeric hemoglobin. These large molecules (2.6×10^6 to 4.0×10^6 daltons) are composed of 12 submultiples, each of which contains 12 to 18 subunits.[8] Many of these polymeric hemoglobins display cooperative oxygen binding. Although considerable heterogeneity has been noted in the size of annelid hemoglobin subunits, it is likely that when maximal denaturing conditions are employed, the polymers ultimately break up into polypeptides of 14,000 to 17,000 daltons, again a confirmation of the Svedberg hypothesis.[22] In most cases, there is structural heterogeneity among the subunits in a particular polymeric hemoglobin. Furthermore, there is a poor stoichiometric relationship between iron content and subunit size. Most annelid hemoglobins contain one heme per 22,000- to 27,000-dalton protein. It is possible that some of the globin subunits lack heme groups or (less likely) that one heme binds to two subunits.[8] Alternatively, heme may be lost during purification of the protein. The primary sequence of one subunit of earthworm (*Lumbricus terrestris*) hemoglobin is thus far the only structural information on polymeric hemoglobins.[23] As with the monomeric *Glycera* hemoglobin, the earthworm hemoglobin subunit shows significant structural homology with vertebrate hemoglobins. Moreover, inferences on secondary structure from primary sequence suggest similarity with vertebrate globins. Circular dichroism measurements of earthworm hemoglobin suggest the presence of only 40 per cent α helix compared with 70 per cent in vertebrate hemoglobins.[30] However, the large size of these molecules may preclude an accurate assessment of α-helical content by optical measurements.

The quaternary structure of annelid hemoglobins has considerable aesthetic appeal. Electron micrographs (Fig. 6–11) reveal regular hexagonal structures (240 Å in diameter) with a hollow central channel.[8, 31] Side views show two stacked discs superimposed directly on one another with no twist (160 Å in height). Each of the 12 spherical units contained in the polymer has a diameter of about 70 Å and corresponds to the 250,000-dalton submultiple, determined from analysis by ultracentrifugation or gel filtration.[8] Although the structure just described is shared by a number of annelid hemoglobins that have been examined to date, alternate or additional features have been noted. Some polymers lack a hollow center.[31] In others, the shape of the submultiple appears to be triangular or kite-like rather than spherical.

The annelid hemoglobins show a striking diversity of function. By necessity, the monomeric hemoglobins bind oxygen noncooperatively. The polymeric hemoglobins may have marked subunit cooperativity. For example, the hemoglobin of *Arenicola marina* has an *n*

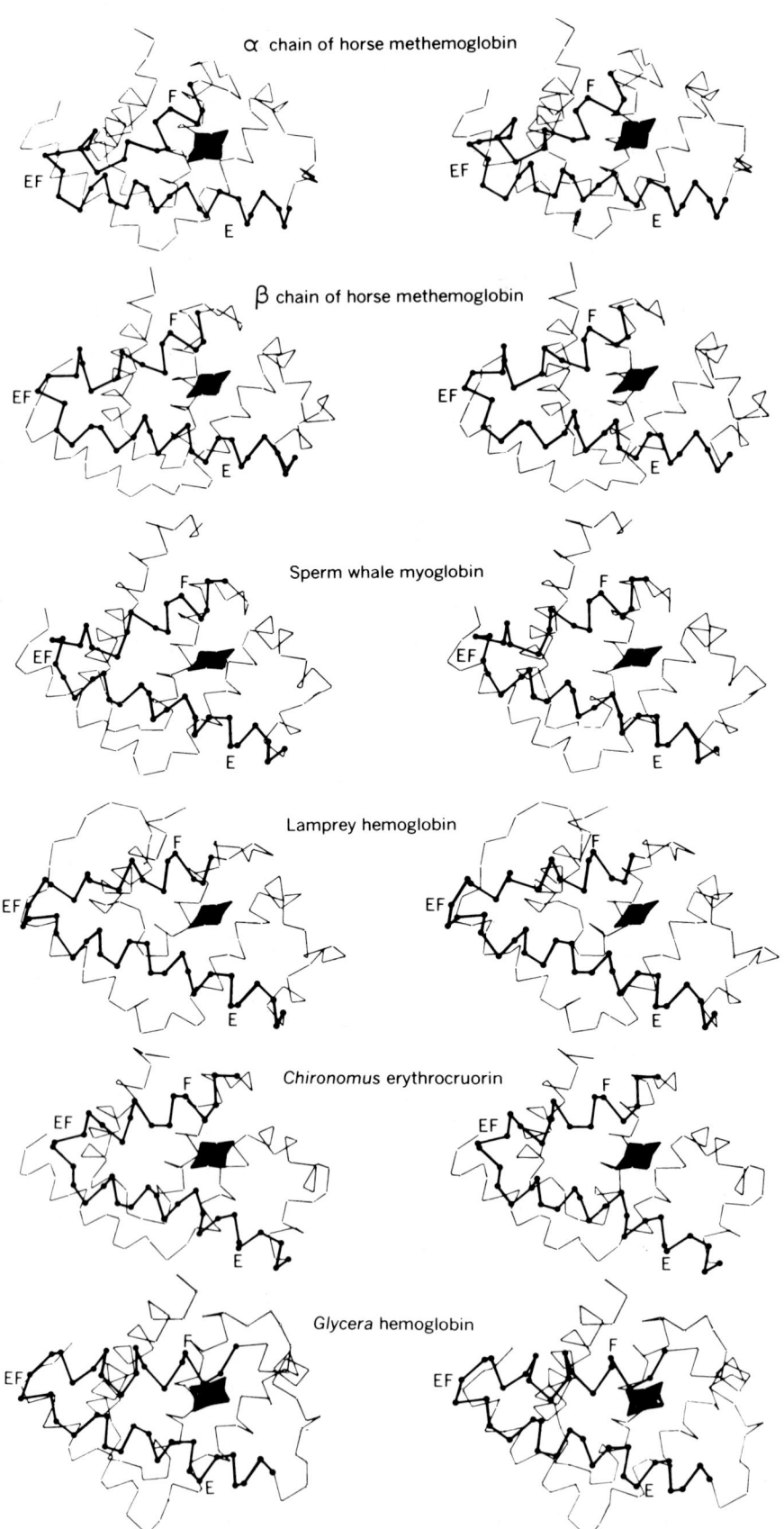

Figure 6–9. See legend on opposite page.

ANIMAL HEMOGLOBINS 137

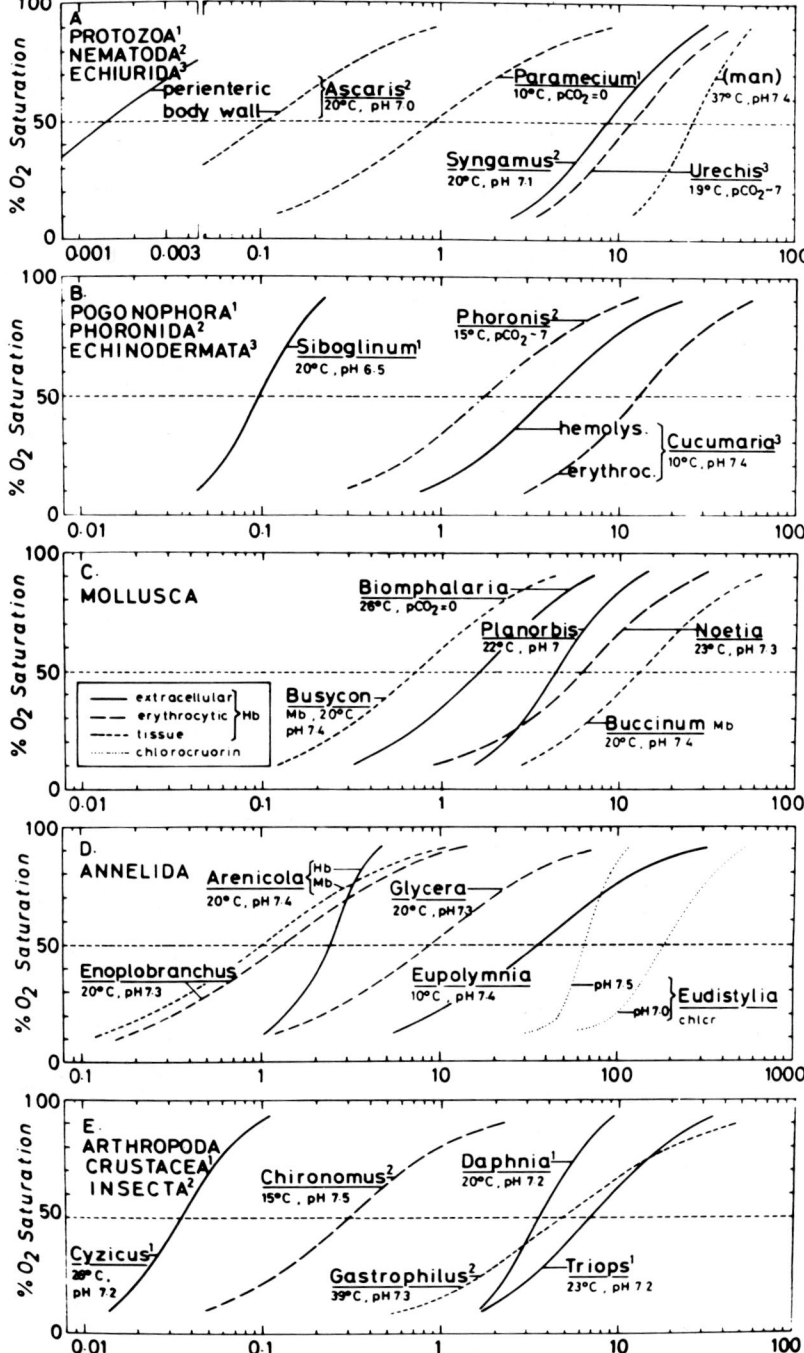

Figure 6–10. Oxygen binding curves of hemoglobins from various invertebrates: polymeric extracellular hemoglobins (———); oligomeric hemoglobins (usually erythrocytic) (— — —); chlorocruorin (. . . . .); tissue proteins (- - - - - -). Note differences in PO_2 scales. (From Weber, R. E.: Am. Zool. 20:79, 1980.)

Figure 6–9. Stereodiagram of carbon-carbon backbones of vertebrate and invertebrate hemoglobins showing similarities in three-dimensional structures and the typical myoglobin fold. (From Dickerson, R. E., and Geis, I.: Hemoglobin: Structure, Function, Evolution and Pathology. Menlo Park, California, Benjamin-Cummings, 1983.)

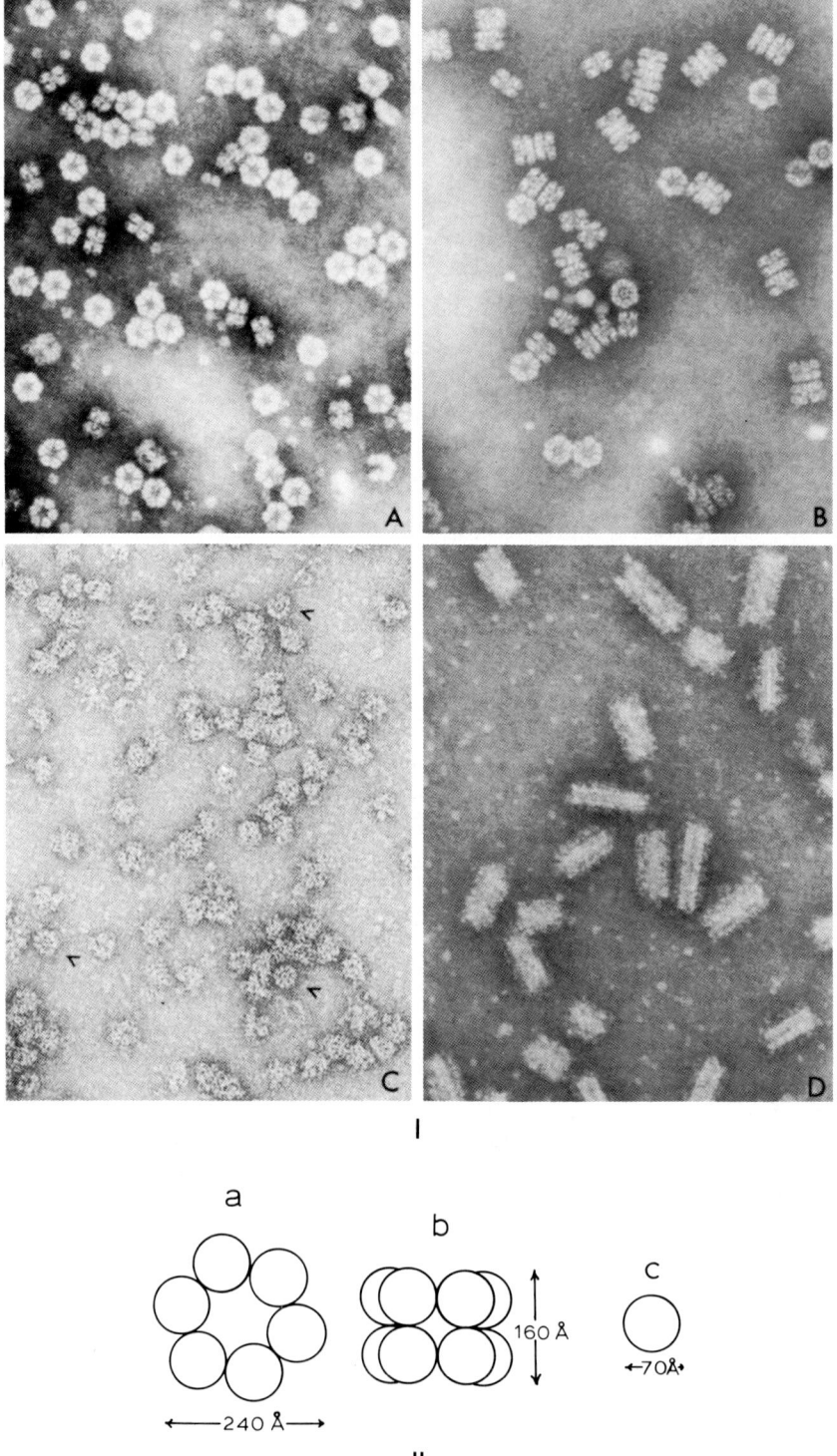

Figure 6–11. I, Electron micrographs of negatively stained invertebrate hemoglobins. *A*, *Eudistylia* chlorocruorin (annelid worm). *B*, *Euzonus* hemoglobin (annelid worm). *C*, *Helisoma* hemoglobin (snail-mollusc). *D*, *Cardita* hemoglobin (clam-mollusc). From Terwilliger, R. C.: Am. Zool. *20*:53, 1980.) *II*, Diagram of quaternary structure of typical annelid polymeric hemoglobin (70 Å diameter sphere corresponds to 25,000-dalton submultiple). (From Garlick, R. L.: Am. Zool. *20*:69, 1980.)

value of 4.8 (Fig. 6–10) and sufficiently low oxygen affinity for the efficient transfer of oxygen to high-affinity monomeric myoglobin. The oxygen affinity of *Arenicola* hemoglobin is sensitive to cations,[32] in striking contrast to the vertebrate hemoglobins, which are regulated by anions (see below).

Molluscan Hemoglobins. As in some of the other phyla, molluscan hemoglobins consist of intracellular low–molecular-weight heme proteins as well as large extracellular hemoglobins. Monomeric heme proteins (15,000 to 17,000 daltons) are abundant in radicular muscles and in nerve and heart tissue of many snails (gastropods). In some of these animals, the myoglobin is dimeric and possesses some subunit cooperativity.[7] A thorough examination of structure-function relationships in these homodimers would be of considerable interest. Some arcid clams have dimeric and tetrameric hemoglobins inside red blood cells. These molecules may show marked subunit cooperativity but are not responsive to allosteric effectors. The hemoglobins of some arcid clams *(Anadara)* have a reverse temperature dependency: Oxygen affinity increases directly with temperature.[33] This anomalous behavior may help preserve adequate oxygen uptake when the clam languishes in warm water shoals that have a significant reduction in dissolved oxygen.

Two types of large extracellular hemoglobins of molluscs have been thoroughly investigated: those of planorbid snails and of the clams *Artarte* and *Cardita*. The planorbid hemoglobins have a molecular weight of 1.3×10^6 to 1.7×10^6 daltons, about half the size of the giant annelid hemoglobins. Their 170,000- to 200,000-dalton subunits, are about 10 times larger than those found in most polymeric hemoglobins, and each has about 10 oxygen binding domains.[7, 34] The clam hemoglobins also have large (290,000- to 300,000-dalton) subunits that have 18 to 20 oxygen binding domains.[7] The subunits of these molluscan hemoglobins are another exception to Svedberg's rule, and, like the molluscan hemocyanins, also resemble beads on a string with spherical heme binding domains and interdomain segments. However, as shown in Figure 6–11, the quaternary structure of *Cardita* hemoglobin is radically different, consisting of rod-like polymers measuring 210 to 365 Å in diameter and having a variable length (360 to 1200 Å). It will be of considerable interest to investigate the arrangement and structure of globin genes coding for the larger molluscan hemoglobin and hemocyanin subunits that have multiple oxygen binding domains. It may be that they arose by means of gene duplication.

Despite their large size, extracellular snail and clam hemoglobin polymers tend to lack subunit cooperativity or response to allosteric effectors (Fig. 6–10).

Arthropod Hemoglobins. Within the enormous phylum Arthropoda, hemoglobins have been encountered in certain groups of insects (Diptera [*Chironomus, Gastrophilus*] and Hemiptera [*Buenoa*]) as well as in a number of branchiopod crustaceans.

The insect hemoglobins are either monomers or dimers and have heme-containing subunits of about 15,000 daltons. Braunitzer's group has determined the primary sequences of a number of *Chironomus* hemoglobins.[25] There is about 20 per cent homology with sperm whale myoglobin and with vertebrate hemoglobin chains. X-ray analysis reveals the presence of a myoglobin-like fold[27] (Fig. 6–9). The oxygen affinities of insect hemoglobins vary considerably, but as expected from their structure, they bind oxygen noncooperatively (Fig. 6–10).

In contrast, the branchiopod hemoglobins are large (250,000- to 680,000-dalton) polymers consisting of subunits of widely varying size. Some have the commonplace 15,000- to 17,000-dalton heme-containing subunits. Two branchiopods (*Lepidurus* and *Daphnia pulex*) have 34,000-dalton subunits containing two hemes.[7] Here is yet another variation on Svedberg's proposal that a 17,000-dalton protein is the basic heme-containing unit. These hemoglobins also have marked (100-fold) variability in oxygen affinity, but unlike the insect hemoglobins, these multisubunit hemoglobins display marked cooperativity (Fig. 6–10).

One of the most dramatic and fascinating phenomena in biology is the marked change in hemoglobin synthesis that can occur with changing ambient oxygen tension. When placed in a hypoxic environment, the water flea *Daphnia* changes from colorless to bright red, owing to a sudden surge in hemoglobin synthesis.[35] This has also been observed in other insects, such as *Moina*, the polychete (annelid) *Neanthes,* and *Chironomus* larvae.[9] These animals provide interesting models in which to study the environmental control of gene expression.

Echinoderm Hemoglobins. Thus far, discussion in this chapter has focused on oxygen-carrying proteins from invertebrate phyla in the subkingdom Protostomia, which comprises the great majority of invertebrates. As shown in Figure 6–1, the protostomes and deuterostomes diverged from a common ancestor very early in animal evolution. The deuterostome lineage gave rise to echinoderms and eventually to lower chordates and vertebrates. Thus, the echinoderms may be viewed as a link between invertebrates and vertebrates. The hemoglobins of the echinoderm sea cucumbers *Cucumaria minata* and *Molpodia arenicola* display ligand-linked subunit aggregation[36, 36a] similar to that found in the most primitive vertebrates, the cyclostomes (see below). The oxygenated hemoglobin is a dimer composed of two 18,000-dalton subunits. Upon deoxygenation, dimers combine to form higher-order aggregates. Moreover, these hemoglobins have significant cooperative behavior ($n = 1.8$) (Fig. 6–10). Thus, these echinoderms have hemoglobins of intermediate complexity. It is not yet clear whether the 36,000-dalton dimer is composed of identical or dissimilar subunits. In any event, these echinoderm hemoglobins are an interesting prototype of vertebrate hemoglobin.

Chlorocruorins

A few families of polychete annelid worms* have a red-green polymeric respiratory pigment that Lankester[20] called chlorocruorin. The prosthetic group differs from heme in that the vinyl group on the 2 position of the porphyrin ring has been oxidized to a formyl group.[37] Chlorocruorin is dichroic, being red when concentrated and green when dilute.[38] Its absorption spectra are similar to those of hemoglobin but are shifted toward higher wavelengths. The chlorocruorins are remarkably similar to the large annelid hemoglobins discussed earlier: they have a molecular weight of about 3×10^6 daltons and are composed of 12 submultiples arranged in two hexagonal discs stacked on top of one another[7] (Fig. 6–11*II*). Like the hemoglobin polymers, the chlorocruorins lack a firm stoichiometric relationship between subunit composition and porphyrin content: one oxygen binds per 25,000 to 30,000 daltons of protein.

Chlorocruorins tend to have low oxygen affinity and often display marked subunit cooperativity. As shown in Figure 6–10, *Eudistylia* chlorocruorin has a P_{50} of between 60 and 180 mm Hg, an n value of around 2.5, and a normal Bohr effect.[39] It is unlikely that this protein is ever fully saturated with oxygen. Nevertheless, its high degree of cooperativity should enable it to unload oxygen effectively. Furthermore, the high concentration of chlorocruorin in the worm's blood (exceeding the concentration of respiratory protein in nearly all other invertebrates) also helps to maintain effective oxygen transport.

The adaptational significance of chlorocruorins remains elusive. In *Serpula*, hemoglobin and chlorocruorin coexist within the same animal and perhaps within the same polymer. Younger *Serpula* have more of the former, and older ones have more of the latter.[37] It would be of considerable interest to examine the enzyme(s) responsible for porphyrin synthesis in this animal as well as other polychetes that have either of the two respiratory pigments but not both.

VERTEBRATES

In contrast to the variation in prosthetic groups and molecular size among the invertebrate oxygen transport proteins, all vertebrates have hemoglobins in which a heme (ferroprotoporphyrin IX) is bound to a globin subunit. Vertebrate hemoglobins (except that of the cyclostomes) are highly cooperative 64,000-dalton heterotetramers that have the formula $\alpha_2\beta_2$. These hemoglobins are located inside circulating red cells. As shown in Figure 6–12, the red cells of vertebrates vary enormously in size and shape. Only mammalian red cells lack nuclei. The intracellular concentration of hemoglobin is generally higher than that in invertebrate red cells. Hemoglobin function within the red blood cell is determined not only by the intrinsic properties of the hemoglobin per se but also by its interaction with intracellular cofactors. The oxygen affinities of most vertebrate hemoglobins are strongly pH-dependent. As discussed in Chapters 3 and 5, this phenomenon, the "Bohr effect," has considerable physiologic importance, enabling the animal to exchange O_2 and CO_2 at both pulmonary and tissue levels. In addition to protons, intracellular hemoglobin function is also mediated by organic phosphates. As illustrated in Figure 6–13, the primary intracellular mediator varies among the different classes of vertebrates. In erythrocytes of elasmobranchs,

---

*Sabellidae, Serpulidae, Chlorohaemidae, and Ampharetidae.

ANIMAL HEMOGLOBINS 141

teleost fish, and reptiles, adenosine triphosphate (ATP) is the most abundant organic phosphate, and in fish and reptiles, hemoglobin function is markedly sensitive to changes in ATP concentration. Both ATP and 2,3-diphosphoglycerate (2,3-DPG) appear to regulate hemoglobin function in amphibian red blood cells, whereas the primary effector in avian erythrocytes is inositol pentaphosphate (IPP). As indicated in Figure 6–13, 2,3-DPG is the important regulator in mammalian red cells.

Thus, except for the cyclostomes, all vertebrate hemoglobins are intracellular tetramers of the type $\alpha_2\beta_2$. They have marked subunit cooperativity and are regulated by both protons (Bohr effect) and intracellular organic phosphates. Within these constraints, however, there is a broad and fascinating diversity in structure, function, and adaptational roles.

Cyclostomes

The class Agnatha comprises primitive fish that lack jaws or paired fins. The lamprey and hagfish are the primary surviving members of this group. Fossil evidence suggests that lampreys diverged as early as the Paleozoic era (500 MyBP)* and have changed little since mid-Pennsylvanian times (320 MyBP). Studies on lamprey hemoglobin have provided valuable insights into the general relationship between ligand binding and subunit interactions. Early measurements indicated that lamprey hemoglobin was a 17,000 dalton monomeric hemoglobin[40] yet it bound oxygen with a small degree of cooperativity.[41] In a more compre-

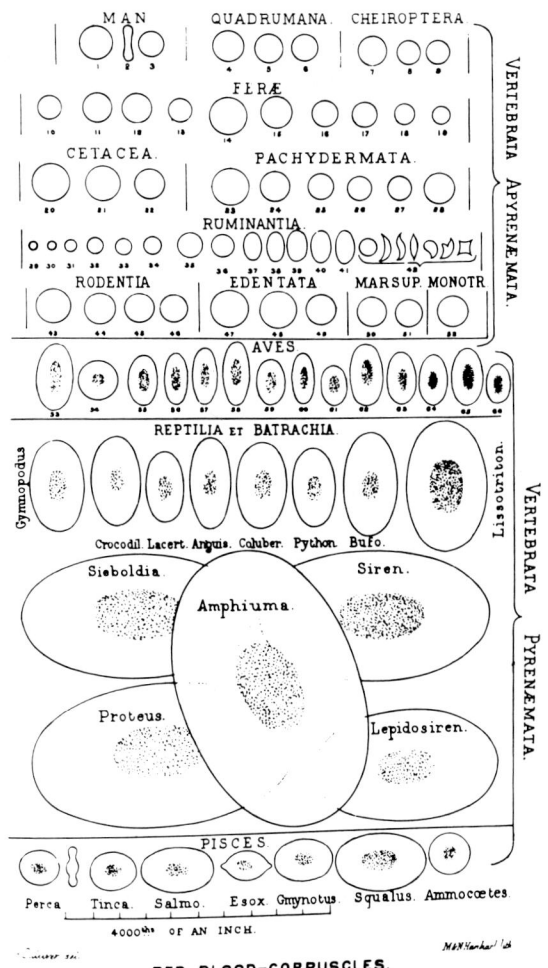

Figure 6–12. A century-old drawing of red blood cells from a variety of animals. At the top, red cells from 52 species of mammals are shown. All these cells lack nuclei. In contrast, the red cells of all other vertebrate classes are nucleated and are generally much larger than mammalian red cells. (From Gulliver, G.: Proc. Zool. Soc. Lond. p. 474, 1875.)

*MyBP = millions of years before the present.

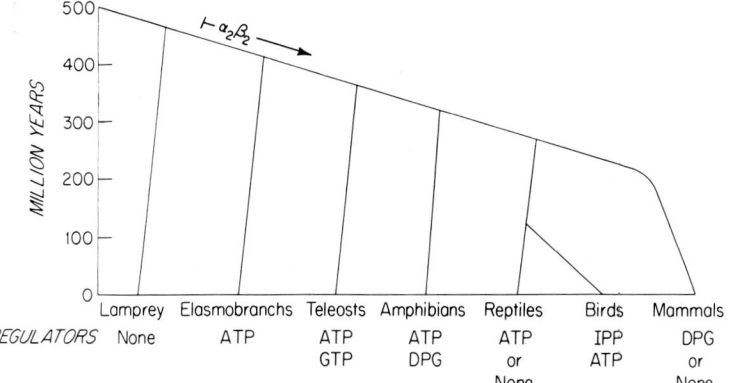

Figure 6–13. Simplified phylogenetic tree of vertebrates showing the emergence of hemoglobin heterotetramers and the principal mediators of hemoglobin function. (From Bunn, H. F.: Am. Zool. 20:199, 1980.)

hensive study, Briehl[42] showed that the oxygen affinity decreased significantly both at lower pH (the Bohr effect) and also with increasing hemoglobin concentration Furthermore, at high concentration and low pH, increasing cooperativity between subunits was noted. These findings suggested that oxygen binding was affected by the aggregation of subunits. Sedimentation velocity measurements demonstrated that with increasing concentration, only deoxygenated hemoglobin aggregated and that the extent of aggregation was markedly enhanced with decreasing pH. Briehl[42] formulated these results in terms of linked functions, similar to those developed by Wyman for tetrameric hemoglobin (see Chapter 3). The data suggested that monomers of lamprey hemoglobins can undergo a conformational isomerization. One conformer has a high oxygen affinity and fails to aggregate. The other conformer has a low oxygen affinity and is stabilized both by protons and by aggregation. These findings attracted considerable interest because they have clear implications for understanding the behavior of both normal tetrameric hemoglobins (see Chapter 3) and sickle hemoglobin (see Chapter 11). Moreover, lamprey hemoglobin resembles those hemocyanins, mentioned previously, that have tight linkage between oxygenation and subunit assembly.

The three-dimensional structure of lamprey hemoglobin (component V from *Petromyzon marinus*) has been solved at 2 Å resolution.[43] The cyanmet derivative has the same overall tertiary structure as myoglobin. Of note is an extended nine-residue sequence at the N terminus[44, 44a] that folds along the H helix. Unfortunately, there are no clues from the x-ray analysis of lamprey hemoglobin as to why the monomers aggregate when deoxygenated and protonated. The oxygen-linked proton binding has a pK of about 6. Thus far, structural analyses reveal no specific residues that would be responsible for this property.

Elasmobranchs

Sharks, rays, and skates are cartilaginous fish that form the class chondrichthyes (elasmobranchs). Marine forms are able to maintain an osmolarity in their blood and tissue as great as that of sea water. This is achieved by a build-up of nitrogenous waste products such as urea and trimethylamine oxide. While swimming in the ocean, sharks have a blood urea level of about 0.45 M; sharks acclimated to fresh water have a urea concentration of 0.001 M, comparable to that of man. Elasmobranchs have evolved hemoglobins that are resistant to the denaturing effects of high concentrations of urea. The oxygen affinities of skate, ray, and dogfish hemoglobins are not affected by up to 5 M of urea, whereas the oxygen affinity of human hemoglobin increases steadily.[45] Moreover, subunit cooperativity, the Bohr effect, and tetrameric stability of elasmobranch hemoglobins are all preserved despite the presence of a high concentration of urea.

Teleosts (Bony Fish)

Fish hemoglobins have been enthusiastically investigated by biochemists and physiologists. Hemoglobin fulfills two very different functions in fish. First, it assumes the conventional role of transporting oxygen to peripheral tissues. This problem is a formidable challenge for most aquatic animals. A few families of fish breathe air by means of lungs roughly similar to those of terrestrial animals. In contrast, the vast majority of fish depend on culling oxygen that is dissolved in water in low concentrations. As water rushes through the gills, a large surface area of capillaries facilitates the binding of oxygen to hemoglobin. The oxygen content in water is highly variable. Oxygen is less soluble in warm water and becomes progressively more scarce with increasing depth and in the absence of flora capable of photosynthesis. Second, as will be discussed in detail, fish hemoglobins may also be utilized to fill the swim bladder with oxygen against a pressure gradient. This phenomenon helps the fish control its buoyancy. Like many classes of vertebrates, a given species of fish will often have multiple hemoglobins. One type of hemoglobin may be utilized for oxygen transport and the other to fill the swim bladder and provide adequate oxygenation of the retina. Moreover, multiple hemoglobins may help to prevent precipitation or crystallization inside the red cell. The multiplicity of bands that appear during electrophoresis of fish hemoglobin is more apparent than real. Some of these bands are asymmetrical hybrid tetramers of the type $\alpha_2\beta^A\beta^B$. Such hybrids are present in mammalian red cells but do not appear on electrophoresis or chromatography because the tetramer readily dissociates into unlike dimers ($\alpha\beta^A$ and $\alpha\beta^B$) during the analysis (see Chapter 10). In contrast, fish hemoglobins have much more stable tetramers that do not readily dissociate into dimers.[46] Therefore, they appear as additional components.[47, 48]

In this section, the functional behavior of fish hemoglobins and how their properties are

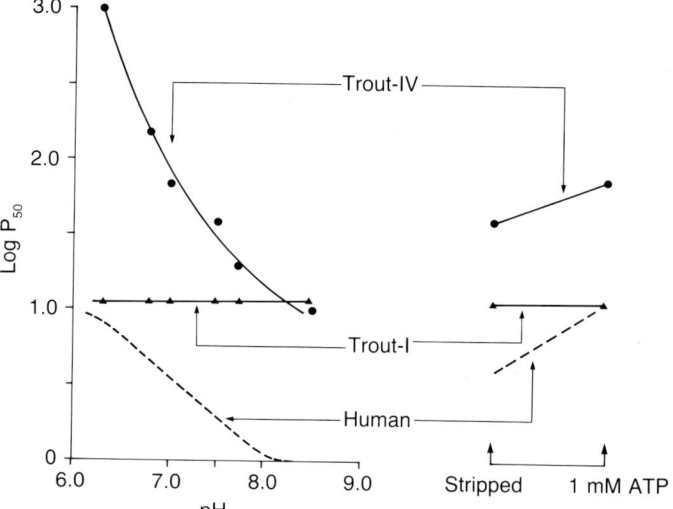

Figure 6–14. Comparison of functional properties of trout hemoglobins: Hb Trout-I (▲) and Hb Trout-IV (●). *Left,* Effect of pH on oxygen affinity, 20°C. Note that Hb Trout-I has no Bohr effect, whereas Hb Trout-IV has an exaggerated Bohr effect, i.e., Root effect. For comparison, comparable data for human hemoglobin are shown by the interrupted line. *Right,* Effect of ATP on oxygen affinity, pH 7.0, 20°C. Note that Hb Trout-I is unaffected by ATP, whereas the affinity of Hb Trout-IV is markedly lowered by ATP. (Prepared from data of Brunori and colleagues.[49,51])

determined by specific structural features will be described. Rather than catalogue the vast array of fish hemoglobins that have been investigated all over the world, the focus will be on two genera, the trout *(Salmo)* and the carp *(Cyprinus)*, whose structures and functional properties have been most exhaustively studied. The section will end with a consideration of how intracellular hemoglobin function can be modified in response to environmental challenges.

Trout Hemoglobins. When hemolysate of the European rainbow trout *Salmo irideus* is analyzed by electrophoresis or ion-exchange chromatography, three major components and a minor one are detected. Designated in order of decreasing isoelectric point, they are I (15% to 20%), II (15% to 20%), III (~3%), and IV (60% to 70%).[49] Brunori[49] and colleagues in Rome have completed an extensive examination of the properties of these hemoglobins. Their results agree very well with similar studies on hemoglobins of the American rainbow trout, *Salmo gairdneri.*[50] This collective body of information is of considerable interest because the functional properties of the trout hemoglobins appear to have a plausible structural explanation and because these hemoglobins play well-defined physiologic roles.

Hb Trout-I displays good subunit cooperativity ($n = 2.5$) but is totally unresponsive to organic allosteric modulators (Fig. 6–14). It lacks a Bohr effect, and its oxygen affinity is totally unaffected by ATP, the major organic phosphate in trout erythrocytes, and even by the more potent polyanion, inositol hexaphosphate (IHP).[51] However, the oxygen affinity of Hb Trout-I is lowered by chloride ion. The fact that a hemoglobin such as Hb Trout-I can possess full subunit cooperativity and yet fail to respond to heterotropic effectors suggests that its deoxy (T) quaternary structure is stabilized by interactions other than protons and polyanions. These interesting properties can be explained in structural terms.[52–54a] The critical residues responsible for the Bohr effect and interaction with organic phosphates are shown in Table 6–2. The β chain of Hb Trout-

Table 6–2. **FUNCTIONALLY IMPORTANT AMINO ACID REPLACEMENTS IN β CHAINS OF SELECTED VERTEBRATE HEMOGLOBINS***

Hemoglobin	NA1	NA2	EF6	F9	FG1	H21	HC3
Trout-I	NH$_2$–Val	Glu	*Leu*†	Ala	*Asn*	Ser	*Phe*
Trout-IV	NH$_2$–Val	Asp	Lys	Ser	Glu	Arg	His
Carp	NH$_2$–Val	Glu	Lys	Ser	Glu	Arg	His
Tadpole III	NH$_2$–Val	His	Lys	Ala	Asn	His	His
Frog C.	—	—	Lys	Ser	*Gly*	Lys	His
Crocodile: Caiman	NH$_2$–Ser	Pro	Lys	*Phe*	Glu	*Ala*	His
Nile	Ac–Ala	Ser	Lys	Cys	Glu	*Ala*	His
Mississippi	Ac–Ala	Ser	Lys	Cys	Glu	*Ala*	His
Human	NH$_2$–Val	His	Lys	Cys	Asp	His	His

*Modified from Perutz, M. F.: Mol. Biol. Evol. *1*:1, 1983.
†Italicized residues indicates that replacement has critical effect on function.

144 ANIMAL HEMOGLOBINS

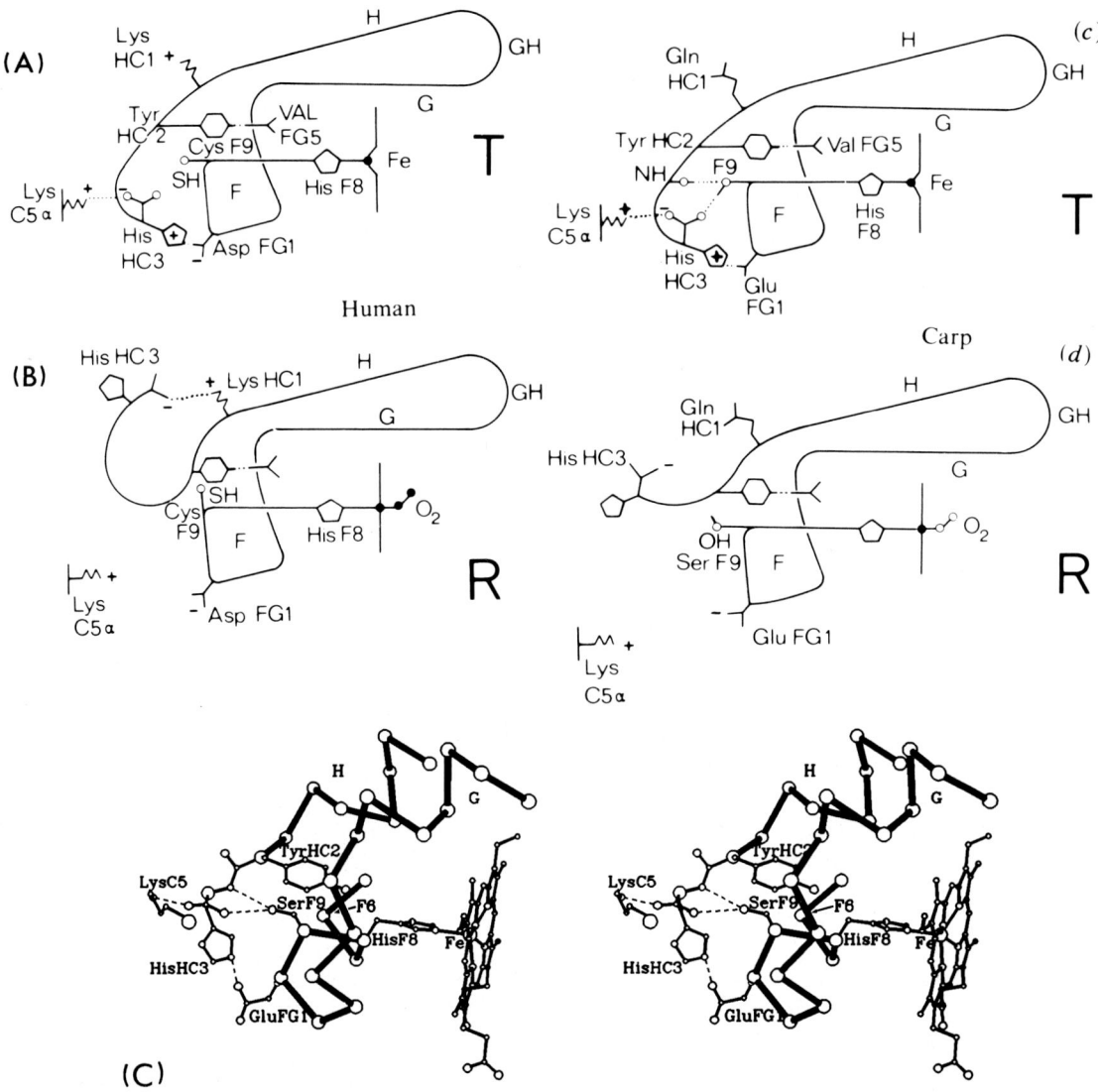

Figure 6–15. Molecular basis of the Root effect of fish hemoglobin. A and B, Diagrams comparing the R and T structures of mammalian (human) and fish (carp) hemoglobins. In the carp T structure, the β F9 Ser forms hydrogen bonds with β HC3 His, thereby providing additional stability to the T structure. C, Stereodiagram of these interactions in the T structure of carp hemoglobin. (From Perutz, M. F.: Mol. Biol. Evol. 1:1, 1983.)

I has Phe instead of His at the C terminus and therefore cannot make the oxygen-linked salt linkage that is an important contributor to the Bohr effect in most vertebrates. Furthermore, at β F9, Hb Trout-I has Ala instead of Ser, which, as will be explained in detail later, may be responsible for the exaggerated Bohr effect found in many of the fish hemoglobins. The failure of Hb Trout-I to respond to organic phosphates can be explained by the fact that at two sites normally involved in polyanion binding, it has uncharged amino acids in place of positively charged ones: β EF6 Leu and β H21 Ser.

The Root Effect. In contrast to Hb Trout-I, Hb Trout-IV (as well as Hb Trout-III[50]) is very sensitive to pH and organic phosphates. The exaggerated alkaline Bohr effect, commonly called the Root effect, is shared by a number of fish hemoglobins. As shown in Figure 6–14, the effect of pH on the P_{50} of Hb Trout-IV is much more marked than that on the P_{50} of human hemoglobin. Moreover, the oxygen affinity of Hb Trout-IV is decreased markedly by the addition of organic polyanions such as ATP or IHP. At pH 6.0, in the presence of 1 mM of ATP, Hb Trout-IV has such low oxygen affinity that it is less than 10 per cent saturated by air at room temperature. Moreover, under these conditions, the hemoglobin has lost nearly all of its subunit cooperativity. In fact, at about 50 per cent oxygen saturation, Hill's n is less than 1.0 owing to differences in the oxygen affinities of α and β chains. Under these circumstances, the T quaternary structure is so stabilized that the tetramer fails to flip into the R structure even when fully oxygenated.

The carp *(Cyprinus carpio)* has three structurally distinct hemoglobins whose functional properties are nearly identical to one another[55, 56] and strongly resemble those of Hb Trout-IV. Thus, carp hemoglobin has a Root effect and interacts strongly with organic phosphates.[53, 54] Like Hb Trout-IV, cooperativity between the subunits of carp hemoglobin disappears both at low pH, in the presence of organic phosphate, in which hemoglobin remains primarily in the T structure, and at high pH, in which the R structure predominates. The MWC two-state allosteric model (see Chapter 3) provides a useful framework for interpreting the properties of these fish hemoglobins, but precise oxygenation data cannot be fitted to the simplest form of this model.[57]

Primary sequence analyses of Hb Trout-IV and carp hemoglobin (Table 6–2) permit a stereochemical explanation of why they are so responsive to heterotropic modifiers.[49, 54] β HC3 His is probably a substantial contributor to the Root effect of Hb Trout-IV and carp hemoglobin, just as it appears to account for a significant amount of the Bohr effect in human hemoglobin. Moreover, Perutz[54] has concluded that β F9 Ser is another important contributor, thereby accounting for the exaggerated Bohr effect in fish hemoglobin. The hydroxyl group of the serine is likely to donate a hydrogen bond to the terminal oxygen atom of β HC 3 His and to accept a hydrogen bond from the peptide NH of the same residue (Fig. 6–15). These interactions would confer increased stability on the T quaternary structure.

Interaction with Organic Phosphates. The most abundant organic phosphates in fish red cells are ATP and guanosine triphosphate (GTP).[58–61] Occasionally, other polyphosphates such as inositol pentaphosphate, inositol diphosphate, and 2,3-DPG have been detected in fish red cells but in lesser amounts than ATP or GTP.[60, 61] The latter compounds serve as important mediators of intracellular hemoglobin function. In contrast to observations on mammalian hemoglobins, ATP is a more potent allosteric modifier of some and perhaps most fish hemoglobins than is 2,3-DPG.[58] Moreover, in certain fish, GTP may be more effective than ATP.[62, 63]

Perutz[54] has provided a stereochemical explanation for the enhanced interaction of nucleotide triphosphates with fish hemoglobins. As shown in Table 6–2, teleost fish have a negatively charged residue at β NA2 rather than the hydrogen donor sites (His, Gln, or Asn) found at β NA2 in mammalian hemoglobins. This difference in structure allows the N-6 amino group of the adenine in ATP to form a hydrogen bond with the carboxyls of β NA2 Glu or Asp (Fig. 6–16). GTP can also bind here in a stereochemically favorable fashion.

Physiologic Implications of Allosteric Modifiers. The Root effect is one of the most striking properties found among the vertebrate hemoglobins. The prevalence and magnitude of the Root effect among hemoglobin components of various fish can be analyzed by com-

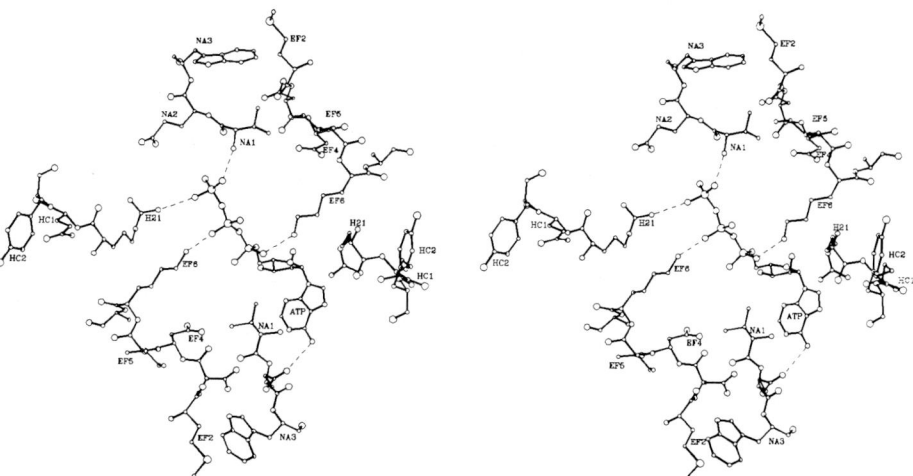

Figure 6–16. Stereodiagram showing suggested ATP binding site of fish hemoglobins. The N6 atom of the adenine donates a hydrogen bond to the carboxyl group of β NA2 Glu. (From Perutz, M. F.: Mol. Biol. Evol. *1*:1, 1983.)

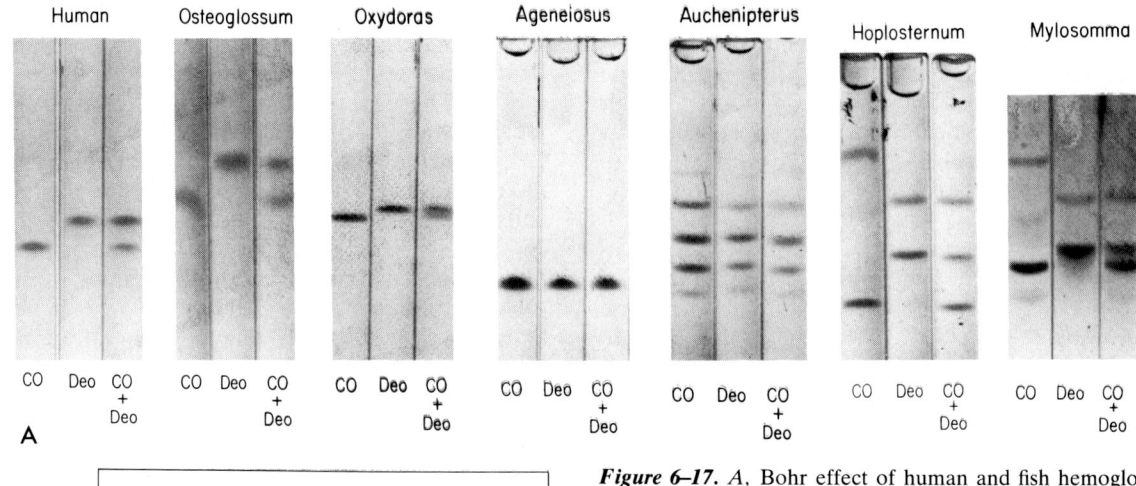

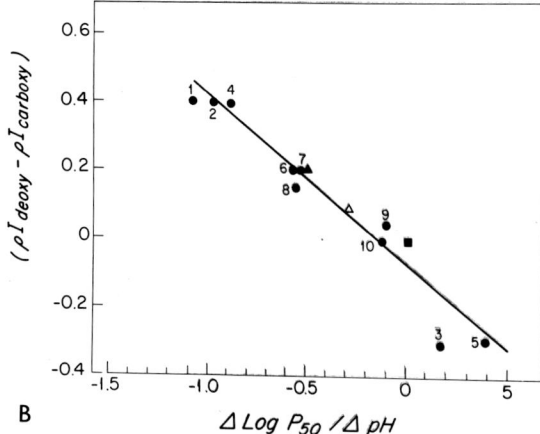

Figure 6–17. A, Bohr effect of human and fish hemoglobins estimated by gel electrofocusing of deoxygenated hemolysates and hemolysates saturated with carbon monoxide. The change in isoelectric point (pI) of each hemoglobin component provides a measure of its Bohr effect. An increase in pI upon deoxygenation indicates a "normal" Bohr effect ($\Delta \log P_{50}/\Delta$ pH < O). Note that *Hoplosternum* and *Mylossoma* each have a hemoglobin component with a "normal" Bohr effect and one with a "reverse" Bohr effect ($\Delta \log P_{50}/\Delta$ pH > O). B, Relationship between Bohr effect estimated from gel electrofocusing data (pI deoxy − pI carboxy) with that determined by oxygen equilibria ($\Delta \log P_{50}/\Delta \log$ pH) (● = fish hemoglobins; ▲ = normal human hemoglobin; △ = human hemoglobin Syracuse [β 143 His→Pro]; ■ = amphibian hemoglobin [*Typhlonectes*]). The $\Delta \log P_{50}/\Delta \log$ pH was calculated at pI of the hemoglobin component. (1 = *Prochilodus*; 2 = *Pterygoplichthys* (anodal component); 3 = *Pterygoplichthys* (cathodal component); 4 = *Hoplosternum* (anodal component); 5 = *Hoplosterum* (cathodal component); 6 = *Osteoglossum;* 7 = *Arapaima;* 8 = *Mylosomma* (anodal component); 9 = *Pseudodoras;* 10 = *Lepidosiren.*) The isoelectric points were determined at 4°C, and the oxygen equilibria were done at 20°C. (From Bunn, H. F., and Riggs A.: Comp. Biochem. Physiol. *62A*:95, 1979.)

paring the electrophoretic patterns of oxygenated and deoxygenated hemolysates.[64] If $\Delta \log P_{50}/\Delta$pH < 0, hemoglobin will bind protons upon deoxygenation and become more positively charged. As shown in Figure 6–17, a variety of patterns have been noted among freshwater fish. Some have hemoglobins that lack a Bohr effect. Others have one component with an exaggerated Bohr effect (Root effect) along with another component with a reverse Bohr effect ($\Delta \log P_{50}/\Delta$pH > 0).

The adaptational significance of these combinations of hemoglobins with absent, normal, and reverse Bohr effects is far from obvious. However, a few generalizations can be made. In many fish, oxygen is secreted against a concentration gradient into the swim bladder, enabling control of buoyancy. As illustrated in Figure 6–18, the swim bladder is surrounded by an elaborate vascular network, the *rete mirabile,* in which a countercurrent circulation

enables the secretion of hydrogen ions against a concentration gradient. Therefore, as local pH falls, oxygen is released at high pressure from hemoglobin having a Root effect. In this way, oxygen pressures of up to 50 Atm can be maintained in the swim bladder, while the remaining parts of the fish may have marginal oxygenation. Hemoglobins with a Root effect can be viewed as a macromolecular transducer[65] that works by coupling the concentration gradients of two ligands, H^+ and O_2, which bind to hemoglobin with strong linkage. Despite its elegance, this system is not sufficient for the control of buoyancy in some and perhaps most fish. Hemoglobin with a Root effect is not able to generate sufficient oxygen pressure in fish living in very deep water.[66] Under extreme pressure, oxygen and other gases have such high density that lipid becomes a superior hydrostatic device.

In like manner, hemoglobin having a Root

effect may facilitate transfer of oxygen across the choroid rete of the eye, allowing adequate oxygenation of the metabolically active cells in the retina.

The level of nucleotide triphosphates in fish red cells plays a vital role in adaptation to hypoxia. A variety of fish acquire an increase in red cell oxygen affinity when placed in hypoxic water.[67-69] As shown in Figure 6–19, this shift to the left in the oxyhemoglobin dissociation curve can be attributed to a decrease in the level of nucleotide triphosphates. The most abundant organic phosphate in the red cells of killifish[70] and trout[69] is ATP, whereas in carp[68] and eels[67] it is GTP. Moreover, the hemoglobins of carp and eels are more responsive to GTP than to ATP.[67, 68] The level of red cell nucleotide triphosphates falls within a few days after fish are exposed to hypoxic water.[68, 70] Conversely, when benthic

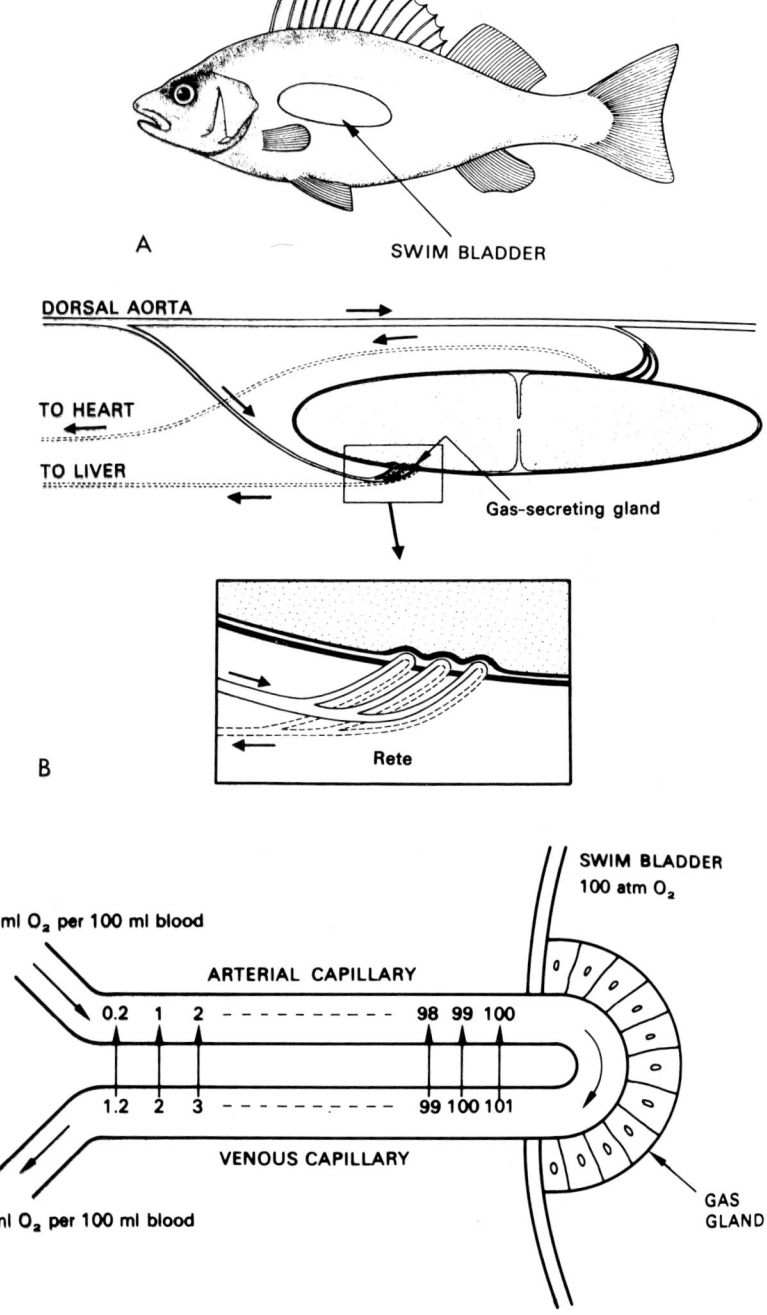

Figure 6–18. *A*, The swim bladder of teleost fish is located in the abdominal cavity, just below the vertebral column. Although the shape of the swim bladder varies considerably among species, its volume is above 5% of body volume in marine fish and 7% in freshwater fish. This volume of gas will decrease the specific gravity of the fish so that it can achieve neutral buoyancy. *B*, Diagram of circulation to the swim bladder. Blood reaches the organ through a set of parallel capillaries of very high surface area called the *rete mirabile* (inset). *C*, Diagram of parallel capillaries in the *rete mirabile*, which constitutes a countercurrent multiplier. This device allows the maintenance of very high gas pressures in the distal arterial capillary and adjacent venous capillary, while the blood entering and leaving the rete has much lower gas tension. The secretion of lactic acid by the gas gland at the tip of the rete allows the marked unloading of oxygen from fish hemoglobins that possess a Root effect. Thus, the blood in the capillary veins of the rete has a lower oxygen *content* but a higher oxygen *tension* than that in the adjacent arterial capillary. (From Schmidt-Nielsen, K.: Animal Physiology; Adaptation and Environment. Cambridge, Cambridge University Press, 1975, pp. 552–561. This text provides an excellent account of the physiology of the swim bladder.)

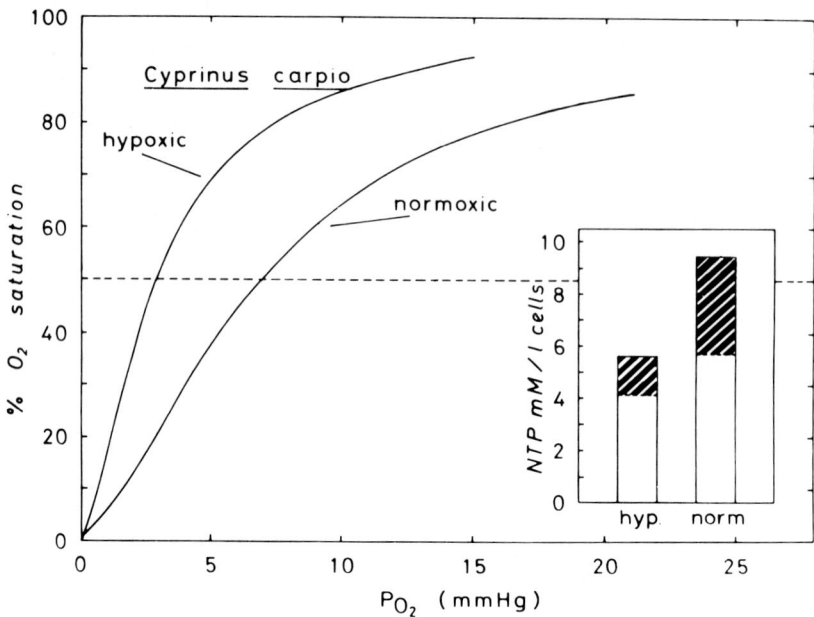

Figure 6–19. Oxygen binding curves of blood of carp acclimated to hypoxic and normoxic water, measured at 20°C and pH 7.9. *Inset,* Levels of red cell ATP (open histograms) and GTP (hatched histograms) in carp acclimated to hypoxic and normoxic water. (From Weber, R. E., and Lykkeboe, G.: J. Comp. Physiol. *128*:127, 1978.)

fish are changed from their hypoxic deep-water habitat to normoxic water, the level of ATP in their red cells rises.[71] This ATP-mediated increase in oxygen affinity constitutes an important mode of adaptation to hypoxia. In contrast, when man and other mammals are subjected to hypoxic stress, the level of red cell organic phosphates rises. However, this response is sometimes maladaptive (see below). As is the case of 2,3-DPG in red cells of man (see Chapter 5) and other mammals, ATP and GTP in fish red cells modulate oxygen affinity not only by interacting with hemoglobin but also by lowering intracellular pH and thereby decreasing oxygen affinity through the Bohr effect. The mechanism responsible for the alterations in red cell nucleotide triphosphates that accompany changes in P_{O_2} is not well understood. Rapid reduction in ATP has been noted following *in vitro* incubation of red cells in a totally anaerobic environment.[69, 70] However, ATP in fish red cells is derived primarily from oxidative metabolism. It is unlikely that partial reduction in P_{O_2}, as occurs *in vivo*, would significantly affect the rate of oxidative phosphorylation; in fact, incubation of red cells under these conditions does not lower the level of ATP.[70] Thus, it is likely that the control of red cell ATP in response to P_{O_2} is at the organismal rather than the cellular level.[69]

Temperature. Oxygen transport in fish is strongly dependent on the temperature of their habitat. The vast majority of fish are poikilotherms—their body temperature matches that of the water in which they are swimming. Thus, the overall rate of cellular and oxygen metabolism varies directly with ambient temperature. However, the oxygen content of water decreases in a nearly linear fashion with increasing temperature: at atmospheric pressure, 7 mg of oxygen can be dissolved in 100 ml of cold water (0°C), but only 3 mg of oxygen are soluble in warm water (40°C).[72] Moreover, the affinity of most fish hemoglobins for oxygen declines with rising temperature. Therefore, when fish are exposed to warm water, the oxygenation of blood is compromised, whereas oxygen demand is apt to be maximal. This potential problem can be offset by several kinds of adaptations.[73] In a comprehensive study of catostomid fish, Powers[72, 74] has shown that during the warm summer months, there is a 50 per cent increase in the hematocrit. The intracellular hemoglobin concentration remains constant. Therefore, the oxygen-carrying capacity of the blood varies directly with the hematocrit. Moreover, red cell ATP decreases 50 per cent during acclimation to warm water. The resulting increase in oxygen affinity allows enhanced oxygen extraction.

Unlike the muscles of nearly all other fish that are poikilothermic, the muscles of the tuna are maintained up to 15°C warmer than water temperature. This is achieved by a countercurrent circulation in which metabolic heat from the venous blood of muscles is transferred to arterial blood going from the gills to the muscles.[75] If the tuna had hemoglobin with a normal temperature coefficient for oxygen binding, the arterial blood, as it is gradually warmed during passage through the countercurrent multiplier, would transfer its oxygen to the veins, and the blood arriving at the muscle capillaries would be poorly saturated with oxygen. This problem is circumvented by the evolution of a hemoglobin with a reverse temperature coefficient: its oxygen affinity increases as temperature rises[75a] (similar to that of the arcid clam, discussed previously). In all hemoglobins, heat is liberated with oxygenation of each of the four hemes. However, in tuna hemoglobin, the transition from the T to R quaternary structure absorbs so much heat that the overall oxygenation process is endothermic.[76] Perutz[54] has concluded that an additional set of hydrogen bonds is probably involved in the stabilization of the T structure of tuna hemoglobin.

Maternal-Fetal Oxygen Transport. Throughout this survey of vertebrate hemoglobins, differences in the oxygenation of maternal and fetal blood will be noted. The higher oxygen affinity of fetal blood compared with maternal blood appears to be a general phenomenon in vertebrate biology, occurring in teleosts, amphibians, birds, and mammals. It is likely that this phenomenon facilitates the transport of oxygen to the fetus. In the sea perch, *Embiotoca lateralis*, there appears to be a dual mechanism for the higher oxygen affinity of fetal red cells.[77] First, these animals have structurally distinct fetal hemoglobin whose intrinsic oxygen affinity is higher than that of adult hemoglobin. Second, fetal red cells have lower concentrations of organic phosphates.

Amphibians

All vertebrates undergo transitions of hemoglobin production during development. In amphibians, this process assumes particular interest because these animals experience a metamorphosis in which they pass from an aquatic to a terrestrial existence. Therefore, it is worth determining whether this abrupt change in life style is accompanied by appropriate changes in hemoglobin function.

The bullfrog *(Rana catesbeiana)* has been thoroughly investigated as a model of hemoglobin switching during ontogeny. As shown in Figure 6–20, primitive red cells are produced in ventral blood islands during embryonic development. In the larval (tadpole) period,

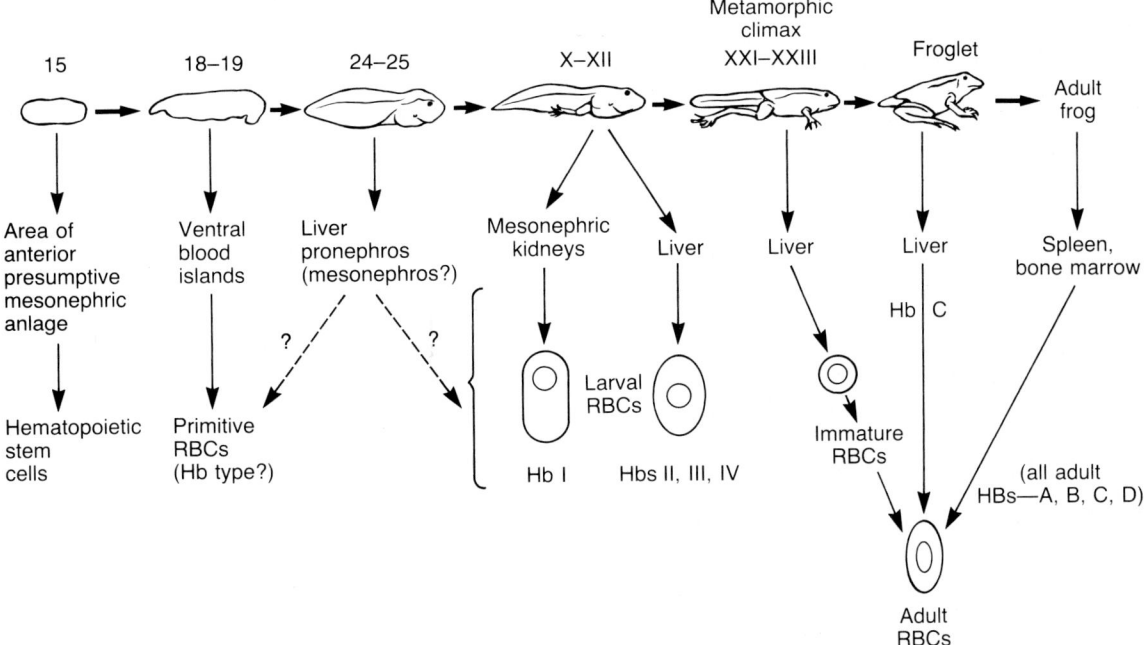

Figure 6–20. Ontogeny of erythropoiesis and hemoglobin synthesis in the bullfrog. The Arabic numbers at the top refer to embryonic stages. The Roman numerals refer to larval and metamorphic stages. (From Broyles, R. H.: Changes in the blood during amphilbian metamorphosis. *In* Gilbert, L. I., and Frieden, E. (eds.): Metamorphosis: A Problem in Developmental Biology. 2nd ed. New York, Plenum Publishing Corp., 1981, p. 461.)

large, oval red cells are made in the kidney, whereas smaller elliptical cells are made in the liver.[78] The kidney erythrocytes contain one type of larval hemoglobin (Hb I = $\alpha_2^1\beta_2^1$), whereas the liver cells contain three major components composed of two α and two β chains not shared by component I—Hbs II, III, and IV. Hbs I and II, the major components in young tadpoles, have substantially higher oxygen affinity than Hbs III and IV,[78a] which compose about two thirds of the tadpole hemoglobin just prior to metamorphosis. In the absence of organic phosphates, tadpole hemoglobins have an absent or reverse alkaline Bohr effect ($\Delta \log P_{50}/\Delta pH \geq 0$). This can be explained by analysis[54, 79] of primary sequence[79, 80] of component III, which reveals alterations in residues that normally make a substantial contribution to the Bohr effect: (a) the NH_2 terminus of the α chain is acetylated; (b) β FG1, which is normally aspartic or glutamic acid and forms a salt bond with the β C-terminal histidine, is asparagine; and (c) β F9, normally serine in hemoglobins with a Root effect, is alanine (Table 6–2).

Following metamorphosis, the red cells of the froglet are made primarily in the liver (Fig. 6–20). However, in the adult frog, erythropoiesis shifts to the spleen and bone marrow.[81] Frog red cells contain two major hemoglobin components (B and C) and two minor components (A and D). Apparently, the two major components are composed of four distinct subunits ($\alpha_2^B\beta_2^B$ and $\alpha_2^C\beta_2^C$). None of the adult globin chains are shared by any of the tadpole components. Hb C is the predominant component in the froglet. Its oxygen affinity is substantially higher than that of Hb B but is lower than those of the tadpole hemoglobins.[82] Moreover, the Bohr effect of Hb C is half as large as that of Hb B but, again, is greater than that of tadpole hemoglobins. Finally, frog Hb C has a tendency to polymerize owing to disulfide bond formations. The first six residues of the β chain of Hb C are deleted.[83] Its weak Bohr effect is probably due in part to the presence of glycine rather than glutamic or aspartic acid at β FG1[54] (Table 6–2).

Organic Phosphates. Hemoglobin function in the red cells of the bullfrog as well as other amphibians is regulated by organic phosphates. The predominant contributors are ATP and 2,3-DPG.[60] In addition, a small amount of inositol polyphosphate has been found.[84] The red cells of the bullfrog tadpole contain 2.7 mM of ATP, 2.5 mM of GTP, and 2 mM of 2,3-DPG, whereas in the adult bullfrog the concentrations are 3.9 mM of ATP, 0.2 mM of GTP, and 1.7 mM of 2,3-DPG.[60] The hemoglobins of the tadpole and frog show interesting differences in their responses to organic phosphate.[84] The oxygen affinity of frog hemoglobin is more responsive than that of tadpole hemoglobin to the addition of 2,3-DPG but less sensitive to the addition of ATP. Moreover, frog hemoglobin has the unusual property of being totally unresponsive to the most potent of all the organic phosphate regulators, inositol hexaphosphate.

In summary, there is a sequence of changes in hemoglobin function throughout bullfrog development. During the maturation from young tadpole to adult frog, there is a four-step decrease in oxygen affinity. In addition, there is a three-step increase in the alkaline Bohr effect. For reasons discussed elsewhere in this chapter, it is likely that these alterations are adaptive in the transition from an aquatic to a terrestrial environment.

The hemoglobin of another anuran amphibian, *Xenopus laevis*, has also been extensively investigated. Neither a frog nor a toad, *Xenopus* is completely aquatic except during droughts, when the animal escapes dehydration by burrowing in mud and entering aestivation. Like frogs, the *Xenopus* tadpole is a water-breather. The adult animal, despite its aquatic environment, breathes air through its lungs and also its skin. The functional properties of *Xenopus* tadpole hemoglobin have not yet been investigated, but a weak Bohr effect would be expected owing to the presence of Phe in place of His at the C terminus of the β chain.[54] In contrast, hemoglobin from the adult animal has a substantial Bohr effect, about threefold greater than that of the major component of *Rana catesbeiana* hemoglobin, owing in part to β F9 Ser, which is thought to contribute to the Root effect in fish hemoglobins.* The oxygen affinity of the adult *Xenopus* hemoglobin is higher than that of the other anurans.[85] This property, along with the substantial Bohr effect, may help the animal adapt to its relatively hypoxic aqueous environment.[86]

During exposure to increased salinity as well as during aestivation, the oxygen affinity of *Xenopus* red cells increases, again an adaptive response. In both cases, the shift to the left in the oxygen dissociation curve appears to be due to a proportional increase in the concentration of urea in the plasma and red cell. As mentioned previously, urea does not alter the

---

*Hemoglobins of *Rana catesbeiana* and *Rana esculanta* also have β F9 Ser, but their Bohr effects appear to be weakened by the absence of negatively charged Glu at β FG1 that forms a salt bridge with the β C-terminal His.[54]

oxygenation of elasmobranch hemoglobin[45] and causes only a small increase in the oxygen affinity of human hemoglobin. In contrast, urea markedly increases the oxygen affinity of *Xenopus* hemoglobin. Unlike its effect in most other vertebrates, the level of red cell organic phosphates does not appear to play a regulatory role in *Xenopus* red cells.

As in mammals and birds, discussed later in this chapter, an increase in oxygen affinity may help amphibians adapt to high altitude. Red cells from the frog *Telmatobius culeus*, which lives in Lake Titicaca in the Andes at 3800 M, have a higher oxygen affinity than those of any other frog.[87] When the salamander *Ambystoma tigrinum* is exposed to experimental hypoxia, an increase in oxygen affinity is also observed,[87a] owing in part to a decrease in red cell organic phosphates.

The caecilians constitute a separate order of amphibians *(Apoda)*. As in so many other animals discussed in this chapter, fetal red cells from *Typhlonectes* have higher oxygen affinity than those from the mother. Unlike the sea perch,[77] this *Apoda* lacks a distinct fetal hemoglobin. The higher oxygen affinity of its fetal red cells can be explained by a single mechanism: a decreased concentration of red cell organic phosphates.[88]

Reptiles

The reptiles are divided into three orders, Chelonia (turtles), Crocodilia (crocodilians), and Squamata (lizards and snakes), which diverged from one another almost as long ago as the phylogenetic line that led to birds and mammals. Therefore, it is no surprise that the reptiles are a diverse group of animals. Some live exclusively on land, some live exclusively in water, and some are amphibious. They are ectotherms and therefore utilize external sources of energy to raise their body temperature to levels required for various activities. In contrast to mammals, reptiles have a rather sluggish basal metabolism and rely on anaerobic metabolism during spurts of exercise. Accordingly, both oxygen availability and oxygen utilization vary enormously among these animals. The measurement of oxygen binding to hemoglobin in the blood of reptiles has physiologic relevance only if it is performed at the temperature at which the animal is active. The P_{50} of reptile red cells, like that of mammals (see below), varies inversely with the size of the animal. However, this relationship does **not** pertain with snakes. In general, both oxygen affinity and the Bohr effect are lower in red cells of reptiles than in those of mammals. However, among reptiles, both these measurements vary widely, and their adaptational significance is often unclear.

The hemoglobins of reptiles appear to differ from other vertebrate hemoglobins in two interesting respects. In several species of turtles, snakes, lizards, and crocodilians, the hemoglobin tetramers form disulfide bridges with each other. It is not always clear to what extent this phenomenon affects intracellular hemoglobin function or whether it may at times be merely an *in vitro* artifact. Polymerization due to disulfide bonds has also been noted in mouse and frog hemoglobins as well as in the human variant Hb Porto Alegre (β 9 Ser→ Cys), but in general, the phenomenon is much more commonly observed in reptiles. High levels of methemoglobin have also been frequently observed in blood of a number of different reptiles, including snakes and turtles. Methemoglobinemia of up to 50 per cent has been noted in freshly drawn specimens. The activity of methemoglobin reductase appears to be adequate in red cells of reptiles. Although methemoglobinemia may play a functional role during anaerobic metabolism,[89] the overall significance of this phenomenon is not well understood and deserves further exploration.

ATP is the primary regualtor of oxygen affinity in reptilian red cells.[60, 61] Concentrations range from 2 to 8 mM. Much smaller amounts of GTP and inositol pentaphosphate have also been detected in adult red cells. The responsiveness of reptilian hemoglobins to different organic phosphates is variable. The compound that is most abundant in the reptile's red cells is not necessarily the one with the greatest effect in lowering the oxygen affinity of its hemoglobin.[90]

Like many other vertebrates mentioned previously, reptiles display a significant decrease in red cell oxygen affinity during ontogeny. Prior to hatching, the red cells of fetal reptiles, like fetal bird red cells (see below), contain substantial amounts of 2,3-DPG.[60, 61] However, the 2,3-DPG disappears within a few weeks after hatching. In general, the level of organic phosphates in fetal red cells of reptiles is at least as high as in those of the adult[60, 61] and, therefore, cannot explain the decrease in oxygen affinity during ontogeny. There do not appear to be structurally distinct fetal hemoglobins in reptiles. In some snakes, the high oxygen affinity of fetal red cells may be due to increased methemoglobin.[91] In general, however, the phenomenon is not explained.

Crocodilians. The hemoglobin function of alligators and crocodiles differs from that of other reptiles and, indeed, other vertebrates in two interesting ways.[92] First, their red cells are almost devoid of organic phosphates. Second, crocodile hemoglobin is not responsive to the usual organic phosphates. Instead, the primary regulator appears to be bicarbonate ion: HCO_3^- is as potent in lowering the oxygen affinity of crocodilian hemoglobin as inositol hexaphosphate is in lowering the oxygen affinity of human hemoglobin. Two molecules of bicarbonate bind to each tetramer of crocodilian hemoglobin. In contrast, CO_2 has very little effect on the oxygen affinity. Note that the opposite situation pertains in mammalian hemoglobins: CO_2 lowers oxygen affinity by forming a carbamino complex (see Chapter 3); in contrast, the bicarbonate anion is no more effective than other monovalent anions.

These functional properties of crocodilian hemoglobins can be explained by specific alterations in primary structure.[54, 93, 94] The loss of regulation by organic phosphates is due to replacements of Pro or Ser for His at β NA2 and replacement of Ala for His at β H21 (Table 6–2). Furthermore, the N terminus of the β chain of two crocodilian hemoglobins (Hbs Nile and Mississippi) is blocked by an acetyl group. In Caiman hemoglobin, proline at β NA2 creates a bend that prevents the formation of a stable bond of the N-terminal amino with organic phosphates. These alterations at the β N terminus also impair the oxygen-linked carbamate binding. Model building indicates that the bicarbonate ion binds in a stereospecific site where organic phosphates and carbamino CO_2 are bound in other species.[54, 94] As illustrated in Figure 6–21, each HCO_3^- binds to β EF6 lysine and HCl glutamic acid of one β chain and the N-terminal amino of the other β chain. The alterations mentioned previously at the β N terminus of the three crocodilian hemoglobins analyzed to date allow additional hydrogen bonds with the bicarbonate anion. The precise stereochemical fit between bicarbonate anion and the β chains of crocodilian hemoglobins appears to have been "created" by only three mutations.[54, 94]

It is tempting to conclude that this exploitation of a common anion as an allosteric effector is of adaptive significance. Even though they are obligate air-breathers, crocodilians are able to remain submerged for up to an hour. However, unlike diving mammals and birds, they are unable to store oxygen in muscle myoglobin.[54] The bicarbonate generated from respiring tissues binds to hemoglobin reciprocally with oxygen and therefore enables maximal unloading of oxygen. This slow release of oxygen may allow the animal to maintain an adequate oxygen supply to its vital organs until it has to come up for air.

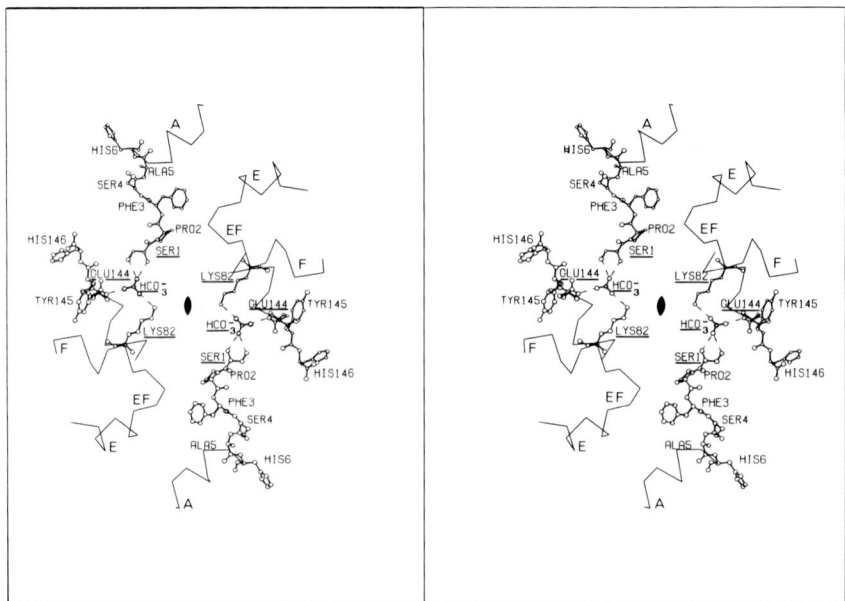

Figure 6–21. Stereodiagram of the proposed bicarbonate binding site between the two β chains of caiman deoxyhemoglobin. The central sign marks the dyad axis of symmetry. Bicarbonate ions and the residues to which they bind are underlined. (From Perutz, M. F.: Mol. Biol. Evol. *1*:1, 1983.)

Birds

Like other groups of animals, birds have special adaptational requirements that are met in part by alterations in intracellular hemoglobin function. Many types of birds are subject to wide fluctuations in ambient temperature as well as degree of hydration and blood pH. Moreover, rates of oxygen utilization vary considerably with the duration and intensity of muscle activity. Despite these vicissitudes, the oxygenation of avian red cells is quite similar to that of mammals. The oxygen affinity of various bird hemoglobins tends to be somewhat lower, but there is a surprising degree of variability of P_{50} values within a given species, particularly domestic fowl.[95] There is no significant relationship between P_{50} and body weight.[96] The Bohr effect of bird red cells is quite similar to that of mammals. However, unlike its effect in mammals, CO_2 causes only a minimal reduction in the oxygen affinity of bird red cells[96] and in some species may even increase oxygen affinity.[95] This phenomenon may have adaptive significance. As air rushes through the bird's posterior lung, the PCO_2 drops nearly to zero. If this caused a further increase in oxygen affinity, as it would in mammalian red cells, oxygen transport to tissues would be compromised.

Like so many animals, birds tend to have multiple hemoglobins. The biosynthesis of certain avian hemoglobins, particularly those of the chicken, has been subjected to exhaustive investigations. As explained in detail in Chapter 7, studies of the structure and function of embryonic and adult globin genes in the chicken have lead to valuable insights into the control of gene expression. In general, however, little is known about the functional or adaptive significance of multiple hemoglobins in avian erythrocytes. When individual components from a particular species have been isolated and studied, they tend to have similar oxygen binding. Unlike the red cells of reptiles and certain fish, there is very little methemoglobin in avian red cells.[97]

For a long time (1940 to 1973), avian cells were thought to be rich in inositol hexaphosphate (phytic acid),[98] a compound that is ubiquitous in plants. It is now known that inositol pentaphosphate is the most abundant organic phosphate and primary regulator of hemoglobin function.[60, 61, 98] In some birds, such as the ostrich, inositol tetraphosphate is the principal red cell organic phosphate.[99] As in other animals, the sensitivity of avian hemoglobins to organic phosphates does not correlate with the compounds that are present in the red cell. In general, relative responsiveness is in the order 2,3-DPG < ATP < inositol tetraphosphate < inositol pentaphosphate < inositol hexaphosphate.[99, 100] The interaction of avian hemoglobins with the inositol polyphosphates is enhanced by the substitution of additional positively charged residues on the β chain: H13 Ala → Arg and H17 Asn → His.[54, 101] These sites may be too far from the effector to form direct bonds with its phosphates, but they would neutralize its negative charge and therefore contribute indirectly to the binding energy.[54]

As in the red cells of other vertebrates, there is a marked change in the composition of organic phosphates in avian red cells during ontogeny. The principal mediator in embryonic red cells is 2,3-DPG.[102, 103] Just before or soon after hatching, ATP begins to rise and for about a week or so becomes the most abundant organic phosphate in the red cell.[60, 104] Thereafter, inositol pentaphosphate becomes predominant. This intriguing sequence in the levels of phosphorylated intermediates, depicted in Figure 6–22, attests to a complex but well-regulated series of enzymatic steps that is at present poorly understood. The overall process appears to be common if not universal among birds[105] and is likely to have adaptive significance. The sequence of intermediates of increasing allosteric potency permits a smooth increase in P_{50} during ontogeny, a phenomenon common in other kinds of animals but solved in such a special way by birds.

Unlike 2,3-DPG, inositol pentaphosphate is a rather stable compound that apparently turns over very slowly and may persist throughout the life span of the red cell.[106] Nevertheless, young avian red cells appear to have higher levels of this compound than older cells. When chickens were subjected to acute blood loss, a significant rise in inositol pentaphosphate and ATP was noted.[107] Changes in the levels of organic phosphates may account for some of the variability in the oxygen affinity of bird red cells noted earlier.

Like many mammals and at least one amphibian, birds may adapt to high altitude by an increase in red cell oxygen affinity. The bar-headed goose, which breeds in the highlands of Central Asia at altitudes of about 4000 M, has a significantly lower whole blood P_{50} than its lowland relatives, greylag and Canada geese. This difference can be explained by a slightly higher intrinsic oxygen affinity in the hemoglobin of the bar-headed goose (1.3 mm Hg), which is magnified 10-fold in the presence

154 ANIMAL HEMOGLOBINS

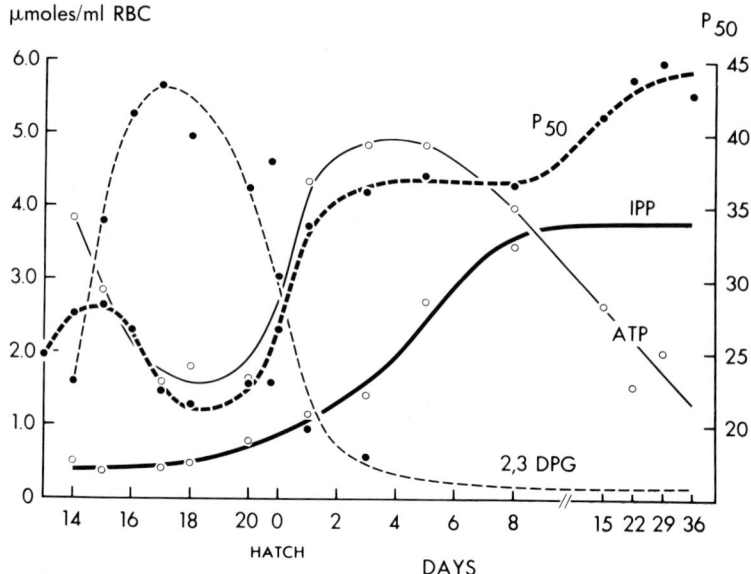

Figure 6–22. Correlation of whole blood P_{50} with 2,3-DPG, inositol-P_5 (IPP), and ATP content of erythrocytes from chick embryos and young chicks. (From Isaacks, R. E., et al.: Comp. Biochem. Physiol. 53A:151, 1976.)

of inositol hexaphosphate.[108] Like humans and rats (see Chapter 5), birds whose red cells have relatively high oxygen affinity display improved cardiovascular and behavioral responses when challenged with hypoxia.[109]

Mammals

In general, mammals are subjected to far less variability in environmental conditions than other vertebrates: they maintain body temperature, as well as blood pH, PCO_2, and osmolarity, within narrowly defined limits and, with few exceptions, inhale a generous supply of oxygen. Nevertheless, there are interesting and meaningful differences in the functional behavior of hemoglobins among mammals. In nearly all cases, these differences have a sound stereochemical explanation. However, their adaptive significance is often less well understood.

Unlike red cells of all other vertebrates, mammalian red cells lack nuclei. This feature enables the cell to be considerably more pliable, so that it can effectively traverse narrow-bore capillaries. The size, shape (Fig. 6–11), and life span of mammalian red cells vary widely among different species. Nevertheless, these cells have a number of common properties. As explained in Chapter 5, they have a much simpler metabolism than nucleated red cells. Moreover, they appear to be more efficient oxygen-carrying units. They tend to have a higher intracellular concentration of hemoglobin, which remains fully functional throughout its life span, free of significant methemoglobin formation. Virtually all mammalian hemoglobins have a substantial Bohr effect.[110] The residues that contribute to the alkaline Bohr effect in human hemoglobin (see Chapter 3) are highly conserved in other mammals. There is a small degree of variability in the Bohr effect among mammals, owing in part to differential proton binding that accompanies their interaction with organic phosphates and in part to other intrinsic differences among hemoglobins.[110, 111]

Regulation of Hemoglobin Function by 2,3-DPG. As discussed in Chapters 2, 3, and 5, the molecular interaction of 2,3-DPG with human hemoglobin has been thoroughly worked out. The negatively charged groups of 2,3-DPG form electrostatic bonds with specific positively charged residues on the β chains of deoxyhemoblobin A: N-terminal Val, NA2 His, EF6 Lys, and H21 His.[112] A comparison of the primary structure of the β globin chains of more than 50 mammals shows that these residues are highly conserved.[113, 114]

The most abundant organic phosphate in the red cells of most mammals is 2,3-DPG. Its concentration ranges from 4 to 13 mmoles/liter of packed red cells.[115–118] In contrast, this compound is present in only micromolar amounts in other tissues. The control of 2,3-DPG concentration in mammalian red cells is still poorly understood. As discussed in Chapter 5, one enzyme molecule is responsible for both synthesis and hydrolysis of 2,3-DPG. The level of this enzyme is high in red cells of most mammals.[116] A complex array of cofactors govern the relative activities of this bifunctional enzyme. The emergence of 2,3-DPG as the dominant organic phosphate in mammalian red cells may be related to the fact that these anucleated cells are deprived of oxidative metabolism and, therefore, produce limited amounts of ATP (about 1 mM).[119] In contrast, the levels of ATP in the nucleated red cells from other vertebrates tend to be considerably higher. As mentioned previously, the hemoglobins from all these animals show little specificity in their reactivity toward organic phosphates. For example, mammalian hemoglobins are markedly affected by inositol polyphosphates, compounds absent in mammalian red cells.

In order to determine the extent to which 2,3-DPG affects the functional behavior of mammalian red cells, it is necessary to measure the compound in as wide a variety of species as possible and to determine its effect on the animal's hemoglobin. Figure 6–23 presents initial observations made by Bunn[120] on domestic mammals. The animals could be divided into two distinct groups. The ruminants (sheep, goat, cow) and the cat had very low levels of red cell 2,3-DPG and hemoglobins that had intrinsically low oxygen affinity and were un-

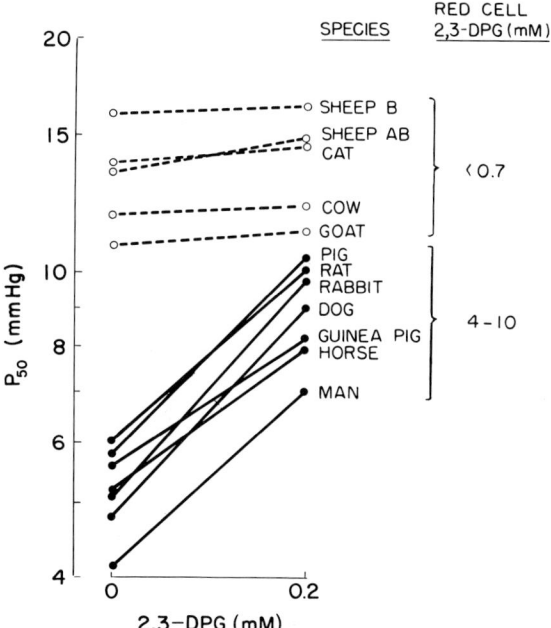

Figure 6–23. The effect of 2,3-DPG on the oxygen affinity of hemoglobins from domestic mammals. P_{50} is the partial pressure of oxygen at which hemoglobin was half-saturated. Oxygen equilibria were done in 0.05 mM hemoglobin (tetramer) in 0.1 M NaCl, 0.05 M bis-TRIS, pH 7.2, 20°C. The concentration range of red cell 2,3-DPG (mmoles/liter of red cells) for the two groups of animals is shown on the right. (From Bunn, H. F.: Science 172:1049, 1971.)

responsive to the addition of 2,3-DPG. In contrast, the other six animals tested had much higher amounts of red cell 2,3-DPG and hemoglobins of higher oxygen affinity that was markedly lowered by the addition of 2,3-DPG.

Subsequent measurements were made on a diverse group of 71 mammalian species, representing 14 orders.[118] Two other orders have also been examined.* All of these mammals had high levels of red cell 2,3-DPG and responsive hemoglobin, except for two groups, corresponding to earlier observations in domestic mammals.[120] In nine species of *Feloidea*, including the cats, civets, and hyenas, results were very similar to those in the common domestic cat. Figure 6–24 shows the phylogenetic relationship among the carnivores and other mammals. The divergence of carnivores that have abundant 2,3-DPG and those that lack this mediator occurred in the early Eocene, about 50 million years ago. Among the artiodactyls, the *Bovidae* and *Cervidae* have even lower levels of red cell 2,3-DPG than the *Feloidea* and also have low-affinity hemoglobins unresponsive to this compound. The pronghorn antelope[124] and the giraffe[125] also have low levels of 2,3-DPG. The dichotomy in this order occurred in the late Paleocene, about 60 million years ago (Fig. 6–24).

These observations suggest that animals can get along without an intracellular modifier but only if their hemoglobins have low enough oxygen affinity to function physiologically for optimal oxygen unloading. Conversely, animals having high levels of 2,3-DPG need this cofactor to lower the oxygen affinity of their red cells to a point at which they can achieve optimal oxygen unloading.

The loss of 2,3-DPG regulation in these two groups of mammals is an interesting example of convergent evolution. The inability of these mammals to synthesize abundant red cell 2,3-DPG can be attributed to a marked decrease in diphosphoglycerate mutase.[116] The molecular basis for the acquisition of intrinsically low oxygen affinity is not known. X-ray analysis of these hemoglobins will be necessary to ascertain which amino acid substitutions are responsible for the presumed increased stability of the deoxy quaternary structure. Perutz[54, 126] has observed that the mammalian hemoglobins with intrinsically low oxygen affinity have hydrophobic residues at position β NA2, whereas mammals with high-affinity hemoglobin have

---

*Asian and African elephants, representing Proboscidea,[121] and the manatee, representing Sirenia.[122, 123]

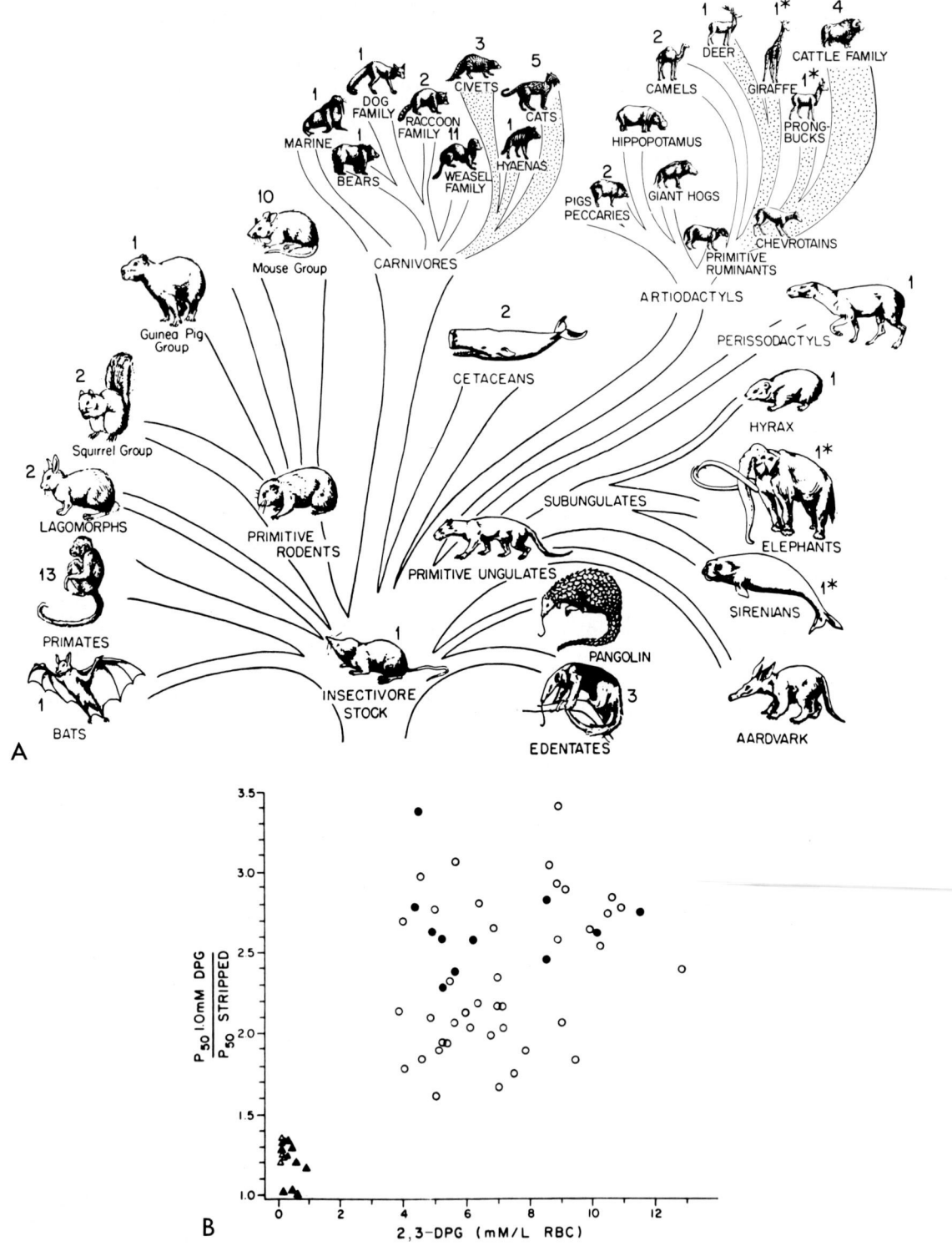

Figure 6–24. *A*, Simplified phylogenetic tree of mammals. The numbers indicate how many species in each mammalian order were studied by Scott and associates.[117] The number with asterisks (*) indicate animals studied by others. The stippled areas represent the development of animals having low red cell 2,3-DPG and low-affinity nonresponsive hemoglobins. Prepared from diagrams of A. S. Romer. (From Bunn. H. F.: Blood 58:189, 1981.) *B*, Relationship between red cell 2,3-DPG and the response of the stripped hemolysates to the addition of 1 mM 2,3-DPG. Conditions are the same as those in Figure 6–21. (Feloidea (▲), ruminants (△), primates (●), and other mammals (○). (From Scott, A. F., et al.: J. Exp. Zool. *201*:269, 1977.)

Table 6–3. CHANGES IN PRIMARY STRUCTURE OF THE β CHAIN AT THE 2,3-DPG BINDING SITE

Hemoglobin	Reactivity with 2,3-DPG	NA1	NA2	NA3	EF6	H21
Human A	+++	H_3N^+—	Val—	His—Leu	... Lys	... His ...
Human F	+	H_3N^-—	Gly—	His—Leu	... Lys	... Ser ...
Lemur	+	H_3N^+—	Thr—	*Leu*—Leu	... Lys	... His ...
Horse	+++	H_3N^+—	Val—	Gln—Leu	... Lys	... His ...
Llama	+	H_3N^+—	Val—	*Asn*—Leu	... Lys	... His ...
Ruminants	0		H_3N^+—	*Met*—Leu	... Lys	... His ...
Cat A	+	H_3N^+—	Gly—	*Phe*—Leu	... Lys	... His ...
Cat B	0	*Acetyl*-N—	Ser—	*Phe*—Leu	... Lys	... His ...

a hydrophilic residue at β NA2 (Table 6–3). He has proposed that the hydrophobic residues at this position are directed into the interior of the molecule in such a way that the deoxy conformation is stabilized, leading to lowered O_2 affinity.

The molecular mechanisms responsible for loss of response to 2,3-DPG are reasonably well understood and differ in the two groups. The red cells of the cat family contain two hemoglobins, A and B. These hemoglobins differ only in their β chains, which are encoded by nonallelic genes. The total failure of cat Hb B to respond to 2,3-DPG[120, 127, 128] can be explained by its lacking two positively charged residues that in other mammals are responsible for the binding of 2,3-DPG. The N-terminal serine residue is blocked by an acetyl group, and the second residue is phenylalanine rather than histidine (Table 6–3). The partial response of cat Hb A to 2,3-DPG is probably due to the free N-terminal glycine balanced against the absence of hisitidine at NA2. The failure of ruminant hemoglobins to respond to 2,3-DPG can be explained by an entirely different mechanism. The β chains of these hemoglobins contain only 145 residues rather than 146. A single residue has been deleted at the N-terminal segment of the β chain.* As a result, it is likely that in the native deoxygenated hemoglobin, the N termini are too far apart (about 22 Å) to bind the 2,3-DPG molecule.[131]

The lemur, a primitive primate, has red cell function midway between that of the two groups of mammals just described. The concentration of 2,3-DPG in lemur red cells is considerably lower than that of other primates but higher than that of the cats and ruminants.[132] The low oxygen affinity of lemur red cells can be attributed to the functional behavior of the hemoglobin per se. Its intrinsically low O_2 affinity and its impaired interaction with 2,3-DPG may both be explained by the presence of leucine rather than histidine at β NA2. This hydrophobic residue may stabilize the deoxyhemoglobin (see previous discussion) and would reduce the binding of 2,3-DPG.

It is difficult to assign a temporal order to the changes in red cell metabolism and hemoglobin function noted in the ruminants and *Feloidea*. The development of intrinsically low O_2 affinity may have occurred first, a "pre-adaptation" allowing the loss of 2,3-DPG modulation.[133] Despite evidence to the contrary,[134] the binding of 2,3-DPG to hemoglobin may affect its rate of synthesis.[135] If so, the impaired reactivity of these hemoglobins to 2,3-DPG owing to structural mutations probably preceded the marked reduction in 2,3-DPG synthesis.

Does the phenomenon we have observed in ruminants and *Feloidea* have any adaptive significance? These two groups of animals tend to be sprinters, dependent on sudden bursts of energy. During such spurts of exercise, the body temperature increases and pH falls as an oxygen debt develops. Both of these factors lower oxygen affinity and, therefore, facilitate oxygen unloading.[136] It is unclear what adaptational advantage was gained by the loss of 2,3-DPG regulation. These animals are likely to be more restricted physiologically than the larger group of mammals whose hemoglobin function can be regulated over a much wider range in response to alterations in body size, metabolic rate, and oxygen availability.[133]

Knowledge of the intrinsic oxygen affinity of an animal's hemoglobin and its response to 2,3-DPG and of the level of red cell 2,3-DPG permits a reasonably good prediction of the animal's whole blood oxygen affinity.[118] Direct measurements have revealed striking variability among different species (Fig. 6–25). It is unclear whether there is adaptive significance in these wide differences in oxygen affinity.

---

*A human hemoglobin variant (Hb Leiden) with a deletion of one amino acid near the N terminus of the β chain also has impaired reactivity with 2,3-DPG.[129, 130]

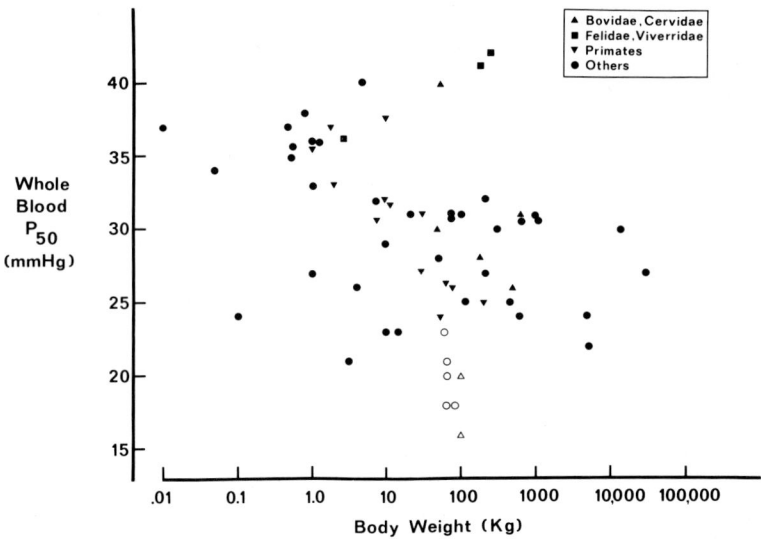

Figure 6–25. The relationship between a mammal's body weight and whole blood P_{50} (pH 7.4, 37°C). Open symbols represent animals adapted to high altitude. (From Bunn, H. F., et al.: Ann. N.Y. Acad. Sci. *241*:498, 1974.)

Despite the fact that these data points are considerably scattered, P_{50} appears to vary inversely with body weight.[137] It may be that smaller animals, with their relatively active metabolism, would benefit from enhanced oxygen unloading.

Adaptation to Hypoxia. As shown in Figure 6–25, animals adapted to high altitude tend to have increased whole blood oxygen affinity (reduced P_{50}). Furthermore, diving mammals[138] and some burrowing mammals[139] also have slightly higher oxygen affinity compared with other mammals of comparable body weight. This alteration is likely to be beneficial to the hypoxic animal, enabling it to have enhanced oxygenation of arterial blood. As discussed in Chapter 5, there is experimental support for the adaptive value of increased oxygen affinity in hypoxic hypoxia.

The whole blood oxygen affinities of high-altitude Camelidae (vicuña, alpaca, llama, and guanaco) appear to be significantly higher than those of their lowland relatives,[140] although conflicting data have been reported.[141, 142] Increased oxygen affinity may be due in part to reduced levels of red cell 2,3-DPG in these animals at high altitude.[116] In addition, the hemoglobins of the llama[117] and the guanaco[143] have lower reactivity toward 2,3-DPG compared with hemoglobins of other mammals. These results can be explained by the presence of asparagine at position β NA2 instead of histidine, one of the residues normally responsible for the binding of 2,3-DPG (Table 6–3). Horse hemoglobin has glutamine at this position and yet has normal reactivity with 2,3-DPG.[144] From molecular model fitting, Perutz[54] has concluded that the amide group of the horse β NA2 glutamine can form a hydrogen bond with a phosphate of 2,3-DPG, whereas this interaction is not possible with NA2 asparagine of the llama β chain.

Increased whole blood oxygen affinity has also been observed in deer mice that have adapted to high altitude. This is primarily due to decreased red cell 2,3-DPG.[145, 146] The disparate levels of 2,3-DPG in highland and lowland deer mice appear to be genetically determined. Genetic modulation of red cell 2,3-DPG has also been demonstrated in a strain of rats.[147]

The mole *Talpa europea* adapts to a hypoxic subterranean environment by having increased whole blood oxygen affinity.[139] As with the llama, the mole has hemoglobin with impaired reactivity to 2,3-DPG.

When humans are subjected to various types of hypoxia, oxygen affinity usually decreases because of an increase in red cell 2,3-DPG (see Chapter 5). This effect may be partly or completely offset by accompanying alkalosis, which increases oxygen affinity. A similar increase in red cell 2,3-DPG has also been noted in rats,[134, 148] guinea pigs,[148] and mice[145, 146] following hypoxic stress. For high-altitude exposure, this change may be maladaptive for reasons stated previously and in Chapter 5. In contrast, individuals with anemia derive significant benefit from a decrease in oxygen affinity because they have nearly normal arterial oxygen saturation and therefore gain significant improvement in oxygen unloading.

Some animals undergo a change in hemoglobin phenotype when they become anemic. Anemic cats have increased synthesis of Hb B, which has a higher oxygen affinity than Hb A.[149] This is offset by an increase in red cell ATP and 2,3-DPG, so that the anemic cat has a somewhat lower red cell oxygen affinity than normal. A comparable phenomenon is observed in sheep. When sheep with Hb A become anemic, they produce Hb C,[150, 151] which has a somewhat higher oxygen affinity than Hb A.[118, 152] Anemia also induces a significant increase in red cell 2,3-DPG in sheep.[153] As mentioned previously, sheep (and cat) hemoglobins are unresponsive to 2,3-DPG. Nevertheless, the rise in red cell organic phosphates induced by anemia reduces oxygen affinity by lowering intracellular pH (see Chapter 5). The red cell oxygen affinity is unchanged when sheep with Hb A become anemic[154] because the effect of Hb C is offset by the decrease in intracellular pH. In contrast, sheep with Hb B do not undergo an alteration in hemoglobin when they become anemic. The low oxygen affinity of sheep with Hb B is reduced even further during anemia[154] by the increase in red cell 2,3-DPG. It is noteworthy that sheep with Hb B tolerate anemia better than those with the higher-affinity hemoglobins, A and C.[155]

A decrease in red cell 2,3-DPG and a corresponding increase in oxygen affinity have been observed in a variety of hibernating mammals: hedgehog,[156] ground squirrel,[157, 158] woodchuck,[159] and hamster.[160] It is uncertain whether this change has any adaptive value. The decrease in body temperature that accompanies hibernation would contribute much more than the reduction in 2,3-DPG in raising oxygen affinity.

Maternal-Fetal Oxygen Transport. The maintenance of adequate oxygen transport across the placenta is crucial to the development of the fetus of mammals as well as of other vertebrates discussed earlier in this chapter. Several independent factors determine transplacental oxygen flux,[161] including placental blood flow, the diffusion of oxygen across the placenta, the oxygen-carrying capacity of maternal and fetal blood, and their relative affinities for oxygen. Significantly higher oxygen affinity of fetal blood is found almost universally among mammals. The only exception that has been noted to date is the domestic cat.[162] This observation suggests that the higher oxygen affinity of fetal blood has adaptive significance, permitting enhanced transport of oxygen across the placenta. This claim is supported by observations in pregnant rats.[163, 164]

In most species that have been examined, red cells in the early embryo contain structurally distinct hemoglobins. Embryonic hemoglobins of man (see Chapter 4), mouse,[165] and rabbit[166] have higher oxygen affinities compared with adult hemoglobins. In some animals, such as primates and ruminants, embryonic hemoglobins are succeeded by distinct fetal hemoglobins, which become the primary constituent of red cells during middle and late fetal development.

There are three distinct mechanisms by which fetal red cells have higher oxygen affinity than maternal red cells (Table 6–4).[144, 167, 168] Ruminants have fetal hemoglobin that has significantly higher oxygen affinity than that of the corresponding adult hemoglobin. These fetal hemoglobins resemble their adult counterparts in their unresponsiveness to 2,3-DPG. Furthermore, like adult red cells, fetal red cells of ruminants contain only small amounts of 2,3-DPG. Following birth, there is a switch to production of adult hemoglobin. During this transition, the red cells of the newborn sheep and goats temporarily acquire significant amounts of red cell 2,3-DPG,[169] which cause a lowering of oxygen affinity by virtue of reduction of intracellular pH. This phenomenon gives the newborn animals a prompt decrease in oxygen affinity that tides them over until they have acquired adult hemoglobin. In addition, sheep with Hb A produce Hb C during the newborn period.[170] This may reflect a response to hypoxic stress, as discussed earlier.

Primates solve the problem of differential maternal-fetal oxygen affinity in a different way. In the absence of organic phosphate, their fetal hemoglobin has about the same oxygen affinity as that of the adult hemoglobin. However, the adult hemoglobin is much more sensitive to 2,3-DPG,[171–173] so that fetal red cells that contain Hb F and normal levels of 2,3-

Table 6–4. INCREASED O_2 AFFINITY OF FETAL RED CELLS

Structurally Distinct Fetal Hemoglobin	Mechanism	Examples
Yes	Fetal Hb has ↑ O_2 affinity	Ruminants
Yes	Fetal Hb has ↓ reactivity with 2,3-DPG	Primates
No	Decreased fetal RBC 2,3-DPG	Dog, horse, pig, rabbit, guinea pig, mouse, rat, opossum, seal

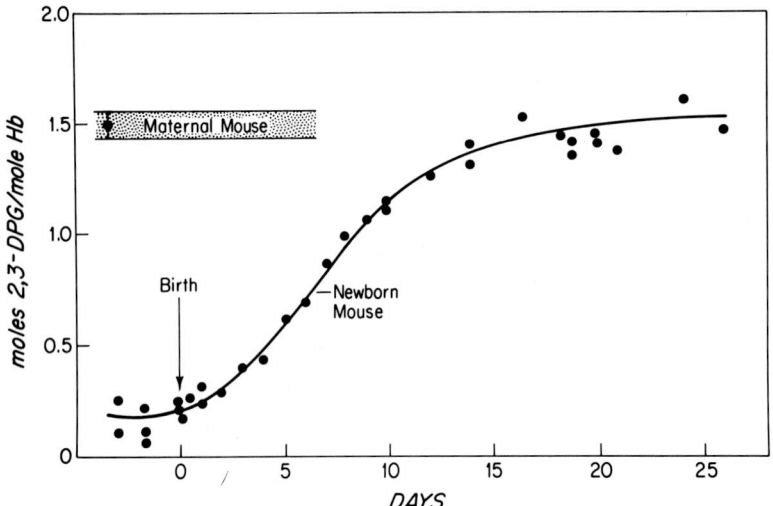

Figure 6–26. Change in the level of red cell 2,3-DPG in a mouse before and after birth. (Drawn from data of Petschow, R., et al.: Respir. Physiol. *35*:271, 1978.)

DPG have significantly higher oxygen affinity than adult red cells containing Hb A. The molecular basis for this difference in response to 2,3-DPG is shown in Table 6–3. Human Hb F has serine instead of histidine at H21, one of the sites at which 2,3-DPG binds.

Most mammals lack a structurally distinct fetal hemoglobin and achieve higher oxygen affinity in fetal red cells by a reduced concentration of 2,3-DPG. Examples include the pig,[174–177] guinea pig,[168] dog,[168] horse,[144] rabbit,[178] opossum,[179] mouse,[180] rat,[181] and seal.[182] Immediately after birth, red cell 2,3-DPG begins to rise, giving the newborn animal a normal or even decreased oxygen affinity. Data on newborn mice are shown in Figure 6–26.[180] During the first 15 days following birth, the 2,3-DPG in newborn red cells rises to a level comparable to that of maternal 2,3-DPG. The low levels of 2,3-DPG in red cells of rabbit, guinea pig, and dog fetuses can be attributed to enhanced activity of pyruvate kinase.[183, 184] In rabbits, this is due to a fetal isoenzyme.[185] In rodents of the subclass Myomorpha, DPG synthase is reduced in fetal cells and therefore also contributes to this low level of 2,3-DPG.[181, 186] This phenomenon is another example of how intracellular hemoglobin function can be modulated by alterations in glycolytic enzymes.

Molecular Evolution*

There is rapidly growing information about the primary structure of globin subunits from a large variety of animals. These data have permitted an increasingly clear understanding of the molecular evolution of hemoglobin. At present, primary sequences have been determined on 126 hemoglobin subunits from 66 animals.[113] This information has been used to deduce probable sequences of ancestor subunits that provide independent determinations of phylogenetic lineages. The approach most commonly used is the calculation of maximum parsimony,[187] i.e., the smallest number of base changes in the corresponding DNA of ancestor sequences to allow for the observed contemporary sequences.

Figure 6–27 shows the application of such an analysis on globin sequences from a variety of animals.[188] This phylogenetic tree displays a number of interesting features. First, the relationships shown here bear striking resemblance to those derived from classic morphological and paleontological data. Indeed, from analyses of sequences of globins, myoglobin, cytochrome c, fibrinopeptides and lens crystallins, Goodman[187] has constructed a phylogenetic tree whose branch points agree remarkably well with those obtained from classic fossil evidence. Most of these lineages are orthologous, i.e., they split at the time of speciation. In contrast, some lineages are paralogous; they arose by gene duplication prior to speciation. The lineages shown in Figure 6–27 permit accurate estimates of when globin genes duplicated. For example, the β globin gene was duplicated from a mammalian ancestor about 220 million years ago (MyBP or millions of years before the present), enabling the emergence of embryonic-fetal genes. About 150 MyBP, another duplication took place, giving rise to the precursors of the human embryonic (ε) and fetal (γ) globin genes. Note that the human γ chains are much more similar to the

---

*Dickerson and Geis[113] have recently presented a comprehensive and thoughtful review of this topic.

macaque γ chain than they are to the human β chain, an example of paralogous radiation. Another instance is the β chains of the frog and tadpole which diverged over 400 MyBP and therefore, as mentioned previously, are each as similar to the human β chain as they are to each other. A third example is the very early duplication of the α-chain gene (350 MyBP), giving rise to the human ζ and chicken π chains. These embryonic chains resemble each other more closely than they resemble the adult α chains of the same species. As a final example, protein sequence data have led to the conclusion that vertebrate myoglobins arose entirely independently from invertebrate myoglobin and 200 MyBP later.[188, 188a]

These analyses of primary sequence provide powerful independent information not only on phylogenetic branch points but also on rates of molecular evolution. This information may help to settle a vigorous debate that has been raging in recent years between neutralists and selectionists (Darwinians). The former group, represented by Kimura[189] and Jukes,[190] claim that the vast bulk of structural changes in proteins are the result of random fixation (genetic drift) and are therefore adaptively neutral. Accordingly, the rate of these changes has been relatively constant and can be utilized as a "molecular clock." In contrast, Goodman[187, 191] and other proponents of Darwinian molecular evolution have concluded that in order for a structural alteration to become fixed, it is likely to have a selective advantage. They have presented evidence that the rate of these structural alterations is far from uniform. This argues against random fixation. For example, the rate at which the globin genes evolved was relatively rapid about 425 MyBP ago, when gene duplication permitted the formation of a cooperative heterotetramer ($\alpha_2\beta_2$). Indeed, residues at subunit interfaces, which are responsible for cooperativity, evolved four times more rapidly than exterior residues, which are less important to hemoglobin function. The rapid evolution of the globin

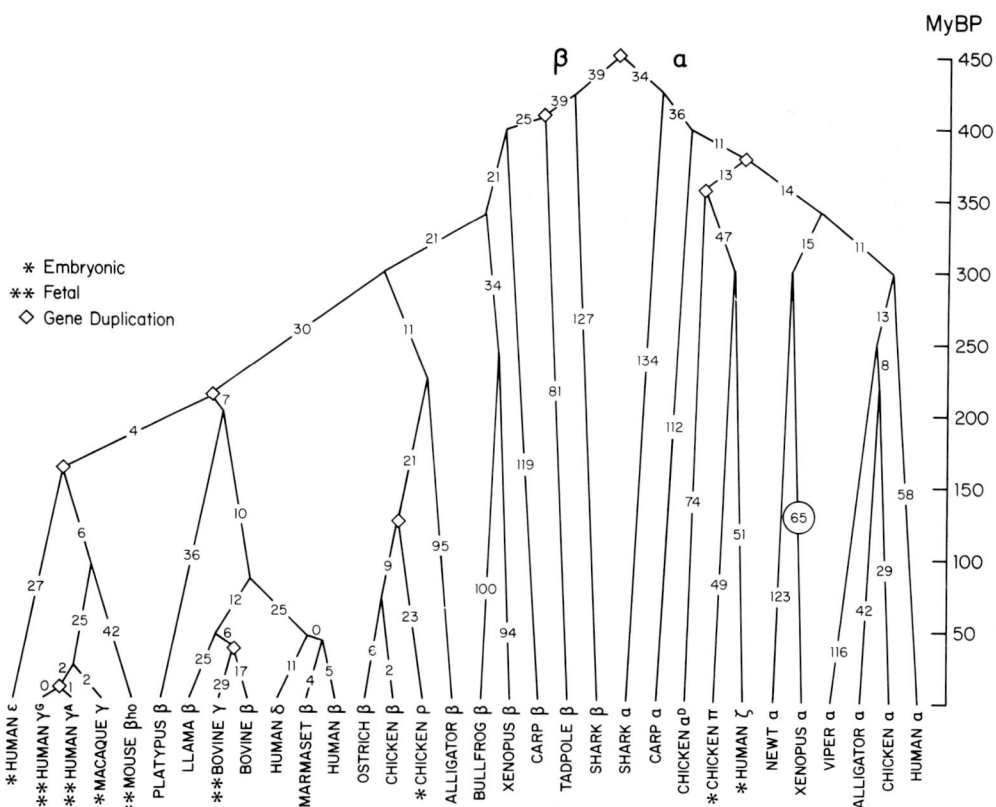

Figure 6–27. Phylogenetic tree of the hemoglobin family determined by Goodman and associates utilizing analyses by augmented parsimony. The vertical axis is millions of years before present (MyBP), as deduced from the paleontological record and not from the sequences themselves. The numbers along the lines of descent indicate augmented nucleotide replacements, taking into account invisible events such as superimposed mutations at the same locus, silent mutations involving degeneracy of the genetic code, and back mutations to the original amino acid. The diamonds represent postulated gene duplications (From Goodman, M., et al.: *Systematic Zoology* 31:376, 1982.)

to functional domains. For example, protein coded by the central exon can bind heme.[192] The exon may have been duplicated many times, providing a binding site for a variety of heme proteins.[193–195] The C-terminal exon may be critical for the assembly of subunits.[196] More recently, about 85 MyBP, there appears to have been another spurt in the rate of sequence change of globin chains, during the evolution of primates from their eutherian ancestors. The molecular rationale for this recent acceleration of molecular evolution is not clear because there are no clear-cut differences in the properties of primate hemoglobins compared with those of other mammals.

The relative importance of adaptive versus neutral fixations in hemoglobin structure is difficult to resolve. There is little doubt that certain residues in α and β chains are crucial to proper physiologic function and hence "invariant" throughout molecular evolution. It is fair to conclude that the evolution of these key structural sites was highly adaptive. Moreover, Perutz[54] has shown that hemoglobin can acquire new functions of adaptive significance, such as the Root effect in fish or the HCO_3^- binding site in crocodilians, by means of mutations at a few (three to four) sites. Conversely, a large number of fixations of globin structure have no apparent adaptive importance. However, the fact that these sites are not involved in heme or subunit interactions or binding to allosteric effectors by no means proves that they are adaptively neutral. There are a number of other constraints on the molecular engineering of the hemoglobin molecule besides its oxygen binding properties. In the red cells of many animals, hemoglobin is crowded into a very confined space: its concentration falls just short of its maximum solubility. Therefore, structural alterations at the surface could have a significant effect on solubility.[110, 197] Mutations such as sickle hemoglobin (β 6 Glu → Val) are clearly deleterious, leading to decreased solubility. Other surface alterations could enhance solubility and therefore could be of selective advantage. Additional constraints that may have bearing on the evolution of globin chains include the role of surface charge on subunit assembly (see Chapter 10) and on intracellular pH by way of the Gibbs-Donnan equilibrium (see Chapter 5). Relative susceptibility to proteolysis may be yet another factor influencing the fixation of globin chain mutations. Finally, there are a number of constraints at the level of base sequences such as secondary structure and stability of DNA and RNA. The rate of fixation of mutations of globin genes appears to depend on the interplay of a complex array of independent factors. The next chapter will provide further insights into globin gene evolution at the level of DNA structure.

References

1. Klippenstein, G. L.: Structural aspects of hemerythrin and myohemerythrin. Am. Zool. *20*:39, 1980.
2. Bonaventura, J., and Bonaventura, C.: Hemocyanins: Relationships in their structure, function and assembly. Am. Zool. *20*:7, 1980.
3. Bonaventura, J., Bonaventura, C., and Sullivan, B.: Hemoglobins and hemocyanins: Comparative aspects of structure and function. J. Exp. Zool. *194*:155, 1975.
4. Van Holde, K. E., and Miller, K. I.: Hemocyanins. Q. Rev. Biophys. *15*:1, 1982.
5. Mangum, C. P.: Respiratory function of the hemocyanins. Am. Zool. *20*:19, 1980.
6. van Bruggen, E. F. J.: Hemocyanin: The mystery of blue blood. Trends Biochem. Sci. *7*:185, 1980.
7. Terwilliger, R. C.: Structures of invertebrate hemoglobins. Am. Zool. *20*:53, 1980.
8. Garlick, R. L.: Structure of annelid high molecular weight hemoglobins (erythrocruorins). Am. Zool. *20*:69, 1980.
9. Weber, R. E.: Functions of invertebrate hemoglobins with special reference to adaptations to environmental hypoxia. Am. Zool. *20*:79, 1980.
10. Antonini, E., and Chiancone, E.: Assembly of multisubunit respiratory proteins. Ann. Rev. Biophys. Bioeng. *6*:239, 1977.
11. Davis, R. H., and Steers, E.: Myoglobin from the ciliate protozoan *Paramecium aurelia*. Comp. Biochem. Physiol. *54B*:141, 1976.
12. Klippenstein, G. L., Cote, J. L., and Ludlam, S. E.: The primary structure of myohemerythrin. Biochemistry *15*:1128, 1976.
13. Ward, K. B., Hendrickson, W. A., and Klippenstein, G. L.: Quaternary and tertiary structure of haemerythrin. Nature *257*:818, 1975.
14. Stenkamp, R. E., Sieker, L. C., Jensen, L. H., and McQueen, J. E., Jr.: Structure of methemerythrin at 2.8 Å resolution: Computer graphics fit of an averaged electron density map. Biochemistry *17*:2499, 1978.
15. Klotz, I. M., Klippenstein, G. L., and Hendrickson, W. A.: Hemerythrin: Alternative oxygen carrier. Science *192*:335, 1976.
15a. Klotz, I.M., and Kurtz, D. M.: Binuclear oxygen carriers: Hemerythrin. Accounts of Chemical Research *17*:16, 1984.
16. Mellema, J. E., and Klug, A.: Quaternary structure of gastropod hemocyanin. Nature *239*:146, 1972.
17. Brouwer, M., Ryan, M., Bonaventura, J., and Bonaventura, C.: Functional and structural properties of *Murex fulvescens* hemocyanin: Isolation of two different subunits required for reassociation of a molluscan hemocyanin. Biochemistry *17*:2810, 1978.
17a. Yokota, E., and Riggs, A. F.: The structure of the hemocyanin from the horseshoe crab *Limulus polyphemus:* The amino acid sequence of the largest cyanogen bromide fragment. J. Biol. Chem. *259*:4739, 1984.
18. Bonaventura, C., Sullivan, B., Bonaventura, J., and Bourne, S.: CO binding by hemocyanins of *Limulus polyphemus, Busycon carica* and *Callinectes sapidus*. Biochemistry *13*:4784, 1974.
19. Mangum, C. P., and Lykkeboe, G.: The influence

of inorganic ions and pH on oxygenation properties of the blood in the gastropod mollusc *Busycon canaliculatum*. J. Exp. Zool. *207*:417, 1979.
20. Lankester, E. R.: A contribution to the knowledge of haemoglobin. Proc. R. Soc. Lond. B *21*:70, 1872.
20a. Grinich, N. P., and Terwilliger, R. C.: The quaternary structure of an unusual high-molecular weight intracellular haemoglobin from the bivalve mollusc *Barbatia reeveona*. Biochem. J. *189*:1, 1980.
21. Keilin, D., and Hartree, E. F.: Relationship between haemoglobin and erythrocruorin. Nature *168*:266, 1951.
22. Svedberg, T.: Sedimentation constants, molecular weights and isoelectric points of the respiratory proteins. J. Biol. Chem. *103*:311, 1933.
23. Garlick, R. L., and Riggs, A. F.: The amino acid sequence of a major polypeptide chain of earthworm hemoglobin. J. Biol. Chem. *257*:9005, 1982.
24. Imamura, T., Baldwin, T. O., and Riggs, A.: The amino acid sequence of the monomeric hemoglobin component from the blood worm, *Glycera dibranchiata*. J. Biol. Chem. *247*:2785, 1972.
25. Aschauer, H., and Braunitzer, G.: Aminosaeuresequenz eines dimeren hamoglobins (Erythrocruorin) von *Chironomus thummi thummi*: Komponente CTT VIII. Hoppe-Seyler's Z. Physiol. Chem. *362*:409, 1981.
26. Padlan, E. A., and Love, W. E.: Three-dimensional structure of hemoglobin from the polychaete annelid, *Glycera dibranchiata* at 2.5 Å resolution. J. Biol. Chem. *249*:4067, 1974.
27. Huber, R., Epp, O., and Formanek, H.: Structure of deoxy- and carbonmonoxyerythrocruorin. J. Mol. Biol. *52*:349, 1970.
28. Tuchschmid, P. E., Kunz, P. A., and Wilson, K. J.: Isolation and characterization of the hemoglobin from the lanceolate fluke *Dicrocoelium dendriticum*. Eur. J. Biochem. *88*:387, 1978.
29. Okazaki, T., and Wittenberg, J. B.: The hemoglobin of *Ascaris* perienteric fluid. III. Equilibria with oxygen and carbon monoxide. Biochim. Biophys. Acta *111*:503, 1965.
30. Harrington, J. P., Pandolfelli, E., and Herskovits, T.: Solution studies on heme proteins: Circular dichroism and optical rotation of *Lumbricus terrestris* and *Glycera dibranchiata* hemoglobin. Biochim. Biophys. Acta *328*:61, 1973.
31. Vinogradov, S. N., Kapp, O. H., and Ohtsuki, M.: The extracellular hemoglobins and chlorocruorins of annelids. In Harris, J. R. (ed.): Electron Microscopy of Proteins. Vol. 3. New York, Academic Press, pp. 135–164, 1981.
32. Weber, R. E.: Cationic control of O_2 affinity in lugworm erythrocruorin. Nature *292*:386, 1981.
33. Collett, L. C., and O'Gower, A. K.: Molluscan hemoglobins with unusual temperature-dependent characteristics. Comp. Biochem. Physiol. *41A*:843, 1972.
34. Terwilliger, N. B., Terwilliger, R. C., and Schabtach, E.: The quaternary structure of a molluscan (*Helisoma trivolvis*) extracellular hemoglobin. Biochim. Biophys. Acta *453*:101, 1976.
35. Fox, H. M., and Phear, E. A.: Factors influencing haemoglobin synthesis in *Daphnia*. Proc. R. Soc. Lond. B *141*:179, 1953.
36. Bonaventura, C., Bonaventura, J., Kitto, B., Brunori, M., and Antonini, E.: Functional consequences of ligand linked dissociation in hemoglobin from the sea cucumber *Malpodia arenicola*. Biochim. Biophys. Acta *428*:779, 1976.
36a. Terwilliger, R. C.: Oxygen equilibrium and subunit aggregation of a holothurian hemoglobin. Biochim. Biophys. Acta *386*:62, 1975.
37. Fischer, H., and vonSeemann, C.: Die Konstitution des Spirographishämins. Hoppe-Seyler's Z. Physiol. Chem. *242*:133, 1936.
38. Fox, H. M.: Chlorocruorin. In Barcroft Symposium on Respiratory Proteins. New York, Interscience, 1948, p. 291.
39. Manwell, C.: Chemistry, genetics and function of invertebrate respiratory pigments—configurational changes and allosteric effects. In Dickens, F., and Neil, E. (eds.): Oxygen in the Animal Organism. I.U.B. Symposium series, No. 31, 1964, pp. 49–119.
40. Svedberg, T., and Pederson, K. O.: The Ultracentrifuge. New York, Oxford University Press, 1940.
41. Wald, G., and Riggs, A.: The hemoglobin of the sea lamprey *Petromyzon marinus*. J. Gen. Physiol. *35*:45, 1951.
42. Briehl, R. W.: The relation between the oxygen equilibrium and aggregation of subunits in lamprey hemoglobin. J. Biol. Chem. *238*:2361, 1963.
43. Love, W. E., Klock, P. A., Lattman, E. E., Padlan, E. A., Ward, K. B., and Hendrickson, W. A.: The structures of lamprey and bloodworm hemoglobins in relation to their evolution and function. Symp. Quant. Biol. *36*:349, 1971.
44. Li, S. L., and Riggs, A.: The amino acid sequence of hemoglobin V from the lamprey. J. Biol. Chem. *245*:6749, 1970.
44a. Hombrados, I., Rodewald, K., Neuzil, E., and Braunitzer, G.: Haemoglobins, LX. Primary Structure of the major haemoglobin of the sea lamprey *Petromyzon marinus* (var. Garonne, Loire). Biochemie *65*:247, 1983.
45. Bonaventura, J., Bonaventura, C., and Sullivan, B.: Urea tolerance as a molecular adaptation of elasmobranch hemoglobin. Science *186*:57, 1974.
46. Brunori, M., Giardina, B., Chiancone, E., Spagnuola, C., Binotti, I., and Antonini, E.: Studies on the properties of fish hemoglobins. Molecular properties and interaction with third components of the isolated hemoglobins from the trout (*Salmo irideus*). Eur. J. Biochem. *39*:563, 1973.
47. Mied, P. A., and Powers, D. A.: Hemoglobins of the killifish *Fundulus heteroclitus*. J. Biol. Chem. *253*:3521,1978.
48. Shimada, T., Okihama, Y., Okazaki, T., and Shukuya, R.: The multiple hemoglobins of the Japanese eel, *Anguilla japonica*. J. Biol. Chem. *255*:7912, 1980.
49. Brunori, M.: Molecular adaptation to physiological requirements: The hemoglobin system of trout. Curr. Top. Cell. Regul. *9*:1, 1975.
50. Herbert, K., Lau, F., Wallach, D. E., Pennelly, R. R., and Noble, R. W.: Ligand binding properties of hemoglobin 3 of the trout, *Salmo gairdneri*. J. Biol. Chem. *250*:1400, 1975.
51. Brunori, M., Falcioni, G., Fortuna, G., and Giardina, B.: Effect of anions on the oxygen binding properties of the hemoglobin components from trout (*Salmo irideus*). Arch. Biochem. Biophys. *168*:512, 1975.
52. Bossa, F., Barra, D., Coletta, M., Martini, F., Liverzani, A., Petruzzelli, R., Bonaventura, J., and Brunori, M.: Primary structure of hemoglobins from trout (*Salmo irideus*). Partial determination of amino acid sequence of Hb Trout IV. FEBS Lett *64*:76, 1976.
53. Bossa, F., Barra, D., Petruzzelli, R., Martini, F.,

and Brunori, M.: Primary structure of hemoglobin from trout (*Salmo irideus*). Amino acid sequence of α chain of Hb Trout I. Biochim. Biophys. Acta *536*:298, 1978.
54. Perutz, M. F.: Species adaptation in a protein molecule. Mol. Biol. Evol. *1*:1, 1983.
54a. Barra, D., Petruzelli, R., Bossa, A., and Brunori, M.: Primary structure of hemoglobin from trout (*Salmo irideus*)—amino acid sequence of the beta-chain of trout Hb-I. Biochem. Biophys. Acta *742*:72, 1983.
55. Gillen, R. G., and Riggs, A.: Structure and function of the hemoglobins of the carp, *Cyprinus carpio*. J. Biol. Chem. *247*:6039, 1972.
56. Tan, A. L., Noble, R. W., and Gibson, Q. H.: Conditions restricting allosteric transitions in carp hemoglobin. J. Biol. Chem. *248*:2880, 1973.
57. Mayo, K. H.: Carp hemoglobin. J. Mol. Biol. *146*:589, 1981.
58. Gillen, R. G., and Riggs, A.: The hemoglobins of a fresh-water teleost, *Cichlasoma cyanoguttatum* (Baird and Cirard)-I. The effects of phosphorylated organic compounds upon the oxygen equilibria. Comp. Biochem. Physiol. *38B*:585, 1971.
59. Geoghegan, W. D., and Poluhowich, J. J.: The major erythrocytic organic phosphates of the American eel, *Anguilla rostrata*. Comp. Biochem. Physiol. *49B*:281, 1974.
60. Bartlett, G. R.: Phosphate compounds in vertebrate red blood cells. Am. Zool. *20*:103, 1980.
61. Issacks, R. E., and Harkness, D. R.: Erythrocyte organic phosphates and hemoglobin function in birds, reptiles, and fishes. Am. Zool. *20*:115, 1980.
62. Kaloustian, K. V., and Poluhowich, J. J.: The role of organic phosphates in modulating the oxygenation behavior of eel hemoglobin. Comp. Biochem. Physiol. *53A*:245, 1976.
63. Torracca, A. M. V., Raschetti, R., Salvioli, R., Ricciardi, G., and Winterhalter, K. H.: Modulation of the Root effect in goldfish by ATP and GTP. Biochim. Biophys. Acta *496*:367, 1977.
64. Bunn, H. F., and Riggs, A.: The measurement of the Bohr effect of fish hemoglobins by gel electrofocusing. Comp. Biochem. Physiol. *62A*:95, 1979.
65. Brunori, M., Coletta, M., Giardina, B., and Wyman, J.: A macromolecular transducer as illustrated by trout hemoglobin IV. Proc. Natl. Acad. Sci. USA *75*:4310, 1978.
66. Noble, R. W., Pennelly, R. R., and Riggs, A.: Studies of the functional properties of the hemoglobin from the benthic fish, *Antimora rostrata*. Comp. Biochem. Physiol. *52B*:75, 1975.
67. Weber, R. E., Lykkeboe, G., and Johansen, K.: Biochemical aspects of the adaptation of hemoglobin-oxygen affinity of eels to hypoxia. Life Sci. *17*:1345, 1975.
68. Weber, R. E., and Lykkeboe, G.: Respiratory adaptations in carp blood: Influences of hypoxia, red cell organic phosphates, divalent cations and CO_2 on hemoglobin-oxygen affinity. J. Comp. Physiol. *128*:127, 1978.
69. Tetens, V., and Lykkeboe, G.: Blood respiratory properties of rainbow trout, *Salmo gairdneri*: Responses to hypoxia acclimation and anoxic incubation of blood *in vitro*. J. Comp. Physiol. *145*:117, 1981.
70. Greaney, G. S., and Powers, D. A.: Cellular regulation of an allosteric modifier of fish haemoglobin. Nature *270*:73, 1977.
71. Wood, S. C., Johansen, K., and Weber, R. E.: Effects of ambient PO_2 on hemoglobin-oxygen affinity and red cell ATP concentrations in a benthic fish, *Pleuronectes platessa*. Respir. Physiol. *25*:259, 1975.
72. Powers, D. A.: Structure, function, and molecular ecology of fish hemoglobins. Ann. N. Y. Acad. Sci. *241*:472, 1974.
73. Wood, S. C.: Adaptation of red blood cell function to hypoxia and temperature in ectothermic vertebrates. Am. Zool. *20*:163, 1980.
74. Powers, D. A.: Molecular ecology of teleost fish hemoglobins: Strategies for adapting to changing environments. Am. Zool. *20*:139, 1980.
75. Carey, F. G., and Lawson, K. D.: Temperature regulation in free-swimming blue-fin tuna. Comp. Biochem. Physiol. *44A*:375, 1973.
75a. Rossi-Fanelli, A., and Antonini, E.: Oxygen equilibrium of hemoglobin from *Thunnus thynnus*. Nature *186*:895, 1960.
76. Carey, F. G., and Gibson, Q. H.: Reverse temperature dependence of tuna hemoglobin oxygenation. Biochem. Biophys. Res. Commun. *78*:1376, 1977.
77. Ingermann, R. L., and Terwilliger, R. C.: Intraerythrocytic organic phosphates of fetal and adult seaperch (*Embiotoca lateralis*): Their role in maternal-fetal oxygen transport. J. Comp. Physiol. *144*:253, 1981.
78. Broyles, R. H., Johnson, G. M., Maples, P. B., and Kindell, G. R.: Two erythropoietic microenvironments and two larval red cell lines in bullfrog tadpoles. Dev. Biol. *81*:299, 1981.
78a. Watt, K. W. K., and Riggs, A.: Hemoglobins of the tadpole of the bullfrog *Rana catesbeiana*: Structure and function of isolated components. J. Biol. Chem. *250*:5934, 1975.
79. Watt, K. W. K., Maruyama, T., and Riggs, A.: Hemoglobins of the tadpole of the bullfrog, *Rana catesbeiana*. J. Biol. Chem. *255*:3294, 1980.
80. Maruyama, T., Watt, K. W. K., and Riggs, A.: Hemoglobins of the tadpole of the bullfrog, *Rana catesbeiana*. J. Biol. Chem. *255*:3285, 1980.
81. Broyles, R. H.: Changes in the blood during amphibian metamorphosis. *In* Gilbert, L. I., and Frieden, E. (eds.): Metamorphosis: A Problem in Developmental Biology. 2nd ed. New York, Plenum Publishing Corp., 1981, p. 461.
82. Aggarwal, S. J., and Riggs, A.: The hemoglobins of the bullfrog *Rana catesbeiana*. I. Purification amino acid composition and oxygen equlibria. J. Biol. Chem. *244*:2372, 1969.
83. Baldwin, T. O., and Riggs, A.: The hemoglobins of the bullfrog, *Rana catesbeiana*. J. Biol. Chem. *249*:6110, 1974.
84. Araki, T., Kajita, A., and Shukuya, R.: The effect of organic phosphates on the allosteric property of *Rana catesbeiana* hemoglobins. Biochem. Biophys. Res. Commun. *43*:1179, 1971.
85. Jokumsen, A., and Weber, R. E.: Haemoglobin-oxygen binding properties in the blood of *Xenopus laevis*, with special reference to the influences of aestivation and of temperature and salinity acclimation. J. Exp. Biol. *86*:19, 1980.
86. Lenfant, C., and Johansen, K.: Respiratory adaptations in selected amphibians. Respir. Physiol. *2*:247, 1967.
87. Hutchinson, V. H., Haines, H. B., and Engbretson, G.: Aquatic life at high altitude: Respiratory adaptations in the Lake Titicaca frog *Telmatobius culeus*. Respiro. Physiol. *27*:115, 1976.
87a. Wood, S. C., Hoyt, R. W., and Burggren, W. W.: Control of hemoglobin function in the salamander, *Ambystoma tigrinum*. Mol. Physiol. *2*:263, 1982.

88. Garlick, R. L., Davis, B. J., Farmer, M., Fyhn, H. J., Fyhn, V. E. H., Noble, R. W., Powers, D. A., Riggs, A., and Weber, R. E.: A fetal-maternal shift in the oxygen equilibrium of hemoglobin from the viviparous caecilian *Typhlonectes compressicauda*. Comp. Biochem. Physiol. *62A*:239, 1979.
89. Pough, F. H.: Blood oxygen transport and delivery in reptiles. Am. Zool. *20*:173, 1980.
90. Coates, M.: Studies on the interaction of organic phosphates with haemoglobin in an amphibian (*Bufo marinus*), a reptile (*Trachydosaurus rugosus*) and man. Aust. J. Biol. Sci. *28*:367, 1975.
91. Pough, F. H.: Ontogenetic change in molecular and functional properties of blood of garter snakes, *Thamnophis sirtalis*. J. Exp. Zool. *201*:47, 1977.
92. Bauer, C., Forster, M., Gros, G., Mosca, A., Perrella, M., Rollema, H. S., and Vogel, D.: Analysis of bicarbonate binding to crocodilian hemoglobin. J. Biol. Chem. *256*:8429, 1981.
93. Leclerq, F., Schnek, A. G., Braunitzer, G., Stangl, A., and Schrank, B.: Direct reciprocal allosteric interaction of oxygen and hydrogen carbonate sequence of the haemoglobins of the Caiman (*Caiman crocodylus*), the Nile crocodile (*Crocodylus niloticus*) and the Mississippi crocodile (*Alligator mississippiensis*). Hoppe-Seyler's Z. Physiol. Chem. *362*:1151, 1981.
94. Perutz, M. F., Bauer, C., Gros, G., Leclerq, F., Vandecasserie, C., Schnek, A. G., Braunitzer, G., Friday, A. E., and Joysey, K. A.: Allosteric regulation of crocodilian haemoglobin. Nature *291*:682, 1981.
95. Lutz, P. L.: On the oxygen affinity of bird blood. Am. Zool. *20*:187, 1980.
96. Baumann, F. H., and Baumann, R.: A comparative study of the respiratory properties of bird blood. Respir. Physiol. *31*:333, 1977.
97. Board, P. G., Agar, N. S., Gruca, M., and Shine, R.: Methaemoglobin and its reduction in nucleated erythrocytes from reptiles and birds. Comp. Biochem. Physiol. *57B*:265, 1977.
98. Vandecasserie, C., Paul, C., Schnek, A. G., and Leonis, J.: Oxygen affinity of avian hemoglobins. Comp. Biochem. Physiol. *44A*:711, 1973.
99. Isaacks, R., Harkness, D., Sampsell, R., Adler, J., Roth, S., Kim, C., and Goldman, P.: Studies on avian erythrocyte metabolism. Inositol tetrakis phosphate: The major phosphate compound in the erythrocytes of the ostrich (*Struthio camelus camelus*). Eur. J. Biochem. *77*:567, 1977.
100. Isaacks, R. E., Harkness, D. R., Adler, J. L., and Goldman, P. H.: Studies on avian erythrocyte metabolism. Effect of organic phosphates on oxygen affinity of embryonic and adult type hemoglobins of the chick embryo. Arch. Biochem. Biophys. *173*:114, 1976.
101. Oberthur, W., Voelter, W., and Braunitzer, G.: Die sequenz der hamoglobine von Streifengans (*Anser indicus*) und Strauss (*Struthio camelus*). Inositpentaphosphat als modulator der evolutionsgeschwindigkeit: Die uberraschende sequenz α 63 (E12) Valin. Hoppe-Seyler's Z. Physiol. Chem. *361*:969, 1980.
102. Isaacks, R. E., and Harkness, D. R.: 2,3-Diphosphoglycerate in erythrocytes of chick embryos. Science *189*:393, 1975.
103. Borgese, T. A., and Lampert, L. M.: Duck red cell 2,3-diphosphoglycerate: Its presence in the embryo and its disappearance in the adult. Biochem. Biophys. Res. Commun. *65*:822, 1975.
104. Isaacks, R. E., Harkness, D. R., Froeman, G. A., Goldman, P. H., Adler, J. L., Sussman, S. A., and Roth, S.: Studies on avian erythrocyte metabolism—II. Relationship between the major phosphorylated metabolic intermediates and oxygen affinity of whole blood in chick embryos and chicks. Comp. Biochem. Physiol. *53A*:151, 1976.
105. Isaacks, R. E., Harkness, D. R., Sampsell, R. N., Adler, J. L., Kim, C. Y., and Goldman, P. H.: Studies on avian erythrocyte metabolism—IV. Relationship between the major phosphorylated metabolic intermediates and oxygen affinity of whole blood in adults and embryos in several galliforms. Comp. Biochem. Physiol. *55A*:29, 1976.
106. Oshima, M., and Taylor, T. G.: Phytic acid in chicken erythrocytes. Biochem. J. *83*:13, 1963.
107. Jones, S. R., Smith, J. E., and Board, P. B.: Changes in erythrocyte metabolism following acute blood loss in chickens. Poultry Sci. *57*:1667, 1978.
108. Rollema, H. S., and Bauer, C.: The interaction of inositol pentaphosphate with the hemoglobins of highland and lowland geese. J. Biol. Chem. *254*:12038, 1979.
109. Black, C. P., and Tenney, S. M.: Oxygen transport during progressive hypoxia in high-altitude and sea-level waterfowl. Respir. Physiol. *39*:217, 1979.
110. Riggs, A.: Factors in the evolution of hemoglobin function. Fed. Proc. *35*:2115, 1976.
111. Tomita, S., and Riggs, A.: Studies of the interaction of 2,3-diphosphoglycerate and carbon dioxide with hemoglobins from mouse, man, and elephant. J. Biol. Chem. *246*:547, 1971.
112. Arnone, A.: X-ray diffraction study of binding of 2,3-diphosphoglycerate to human deoxyhemoglobin. Nature *237*:146, 1972.
113. Dickerson, R. E., and Geis, I.: Hemoglobin: Structure, Function, Evolution and Pathology. Menlo Park, California, Benjamin-Cummings, 1983.
114. Dayhoff, M. O.: Atlas of Protein Sequence and Structure. Vol. 5, Suppl. 3. Washington, D.C., National Biomedical Research Foundation, Georgetown University Medical Center, 1978.
115. Rapoport, S., and Guest, G. M.: Distribution of acid soluble phosphorus in the blood of various vertebrates. J. Biol. Chem. *138*:269, 1941.
116. Harkness, D. R., Ponce, J., and Grayson, V.: A comparative study of the phosphoglyceric acid cycle in mammalian erythrocytes. Comp. Biochem. Physiol. *28*:129, 1969.
117. Bartlett, G. R.: Patterns of phosphate compounds in red blood cells of man and animals. *In* Brewer, G. J. (ed.): Red Cell Metabolism and Function. New York, Plenum Press, 1970.
118. Scott, A. F., Bunn, H. F., and Brush, A. G.: The phylogenetic distribution of red cell 2,3-diphosphoglycerate and its interaction with mammalian hemoglobins. J. Exp. Zool. *201*:269, 1977.
119. Coates, M. L.: Hemoglobin function in the vertebrates: An evolutionary model. J. Mol. Evol. *6*:285, 1975.
120. Bunn, H. F.: Differences in the interaction of 2,3-diphosphoglycerate with certain mammalian hemoglobins. Science *172*:1049, 1971.
121. Dhindsa, D. S., Sedgwick, C. J., and Metcalfe, J.: Comparative studies of the respiratory functions of mammalian blood. VIII. Asian elephant (*Elephas maximus*) and African elephant (*Loxodonta africana*). Respir. Physiol. *14*:332, 1972.
122. White, J. R., Harkness, D. R., Isaacks, R. E., and Duffield, D. A.: Some studies on blood of the Florida manatee *Trichechus manatus latrostris*. Comp. Biochem. Physiol. *55A*:413, 1976.
123. Farmer, M., Weber, R. E., Bonaventura, J., Best, R. C., and Domning, D.: Functional properties of

hemoglobin and whole blood in an aquatic mammal, the Amazonian manatee (*Trichechus inunguis*). Comp. Biochem. Physiol. *62A*:231, 1979.
124. Dhindsa, D. S., Metcalfe, J., McKean, R., and Thorne, T.: Comparative studies of the respiratory functions of mammalian blood. XI. Pronghorn antelope (*Antilocapra americana*). Respir. Physiol. *21*:297, 1974.
125. Charache, S., Bush, M., and Winslow, R.: Oxygen transport in the giraffe. (Abstract.) In ASH 18th Annual Meeting, Dallas, Texas, 1975, p. 154.
126. Perutz, M. F., and Imai, K.: Regulation of oxygen affinity of mammalian haemoglobins. J. Mol. Biol. *136*:183, 1980.
127. Taketa, F., Mauk, G., and Lessard, J. L.: Beta chain amino termini of the cat hemoglobins and the response to 2,3-diphosphoglycerate. J. Biol. Chem. *246*:4471, 1971.
128. Taketa, F.: Structure of the Felidae hemoglobins and response to 2,3-diphosphoglycerate. Comp. Biochem. Physiol. *45B*:813, 1973.
129. Nagel, R. L., Reider, R. F., Bookchin, R. M., and James, G. W.: Some functional properties of hemoglobin Leiden. Biochem. Biophys. Res. Commun. *53*:1240, 1973.
130. Bonaventura, J., Bonaventura, C., Amiconi, G., Amiconi, E., Antonini, E., and Brunori, M.: Functional properties of hemoglobin Leiden (β 6 or 7 glu deleted). Arch. Biochem. Biophys. *161*:328, 1974.
131. Perutz, M. F.: Stereochemistry of cooperative effects in haemoglobin. Nature *228*:726, 1970.
132. Dhindsa, D. S., Metcalfe, J., and Hoversland, A. S.: Comparative studies of the respiratory functions of mammalian blood. IX. Ring-tailed lemur (*Lemur catta*) and black lemur (*Lemur macaco*). Respir. Physiol. *15*:331, 1972.
133. Scott, A. F., Bunn, H. F., and Brush, A. H.: Functional aspects of hemoglobin evolution in the mammals. J. Mol. Evol. *8*:311, 1976.
134. Duhm, J., and Gerlach, E.: On the mechanism of the hypoxia induced increase of 2,3-diphosphoglycerate in erythrocytes. Pfluegers Arch. *326*:254, 1971.
135. Oski, F. A., Gottlieb, A. J., Miller, W. W., and Deliveria-Papadopoulos, M.: The effects of deoxygenation of adult and fetal hemoglobin as the synthesis of red cell 2,3-diphosphoglycerate and its *in vivo* consequences. J. Clin. Invest. *49*:400, 1970.
136. Kay, F. R.: 2,3-Diphosphoglycerate, blood oxygen dissociation and the biology of mammals. Comp. Biochem. Physiol. *57A*:309, 1977.
137. Schmidt-Nielsen, K., and Larimer, J. L.: Oxygen dissociation curves of mammalian blood in relation to body size. Am. J. Physiol. *195*:424, 1958.
138. Dhindsa, D. S., Metcalfe, J., Hoversland, A. S., and Hautman, R. A.: Comparative studies of the respiratory functions of mammalian blood. X. Killer whale (*Orcinus orca*) and beluga whale (*Delphinapterus leucas*). Respir. Physiol. *20*:93, 1974.
139. Jelkmann, W., Oberthur, W., Kleinschmidt, T., and Braunitzer, G.: Adaptation of hemoglobin function to subterranean life in the mole, *Talpa europaea*. Respir. Physiol. *46*:7, 1981.
140. Chiodi, H.: Comparative study of the blood gas transport in high altitude and sea level Camelidae and goats. Respir. Physiol. *11*:84, 1970–71.
141. Bartels, H., Hilpert, P., Barbey, K., Betke, K., Riegel, K., Lang, E. M., and Metcalfe, J.: Respiratory functions of blood of the yak, llama, camel, Dybowski deer, and African elephant. Am. J. Physiol. *205*:331, 1963.
142. Bauer, C., Rollema, H. S., Till, H. W., and Braunitzer, G.: Phosphate binding by llama and camel hemoglobin. J. Comp. Physiol. *136*:67, 1980.
143. Petschow, D., Wurdinger, I., Baumann, R., Duhm, J., Braunitzer, G., and Bauer, C.: Causes of high blood O_2 affinity of animals living at high altitude. J. Appl. Physiol. *42*:139, 1977.
144. Bunn, H. F., and Kitchen, H.: Hemoglobin function in the horse. The role of 2,3-diphosphoglycerate in modifying the oxygen affinity of maternal and fetal blood. Blood *42*:471, 1973.
145. Snyder, L. R. G.: 2,3-Diphosphoglycerate in high- and low-altitude populations of the deer mouse. Respir. Physiol. *48*:107, 1982.
146. Snyder, L. R. G., Born, S., and Lechner, A. J.: Blood oxygen affinity in high- and low-altitude populations of the deer mouse. Respir. Physiol. *48*:89, 1982.
147. Noble, N. A., and Brewer, G. J.: Studies of the metabolic basis of the ATP-DPG differences in genetically selected high and low ATP-DPG rat strains. In Brewer, G. J. (ed.): Hemoglobin and Red Cell Structure and Function. New York, Plenum Press, 1972, pp. 155–164.
148. Baumann, R., Bauer, C., and Bartels, H.: Influence of chronic and acute hypoxia on oxygen affinity and red cell 2,3-diphosphoglycerate of rats and guinea pigs. Respir. Physiol. *11*:135, 1971.
149. Mauk, A. G., Whelan, H. T., Putz, G. R., and Taketa, F.: Anemia in domestic cats: Effect on hemoglobin components and whole blood oxygenation. Science *185*:447, 1974.
150. Blunt, M. H., and Evans, J. V.: Changes in the content of potassium and in haemoglobin type in merino sheep under a severe anemic stress. Nature *200*:1215, 1963.
151. VanVliet, G., and Huisman, T. H. J.: Changes in the haemoglobin types of sheep as a response to anemia. Biochem. J. *93*:401, 1964.
152. Vaccaro-Torracca, A. M., Vestri, R., and Salmaso, S.: Higher oxygen affinity of sheep Hb C compared to Hb A and Hb B_1. Experientia *36*:559, 1980.
153. Agar, N. S., Harley, J. D., Cruca, M. A., and Roberts, J.: Erythrocyte 2,3-diphosphoglycerate in anaemic sheep. Experientia *33*:275, 1977.
154. Huisman, T. H. J., and Kitchens, J.: Oxygen equilibria studies of the hemoglobins from normal and anemic sheep and goats. Am. J. Physiol. *215*:140, 1968.
155. Dawson, T. J., and Evans, J. V.: Effect of anaemia on oxygen transport in sheep with different haemoglobin types. Aust. J. Exp. Biol. Med. Sci. *45*:437, 1967.
156. Bartels, H., Schmelzle, R., and Ulrich, S.: Comparative studies of the respiratory function of mammalian blood. V. Insectivora: Shrew, mole and hibernating and non-hibernating hedgehog. Respir. Physiol. *7*:278, 1969.
157. Burlington, R. F., and Whitten, B. K.: Red cell 2,3-diphosphoglycerate in hibernating ground squirrels. Comp. Biochem. Physiol. *38*:469, 1971.
158. Larken, E. C.: The response of erythrocyte organic phosphate levels of active and hibernating ground squirrels (*Spermophilus mexacanus*) to isobaric hypoxia. Comp. Biochem. Physiol. *45A*:1, 1973.
159. Harkness, D. R., Roth, S., and Goldman, P.: Studies on the red cell oxygen affinity and 2,3-diphosphoglyceric acid in the hibernating woodchuck (*Marmota monax*). Comp. Biochem. Physiol. *48A*:591, 1974.
160. Tempel, G. E., and Musacchia, X. J.: Erythrocyte 2,3-diphosphoglycerate and concentrations in hi-

bernating, hypothermic and rewarming hamsters. Proc. Soc. Exp. Biol. Med. *148*:588, 1975.
161. Bartels, H.: Prenatal Respiration. Amsterdam and London, North Holland Publishing Co., 1970, p. 89.
162. Novy, M. J., and Parer, J. T.: Absence of high blood oxygen affinity in the fetal cat. Respir. Physiol. *6*:144, 1969.
163. Hebbel, R. P., Berger, E. M., and Eaton, J. W.: Effect of increased maternal hemoglobin oxygen affinity on fetal growth in rats. Blood 55:969, 1980.
164. Bauer, C., Jelkmann, W., and Moll, W.: High oxygen affinity of maternal blood reduces fetal weight in rats. Respir. Physiol. *43*:169, 1981.
165. Bauer, C., Tamm, R., Petschow, D., Bartels, R., and Bartels, H.: Oxygen affinity and allosteric effects of embryonic mouse haemoglobins. Nature *257*:333, 1975.
166. Jelkmann, W., and Bauer, C.: Embryonic hemoglobins: Dependency of functional characteristics on tetramer composition. Pfluegers Arch. *377*:75, 1978.
167. Metcalfe, J., Dhindsa, D. S., and Novy, M. J.: General aspects of oxygen transport in maternal and fetal blood. *In* Longo, L. D., and Bartels, H. (eds.): Respiratory Gas Exchange and Blood Flow in the Placenta. Proceedings of the Satellite Symposium on Placental Gas Exchange, Hanover, Germany. Bethesda, Maryland, USPHS, 1971.
168. Dhindsa, D. A., Hoversland, A. S., and Templeton, J. W.: Postnatal changes in oxygen affinity and concentrations of 2,3-diphosphoglycerate in dog blood. Biol. Neonate *20*:226, 1972.
169. Blunt, M. H., Kitchens, J. L., Mayson, S. M., and Huisman, T. H. J.: Red cell 2,3-diphosphoglycerate and oxygen affinity in newborn goats and sheep. Proc. Soc. Exp. Biol. Med. *138*:800, 1971.
170. Huisman, T. H. J., Lewis, J. P., Blunt, M. H., Adams, H. R., Miller, A., Dozy, A. M., and Boyd, E. M.: Hemoglobin C in newborn sheep and goats: A possible explanation for its function and biosynthesis. Pediatr. Res. *3*:189, 1969.
171. Bauer, C., Ludwig, I., and Ludwig, M.: Different effects of 2,3-diphosphoglycerate and adenosine triphosphate on the oxygen affinity of adult and foetal human haemoglobin. Life Sci. *7*:1339, 1968.
172. Tyuma, I., and Shimizu, K.: Different response to organic phosphates of human fetal and adult hemoglobins. Arch. Biochem. Biophys. *129*:404, 1969.
173. Takenaka, O., and Morimoto, H.: Oxygen equilibrium characteristics of adult and fetal hemoglobin of Japanese monkey (*Macada fuscata*). Biochim. Biophys. Acta *446*:457, 1976.
174. Kutas, F., and Stuzel, M.: The organic acid soluble phosphate contents of mammalian and avian erythrocytes at the beginning of postnatal life. Experientia *14*:214, 1958.
175. Baumann, R., Teischel, F., Zoch, R., and Bartels, H.: Changes in red cell diphosphoglycerate concentration as cause of the postnatal decrease in pig blood oxygen affinity. Respir. Physiol. *19*:153, 1973.
176. Tweeddale, P. M.: DPG and the oxygen affinity of maternal and foetal pig blood and haemoglobins. Respir. Physiol. *19*:12, 1973.
177. Novy, M. J., Hoversland, A. S., Dhindsa, D. S., and Metcalfe, J.: Blood oxygen affinity and hemoglobin type in adult, newborn and fetal pigs. Respir. Physiol. *19*:1, 1973.
178. Jelkmann, W., and Bauer, C.: Oxygen affinity and phosphate compounds of red blood cells during intrauterine development of rabbits. Pfluegers Arch. *372*:149, 1977.
179. Murphy, W. S., Metcalfe, J., Hoversland, A. S., and Dhindsa, D. S.: Postnatal changes in blood respiratory characteristics in an American opossum (*Sidelphis virginiana*). Respir. Physiol. *29*:73, 1977.
180. Petschow, R., Petschow, D., Bartels, R., Baumann, R., and Bartels, H.: Regulation of oxygen affinity in blood of fetal, newborn and adult mouse. Respir. Physiol. *35*:271, 1978.
181. Jelkmann, W., and Bauer, C.: Regulation of red cell DPG metabolism in fetuses and adults. Acta Biol. Med. Ger. *40*:661, 1981.
182. Qvist, J., Weber, R. E., and Zapol, W. M.: Oxygen equilibrium properties of blood and hemoglobin of fetal and adult Weddell seals. J. Appl. Physiol. *50*:999, 1981.
183. Jelkmann, W., and Bauer, C.: High pyruvate kinase activity causes low concentration of 2,3-diphosphoglycerate in fetal rabbit red cells. Pfluegers Arch. *375*:189, 1978.
184. Mueggler, P. A., and Black, J. A.: The hematology and biochemistry of canine postnatal anemia. *In* Brewer, G. (ed.): The Red Cell: 5th Ann Arbor Conference. New York, Liss, 1981, p. 245.
185. Franzke, R., and Jelkmann, W.: Characterization of the pyruvate kinase which induces the low 2,3-DPG level of fetal rabbit red cells. Pfluegers Arch. *394*:21, 1982.
186. Jelkmann, W., and Bauer, C.: 2,3-DPG levels in relation to red cell enzyme activities in rat fetuses and hypoxic newborns. Pfluegers Arch. *389*:61, 1980.
187. Goodman, M.: Decoding the pattern of protein evolution. Prog. Biophys. Mol. Biol. *37*:105, 1981.
188. Goodman, M., Weiss, M. L., and Czelusniak, J.: Molecular evolution above the species level: Branching pattern, rates, and mechanisms. Systematic Zoology *31*:376, 1982.
188a. Goodman, M., Romero-Herrera, A. E., Dene, H., Czelusniak, J., and Tashian, R. E.: Amino acid sequence evidence on the phylogeny of primates and other eutherians. *In* Goodman, M. (ed.): Macromolecular Sequence in Systematic and Evolutionary Biology. New York, Plenum Press, 1982, pp. 115–191.
189. Kumura, M.: Model of effectively neutral mutations in which selective constraint is incorporated. Proc. Natl. Acad. Sci. USA *76*:3440, 1979.
190. Jukes, T. H.: Silent nucleotide substitutions and the molecular evolutionary clock. Science *210*:973, 1980.
191. Goodman, M. G., Moore, W., and Matsuda, G.: Darwinian evolution in the geneology of haemoglobin. Nature *253*:603, 1975.
192. Craik, C. S., Buchman, S. R., and Beychok, S.: Characterization of globin domains: Heme binding to the central exon product. Proc. Natl. Acad. Sci. USA *77*:1384, 1980.
193. Gilbert, W.: Why genes in pieces? Nature *271*:501, 1978.
194. Darnell, J. E.: Implications of RNA-RNA splicing in evolution of eukaryotic cells. Science *202*:1257, 1978.
195. Crick, F.: Split genes and RNA splicing. Science *204*:264, 1979.
196. Eaton, W. A.: The relationship between coding sequences and function in haemoglobin. Nature *284*:183, 1980.
197. Coates, M., and Riggs, A.: Perspectives on the evolution of hemoglobin. Tex. Rep. Biol. Med. *40*:9, 1980–81.

TOM MANIATIS

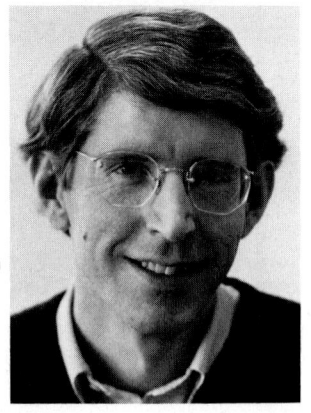

The virtual explosion of new knowledge that has accumulated in recent years concerning the molecular genetics of normal and abnormal human hemoglobins has been fueled by the breakthroughs of recombinant DNA technology. Tom Maniatis has consistently been at the forefront of this rapidly moving field and has played a pivotal role in many of the major accomplishments that have led to the detailed molecular characterization of the human globin gene system.

Maniatis obtained his Ph.D. in Molecular Biology at Vanderbilt University in Nashville, Tennessee, where he worked on the x-ray crystallography of DNA in the laboratory of Leonard Lerman. He then did postdoctoral work in the laboratory of Mark Ptashne at Harvard University Biological Laboratories, studying the mechanisms of gene regulation in bacteriophage λ. At Harvard, he met Arg Efstratiadis and Fotis Kafatos, and the three began a collaboration studying the molecular genetics of globin as a model for gene regulation. They soon succeeded in synthesizing full-length single-stranded and then double-stranded cDNA copies of rabbit globin mRNA. The next experiment was to insert the cDNA into a bacterial plasmid for cloning by recombinant DNA technology, but there was an obstacle for continuing the work at Harvard.

In 1975 and 1976, the "recombinant DNA debate" over the potential biohazards of the technology was raging, and the NIH established a committee that issued strict guidelines for the conduct of such research. In Cambridge, however, it became virtually impossible to do recombinant DNA work, even under the NIH guidelines. Following a public debate over plans by Harvard to build a high level (P3) containment laboratory for recombinant DNA research, the Cambridge City Council declared a moratorium on all such research and then issued its own set of recommendations, which contained more restrictions and requirements than did the NIH guidelines. Being unable to clone the rabbit globin cDNA at Harvard, Maniatis moved to the Cold Spring Harbor Laboratories, and the cloning was successfully accomplished there.

Subsequently, Maniatis accepted a faculty position in the Division of Biology at Caltech, where he developed and refined the technique for isolating single copy genes from "libraries" of total cellular DNA. Using the cloned rabbit β globin cDNA as a probe, he isolated recombinant bacteriophage containing the genomic rabbit β globin gene. This work was a major accomplishment, as it established for the first time the feasibility of purifying single copy genes from complex eukaryotic genomes without prior enrichment of DNA for the target gene.

Transferring the globin cDNA and gene cloning technology to the human gene system was fraught with administrative difficulties. The initial NIH guidelines allowed for cloning of nonembryonic primate tissue only under conditions of physical and biological containment that were not readily available. However, "embryonic" primate tissue could be cloned under the same conditions of containment as allowed for other mammalian tissue. Bernard Forget, Sherman Weissman, and colleagues at Yale University applied to their institutional biohazard committee to have cord blood and fetal liver approved as "embryonic" tissues. When approval was granted, human α, β, and γ globin cDNAs were prepared in collaboration with Efstratiadis and associates, and were subsequently cloned at the P3 facility at Yale. Human fetal liver DNA was provided to Maniatis at Caltech, and the first library of human genomic DNA was constructed, from which not only human globin genes but also a varied assortment of other human genes were subsequently purified. This pioneer work provided the cornerstone and reagents for the large body of future work by numerous laboratories on the structure and function of normal and thalassemic globin genes.

Maniatis recently returned to Harvard, where he is now Professor of Biochemistry and Molecular Biology. His laboratory has maintained its leadership in the field and has focused its work most recently on the study of globin gene expression following transfer into tissue culture cells and on the analysis of the mechanism of processing or splicing of precursor globin mRNA molecules.

MOLECULAR GENETICS AND BIOSYNTHESIS OF HEMOGLOBIN

7

A number of newer molecular biology techniques have contributed a great deal in recent years to our precise understanding of the fine structure and chromosomal arrangement of the human globin genes and to our knowledge of the various molecular processes involved in globin gene expression and hemoglobin synthesis. These technologies include molecular hybridization assays using radioactive synthetic DNA copies (cDNAs) of globin messenger RNA (mRNA); gene mapping by restriction endonuclease digestion of DNA, and the gel blotting procedure of Southern; the actual isolation or cloning of human globin genes and adjacent flanking DNA by recombinant DNA technology; the nucleotide sequence analysis of isolated human globin genes by rapid DNA sequencing techniques; and study of gene transcription and post-transcriptional processes in gene transfer/gene expression systems utilizing tissue culture cells. The general principles of this methodology will be discussed in Chapter 8. In this chapter, we will summarize the currently available information, obtained by these various techniques, concerning the fine structure, chromosomal organization, and mechanisms of expression of the normal human globin genes.

GENERAL PROCESSES INVOLVED IN GENE EXPRESSION AND PROTEIN SYNTHESIS

The major steps involved in gene expression and protein synthesis are illustrated schematically in Figure 7–1 and pertain to the synthesis of hemoglobin as well as that of any other protein. The genetic information for the structure of a given protein is encoded in the nucleotide sequence of the DNA, which makes up a gene located on a chromosome within the cell nucleus. Each amino acid is specified by a sequence of three nucleotide bases called a codon (Table 7–1). A given amino acid may have many different codons, but each is spe-

170 MOLECULAR GENETICS AND BIOSYNTHESIS OF HEMOGLOBIN

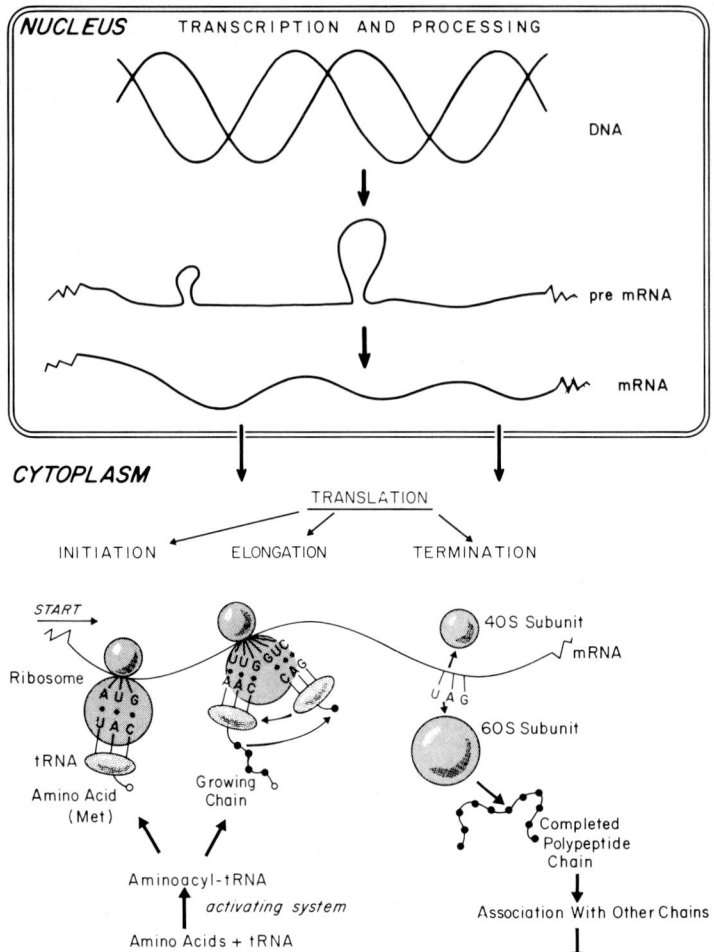

Figure 7–1. Schematic representation of the mechanism of polypeptide-chain biosynthesis.

cific for only one amino acid and for a different specific transfer RNA (tRNA) molecule necessary for binding and transporting that amino acid. The genetic information is relayed to the cytoplasm of the cell, where protein synthesis must occur, by the synthesis of a strand of RNA called messenger RNA, or mRNA. The mRNA is a mirror image of the nucleotide sequence of the DNA of the gene resulting from copying of the coding strand of the gene DNA into RNA by the enzyme RNA polymerase in the process called transcription. The nucleotides of the DNA are represented in the mRNA as complementary nucleotides according to Watson-Crick base pairing: C in the DNA is represented as G in the RNA, G as C, A as U, and T as A. After processing in the nucleus (to be discussed in later sections) and transport from nucleus to cytoplasm, the mRNA molecule is the template on which amino acid residues are sequentially joined to one another by peptide bonds to form polypeptide chains in a complex set of enzymatic reactions involving the interactions of cellular ribosomes, transfer RNA, and numerous other factors in the process called translation. The initial step of mRNA binding to ribosomes is called initiation: It is a complex enzymatic reaction that brings together the mRNA; the smaller (40s) ribosomal subunit; a special initiator tRNA, which carries the amino acid methionine; and the larger (60s) ribosomal subunit. The reaction requires a number of separate protein factors (initation factors), GTP, and ATP. The initiator codon AUG of the mRNA, which precisely signals the starting point for mRNA translation, also constitutes the only codon for the amino acid methionine. Thus, in mammalian systems, just as in bacterial systems, the first amino acid incorporated into a protein chain is methionine; but contrary to the bacterial systems, this initial amino acid does not have a blocked (formylated) amino group, and it is later cleaved **from** the nascent polypeptide chain during its elongation. The completed mammalian polypeptide chain therefore does not necessarily have an N-terminal methionine.

Once initiated, the synthesis of a protein chain continues by the process of elongation, which involves the sequential addition of amino acids to the initial amino acid by peptide bond formation, resulting in gradual lengthening of the polypeptide chain. The initiator codon AUG sets the phase or reading frame of the mRNA, so that subsequent triplet nucleotide codons following the AUG are read in a linear fashion without skips and are translated into amino acids until a termination codon is encountered, which signals the end of polypeptide chain synthesis. Translation of the mRNA proceeds in a 5' (N-terminal coding) to 3' (C-terminal coding) direction. Each amino acid is brought to its position by a specific tRNA to which it is attached (the complex is called amino-acyl tRNA). The amino-acyl tRNA binds to the ribosome and the specific codon sequence of the mRNA by a complementary trinucleotide sequence of its own, called the anti-codon, which is located in a specific site of the tRNA. The nascent peptide chain that is attached to the previous tRNA is transferred to the new tRNA and a peptide bond is formed with the new amino acid. This new peptidyl-tRNA complex then moves to the position of the previous tRNA, which is released as the ribosome moves along to the next codon. A new amino-acyl tRNA binds to this new codon, and the process is repeated. This process involves a complex set of reactions that require many enzymes and cofactors such as GTP. Chain elongation continues until the ribosome, traveling down the messenger RNA in "ticker tape" fashion, encounters a specific nucleotide codon (UAA, UAG, or UGA) that signals chain termination. The polypeptide chain is then released as the ribosome dissociates into its two subunits and

Table 7–1. THE MESSENGER RNA CODONS FOR THE VARIOUS AMINO ACIDS

Alanine	Arginine	Asparagine	Aspartic acid	Cysteine
GCU	CGU	AAU	GAU	UGU
GCC	CGC	AAC	GAC	UGC
GCA	CGA			
GCG	CGG			
	AGA			
	AGG			

Glutamic acid	Glutamine	Glycine	Histidine	Isoleucine
GAA	CAA	GGU	CAU	AUU
GAG	CAG	GGC	CAC	AUC
		GGA		AUA
		GGG		

Leucine	Lysine	Methionine	Phenylalanine	Proline
UUA	AAA	AUG	UUU	CCU
UUG	AAG		UUC	CCC
CUU				CCA
CUC				CCG
CUA				
CUG				

Serine	Threonine	Tryptophan	Tyrosine	Valine
UCU	ACU	UGG	UAU	GUU
UCC	ACC		UAC	GUC
UCA	ACA			GUA
UCG	ACG			GUG
AGU				
AGC				

SPECIAL CODONS

Chain initiation	Chain terminaton (nonsense codons)
AUG	UAA
	UAG
	UGA

The first letter shown for each triplet codon represents the 5' end of the mRNA codon. Note that AUG serves both as chain initiation codon and as methionine codon.
From Bunn, Forget & Ranney: *Human Hemoglobins*, 1977, p. 113.

separates from the mRNA. The polypeptide chain then assumes its secondary and tertiary structure and may bind to other polypeptide subunits and other cellular components to form a mature protein. The details of these general processes have been extensively reviewed elsewhere.[1,2]

The synthesis of hemoglobin is accomplished by this same basic mechanism. In fact, much of the process of eukaryotic protein synthesis was elucidated by the study of globin synthesizing cells and cell-free systems. Once synthesized, the globin chains bind heme and combine with one another to form appropriate tetramers of complete hemoglobin molecules.

NORMAL HUMAN GLOBIN GENE STRUCTURE AND ORGANIZATION

Genetic Analysis of Globin Gene Number and Organization

Prior to precise knowledge of globin gene organization by gene mapping and gene cloning procedures, a general picture of the number and arrangement of the normal human globin genes had emerged from the genetic analysis of normal and abnormal hemoglobins and their pattern of inheritance. The structure and number of different normal human hemoglobins (see Table 4–1) required that, at a minimum, there must be at least one different globin gene for each of the different globin chains: α, β, γ, δ, ε, and ζ. From the study of hemoglobin variants and the analysis of the biochemical heterogeneity of the γ chains in Hb F, evidence showed that the α and γ globin genes were duplicated. Individuals were identified whose red cells contained more than two structurally different α globin chains, which could be best explained by duplication of the α globin gene locus, and the characterization of the structurally different $^G\gamma$ and $^A\gamma$ globin chains of Hb F (see Chapter 4) imposed a requirement for duplication of the γ globin gene locus.[3]

From the study of the pattern of inheritance of Hb variants from individuals carrying both an α-chain and a β-chain variant, it became clear early on that the α and β globin genes must be on different chromosomes or, at the very least, very widely separated if on the same chromosome: α and β Hb variants were always observed to segregate independently in offspring of doubly affected parents. However, linkage of the various non–α globin genes to one another was established from the study of interesting Hb variants that contained fused globin chains presumably resulting from non-homologous crossing over between non–α globin gene loci. Thus, the characterization of Hb Lepore, with its δβ fusion chain, established that the δ globin gene was linked to and located on the 5' (or N-terminal) side of the β globin gene, whereas the analysis of Hb Kenya, with its $^A\gamma\beta$ fusion chain, provided evidence for linkage of the $^A\gamma$ gene, and presumably the $^G\gamma$ gene as well, to the 5' side of the δ and β globin genes (for detailed discussions of Hb Lepore and Hb Kenya, see Chapters 8, 9, and 10). Thus, the general concept of the arrangement of the globin genes that emerged from these various genetic analyses can be represented as illustrated in Figure 7–2. Although the $^G\gamma$ globin gene is shown on the 5' side of the $^A\gamma$ globin gene as the most likely or logical arrangement, traditional genetic analyses could not rule out the possibility that the $^G\gamma$ globin gene was in fact located to the 3' (or C-terminal) side of the β globin gene. It was also assumed, although unsupported by any genetic evidence, that the embryonic α-like (ζ) and β-like (ε) globin genes were likely to be linked to the loci for their adult counterparts. The actual distance separating the linked γ, δ, and β genes could not be accurately estimated by genetic analysis other than by the study of recombination frequencies, which indicated that the genes were "very close" to one another in genetic terms but nevertheless could still be separated by hundreds of thousands of nucleotides.

Chromosomal Localization of Globin Genes

By the use of rodent/human somatic hybrid cells containing only one or a limited number of human chromosomes, Deisseroth and co-workers clearly established that the human α and β globin genes resided on different chromosomes[4] and that the α genes were located on chromosome 16,[5] whereas the β-like genes were located on chromosome 11.[6] The latter results were obtained by liquid hybridization assays (Cot curve analyses) of total cellular DNA from the various somatic hybrid cells hybridized to radioactive cDNA synthesized from α and β globin mRNA by use of the enzyme reverse transcriptase from avian myeloblastosis virus (see Chapter 8 for description of methodology).

These results were later confirmed and extended by various groups using the gene mapping procedure of Southern (see Chapter 8 and Fig. 8–16 for a description of the procedure) with DNA from various hybrid cell lines containing different translocations or deletions of the involved chromosomes. These studies thus led to the regional localization of the globin gene loci on their respective chromosomes—the β globin gene cluster to the short arm[7-11] of chromosome 11 and the α globin gene loci to the short arm of chromosome 16.[12] These chromosomal assignments were further confirmed by in situ hybridization of radioactive cloned globin gene probes to metaphase chromosomes.[13-15] By the analysis of recombination frequencies between polymorphic markers of various genes known to be linked to the β globin gene cluster, it has been possible to locate the β globin gene cluster in relation to other genes on the short arm of chromosome 11. Thus, it has been established that the β globin gene cluster is much more tightly linked to the parathyroid hormone (PTH) gene[16] than to the insulin gene[16-17a] and that the order of these genes going from centromere to chromosome tip is: PTH → β globin → insulin.[16] There are conflicting data concerning the precise subregion of the short arm of chromosome 11 that carries the β globin gene cluster. Gene mapping studies of DNA derived from cell hybrids containing X-irradiation–induced deletions of chromosome 11[7] as well as in situ hybridization studies[13] initially suggested that the β cluster was located close to the centromere on the short arm, between bands p11 and p12. However, gene mapping studies of DNA from cell lines carrying various naturally occurring translocations of chromosome 11 have located the β gene cluster further away from the centromere, in the distal third of the short arm[17, 18] beyond band p14.[18] This result has been confirmed by subsequent in situ hybridization studies.[18a]

Detailed Chromosomal Organization of Human Globin Genes

A very precise picture of the chromosomal organization of the α-like and non–α-like human globin gene clusters, with respect to the number of structural loci and intergene distances, has recently been obtained through the use of the technique of restriction endonuclease mapping using the gel blotting procedure of Southern as well as through the actual isolation and characterization of large fragments of human DNA containing the various globin genes by recombinant DNA technology. Sets of overlapping genomic DNA fragments spanning the entire α and non–α globin gene clusters have been obtained by gene cloning, initially in bacteriophage lambda[19-21] and more recently as larger fragments in cosmid vectors.[22-25] Detailed analysis of these recombinant DNA clones has led to the determination of the gene organization illustrated in Figure 7–3. Some of the results were expected, such as the finding of single δ and β globin gene loci and duplication of the α and γ globin gene loci. In addition, single loci for the embryonic ζ and ε globin chains were found to be linked to the α and β globin gene clusters, respectively. However, a somewhat unexpected finding was the presence in the globin gene clusters of additional gene-like structures with structural homology to the authentic globin genes—one in the β gene cluster, between the $^A\gamma$ and δ globin genes, and two in the α gene cluster, between the ζ and authentic α globin genes. These structures have been termed ψ or pseudogenes and will be discussed later. Another noteworthy feature of the chromosomal organization of the α and non–α globin gene clusters is that the different genes or gene pairs are arrayed on the chromosome from N-terminal coding (5′) to C-terminal coding (3′) sequences in the same order that they are expressed developmentally: ε → γ → δ + β and

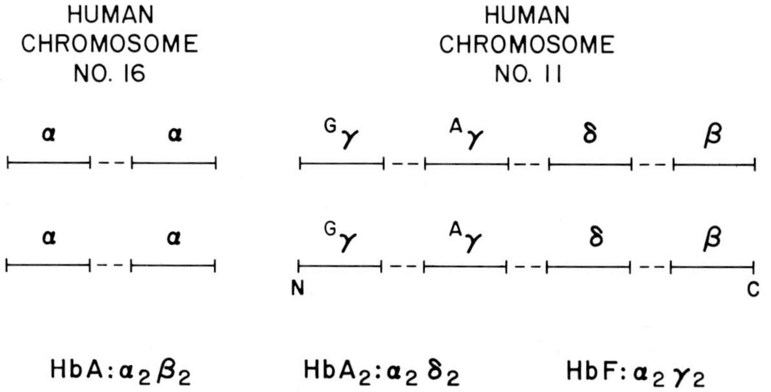

Figure 7–2. Genetic map of the human globin gene complex based on information available before recombinant DNA studies of the system. (From Forget, B. G., et al.: ICN-UCLA Symp. Mol. Cell. Biol. *14*:367, 1979.)

HUMAN CHROMOSOME NO. 16

HUMAN CHROMOSOME NO. 11

HbA: $\alpha_2\beta_2$ HbA$_2$: $\alpha_2\delta_2$ HbF: $\alpha_2\gamma_2$

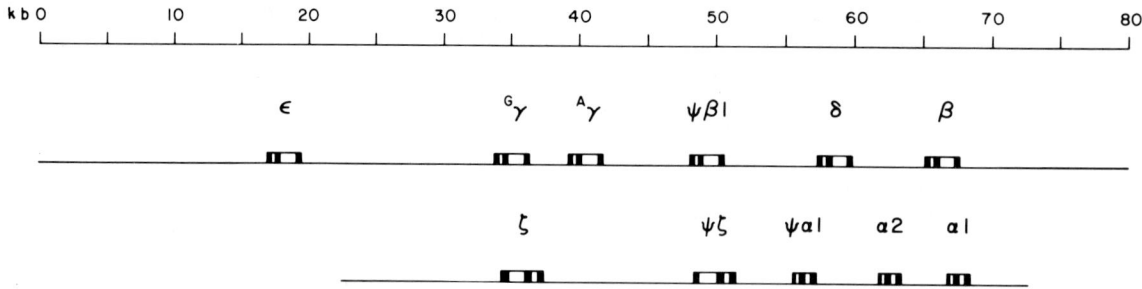

Figure 7–3. Genetic map of the human α and non-α globin gene complexes based on information obtained through gene cloning using recombinant DNA technology.

ζ → α, respectively. The significance of this organization in relation to the control of the switches in globin gene expression that occur during embryonic and fetal development is not known. Although this same general spatial organization of the different globin genes is usually maintained in other animal species, there are notable expections, such as in the chicken and the goat, in which embryonic or fetal globin genes are located to the 3' side of the adult globin genes.[26]

With regard to intergene distances, a general pattern can be observed in the organization of the globin gene clusters: Globin gene pairs that resulted from relatively recent gene duplication events are spaced relatively closely to one another, such as the two α loci, the δ and β globin gene pair, and the $^G\gamma$ and $^A\gamma$ globin gene pair, whereas larger distances separate the genes or gene pairs that are expressed at different developmental times and are evolutionarily more distantly related. Thus, in the β gene cluster, the members of the δ/β gene pair and γ gene pair are separated from one another by approximately 5000 to 6000 nucleotides (5 to 6 kilobases, or kb), whereas considerably longer distances of 15 to 18 kb separate the δ/β gene pair from the $^G\gamma/^A\gamma$ gene pair and the $^G\gamma/^A\gamma$ genes from the ε gene.[20] In the α gene cluster, approximtely 4 kb separate the two functional α1 and α2 globin genes, whereas more than 20 kb of DNA separate the functional embryonic ζ globin gene from the α globin gene pair.[21] It should be noted, however, that the evolutionarily closely related ζ/ψζ gene pair does not follow the general pattern of globin gene organization: More than 10 kb of DNA separate these two genes,[21] and there is considerable heterogeneity in the precise length of this region of intergene DNA from individual to individual, owing to variable numbers of a tandemly repeated 36 base-pair DNA sequence,[27, 28] which will be discussed in more detail later. It would appear that following the ζ/ψζ gene duplication event, there occurred an insertion of new DNA between the two loci. It is not known if the latter phenomenon was facilitated by the fact that the ψζ gene is nonfunctional and nonessential. As discussed in Chapter 8, deletion of the ψζ gene does not affect the production of Hb Portland ($\zeta_2\gamma_2$) in Mediterranean infants with hydrops fetalis that is due to homozygosity for a gene deletion encompassing both α globin genes and the ψζ gene[29] (see Fig. 8–21).

Although the usual organization of the human α globin gene cluster is as shown in Figure 7–3, a surprisingly high prevalence has been found in normal individuals of chromosomes bearing either one or three ζ-like globin genes instead of the usual two, presumably as a result of nonhomologous crossing over between the ζ and ψζ globin gene loci: The incidence of a single ζ locus was found to be 0.4 per cent in one study[30] and 2.3 per cent in another,[30a] and that of triplicated ζ-like loci was found to be 1.3 per cent.[30] In the triplicated locus, the restriction endonuclease map is consistent with duplication of the ψζ gene rather than of the functional ζ gene. In the case of the single locus, it is likely to be a fusion gene with the 5' end of the functional ζ gene and the 3' end of the ψζ gene. Because of the near-normal structure of the ψζ gene (to be discussed later), such a fusion gene would be functional and capable of producing ζ globin chains as long as the crossover occurred beyond (i.e., to the 3' side of) codon 6 of the functional ζ globin gene. However, individuals have not yet been identified who are homozygous for the single ζ locus, giving rise to the possibility that such an occurrence might not be compatible with normal embryonic development. At least two different crossover events have been identified that are associated with deletions of different sizes.[30] This is presumably due to crossing over between different regions of the ζ and ψζ genes that have intervening sequences of different sizes, as discussed in the next section. Crossing over between the duplicated α or γ genes has also resulted in the generation of loci with single or triplicated α or γ genes in different individuals, as discussed in Chapter 8.

Rare individuals have been identified in whom both γ globin genes are of either the $^G\gamma$ or $^A\gamma$ type.[30b] This phenomenon could have occurred by point mutation or by gene conversion events that are thought to occur between the linked γ globin genes.[26]

Fine Structure of Human Globin Genes

Intervening Sequences

General Features. Until mid 1977, it was believed that the DNA sequence containing the coding information of globin and other genes in animal cells was colinear with the nucleotide sequence of the messenger RNA and the amino acid sequence of the encoded protein. Then, the very unexpected and surprising discovery was made that the coding region of globin genes was in fact interrupted by considerable stretches of noncoding DNA that were termed "intervening sequences" or "introns." This initial observation, which revolutionized the field by drastically changing pre-existing concepts of gene structure and gene expression, was made independently by investigators in two different laboratories, with one group studying the mouse β globin gene by gene cloning and electron microscopy of hybrids formed between mouse β globin cDNA and the genomic DNA,[31] and the other group studying the arrangement of the cellular rabbit β globin gene[32] by the gene mapping procedure of Southern. Subsequently, introns were also demonstrated in the human δ and β globin genes by gene mapping[33, 34] and gene cloning procedures.[19]

The coding region of the globin genes of man and other animals is interrupted at two positions. In the non–α globin genes, the intervening sequences interrupt the sequence between codons 30 and 31 and between codons 104 and 105; in the α globin gene family, the intervening sequences interrupt the coding sequence between codons 31 and 32 and between codons 99 and 100 (Fig. 7–4). Although the precise codon position numbers at which the interruption occurs differ between α and non–α globin genes, it is noteworthy that the introns occur at precisely the same position with regard to the regions of the primary structure of the α and non–α globin chains that are homologous and can be aligned if it is assumed that the α and β globin gene families originally evolved from a single ancestral globin gene. It can be noted from Figure 7–4 that the first intervening sequence (IVS-1) is shorter than the second intervening sequence (IVS-2) in both α and β globin genes but that IVS-2 of the human α globin gene is considerably shorter than that of the human β globin gene. The precise lengths of these intervening sequences, determined by direct nucleotide sequence analysis of cloned globin genes, are listed in Table 7–2. In the case of the ζ-like globin genes, the structure and pattern of intron sizes are rather different from those of the α-like and other globin genes: Whereas the introns in the α and ψα genes are rather small (<150 bp), those of the ζ and ψζ genes are considerably larger and, furthermore, IVS-1 is much larger than IVS-2, being 8 to 10 times larger than the IVS-1 of any other globin gene. The introns of the ψζ gene are significantly larger than those of the ζ gene; this is due to higher numbers in the ψζ gene of tandemly repeated 14-bp and 5-bp sequences that make up the bulk of IVS-1 and IVS-2, respectively, in the ζ-like globin genes.[35] The 14-bp repeated sequence of the ζ IVS-1 bears striking homology to a similar simple repeated sequence located in the DNA flanking the 5′ end of the human insulin gene.[36, 37] The em-

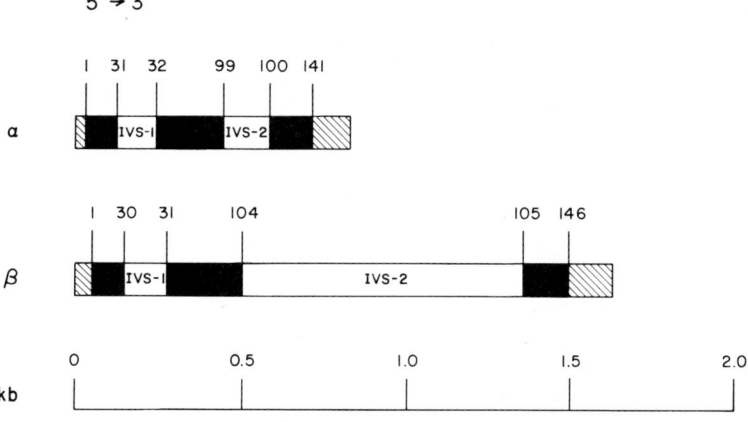

Figure 7–4. Fine structure of human α and β globin genes. The *filled blocks* represent the coding regions of the gene; the *hatched blocks* at either end represent the 5′ and 3′ untranslated sequences; IVS-1 and IVS-2 are the intervening sequences (introns) that interrupt the coding sequences of the genes. The numbers above the diagram indicate the amino acid codon positions of the coding sequence. (Modified from Forget, B. G.: *In* Goldwasser, E. (ed.): Regulation of Hemoglobin Biosynthesis. New York, Elsevier Science Publishing Co., Inc., 1983, p. 27.)

Table 7–2. SIZES OF INTERVENING SEQUENCES OF HUMAN GLOBIN GENES

Gene	IVS-1	IVS-2
β	130	850
δ	128	889
$^A\gamma$	122	866, 876
$^G\gamma$	122	886, 904
ε	122	850
α1	117	149
α2	117	140, 142
ψα1	127	134
ζ	886	239
ψζ	1264	324

The sizes are given in nucleotide base pairs (bp). The two different sizes listed for the IVS-2 of the α2, $^G\gamma$, and $^A\gamma$ genes are the results of nucleotide sequence analysis of different genes.

bryonic α-like π' globin gene of the chicken demonstrates the same pattern as the ζ and ψζ genes with regard to a larger IVS-1 (577 bp) than IVS-2 (294 bp), but in this case, the introns do not contain a simple repeated sequence.[38]

The lengths of the large introns (IVS-2) of each of the human non–α globin genes (β, δ, $^A\gamma$, $^G\gamma$, and ε) are quite similar (see Table 7–2). Nevertheless, sequence analysis[39–44] and hybridization experiments[19] have shown that despite the homology in coding sequences of these genes, the nucleotide sequences of their large intervening sequences have diverged considerably from one another and share very little homology except in the case of the duplicated $^G\gamma$ and $^A\gamma$ globin genes.[44] On the other hand, there has been considerably more conservation of the nucleotide sequence of IVS-1 between some, but not all, of the non–α globin genes. For instance, there is definite homology between IVS-1 sequences in the β/δ, γ/ε, and β/ε gene pair comparisons but not in the β/γ gene pair comparison.[44] In the case of the α globin gene family, there has been considerable conservation of the sequence of IVS-1 and IVS-2 between the duplicated α globin genes and the ψα globin gene,[45–48] but there is little or no homology between the intron sequences of these genes and those of the ζ and ψζ genes,[35] except for the finding of several copies of the sequences CGG and CGGG in IVS-2 of the α globin genes, suggesting an origin for this simple repeat sequence in IVS-2 of the ζ-like genes.[35]

Fate of Intervening Sequences During Globin Gene Expression. The presence of intervening sequences that interrupt the coding sequences of structural genes imposes a requirement for some cellular process to prevent the occurrence of these sequences in the mature mRNA. It has been found that intervening sequences are in fact transcribed into globin (and other) precursor mRNA molecules[49–51] but that they are subsequently excised and the proper ends of the coding sequences religated to yield the mature mRNA. This post-transcriptional processing of mRNA precursors has been termed "splicing" and is illustrated schematically in Figure 7–5. Until recently, very little was known concerning the enzyme(s) and other cofactors involved in splicing. However, recent progress has been achieved in obtaining the synthesis of large amounts of precursor mRNA *in vitro*[52] as well as the splicing of precursor mRNA molecules in cell-free *in vitro* systems.[53–57a] These advances have started to lead to the elucidation of the biochemistry of this fascinating process.

One mechanism that has been postulated to occur during splicing is the association of the precursor mRNA with a low–molecular weight RNA species called U1 RNA that is a component of a small nuclear ribonucleoprotein particle, abbreviated snRNP.[58–61] The interesting feature of U1 RNA is that near its 5' extremity, it contains nucleotide sequences that are complementary to conserved ("consensus") sequences found at the 5' and 3' ends of introns (see later discussion).[62, 63] Thus, it has been proposed that base pairing of U1 RNA to pre-mRNA at its intron/exon junctions may facilitate the approximation or juxtaposition of coding sequences that must be ligated to one another after excision of the intervening sequences.[62–63a] Experimental evidence of a role for U1 RNA or its snRNP in the splicing process has recently begun to accumulate. The most convincing evidence of such an involvement consists of experiments demonstrating that antibodies directed against U1 RNA containing snRNPs, but not those directed against other snRNPs, can inhibit splicing in isolated nuclei[64] or in cell-free systems.[65–65b] Cell-free splicing can also be abolished by removal of the first eight nucleotides of U1 RNA that are thought to base pair with the nucleotides at the 5' splice site of precursor mRNA molecules.[65a] An important role for U1 snRNPs in the splicing process is therefore very likely.

Although some early reports suggested that excision of introns might occur in a stepwise or "piecemeal" fashion,[66–68] more recent analyses of splicing in cell-free systems[68a–68c] indicate that introns are excised in a single piece. Splicing appears to proceed in the following manner[68b–68d] (Fig. 7–5B): initial cleavage of the pre-mRNA at the 5' or donor site of the exon/intron junction, then formation of a peculiar covalent bond between the 5' end of the intron and a region of the intron approximately 18 to 37 nucleotides from the 3' end or acceptor site of the intron, generating a lariat-like or branched RNA structure. The covalent bond formed is a 2' to 5' nucleotide linkage (in contrast to the common 3' to 5' linkage), and it involves the G of the GT dinucleotide at the 5' end of the cleaved intron and the A residue in the recognition sequence

$$ACT^{TT}_{CC} \text{ or } ATC^{TT}_{CC}$$

that is usually located near the 3' end of the intron.[68b, 68e] This recognition sequence tends to be redundant in introns, and its use appears to be relatively nonstringent: Alternative sites can be utilized if the distal site is mutated. The final step in the splicing process is cleavage of the intron at its 3' end, which releases the lariat-like intron fragment, followed by the joining of the adjacent exons.

The enzymes or other cofactors necessary for splicing of globin mRNA precursor molecules are not restricted to erythroid cells; globin precursor mRNA molecules transcribed from heterologous globin genes introduced into monkey kidney cells or mouse fibroblasts are processed normally to yield mature globin mRNA,[69-72] as are globin precursor mRNA molecules microinjected into frog oocyte nuclei.[52] Thus, the splicing apparatus of higher eukaryotic cells appears to be rather universal and shows no evidence of species or tissue specificity. Studies of globin gene expression in the SV40 virus/monkey kidney cell gene transfer system also suggested that splicing may be a necessary process to ensure the synthesis of stable globin mRNA: Transcripts of intronless globin gene constructs did not accumulate to any appreciable degree in cells infected with SV40/globin recombinant viruses.[73, 74] It is possible, therefore, that splicing may be linked to some other process essential for normal mRNA biogenesis such as transport from nucleus to cytoplasm. Nevertheless, splicing is not absolutely essential for the normal expression of all genes in animal cells, since there are a number of examples of intronless genes, such as those for most histones, most heat-shock proteins of *Drosophila*, α and β interferons, and the enzyme thymidine kinase of herpes simplex virus. Gene transfer and expression studies of a number of different intron-containing genes have more recently shown that globin genes appear to be relatively unique in their requirement for splicing to produce stable cytoplasmic mRNA. However, the functional globin genes of the insect *Chironomus thummi thummi* are intronless,[74a] indicating that the requirement for globin precursor mRNA splicing must have been acquired at a point in evolution after the invertebrate/vertebrate divergence.

Preserved Sequences at Junctions Between Coding and Intervening Sequences. A crucial prerequisite for the proper splicing of globin (and other) precursor mRNA molecules is the presence of specific nucleotide sequences at the junctions between coding sequences (exons) and intervening sequences (introns).

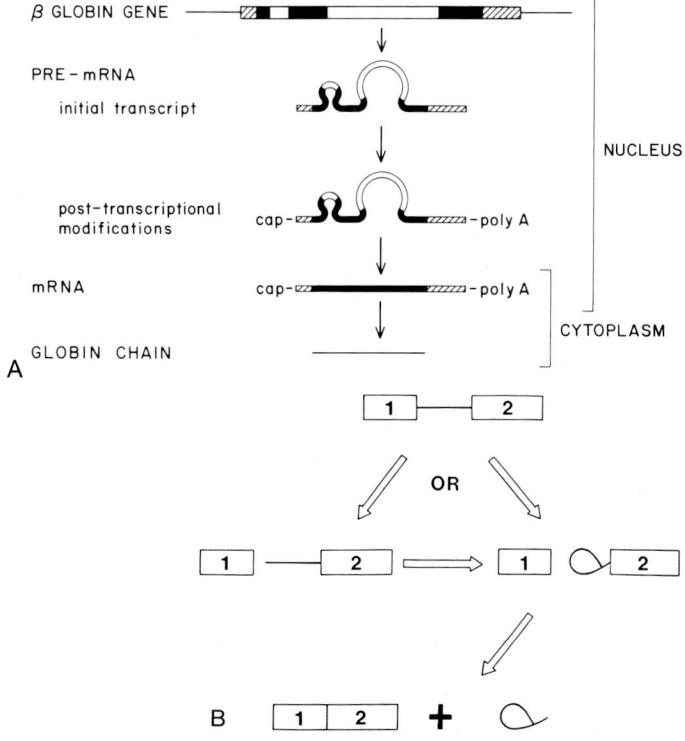

Figure 7–5. Schematic representation of the process of β globin gene expression. *A*, Overall process. *B*, Steps in excision of intron between exon 1 and exon 2. (*B*, from Ruskin, B., et al.: Cell *38*:317, 1984.)

Comparison of these sequences in many different genes has permitted the derivation of two different "consensus" sequences that are universally found at the 5' and 3' ends, respectively, of introns.[75] The specific sequences thus derived are as follows:

$$(5')^C_A AG\underline{GT}^A_G AGT ----- \begin{pmatrix} T \\ C \end{pmatrix}_n N^C_T \underline{AG}G (3')$$

where "N" represents any nucleotide and "n" a variable number of pyrimidine nucleotides equal to or greater than 11. The arrows indicate the sites within the consensus sequences where cleavage or splicing actually occurs. The 5' sequence is sometimes called the "donor" splice site, and the 3' sequence is known as the "acceptor" splice site. The underlined dinucleotides GT and AG, at the very 5' and 3' ends, respectively, of the intron, are essentially invariant and are thought to be absolutely required for proper splicing—the so-called "GT-AG rule."[76] The importance or significance of these consensus sequences is underscored by the fact that mutations that alter these normal consensus sequences or mutations that create consensus sequences at new sites in a globin gene lead to abnormal processing of globin mRNA precursors and constitute the molecular basis for many of the thalassemia syndromes, hereditary disorders characterized by decreased synthesis of α or β globin chains (see Chapter 8). Nevertheless, there is one example of a functional globin gene in the chicken with an intron that has a GC rather than a GT at its 5' splice site.[76a] As noted previously, another important conserved sequence near the 3' end of introns is the sequence

$$ACT^{TT}_{CC} \text{ or } ATC^{TT}_{CC},$$

which tends to be redundant and is involved in the formation of the branched RNA intermediate in the splicing reaction.[68b, 68e]

The requirement of internal sequences within IVS-2 of the β globin gene for proper precursor mRNA splicing has been thoroughly analyzed in deletion mutation experiments performed on the rabbit β globin gene[76b] and the human $^G\gamma$ globin gene.[76c] In separate 3' and 5' deletion mutants, it was found that a minimum of 6 bp at the 5' end of the intron and 20 to 24 bp at the 3' end of the intron were required for accurate and efficient splicing to occur. However, with a rabbit β globin minigene containing only these 6 5' and 24 3' nucleotides of the intron, no correctly spliced globin mRNA was obtained unless an additional 50 bp of nonspecific foreign DNA were inserted between the two ends of the intron. Therefore, it appears from these studies that no specific internal intron sequences are absolutely required for the normal accumulation of properly spliced globin mRNA but that a minimal intron length of at least 80 bp is an important requirement for splicing.

Functional and Evolutionary Implications of Intervening Sequences. There has been considerable discussion, speculation, and debate concerning the role and significance of intervening sequences in eukaryotic gene evolution and function. In other words: "Why genes in pieces?" A number of theories have been put forth to explain the "raison d'être" of this unusual phenomenon. A hypothesis was first presented by Gilbert,[77] then extended by Blake,[78] that introns separate regions of genes encoding different functional domains of proteins. From an evolutionary point of view, the ability of eukaryotic cells to splice out intervening sequences can permit and facilitate the juxtaposition and joint expression of DNA sequences previously more widely separated in the genome and brought together by various "illegitimate" recombination events. Thus, splicing can accelerate the rate at which selection during evolution can be exerted on the genome for favorable recombination events leading to the formation of fused proteins made possible by the permissive process of RNA splicing. This phenomenon has been called "exon shuffling."

In the case of globin and many other proteins, introns do in fact subdivide the gene into exons encoding distinct functional regions of the protein. Thus, the central exon of the different globin genes would appear to encode the entire heme-binding region, or heme "pocket," of the globin chain, whereas the two flanking exons encode non–heme-binding regions of the globin chain. A number of analyses have been performed to examine this possibility and have led to the conclusion that the peptide encoded by the central globin gene exon is, in fact, capable of performing essentially all of the major heme-binding functions of the complete globin chain[79, 80] and that it contains, as well, all of the $\alpha_1\beta_2$ intersubunit contacts.[79] However, the central exon peptide is not able, by itself, to maintain a stable complex of ferrous heme with molecular oxygen and requires the side exon products and the complementary heme-containing subunit to perform this function.[81]

A second theory, proposed by Go,[82] states that introns may interrupt a gene not necessarily between functional domains of the encoded protein but between modular structural subunits (subdomains or compact regions) of the protein based on a plot of the distances between α carbon atoms.[83–85] The analysis of such a plot of the structure of the β globin chain revealed the presence of four rather than three subdomains and suggested that there must have existed an ancestral globin or globin-like gene with a third intron, located in the center of the exon encoding the heme-binding domain and later lost during evolution.[82] Shortly after the publication of this theory, it was shown that the soybean leghemoglobin gene does in fact contain a third intron[86–88] precisely at the position predicted by the model of Go.

Preserved Sequences in 5'-Flanking DNA of Globin Genes

The DNA sequences flanking the 5' extremity of the human globin genes contain three sets of sequences that are common to all of these genes and are situated at relatively similar distances from the site of initiation of transcription of the globin genes (the 5' cap site of globin mRNA; see later discussion). The first preserved sequence is ATAA, which constitutes the so-called "ATA" box situated approximately 30 nucleotides from the cap site.[35, 44, 45, 48] The second preserved sequence is CCAAT, situated approximately 70 to 80 nucleotides from the cap site.[35, 44, 45, 48] In the case of the human δ globin gene, there are three CCAAT-like sequences, but none has the perfect "canonical" sequence; the closest is CCAAC.[42, 44, 45] In the case of both γ globin genes, the CCAAT sequence is duplicated.[40, 41, 44] The third preserved 5'-flanking sequence is somewhat more variable and is located approximately 80 to 100 nucleotides from the cap site: It has the general structure GGGGG^C_TG or the inverted form C^A_GCCCCC and may be duplicated in either a direct or inverted orientation.[26]

Similar conserved sequences have been found in the 5'-flanking DNA of a large number of other nonglobin eukaryotic genes and have been shown to be essential for normal gene transcription. They presumably constitute binding sites or other regulatory signals for RNA polymerase II. The role of these sequences in gene transcription has been tested in various cell-free and tissue culture cell systems capable of transcribing cloned gene fragments. Site-directed mutagenesis and deletion of specific 5'-flanking sequences have demonstrated their importance for the efficiency and/or accuracy of the transcription process.[89] In the case of globin genes specifically, the ATA box appears to be essential for high levels of transcription in cell-free systems[90, 91] but less so in intact cells, where its deletion or alteration seems to have an effect more on the accuracy of the site of transcription initiation than on the overall level of transcription.[92, 93]

In the case of the CCAAT box, it does not appear to be essential for cell-free transcription of globin genes[91] but is extremely important for efficient transcription of globin genes transferred into tissue culture cells,[92, 93] as are the conserved sequences further upstream between residues −80 to −100 from the cap site.[94, 95] As noted previously, the normal human δ globin gene does not have a perfectly conserved CCAAT sequence, and it has been proposed that this abnormality may be responsible, at least in part, for the normally low level of δ globin gene expression that occurs *in vivo*. Interestingly, transcription of cloned δ globin gene DNA in a cell-free system that depends essentially on an intact ATA box is not greatly diminished compared with other non-α globin gene DNA,[96] in contrast to the situation following gene transfer and CCAAT-box–dependent expression in tissue culture cells, where much lower levels of δ mRNA than of β mRNA are detected.[97]

The importance of these various 5'-flanking sequences for normal globin gene expression is also underscored by the fact that decreased expression of the β globin gene in certain forms of β thalassemia has been found to be due to nucleotide base substitutions in these sequences, specifically in and around the ATA box and the −80 to −100 region (see Chapter 8).

Globin mRNA Encoding Sequences

Untranslated Sequences. The transcript of the human globin genes that is represented in mature globin mRNA contains, in addition to the information required to encode the globin polypeptide chains, additional sequences at both extremities of the mRNA. These additional untranslated nucleotides account for approximately 30 per cent of the length of the globin mRNA. The 3' (C-terminal) untranslated sequences are two to three times the length of the 5' (N-terminal) untranslated sequences. The lengths of these sequences in the

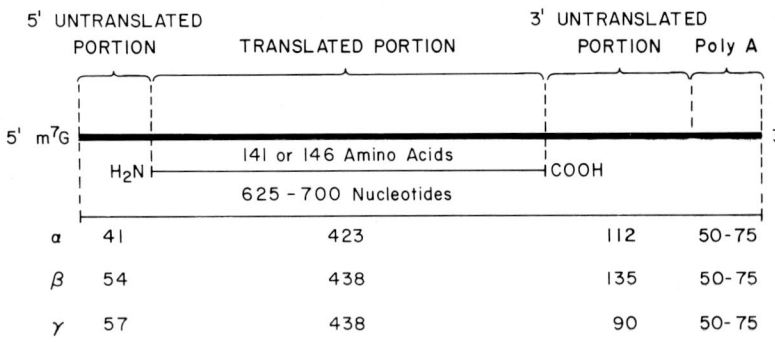

Figure 7–6. Relative sizes of translated and untranslated regions of the major human globin messenger RNAs. (From Forget, B. G.: Ann. Intern. Med. *91*:605, 1979.)

major human globin mRNAs are illustrated in Figure 7–6. Besides the nucleotides that are transcribed from the globin gene, the globin mRNA contains other nucleotides that are added to it in the nucleus following transcription—a methylated guanylic acid (m⁷G cap structure) at the 5′ extremity and a number of adenylic acid residues constituting the poly(A) at the 3′ extremity of the mRNA. The precise functions of these untranslated sequences in globin and other mRNAs are not completely known. However, the 5′ methylated cap structure appears to be important for the initiation of polypeptide chain synthesis through its interaction with specific initiation factors as well as for accurate splicing of the precursor mRNA molecules. The poly(A) tail of mRNAs appears to contribute to the stability of the mRNA.

5′ Untranslated Sequences. The very 5′ terminus of globin and other eukaryotic mRNAs is occupied by a group of two or three modified nucleotides linked to one another in an unusual manner and commonly referred to as a "cap." This cap structure has the following composition: It consists of a guanylic acid residue methylated in the number 7 position of the purine ring (m⁷G) bound to the following nucleotide in a reversed (5′–5′) pyrophosphate linkage. The m⁷G is added post-transcriptionally, but the adjacent (second) nucleotide is derived from the site of initiation of transcription of the gene. The second nucleotide of the mRNA, and occasionally the third nucleotide as well, may also be methylated post-transcriptionally in its ring structure or its ribose, hence the designation of the overall 5′ terminal structure—m⁷GppmNmNmN. There is convincing evidence that the 5′ cap is important for optimal mRNA function. Removal of the cap by various chemical or enzymatic treatments markedly decreases the ability of the mRNA to initiate protein synthesis in various cell-free protein synthesizing systems. The cap has been shown to combine to a specific initiation factor required for protein synthesis, and synthetic analogues of the cap can inhibit the function of this initiation factor *in vitro*.[97a] Although the cap structure is important for optimal mRNA function, it is probably not an absolute requirement for initiation of protein synthesis by most cellular mRNAs. A role for the cap in the metabolism and processing of nuclear precursor mRNA molecules has also been recognized recently. The cap appears to be important for the maintenance of stability of precursor mRNAs injected into frog oocyte nuclei.[52] In different cell-free splicing systems, the cap also appears to be required for efficient splicing[97b] and for the prevention of aberrant splicing.[57a]

The 5′ untranslated sequences of the various globin genes and their corresponding mRNAs contain additional preserved nucleotide sequences. The dinucleotide AC is found immediately following the cap site in all of the globin genes except the ε gene, where AT is found. This dinucleotide, however, is not universally present in other nonglobin eukaryotic mRNAs and is therefore not a true capping signal analogous to the consensus splicing signals described previously. Another preserved sequence in the 5′ noncoding region of globin mRNAs is the hexanucleotide sequence CTTCTG (or CTTCCG in the ε gene), which is found starting at a point eight nucleotides to the 3′ side of the cap site in the various non–α globin genes. In the human α globin genes, the corresponding sequence is found starting at a point four nucleotides from the cap site, but in the ζ globin gene, this exact sequence is not found, although a somewhat homologous sequence, GTCCTG, is located at a point starting 11 nucleotides from the cap site. Analysis of the nucleotide sequence of the 5′ noncoding regions of many different eukaryotic mRNAs has revealed the frequent, although not invariant, presence of the sequence $CTT{}^{C}_{T}TG$.[98] It has been postulated that this sequence, which is complementary to a sequence at the 3' end of 18S ribosomal RNA, might play a role in the binding of mRNAs to the small ribosomal subunit;[99, 99a] an analogous ribosome-binding sequence has been shown to be very important for the function of prokaryotic mRNAs.[100] Comparison of the 5' noncoding sequences of many different eukaryotic mRNAs reveals that a number of them lack the presumed binding sequence yet function perfectly well.[98, 101] The initiator codon (AUG) and adjacent nucleotides forming the sequence

$$CC^A_GCCAUGG^{102}$$ appear to constitute the

only recognizable signal or consensus sequence in the 5' noncoding sequence of eukaryotic mRNAs, and it has been proposed that this sequence may constitute the ribosome-binding sequence as well as the signal for initiation of mRNA translation.[98, 102, 103]

3' Untranslated Sequences. In newly synthesized mRNAs the 3' terminal poly(A) tail consists of approximately 200 nucleotides. In reticulocytes, the steady state globin mRNA has a long half-life, and its poly(A) tail is considerably shorter and variable in length, consisting of approximately 50 to 75 nucleotides. The precise function of the poly(A) tail is not known. It is clear, however, that it and the entire 3' noncoding region are not essential for translation of globin mRNA because RNA transcripts of globin cDNA lacking these sequences are effectively translated *in vitro*.[104] On the other hand, a number of studies have demonstrated that absence of poly(A) from globin mRNA drastically decreases the stability of the mRNA and shortens its effective half-life, at least when translation of the mRNA is studied after its microinjection into *Xenopus* oocytes.[105] Increased stability may be conferred on the mRNA by the poly(A) because of changes in the secondary structure of the mRNA or because of binding of specific proteins to the poly(A) sequence. Not all mRNAs, however, contain poly(A). Histone mRNA is a notable exception, and total cellular mRNA of animal cells also contains a class of poly(A)$^-$ mRNA species distinct from the poly(A)$^+$ mRNA species.

The 3' noncoding sequences of globin mRNA that are transcribed from the globin genes themselves constitute the region of the mRNA structure that varies the most between different globin mRNA species. Even the closely related $^G\gamma$ and $^A\gamma$ globin genes show 7 per cent divergence of nucleotide sequence in their 3' noncoding regions.[44] In the case of the two α globin genes, the divergence is even greater (21 per cent),[45, 46, 48, 106] and this finding has been used to devise molecular assays that permit the identification and differentiation of the specific mRNA transcripts of the α1 and α2 globin genes.[107-108a] The one common feature of the 3' noncoding sequence of globin and other mRNAs (except for nonpolyadenylated histone mRNAs) is the presence of a hexanucleotide AAUAAA approximately 20 nucleotides from the poly(A) tail.[109] It was initially assumed[109] and subsequently demonstrated experimentally that this consensus sequence constitutes a necessary signal for the proper processing and polyadenylation of the 3' end of mRNA transcripts.[110, 110a] Base substitutions in this consensus sequence have also been shown to be responsible for certain types of thalassemia due to faulty processing and polyadenylation of globin mRNA transcripts (see Chapter 8). It appears that the AAUAAA and a second downstream sequence[110b, 110c] are signals not only for poly(A) addition but also, perhaps more importantly, for the proper cleavage of the primary RNA transcripts of globin (and other) genes that normally extend beyond the site of polyadenylation (as discussed later).[110c] The nucleotide immediately preceding the site of poly(A) addition in globin and other mRNAs is almost always C, and GC is the most common, although not invariant, dinucleotide at this site.

Coding Sequences. The complete nucleotide sequences of the coding as well as noncoding regions of the human α2, β, and $^G\gamma$ mRNAs are shown in Figure 7–7. These sequences were determined initially from the analysis of synthetic DNA copies (cDNAs) made from the mRNAs by viral reverse transcriptase enzyme and sequenced either directly or after cloning and amplification in bacterial plasmids.[111] The sequences were subsequently confirmed, and in some cases revised, after the analysis of the cloned chromosomal genes,[35, 39-47] which also provided sequence information of the human δ, ε, and ζ globin encoding sequences; ζ globin cDNA was also cloned,[112] and its sequence agreed with the genomic ζ globin gene sequence.[35]

A striking and initially surprising feature that was noted from the analysis of the nucleotide sequence of the coding portion of various globin mRNAs was the presence of a marked bias in the use of certain codons for certain amino acids. This finding was first observed in the case of the human and rabbit β globin mRNAs that were the first to be sequenced[113, 114] and has been a consistent feature of all globin mRNAs as well as of other nonglobin eukaryotic mRNAs. The codon usage

182 MOLECULAR GENETICS AND BIOSYNTHESIS OF HEMOGLOBIN

```
                                          -10                    -5                           0
                         m⁷GpppA  CUC  UUC  UGG  UCC  CCA  CAG  ACU  CAG  AGA  GAA  CCC  ACC  [AUG]
                1                       5                       10                      15                      20
                Val  Leu  Ser  Pro  Ala  Asp  Lys  Thr  Asn  Val  Lys  Ala  Ala  Trp  Gly  Lys  Val  Gly  Ala  His
                GUG  CUG  UCU  CCU  GCC  GAC  AAG  ACC  AAC  GUC  AAG  GCC  GCC  UGG  GGC  AAG  GUU  GGC  GCG  CAC
                21                      25                      30                      35                      40
                Ala  Gly  Glu  Tyr  Gly  Ala  Glu  Ala  Leu  Glu  Arg  Met  Phe  Leu  Ser  Phe  Pro  Thr  Thr  Lys
                GCU  GGC  GAG  UAU  GGU  GCG  GAG  GCC  CUG  GAG  AGG  AUG  UUC  CUG  UCC  UUC  CCC  ACC  ACC  AAG
                41                      45                      50                      55                      60
                Thr  Tyr  Phe  Pro  His  Phe  Asp  Leu  Ser  His  Gly  Ser  Ala  Gln  Val  Lys  Gly  His  Gly  Lys
                ACC  UAC  UUC  CCG  CAC  UUC  GAC  CUG  AGC  CAC  GGC  UCU  GCC  CAG  GUU  AAG  GGC  CAC  GGC  AAG
                61                      65                      70                      75                      80
                Lys  Val  Ala  Asp  Ala  Leu  Thr  Asn  Ala  Val  Ala  His  Val  Asp  Asp  Met  Pro  Asn  Ala  Leu
                AAG  GUG  GCC  GAC  GCG  CUG  ACC  AAC  GCC  GUG  GCG  CAC  GUG  GAC  GAC  AUG  CCC  AAC  GCG  CUG
                81                      85                      90                      95                     100
                Ser  Ala  Leu  Ser  Asp  Leu  His  Ala  His  Lys  Leu  Arg  Val  Asp  Pro  Val  Asn  Phe  Lys  Leu
                UCC  GCC  CUG  AGC  GAC  CUG  CAC  GCG  CAC  AAG  CUU  CGG  GUG  GAC  CCG  GUC  AAC  UUC  AAG  CUC
                101                     105                     110                     115                     120
                Leu  Ser  His  Cys  Leu  Leu  Val  Thr  Leu  Ala  Ala  His  Leu  Pro  Ala  Glu  Phe  Thr  Pro  Ala
                CUA  AGC  CAC  UGC  CUG  CUG  GUG  ACC  CUG  GCC  GCC  CAC  CUC  CCC  GCC  GAG  UUC  ACC  CCU  GCG
                121                     125                     130                     135                     140
                Val  His  Ala  Ser  Leu  Asp  Lys  Phe  Leu  Ala  Ser  Val  Ser  Thr  Val  Leu  Thr  Ser  Lys  Tyr
                GUG  CAC  GCC  UCC  CUG  GAC  AAG  UUC  CUG  GCU  UCU  GUG  AGC  ACC  GUG  CUG  ACC  UCC  AAA  UAC
                141         Term        145                     150                     155                     160
                Arg  [UAA]  Ala  Gly  Ala  Ser  Val  Ala  Val  Pro  Pro  Ala  Arg  Trp  Ala  Ser  Gln  Arg  Ala  Leu
                CGU  [CAA]  GCU  GGA  GCC  UCG  GUA  GCC  GUU  CCU  CCU  GCC  CGC  UGG  GCC  UCC  CAA  CGG  GCC  CUC
                       Gln
                161                     165                     170                     175
                Leu  Pro  Ser  Leu  His  Arg  Pro  Phe  Leu  Val  Phe  Glu   Term
                CUC  CCC  UCC  UUG  CAC  CGG  CCC  UUC  CUG  GUC  UUU  G[AA  UAA]  AGU  CUG  AGU  GGG  CGG  C-Poly(A)
A
```

```
                                               -15                              -10
                                m⁷GpppAC  AUU  UGC  UUC  UGA  CAC  AAC  UGU  GUU  CAC
             -5                           0                        5                            10
        UAG  CAA  CCU  CAA  ACA  GAC  ACC  [AUG]  GUG  CAC  CUG  ACU  CCU  GAG  GAG  AAG  UCU  GCC  GUU
                         15                           20                           25                           30
        ACU  GCC  CUG  UGG  GGC  AAG  GUG  AAC  GUG  GAU  GAA  GUU  GGU  GGU  GAG  GCC  CUG  GGC  AGG
                              35                           40                           45
        CUG  CUG  GUG  GUC  UAC  CCU  UGG  ACC  CAG  AGG  UUC  UUU  GAG  UCC  UUU  GGG  GAU  CUG  UCC
        50                           55                           60                           65
        ACU  CCU  GAU  GCU  GUU  AUG  GGC  AAC  CCU  AAG  GUG  AAG  GCU  CAU  GGC  AAG  AAA  GUG  CUC
        70                           75                           80                           85
        GGU  GCC  UUU  AGU  GAU  GGC  CUG  GCU  CAC  CUG  GAC  AAC  CUC  AAG  GGC  ACC  UUU  GCC  ACA
             90                           95                           100                          105
        CUG  AGU  GAG  CUG  CAC  UGU  GAC  AAG  CUG  CAC  GUG  GAU  CCU  GAG  AAC  UUC  AGG  CUC  CUG
                  110                          115                          120                               125
        GGC  AAC  GUG  CUG  GUC  UGU  GUG  CUG  GCC  CAU  CAC  UUU  GGC  AAA  GAA  UUC  ACC  CCA  CCA
                       130                          135                          140
        GUG  CAG  GCU  GCC  UAU  CAG  AAA  GUG  GUG  GCU  GGU  GUG  GCU  AAU  GCC  CUG  GCC  CAC  AAG
        145                          150                          155                          160
        UAU  CAC  [UAA]  GCU  CGC  UUU  CUU  GCU  GUC  CAA  UUU  CUA  UUA  AAG  GUU  CCU  UUG  UUC  CCU
             165                          170                          175                          180
        AAG  UCC  AAC  UAC  UAA  ACU  GGG  GGA  UAU  UAU  GAA  GGG  CCU  UGA  GCA  UCU  GGA  UUC  UGC
        CU[A  AUA  AA]A  AAC  AUU  UAU  UUU  CAU  UGC  POLY A
B
```

Figure 7–7. Nucleotide sequences of the major human globin mRNAs. The initiation codon, termination codon, and polyadenylation signal of each mRNA are enclosed in boxes. *A*, α2 globin mRNA, showing mutation and readthrough product of chain termination mutant Hb Constant Spring. *B*, β globin mRNA.

Illustration continued on opposite page

m7GpppAC ACU CGC UUC UGG AAC GUC UGA GGU UAU CAA UAA GCU CCU AGU CCA GAC GCC [AUG]

```
 1               5                          10                         15                         20
Gly His Phe Thr Glu Glu Asp Lys Ala Thr Ile Thr Ser Leu Trp Gly Lys Val Asn Val
GGU CAU UUC ACA GAG GAG GAC AAG GCU ACU AUC ACA AGC CUG UGG GGC AAG GUG AAU GUG

21                          25                         30                         35                         40
Glu Asp Ala Gly Gly Glu Thr Leu Gly Arg Leu Leu Val Val Tyr Pro Trp Thr Gln Arg
GAA GAU GCU GGA GGA GAA ACC CUG GGA AGG CUC CUG GUU GUC UAC CCA UGG ACC CAG AGG

41                          45                         50                         55                         60
Phe Phe Asp Ser Phe Gly Asn Leu Ser Ser Ala Ser Ala Ile Met Gly Asn Pro Lys Val
UUC UUU GAC AGC UUU GGC AAC CUG UCC UCU GCC UCU GCC AUC AUG GGC AAC CCC AAA GUC

61                          65                         70                         75                         80
Lys Ala His Gly Lys Lys Val Leu Thr Ser Leu Gly Asp Ala Ile Lys His Leu Asp Asp
AAG GCA CAU GGC AAG AAG GUG CUG ACU UCC UUG GGA GAU GCC AUA AAG CAC CUG GAU GAU

81                          85                         90                         95                        100
Leu Lys Gly Thr Phe Ala Gln Leu Ser Glu Leu His Cys Asp Lys Leu His Val Asp Pro
CUC AAG GGC ACC UUU GCC CAG CUG AGU GAA CUG CAC UGU GAC AAG CUG CAU GUG GAU CCU

101                        105                        110                        115                        120
Glu Asn Phe Lys Leu Leu Gly Asn Val Leu Val Thr Val Leu Ala Ile His Phe Gly Lys
GAG AAC UUC AAG CUC CUG GGA AAU GUG CUG GUG ACC GUU UUG GCA AUC CAU UUC GGC AAA

121                        125                        130                        135                        140
Glu Phe Thr Pro Glu Val Gln Ala Ser Trp Gln Lys Met Val Thr Gly Val Ala Ser Ala
GAA UUC ACC CCU GAG GUG CAG GCU UCC UGG CAG AAG AUG GUG ACU GGA GUG GCC AGU GCC

141                        145
Leu Ser Ser Arg Tyr His
CUG UCC UCC AGA UAC CAC [UGA] GCU CGC UGC CCA UGA UGC AGA GCU UUC AAG GAU AGG CUU

UAU UCU GCA AGC AAU ACA AAU [AAU AAA] UCU AUU CUG CUA AGA GAU CAC polyA
C
```

Figure 7–7. *Continued. C,* $^G\gamma$ *globin mRNA.*

in the human α, β, and γ mRNAs is shown in Figure 7–8. In the case of certain amino acid codons in a given globin mRNA, there does not appear to be any preferential use of codons; all possible codons for a given amino acid are utilized in an apparently random fashion or at least without a statistically significant bias. For example, in the case of human β and γ mRNAs (but not α mRNA), the two possible codons for phenylalanine are both used with approximately equal frequency. On the other hand, in the case of other amino acids, in particular the amino acids that are the most abundant in globin chains, such as leucine and valine, there is a marked preference in all three human globin mRNAs for use of one particular codon out of the possible four or six—CUG in the case of leucine, which is utilized 41 times out of 53 possible opportunities, and GUG for valine, which is utilized 31 times out of 44 possible opportunities (see Fig. 7–8).

There is one notable aspect in which codon usage in α (and ζ) globin mRNA differs significantly from that in the non–α globin mRNAs, probably as a result of the somewhat unusual overall base composition of α globin mRNA. In total human DNA, the C + G base composition is approximately 40 per cent, and as in most eukaryotic mRNAs, there is a bias against the occurrence of CG dinucleotides. Human α globin mRNA, on the other hand, has a C + G content of 64.7 per cent (versus approximately 51 per cent for β and γ mRNAs) and manifests no bias against CG dinucleotides, which occur at or above the expected frequency for the base composition of the mRNA. As a result, codons containing C or G in the third position or containing the CG dinucleotide sequence occur much more frequently in the α mRNA than in the non–α mRNAs. For example, the codons CCG for proline and GCG for alanine are used in 2 out of 7 and in 7 out of 21 possible opportunities, respectively, in human α mRNA but are not found in a total of 11 and 26 opportunities, respectively, in β and γ mRNAs (see Fig. 7–8). In the case of arginine, which has six possible codons (four CGN codons, AGA, and AGG), two of three codons in human α mRNA are CGN-containing codons and one is AGG, whereas in β and γ mRNAs, all four possible CGN codons are avoided, and of the six arginine codons, five are AGG and one is AGA.

The causes or potential advantages to the organism of bias in codon usage for globin and other mRNAs are not immediately evident. Although the specific characteristics of the bias can vary somewhat from one specialized tissue

1 \ 2		U	α	β	γ		C	α	β	γ		A	α	β	γ		G	α	β	γ	2/3
U	Phe	UUU	0	5	3	Ser	UCU	3	1	2	Tyr	UAU	1	2	0	Cys	UGU	0	2	1	U
		UUC	7	3	5		UCC	4	2	5		UAC	2	1	2		UGC	1	0	0	C
	Leu	UUA	0	0	0		UCA	0	0	0	Term	UAA	1	1	0	Term	UGA	0	0	1	A
		UUG	0	0	2		UCG	0	0	0		UAG	0	0	0	Trp	UGG	1	2	3	G
C	Leu	CUU	1	0	1	Pro	CCU	2	5	2	His	CAU	0	2	4	Arg	CGU	1	0	0	U
		CUC	2	3	3		CCC	3	0	1		CAC	10	7	3		CGC	0	0	0	C
		CUA	1	0	0		CCA	0	2	1	Gln	CAA	0	0	0		CGA	0	0	0	A
		CUG	14	15	11		CCG	2	0	0		CAG	1	3	4		CGG	1	0	0	G
A	Ileu	AUU	0	0	0	Thr	ACU	0	3	3	Asn	AAU	0	1	2	Ser	AGU	0	2	2	U
		AUC	0	0	3		ACC	9	3	5		AAC	4	5	3		AGC	4	0	2	C
		AUA	0	0	1		ACA	0	1	2	Lys	AAA	1	3	2	Arg	AGA	0	0	1	A
	Met	AUG	2	1	2		ACG	0	0	0		AAG	10	8	8		AGG	1	3	2	G
G	Val	GUU	1	3	2	Ala	GCU	2	6	3	Asp	GAU	0	5	5	Gly	GGU	2	4	1	U
		GUC	3	2	2		GCC	12	9	6		GAC	8	2	3		GGC	5	8	6	C
		GUA	0	0	0		GCA	0	0	2	Glu	GAA	0	2	4		GGA	0	0	6	A
		GUG	9	13	9		GCG	7	0	0		GAG	4	6	4		GGG	0	1	0	G

Figure 7–8. Codon usage in the human α2, β, and $^G\gamma$ globin mRNAs.

to another where one protein is the major gene product expressed, in general the bias is similar in different related organisms, i.e., the same general codon bias is observed in all mammalian mRNA species, but a different bias is observed in lower eukaryotes and in animal viruses.[115] Therefore, it appears that codon bias is specific for related genome types and may constitute part of a genome "strategy" for the modulation of gene expression.[116]

An interesting corollary to the phenomenon of bias in mRNA codon usage is the finding that the distribution of various tRNA isoacceptor species for a given amino acid in total reticulocyte tRNA shows a pronounced preponderance of certain isoacceptor species of tRNA over other possible species.[117, 118] Those isoacceptor tRNA species that are most abundant in reticulocyte tRNA are those in which the anticodons are complementary to the codons that are most frequently utilized in the globin mRNAs: For instance, the isoacceptor tRNA species for leucine that is the most abundant in reticulocyte tRNA is the one that responds to the codon CUG. A similar pattern is found for the relative abundance of specific isoacceptor tRNA species for other amino acid codons. One can consider this phenomenon in two general ways. First, the selection of the various tRNA isoacceptor species could be an adaptative phenomenon that occurs during differentiation of the cell and specialization of its protein synthetic functions. In other words, since many tRNA isoacceptor species are not required for globin synthesis owing to selection or bias in codon usage at the globin mRNA level, these corresponding tRNA species may not accumulate or persist within the reticulocyte. Either they are not transcribed from their respective genes as abundantly as in other less specialized cells, or the tRNAs are initially synthesized in normal amounts but are then degraded and disappear from the cell because of lack of use. Alternatively, the synthesis of certain tRNA species in a selective manner within erythroid cells may be a specific characteristic and requirement of erythroid cell differentiation and may have resulted in selective pressure for certain codons to selectively accumulate and persist within globin genes during the process of evolution. There are currently insufficient data to prefer one hypothesis over the other.

The availability of the precise nucleotide sequence of the coding sequences of the various globin genes has also made possible a more thorough analysis of the evolutionary relationships between these genes than is possible from comparisons of amino acid sequences alone. This topic will be discussed in a separate section.

Pseudogenes

Detailed analysis of various cloned fragments of human globin gene DNA has revealed that between the known functional human globin genes, there are additional DNA sequences that share sequence homology with the well-characterized globin loci. These sequences constitute additional genes or gene-like structures that do not correspond to known globin polypeptide chains, and they have been termed "pseudogenes." A similar phenomenon has been identified in the globin gene clusters of other animal species such as the rabbit, mouse, goat, and sheep, as well as in nonglobin gene systems. Structural analysis of globin pseudogenes has revealed the presence of a number of structural anomalies that would prevent normal expression of these genes (reviewed in ref. 119). In the case of the human globin genes, two presumed pseudogenes were initially identified in the non-α globin gene cluster[20]—one between the $^A\gamma$ gene and the δ globin gene (ψβ1) and another situated 5' to the ε gene that was tentatively called ψβ2. Nucleotide sequence analysis of ψβ1 has confirmed it to be a typical pseudogene with nonsense mutations in the coding region as well as other mutations involving the initiation codon and the 5'-flanking consensus sequences important for gene transcription.[120, 121] On the other hand, ψβ2 was found not to be a true pseudogene but to consist of a long stretch of A + T residues[122] that must have been responsible for the hybridization signal obtained with the AT-tailed globin cDNA probe that was used in the initial analysis.

In the human α-like globin gene cluster, one pseudogene (ψα1) was initially identified 5' to the α2 globin gene,[21] and its nucleotide sequence has been determined.[47] This ψα1 is a typical pseudogene and contains a number of structural anomalies that would prevent its normal expression. These include (1) the sequence GTG instead of ATG at the position of the initiation codon; (2) a 20-nucleotide deletion in the coding sequence that abolishes the codons for amino acids 38 to 45 and generates, by frameshift, three in-phase termination codons in the remainder of the coding sequence; (3) replacement of the normal dinucleotide sequence GT at the 5' extremity of both intervening sequences by the dinucleotides GC and GA, respectively; (4) deletion of 23 nucleotides between the CCAAT and ATA boxes in the 5'-flanking DNA; and (5) mutation of the polyadenylation signal AATAAA to AATGAA. Functional studies of the ψα1 gene have been performed in cell-free transcription systems as well as after gene transfer into tissue culture cells:[96, 123] The transcriptional capacity of the gene was decreased 3- to 10-fold compared with a normal α globin gene, and there was total failure of polyadenylation at the normal site. The ζ-like gene situated close to the 5' side of the ψα1 gene was initially thought to represent a functional duplicated ζ globin gene,[21] but subsequent nucleotide sequence analysis revealed that it was in fact a pseudogene.[35] In contrast to other pseudogenes, however, it does not have a large number of abnormalities. It contains one nonsense mutation (at codon position 6) and only two additional base substitutions compared with the normal ζ coding sequence, causing two amino acid replacements.[35] This pseudogene has therefore presumably developed only in the relatively recent evolutionary past.

The majority of globin pseudogenes appear to have arisen by gene duplication events within the globin gene clusters, followed by mutation and inactivation of the duplicated gene and subsequent accumulation of additional mutations through loss of selective pressure. However, a second mechanism has been implicated in the generation of globin (and other) pseudogenes that are found at chromosomal locations different from those of the normal genes—the synthesis in the cell of cDNA copies of the mature mRNA followed by their integration at apparently random sites within the genome. Such pseudogenes have been called "processed genes" and are characterized by the absence of the usual intervening sequences and the presence within the DNA sequence of a poly(dA) stretch at the 3' end of the gene in the position corresponding to the normal poly(A) site of the mRNA.[123a] A processed α globin pseudogene has been identified in the mouse[119, 123a, 123b] but not in man. As noted previously, the normal globin genes of an insect lack introns,[74a] but these genes probably lost their introns by a recombination event (gene conversion) and not by the mechanism leading to processed pseudogenes.

Intergene DNA

Size of Duplication Units of Closely Related Globin Genes. Analysis of different human

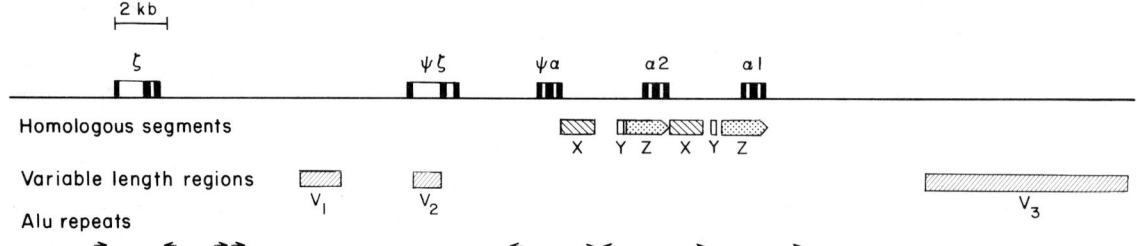

Figure 7–9. Structural features of the human α globin gene cluster. The homologous sequence segments X, Y, and Z presumably arose as a result of a gene duplication event involving the single ancestral α globin gene and its flanking DNA. The nature of the variable length regions V_1, V_2, and V_3 is discussed in the text. (Modified from Collins, F. S., and Weissman, S. M.: Prog. Nucleic Acid Res. Mol. Biol. *31*:315, 1984.)

globin gene fragments by hybridization to one another (so-called heteroduplex formation) and by restriction endonuclease analysis has permitted the definition of the degree of sequence homology in the flanking DNA of closely related globin genes that evolved from one another by relatively recent gene duplication events. In the case of the human δ/β globin gene pair, there is very little homology of the flanking DNA to either side of the actual structural gene regions; similarly, the large intervening sequences of these genes share little or no sequence homology. In contrast, in the case of the $^G\gamma/^A\gamma$ and α1/α2 globin gene pairs, not only do the intervening sequences share considerable sequence homology but so do substantial lengths of the flanking DNA adjacent to these genes. These gene pairs therefore consist of duplication units of structural gene sequences plus flanking DNA. In the case of the γ globin genes, the duplication unit is approximately 5 kb in length,[40, 41] and in the case of the α globin genes, it is approximately 4 kb.[21, 48] However, in contrast to the situation in the γ globin gene duplication unit, the α globin gene duplication unit is interrupted at two points by nonhomologous sequences[21, 48] (see Fig. 7–9). The flanking DNA to the 3' side of the ψα1 gene also shares considerable homology with the 3'-flanking DNA of the α2 (but not the α1) globin gene (Fig. 7–9), suggesting that this pseudogene originated from a duplication event of the normal α2 globin gene.[47] This 5' homology block (X in Figure 7–9) demonstrates a gradient of sequence divergence in the 5' to 3' direction.[123c]

Such duplication units probably resulted from a process of gene matching or gene conversion during evolution that allowed for recombination between duplicated genes and provided a mechanism for correction of the nucleotide sequence of one gene against that of another and for maintenance of gene numbers.[21, 40, 96, 124] However, this type of gene structure could also lead to loss of globin genes by nonhomologous crossing-over events. Such events have in fact been observed during propagation of recombinant DNA clones *in vitro*[20, 21] and have been implicated as the molecular basis for certain forms of α and γ thalassemia as well as for triplication events of the α and γ globin genes (see Chapter 8).

Repetitive DNA Sequences. *Alu I Family Sequences*. Analysis of cloned gene fragments has also revealed the presence, within the human globin gene clusters, of short repetitive DNA sequences that are found interspersed in many other sites of the human genome. These repetitive DNA sequences occur as single copies or as double copies in an inverted-repeat orientation. In the non–α gene cluster, they are found to the 5' side of the ε gene and to either side of the γ gene pair and of the δ/β gene pair[20, 125–130] (Fig. 7–10). In the α gene cluster, they are found to either side of each of the α and other α-like globin genes[21, 131, 132] (see Fig. 7–9). The precise role of these repetitive DNA sequences is unknown. However, it has been shown that the repetitive DNA sequences isolated from the human globin gene clusters can be transcribed *in vitro* by RNA polymerase III to yield discrete, low–molecular weight (and rarely larger) RNA species of unknown function.[125–128, 131–133b] Nucleotide sequence analysis of these repetitive DNA segments[134] has confirmed that they belong to the Alu I family of repetitive DNA sequences,[135] so called because of the presence of a recognition site for this restriction endonuclease in the center of the repeat sequence.[136, 136a] These repetitive sequences are approximately 300 nucleotides in length and occur approximately 300,000 times within the human genome. The various Alu I family sequences within the genome share approximately 80 per cent homology, and some of these sequences are transcribed *in vivo* since RNA sequences have been isolated from nuclear and cytoplasmic RNA of human cells that are, at least in part, complementary to Alu I family repetitive sequence DNA.[137–140a] There is even evidence that certain Alu I sequences in the human non-α globin gene cluster are in fact transcribed specifically in erythroid cells that are expressing the adjacent globin gene.[141, 142] Alu I family sequences are usually flanked by short, direct repeat sequences of DNA, a finding that is consistent with Alu I DNA sequences being a form of transposable DNA element, and it has been suggested that these DNA elements may have been generated by reverse transcription of RNA transcripts followed by integration of the DNA copies into the genome.[143–145] They may represent processed pseudogenes of an abundant cytoplasmic RNA (7SL RNA).[145a] The involvement and possible role of these sequences in various globin gene deletion syndromes will be discussed in Chapter 8.

Kpn I Family Sequences. In addition to the short, interspersed, repetitive sequences of Alu I family DNA, longer stretches of less frequently reiterated repetitive DNA sequences have also been found in the human non-α globin gene cluster. These sequences are located to the 3' side of the β gene[146, 147] and to the 5' side of the $^G\gamma$ gene[148, 149] (Fig. 7–10) and have been shown[150] to be members of a family of repetitive DNA sequences called the Kpn I family, so called because of the frequent occurrence in these sequences of recognition sites for this restriction endonuclease.[26, 136a, 151, 152] The general structure of this family of repetitive DNA sequences consists of a stretch of DNA, ranging in length from 1.5 to over 6 kb, in which there are subsets of repetitive DNA sequences that can be arranged in different ways in different individual 6-kb units. For instance, as shown in Figure 7–10, the two long stretches of Kpn I family DNA in the non-α globin gene cluster share two subsets of sequences in common, whereas they differ in a third subset. Shorter versions of Kpn I family repetitive DNA sequences are also found in the non-α gene cluster further to the 3' side of the β globin gene[149, 150] (see Fig. 7–10) and to the 5' side of the ε globin gene.[26, 122]

As in the case of the Alu I family repetitive DNA sequences, the function of the Kpn I family repetitive DNA is unknown. These sequences are transcribed into RNA molecules of various sizes,[153–154b] which are found virtually exclusively in the nucleus of cells[153] and have as yet an undefined role. Nucleotide sequence analysis of a Kpn I repeat in man and an analogous sequence in the mouse has revealed the presence of a long open reading frame potentially capable of encoding a protein.[154c, 154d] A characteristic feature of the structure of the Kpn I family repetitive DNA sequences is the presence of a poly(dA) sequence at one extremity.[155, 155a] This finding has been interpreted as evidence that these DNA sequences originated as cDNA copies of polyadenylated RNA species that were then integrated into the genome in the manner of transposable DNA elements.[155] The finding of directly repeated DNA sequences to either side of some Kpn I family repetitive DNA elements that have been totally sequenced[156, 156a] gives added credence to this thesis. However, not all Kpn I family repetitive DNA elements are flanked by direct repeats.[155a]

Other Repetitive DNA Sequences. A third type of repetitive DNA sequence has been identified in the intergene DNA between the δ and β globin genes. This sequence, which has a length of approximately 250 bp, shares sequence homology with the nontranscribed spacer DNA located between the repeated ribosomal RNA genes of the mouse.[157] It is not usually recognized as a repetitive DNA sequence in gene mapping studies using the method of Southern because of the standard use, in the molecular hybridization step of this technique, of "carrier" salmon sperm DNA, which effectively competes with this repetitive sequence for hybridization sites owing to shared sequence homology. This repetitive DNA sequence has been highly conserved dur-

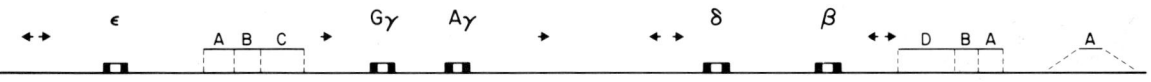

Figure 7–10. Location of repetitive DNA sequences in the human non-α globin gene cluster. Alu I family repetitive DNA sequences are represented by the *short arrows*, whereas different members of the Kpn I family of repetitive DNA sequences are indicated by the *lettered bars*.

ing evolution, and cross-hybridizing sequences have been detected in the genomes of lower eukaryotes such as the slime mold and yeast.[157]

Another noteworthy feature of this repetitive DNA sequence is the presence within it of a tandem repeat of 16 or 17 TG dinucleotides.[157, 157a] A similar sequence is present in IVS-2 of the γ globin genes, and it has been proposed that this sequence serves as a "hot spot" for recombination between the two γ globin genes, leading to a gene conversion event that corrects the nucleotide sequence of one gene against that of the other.[40, 41] It has been suggested that the similar sequence in the inter-δβ globin gene DNA might serve as a "hot spot" for recombination within the non–α globin gene cluster, accounting for the patterns of restriction fragment length polymorphisms observed within the cluster (discussed later).

Other Features of Intergene DNA. The interglobin gene DNA has some additional noteworthy features—regions of simple sequence DNA and regions of sequence variability.

Simple Sequence DNA. The regions of simple sequence DNA include stretches of 200-bp and 40-bp DNA situated to the 5' side of the $^G\gamma$ and δ globin genes, respectively, that are composed almost exclusively of pyrimidines (C or T) on one strand and complementary purines (G or A) on the other.[148, 157a] To the 5' side of the β globin gene, there is a region containing variable numbers of the simple repeated sequence ATTTT.[157a, 158]

In the α globin gene cluster, a 90-bp region of alternating purines and pyrimidines has been identified between the α1 and α2 globin genes, near the 5' end of the α1 globin gene duplication unit[159] (between Y and Z in Figure 7-9). This region of DNA has been shown to develop regions of single strandedness in vitro that are susceptible to cleavage by the enzyme S1 nuclease.[159] Regions of DNA with alternating purine/pyrimidine nucleotides have also been shown to be capable of adopting a left-handed or Z-DNA conformation that may have various functions, including roles in chromosome organization and genome rearrangement.[160, 160a] It is noteworthy that this region of in vitro S1 sensitivity in the inter–α1/α2 globin gene DNA coincides with one of the three sites within the α globin gene cluster where recombination events have occurred and resulted in either gene deletion or gene duplication events (see Chapter 8). A somewhat analogous 52-bp stretch of alternating purine/pyrimidine residues has been identified in the inter-δβ globin gene DNA.[157a] It is also capable of forming a region of S1 nuclease sensitivity in vitro[160b] and may constitute a "hot spot" for recombination in the non–α globin gene cluster (see next section). Another analogous sequence in the 5'-flanking DNA of the mouse β major globin gene has been shown to exert a negative regulatory influence on globin gene promoter function in nonerythroid cells.[160c]

As noted previously, simple sequence DNA has also been identified within the intervening sequences of the ζ and ψζ genes, IVS-2 of the γ globin genes (which can adopt the Z-DNA conformation[160d]), and the short repetitive DNA sequence in the inter-δβ globin gene DNA. The presence of variable numbers of a repeated simple DNA sequence between the ζ and ψζ globin genes also accounts for restriction fragment length polymorphism in this region of DNA, as discussed in the next section.

Sequence Variability and Restriction Fragment Length Polymorphisms. In contrast to mRNA encoding sequences, which show little or no variability between individuals, the intergene DNA and intervening sequence DNA can vary significantly in their nucleotide sequence from one person to another. It has been estimated that approximately one out of every 200 to 400 nucleotides of "extragenic" DNA may be different in any two individuals. This remarkable fact is probably explained by the lack of functional constraints on the sequence of extragenic DNA, which can "evolve" or change without causing deleterious consequences to the organism. As a result, numerous changes or differences can be maintained in the "extragenic" DNA of the organism without negative bias due to natural selection. Such sequence variability has proved to be very informative in a number of genetic studies or analyses because of the fact that it provides a type of marker or fingerprint for an individual's genome. Applications have included prenatal diagnosis and population genetics (see Chapter 8).

Sequence variability is detected most frequently by gene mapping procedures using restriction endonuclease enzymes, which cleave DNA at specific recognition sequences (see Chapter 8). The generation of DNA fragments of different sizes in different individuals provides evidence for sequence variability in the region of DNA tested, called restriction fragment length polymorphism. There are two general causes of restriction fragment length polymorphism: (1) a base substitution (or other change) within the recognition sequence for the restriction endonuclease—in this case, the restriction fragment length polymorphism is detected only by the enzyme(s) specifically recognizing the target sequence; and (2) variation in the length of DNA present in different individuals between two consecutive restriction endonuclease sites—in this case, the restriction fragment length polymorphism can usually be detected by a number of different enzymes with varied recognition sequence specificities.

In the non–α globin gene cluster, a number of polymorphisms have been identified that are of the first type, i.e., due to alterations of specific restriction endonclease sites. They are found in intergene as well as intervening sequence DNA, and one polymorphism is even present in the coding sequence of the β globin gene but does not cause a change in amino acid sequence. The location and nature of these restriction site polymorphisms are illustrated in Figure 7–11.[161, 161a] A number of these polymorphisms are clustered in the Kpn I family repetitive DNA sequence located 3' to the β globin gene. Most of the polymorphisms in the non–α globin gene cluster are quite common and widely distributed among different racial groups. In contrast, other polymorphisms are relatively rare, such as the Pst I site in IVS-2 of the δ globin gene,[19, 162] or are virtually restricted to certain racial groups, such as the absence of the Hpa I site 3' to the β globin gene,[163] which is tightly linked to a β globin gene bearing the sickle or $β^C$ mutations and is therefore found virtually only in blacks or in Mediterraneans carrying the $β^S$ or $β^C$ genes.[164]

These polymorphisms do not occur in association with one another in a totally random fashion. Thus, a number of specific combinations or groupings of polymorphisms, called haplotypes, have been identified at a high frequency in different population groups.[161, 165] The analysis of haplotypes has been most useful in studies of the genetics of hereditary disorders affecting the globin genes. In particular, the establishment of linkage between a given haplotype and a β-thalassemic globin gene in a given family has provided the ability for prenatal diagnosis of thalassemia by analysis of DNA obtained by amniocentesis or chorionic villus biopsy (see Chapter 8). Haplotype analysis has also facilitated studies of the molecular basis of β thalassemia by identifying individuals likely to carry novel mutations (see Chapter 8) and has shed light on the extraordinary heterogeneity of chromosomes bearing the $β^S$ globin gene, suggesting the occurrence of multiple separate mutations as the basis for this disorder[166–168a] (see Chapter 12).

Studies of haplotypes have also suggested an unexpectedly high frequency of presumed crossover or recombination events between the 5' and 3' ends of the non–α globin gene cluster.[161, 167, 169, 170] It has been proposed that there exists a "hot spot" for recombination somewhere between the 5' end of the δ globin gene and the 5' end of the β globin gene.[161, 169, 170] A candidate for such a recombination "hot spot" is the block of tandemly repeated TG dinucleotides within the short repetitive sequence, discussed earlier, that is located approximately at the midpoint of the inter-δβ globin gene DNA.[157] Other candidate

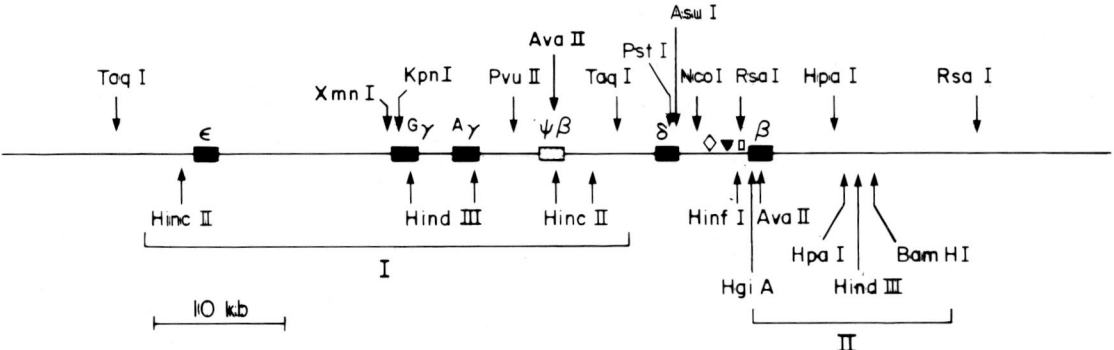

Figure 7–11. Restriction endonuclease site polymorphisms in the human non-α globin gene cluster. The sites shown below the line have been studied most intensively and are commonly utilized to define chromosomal haplotypes in genetic analyses. Polymorphisms at the sites encompassed in brackets I and II are usually in linkage disequilibrium with one another within each bracketed area, but random combinations or associations occur between polymorphisms of group I and those of group II. The symbols shown 5' to the β globin gene indicate the location of various strucures that may be "hot spots" for recombination between the 5' (I) and 3' (II) regions of the cluster (see text). (◇ = $(TG)_n$ simple repeat; ▼ = $(ATTT)_n$ repeat; ☐ = alternating purine/pyrimidine sequence.) (Modified from Collins, F. S. and Weissman, S. M., Prog. Nucl. Acids. Res. and Mol. Biol. *31*:315, 1984.)

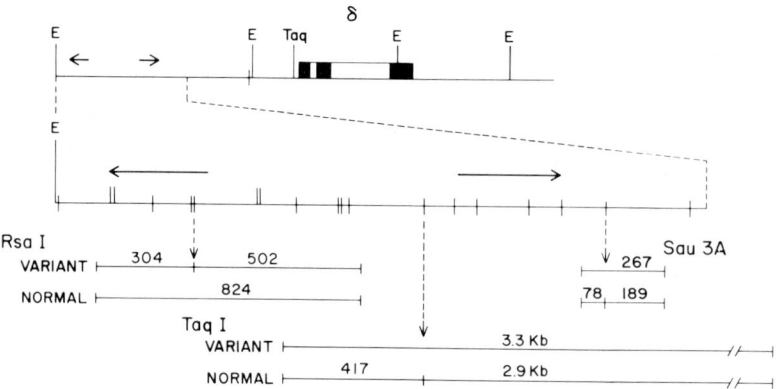

Figure 7–12. Nucleotide sequence variability in the region 5' to the human δ globin gene. Normal individuals have one of two different sequences on a given chromosome, differing by 19 nucleotides over a region of approximately 2 kb: 15 base substitutions, shown as vertical bars crossing the baseline, and four base insertions, shown as vertical bars above the baseline. Three of the base substitutions create restriction fragment length polymorphisms, as indicated, for the enzymes Rsa I, Sau 3A, and Taq I. The *horizontal arrows* indicate the position of a pair of Alu I repetitive DNA sequences. (From Forget, B. G., et al.: *In* Stamatoyannopoulos, G., and Nienhuis, A. W. (eds.): New York, Alan R. Liss, Inc., 1983, p. 65.)

sequences in this region of intergene DNA include the previously discussed ATTTT tandem repeat[158] and a 52-bp stretch of alternating purine and pyrimidine residues.[157a] Three different restriction site polymorphisms occur within this region of DNA in different positions relative to these three defined structures (see Fig. 7–11). The random pattern of segregation of these polymorphisms with regard to either the 5' or 3' subsets of polymorphisms in the gene cluster suggests that recombination events have occurred throughout this region rather than in one of these specific structures.

Direct nucleotide sequence analysis has also revealed clusters in which there are multiple nucleotide sequence differences between individuals. These regions include the 5' end of IVS-2 of the $^A\gamma$ globin gene[40] and an area of approximately 2 kb located at a site between 2 kb and 4 kb to the 5' side of the δ globin gene[157a, 171, 172] (Fig. 7–12). The functional or evolutionary implications of these "hyperpolymorphic" regions of DNA are poorly understood.

In the human α globin gene cluster, restriction fragment length polymorphisms are due to a different phenomenon—the presence of variable amounts or lengths of DNA in the intergene DNA between the ζ and ψζ globin genes as well as in the DNA to the 3' side of the α1 globin gene[27, 28] (regions V_1 and V_3 in Figure 7–9). This type of polymorphism is usually due to the insertion or deletion of various numbers of a simple repeat sequence, such as that initially characterized in the DNA flanking the 5' end of the human insulin gene.[36, 37] The hypervariable region between the ζ and ψζ genes has been characterized by cloning and nucleotide sequencing.[28] It contains variable numbers of a tandemly repeated 36-bp sequence that can be subdivided into two 14-bp domains that are closely related to one another and share sequence homology with the tandemly repeated sequences found in the 5'-flanking DNA of the insulin gene and in IVS-1 of the ζ and ψζ globin genes.[28] Nucleotide sequence analysis of the hypervariable region to the 3' side of the α1 globin gene has not yet been reported.

PROCESS OF NORMAL GLOBIN GENE EXPRESSION

Biogenesis of Globin mRNA

The general process of eukaryotic gene expression and mRNA biogenesis has been reviewed elsewhere,[173] and in the previous section, we have discussed the various structural elements of the globin genes that are required for their normal expression. In this section, we will emphasize the various features that have been characterized in the process of globin mRNA formation.

Site of Transcription Initiation

Transcription of the globin genes is initiated at the "cap site," which constitutes the 5' end of the mature cytoplasmic globin mRNA. The 5' terminus of high–molecular weight precursor β globin mRNA was shown some years ago to be the same as that of the mature cytoplasmic mRNA.[174] However, more recent reports have identified minor subpopulations of human precursor ε, γ, and β globin mRNA molecules that have 5' termini originating from sites located further to the 5' side of the cap site.[175–179] The functional significance of these atypical globin mRNA transcripts is not known. They are present not only in nuclear RNA of erythroid precursor cells but also in cytoplasmic and reticulocyte RNA, where they can constitute up to 10 per cent of the globin mRNA molecules. Where it has been studied, these transcripts have a 5'-methylated cap structure, are polyadenylated, and appear to be properly processed or spliced. In studies that utilized various inhibitors of RNA polymerases,[177, 177a] it appeared that the atypical β globin RNAs were transcribed by RNA polymerase III (pol. III) rather than by RNA polymerase II, which normally transcribes the globin genes. Pol. III is the polymerase that normally transcribes tRNA and 5S RNA genes as well as Alu I repetitive DNA sequences. In fact, one of the atypical ε globin gene transcripts has its 5' terminus close to a putative pol. III promoter sequence of an upstream Alu I family repetitive DNA sequence.[176] In the 5'-flanking DNA of the non–α globin genes, a number of sequences can also be found that resemble the consensus sequences for pol. III promoters as well as sequences homologous to the CCAAT and ATA boxes of RNA polymerase II promoters,[177–179] which may serve as atypical sites for initiation of globin gene transcription. In gene transfer experiments, the site of transcription initiation of the ε globin gene can be influenced by *cis*- as well as *trans*-acting factors.[179a]

Precursor Globin mRNA Molecules

As noted previously, precursor globin mRNA molecules in the nucleus of erythroid precursor cells are larger than the mature cytoplasmic globin mRNA.[180–192] The additional sequences can be entirely accounted for by the lengths of the intervening sequences of the globin genes that are transcribed into precursor mRNA molecules[49–51] and subsequently removed by the process of RNA splicing (see previous section on intervening sequences). The finding in nucleated cells of RNA species of intermediate sizes between mature globin mRNA and full-length precursor mRNA in man[193] as well as in other animal species[66–68, 68d] suggests that the two intervening sequences are removed sequentially rather than simultaneously.

Site of Transcription Termination

The primary transcript of the globin genes is in all likelihood larger than that observed in the discrete globin precursor mRNA species that have been characterized. Recent evidence has accumulated indicating that transcription of globin (and other) genes extends well beyond the site of poly(A) addition and that polyadenylation occurs only after the cleavage of a higher–molecular weight RNA species at a point 10 to 20 bp distal to the consensus polyadenylation signal (AATAAA) in the 3' noncoding portion of the mRNA.[110–110c]

In the case of globin genes, the 3' end of the primary transcript has been most extensively studied in the case of the β globin gene of cultured mouse erythroleukemia (MEL) cells; these studies utilized the "run off" transcription assay in which isolated nuclei are incubated *in vitro* in the presence of ^{32}P-labeled nucleotide triphosphates. In such assays, transcripts that were initiated in the intact cell are completed *in vitro* but are not further processed or polyadenylated. Thus, it is possible to detect labeled precursor molecules that are presumably analogous to authentic primary transcripts prior to processing. The results of such experiments indicated that in MEL cell nuclei, the primary transcript of the β globin gene extends for a distance of approximately 1.0 kb beyond the 3' end of the gene.[194, 195] Similar studies performed with nuclei from various cultured human cells that express different globin genes have demonstrated the same phenomenon of transcription well beyond the polyadenylation site of the various human globin genes.[196] There is also evidence of presumed primary gene transcripts of very large size in nucleated avian erythroid cells.[197]

Additional evidence of primary transcription beyond the site of poly(A) addition is provided by two thalassemia mutations consisting of base substitutions in the consensus polyadenylation signal AAUAAA.[198, 199] In the case of the α-thalassemia mutation,[198] elongated transcripts were not observed in RNA isolated from peripheral blood reticulocytes but were observed following transfer and expression of the mutant gene in tissue culture cells (see Chapter 8). In the case of the β-thalassemia gene,[199] elongated β gene transcripts were actually identified in RNA isolated from erythroid cells of the affected patient.

Post-transcriptional Processing

The post-transcriptional processes of 5' capping and 3' polyadenylation occur very rapidly and precede the process of excision or splicing out of intervening sequences.[173] Very little is known concerning the process of transport of the nascent mRNA from nucleus to cytoplasm. As mentioned previously, splicing appears to be required for the accumulation of cytoplasmic globin mRNA in gene transfer/gene expression studies in tissue culture cells.[73, 74] Thus, it is possible that normal globin mRNA splicing and transport of the mRNA from nucleus to cytoplasm are linked in an as-yet-to-be-determined fashion. This notion is also supported by the observation that abnormal globin mRNA splicing in at least one form of β thalassemia appears to be associated with a lesion in transfer of nascent globin mRNA from nucleus to cytoplasm.[200, 201] The association of precursor and mature globin mRNA with various proteins to form mRNP particles[202, 203] may also play an important role in mRNA processing, transport, stability, and function.

Regulation of Globin Gene Expression

The specific factors that activate globin gene expression in erythroid cells and suppress it in nonerythroid cells are not known. Nevertheless, a number of features characterize active versus inactive globin genes and provide some insight on the prerequisites for globin gene expression.

DNA Methylation

It is clear that the state of methylation of the DNA of a gene influences its ability to be expressed.[26, 204-210] In general, genes that are being actively transcribed are almost always hypomethylated, whereas inactive genes are usually, although not necessarily, hypermethylated. Methylation of DNA usually involves position 5 of the pyrimidine ring of cytidine residues and is found mostly in CG dinucleotide sequences (designated ^mCG). In human DNA, approximtely 5 per cent of all C residues and 70 per cent of all CG dinucleotides are methylated. The methylation of cytidine occurs after incorporation of the nucleotide into the DNA chain and is performed by enzymes called DNA methyltransferases, of which there is more than one type. Methylation of specific sites in DNA can be assessed by the gene mapping procedure of Southern (see Chapter 8), using different restriction endonucleases that have specificities influenced by DNA methylation. For example, the enzyme Hpa II will cleave DNA at the sequence CCGG but not at C^mCGG; on the other hand, the enzyme Msp I will cleave the sequence CCGG whether the second C is methylated or not (except in the case of the sequence GGC^mCGG). Thus, the presence or degree of methylation at such sequences in and around a given gene can be assessed by comparing the pattern of DNA cleavage with these two enzymes in gene mapping experiments. However, it should be noted that analysis of DNA in this fashion provides information only on the methylation status of CCGG sequences and not that of other important potentially methylated C or CG residues in other sequence environments.

The methylation status of globin genes has been studied in various human and nonhuman tissues as well as in erythroid cells at different stages of development.[26, 210] In nonerythyroid tissues, the globin genes are generally extensively methylated, as expected for inactive genes. In nucleated erythyroid cells, the globin genes that are being expressed are generally undermethylated relative to the nonexpressed globin genes, such as the embryonic versus adult globin genes in yolk sac–derived erythroid cells. CCGG sequences in the 5'-flanking DNA of various globin genes demonstrate the most striking correlation between hypomethylation and gene expression.

In the case of the human globin genes, the most remarkable association between hypomethylation and gene activity can be found in the DNA flanking the 5' end of the fetal γ globin genes. The 5'-flanking DNA of both $^G\gamma$ and $^A\gamma$ globin genes contains a CCGG sequence at position -54 from the cap site, roughly midway between the CCAAT and ATA boxes. Both of these sites are hypomethylated in fetal liver erythroid cells that have active γ globin genes but are fully methylated in erythroid cells of adult bone marrow where γ globin genes are not expressed to any significant degree.[211, 212] In an interesting set of gene transfer/gene expression studies in tissue culture cells, γ globin genes were modified by methylation at various sites and were then studied for their ability to be expressed in the recipient host cell, where the methylation status of the transferred DNA was maintained even after DNA replication. Methylation in the 5'-flanking region of DNA (residues -760 to $+100$) but not in the remainder of the γ globin gene prevented its expression in the transfected tissue culture cells.[213]

Hypomethylation of the immediate 5'-flanking DNA of the γ globin genes therefore appears to be a prerequisite for their normal expression. These observations provided the rationale for attempts to reactivate γ globin gene expression in adult erythroid marrow cells by the administrtion of 5-azacytidine, an inhibitor of DNA methyltransferase enzymes (see Chapter 9).

Although DNA hypomethylation in 5'-flanking DNA may be a prerequisite for gene expression, it is probably not the primary event responsible for the activation of specialized genes such as the globin genes, because there are many situations in which globin or other genes are hypomethylated but not expressed. Other factors must be responsible for triggering gene expression once the gene is in a state capable of being expressed. In addition, other events or factors must be required to cause undermethylation of specific regions of a given gene in specific tissues at specific times in development, but these are not understood.

Chromatin Structure

DNA does not exist in the cell as a naked strand but is associated with various proteins to form chromatin. The structure or physical state of chromatin can vary in regions where the DNA is being actively transcribed. In general, active genes are packaged in an altered form of chromatin that displays increased susceptibility to digestion by various nucleases such as DNase I.[214] In some respects, DNase I sensitivity of a given gene appears to be another prerequisite for gene expression and generally correlates with gene activity in a manner analogous to that previously discussed in the case of DNA hypomethylation.

In the globin gene system, DNase I sensitivity has been most extensively studied in the chicken,[215–220] in which it is possible to study nucleated erythroid cells at various stages of development. At least three different levels or degrees of DNase I sensitivity have been defined in this and other gene systems:

1. Moderate or intermediate DNase I sensitivity that affects the entire region or domain in which an active gene is located. This state of sensitivity reflects the general potential for transcription of a specific gene region in a given cell type.

2. Marked or very high DNase I sensitivity that usually affects the structural gene itself and correlates well with active transcription of the gene.

3. DNase I hypersensitive sites, which are discrete regions of DNA that manifest even more pronounced sensitivity to digestion by DNase I and probably constitute the sites of the "first hits" by the enzyme. These hypersensitive sites are usually, but not exclusively, located in the 5'-flanking DNA of genes that are being actively transcribed.[222, 222a]

In 20-hour-old chicken embryos, the globin genes of cells that are the presumed precursors (i.e., stem cells) of the embryonic erythroid cells are packaged in chromatin that is resistant to digestion by DNase I,[219] i.e., in the "closed" conformation of chromatin characteristic of inactive genes. However, with the onset of hemoglobin synthesis at 35 hours of embryogenesis, the globin gene domain of the early embryonic erythroid cells manifests a moderate sensitivity to digestion by DNase I,[219] consistent with the "open" configuration of chromatin characteristic of active genes. The region of moderate DNase I sensitivity of the globin gene clusters in chicken erythroid cells extends at least 8 kb to the 3' side of both the α and β gene clusters and approximately 7 kb to the 5' side of the β gene cluster, where a definite transition to a DNase I–resistant domain occurs.[216]

In embryonic erythroid cells, both the embryonic and adult non–α globin genes are very sensitive to DNase I digestion, but in adult erythroid cells, only the adult β globin gene remains highly sensitive; the embryonic globin gene becomes relatively more resistant but still retains moderate sensitivity similar to that of the overall domain.[215, 216] The state of marked sensitivity to DNase I appears to be conferred by the binding to the gene of a particular set of nonhistone proteins called HMG (high mobility group) 14 and 17.[214] These proteins are not specific for globin genes but constitute abundant components in the nucleus of all cell types that bind specifically to active chromatin. For instance, HMG 14 and 17 from the brain can confer marked DNase I sensitivity to globin genes in erythroid cell chromatin, but HMG 14 and 17 from erythyroid cells do not affect the DNase I sensitivity of globin genes in brain chromatin.

More recently, attention has focused on DNase I hypersensitive sites in active chromatin. A very good correlation has been established between the presence of such sites, especially in the 5'-flanking DNA of a gene, and active transcription of that gene.[222, 222a] In the chicken globin gene system, such hypersensitive sites are found in the 5'-flanking

DNA of the adult β globin genes in adult erythroid cells[216, 221, 223, 224] and in the 5'-flanking DNA of embryonic β-like globin genes in embryonic erythroid cells;[216, 219] similar sites are also present in the α globin gene cluster.[220] The nature of these sites has been examined in some detail, and it has been found that the same general region of DNase I hypersensitivity also contains sites that are cleaved by S1 nuclease,[223] which specifically cleaves single-stranded DNA. It has therefore been proposed that the DNA within a DNase I hypersensitive site has a peculiar conformation and that the sensitivity to S1 nuclease digestion is probably related to supercoiling of the DNA,[225–227] since bacterial plasmids containing these cloned regions of DNA can also be cleaved by S1 nuclease but only when the DNA supercoiled. It is noteworthy that sites of S1 and DNase I hypersensitivity tend to occur in regions of DNA containing homopurine-homopyrimidine stretches that are theoretically capable of adopting the Z or left-handed helical configuration of DNA.[159, 160b, 160d, 227a, 227b]

Somewhat similar but less extensive studies have been performed in the case of the human globin gene system,[228–229a] using normal human erythroid cells as well as human erythroleukemia cells that have unusual patterns of globin gene expression—the K562 and HEL cell lines that synthesize varied levels of α, ζ, ε, $^G\gamma$ and $^A\gamma$ globin chains, but no β chains. In normal human erythroid cells as well as in the erythroleukemia cells, the entire non–α globin gene domain was found to manifest moderate DNase I sensitivity, including the region of the nonexpressed β globin gene in the leukemic cells. In fetal liver erythroid cells, DNase I hypersensitive sites were found in the immediate 5'-flanking DNA (<200 bp from the cap site) of the $^G\gamma$, $^A\gamma$, δ, and β globin genes, but in adult bone marrow cells, these sites were retained only in the case of the δ and β globin genes.[229] The erythroleukemia cells displayed hypersensitive sites 5' to the ε and both γ globin genes,[228–229b] but some differences were noted in the pattern of DNase I hypersensitive sites adjacent to the δ and β globin genes. In K562 cells that synthesize some δ[230] but no β globin mRNA,[230–231a] a DNase I hypersensitive site was detected adjacent to the δ globin gene[229] but not the β globin gene.[228, 229] In HEL cells, there is no synthesis of either δ or β globin mRNA,[229] yet DNase I hypersensitive sites are found in the 5'-flanking DNA of both the δ and β globin genes of these cells.[229] The presence of DNase I hypersensitive sites is therefore not an absolute indication of active gene transcription but may reflect a preactivation state of a gene that requires additional regulatory factors for its expression or that can be inhibited from being expressed by other factors.

Another model system in which hypersensitive sites adjacent to globin genes are not associated with gene expression consists of the chicken globin genes in erythroblasts transformed by a temperature-sensitive avian erythroblastosis virus[232] and in fibroblasts infected with a temperature-sensitive Rous sarcoma virus or "shocked" by exposure to high concentrations of NaCl.[233]

In summary, the various studies we have discussed provide evidence that globin genes must be in a particular chromatin configuration in order to be expressed. However, these changes in chromatin structure appear to precede gene transcription and do not seem to trigger transcription itself or to result from active transcription, since most of these changes can occur in the absence of actual globin gene transcription. As in the case of DNA hypomethylation, one is dealing with a permissive state of the gene that has resulted through the action of unknown factors and that requires additional unknown factors for activation of transcription.

Other Factors Influencing Gene Expression

Association with the Nuclear Matrix. Another feature of actively transcribed genes is that they tend to be preferentially associated with a lattice-like filamentous structure within the nucleus called the nuclear matrix.[234–237] This phenomenon has been especially studied in the case of the ovalbumin gene in chicken oviduct cells,[238, 239] but the β globin gene is also preferentially associated with the nuclear matrix in chicken erythroid cells.[240] A similar phenomenon was observed in the case of the human γ globin gene in K562 erythroleukemia cells, but the unexpressed insulin gene was also preferentially associated with the nuclear matrix in these cells.[241] However, in gene transfer systems using nonerythroid cells, expressed globin genes are not preferentially associated with the nuclear matrix.[241a] In HeLa cells, the human γ and β globin genes are not preferentially associated with the matrix, as expected, but the human α globin genes, for unknown reasons, do display significant attachment to the matrix.[242] It has also been observed that intranuclear globin mRNA sequences are preferentially associated with the nuclear matrix in avian erythroid cells.[243,244]

Trans-Acting Factors. Relatively little progress has been achieved in identifying specific protein or other soluble factors that may be responsible for activation or inactivation of globin or other genes that are otherwise capable of being expressed in a differentiated cell type such as erythroid cells. As mentioned previously, the HMG 14 and 17 nonhistone proteins are associated with active genes and confer increased DNase I sensitivity, but these proteins are not tissue-specific. However, certain nonhistone proteins in mouse erythroleukemia cells have been shown to bind specifically to cloned mouse β-globin gene DNA.[244a] In chicken erythroid cells, a protein factor has been identified that specifically binds and confers DNase I hypersensitivity to the 5'-flanking DNA of the β globin gene.[245] The factor can be isolated from erythroid cells of 9-day-old chickens that synthesize β globin chains but not from earlier embryonic erythroid cells in which the β globin gene is not expressed.[245] The factor has been only partially purified. It is inactivated by protease digestion and has an apparent molecular weight of 60 kilodaltons.[245]

Less well characterized factors appear to exert a negative regulatory influence on human globin genes in different model systems. As discussed earlier, the β globin genes of K562 and HEL cells are not expressed, even though they are in a permissive chromatin configuration. However, β globin genes from K562 and HEL cells are expressed normally in various gene transfer/gene expression systems.[246–247a] Furthermore, normal β globin genes introduced into K562 cells are not expressed.[247] It therefore appears that K562 cells contain a factor capable of suppressing normal β globin genes. Alternatively, these cells may be deficient in a positive regulatory factor that is essential for β globin gene expression. Hybrid mouse erythroleukemia (MEL) cells obtained by cell fusion and containing chromosome 16 from K562 cells, which actively synthesize ζ globin genes, express the transferred human α globin genes but not the ζ globin gene after induction by DMSO[248]; similar results were obtained with other types of human donor cells.[248a] These results could be interpreted as indicating the presence of a factor in the MEL cells that is capable of suppressing ζ gene expression, or the need for specific positive regulatory factors to allow embryonic ζ globin gene expression in an adult intracellular environment. Yet another set of experiments in fact suggests that the latter may be the case: After transfer of the cloned human ζ globin gene into various cell types, expression of the gene was obtained only in embryonic frog oocytes and not in other adult-type cells.[248b]

Analysis of the expression of cloned globin genes transferred into MEL cells has provided additional insight on the differential expression and potential requirement of trans-acting factors for human α, β, and γ globin gene expression, as well as information on the regions of the genes that might interact with such factors.[248c–248f] Cloned human α globin genes, after transfer into MEL cells, are expressed constitutively at a high level that does not increase further after DMSO induction. For expression in their new environment, these transferred α globin genes therefore do not require additional trans-acting factors that might be produced after the exposure of the MEL cells to DMSO or other inducing agents. On the contrary, cloned human β globin genes, after transfer into MEL cells, are highly responsive to induction by DMSO and other agents and are therefore thought to respond to the action of trans-acting factors produced during induction. In contrast, transferred human γ globin genes are not inducible in MEL cells but are expressed at very low constitutive levels or not at all. By making various hybrid genes containing either the promoter (5'-flanking) or structural region of the β globin gene, the remarkable observation was made that not only the promoter region but also the structural region, or "body," of the human β globin gene is responsive to the factors that are responsible for conferring inducibility of globin gene expression in MEL cells. Similarly, the high constitutive level of expression of human α globin genes in MEL cells is promoter-independent and appears to be a property of the body of the gene itself.

Another approach to the identification of red cell–specific regulatory proteins has been to produce and characterize monoclonal antibodies that react with nuclear preparations of avian erythroid cells.[249] A number of such antibodies have been isolated and shown to be red cell–specific,[249] but the characterization of the proteins against which they react has not yet been reported.

Finally, any discussion of trans-acting factors should include mention of the fact that enhancer elements appear to interact with trans-acting factors,[249a–249d] which may account for the tissue specificity of some enhancers. Furthermore, it has been shown that the product of the E1A gene of adenovirus, directly or indirectly, has a positive effect on the expression of globin[249e, 249f] and other genes.

The Fetal to Adult Hemoglobin Switch

The pattern of human globin gene expression during development has been discussed in Chapter 4 (see Fig. 4–4). The mechanism by which erythroid cells switch from the synthesis of Hb F to that of Hb A during the neonatal period has been the subject of much study and speculation. The issue has generated a great deal of interest because it constitutes an excellent model system for study of the developmental regulation of gene expression and also because of the practical consideration that reactivation, or prevention of suppression, of γ globin gene expression could potentially constitute a form of gene therapy for serious β-chain hemoglobinopathies such as sickle cell anemia and β thalassemia (see Chapters 8 and 12).

Despite a tremendous amount of work on this topic, the precise mechanism that regulates the normal "switch" from γ to β globin gene expression remains essentially unknown. The switch seems to be regulated more by a developmental "clock" and gestational age than by intrauterine or extrauterine environmental factors, since prematurity has little effect on the process.[250, 251] Nevertheless, some modulation of the process can occur such as in the case of intrauterine growth retardation,[252] maternal anoxia,[253] the D_1 trisomy syndrome,[254–256] and hyperinsulinemia secondary to maternal diabetes mellitus,[256a] in which there seems to be some delay in the switch. Conversely, in some cases of Down's syndrome (trisomy 21)[257] and the C/D chromosomal translocation syndrome,[258] there appears to be an acceleration of the switch.

The developmental programming of fetal versus adult globin gene expression, independent of environmental factors, is illustrated by a number of transplantation experiments betweeen fetal and adult donor/recipient pairs in sheep as well as in man. When fetal liver cells were transplanted into lethally irradiated adult sheep, the initial experiments revealed the subsequent appearance, in one treated animal, of substantial amounts of Hb A, which could only be derived from the progeny of the transplanted fetal erythroid progenitor cells.[259]

These results suggested an environmental influence on the fetal to adult hemoglobin switch. However, subsequent analogous experiments by different investigators[260, 260a] failed to demonstrate any substantial difference between the pattern of hemoglobin synthesis in a number of reconstituted animals and that expected for fetal liver erythroid cells of a fetal lamb of the same gestational age as the donor: There was substantial synthesis of Hb F and rarely earlier or more than expected Hb A synthesis for the age of the donor cells. It is difficult to totally reconcile the differences in the results of the two studies, but a partial explanation may be provided by the fact that the fetal to adult hemoglobin switch occurs more abruptly and progresses more rapidly in sheep than in man.[261] Thus, the Hb A observed in the first study may have resulted from only slightly earlier than expected switching for the gestational age of the donor fetal cells. Results somewhat analogous to those of the second study were obtained when human fetal liver cells (instead of bone marrow) were transplanted in children following marrow ablation for therapy of acute leukemia: The pattern of hemoglobin synthesis after engraftment was similar to that expected for the donor cells.[262, 262a]

The reverse experiment was also performed, in which adult bone marrow cells were transplanted into fetal lambs *in utero* at a time when they synthesized only Hb F; the transplanted cells were derived from animals who were homozygous for adult Hb B, whereas the recipient animals were homozygous for adult Hb A.[263] Repeated sampling of the blood of the transplanted fetuses revealed the appearance of substantial amounts of $β^B$ globin chains at a time preceding the appearance of $β^A$ globin chains resulting from the fetal to adult switch in the recipient's endogenous erythroid cells.[263] The results were consistent with the lack of influence of the fetal environment on the pattern of β (or γ) globin gene expression of adult erythroid cells.

Taken together, these various transplantation experiments provide convincing evidence for a predetermined program of γ and β globin gene expression that is intrinsic to erythroid precursor cells derived from different developmental stages or ages and that cannot be significantly altered by transferring the cells to a different developmental environment. The intrinsic programming of erythroid progenitor cells during the period of the fetal to adult hemoglobin switch is also illustrated by the fact that the pattern of γ to β globin gene expression observed in *in vitro* cultures of erythroid colonies derived from fetal and neonatal progenitor cells is very similar to that observed in the erythroid cells of the intact animal at the same time of development *in vivo*.[264-267]

Another issue related to the developmental program of hemoglobin switching is whether or not fetal and adult erythroid cells derive from the same family of erythroid progenitor or stem cells. This issue is the subject of some controversy and is not totally resolved. One hypothetical model (the "clonal" model) for the mechanism of the fetal switch would be the progressive replacement of cells derived from a fetal stem cell lineage by cells derived from an adult stem cell lineage. The fairly good correlation between the switch in the site of erythropoiesis, from liver to bone marrow, and the switch in type of hemoglobin synthesized, from Hb F to Hb A, initially suggested the possibility of different, organ-specific, erythroid cell populations with different programs of hemoglobin synthesis. However, the available data suggest no clear-cut difference in the lineage of marrow-derived versus liver- or spleen-derived erythroid cells. Throughout fetal development, the ratio of γ to β globin chain synthesis is the same in erythroid cells isolated from different sites of erythropoiesis,[268, 269] indicating the presence of a common progenitor cell population in the fetal liver, spleen, and bone marrow. Furthermore, during the perinatal switching period, virtually all of the red cells contain both Hb F and Hb A in variable amounts, consistent with a gradual and progressive change in the program of globin gene expression in a continuum of related progenitor cells. If the switch were due to the differential proliferation or output of two totally distinct progenitor cell pools (one strictly fetal and the other strictly adult), one would expect to find variable admixtures of two different red cell populations during the perinatal switch—one containing exclusively (or predominantly) Hb F and the other containing Hb A. Such a phenomenon is not observed, and the postnatal decline in Hb F synthesis is generally smooth and gradual.[250, 251]

Nevertheless, there is some evidence for a change in the erythroid progenitor cell population at the time of the neonatal hemoglobin switch in man. Analysis of the time course of the transition from Hb F to Hb A production in the postnatal period has revealed two distinct phases: In the first phase, from birth to 6 weeks, erythropoiesis is markedly suppressed but the proportion of Hb F remains relatively constant; in the second phase, following the reactivation of erythropoiesis, the proportion of Hb A rapidly increases.[270, 271] Earlier histochemical studies of the distribution of Hb F in neonatal red cells also revealed the relatively sudden appearance of cells containing predominantly Hb A at about 2 months of age, following recovery from the neonatal period of suppression of erythropoiesis.[272]

The most convincing evidence for a change in progenitor cell population during the neonatal period has been obtained from the study of hemoglobin synthesis in erythroid colonies derived from the blood of newborn infants. By analyzing the characteristics of globin chain synthesis in individual colonies that developed at different times in culture, two different populations of colonies were identified—colonies unique to cord blood (fetal colonies), in which there was a strong negative correlation of $^G\gamma$ with β globin chain synthesis, and colonies analogous to those found in adults (adult colonies), in which the proportion of $^G\gamma$ synthesis did not correlate with the proportion of γ (or β) synthesis.[273] Qualitatively, different progenitor cell populations were also identified by the same investigators in studies of the fetal hemoglobin switch in rhesus monkeys.[274] The results of these various studies were interpreted as being consistent with a clonal model for hemoglobin switching in which fetal progenitors are gradually replaced during ontogeny by adult progenitors. It is not clear, however, whether these different populations of progenitors derive from distinct populations of pluripotential stem cells or whether they result from qualitative differences in the pattern of maturation or differentiation among the progeny of a single population of pluripotential stem cells.

Considerable speculation has focused on the possibility that some hormonal or humoral factor(s) may regulate the switch, but there is little or no evidence to support this contention, except in a very circumstantial fashion. The various observations that have suggested the possible influence of humoral or hormonal factors on hemoglobin switching include increased maternal synthesis of Hb F during pregnancy,[275-277] shortly following the time of peak secretion of chorionic gonadotropin (HCG) by the placenta; increased Hb F production in patients with HCG-producing germline tumors[278, 279] or with thyrotoxicosis;[280] and increased production of Hb F in non-human primates after the administration of D-thyroxine, which was observed in one study[281] but not another.[282] However, the increased Hb F production in these various circumstances, as in other situations associated with increased Hb F synthesis in adults, is characterized by a relative increase in the production and/or accumulation of F cells, probably due to erythropoietic stress (see next section), and not by a reversal of the switch in the majority of erythroid cells, as would be expected if a specific humoral effect were being exerted on the mechanism of globin gene expression in the whole erythron. The increased production of F cells in the face of erythropoietic stress is probably mediated to some degree by increased erythropoietin levels,[283] but there is no evidence that the physiologic neonatal fetal to adult hemoglobin switch is induced by changes in the amount or type of erythropoietin produced. The strongest evidence against a role of one of the traditional hormones in the switch was provided by pituitary ablation experiments in fetal sheep:[261] Hypophysectomy *in utero* did not affect the time of onset of the fetal to adult hemoglobin switch but did result in a moderate slowing of the rate at which switching occurred, concomitant with an overall delay in the development of the animals.[261] On the other hand, a factor in "pre-switch" fetal sheep serum has been identified that can influence the ratio of Hb F to Hb A synthesis in erythroid cell colonies derived from adult progenitor cells cultured *in vitro* (see next section), but the relevance of this factor to normal perinatal hemoglobin switching remains to be determined.

As discussed in the prior sections on DNA methylation and chromatin structure, changes in the degree of hypomethylation and DNase I hypersensitivity of the 5'-flanking DNA of the γ and β globin genes accompany the changes in the level of expression of these genes in adult versus fetal erythroid cells. However, the factors that mediate these changes are not known.

Finally, there has been a great deal of speculation regarding the presence of regulatory DNA sequences in the inter-γδ gene region that might be responsible for mediating the fetal to adult switch. The models are discussed in detail in Chapter 8 and are based primarily on comparisons of the different deletions causing hereditary persistence of fetal hemoglobin (HPFH) and δβ thalassemia. The models are totally speculative, and although they may explain the differences in the phenotype of Hb F expression in these different genetic syndromes, they do not necessarily shed light on the process of the normal switch. In particular, the ratio of $^G\gamma$ to $^A\gamma$ globin chain synthesis in the common deletion type of HPFH is characteristic of that observed in adult rather than fetal erythroid cells, and furthermore, in homozygotes, there is less synthesis of γ chains than α chains ($\gamma/\alpha \approx 0.5$) instead of equal synthesis ($\gamma/\alpha = 1.0$) as occurs in normal fetal cells. Therefore, this form of HPFH should probably not be considered simply a condition in which the switching process has been totally arrested, and thus, it may not constitute a valid model for the physiologic switch.

In summary, it should be obvious from the preceding discussion that the factors responsible for the perinatal switch from fetal to adult hemoglobin synthesis remain a total mystery.

Increased Production of Hb F in Adult Life and in *In Vitro* Cultures of Adult Erythroid Cell Colonies

As discussed in Chapter 4, the small amount of Hb F that is normally present in adults is restricted to a minor subpopulation of red cells called F cells.[284, 285] With the exception of HPFH (see previous discussion and Chapter 8), when Hb F levels are increased in adults owing to various hereditary or acquired disorders, the cause is an increased production and/or selective survival of this subpopulation of F cells.[286, 287] The phenomenon of increased Hb F in adults is therefore not analogous to a reversal of the normal hemoglobin switching process. One exception to this general rule is the abnormal erythropoiesis that occurs during the course of juvenile chronic myelogenous leukemia. In that disorder, there is often progressive replacement of normal erythroid cells by a clone of malignant erythroid cells that have many fetal characteristics, not only from the point of view of hemoglobin synthesis but also the pattern of synthesis of other nonglobin proteins such as carbonic anhydrase B and "i" antigen.[288, 289]

The source or origin of F cells has been the subject of some debate and speculation as to whether or not F cells derive from the same or a totally different pluripotential marrow stem cell from that which gives rise to non-F or A cells.[286, 290] The evidence for and against the "clonal" model of fetal hemoglobin switching during the neonatal period was discussed in the preceding section. There is general agreement, however, based on studies of patients with clonal disorders of hematopoiesis,[291-293] that F cells and A cells in adults derive from the same population or pool of pluripotential stem cells.

The type of erythroid progenitor cell that gives rise to F cells has been elucidated to some degree by studies of hemoglobin synthesis in erythroid cell colonies grown *in vitro* from cultures of human bone marrow and peripheral blood mononuclear cells.[264-267, 294, 295] The initial observation of increased Hb F synthesis in such cultures[296, 297] subsequently led to a large number of studies by many different investigators in an attempt to elucidate the mechanism of this unexpected finding. It is beyond the scope of this chapter to review this large body of work; thus, we will only summarize briefly the general conclusions that have been drawn from this research.

The studies of Stamatoyannopoulos, Papayannopoulou, and coworkers[294, 295] revealed that the level of Hb F synthesis is generally higher in erythroid colonies derived from the more immature progenitor cells, called BFU-Es, than in those derived from the more mature progenitor cells, called CFU-Es. Also, by immunofluorescent staining, using anti–Hb F antibodies, erythroid cells in CFU-E–derived colonies virtually always stain uniformly for Hb F (or not at all), whereas in BFU-E–derived colonies, there may be a sectored pattern of staining in which some, but not all, of the erythroid cells in a given colony stain positively for Hb F. The model proposed by these investigators on the basis of their observations is illustrated in Figure 7–13 and can be described as follows: Progenitor cells at the early or BFU-E stage of committed erythroid stem cell maturation have the potential to express both Hb F and Hb A, but during the progressive maturation of these progenitor cells from BFU-Es to CFU-Es, the majority of the progenitors lose their potential for γ globin gene expression and their progeny become predominantly A cells, with relatively few progenitors giving rise to F cells (which should be more accurately designated as "A + F" cells). A hypothetical corollary of this model is that F cells may in fact derive directly from BFU-E progenitor cells that "short-circuit" the normal pathway of progenitor cell maturation through the CFU-E stage and give rise somewhat prematurely to differentiated erythroid cell progeny that manifest the early potential of their immediate progenitors and contain both Hb F and Hb A (see Fig. 7–13,

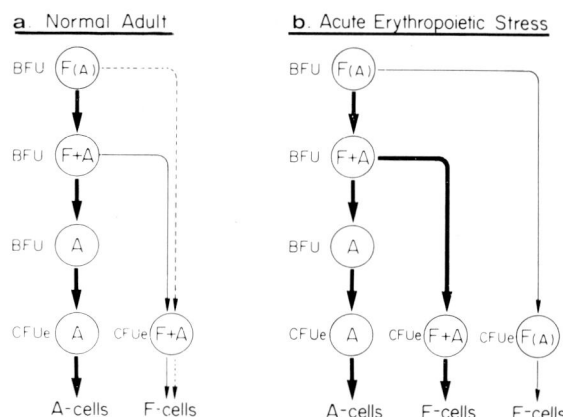

Figure 7–13. Model for the origin of F cells based on differential maturation of erythroid progenitor cells. A minor "short circuit" pathway of maturation giving rise to F cells in normal adults becomes enhanced during erythropoietic stress. (From Stamatoyannopoulos, G., and Papayannopoulou, T.: *In* Stamatoyannopoulos, G., and Nienhuis, A. W. (eds.): Cellular and Molecular Regulation of Hemoglobin Switchings. New York, Grune and Stratton, Inc., 1979, p. 323.)

pathway designated by dashed line). This model is very attractive because it reconciles both the results of *in vitro* culture experiments and the *in vivo* observations of increased F-cell production in conditions associated with erythropoietic stress. The model proposes that under conditions of erythropoietic stress, the "short-circuit" pathway of progenitor cell maturation becomes favored and quantitatively more significant, thereby resulting in the production of increased numbers of erythroid cells containing Hb F (see Fig. 7–13, right panel). Thus, the increased levels of Hb F synthesis by normal adult erythroid cells in the *in vitro* culture systems could be considered as the laboratory equivalent of erythropoietic stress *in vivo*.

There are, however, some opposing viewpoints to the preceding theory. In particular, a number of investigators have not detected a significant difference in the amount of Hb F synthesized by less mature (BFU-E–derived) versus more mature (CFU-E–derived) erythroid colonies.[298, 299] In another study,[300] it was determined that the percentage of F cells was similar in CFU-E– versus BFU-E–derived colonies but that the amount of Hb F/F cell was higher in the BFU-E–derived F cells than in the CFU-E–derived F cells. A number of investigators have also found variable levels of Hb F synthesis in virtually all BFU-E–derived erythroid colonies from adult blood that were individually analyzed,[273, 301–303] suggesting that commitment to Hb F production is ongoing, on a somewhat random basis, throughout colony formation in culture. Thus, an alternative, although less satisfying, model for F-cell production in adults is that a program for Hb F synthesis is present in many, if not all, erythroid progenitor cells but that the actual expression of Hb F by their progeny *in vivo* occurs in only a small number of cells, either on a random basis or owing to regulatory influences or factors that are poorly understood.

A fascinating observation has resulted from comparisons of the levels of Hb F synthesis in adult human erythroid cell colonies when grown in the presence of different types of additives to the culture. When the tissue culture medium was supplemented by "preswitch" serum from fetal sheep of 80 to 120 days of gestation instead of the usual fetal calf serum, the level of Hb F synthesis in cultured colonies was very low and was similar to that in erythroid cells of the adult individual *in vivo*[304, 305] There was thus a reversion to a more physiological pattern of Hb F synthesis by erythroid colonies grown *in vitro* in the presence of serum isolated from fetal sheep about to undergo the fetal to adult hemoglobin switch *in utero*. This reversion to the physiological adult pattern of hemoglobin synthesis occurred not only in erythroid colonies derived from normal adult progenitor cells but also in those derived from progenitor cells of individuals with activated Hb F synthesis *in vivo*, such as patients with sickle cell anemia and β thalassemia.[304] Even more remarkable is the observation that Hb F synthesis was reduced to normal or near-normal levels in cultured erythroid colonies derived from progenitor cells of individuals with nondeletion as well as deletion types of pancellular hereditary persistence of fetal hemoglobin (HPFH)[304, 306] (see Chapter 8). Individuals with pancellular HPFH have mutations that are assumed to result in the permanent failure of suppression of γ-chain synthesis after birth and, as a result, continued synthesis of Hb F, at a high level, in all adult erythroid cells. These results indicate that mutations affecting the developmental expression of globin genes can be influenced by exogenous, *trans*-acting, regulatory factors.

The activity in fetal sheep serum responsible for the restoration of the physiological pattern of Hb F synthesis in erythroid cell colonies derived from adult progenitor cells has been termed "switching factor," but its precise nature or physiological role in the perinatal fetal to adult hemoglobin switch has not yet been characterized. It is noteworthy that fetal sheep serum had no effect on the ratio of Hb F to Hb A synthesis in cultures of erythroid cells derived from human fetal liver, but it did appear to accelerate somewhat the switch from Hb F to Hb A synthesis in erythroid colonies derived from cord blood of newborn infants.[304] In replating or transfer experiments the "switching factor" activity could also be demonstrated to influence the pattern of Hb F synthesis in the progeny of erythroid progenitor cells that were exposed to the factor at both early and late stages of progenitor cell development.[305] The optimal effect was obtained when the factor was present throughout the development of the progenitor cells.

Studies of hemoglobin synthesis in erythroid cell colonies grown *in vitro* have also revealed another noteworthy feature of Hb F synthesis in adult erythroid cells, namely the asynchrony of its synthesis in relation to that of Hb A during erythroid cell maturation. By measuring the ratio of Hb F to Hb A synthesis in erythroid cells at progressively increasing different times in culture (and therefore at increasing degrees of maturity), it was discovered that the most immature erythroid cells synthesized proportionally more Hb F than did more mature erythroid cells and that the ratio of Hb F to Hb A synthesis decreased progressively during erythroid cell maturation.[307–310] Similar observations were also made in erythroid cells derived directly from *in vivo* sources.[311] Thus, the level of Hb F synthesis as a percentage of total hemoglobin synthesis can differ substantially depending on the stage of erythroid cell maturation at which it is assayed in erythroid colonies grown *in vitro*. This phenomenon may explain some of the discrepancies in the levels of Hb F synthesis observed in different earlier studies of hemoglobin synthesis in adult erythroid cell colonies grown *in vitro*. However, the particular relevance of this phenomenon to F-cell biology or to the general process of perinatal fetal to adult hemoglobin switching remains to be determined.

In summary, studies of hemoglobin synthesis in erythroid cell colonies derived from normal adult erythroid progenitor cells have revealed some interesting phenomena relating to Hb F synthesis that have led to the formulation of models to explain the basis for increased F-cell production in adults during various states of erythropoietic stress, but as interesting as those observations may be, they have not shed any significant light on the mystery of the basic mechanism of the perinatal fetal to adult hemoglobin switch.

EVOLUTIONARY CONSIDERATIONS

As discussed in Chapter 6, a comparison of the structure of various animal globin chains has allowed the construction of phylogenetic trees illustrating the evolutionary relatedness of the globin genes in different animal species (see Fig. 6–27). The recent availability of complete nucleotide sequence information on a large number of different cloned animal globin genes, including introns as well as exons, has permitted an even more detailed and precise comparison of evolutionary relationships between various globin genes in the animal kingdom. In addition, comparison of the precise chromosomal organization of the globin genes in different animal species has provided further information on the evolution of the globin genes following their presumed origin from a single ancestral gene. We will briefly summarize here the results of these analyses. The topic has been reviewed extensively elsewhere.[26, 44, 312, 313]

Changes in Chromosomal Organization of Globin Genes During Evolution

Various estimates place the time of duplication of the α and β globin genes from their single ancestral gene during early vertebrate evolution at approximately 450 million years ago.[312–314] In most vertebrates, the α and β globin gene clusters have subsequently become separated from one another and are found on different chromosomes. However, in the frog, the lowest vertebrate studied thus far, the α and β globin genes are still linked on the same chromosome. In some species of frogs, there is a single such cluster,[315] whereas in other species, such as *Xenopus laevis*, there are two similar unlinked clusters[315–317] that probably arose because of tetraploidization. In the frog globin cluster, the order of the genes, in the 5' → 3' direction of transcription, is as follows: two larval (embryonic) α-like genes, one adult α gene, one adult β gene, and two larval (embryonic) β-like genes (Fig. 7–14).

In birds and mammals, the α and β globin gene clusters have become dispersed to separate chromosomes. The mechanism(s) by which this separation occurred is not known. It is interesting to note, however, that in man, the myoglobin gene, which presumably arose from the same ancestral gene as the α and β globin genes, is located on yet a different chromosome (No. 22) from those bearing the α and β globin gene clusters.[318]

A general feature of the chromosomal organization of globin gene clusters in mammals is the arrangement of the genes in the general order (5' → 3') in which they are expressed during development: embryonic → fetal → adult (see Fig. 7–14). However, as noted previously, the frog larval β-like genes (expressed in tadpoles) are located 3' to the adult β gene, and in the chicken, there is a second embryonic gene located 3' to the adult β gene.[319, 320] These exceptions indicate that the precise arrangement of the globin genes in the order of their developmental expression has not been strictly conserved throughout evolution and therefore is not an absolute requirement for the normal pattern of regulation of globin gene expression during development. There are even minor exceptions in mammals. In the goat, the β globin gene cluster is triplicated. Within each of the three "subclusters," there are two embryonic genes, a pseudogene, and one of the following: an adult $β^A$ gene, a "juvenile" $β^C$ gene, or a fetal γ gene. Within each of the three "subclusters," the genes are arranged in the expected order listed above; however, the subcluster containing the fetal γ globin gene is situated to the far 3' side rather than the 5' side of the overall cluster.[321, 321a] In the mouse, the βh0 and βh1 genes that are expressed in early embryonic development are located to the 3' side of the embryonic y gene that is expressed later in embryonic development.[322] Similarly, in the rabbit, the embryonic β4 globin gene is expressed for a longer time in embryonic development than the embryonic β3 globin gene that is situated to its 3' side.[322a]

Another noteworthy constant feature of the mammalian β gene cluster is the presence of one (or more) pseudogenes between the fetal or embryonic genes and the adult β globin genes. The functional significance of this finding with regard to normal globin gene expression or switching is unclear, but in different species, these pseudogenes appear to have different evolutionary origins (see next section). Finally, the distance (in kb of DNA) separating the embryonic ε gene from the other non–α globin genes has increased dramatically between the brown lemur (a prosimian) and the baboon and gorilla, which have a β globin gene organization similar to that of man.[323] It would appear that an insertion of a segment of DNA occurred. In man, this region of DNA contains a repetitive DNA element of the Kpn I family, approximately 6 kb in length, and such elements are known to have characteris-

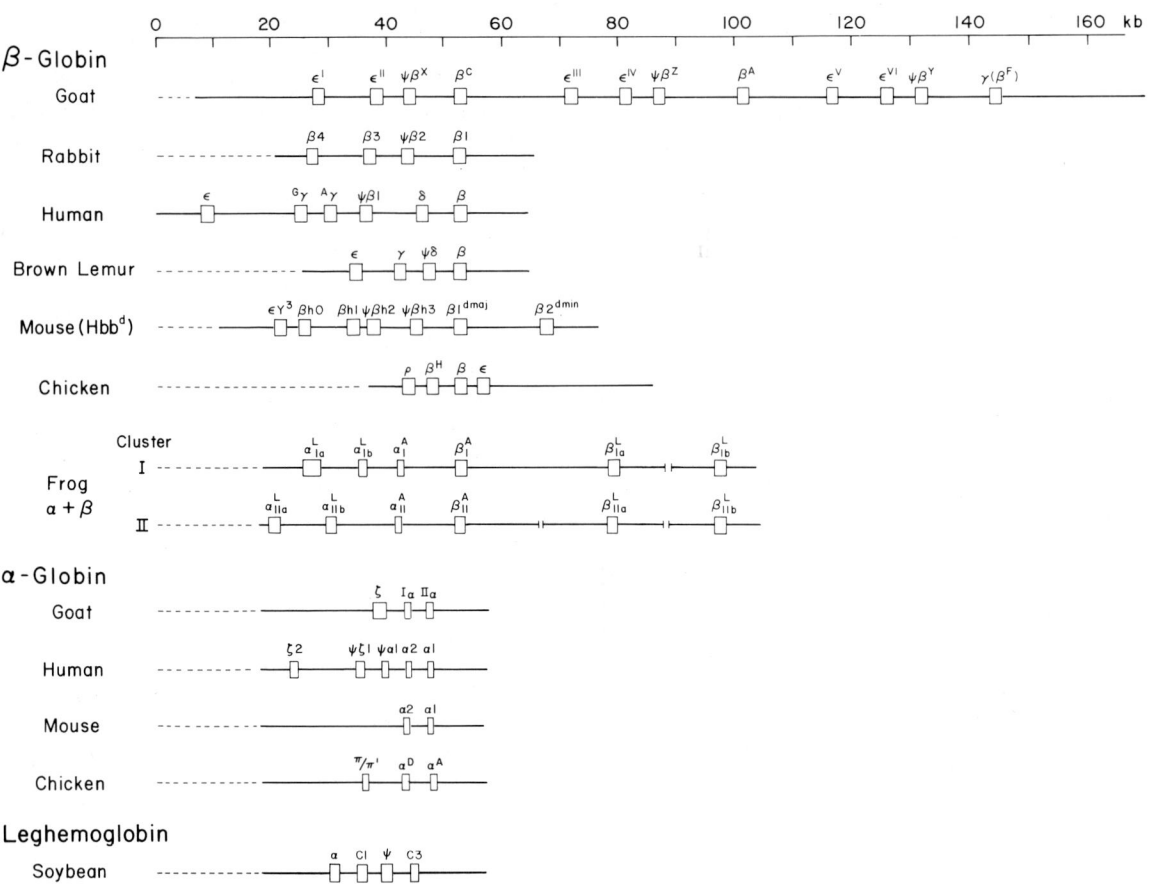

Figure 7–14. Chromosomal organization of the globin gene clusters in various species. (Modified from Collins, F. S., and Weissman, S. M.: Prog. Nucleic Acid Res. Mol. Biol. *31*:315, 1984.)

tics of transposable DNA elements (see preceding section on repetitive DNA sequences).

Evolutionary Relationship Between Individual Globin Genes

As stated previously and as discussed in Chapter 6, the various globin genes presumably arose by gene duplication events from ancestral genes. Orthologous genes are related genes that derived from a common ancestral gene prior to speciation and are found in many different animal species, whereas paralogous genes are those derived by duplication events within a given species. The relatedness between various globin genes can be assessed, on an evolutionary time scale, by the number and types of nucleotide sequence differences in the genes. Two types of nucleotide substitutions can occur—silent substitutions that do not change the encoded amino acid sequence and replacement substitutions that do change

the amino acid sequence of the protein. It has been estimated that silent substitutions occur at a rate of approximately 1 per cent per 1.4 million years (MY), whereas the replacement substitution rate is approximately 1 per cent per 10 MY.[44, 324] Based on these estimates, an evolutionary tree of the human β globin gene family has been derived in which the δ/β divergence is placed at 40 MY ago, the γ/ε divergence at 100 MY ago, and the β,δ/γ,ε divergence at 200 MY ago.[44] Such evolutionary trees are based to a certain extent on the assumption that the rate of evolution is fixed, whereas, in fact, a number of factors can influence the rate, such as the mutation rate and the probability of fixation or persistence of the mutation by the process of natural selection.

To avoid the pitfalls of constructing evolutionary trees on the basis of a fixed rate of evolution, an alternative method, that of maximum parsimony, has been devised that makes no assumptions about the rates of mutation.[312]

It is a geneological analysis in which the evolutionary tree that is constructed is based on the smallest number of independent mutations connecting the various branches. A detailed phylogenetic tree, using this approach to analyze nucleotide sequence data, has been constructed for the globin gene family and is illustrated in Figure 7–15. An example of discordant results, using this method instead of the calculation based on a fixed rate of evolution, is illustrated by the case of the ψα gene in man. By the fixed rate method, the ψα gene was estimated to have diverged from the human α gene 60 MY ago, 20 MY after the divergence between human α and rabbit α.[47] By the maximum parsimony method (see Fig. 7–15), the ψα gene would be more ancient and would have arisen prior to the human/rabbit α divergence.

Another pitfall in constructing evolutionary trees for paralogous genes is the possibility of gene conversion events by which intrachromosomal recombination events between linked genes can result in the "correction" or homogenization of the sequence of one gene by that of another. The best example of this process is illustrated by the sequence analysis of the large introns (IVS-2) of the linked $^G\gamma$ and $^A\gamma$ globin gene in man. The sequence of IVS-2 of a given $^A\gamma$ globin gene is more similar to that of the linked $^G\gamma$ gene on the same chromosome than to that of the $^A\gamma$ gene on the *trans* chromosome.[40, 41] Thus, a gene conversion event can result in the appearance of a closer evolutionary relationship between two genes than is in fact the case. An example of such an occurrence is the case of the human δ/β gene duplication, which was initially estimated to have occurred 40 MY ago.[44] More recent analyses, taking into account sequence information of introns as well as flanking DNA and comparisons of β-like genes in other animal species, have concluded that the δ/β gene duplication is probably much more ancient[326–328] but that a more recent gene conversion event between the δ and β globin genes (40 MY ago) has rendered the coding and 5'-flanking sequences of the δ gene more homologous to those of the β gene. The technique that has been most useful for allowing such comparisons and providing the necessary data for drawing conclusions is the dot matrix com-

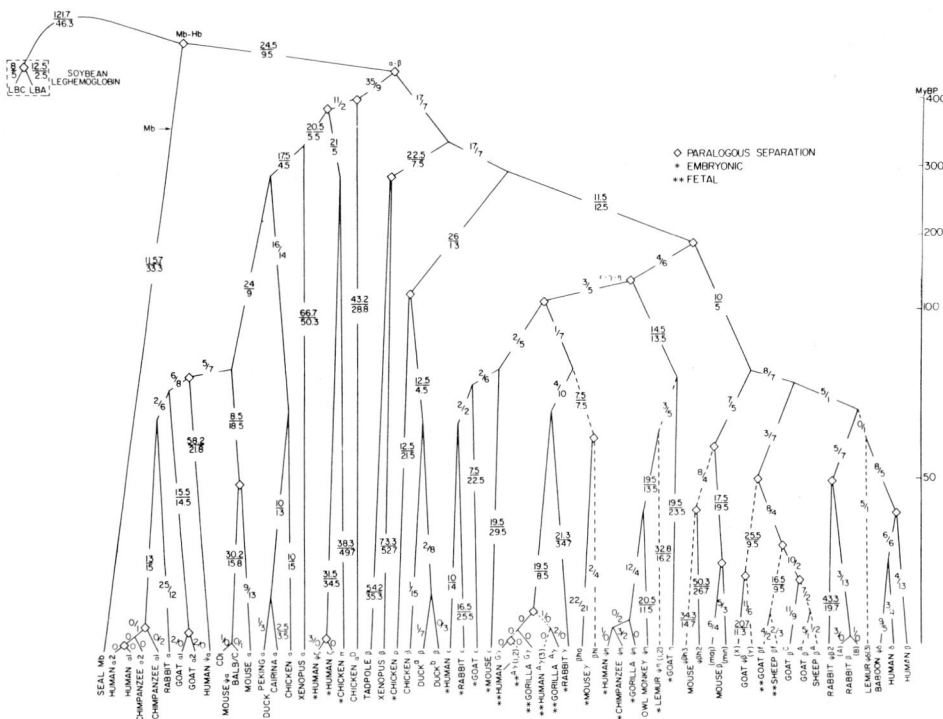

Figure 7–15. Phylogenetic tree of various globin genes constructed by the method of maximum parsimony from the analysis of DNA sequences of the coding portions of the genes. (From Goodman, M., et al.: J. Mol. Biol. *180*:803, 1984.)

puter program[329] that generates a two-dimensional plot of the comparison of two nucleotide sequences. Areas of sequence homology appear as diagonal lines; insertions or deletions simply result in a shift of the position of the diagonal line without a loss in the ability to follow regions of homology between the two sequences that are being compared. Such analyses have proved to be very helpful in defining homologies between distantly related genes.

With this background information on general principles and methodologies, one can summarize some additional results and conclusions, other than those already discussed, regarding the evolutionary history of the globin genes in man and other selected mammalian species. The α-like and β-like embryonic globin genes diverged from their ancestral adult counterparts at surprisingly different times. The human ζ and ψζ genes diverged from the α gene very early in evolution, whereas the ε gene diverged from the other β-like genes much later (see Fig. 7–15). Thus, there is more homology between the human ζ gene and α-like embryonic genes of other animal species than between the human ζ and human α genes.

The teleological or developmental advantages or consequences of this phenomenon, if any, are not clear.

The human ψβ1 gene, located between the ^Aγ and δ globin genes, has an interesting evolutionary history. Although sharing considerable homology with the human ε and γ globin genes, it is most closely homologous to the functional goat ε^II gene and therefore appears to be orthologously related to it.[330] Additional evidence for the origin of the ψβ1 gene earlier in evolution than the primate/nonprimate divergence consists of the finding that the non–α gene cluster of the brown lemur, a prosimian, contains a pseudogene between its single γ gene and its β gene[323, 331] that is a fusion gene, the 5′ end of which is very homologous to the human ψβ1 gene[120, 121] and the 3′ end of which is homologous to the human δ globin gene,[331] and that presumably arose by nonhomologous crossing over between linked ψβ1 and δ gene loci. Thus, it has been proposed that the ψβ1 gene of primates, the ψδ gene of prosimians, and the ε^II gene of the goat all descended from a common ancestral globin gene that is distinct from the other

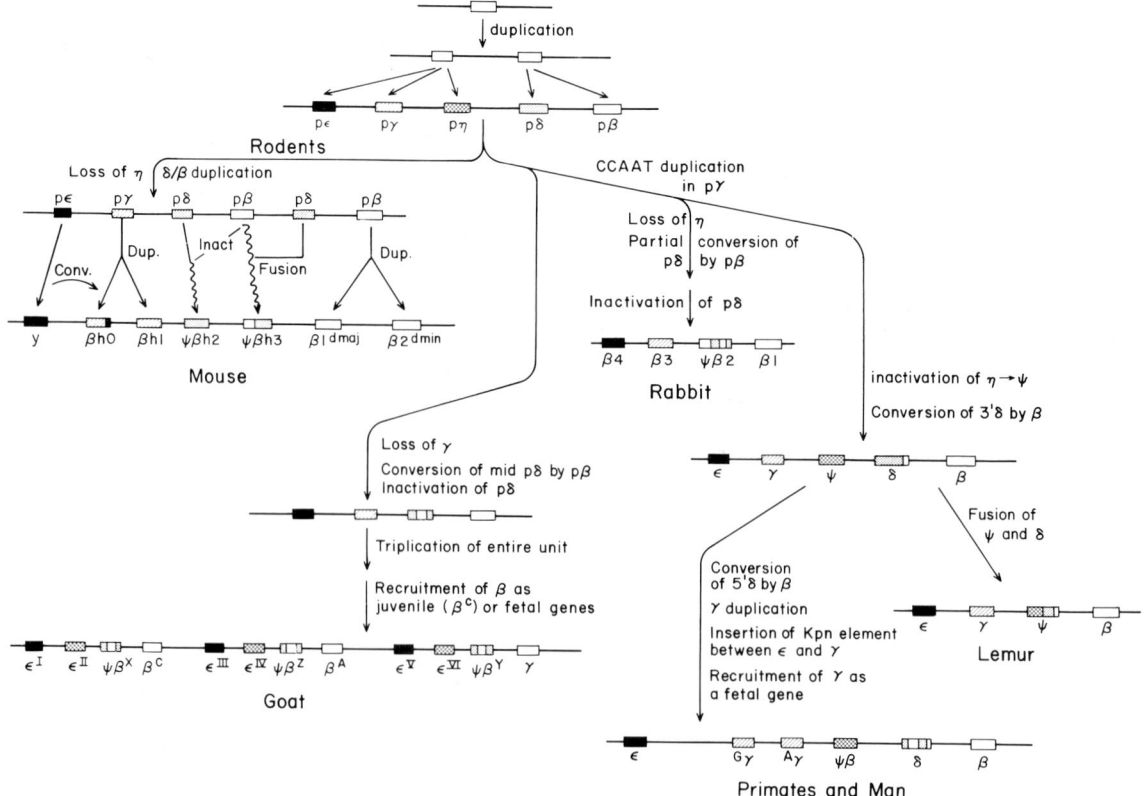

Figure 7–16. Model of the evolution of the β-like globin gene cluster in various animal species. (Modified from Collins, F. S., and Weissman, S. M.: Prog. Nucleic Acid Res. Mol. Biol. *31*:315, 1984.)

ancestral non–α globin genes. This ancestral globin gene has been designated the η gene[330, 331a] for eta, the seventh letter (following zeta) in the Greek alphabet.

Based on nucleotide sequence comparisons and homologies between the various β-like globin genes, it has been possible to derive models for the origin of the non–α globin genes of various mammalian species by a proposed series of gene duplications, gene conversions, and occasional nonhomologous crossovers. These models, generated by a number of different investigators,[321, 325–328, 300, 331a, 332] can be combined into an overall scheme that is illustrated in Figure 7–16. The starting point of the model is duplication of the ancestral single β globin gene into a two-gene cluster, the 5' member of which is the ancestor of the ε, γ, and η globin genes and the 3' member of which is the ancestor of the δ/β globin gene pair. The ancient prototype mammalian non–α globin gene cluster would therefore have consisted of five genes, designated proto-ε, proto-γ, proto-η, proto-δ, and proto-β (see Fig. 7–16). Different perturbations of this basic cluster can explain the current organization of the cluster in the various species that have been studied, such as the mouse,[326, 326a, 332] the rabbit,[327, 328] the goat,[321] and primates,[323, 331a] including man.[20] The various perturbations are indicated in Figure 7–16 and have been discussed in detail elsewhere.[26, 313, 321, 323, 325–328, 330–332] A particularly noteworthy observation is the fact that the γ globin gene expressed during fetal development in the goat appears to be derived from a proto-β globin gene lineage rather than a proto-γ globin gene lineage. Nucleotide sequence analysis of the goat γ globin gene has in fact demonstrated that it shares very close homology with the goat β globin gene,[333] consistent with a much closer evolutionary relationship than exists between the human γ and β globin genes. Therefore, this gene has been more recently referred to as the goat β^F gene.[321a]

Heme: Biosynthesis and Interaction with Globin Synthesis

Mechanism and Control of Heme Synthesis

Heme consists of divalent iron coordinately bound within a protoporphyrin 9 ring; oxidized (or trivalent) iron, when bound to protoporphyrin 9, forms oxidized heme (hemin). The porphyrin moiety of heme is synthesized by the complex metabolic pathway shown in Figure 7–17, the details of which have been reviewed elsewhere.[334] Heme synthesis begins with the condensation of glycine and succinyl CoA to form δ-aminolevulinic acid (ALA). This reaction is catalyzed by the enzyme ALA synthetase in mitochondria of erythroid (or other) cells. This enzymatic reaction requires pyridoxal phosphate as a cofactor and seems to be the rate-limiting step in the heme synthesis pathway. Heme synthesis then proceeds in the cell's cytoplasm by a series of extramitochondrial enzymatic reactions. However, the last three enzymatic reactions in the heme synthetic pathway are again localized to the cell's mitochondria: (1) the synthesis of protoporphyrinogen 9 from coproporphyrinogen III, a reaction that is catalyzed by coproporphyrinogen oxidase, (2) the oxidation of protoporphyrinogen 9 to protoporphyrin 9, and (3) the synthesis of heme from protoporphyrin 9, which involves the binding of iron to the porphyrin ring, a reaction catalyzed by the enzyme heme synthetase (or ferrochelatase). It is not clear whether heme itself is produced initially or whether hemin is first produced and then reduced to heme by the cytochrome b_5 reductase system (see Chapter 17).

It is most interesting that the initial and final enzymatic reactions in the heme synthesis pathway are localized in the cell's mitochondria, an anatomic arrangement well suited to allow heme to control its own synthesis by end-product inhibition. In fact, the synthesis of heme is in great part controlled by the procsses of end-product repression and feedback inhibition of the enzyme ALA synthetase. Heme itself has two effects on this enzyme. First, it interacts directly with ALA synthetase and inactivates it (end-product repression), and second, since ALA synthetase has a short half-life, its cellular level rapidly decreases after its synthesis is suppressed owing to feedback inhibition. Similar mechanisms affecting the activity of heme synthetase may limit the formation of heme from protoporphyrin.[9] Heme may also regulate its own synthesis by inhibiting the uptake or transfer of iron from transferrin into the reticulocyte.[335] Heme synthesis is also controlled to some extent by globin synthesis. When protein synthesis in reticulocytes is inhibited by cycloheximide, heme synthesis is also rapidly and reversibly reduced and the onset of inhibition is too rapid to be due to decreased synthesis of the enzymes responsible for heme production. The inhibition is probably mediated via free heme, which accumulates in the absence of globin synthesis.

IRVING M. LONDON

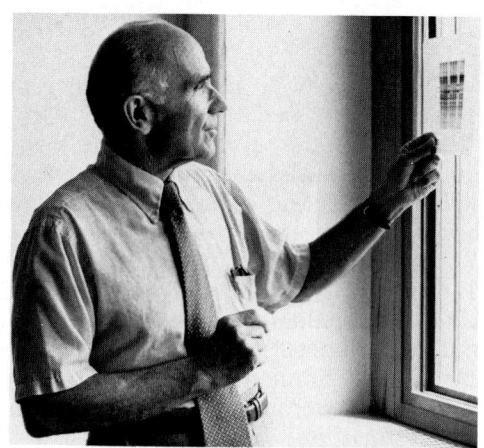

Investigation of the biosynthesis of hemoglobin began in the late 1940s. Since that time, Irving London has continued to be one of the leaders of this important field.

London received a classical education at Harvard College and then went on to Harvard Medical School. World War II disrupted his postdoctoral training but provided the impetus for his debut in biomedical research, investigating the chemotherapy of malaria. This work piqued his career-long interest in erythropoiesis and red cell metabolism.

London joined the faculty of the College of Physicians and Surgeons at Columbia University and began a highly productive collaboration with David Shemin and David Rittenberg in the Biochemistry Department. These scientists were pioneers in the use of newly available isotopes for studying metabolism *in vivo* and *in vitro*. They showed that the incorporation of ^{15}N-labeled glycine into hemoglobin provided the first reliable data on the production, life span, and survival of red blood cells. London extended this work to studies of patients with various hematological disorders and demonstrated enhanced and random red cell destruction in sickle cell anemia and ineffective erythropoiesis in pernicious anemia. These *in vivo* measurements of heme synthesis and turnover provided the first demonstration of early labeled bile pigment. London then directed his attention to the biosynthesis of hemoglobin *in vitro*. He showed that reticulocytes but not mature red cells could convert glycine into heme. Subsequent incubations of nucleated blood cells of birds revealed not only heme synthesis but also, for the first time, the formation of peptide bonds. Studies of polypeptide synthesis led London and E. Dimant to examine the biosynthesis and turnover of glutathione, the versatile tripeptide that figures so prominently in the red cell's defense against oxidant stress.

London found that heme regulates its own synthesis by inhibiting the formation of delta aminolevulinic acid and that it promotes the assembly of the hemoglobin tetramer and the coordinate synthesis of the alpha and beta chains of globin. The role of heme in the translational control of the synthesis of globin and other proteins has been a major focus of much of London's research over the past two decades. The reticulocyte proved to be an ideal model system for investigating the molecular events responsible for the initiation of polypeptide translation. As discussed in the pages that follow, London and his colleagues unraveled the mechanism by which the initiation of protein synthesis is controlled by heme and the heme-regulated protein kinase. This phenomenon has direct bearing on the pattern of globin chain synthesis in the heme-deficient anemias.

Concurrent with his unflagging productivity in the laboratory, Irving London has been one of the nation's leading medical educators and administrators. In 1955, he became the first Chairman of Medicine at the newly created Albert Einstein College of Medicine. During his 15-year tenure, he assembled a truly outstanding department. In addition, he was a founder of the Institute of Medicine of the National Academy of Sciences. He is now completing 15 years as the first director of the Harvard–M.I.T. Division of Health Sciences and Technology. This innovative experiment in medical education has been as pivotal as London's early studies on heme biosynthesis. Two generations of students are in his debt. He remains the urbane and articulate spokesman for the highest standards in science and education.

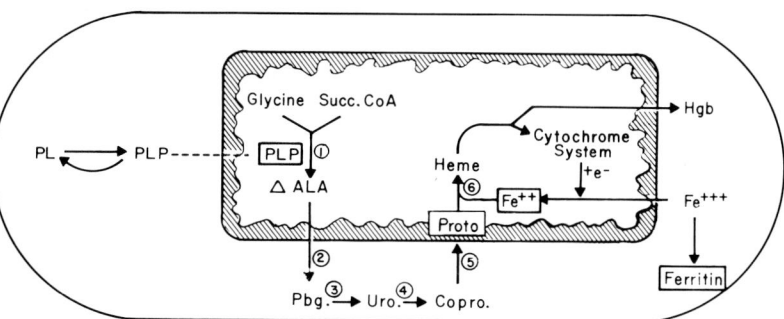

Figure 7-17. Biosynthesis of heme. The central rectangle represents reactons occurring within mitochondria. (PL = pyridoxine; PLP = pyridoxal phosphate; Succ. CoA = succinyl CoA; △ALA = δ-aminolevulinic acid; Pbg. = porphobilinogen; Uro. = uroporphyrinogen III; Copro. = coproporphyrinogen III; Proto = protoporphyrinogen 9. (Courtesy of Dr. L. R. Solomon.)

The abnormal reduction of heme synthesis observed in thalassemia presumably results from a similar mechanism due to the primary decrease in globin synthesis that occurs in this disorder (see Chapter 8). Finally, the level of heme in the cell can be influenced to some degree by the activity of heme oxygenase, the rate-limiting enzyme of the heme catabolism pathway.[336] This enzyme can in fact be induced at the transcriptional level by free heme.[337]

Levels of heme synthetic and degradative enzymes have been measured during erythroid differentiation in erythroid colonies cultured in vitro.[338] Activity of ALA synthetase and ALA dehydrase increases progressively while activity of heme oxygenase progressively decreases over 60 hours, concomitant with the peak of erythroid colony formation and incorporation of ^{14}C ALA into heme. These results appear somewhat contradictory at first glance, since one would expect the increased levels of heme, which accumulate during erythroid differentiation, to have opposite effects on these enzymes in view of the regulatory pathway previously described. Although it is possible that different regulatory mechanisms are operative early in erythroid differentiation, it is probable that with normal levels of globin synthesis, little free heme accumulates in developing erythroid cells and therefore no inhibition of heme synthetic enzymes or induction of heme degradative enzymes occurs until late in erythroid differentiation when globin synthesis slows considerably. Similar results have been observed during induction of erythroid differentiation in mouse erythroleukemia cells.[338a]

A molecular genetic analysis of heme synthesis will soon be possible now that it is possible to clone the genes encoding heme synthetic enzymes.[338b]

Disorders of Heme Synthesis

A number of humoral and pharmacological agents as well as environmental factors affect heme synthesis. Some of these factors, however, influence primarily hepatic heme synthesis. We will limit our discussion to those factors that are particularly relevant to heme synthesis in erythroid cells. An adequate supply of iron, of course, is necessary for normal heme synthesis, and in some circumstances, the availability of iron may be a limiting factor controlling the rate of heme synthesis at the heme synthetase step where iron is essential. Iron deficiency results in decreased utilization of labeled glycine for heme synthesis. Although erythrocyte free protoporphyrin levels are increased in iron deficiency, total porphyrin content is decreased. There is also some evidence that excess protoporphyrins in iron-deficient cells may exert feedback inhibition on earlier steps of the heme synthesis pathway.

The situation is less clear in states of iron overload. Theoretically, excess iron, just as free heme, should induce heme oxygenase and inhibit ALA synthetase,[339, 340] thus resulting in a depression of heme levels in the cell. Mitochondrial damage induced by iron overload could also cause decreased heme synthesis as a secondary phenomenon. However, no clinically evident abnormalities of red cell heme metabolism have been reported in iron overload caused by idiopathic hemochromatosis.

Isoniazid (INH), other antituberculous drugs such as cycloserine and pyrazinamide, and other drugs such as L-dopa, penicillamine, and hydralazine are all potent inhibitors of heme synthesis and probably act via pyridoxine antagonism, thus secondarily inhibiting ALA synthetase activity. It is thought that these drugs act by forming hydrazone derivatives with pyridoxal phosphate, resulting in its removal from apoenzymes and loss via increased urinary excretion. The hydrazones also inhibit phosphorylation of pyridoxine to pyridoxal phosphate. The inhibitory effect of these drugs can be reversed by the administration of pyridoxal phosphate. Lead inhibits the activity of multiple enzymes in the heme synthesis pathway—heme synthetase, ALA dehydrase, coproporphyrinogen oxidase, and possibly ALA synthetase. Ethanol also inhibits heme synthesis, although there is some controversy with regard to the precise mechanism(s) involved. The initial report of inhibition by ethanol of the phosphorylation of pyridoxine to pyridoxal phosphate[341] has not been confirmed in later studies.[342–344] Alternative mechanisms include accelerated degradation of pyridoxal phosphate[342, 345] or generalized mitochondrial damage caused by ethanol leading to secondary changes in heme synthetic enzymes.[344] Chloramphenicol, which specifically inhibits mitochondrial protein synthesis, is another mitochondrial toxin[346] that can produce secondary defects in heme synthetic enzymes, especially ferrochelatase.[347]

Most of these inhibitors of heme synthesis can cause a clinically significant hematologic disorder termed "secondary sideroblastic anemia." This condition, which can also occur as a primary idiopathic disorder, is characterized by anemia, hypochromic red blood cells having a decreased intracellular hemoglobin content, and the presence of ringed sideroblasts in the marrow. Ringed sideroblasts are nucleated erythyroid precursor cells that contain excessive deposits of iron in mitochondria, which usually form a ring around the cell nucleus. The marked increase in mitochondrial iron deposits probably results not only from passive accumulation of iron due to decreased utilization secondary to decreased heme synthesis but also from increased cellular uptake of iron due to loss of inhibition of cellular iron uptake as a result of the heme deficiency.[335, 348, 348a]

The precise mechanism responsible for decreased heme synthesis in the idiopathic variety of this disorder has not been definitively established.[348, 348a] The disorder is quite heterogeneous with regard to abnormalities detected in heme synthetic enzymes, the most common, but not invariable, finding being reduced activity of ALA synthetase.[349] Although rare patients respond to the administration of pyridoxal phosphate,[349, 350] pyridoxine metabolism is normal in most patients.[345, 351] It is possible that, as perhaps in the case of ethanol, the disorder represents a primary mitochondrial disease with alterations of heme synthetic enzymes representing a secondary event. A number of different mitochondrial defects have in fact been described in individuals with this disorder.[352] Finally, it should be noted that although many individuals are exposed to agents that can cause sideroblastic anemia, relatively few in fact develop the disorder. There may therefore be a population at risk, and it has been suggested that individuals who are heterozygous for hemochromatosis (iron overload due to increased gastrointestinal absorption) may be particularly susceptible to both the acquired and idiopathic[353] forms of this disorder.

Effect of Heme Deficiency on Globin-Chain Synthesis

A number of early studies demonstrated a definite degree of coordination of the rates of heme and globin synthesis[354] and an important role for hemin in the maintenance and stimulation of *in vitro* globin chain synthesis in intact rabbit reticulocytes.[355–358] Furthermore, a number of clinical disorders of heme synthesis in man have inhibitory effects on globin chain synthesis. These disorders include iron deficiency, lead poisoning, isoniazid toxicity, and the primary sideroblastic anemias. Although these various disorders are associated with a reduction of total globin chain and hemoglobin synthesis, resulting in a hypochromic microcytic anemia, quantitation of the relative amounts of α and β globin chain synthesis by radiolabeling procedures has revealed in many studies,[359–364] but not all,[365–371] that α globin chain synthesis is more severely affected than β-chain synthesis, with α/β synthetic ratios in the range of those observed in α-thalassemia trait (see Chapter 8). In various studies, the addition of hemin *in vitro* resulted in the restoration of a more normal or balanced α/β globin chain synthetic ratio[359, 363] as well as an overall increase in globin and hemoglobin synthesis.

The cause of unequal suppression of α and β globin chain synthesis in states of heme deficiency can probably be attributed to two interacting phenomena operating at the level of translation of globin mRNA: (1) the presence of an inhibitor of polypeptide chain initiation that is activated when heme is deficient (see next section), and (2) the characteristics of α globin mRNA itself, which is less efficient than β globin mRNA in initiating polypeptide chain synthesis.[372, 373] Thus, in the presence of various inhibitors of chain initiation, α globin chain synthesis is more severely suppressed than β-chain synthesis.[374] As noted in Chapter 4, the low levels of Hb A_2 observed in various disorders associated with heme deficiency are probably due to a post-translational phenomenon in which δ globin chains, initially synthesized in normal amounts, cannot compete as efficiently as the β globin chains for the reduced pool of available α globin chains resulting from the phenomenon of selective inhibition of α globin chain synthesis due to heme deficiency.

Effect of Hemin on Initiation of Polypeptide Chain Synthesis

In cell-free systems prepared from unfractionated rabbit reticulocyte hemolysates, globin is actively synthesized for approximately 5 minutes, and then protein synthesis abruptly ceases. This inactivation of globin chain synthesis has been shown to be due to inhibition of initiation of polypeptide chain synthesis, which can be prevented or considerably delayed by the prior addition of hemin to the cell-free system. Although this effect of hemin was initially thought to be specific for globin chain synthesis, it was subsequently shown that hemin can also influence the rate of synthesis of nonglobin proteins in reticulocytes. The inhibition of protein synthesis in the absence of hemin is due to the activation of a protein inhibitor of polypeptide chain initiation that was initially termed the "hemin-controlled repressor" but that more recently and appropriately has been renamed the "hemin-regulated or hemin-controlled inhibitor" (HRI or HCI).[375-379]

The mechanism of action of the HRI has been progressively elucidated over the last few years, and the current understanding of the process can be summarized as follows.[377, 379] The HRI is a cyclic AMP–independent protein kinase that is activated in the absence of hemin. Activated HCI specifically phosphorylates a single site on the α chain of the initiation factor called eIF-2, which is required for one of the early steps in initiation of protein synthesis—the formation of a ternary complex between eIF-2, GTP, and initiator tRNA (methionyl tRNA) that then binds to the small ribosomal subunit (40S). The inhibition of polypeptide chain initiation is not due to direct inactivation of eIF-2 by phosphorylation, since only a small fraction of eIF-2 is phosphorylated in inactive hemin-deficient lysates, and phosphorylated eIF-2 can be utilized in the formation of the ternary complex. Rather, the inhibition of chain initiation appears to result from the interaction between phosphorylated eIF-2, designated eIF-2(αP), and another protein factor that is involved in the recycling of eIF-2. During the joining of the 48S complex (40S/eIF-2/GTP/Met-tRNA/mRNA) and the 60S ribosomal subunit, the eIF-2/GDP binary complex is formed. The factor required for recycling of eIF-2 catalyzes the dissociation of GDP from eIF-2, thus permitting the binding of GTP by eIF-2 and the formation of the ternary complex which can now be utilized in a subsequent cycle of initiation.[379] This other protein factor has been given various names—reversing factor (RF), eukaryotic initiation factor 2B (eIF-2B), and GDP exchange factor (GEF). When eIF-2 is phosphorylated, it forms a nondissociable complex with RF, and the bound RF is unavailable for the GTP-GDP exchange. Thus, RF becomes depleted and rate-limiting through the formation of an inactive RF/eIF-2(αP) complex. Protein synthesis is inhibited when the amount of available RF is too low to generate sufficient eIF-2/GTP/Met-tRNA to meet the requirements for new cycles of polypeptide chain initiation.

The elucidation of this intricate mechanism by which hemin influences protein synthesis provides additional fascinating information on the role of heme in the molecular biological and biochemical processes of erythroid cells and poses the important question of the generality of this mechanism in other cells.

References

1. Lewin, B.: Genes. New York, John Wiley & Sons, Inc., 1983.
2. Alberts B., Bray, D., Lewis, J., Raff, M., Roberts, R., and Watson, J. D.: Molecular Biology of the Cell. New York, Garland Publishing, Inc., 1983.
3. Bunn, H. F., Forget, B. G., and Ranney, H. M.: Human Hemoglobins. Philadelphia, W. B. Saunders Co., 1977.
4. Deisseroth, A., Velez, R., and Nienhuis, A. W.: Hemoglobin synthesis in somatic cell hybrids: Independent segregation of the human alpha- and beta-globin genes. Science *191*:1262, 1976.
5. Deisseroth, A., Nienhuis, A., Turner, P., Velez, R., Anderson, W. F., Ruddle, F., Lawrence, J., Creagan, R., and Kucherlapati, R.: Localization of the human α-globin structural gene to chromosome 16 in somatic cell hybrids by molecular hybridization assay. Cell *12*:205, 1977.
6. Deisseroth, A., Nienhuis, A., Lawrence, J., Giles, R., Turner, P., and Ruddle, F. H.: Chromosomal localization of human β globin gene on human chromosome 11 in somatic cell hybrids. Proc. Natl. Acad. Sci. USA *75*:1456, 1978.
7. Gusella, J., Varsanyi-Briener, A., Kao, F. T., Jones, C., Puck, T. T., Keys, C., Orkin, S., and Housman, D.: Precise localization of human β-globin gene complex on chromosome 11. Proc. Natl. Acad. Sci. USA *76*:5239, 1979.
8. Jeffreys, A. J., Craig, I. W., and Francke, U.:

Localization of the $^G\gamma$-, $^A\gamma$-, δ- and β-globin genes on the short arm of human chromosome 11. Nature 281:606, 1979.
9. Lebo, R. V., Carrano, A. V., Burkhart-Schultz, K., Dozy, A. M., Yu, L.-C., and Kan, Y. W.: Assignment of human β-, γ-, and δ-globin genes to the short arm of chromosome 11 by chromosome sorting and DNA restriction enzyme analysis. Proc. Natl. Acad. Sci. USA 76:5804, 1979.
10. Sanders-Haigh, L., Anderson, W. F., and Francke, U.: The β-globin gene is on the short arm of human chromosome 11. Nature 283:683, 1980.
11. Scott, A. F., Phillips, J. A., and Migeon, B. R.: DNA endonuclease analysis for localization of human β- and δ-globin genes on chromosome 11. Proc. Natl. Acad. Sci. USA 76:4563, 1979.
12. Koeffler, H. P., Sparkes, R. S., Stang, H., and Mohandas, T.: Regional assignment of genes for human α-globin and phosphoglycollate phosphatase to the short arm of chromosome 16. Proc. Natl. Acad. Sci. USA 78:7015, 1981.
13. Malcolm, S., Barton, P., Murphy, C., and Ferguson-Smith, M. A.: Chromosomal localization of a single copy gene by in situ hybridization—human β globin genes on the short arm of chromosome 11. Ann. Hum. Genet. 45:135, 1981.
14. Gerhard, D. S., Kawasaki, E. S., Bancroft, F. C., and Szabo, P.: Localization of a unique gene by direct hybridization in situ. Proc. Natl. Acad. Sci. USA 78:3755, 1981.
15. Barton, P., Malcolm, S., Murphy, C., and Ferguson-Smith, M. A.: Localization of the human α-globin gene cluster to the short arm of chromosome 16 (16p12-16p-ter) by hybridization in situ. J. Mol. Biol. 156:269, 1982.
16. Antonarakis, S. E., Phillips, J. A. III, Mallonee, R. L., Kazazian, W. H., Jr., Fearon, E. R., Waber, P. G., Kroneberg, H. M., Ullrich, A., and Meyers, D. A.: β-globin locus is linked to the parathyroid hormone (PTH) locus and lies between the insulin and PTH loci in man. Proc. Natl. Acad. Sci. USA 80:6615, 1983.
17. Lebo, R. V., Chakravarti, A., Buetow, K. H., Cheung, M.-C., Cann, H., Cordell, B., and Goodman, H.: Recombination within and between the human insulin and β-globin gene loci. Proc. Natl. Acad. Sci. USA 80:4808, 1983.
17a. White, R., Leppert, M., Bishop D. T., Barker, D., Berkowitz, J., Brown, C., Callahan, P., Holm, T., and Jerominski, L.: Construction of linkage maps with DNA markers for human chromosomes. Nature 313:101, 1985.
18. de Martinville, B., and Francke, U.: The c-Ha-ras1, insulin and β-globin loci map outside the deletion associated with aniridia-Wilms' tumor. Nature 305:641, 1983.
18a. Morton, C. C., Kirsch, I. R., Taub, R., Orkin, S. H., and Brown, J. A.: Localization of the β-globin gene by chromosomal in situ hybridization. Am. J. Hum. Genet. 36:576, 1984.
19. Lawn, R. M., Frisch, E. F., Parker, R. C., Blake, G., and Maniatis, T.: The isolation and characterization of linked δ- and β-globin genes from a cloned library of human DNA. Cell 15:1157, 1978.
20. Fritsch, E. F., Lawn, R. M., and Maniatis, T.: Molecular cloning and characterization of the human β-like globin gene cluster. Cell 19:959, 1980.
21. Lauer, J., Shen, C. K., and Maniatis, T.: The chromosomal arrangement of human α-like globin genes: Sequence homology and α-globin gene deletions. Cell 20:119, 1980.

22. Grosveld, F. G., Dahl, H. H. M., deBoer, E., and Flavell, R. A.: Isolation of β globin–related genes from a human cosmid library. Gene 13:227, 1981.
23. Grosveld, F. G., Lund, T., Murray, E. J., Mellor, A. L., Dahl, H. H. M., and Flavell, R. A.: The construction of cosmid libraries which can be used to transform eukaryotic cells. Nucleic Acids Res. 10:6715, 1982.
24. Lau, Y.-F., and Kan, Y. W.: Versatile cosmid vectors for the isolation, expression, and rescue of gene sequences: Studies with the human α-globin gene cluster. Proc. Natl. Acad. Sci. USA 80:5225, 1983.
25. Collins, F. S., Stoeckert, C. J., Serjeant, G. R., Forget, B. G., and Weissman, S. M.: $^G\gamma\beta^+$ Hereditary persistence of fetal hemoglobin: Cosmid cloning and identification of a specific mutation 5' to the $^G\gamma$ gene. Proc. Natl. Acad. Sci. USA 81:4894, 1984.
26. Collins, F. S., and Weissman, S. M.: The molecular genetics of human hemoglobin. In Cohn, W. E., and Moldave, K. (eds.): Progress in Nucleic Acids Research and Molecular Biology Vol. 31. New York, Academic Press, 1984, pp. 315–437.
27. Higgs, D. R., Goodbourn, S. E. Y., Wainscoat, J. S., Clegg, J. B., and Weatherall, D. J.: Highly variable regions of DNA flank the human α globin genes. Nucleic Acids Res. 9:4213, 1981.
28. Goodbourn, S. E. Y., Higgs, D. R., Clegg, J. B., and Weatherall, D. J.: Molecular basis of length polymorphism in the human ζ-globin gene complex. Proc. Natl. Acad. Sci. USA 80:5022, 1983.
29. Pressley, L., Higgs, D. R., Clegg, J. B., and Weatherall, D. J.: Gene deletions in α-thalassemia prove that the 5'-ζ locus is functional. Proc. Natl. Acad. Sci. USA 77:3586, 1980.
30. Winichagoon, P., Higgs, D. R., Goodbourn, S. E. Y., Lamb, J., Clegg, J. B., and Weatherall, D. J.: Multiple arrangements of the human embryonic zeta globin genes. Nucleic Acids Res. 10:5853, 1982.
30a. Felice, A. E., McKie, V. C., McKie, K., and Huisman, T. H. J.: Deletions and duplications of α or ζ globin genes in children with sickle cell anemia. Blood 64(Suppl. 1):47a, 1984.
30b. Powers, P. A., Altay, C., Huisman, T. H. J., and Smithies, O.: Two novel arrangements of the human fetal globin genes: $^G\gamma$-$^G\gamma$ and $^A\gamma$-$^A\gamma$. Nucleic Acids Res. 12:7023, 1984.
31. Tilghman, S. M., Tiemeier, D. C., Seidman, J. G., Peterlin, B. M., Sullivan, M., Maizel, J. V., and Leder, P.: Intervening sequence of DNA identified in the structural portion of the mouse β globin gene. Proc. Natl. Acad. Sci. USA 75:725, 1978.
32. Jeffreys, A. J., and Flavell, R. A.: The rabbit β globin gene contains a large insert in the coding sequence. Cell 12:1097, 1977.
33. Flavell, R. A., Kooter, J. M., DeBoer, E., Little, P. F. R., and Williamson, R.: Analysis of the $\beta\delta$-globin gene loci in normal and Hb Lepore DNA: Direct determination of gene linkage and intergene distance. Cell 15:25, 1978.
34. Mears, J. G., Ramirez, F., Leibowitz, D., and Bank, A.: Organization of human δ- and β-globin genes in cellular DNA and the presence of intragenic inserts. Cell 15:15, 1978.
35. Proudfoot, N. J., Gil, A., and Maniatis, T.: The structure of the human zeta-globin gene and a closely linked, nearly identical pseudogene. Cell 31:553, 1982.
36. Bell, G. I., Selby, M. J., and Rutter, W. J.: The

37. Ullrich, A., Dull, T. J., Gray, A., Philips, J. A, III, and Peter, S.: Variation in the sequence and modification state of the human insulin gene flanking region. Nucleic Acids Res. 10:2225, 1982.
38. Engel, J. D., Rusling, D. J., McCune, K. C., and Dodgson, J. B.: Unusual structure of the chicken embryonic α-globin gene, pi'. Proc. Natl. Acad. Sci. USA 80:1392, 1983.
39. Baralle, F. E., Shoulders, C. C., and Proudfoot, N. J.: The primary structure of the human ε-globin gene. Cell 21:621, 1980.
40. Slightom, J. L., Blechl, A. E., and Smithies, O.: Human fetal $^G\gamma$ and $^A\gamma$ globin genes: Complete nucleotide sequences suggest that DNA can be exchanged between these duplicate genes. Cell 21:627, 1980.
41. Shen, S.-H., Slightom, J. L., and Smithies, O.: A history of the human fetal globin gene duplication. Cell 26:191, 1981.
42. Spritz, R. A., deRiel, J. K., Forget, B. G., and Weissman, S. M.: Complete nucleotide sequence of the human δ-globin gene. Cell 21:638, 1980.
43. Lawn, R. M., Efstratiadis, A., O'Connell, C., and Maniatis, T.: The nucleotide sequence of the human β globin gene. Cell 21:647, 1980.
44. Efstratiadis, A., Posakony, J. W., Maniatis, T., Lawn, R. M., O'Connell, C., Spritz, R. A., deRiel, J. K., Forget, B. G., Weissman, S. M., Slightom, J. L., Blechl, A. E., Smithies, O., Baralle, F. E., Shoulders, C. C., and Proudfoot, N. J.: The structure and evolution of the human β globin gene family. Cell 21:653, 1980.
45. Liebhaber, S. A., Goossens, M. J., and Kan, Y. W.: Cloning and complete nucleotide sequence of the human 5'-α globin gene. Proc. Natl. Acad. Sci. USA 77:7054, 1980.
46. Liebhaber, S. A., Goossens, M., Kan, Y. W.: Homology and concerted evolution at the α1 and α2 loci of human α globin. Nature 290:26, 1981.
47. Proudfoot, N. J., and Maniatis, T.: The structure of a human α-globin pseudogene and its relationship to α-globin gene duplication. Cell 21:537, 1980.
48. Michelson, A. M., and Orkin, S. H.: Boundaries of gene conversion within the duplicated human α-globin genes: Concerted evolution by segmental recombination. J. Biol. Chem. 258:15245, 1983.
49. Tilghman, S. M., Curtis, P. J., Tiemeier, D. C., Leder, P., and Weissmann, C.: The intervening sequence of a mouse β-globin gene is transcribed within the 15S β-globin mRNA precursor. Proc. Natl. Acad. Sci. USA 75:1309, 1978.
50. Kinniburgh, A. J., Mertz, J. E., and Ross, J.: The precursor of mouse β-globin messenger RNA contains two intervening RNA sequences. Cell 14:681, 1978.
51. Smith, K., and Lingrel, J. B.: Sequence organization of the β-globin mRNA precursor. Nucleic Acids Res. 9:3295, 1978.
52. Green, M. R., Maniatis, T., and Melton, D. A.: Human β-globin pre-mRNA synthesized in vitro is accurately spliced in xenopus oocyte nuclei. Cell 32:681, 1983.
53. Weingartner, B., and Keller, W.: Transcription and processing of adenoviral RNA by extracts from HeLa cells. Proc. Natl. Acad. Sci. USA 78:4092, 1981.
54. Kole, R., and Weissman, S. M.: Accurate in vitro splicing of human β-globin RNA. Nucleic Acids Res. 10:5429, 1982.
55. Goldenberg, C. J., and Hauser, S. D.: Accurate and efficient in vitro splicing. Nucleic Acids Res. 11:1337, 1983.
56. Padgett, R. A., Hardy, S. F., and Sharp, P. A.: Splicing of adenovirus RNA in a cell-free transcription system. Proc. Natl. Acad. Sci. USA 80:5230, 1983.
57. Hernandez, N., and Keller, W.: Splicing of in vitro synthesized messenger RNA precursors in HeLa cell extracts. Cell 35:89, 1983.
57a. Krainer, A. R., Maniatis, T., Ruskin, B., and Green, M. R.: Normal and mutant human β-globin pre-mRNAs are faithfully and efficiently spliced in vitro. Cell 36:993, 1984.
58. Roberts, R.: Small RNAs and splicing. Nature 283:132, 1980.
59. Knowler, J. T., and Wilks, A. F.: Ribonucleoprotein particles and the maturation of eukaryote mRNA. Trends in Biochem. Sci. 268, 1980.
60. Lerner, M. R., and Steitz, J. A.: Snurps and scyrps. Cell 25:298, 1981.
61. Busch, H., Reddy, R., Rothblum, L., and Choi, Y. C.: SnRNAs, SnRNPs, and RNA processing. Ann. Rev. Biochem. 51:617, 1982.
62. Lerner, M. R., Boyle, J. A., Mount, S. M., Wolin, S. L., and Steitz, J. A.: Are snRNPs involved in splicing? Nature 283:220, 1980.
63. Rogers, J., and Wall, R.: A mechanism for RNA splicing. Proc. Natl. Acad. Sci. USA 77:1877, 1980.
63a. Tatei, K., Takemura, K., Mayeda, A., Fujiwara, Y., Tanaka, H., Ishihama, A., and Ohshima, Y.: U1 RNA-protein complex preferentially binds to both 5' and 3' splice junction sequences in RNA or single stranded DNA. Proc. Natl. Acad. Sci. USA 81:6281, 1984.
64. Yang, V. W., Lerner, M. R., Steitz, J. A., and Flint, S. J.: A small nuclear ribonucleoprotein is required for splicing of adenoviral early RNA sequences. Proc. Natl. Acad. Sci. USA 78:1371, 1981.
65. Padgett, R. A., Mount, S. M., Steitz, J. A., and Sharp, P. A.: Splicing of messenger RNA precursors is inhibited by antisera to small nuclear ribonucleoprotein. Cell 35:101, 1983.
65a. Krämer, A., Keller, W., Appel, B., and Lührmann, R.: The 5' terminus of the RNA moiety of U1 small nuclear ribonucleoprotein particles is required for the splicing of messenger RNA precursors. Cell 38:299, 1984.
65b. DiMaria, P. R., Kaltwasser, G., and Goldenberg, C. J.: Partial purification and properties of a pre-mRNA splicing activity. J. Biol. Chem. 260:1096, 1985.
66. Kinniburgh, A. J., and Ross, J.: Processing of the mouse β-globin mRNA precursor: At least two cleavage-ligation reactions are necessary to exise the larger intervening sequence. Cell 17:915, 1979.
67. Grosveld, G. C., Koster, A., and Flavell, R. A.: A transcription map for the β-globin gene. Cell 23:573, 1981.
68. Donaldson, D. S., McNab, A. R., Rovera, G., and Curtis, P. J.: Nuclear precursor molecules of the two β-globin mRNAs in Friend erythroleukemia cells. J. Biol. Chem. 257:8655, 1982.
68a. Grabowski, P. J., Padgett, R. A., and Sharp, P. A.: Messenger RNA splicing in vitro: An excised intervening sequence and a potential intermediate. Cell 37:415, 1984.
68b. Ruskin, B., Krainer, A. R., Maniatis, T., and Green, M. R.: Excision of an intact intron as a novel lariat structure during pre-mRNA splicing in-vitro. Cell 38:317, 1984.

68c. Padgett, R. A., Konarska, M. M., Grabowski, P. J., Hardy, S. F., and Sharp, P. A.: Lariat RNAs as intermediates and products in the splicing of messenger RNA precursors. Science 225:898, 1984.
68d. Zeitlin, S., and Efstratiadis, A.: In vivo splicing products of the rabbit β-globin pre-mRNA. Cell 39:589, 1984.
68e. Keller, E. B., and Noon, W. A.: Intron splicing: A conserved internal signal in introns of animal pre-mRNAs. Proc. Natl. Acad. Sci. USA 81:7417, 1984.
69. Hamer, D. H., and Leder, P.: SV40 recombinants carrying a functional RNA splice junction and polyadenylation site from the chromosomal mouse β^{maj} globin gene. Cell 17:737, 1979.
70. Hamer, D. H., and Leder, P.: Expression of the chromosomal mouse β^{maj}-globin gene cloned in SV40. Nature 281:35, 1979.
71. Mantei, N., Boll, W., and Weissmann, C.: Rabbit β-globin mRNA production in mouse L cells transformed with cloned rabbit β-globin chromosomal DNA. Nature 281:40, 1979.
72. Wold, B., Wigler, M., Lacy, E., Maniatis, T., Silverstein, S., and Axel, R.: Introduction and expression of a rabbit β-globin gene in mouse fibroblasts. Proc. Natl. Acad. Sci. USA 76:5684, 1979.
73. Hamer, D. H., Smith, K. D., Boyer, S. H., and Leder, P.: SV40 recombinants carrying rabbit β-globin gene coding sequences. Cell 17:725, 1979.
74. Hamer, D. H., and Leder, P.: Splicing and the formation of stable RNA. Cell 18:1299, 1979.
74a. Antoine, M., and Niessing, J.: Intron-less globin genes in the insect Chironomus thummi thummi. Nature 310:795, 1984.
75. Mount, S. M.: A catalogue of splice junction sequences. Nucleic Acids Res. 10:459, 1982.
76. Breathnach, R., Benoist, C., O'Hare, K., Gannon, F., and Chambon, P.: Ovalbumin gene: Evidence for a leader sequence in mRNA and DNA sequences at the exon-intron boundaries. Proc. Natl. Acad. Sci. USA 75:4853, 1978.
76a. Fischer, H. D., Dodgson, J. B., Hughes, S. T., and Engel, J. D.: An unusual 5' splice sequence is efficiently utilized in vivo. Proc. Natl. Acad. Sci. USA 81:2733, 1984.
76b. Wieringa, B., Hofer, E., and Weissmann, C.: A minimal intron length but no specific internal sequence is required for splicing the large rabbit β-globin intron. Cell 37:915–925, 1984.
76c. van Santen, V. L., and Spritz, R. A.: Pre mRNA splicing in vivo: Sequence requirements determined by deletion analysis of an intervening sequence. Proc. Natl. Acad. Sci. USA, in press.
77. Gilbert, W.: Why genes in pieces? Nature 271:501, 1978.
78. Blake, C. C. F.: Do genes-in-pieces imply proteins-in-pieces? Nature 273:267, 1978.
79. Eaton, W. A.: The relationship between coding sequences and function in haemoglobin. Nature 284:183, 1980.
80. Craik, C. S., Buchman, S. R., and Beychok, S.: Characterization of globin domains. Heme binding to the central exon product. Proc. Natl. Acad. Sci. USA 77:1384, 1980.
81. Craik, C. S., Buchman, S. R., and Beychok, S.: O_2 binding properties of the product of the central exon of β-globin gene. Nature 291:87, 1981.
82. Go, M.: Correlation of DNA exonic regions with protein structural units in haemoglobin. Nature 291:90, 1981.
83. Blake, C. C. F.: Exons and the structure, function and evolution of haemoglobin. Nature 291:616, 1981.
84. Levin, R.: On the origin of introns. Science 217:921, 1982.
85. Blake, C.: Exons—present from the beginning? Nature 306:535, 1983.
86. Jensen, E. O., Paludan, K., Hyldig-Nielsen, J. J., Jorgensen, J., and Marcker, K. A.: The structure of a chromosomal leghaemoglobin gene from soybean. Nature 291:677, 1981.
87. Hyldig-Nielsen, J. J., Jensen, E. O., Paludan, K., Wiborg, O., Garrett, R., Jorgensen, P., and Marcker, K. A.: The primary structures of two leghemoglobin genes from soybean. Nucleic Acids Res. 10:689, 1982.
88. Brisson, N., Pombo-Gentile, A., and Verma, D. P. S.: Organization and expression of leghaemoglobin genes. Can. J. Biochem. 60:272, 1982.
89. Breathnach, R., and Chambon, P.: Organization and expression of eukaryotic split genes coding for proteins. Ann. Rev. Biochem. 50:349, 1981.
90. Talkington, C. A., Nishioka, Y., and Leder, P.: In vitro transcription of normal, mutant, and truncated mouse α-globin genes. Proc. Natl. Acad. Sci. USA 77:7132, 1980.
91. Grosveld, G. C., Shewmaker, C. K., Jat, P., and Flavell, R. A.: Localization of DNA sequences necessary for transcription of the rabbit β-globin gene in vitro. Cell 25:215, 1981.
92. Dierks, P., van Ooyen, A., Mantei, N., and Weissmann, C.: DNA sequences preceding the rabbit β-globin gene are required for formation in mouse L cells of β-globin RNA with the correct 5' terminus. Proc. Natl. Acad. Sci. USA 78:1411, 1981.
93. Grosveld, G. C., de Boer, E., Shewmaker, C. K., and Flavell, R. A.: DNA sequences necessary for transcription of the rabbit β-globin gene in vivo. Nature 295:120, 1982.
94. Grosveld, G. C., Rosenthal, A., and Flavell, R. A.: Sequence requirements for the transcription of the rabbit β-globin gene in vivo: The -80 region. Nucleic Acids Res. 10:4951, 1982.
95. Dierks, P., van Ooyen, A., Cochran, M. D., Dobkin, C., Reiser, J., and Weissmann, C.: Three regions upstream from the cap site are required for efficient and accurate transcription of the rabbit β-globin gene in mouse 3T6 cells. Cell 32:695, 1983.
96. Proudfoot, N. J., Shander, M. H. M., Manley, J. L., Gefter, M. L., and Maniatis, T.: Structure and in vitro transcription of human globin genes. Science 209:1329, 1980.
97. Humphries, R. K., Ley, T., Turner, P., Moulton, A. D., and Nienhuis, A. W.: Differences in human α, β and δ gene expression in monkey kidney cells. Cell 30:173, 1982.
97a. Shatkin, A. J.: mRNA cap binding proteins: Essential factors for initiating translation. Cell 40:223, 1985.
97b. Konarska, M. M., Padgett, R. A., and Sharp, P. A.: Recognition of cap structure in splicing in vitro of mRNA precursors. Cell 38:731, 1984.
98. Baralle, F. E., and Brownlee, G. G.: AUG is the only recognizable signal sequence in the 5' non-coding regions of eukaryotic mRNA. Nature 274:84, 1978.
99. Haghenbuchle, O., Snater, M., Steitz, J. A., and Mans, R. J.: Conservation of the primary structure at the 3' end of 18S rRNA from eukaryotic cells. Cell 13:551, 1978.
99a. Sargan, D. R., Gregory, S. P., and Butterworth, P. H. W.: A possible novel interaction between

the 3'-end of 18S ribosomal RNA and the 5'-leader sequence of many eukaryotic messenger RNAs. FEBS Lett. *147*:133, 1982.
100. Shine, J., and Dalgarno, L.: Determinant of cistron specificity in bacterial ribosomes. Nature *254*:34, 1975.
101. De Wachter, R.: Do eukaryotic mRNA 5' noncoding sequences base-pair with the 18 S ribosomal RNA 3' terminus? Nucleic Acids Res. *7*:2045, 1979.
102. Kozak, M.: Compilation and analysis of sequences upstream from the translational start site in eukaryotic mRNAs. Nucleic Acids Res. *12*:857, 1984.
103. Kozak, M.: Comparison of initiation of protein synthesis in procaryotes, eucaryotes and organelles. Microbiol Rev. *47*:1, 1983.
104. Kronenberg, H. M., Roberts, B. E., and Efstratiadis, A.: The 3' noncoding region of β-globin mRNA is not essential for *in vitro* translation. Nucleic Acids Res. *6*:153, 1979.
105. Marbaix, G., Huez, G., Burny, A., Cleuter, Y., Hubert, E., Leclercq, M., Chantrenne, H., Soreq, H., Nudel, U., and Littauer, U. Z.: Absence of polyadenylate segment in globin messenger RNA accelerates its degradation in Xenopus oocytes. Proc. Natl. Acad. Sci. USA *72*:3065, 1975.
106. Michelson, A. M., and Orkin, S. H.: The 3'-untranslated regions of the duplicated human α globin genes are unexpectedly divergent. Cell *22*:371, 1980.
107. Orkin, S. H., and Goff, S. C.: The duplicated human α globin genes: Their relative expression as measured by RNA analysis. Cell *24*:345, 1981.
108. Liebhaber, S. A., and Kan, Y. W.: Differentiation of the mRNA transcripts originating from the α1 and α2 globin loci in normals and α-thalassemics. J. Clin. Invest. *68*:439, 1981.
108a. Liebhaber, S. A., and Cash, F. E.: Locus assignment of α-globin structural mutations by hybrid-selected translation. J. Clin. Invest. *75*:64, 1985.
109. Proudfoot, N. J., and Brownlee, G. G.: 3' Noncoding region sequences in eukaryotic messenger RNA. Nature *263*:211, 1976.
110. Proudfoot, N. J.: The end of the message and beyond. Nature *307*:412, 1984.
110a. Wickens, M., and Stephenson, P.: Role of the conserved AAUAAA sequence: Four AAUAAA point mutants prevent messenger RNA 3' end formation. Science *226*:1045, 1984.
110b. Gil, A., and Proudfoot, N. J.: A sequence downstream of AAUAAA is required for rabbit β-globin mRNA 3'-end formation. Nature *312*:473, 1984.
110c. McLauchlan, J., Gaffney, D., Whitton, J. L., and Clements, J. B.: The consensus sequence YGTGTTYY located downstream for the AATAAA signal is required for efficient formation of mRNA 3' termini. Nucleic Acids Res. *4*:1347, 1985.
111. Forget, B. G.: The structure of human globin messenger RNA. Functional, genetic and evolutionary implifications. *In* Piomelli, S., and Yachnin, S. (eds.): Current Topics in Hematology. New York, Alan R. Liss, Inc., Vol. 3, 1980, pp. 1–74.
112. Cohen-Solal, M. M., Authier, B., deRiel, J. K., Murnane, M. J., and Forget, B. G.: Cloning and nucleotide sequence analysis of human embryonic ζ globin cDNA. DNA *1*:355, 1982.
113. Efstratiadis, A., Kafatos, F. C., and Maniatis, T.: The primary structure of rabbit β-globin mRNA as determined from cloned DNA. Cell *10*:571, 1977.
114. Marotta, C. A., Wilson, J. T., Forget, B. G., and Weissman, S. M.: Human β-globin messenger RNA. III. Nucleotide sequences derived from complementary DNA. J. Biol. Chem. *252*:5040, 1977.
115. Grantham, R., Gautier, C., Gouy, M., Jacobzone, M., and Mercier, R.: Codon catalog usage is a genome strategy modulated for gene expressivity. *9*:43, 1981.
116. Grantham, R.: Workings of the genetic code. Trends in Biochem. Sci. *5*:327, 1980.
117. Hatfield, D., Matthews, C. R., and Rice, M.: Amino acyl-transfer RNA populations in mammalian cells, chromatographic profiles and patterns of codon recognition. Biochim. Biophy. Acta *564*:414, 1979.
118. Hatfield, D., Varricchio, F., Rice, M., and Forget, B. G.: The aminoacyl-tRNA population of human reticulocytes. J. Biol. Chem. *257*:3183, 1982.
119. Little, P. F. R.: Globin pseudogenes. Cell *28*:683, 1982.
120. Jagadeeswaran, P., Pan, J., Forget, B. G., and Weissman, S. M.: Sequences of human repetitive DNA, non-α globin genes and major histocompatibility locus genes. Part II. Sequences of non-α globin genes in man. Cold Spring Harbor Symp. Quant. Biol. *47*:1079, 1983.
121. Chang, L.-Y. E., and Slightom, J. L.: Isolation and nucleotide sequence analysis of β-type globin pseudogene from human, gorilla and chimpanzee. J. Mol. Biol., *180*:767, 1984.
122. Shen, S.-H., and Smithies, O.: Human globin ψβ2 is not a globin-related sequence. Nucleic Acids Res. *10*:7809, 1982.
123. Whitelaw, E., and Proudfoot, N. J.: Transcriptional activity of the human pseudogene ψα globin compared with α globin, its functional gene counterpart. Nucleic Acids Res. *11*:7717, 1983.
123a. Marx, J. L.: Is RNA copied into DNA by mammalian cells? Science *216*:969, 1982.
123b. Flavell, R. A.: The mystery of the mouse α-globin pseudogene. Nature *295*:370, 1982.
123c. Hess, J. F., Schmid, C. W., and Shen, C.-K. J.: A gradient of sequence divergence in the human adult α-globin duplication units. Science *226*:67, 1984.
123c. Hess, J. F., Schmid, C. W., and Shen, C.-K. J.: A gradient of sequence divergence in the human adult α-globin duplication units. Science *226*:67, 1984.
124. Zimmer, E. A., Martin, S. L., Beverley, S. M., Kan, Y. W., and Wilson, A. C.: Rapid duplication and loss of genes coding for the α chains of hemoglobin. Proc. Natl. Acad. Sci. USA *77*:2158, 1980.
125. Duncan, C., Biro, P. A., Choudary, P. V., Elder, J. T., Wang, R. R. C., Forget, B. G., deRiel, J. K., and Weissman, S. M.: RNA polymerase III transcriptional units are interspersed among human non-α globin genes. Proc. Natl. Acad. Sci. USA *76*:5095, 1979.
126. Duncan, C. H., Jagadeeswaran, P., Wang, R. R. C., and Weissman, S. M.: Structural analysis of templates and RNA polymerase III transcripts of Alu family sequences interspersed among the human β-like globin genes. Gene *13*:185, 1981.
127. Fritsch, E. F., Shen, C. K., Lawn, R. M., and Maniatis, T.: The organization of repetitive sequences in mammalian globin gene clusters. Cold Spring Harbor Symp. Quant. Biol. *45*:761, 1980.
128. DiSegni, G., Cararra, G., Tocchini-Valentini, G. R., Shoulders, C. C., and Baralle, F. E.: Selective *in vitro* transcription of one of the two Alu family repeats present in the 5'-flanking region of the

human ϵ globin gene. Nucleic Acids Res. 9:6709, 1981.
129. Coggins, L. W., Grindlay, G. J., Vass, J. K., Slater, A. A., Montague, P., Stinson, M. A., and Paul, J.: Repetitive DNA sequences near three human beta-type globin genes. Nucleic Acids Res. 8:3319, 1980.
130. Coggins, L. W., Lanyon, W. G., Slater, A. A., Grindlay, G. J., and Paul, J.: Characterization of Alu family repetitive sequences which flank human β-type globin genes. Biosci. Rep. 1:309, 1981.
131. Shen, C. K., and Maniatis, T.: The organization, structure, and in vitro transcription of Alu family RNA polymerase III transcription units in the human α-like globin gene cluster: Precipitation of in vitro transcripts by lupus anti-1a antibodies. J. Mol. Appl. Genet. 1:343, 1982.
132. Hess, J. F., Fox, M., Schmid, C., and Shen, C. K.: Molecular evolution of the human adult α-globin-like gene region: Insertion and deletion of Alu family repeats and non-Alu DNA sequences. Proc. Natl. Acad. Sci. USA 80:5970, 1983.
133. Manley, J. L., and Colozzo, M. T.: Synthesis in vitro of an exceptionally long RNA transcript promoted by an AluI sequence. Nature 300:376, 1982.
133a. Perez-Stable, C., Ayres, T. M., and Shen, C.-K. J.: Distinctive sequence organization and functional programming of an Alu repeat promoter. Proc. Natl. Acad. Sci. USA 81:5291, 1984.
133b. Hess, J., Perez-Stable, C., Wu, G. J., Weir, B., Tinoco, I., Jr., and Shen, C.-K. J.: End-to-end transcription of an Alu family repeat: A new type of polymerase III–dependent terminator and evolutionary implications. J. Mol. Biol., in press.
134. Jelinek, W. R., Toomey, T. P., Leinwand, L., Duncan, C. H., Biro, P. A., Choudary, P. V., Weissman, S. M., Rubin, C. M., Houck, C. M., Deininger, P. L., and Schmid, C. W.: Ubiquitous, interspersed repeated sequences in mammalian genomes. Proc. Natl. Acad. Sci. USA 77:1398, 1980.
135. Houck, C. M., Rinehart, F. P., and Schmid, C. W.: A ubiquitous family of repeated DNA sequences in the human genome. J. Mol. Biol. 132:289, 1979.
136. Schmid, C. W., and Jelinek, W. R.: The structure and organization of the major interspersed repetitious sequence in mammalian DNA: The Alu sequence. Science 216:1065, 1982.
136a. Jelinek, W. R., and Schmid, C. W.: Repetitive sequences in eukaryotic DNA and their expression. Ann. Rev. Biochem. 51:813, 1982.
137. Weiner, A. M.: An abundant cytoplasmic 7S RNA is complementary to the dominant interspersed middle repetitive DNA sequence family in the human genome. Cell 22:209, 1980.
138. Calabretta, B., Robberson, D. L., Maizel, A. L., and Saunders, G. F.: mRNA in human cells contains sequences complementary to the Alu family of repeated DNA. Proc. Natl. Acad. Sci. USA 78:6003, 1981.
139. Elder, J. T., Duncan, C. H., and Weissman, S. M.: Transcriptional analysis of interspersed repetitive polymerase III transcription units in human DNA. Nucleic Acids Res. 9:1171, 1981.
140. Haynes, S. R., and Jelinek, W. R.: Low molecular weight RNAs transcribed in vitro by RNA polymerase III from Alu-type dispersed repeats in Chinese hamster DNA are also found in vivo. Proc. Natl. Acad. Sci. USA 78:6130, 1981.
140a. Robertson, H. D., and Dickson, E.: Structure and distribution of Alu family sequences or their analogs within heterogeneous nuclear RNA of HeLa, KB, and L cells. Mol. Cell. Biol. 4:310, 1984.
141. Allan, M., and Paul, J.: Transcription in vivo of an Alu family member upstream from the human ϵ-globin gene. Nucleic Acids Res. 12:1193, 1984.
142. Zavodny, P. J., Roginski, R. S., and Skoultchi, A. S.: Regulated expression of human globin genes and flanking DNA in mouse erythroleukemia–human cell hybrids. In Stamatoyannopoulos, G., and Nienhuis, A. W. (eds.): Globin Gene Expression and Hematopoietic Differentiation. New York, Alan R. Liss, Inc., 1983, pp. 53–62.
143. Jagadeeswaran, P., Forget, B. G., and Weissman, S. M.: Short interspersed repetitive DNA elements in eucaryotes: Transposable DNA elements generated by reverse transcription of RNA Pol III transcripts? Cell 26:141, 1981.
144. Van Arsdell, S. W., Denison, R. A., Bernstein, L. B., and Weiner, A. M.: Direct repeats flank three small nuclear RNA pseudogenes in the human genome. Cell 26:11, 1981.
145. Sharp, P. A.: Conversion of RNA to DNA in mammals: Alu-like elements and pseudogenes. Nature 301:471, 1983.
145a. Ullu, E., and Tschudi, C.: Alu sequences are processed 7SL RNA genes. Nature 312:171, 1984.
146. Kaufman, R. E., Kretschmer, P. J., Adams, J. W., Coon, H. C., Anderson, W. F., and Nienhuis, A. W.: Cloning and characterization of DNA sequences surrounding the human γ, δ and β globin genes. Proc. Natl. Acad. Sci. USA 77:4229, 1980.
147. Adams, J. W., Kaufman, R. E., Kretschmer, P. J., Harrison, M., and Nienhuis, A. W.: A family of long reiterated DNA sequences, one copy of which is next to the human β globin gene. Nucleic Acids Res. 8:6113, 1980.
148. Jagadeeswaran, P., Pan, J., Spritz, R. A., Duncan, C. A., Biro, P. A., Tuan, D., Forget, B. G., and Weissman, S. M.: Structures in intergenic DNA of non-α globin genes of man. In Brown, D., and Fox, C. F. (eds.): Developmental Biology Using Purified Genes. ICN-UCLA Symp. Mol. Biol. Vol. XXIII. New York, Academic Press, 1981, pp. 71–84.
149. Forget, B. G., Tuan, D., Biro, P. A., Jagadeeswaran, P., and Weissman, S. M.: Structural features of the DNA flanking the human non-α globin genes: Implications in the control of fetal hemoglobin switching. Trans. Assoc. Am. Physicians 94:204, 1981.
150. Shafit-Zagardo, B., Brown, F. L., Maio, J. J., and Adams, J. W.: Kpn I families of long, interspersed repetitive DNAs associated with the human β-globin gene cluster. Gene 20:397, 1982.
151. Singer, M. F.: SINEs and LINEs: Highly repeated short and long interspersed sequences in mammalian genomes. Cell 28:433, 1982.
152. Rogers, J.: A straight LINE story. Nature 306:113, 1983.
153. Shafit-Zagardo, B., Brown, F. L., Zavodny, P. J., and Maio, J. J.: Transcription of the Kpn I families of long interspersed DNAs in human cells. Nature 304:277, 1983.
154. Kole, L. B., Haynes, S. R., and Jelinek, W. R.: Discrete and heterogeneous high molecular weight RNA's complementary to a long dispersed repeat family (a possible transposon) of human DNA. J. Mol. Biol. 165:256, 1983.
154a. Schmeckpeper, B. J., Scott, A. F., and Smith, K.

D.: Transcripts homologous to a long repeated DNA element in the human genome. J. Biol. Chem. *259*:1218, 1984.
154b. Sun, L. O., Paulson, K. E., Schmid, C. W., Kadyk, L., and Leinwand, L.: Non-alu family interspersed repeats in human DNA and their transcriptional activity. Nucleic Acids Res. *12*:2669, 1984.
154c. Potter, S. S.: Rearranged sequences of a human Kpn I element. Proc. Natl. Acad. Sci. USA *81*:1012, 1984.
154d. Martin, S. L., Voliva, C. F., Burton, F. H., Edgell, M. H., and Hutchison, C. A. III: A large interspersed repeat found in mouse DNA contains a long open reading frame that evolves as if it encodes a protein. Proc. Natl. Acad. Sci. USA *81*:2308, 1984.
155. DiGiovanni, L., Haynes, S. R., Misra, R., and Jelinek, W. R.: Knp I family of long-dispersed repeated DNA sequences of man: Evidence for entry into genomic DNA of DNA copies of poly (A)-terminated Kpn I RNAs. Proc. Natl. Acad. Sci. USA *80*:6533, 1983.
155a. Grimaldi, G., Skowronski, J., and Singer, M. F.: Defining the beginning and end of Kpn I family segments. EMBO J. *3*:1753, 1984.
156. Thayer, R. E., and Singer, M. F.: Interruption of an α-satellite array by a short member of the Kpn I family of interspersed, highly repeated monkey DNA sequences. Mol. Cell Biol. *6*:697, 1983.
156a. Nomiyama, H., Tsuzuki, T., Wakasugi, S., Fukda, M., and Shimada, K.: Interruption of a human nuclear sequence homologous to mitochondrial DNA by a member of the Kpn I 1.8 kb family. Nucleic Acids Res. *12*:5225, 1984.
157. Miesfeld, R., Krystal, M., and Arnheim, N.: A member of a new repeated sequence family which is conserved throughout eucaryotic evolution is found between the human δ and β globin genes. Nucleic Acids Res. *9*:5931, 1981.
157a. Poncz, M., Schwartz, E., Ballantine, M., and Surrey, S.: Nucleotide sequence analysis of the $\delta\beta$-globin gene region in humans. J. Biol. Chem. *258*:11599–11609, 1983.
158. Spritz, R. A.: Duplication/depletion polymorphism 5'-to the human β globin gene. Nucleic Acids Res. *9*:5037, 1981.
159. Shen, C. K.: Superhelicity induces hypersensitivity of a human polypyrimidine-polypurine DNA sequence in the human α2-α1 globin intergenic region to S1 nuclease digestion—high resolution mapping of the clustered cleavage sites. Nucleic Acids Res. *11*:7899, 1983.
160. Kolata, G.: Z-DNA moves toward "real biology." Science *222*:495, 1983.
160a. Rich, A., Nordheim, A., and Wang, A. H.-J.: The chemistry and biology of left-handed Z-DNA. Ann. Rev. Biochem. *53*:791, 1984.
160b. Cockerill, P. N., and Goodwin, G. H.: Demonstration of an S1-nuclease sensitive site near the human β-globin gene, and its protection by HMG 1 and 2. Biochem. Biophys. Res. Comm. *112*:547, 1983.
160c. Gilmour, R. S., Spandidos, D. A., Vass, J. K., Gow, J. W., and Paul, J.: A negative regulatory sequence near the mouse β-maj globin gene associated with a region of potential Z-DNA. EMBO J. *3*:1263, 1984.
160d. Kilpatrick, M. W., Klysik, J., Singleton, C. K., Zarling, D. A., Jovin, T. M., Hanau, L. H., Erlanger, B. F., and Wells, R. D.: Intervening sequences in human fetal globin genes adopt left-handed Z helices. J. Biol. Chem. *259*:7268, 1984.

161. Orkin, S. H., Antonarakis, S., and Kazazian, H. H., Jr.: Polymorphism and molecular pathology of the human beta-globin gene. Prog. Hematol. *13*:49, 1983.
161a. Orkin, S. H., and Kazazian, H. H., Jr.: Mutation and polymorphisms of the human β-globin gene and its surrounding DNA. Am. Rev. Genet. *18*:131, 1984.
162. Jeffreys, A. J.: DNA sequence variants in the $^G\gamma$-$^A\gamma$, δ- and β- globin genes of man. Cell *18*:1, 1979.
163. Kan, Y. W., and Dozy, A. M.: Polymorphism of DNA sequence adjacent to human β-globin structural gene: Relationship to sickle mutation. Proc. Natl. Acad. Sci. USA *75*:5631, 1978.
164. Kan, Y. W., and Dozy, A. M.: Evolution of the hemoglobin S and C genes in world populations. Science *209*:388, 1980.
165. Antonarakis, S. E., Boehm, C. D., Giardina, P. J. V., and Kazazian, H. H., Jr.: Nonrandom association of polymorphic restriction sites in the β-globin gene cluster. Proc. Natl. Acad. Sci. USA *79*:137, 1982.
166. Antonarakis, S. E., Corrinne, D. B., Serjeant, G. R., Theisen, C. E., Dover, G. J., and Kazazian, H. H., Jr.: Origin of the β^s-globin gene in Blacks: The contribution of recurrent mutation or gene conversion or both. Proc. Natl. Acad. Sci. USA *81*:853, 1984.
167. Pirastu, M., Doherty, M., Galanello, R., Cao, A., and Kan, Y. W.: Frequent crossing over in human DNA generates multiple chromosomes containing the sickle and β-thalassemia genes and increases HbF production. Blood *62*(Suppl. 1):75a, 1983.
168. Pagnier, J., Mears, J. G., Dunda-Belkodja, O., Schaefer-Rego, K. E., Beldjord, C., Nagel, R. L., and Labie, D.: Evidence for the multicentric origin of the sickle cell hemoglobin gene in Africa. Proc. Natl. Acad. Sci. USA *81*:1771, 1984.
168a. Wainscoat, J. S., Bell, J. I., Thein, S. L., Higgs, D. R., Serjeant, G. R., Peto, T. E. A., and Weatherall, D. J.: Multiple origins of the sickle mutation: Evidence from beta S globin gene cluster polymorphisms. Mol. Biol. Med. *1*:191, 1983.
169. Kazazian, H. H., Jr., Antonarakis, S. E., Cheng, T.-C., Boehm, C. D., and Waber, P. G.: DNA polymorphisms in the β-globin gene cluster: Use in discovery of mutations and prenatal diagnosis. In Caskey, C. T., and White, R. L. (eds.): Recombinant DNA Applications to Human Disease. New York, Cold Spring Harbor Laboratory, 1983, p. 29.
170. Chakravarti, A., Buetow, K. H., Antonarakis, S. E., Waber, P. G., Boehm, C. D., and Kazazian, H. H., Jr.: Non-uniform recombination within the β-globin gene cluster. Am. J. Hum. Genet., *36*:1239, 1984.
171. Fukumaki, Y., Collins, F., Kole, R., Stoeckert, C. J., Jr., Jagadeeswaran, P., Duncan, C. H., and Weissman, S. M.: Sequences of human repetitive DNA, non-α globin genes and major histocompatibility locus genes. Part I. Repeated-sequence DNA. Cold Spring Harbor Symp. Quant. Biol. *47*:1079, 1984.
172. Maeda, N., Bliska, J. B., and Smithies, O.: Recombination and balanced chromosome polymorphism suggested by DNA sequences 5' to the human δ-globin gene. Proc. Natl. Acad. Sci. USA *80*:5012, 1983.
173. Darnell, J. E., Jr.: Variety in the level of gene control in eukaryotic cells. Nature *297*:365, 1982.
174. Weaver, R. F., and Weissmann, C.: Mapping of

RNA by a modification of the Berk-Sharp procedure: The 5'-termini of 15S β globin mRNA precursor and mature 10S β globin mRNA have identical map coordinates. Nucleic Acids Res. 6:1175, 1979.
175. Alan, M., Grindlay, G. J., Stefani, L., and Paul, J.: Epsilon globin gene transcripts originating upstream of the mRNA cap site in K562 cells and normal human embryos. Nucleic Acids Res. 10:5133, 1982.
176. Alan, M., Lanyon, W. G., and Paul, J.: Multiple origins of transcription in the 4.5 kb upstream of the ε-globin gene. Cell 35:187, 1983.
177. Carlson, D. P., and Ross, J.: Human β-globin promoter and coding sequences transcribed by RNA polymerase III. Cell 34:857, 1983.
177a. Carlson, D. P., and Ross, J.: α-Amanitin-insensitive transcription of mouse $β^{major}$-globin 5'-flanking and structural gene sequences correlates with mRNA expression. Proc. Natl. Acad. Sci. USA 81:7782, 1984.
178. Ley, T. J., and Nienhuis, A. W.: A weak upstream promoter gives rise to long human β-globin RNA molecules. Biochem. Biophys. Res. Comm. 112:1041, 1983.
179. Grindlay, G. J., Lanyon, W. G., Alan, M., and Paul, J.: Alternative sites of transcription initiation upstream of the canonical cap site in human γ-globin and β-globin genes. Nucleic Acids Res. 12:1811, 1984.
179a. Allan, M., Zhu, J.-D., Montague, P., and Paul, J.: Differential response of multiple ε-globin cap sites to cis- and trans-acting controls. Cell 38:399, 1984.
180. Macnaughton, M., Freeman, K. B., and Bishop, J. O.: A precursor to hemoglobin mRNA in nuclei of immature duck red blood cells. Cell 1:117, 1974.
181. Spohr, G., Imaizumi, T., and Scherrer, K.: Synthesis and processing of nuclear precursor-messenger RNA in avian erythroblasts and HeLa cells. Proc. Natl. Acad. Sci. USA 71:5009, 1974.
182. Ross, J.: A precursor of globin messenger RNA. J. Mol. Biol. 106:403, 1976.
183. Curtis, P. J., and Weissmann, C.: Purification of globin messenger RNA from dimethylsulfoxide-induced Friend cells and detection of a putative globin messenger RNA precursor. J. Mol. Biol. 106:1061, 1976.
184. Bastos, R. N., and Aviv, H.: Globin RNA precursor molecules: Biosynthesis and processing in erythroid cells. Cell 11:641, 1977.
185. Strair, R. K., Skoultchi, A. I., and Shafritz, D. A.: A characterization of globin mRNA sequences in the nucleus of duck immature red blood cells. Cell 12:133, 1977.
186. Kwan, S. P., Wood, T. G., and Lingrel, J. B.: Purification of a putative precursor of globin messenger RNA from mouse nucleated erythroid cells. Proc. Natl. Acad. Sci. USA 74:178, 1977.
187. Curtis, P. J., Mantel, N., van dan Berg, J., and Weissmann, C.: Presence of a putative 15S precursor to β-globin mRNA but not to α-globin mRNA in Friend cells. Proc. Natl. Acad. Sci. USA 74:3184, 1977.
188. Ross, J., and Knecht, D. A.: Precursors of alpha and beta globin messenger RNAs. J. Mol. Biol. 119:1, 1978.
189. Knochel, W., and Grundmann, U.: The putative 15S precursor of globin mRNA contains a poly (A) sequence. Biochim. Biophys. Acta 517:99, 1978.
190. Niessing, J.: Globin messenger precursor RNA in duck immature red blood cells. Eur. J. Biochem. 91:587, 1978.
191. Courtney, M., and Williamson, R.: A nuclear precursor to human γ-globin messenger RNA. Nucleic Acids Res. 7:1121, 1979.
192. Farace, M. G., Ullu, E., Fantoni, A., Rossi, G. B., Cioe, L., and Dolei, A.: Nuclear RNA sequences coding for α and β globins in erythroid cells: Evidence for multiple intermediate molecules. Blood 53:134, 1979.
193. Maquat, L. E., Kinniburgh, A. J., Beach, L. R., Honig, G. R., Lazerson, J., Ershler, W. B., and Ross, J.: Processing of the human β globin mRNA precursor to mRNA is defective in three patients with $β^+$-thalassemia. Proc. Natl. Acad. Sci. USA 77:4287, 1980.
194. Hofer, E., and Darnell, J. E., Jr.: The primary transcription unit of the mouse β-major globin gene. Cell 23:585, 1981.
195. Salditt-Georgieff, M., and Darnell, J. E., Jr.: A precise termination site in the mouse $β^{major}$-globin transcription unit. Proc. Natl. Acad. Sci. USA 80:4694, 1983.
196. Skoultchi, A.: Personal communication.
197. Reynaud, C.-A., Imaizumi-Scherrer, M.-T., and Scherrer, K.: The size of the transcriptional units of the avian globin genes defined at the Pre-messenger RNA level. J. Mol. Biol. 140:481, 1980.
198. Higgs, D. R., Goodbourn, S. E. Y., Lamb, J., Clegg, J. B., and Weatherall, D. J.: α-thalassaemia caused by a polyadenylation signal mutation. Nature 306:398, 1983.
199. Orkin, S. H.: Cheng, T.-C., Antonarakis, S. E., and Kazazian, H. H., Jr.: Thalassemia due to a mutation in the cleavage-polyadenylation signal of the human β-globin gene. EMBO J. 4:453, 1985.
200. Benz, E. J., Jr., Scarpa, A. L., Tonkonow, B. L., Pearson, H. A., and Ritchey, A. K.: Post-transcriptional defects in β globin mRNA metabolism in β-thalassemia: Abnormal accumulation of β mRNA precursor sequences. J. Clin. Invest. 68:1529, 1981.
201. Fukumaki, R., Ghosh, P. K., Benz, E. J., Jr., Reddy, V. B., Lebowitz, P., Forget, B. G., and Weissman, S. M.: Abnormally spliced messenger RNA in erythroid cells from patients with $β^+$-thalassemia and monkey cells expressing a cloned $β^+$-thalassemic gene. Cell 28:585, 1982.
202. Vincent, A., Goldenberg, S., Standart, N., Civelli, O., Immaizumi-Scherrer, T., Maundrell, K., and Scherrer, K.: Potential role of mRNP proteins in cytoplasmic control of gene expression in duck erythroblasts. Mol. Biol. Rep. 7:71, 1981.
203. Pederson, T.: Messenger RNA biosynthesis and nuclear structure: RNA:protein particles are sites of messenger RNA processing in the cell nucleus. Am. Scientist 69:76, 1981.
204. Razin, A., and Riggs, A. D.: DNA methylation and gene function. Science 210:604, 1980.
205. Razin, A., and Friedman, J.: DNA methylation and its possible biological roles. Prog. Nucleic Acid Res. Mol. Biol. 25:33, 1981.
206. Lindahl, T.: DNA methylation and control of gene expression. Nature 290:363, 1981.
207. Ehrlich, M., and Wang, R. Y.-H.: 5-Methylcytosine in eukaryotic DNA. Science 212:1350, 1981.
208. Felsenfeld, G., and McGhee, J.: Methylation and gene control. Nature 296:602, 1982.
209. Bird, A. P.: DNA methylation—how important in gene control? Nature 307:503, 1984.
210. Shen, C. K.: DNA methylation and developmental regulation of eukaryotic globin gene transcription. In Razin, A., Cedar, H., and Riggs, A. (eds.): DNA Methylation. New York, Springer-Verlag, 1984.

211. van der Ploeg, L. H. T., and Flavell, R. A.: DNA methylation in the human γδβ-globin locus in erythroid and nonerythroid tissues. Cell *19*:947, 1980.
212. Mavilio, F., Giampaolo, A., Care, A., Migliaccio, G., Calandrini, M., Russo, G., Pagliardi, G. L., Mastroberardino, G., Marinucci, M., and Peschle, C.: Molecular mechanisms of human hemoglobin switching: Selective undermethylation and expression of globin genes in embryonic, fetal, and adult erythroblasts. Proc. Natl. Acad. Sci. USA *80*:6907, 1983.
213. Busslinger, M., Hurst, J., and Flavell, R. A.: DNA methylation and the regulation of globin gene expression. Cell *34*:197, 1983.
214. Weisbrod, S.: Active chromatin. Nature *297*:289, 1982.
215. Stalder, J., Groudine, M., Dodgson, J. B., Engel, J. D., and Weintraub, H.: Hb switching in chickens. Cell *19*:973, 1980.
216. Stalder, J., Larsen, A., Engel, J. D., Dolan, M., Groudine, M., and Weintraub, H.: Tissue-specific DNA cleavages in the globin chromatin domain introduced by DNAase I. Cell *20*:451, 1980.
217. Zasloff, M., and Camerini-Otero, R. D.: Limited DNase I nicking as a probe of gene conformation. Proc. Natl. Acad. Sci. USA *77*:1907, 1980.
218. Bellard, M., Kuo, M. T., Dretzen, G., and Chambon, P.: Differential nuclease sensitivity of the ovalbumin and β-globin chromatin regions in erythrocytes and oviduct cells of laying hen. Nucleic Acids Res. *8*:2737, 1980.
219. Groudine, M., and Weintraub, H.: Activation of globin genes during chicken development. Cell *24*:393, 1981.
220. Weintraub, H., Larsen, A., and Groudine, M.: α-globin-gene switching during the development of chicken embryos: Expression and chromosome structure. Cell *24*:333, 1981.
221. McGhee, J. D., Wood, W. I., Dolan, M., Engel, J. D., and Felsenfeld, G.: A 200 base pair region at the 5′ end of the chicken adult β-globin gene is accessible to nuclease digestion. Cell *27*:45, 1981.
222. Elgin, S. C. R.: DNAase I-hypersensitive sites of chromatin. Cell *27*:413, 1981.
222a. Elgin, S. C. R.: Anatomy of hypersensitive sites. Nature *309*:17, 1984.
223. Larsen, A., and Weintraub, H.: An altered DNA conformation detected by S1 nuclease occurs at specific regions in active chick globin chromatin. Cell *29*:609, 1982.
224. Dolan, M., Dodgson, J. B., and Engel, J. D.: Analysis of the adult chicken β-globin gene. Nucleotide sequence of the locus, microheterogeneity at the 5′ end of β-globin mRNA and aberrant nuclear RNA species. J. Biol. Chem. *258*:3983, 1983.
225. Kohwi-Shigematsu, T., Gelinas, R., and Weintraub, H.: Detection of an altered DNA conformation at specific sites in chromatin and supercoiled DNA. Proc. Natl. Acad. Sci. USA *80*:4389, 1983.
226. Nickol, J. M., and Felsenfeld, G.: DNA conformation at the 5′ end of the chicken adult β-globin gene. Cell *35*:467, 1983.
227. Schon, E., Evans, T., Welsh, J., and Efstratiadis, A.: Conformation of promoter DNA: Fine mapping of S1-hypersensitive sites. Cell *35*:837, 1983.
227a. Evans, T., Schon, E., Gora-Maslak, G., Patterson, J., and Efstratiadis, A.: S1-hypersensitive sites in eukaryotic promoter regions. Nucleic Acids Res. *12*:8043, 1984.
227b. Cantor, C. R., and Efstratiadis, A.: Possible structures of homopurine-homopyrimidine S1-hypersensitive sites. Nucleic Acids Res. *12*:8059, 1984.
228. Lachman, H. M., and Mears, J. G.: DNase I hypersensitivity in the γ-globin gene locus of K562 cells. Nucleic Acids Res. *11*:6065, 1983.
229. Groudine, M., Kohwi-Shigematsu, T., Gelinas, R., Stamatoyannopoulos, G., and Papayannopoulou, T.: Human fetal to adult hemoglobin switching: Changes in chromatin structure of the β-globin gene locus. Proc. Natl. Acad. Sci. USA *80*:7551, 1983.
229a. Tuan, D. and London, I. M.: Mapping of DNase I–hypersensitive sites in the upstream DNA of human embryonic ε-globin gene in K562 leukemia cells. Proc. Natl. Acad. Sci. USA *81*:2718, 1984.
229b. Zhu, J.-D., Allan, M., and Paul, J.: The chromatin structure of the human ε globin gene: Nuclease hypersensitive sites correlate with multiple initiation sites of transcription. Nucleic Acids Res. *12*:9191, 1984.
230. Dean, A., Ley, T. J., Humphries, R. K., Fordis, M., and Schechter, A. N.: Inducible transcription of five globin genes in K562 human leukemia cells. Proc. Natl. Acad. Sci. USA *80*:5515, 1983.
231. Charnay, P., and Maniatis, T.: Transcriptional regulation of globin gene expression in the human erythroid cell line K562. Science *220*:1281, 1983.
231a. Miller, C., Young, K., Dumenil, D., Alter, B. P., Schofield, J. M., and Bank, A.: Specific globin mRNAs in human erythroleukemia (K562) cells. Blood *63*:195, 1984.
232. Weintraub, H., Beug, H., Groudine, M., and Graf, T.: Temperature-sensitive changes in the structure of globin chromatin in lines of red cell precursors transformed by ts-AEV. Cell *28*:931, 1982.
233. Groudine, M., and Weintraub, H.: Propagation of globin DNAase I-hypersensitive sites in absence of factors required for induction: A possible mechanism for determination. Cell *30*:131, 1982.
234. Paulson, J. R., and Laemmli, U. K.: The structure of histone-depleted metaphase chromosomes. Cell *12*:817, 1977.
235. Marsden, M. P. F., and Laemmli, U. K.: Metaphase chromosome structure: Evidence for a radial loop model. Cell *17*:849, 1979.
236. Vogelstein, B., Pardoll, D. M., and Coffey, D. S.: Supercoiled loops and eucaryotic replication. Cell *22*:79, 1980.
237. Pardoll, D. M., Vogelstein, B., and Coffey, D. S.: A fixed site of DNA replication in eucaryotic DNA cells. Cell *19*:527, 1980.
238. Robinson, S. I., Nelkin, B. D., and Vogelstein, B.: The ovalbumin gene is associated with the nuclear matrix of chicken oviduct cells. Cell *28*:99, 1982.
239. Ciejek, E. M., Tsai, M.-J., and O'Malley, B. W.: Actively transcribed genes are associated with the nuclear matrix. Nature *306*:607, 1983.
240. Hentzen, P. C., Rho, J. H., and Bekhor, I.: Nuclear matrix DNA from chicken erythrocytes contains β-globin gene sequences. Proc. Natl. Acad. Sci. USA *81*:304, 1984.
241. High, K. A., Chan, L., Hollifield, K. L., and Benz, E. J., Jr.: Relationship of globin and insulin genes to the nuclear matrix in a human leukemia cell line. Clin. Res. *31*:409A, 1983.
241a. High, K. A., Schneider, J. W., and Benz, E. J., Jr.: Enhancer dependence and activity level of α and β globin gene sequences in Cos-1 cells do not correlate with proximity to the nuclear matrix. Blood *62*(Suppl. 1):67a, 1983.
242. Cook, P. R., and Brazell, I. A.: Mapping sequences in loops of nuclear DNA by their progressive

detachment from the nuclear cage. Nucleic Acids Res. 8:2895, 1980.
243. Maundrell, K., Maxwell, E. S., Puvion, E., and Scherrer, K.: The nuclear matrix of duck erythroblasts is associated with globin mRNA coding sequences but not with the major proteins of 40S nuclear RNP. Exp. Cell Res. 136:435, 1981.
244. Ross, D. A., Yen, R.-W., and Chae, C. B.: Association of globin ribonucleic acid and its precursors with the chicken erythroblast nuclear matrix. Biochemistry 21:764, 1982.
244a. Triadou, P., Crepin, M., Gros, F., and Lelong, J.-C.: Tissue-specific binding of total and β-globin genomic deoxyribonucleic acid to non-histone chromosomal proteins from mouse erythropoietic cells. Biochemistry 21:6060, 1982.
245. Emerson, B. M., and Felsenfeld, G.: Specific factor conferring nuclease hypersensitivity at the 5' end of the chicken adult β-globin gene. Proc. Natl. Acad. Sci. USA 81:95, 1984.
246. Fordis, C. M., Anagnou, N. P., Dean, A., Nienhuis, A. W., and Schechter, A. N.: A β-globin gene, inactive in the K562 leukemic cell, functions normally in an heterologous expression system. Proc. Natl. Acad. Sci. USA 81:4485, 1984.
247. Donovan-Peluso, M., Young, K., Dobkin, C., and Bank, A.: Erythroleukemia (K562) cells contain a functional β globin gene. Mol. Cell. Biol. 4:2553, 1984.
247a. Papayannopoulou, T., Lindsley, D., Kurachi, S., Lewison, K., Hemenway, T., Melis, M., Anagnou, N. P., and Najfeld, V.: Adult and fetal human globin genes are expressed following chromosomal transfer into MEL cells. Proc. Natl. Acad. Sci. USA: 82:780, 1985.
248. Anagnou, N. P., Yuan, T. Y., Lim, E., Helder, J., Wieder, S., Glaister, D., Marks, B., Wang, A., Colbert, D., and Deisseroth, A.: Regulatory factors specific for adult and embryonic globin genes may govern their expression in erythroleukemia cells. Blood 65:705, 1985.
248a. Zeitlin, H. C., and Weatherall, D. J.: Selective expression within the human α globin gene complex following chromosome-dependent transfer into diploid mouse erythroleukaemia cells. Mol. Biol. Med. 1:489, 1983.
248b. Proudfoot, N. I., Rutherford, T. R., and Partington, G. A.: Transcriptional analysis of human zeta globin genes. EMBO J. 3:1533, 1984.
248c. Chao, M. V., Mellon, P., Charnay, P., Maniatis, T., and Axel, R.: The regulated expression of β-globin genes introduced into mouse erythroleukemia cells. Cell 32:483, 1983.
248d. Wright, S., deBoer, G., Grosveld, F. G., and Flavell, R. A.: Regulated expression of the human β-globin gene family in murine erythroleukaemia cells. Nature 305:333, 1983.
248e. Charnay, P., Treisman, R., Mellon, P., Chao, M., Axel, R., and Maniatis, T.: Differences in human α- and β-globin gene expression in mouse erythroleukemia cells: The role of intragenic sequences. Cell 38:251, 1984.
248f. Wright, S., Rosenthal, A., Flavell, R. A., and Grosveld, F.: DNA sequences required for regulated expression of β-globin genes in murine erythroleukemia cells. Cell 38:265, 1984.
249. Kane, C. M., Cheng, P. F., Burch, J. B. E., and Weintraub, H.: Tissue-specific and species-specific monoclonal antibodies to avian red cell nuclear proteins. Proc. Natl. Acad. Sci. USA 79:6265, 1982.

249a. Schöler, H. R., and Gruss, P.: Specific interaction between enhancer-containing molecules and cellular components. Cell 36:403, 1984.
249b. Sassone-Corsi, P., Wildeman, A., and Chambon, P.: A trans-acting factor is responsible for the simian virus 40 enhancer activity in vitro. Nature 313:458, 1985.
249c. Ephrussi, A., Church, G. M., Tonegawa, S., and Gilbert, W.: B lineage-specific interactions of an immunoglobulin enhancer with cellular factors in vivo. Science 227:134, 1985.
249d. Mercola, M., Goverman, J., Mirell, C., and Calame, K.: Immunoglobulin heavy-chain enhancer requires one or more tissue-specific factors. Science 227:266, 1985.
249e. Green, M. R., Treisman, R., and Maniatis, T.: Transcriptional activation of cloned human β-globin genes by viral immediate-early gene products. Cell 35:137, 1983.
249f. Treisman, R., Green, M. R., and Maniatis, T.: Cis and trans activation of globin gene transcription in transient assays. Proc. Natl. Acad. Sci. USA 80:7428, 1983.
250. Bard, H.: Postnatal fetal and adult hemoglobin synthesis in early preterm newborn infants. J. Clin. Invest. 52:1789, 1973.
251. Bard, H., and Prosmanne, J.: Postnatal fetal and adult hemoglobin synthesis in preterm infants whose birth weight was less than 1,000 grams. J. Clin. Invest. 70:50, 1982.
252. Bard, H., Makowski, E. L., Meschia, G., and Battaglia, F.: The relative rates of synthesis of hemoglobin A and F in immature red cells of newborn infants. Pediatrics 45:766, 1970.
253. Bromberg, Y. M., Abrahamov, A., and Salzberger, M.: The effect of maternal anoxaemia on the foetal haemoglobin of the newborn. J. Obstet. Gynaecol. Br. Commonw. 63:875, 1956.
254. Huehns, E. R., Hecht, F., Keil, J. V., and Motulsky, A. G.: Developmental hemoglobin anomalies in a chromosomal triplication: D_1 trisomy syndrome. Proc. Natl. Acad. Sci. USA 51:89, 1964.
255. Wilson, M. G., Schroeder, W. A., Graves, D. A., and Kach, V. D.: Hemoglobin variations in D-trisomy syndrome. N. Engl. J. Med. 277:953, 1967.
256. Bard, H.: Postnatal fetal and adult hemoglobin synthesis in D_1 trisomy syndrome. Blood 40:523, 1972.
256a. Perrine, S. P., Greene, M. F., and Faller, D. V.: Delay in the fetal globin switch in infants of diabetic mothers. N. Engl. J. Med. 312:334, 1985.
257. Wilson, M. G., Schroeder, W. A., and Graves, D. A.: Postnatal change of hemoglobins F and A_2 in infants with Down's syndrome (G trisomy). Pediatrics 42:349, 1968.
258. Weller, S. D. V., Apley, J., and Raper, A. B.: Malformations associated with precocious synthesis of adult hemoglobin. Lancet 1:777, 1966.
259. Zanjani, E. D., McGlave, P. B., Bhakthavathsalan, A., and Stamatoyannopoulos, G.: Sheep fetal haematopoietic cells produce adult haemoglobin when transplanted in the adult animal. Nature 280:495, 1979.
260. Bunch, C., Wood, W. G., Weatherall, D. J., Robinson, J. S., and Corp, M. J.: Haemoglobin synthesis by fetal erythroid cells in an adult environment. Br. J. Haematol. 49:325, 1981.
260a. Wood, W. G., Bunch, C., Kelly, S., Gunn, Y., and Breckon, G.: Control of haemoglobin switching by a developmental clock? Nature 313:320, 1985.
261. Wood, W. G., Pearce, K., Clegg, J. B., Weatherall, D. J., Robinson, J. S., Thorburn, G. D., and

Dawes, G. S.: Switch from foetal to adult haemoglobin synthesis in normal and hypophysectomised sheep. Nature 264:799, 1976.
262. Delfini, C., Saglio, G., Mazza, U., Muretto, P., Filippetti, A., and Lucarelli, G.: Fetal haemoglobin synthesis following fetal liver transplantation in man. Br. J. Haematol. 55:609, 1983.
262a. Papayannopoulou, T., Nakamoto, B., Agnostelli, F., Lucarelli, G., and Stamatoyannopoulos, G.: Fetal to adult hematopoietic cell transplantation in man: Insights to hemoglobin switching. Blood 64:(Suppl. 1):63a, 1984.
263. Zanjani, E. D., Lim, G., McGlave, P. B., Clapp, J. F., Mann, L. I., Norwood, T. H., and Stamatoyannopoulos, G.: Adult haematopoietic cells transplanted to sheep fetuses continue to produce adult globins. Nature 295:244, 1982.
264. Stamatoyannopoulos, G., and Papayannopoulou, T.: The switching from hemoglobin F to hemoglobin A formation in man: Parallels between the observations in vivo and the findings in erythroid cultures. In The Red Cell: Fifth Ann Arbor Conference. New York, Alan R. Liss, Inc., 1981, pp. 665–675.
265. Stamatoyannopoulos, G., Papayannopoulou, T., Brice, M., Kurachi, S., Nakamoto, B., Lim, G., and Farquhar, M. N.: Cell biology of hemoglobin switching. I. The switch from fetal to adult hemoglobin formation during ontogeny. In Stamatoyannopoulos, G., and Nienhuis, A. W. (eds.): Hemoglobins in Development and Differentiation. New York, Alan R. Liss, Inc., 1981, pp. 287–306.
266. Ogawa, M.: Human hemoglobin switching in culture. Am. J. Hematol. 9:127, 1980.
267. Peschle, C., Migliaccio, A. R., Migliaccio, G., Lettieri, F., Maguire, Y. P., Condorelli, M., Gianni, A. M., Ottolenghi, S., Giglioni, B., Pozzoli, M. L., and Comi, P.: Regulation of Hb synthesis in ontogenesis and erythropoietic differentiation: In vitro studies on fetal liver, cord blood, normal adult blood or marrow, and blood from HPFH patients. In Stamatoyannopoulos, G., and Nienhuis, A. W. (eds.): Hemoglobins in Development and Differentiation. New York, Alan R. Liss, Inc., 1981, pp. 359–371.
268. Wood, W. G., and Weatherall, D. J.: Haemoglobin synthesis during human foetal development. Nature 244:162, 1973.
269. Wood, W. G., Nash, J., Weatherall, D. J., Robinson, J. S., and Harrison, F. A.: The sheep as an animal model for the switch from fetal to adult hemoglobins. In Stamatoyannopoulos, G., and Nienhuis, A. W. (eds.): Cellular and Molecular Regulation of Hemoglobin Switching. New York, Grune and Stratton, 1979, p. 153.
270. Colombo, B., Kim, B., Perez Atencio, R., Molina, C., and Terrenato, L.: The pattern of fetal haemoglobin disappearance after birth. Br. J. Haematol. 32:79, 1976.
271. Terrenato, L., Bertilaccio, C., Spinelli, P., and Colombo, B.: The switch from haemoglobin F to A: The time course of qualitative and quantitative variations of haemoglobins after birth. Br. J. Haematol. 47:31, 1981.
272. Shepard, M. K., Weatherall, D. J., and Conley, C. L.: Semi-quantitative estimation of the distribution of fetal hemoglobin in red cell populations. Bull. Johns Hopkins Hosp. 110:293, 1962.
273. Weinberg, R. S., Goldberg, J. D., Schofield, J. M., Lenes, A. L., Styczynski, R., and Alter, B. P.: Switch from fetal to adult hemoglobin is associated with a change in progenitor cell population. J. Clin. Invest. 71:785, 1983.
274. Alter, B. P., Jackson, B. T., Lipton, J. M., Piasecki, G. J., Jackson, P. L., Kudisch, M., and Nathan, D. G.: Control of the simian fetal hemoglobin switch at the progenitor cell level. J. Clin. Invest. 67:458, 1981.
275. Pembrey, M. E., Weatherall, D. J., and Clegg, J. B.: Maternal synthesis of haemoglobin F in pregnancy. Lancet i:1350, 1973.
276. Popat, N., Wood, W. G., Weatherall, D. J., and Turnbull, A. C.: The pattern of maternal F-cell production during pregnancy. Lancet ii:377, 1977.
277. Boyer, S. H., Belding, T. K., Margolet, L., Noyes, A. N., Burke, P. J., and Bell, W. R.: Variations in the frequency of fetal hemoglobin-bearing erythrocytes (F-cells) in well adults, pregnant women, and adult leukemics. Johns Hopkins Med. J. 137:105, 1975.
278. Dainiak, N., and Hoffman, R.: Hemoglobin F production in testicular malignancy. Cancer 45:2177, 1980.
279. Lee, J. C., Hayashi, R. H., and Shepard, M. K.: Fetal hemoglobin in women with normal and with hydatidiform molar pregnancy. Am. J. Hematol. 13:131, 1982.
280. Eng, L.-I. L., Hollander, L., and Fudenberg, H.: Carbonic anhydrase and fetal hemoglobin in thyrotoxicosis. Blood 30:442, 1967.
281. Fuhr, J. E., and Gengozian, N.: Fetal hemoglobin: In vivo stimulation by D-thyroxine in adult marmosets. Blood Cells 5:471, 1979.
282. Koeller, D., Desimone, J., and Heller, P.: Failure of D-thyroxine to increase fetal hemoglobin levels in normal and anemic baboons. Blood Cells 8:187, 1982.
283. Desimone, J., Biel, S. I., and Heller, P.: Stimulation of fetal hemoglobin synthesis in baboons by hemolysis and hypoxia. Proc. Natl. Acad. Sci. USA 75:2937, 1978.
284. Boyer, S. H., Belding, T. K., Margolet, L., and Noyes, A. N.: Fetal hemoglobin restriction to a few erythrocytes (F cells) in normal human adults. Science 188:361, 1975.
285. Wood, W. G., Stamatoyannopoulos, G., Lim, G., and Nute, P. E.: F-cells in the adult: Normal values and levels in individuals with hereditary and acquired elevations of Hb F. Blood 46:671, 1975.
286. Wood, W. G., Clegg, J. B., and Weatherall, D. J.: Developmental biology of human hemoglobins. Prog. Hematol. 10:43, 1977.
287. Weatherall, D. J., Wood, W. G., and Clegg, J. B.: Genetics of fetal hemoglobin production in adult life. In Stamatoyannopoulos, G., and Nienhuis, A. W. (eds.): Cellular and Molecular Regulation of Hemoglobin Switching. New York, Grune and Stratton, 1979, p. 3.
288. Weatherall, D. J., Edwards, J. A., and Donohoe, W. T. A.: Haemoglobin and red cell enzyme changes in juvenile myeloid leukaemia. Br. Med. J. i:679, 1968.
289. Weatherall, D. J., Clegg, J. B., Wood, W. G., Callendar, S. T., Sheridan, B. L., and Pritchard, J.: Foetal erythropoiesis in human leukaemia. Nature 257:710, 1975.
290. Weatherall, D. J., Clegg, J. B., and Wood, W. G.: A model for the persistence of reactivation of fetal haemoglobin production. Lancet ii:660, 1976.
291. Papayannopoulou, T., Bunn, H. F., and Stamato-

yannopoulos, G.: Cellular distribution of hemoglobin F in a clonal hemopoietic stem-cell disorder. N. Engl. J. Med 298:72, 1978.
292. Bunch, C., Wood, W. G., Weatherall, D. J., and Adamson, J. W.: Cellular origins of the fetal-haemoglobin–containing cells of normal adults. Lancet i:1163, 1979.
293. Hoffman, R., Papayannopoulou, T., Landaw, S., Wasserman, L. R., DeMarsh, Q. B., Chen, P., and Stamatoyannopoulos, G.: Fetal hemoglobin in polycythemia vera: Cellular distribution in 50 unselected patients. Blood 53:1148, 1979.
294. Stamatoyannopoulos, G., and Papayannopoulou, T.: Fetal hemoglobin and the erythroid stem cell differentiation process. In Stamatoyannopoulos, G., and Nienhuis, A. W. (eds.): Cellular and Molecular Regulation of Hemoglobin Switching. New York, Grune and Stratton, 1979, pp. 323–350.
295. Papayannopoulou, T., Nakamoto, B., Kurachi, S., Kurnit, D., and Stamatoyannopoulos, G.: Cell biology of hemoglobin switching. II. Studies on the regulation of fetal hemoglobin synthesis in human adults. In Stamatoyannopoulos, G., and Nienhuis, A. W. (eds.): Hemoglobins in Development and Differentiation. New York, Alan R. Liss, Inc., 1981.
296. Papayannopoulou, T., Brice, M., and Stamatoyannopoulos, G.: Stimulation of fetal hemoglobin synthesis in bone marrow cultures from adult individuals. Proc. Natl. Acad. Sci. USA 73:2033, 1976.
297. Papayannopoulou, T., Brice, M., and Stamatoyannopoulos, G.: Hemoglobin F synthesis in vitro: Evidence for control at the level of primitive erythroid stem cells. Proc. Natl. Acad. Sci. USA 74:2923, 1977.
298. Comi, P., Giglioni, B., Pozzoli, M. L., Ottolenghi, S., Gianni, A. M., Migliaccio, A. R., Migliaccio, G., Lettieri, F., and Peschle, C.: Biosynthesis of globin chains in fetal liver and adult marrow cultures. Exp. Cell Res. 133:347, 1981.
299. Friedman, A. D., Linch, D. C., Miller, B. A., Lipton, J. M., Javid, J., and Nathan, D. G.: Determination fo the hemoglobin F program in human progenitor derived erythroid cells. J. Clin. Invest., in press.
300. Dover, G. J., Chan, T., and Sieber, F.: Fetal hemoglobin production in cultures of primitive and mature human erythroid progenitors: Differentiation affects the quantity of fetal hemoglobin produced per fetal-hemoglobin–containing cell. Blood 61:1242, 1983.
301. Kidoguchi, K., Ogawa, M., and Karam, J. D.: Hemoglobin biosynthesis in individual erythropoietic bursts in culture. J. Clin. Invest. 63:804, 1979.
302. Peschle, C., Migliaccio, G., Covelli, A., Lettieri, F., Migliaccio, R., Condorelli, M., Comi, P., Pozzoli, M. L., Giglioni, B., Ottolenghi, S., Cappellini, M. D., Polli, E., and Gianni, A. M.: Hemoglobin synthesis in individual bursts from normal adult blood: All bursts and subcolonies synthesize $^G\gamma$- and $^A\gamma$-globin chains. Blood 56:218, 1980.
303. Dover, G. J., and Ogawa, M.: Cellular mechanisms for increased fetal hemoglobin production in culture. J. Clin. Invest. 66:1175, 1980.
304. Papayannopoulou, T., Kurachi, S. Nakamoto, B., Zanjani, E. D., and Stamatoyannopoulos, G.: Hemoglobin switching in culture: Evidence for a humoral factor that induces switching in adult and neonatal but not fetal erythroid cells. Proc. Natl. Acad. Sci. USA 79:6579, 1982.
305. Stamatoyannopoulos, G., Nakamoto, B., Kurachi, S., and Papayannopoulou, T.: Direct evidence of interaction between human erythroid progenitor cells and a hemoglobin switching activity present in fetal sheep serum. Proc. Natl. Acad. Sci. USA 80:5650, 1983.
306. Papayannopoulou, T., Tatsis, B., Kurachi, S., Nakamoto, B., and Stamatoyannopoulos, G.: A haemoglobin switching activity modulates hereditary persistence of fetal haemoglobin. Nature 309:71, 1984.
307. Papayannopoulou, T., Kalmantis, T., and Stamatoyannopoulos, G.: Cellular regulation of hemoglobin switching: Evidence for inverse relationship between fetal hemoglobin synthesis and degree of maturity of human erythroid cells. Proc. Natl. Acad. Sci. USA 76:6420, 1979.
308. Chui, D. H. K., Wong, M., Enkin, M. W., Patterson, M., and Ives, R. A.: Proportion of fetal hemoglobin synthesis decreases during erythroid cell maturation. Proc. Natl. Acad. Sci. USA 77:2757, 1980.
309. Gianni, A. M., Comi, P., Giglioni, B., Ottolenghi, S., Migliaccio, A. R., Migliaccio, G., Lettieri, F., Maguire, P., and Peschle, C.: Biosynthesis of Hb in individual fetal liver bursts. Exp. Cell Res. 130:345, 1980.
310. Darbre, P. D., Lauckner, S. M., Adamson, J. W., Wood, W. G., and Weatherall, D. J.: Haemoglobin synthesis in human erythroid bursts during ontogeny: Reproducibility and sensitivity to culture conditions. Br. J. Haematol. 48:237, 1981.
311. Dover, G. J., and Boyer, S. H.: Quantitation of hemoglobins within individual red cells: Asynchronous biosynthesis of fetal and adult hemoglobin during erythroid maturation in normal subjects. Blood 56:1082, 1980.
312. Czelusniak, J., Goodman, M., Hewett-Emmett, D., Weiss, M. L., Venta, P. J., and Tashian, R. E.: Phylogenetic origin and adaptive evolution of avian and mammalian haemoglobin genes. Nature 298:297, 1982.
313. Jeffreys, A. J., Harris, S., Barrie, P. A., Wood, D., Blanchetot, A., and Adams, S. M.: In Bendall, D. S. (ed.): Evolution from Molecules to Men. New York, Cambridge University Press, 1983, pp. 175–195.
314. Hunt, T. L., Hurst-Calderone, S., and Dayhoff, M. O.: In Dayhoff, M. O. (ed.): Atlas of Protein Sequence and Structure. Washington D.C., National Biomedical Research Foundation, 1978, pp. 229–251.
315. Jeffreys, A. J., Wilson, V., Wood, D., Simons, J. P., Kay, R. M., and Williams, J. G.: Linkage of adult α- and β-globin genes in Xenopus laevis and gene duplication by tetraploidization. Cell 21:555, 1980.
316. Patient, R. K., Elkington, J. A., Kay, R. M., and Williams, J. G.: Internal organization of the major adult α- and β-globin genes of X. laevis. Cell 21:565, 1980.
317. Hosbach, H. A., Wyler, T., and Weber, R.: The xenopus laevis globin gene family: Chromosomal arrangement and gene structure. Cell 32:45, 1983.
318. Jeffreys, A. J., Wilson, V., Blanchetot, A., Weller, P., van Kessel, A. G., Spurr, N., Solomon, E., and Goodfellow, P.: The human myoglobin gene: A third dispersed globin locus in the human genome. Nucleic Acids Res. 12:3235, 1984.
319. Dolan, M., Sugarman, B. J., Dodgson, J. B., and Engel, J. D.: Chromosomal arrangement of the chicken β-type globin genes. Cell 24:669, 1981.

320. Villeponteau, B., and Martinson, H.: Isolation and characterization of the complete chicken β-globin gene region: Frequent deletion of the adult β-globin genes in λ. Nucleic Acids Res. *9*:3731, 1981.
321. Townes, T. M., Shapiro, S. G., Wernke, S. M., and Lingrel, J. B.: Duplication of a four-gene set during the evolution of the goat β-globin locus produced genes now expressed differentially in development. J. Biol. Chem. *259*:1896, 1984.
321a. Townes, T. M., Fitzgerald, M. C., and Lingrel, J. B.: Triplication of a four-gene set during evolution of the goat β-globin locus produced three genes now expressed differentially during development. Proc. Natl. Acad. Sci. USA *81*:6589, 1984.
322. Farace, M. G., Brown, B. A., Raschella, G., Alexander, J., Gambari, R., Fantoni, A., Hardies, S. C., Hutchison, C. A. III, and Edgell, M. H.: The mouse βh1 gene codes for the z chain of embryonic hemoglobin. J. Biol. Chem. *259*:7213, 1984.
322a. Rohrbaugh, M. L., and Hardison, R. C.: Analysis of rabbit β-like globin gene transcripts during development. J. Mol. Biol. *164*:395, 1983.
323. Barrie, P. A., Jeffreys, A. J., and Scott, A. F.: Evolution of the β globin gene cluster in man and the primates. J. Mol. Biol. *149*:319, 1981.
324. Perler, F., Efstratiadis, A., Lomedico, P., Gilbert, W., Kolodner, R., and Dodgson, J.: The evolution of genes: The chicken preproinsulin gene. Cell *20*:555, 1980.
325. Martin, S. L., Vincent, K. A., and Wilson, A. C.: Rise and fall of the delta globin gene. J. Mol. Biol. *164*:513, 1983.
326. Hardies, S. C., Edgell, M. H., and Hutchison, C. A. III: Evolution of the mammalian β-globin gene cluster. J. Biol. Chem. *259*:3748, 1984.
326a. Hutchinson, C. A., III, Hardies, S. C., Padgett, R. W., Weaver, S., and Edgell, M. H.: The mouse globin pseudogene βh3 is descended from a pre-mammalian δ-globin gene. J. Biol. Chem. *259*:12881, 1984.
327. Hardison, R. C.: Comparison of the β-like globin gene families of rabbits and humans indicates that the gene cluster 5'-ε-γ-δ-β-3' predates the mammalian radiation. Mol. Biol. Evol. *1*:390, 1984.
328. Hardison, R. C., and Margot, J. B.: Rabbit globin pseudogene ψβ2 is a hybrid of δ- and β-globin gene sequences. Mol. Biol. Evol. *1*:302, 1984.
329. Konkel, D. A., Maizel, J. V., Jr., and Leder, P.: The evolution and sequence comparison of two recently diverged mouse chromosomal β-globin genes. Cell *18*:865, 1979.
330. Goodman, M., Koop, B. F., Czelusniak, J., and Weiss, M. L.: The η-globin gene: Its long evolutionary history in the β-globin gene family of mammals. J. Mol. Biol., *180*:803, 1984.
331. Jeffreys, A. J., Barrie, P. A., Harris, S., Fawcett, D. H., Nugent, Z. J., and Boyd, A. C.: Isolation and sequence analysis of a hybrid δ globin pseudogene from the brown lemur. J. Mol. Biol. *156*:487, 1982.
331a. Harris, S., Barrie, P. A., Weiss, M. L., and Jeffreys, A. J.: The primate ψβ1 gene: An ancient β-globin pseudogene. J. Mol. Biol., *180*:785, 1984.
332. Hill, A., Hardies, S. C., Phillips, S. J., Davis, S. J., Hutchison, C. A. III, and Edgell, M. H.: Two mouse early embryonic β-globin gene sequences: Evolution of the nonadult β-globins. J. Biol. Chem. *259*:3739, 1984.
333. Schon, E. A., Cleary, M. L., Haynes, J. R., and Lingrel, J. B.: Structure and evolution of goat γ-, $β^C$- and $β^A$-globin genes: Three developmentally regulated genes contain inserted elements. Cell *27*:359, 1981.
334. Gidari, A. S., and Levere, R. D.: Enzymatic formation and cellular regulation of heme synthesis. Semin. Hematol. *14*:145, 1977.
335. Ponka, P., and Neuwirt, J.: Haem synthesis and iron uptake by reticulocytes. Br. J. Haematol. *28*:1, 1974.
336. Tenhunen, R.: The enzymatic degradation of heme. Semin. Hematol. *9*:19, 1972.
337. Shibahara, S., Yoshida, T., and Kikucki, G.: Mechanism of increase of heme oxygenase activity induced by hemin in cultured pig alveolar macrophages. Arch. Biochem. Biophys. *197*:607, 1979.
338. Ibrahim, N. G., Lutton, J. D., and Levere, R. D.: The role of haem biosynthetic and degradative enzymes in erythroid colony development: The effect of haemin. Br. J. Haematol. *50*:17, 1982.
338a. Sassa, S.: Heme biosynthesis in erythroid cells: Distinctive aspects of the regulatory mechanism. In Goldwasser, E. (ed.): Regulation of Hemoglobin Biosynthesis. New York, Elsevier Science Publishing Co., Inc., 1983, p. 359.
338b. Grandchamp, B., Romeo, P.-H., Dubart, A., Raich, N., Rosa, J., Nordmann, Y., and Goossens, M.: Molecular cloning of a cDNA sequence complementary to porphobilinogen deaminase mRNA from rat. Proc. Natl. Acad. Sci. USA *81*:5036, 1984.
339. Maines, M. D., and Kappas, A.: Metals as regulators of heme metabolism. Science *198*:1215, 1977.
340. Maines, M. D., and Kappas, A.: Prematurely evoked synthesis and induction of δ-aminolevulinate synthetase in neonatal liver: Evidence for metal ion repression of enzyme formation. J. Biol. Chem. *253*:2321, 1978.
341. Hines, J. D., and Cowan, D. H.: Studies on the pathogenesis of alcohol-induced sideroblastic bone-marrow abnormalities. N. Engl. J. Med. *283*:441, 1970.
342. Lumeng, L., and Li, T.-K.: Vitamin B_6 metabolism in chronic alcohol abuse: Pyridoxal phosphate levels in plasma and the effects of acetaldehyde on pyridoxal phosphate synthesis and degradation in human erythrocytes. J. Clin. Invest. *53*:693, 1974.
343. Chillar, R. K., Johnson, C. S., and Beutler, E.: Erythrocyte pyridoxine kinase levels in patients with sideroblastic anemia. N. Engl. J. Med *295*:881, 1976.
344. Solomon, L. R., and Hillman, R. S.: Vitamin B_6 metabolism in anaemic and alcoholic man. Br. J. Haematol. *41*:343, 1979.
345. Lumeng, L.: The role of acetaldehyde in mediating the deleterious effect of ethanol on pyridoxal 5'-phosphate metabolism. J. Clin. Invest. *62*:286, 1978.
346. Abou-Khalil, S., Salem, Z., and Yunis, A. A.: Mitochondrial metabolism in normal, myeloid, and erythroid hyperplastic rabbit bone marrow: Effect of chloramphenicol. Am. J. Hematol. *8*:71, 1980.
347. Manyan, D. R., and Yunis, A. A.: The effect of chloramphenicol treatment on ferrochelatase activity in dogs. Biochem. Biophys. Res. Commun. *41*:926, 1970.
348. Bottomley, S. S.: Porphyrin and iron metabolism in sideroblastic anemia. Semin. Hematol. *14*:169, 1977.
348a. Bottomley, S.: Sideroblastic anaemia. Clin. Haematol. *11*:389, 1982.

349. Konopka, L., and Hoffbrand, A. V.: Haem synthesis in sideroblastic anaemia. Br. J. Haematol. *42*:73, 1979.
350. Aoki, Y., Muranaka, S., Nakabayashi, K., and Ueda, Y.: δ-aminolevulinic acid synthetase in erythroblasts of patients with pyridoxine-responsive anemia. J. Clin. Invest. *64*:1196, 1979.
351. Solomon, L. R., and Hillman, R. S.: Vitamin B_6 metabolism in idiopathic sideroblastic anaemia and related disorders. Br. J. Haematol. *42*:239, 1979.
352. Aoki, Y.: Multiple enzymatic defects in mitochondria in hematological cells of patients with primary sideroblastic anemia. J. Clin. Invest. *66*:43, 1980.
353. Cartwright, G. E., Edwards, C. Q., Skolnick, M. H., and Amos, D. B.: Association of HLA-linked hemochromatosis with idiopathic refractory sideroblastic anemia. J. Clin. Invest. *65*:989, 1980.
354. Kruh, J., and Borsook, H.: Hemoglobin synthesis in rabbit reticulocytes in vitro. J. Biol. Chem. *220*:905, 1956.
355. Bruns, G. P., and London, I. M.: The effect of hemin on the synthesis of globin. Biochem. Biophys. Res. Commun. *18*:236, 1965.
356. Waxman, H. S., and Rabinovitz, M.: Iron supplementation in vitro and the state of aggregation and function of reticulocyte ribosomes in hemoglobin synthesis. Biochem. Biophys. Res. Commun. *19*:538, 1965.
357. Grayzel, A. I., Horchner, P., and London, I. M.: The stimulation of globin synthesis by heme. Proc. Natl. Acad. Sci. USA *55*:650, 1966.
358. Waxman, H. S., and Rabinovitz, M.: Control of reticulocyte polyribosome content and hemoglobin synthesis by heme. Biochem. Biophys. Acta *129*:369, 1966.
359. White, J. M., Brain, M. C., and Ali, M. A. M.: Globin synthesis in sideroblastic anaemia. I. α and β peptide chain synthesis. Br. J. Haematol. *20*:263, 1971.
360. White, J. M., and Harvey, D. R.: Defective synthesis of α and β globin chains in lead poisoning. Nature *236*:71, 1972.
361. White, J. M., and Ali, M. A. M.: Globin synthesis in sideroblastic anaemia. Br. J. Haematol. *24*:481, 1973.
362. Ben-Bassat, I., Mozel, M., and Ramot, B.: Globin synthesis in iron-deficiency anemia. Blood *44*:551, 1974.
363. White, J. M., and Hoffbrand, A. V.: Haeme deficiency and chain synthesis. Nature *248*:88, 1974.
364. El-Hazmi, M. A. F., and Lehmann, H.: Interaction between iron deficiency and α-thalassaemia: The "in vitro" effect of haemin on α-chain synthesis. Acta Haematol. *60*:1, 1978.
365. Piddington, S. K., and White, J. M.: The effect of lead on total globin and α- and β-chain synthesis; in vitro and in vivo. Br. J. Haematol. *27*:415, 1974.
366. Kan, Y. W., Schwartz, E., and Nathan, D. G.: Globin chain synthesis in the alpha thalassemia syndromes. J. Clin. Invest. *47*:2515, 1968.
367. Tavill, A. S., Grayzel, A. I., London, I. M., Williams, M. K., and Vanderhoff, G. A.: The role of heme in the synthesis and assembly of hemoglobin. J. Biol. Chem. *243*:4987, 1968.
368. Franco, R. S., Hogg, J. W., and Martelo, O. J.: The effect of INH-inhibited heme synthesis on globin synthesis. J. Lab. Clin. Med. *93*:679, 1979.
369. Walford, D. M., and Deacon, R.: Globin chain biosynthesis in iron deficiency. Br. J. Haematol. *44*:201, 1980.
370. Zago, M. A., and Bottura, C.: Bone marrow and peripheral blood globin chain biosynthesis in iron deficiency. Blut *44*:159, 1982.
371. Peters, R. E., May, A., and Jacobs, A.: Globin chain synthesis ratios in sideroblastic anaemia. Br. J. Haematol. *53*:201, 1983.
372. Lodish, H. F., and Jacobsen, M.: Regulation of hemoglobin synthesis: Equal rates of translation and termination of α- and β-globin chains. J. Biol. Chem. *247*:3622, 1972.
373. Lodish, H. F.: Alpha and beta globin messenger ribonucleic acid: Different amounts and rates of initiation of translation. J. Biol. Chem. *246*:7131, 1971.
374. Lodish, H. F.: Model for the regulation of mRNA translation applied to haemoglobin synthesis. Nature *251*:385, 1974.
375. Gross, M.: The control of protein synthesis by hemin in rabbit reticulocytes. Mol. Cell Biochem. *31*:25, 1980.
376. Jagus, R., Crouch, D., Konieczny, A., and Safer, B.: The role of phosphorylation in the regulation of eukaryotic initiation factor 2 activity. Curr. Top. Cell Regul. *21*:35, 1982.
377. Safer, B.: 2B or not 2B: Regulation of the catalytic utilization of eIF-2. Cell *33*:7, 1983.
378. Ochoa, S.: Regulation of protein synthesis initiation in eucaryotes. Arch. Biochem. Biophys. *223*:325, 1983.
379. Matts, R. L., Levin, D. H., Petryshyn, R., Thomas, N. S., and London, I. M.: Translational control of protein synthesis in reticulocyte lysates by eIF-2α kinases. *In* Bermek, E. (ed.): Mechanisms of Protein Synthesis. Berlin, Springer-Verlag, 1984, p. 144.

THE THALASSEMIAS: MOLECULAR PATHOGENESIS

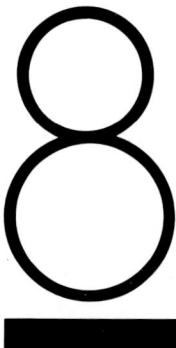

Over the years, the thalassemia syndromes have served as the prototype system for gaining insights into the factors that can regulate or disrupt normal gene expression. The thalassemias constitute a heterogeneous group of naturally occurring, inherited mutations characterized by abnormal globin gene function resulting in total absence or quantitative reduction of α or β globin chain synthesis in human erythroid cells. Alpha thalassemia involves absent or decreased production of α chains, while in the β thalassemias, there is absent or decreased production of β chains. In those cases in which some of the affected globin chain is synthesized, early studies demonstrated no evidence of an amino acid substitution.[1-4] However, in all cases in which genetic evidence was available, the thalassemia gene appeared to be allelic to the structural gene for the α or β globin gene[5] (see Chapter 9). The elucidation of the nature of the various molecular lesions in thalassemia has been a fascinating process, full of surprises, which has closely followed, and depended on, progress and technical breakthroughs in the fields of biochemistry and molecular biology. In recent years, recombinant DNA technology has contributed to a virtual explosion of new information on the precise molecular basis of most forms of thalassemia. The accrual of this knowledge has, to a great degree, paralleled the acquisition of new, detailed information on the structure, organization, and function of the normal human globin genes (see Chapter 7). Historically, as new techniques have been developed for the study of protein synthesis and gene expression, they have been rapidly applied to the study of normal human hemoglobin synthesis and thalassemia. As a result, there has gradually emerged a progressively clearer and increasingly complex picture of the molecular pathology of this group of genetic disorders. One major conclusion that can be drawn from this unfolding mystery is that a

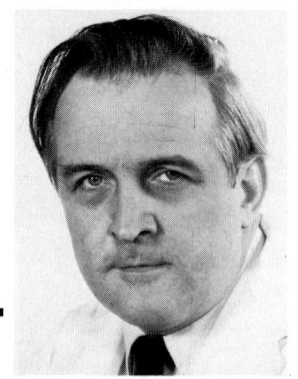

DAVID J. WEATHERALL

After David Weatherall completed his medical training at the University of Liverpool, he was obliged to enter the armed forces for two years of national service. Because of his distaste for flying, bullets, and snakes, he volunteered to serve somewhere in the United Kingdom and therefore was immediately posted to Singapore, where he was put in charge of the children's ward at the Military Hospital. One of his first patients was a severely anemic Ghurka baby from Nepal. This baby, who was being kept alive by regular blood transfusion, had defied the diagnostic efforts of all the army specialists in Malaysia and Singapore. Together with Frank Vella in the Biochemistry Department in the University of Singapore, Weatherall showed that this baby was a β-thalassemia homozygote. The major reward for this effort was a severe reprimand from the Army for not asking permission from the War Office to publish the case. After this auspicious start, he went on to analyze hemoglobin types of a variety of children in Singapore and Malaysia, using fairly primitive equipment, including an electrophoretic set-up powered by car batteries. After 2 years in Southeast Asia, it became apparent that thalassemia was very common in this population.

Weatherall came out of the army and obtained a postdoctoral fellowship with Victor McCusick at Johns Hopkins Hospital. Working with S. H. Boyer, he defined the genetic regulation of α chains of human hemoglobin and then went on to study α thalassemia in black infants. After a brief spell back in England, he returned to Johns Hopkins and worked on the pathophysiology of thalassemia from 1963 to 1965. Early studies using radiolabeling of hemoglobin in reticulocyte preparations were hampered by the lack of a quantitative method for measuring globin-chain synthesis. At that particular time another Englishman, John Clegg, arrived at Johns Hopkins to work on the biosynthesis of insulin. Hearing that the major difficulty was separating globin chains, Clegg suggested that it might be worth trying an adaptation of a method that he had used in his doctoral thesis for fractionating fibrinogen. It worked almost the first time. Radioactively labeled thalassemic material was removed from the deep freeze, and it was convincingly shown that a quantitative method for globin chain synthesis was available at last. In subsequent years, it became possible to define most of the thalassemia syndromes by *in vitro* globin chain synthesis studies using this approach.

On returning to Great Britain in 1966, Weatherall set up a hemoglobin research group in Liverpool and was later joined by John Clegg. Together they characterized the biosynthetic defect in homozygous α thalassemia and discovered the first chain termination mutants as well as a series of different forms of hereditary persistence of fetal hemoglobin.

In 1974, Weatherall became Nuffield Professor of Clinical Medicine at Oxford. Here, he built up a larger research group and obtained a Medical Research Council Unit in 1979. The work of the Unit has been built around the molecular pathology of the hemoglobin disorders, developmental aspects of human hemoglobin, and the interaction between *P. falciparum* malaria and the red cell. The Weatherall laboratory remains at the forefront of thalassemia research, having made a smooth and productive transition from studies of globin chain biosynthesis and hemoglobin biochemistry to molecular analyses of globin genes and globin mRNA. Much of the work on thalassemia has been summarized in the excellent monograph "The Thalassaemia Syndromes" written in collaboration with J. B. Clegg, which is now in its third edition and which constitutes the most thorough and comprehensive description of thalassemia currently in the literature.

fairly homogeneous phenotype can result from a surprisingly large number of varied genotypes.

The discussion of the molecular pathogenesis of thalassemia will be divided into different sections that will illustrate the chronological development of scientific progress in this field and the intimate dependence between the progressive acquisition of new information and the availability, at the time, of certain critical, recently developed, technological tools and processes.

STUDIES OF GLOBIN-CHAIN SYNTHESIS IN INTACT THALASSEMIC ERYTHROID CELLS

Peripheral Blood Reticulocytes

The imbalance of globin-chain synthesis, which is characteristic of thalassemia, was first directly demonstrated in thalassemic cells by three different laboratories between 1964 and 1966.[6-9] These observations were made possible by the development, in the early 1960's, of new techniques for the separation of globin chains[10] and for the measurement of incorporation of radioactive amino acid precursors into newly synthesized globin chains. The procedure consists of incubating peripheral blood reticulocytes for 1 to 2 hours in the presence of a radioactive amino acid precursor, usually leucine or valine. Globin is then prepared from the total cell lysate or from the Hb A purified from the lysate by column chromatography. The globin is fractionated by carboxymethylcellulose column chromatography in the presence of 8 M urea, which separates the α, β, and γ globin chains. An example of a chromatogram obtained with globin isolated from normal nonthalassemic peripheral blood reticulocytes is shown in Figure 8–1A. It can be seen that roughly equal amounts of radioactive, newly synthesized α and β chains are found under the α and β globin chain optical density peaks. One can thus obtain a quantitative ratio of β to α globin chain synthesis (β/α synthetic ratio), which, in a normal cell, is equal to 1.0. When applied to the study of thalassemic reticulocytes, the initial studies all demonstrated a decrease in incorporation of radioactivity into the β chain of Hb A in β thalassemic reticulocytes. Similar studies were subsequently repeated in a number of different laboratories and the results of these studies all indicated a marked decrease of β-chain syn-

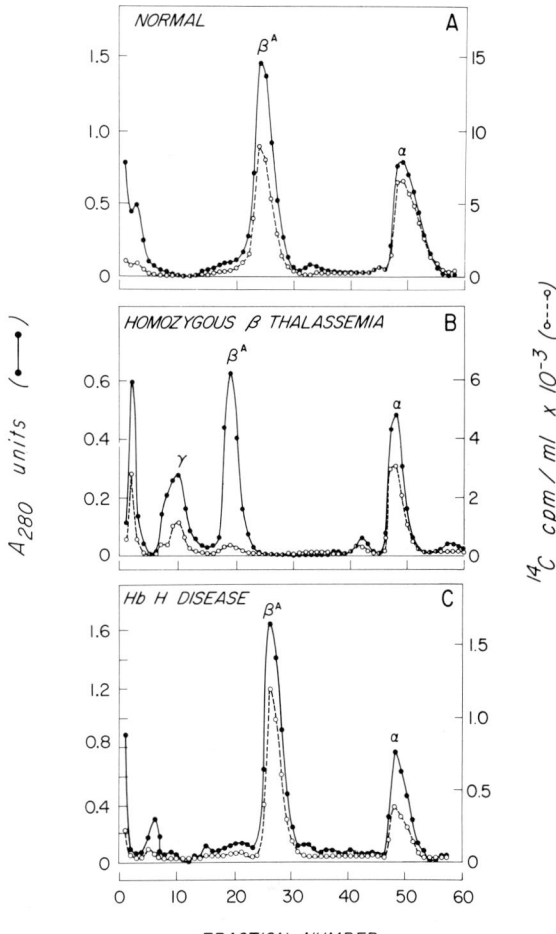

Figure 8–1. Globin synthesis in reticulocytes of patients with nonthalassemic hemolytic anemia, homozygous β+ thalassemia, and Hb H disease. Peripheral blood was incubated with ^{14}C-leucine; globin was then prepared from the red cells and fractionated by carboxymethylcellulose column chromatography. ●–● represents optical density of globin chains. The patient with homozygous β+ thalassemia was transfusion dependent, and therefore, the majority of the unlabeled β globin in *B* is derived from transfused red blood cells. ○---○ represents radioactivity incorporated into newly synthesized globin chains.

thesis relative to α-chain synthesis in β thalassemia.[11-15]

In the usual heterozygotes for β thalassemia, approximately half as much radioactivity is incorporated into β chains as into α chains, but in blacks with β-thalassemia trait, the β/α ratio can be virtually normal.[16-19] In homozygotes for β thalassemia, there is either total absence of β-chain radioactivity (β0 thalassemia) or a marked decrease in β-chain radioactivity (β+ thalassemia) with β/α ratios of 0.1 to 0.3 (Fig. 8–1*B*).

It should be pointed out that the technique

for analysis of globin-chain biosynthesis does not measure absolute rates of α- and β-chain synthesis but expresses only a ratio of one to the other. An attempt has been made to express the data in terms of absolute rates,[20] and the findings are consistent with a normal rate of α-chain synthesis in β thalassemia; therefore, the low β/α ratio is due to decreased β-chain synthesis rather than to increased α-chain synthesis.

The same techniques for the *in vitro* study of globin-chain synthesis were applied to the analysis of α thalassemia.[7, 15, 21–22] In severe homozygous α thalassemia (hydrops fetalis with Hb Bart's), there is a total absence of α-chain synthesis.[23] In Hb H disease, a less severe α-thalassemia syndrome, the globin synthesis profile reveals decreased incorporation of radioactivity into α chains compared with β chains (Fig. 8–1C), with an α/β ratio of 0.3 to 0.6.[15, 21, 22] When globin-chain synthesis is studied in α-thalassemia heterozygotes, a less striking imbalance in globin-chain synthesis is observed in comparison with the β-thalassemia heterozygotes. In the phenotypically obvious form of heterozygous α thalassemia (α thalassemia 1 trait), the α/β ratio is 0.70 to 0.80,[15, 22] whereas in the mild form of heterozygous α thalassemia (the "silent carrier" state or α thalassemia 2 trait), it is 0.80 to 0.95.[22] In American blacks, α thalassemia does not demonstrate as marked or as consistent an imbalance in globin-chain synthesis.[24]

The range of β/α ratios obtained in a large series of patients with various α- and β-thalassemia syndromes is shown in Figure 8–2.

Bone Marrow

Homozygous β Thalassemia. When globin-chain synthesis was studied in the marrow of patients with β thalassemia, interesting observations were made. In homozygous β thalassemia, the β/α synthetic ratio was still abnormal, but the value was closer to normal than in the peripheral blood of the same patient.[16, 25] Although this observation was confirmed in a number of different studies,[26–28a] other studies did not demonstrate as striking or as consistent a difference between marrow and peripheral blood globin synthesis in β thalassemia.[29, 30] The discrepancies among the various studies and the general phenomenon of differences in globin-chain synthesis between marrow and peripheral blood in homozygous β thalassemia can be best explained by a number of variables. These include (1) differences in the erythroid cell populations between marrow and peripheral blood due to selective survival of Hb F–containing cells (see Pathophysiology of β Thalassemia in Chapter 9); the process of cell selection, by itself, would be expected to especially influence the γ/α ratio[28a] but not necessarily the β/α ratio if the β-thalassemic defect is quantitatively similar at all stages of eryth-

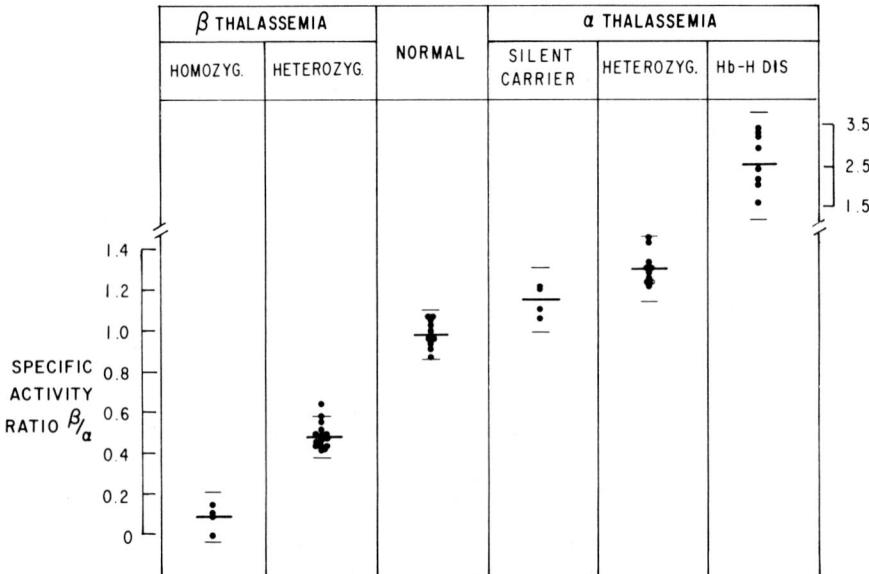

Figure 8–2. Range of values obtained for the ratio of β- to α-chain synthesis in nonthalassemic reticulocytes and reticulocytes of patients with various α- and β-thalassemia syndromes. (From Nathan, D. G.: N. Engl. J. Med. *286*:586, 1972.)

roid maturation; (2) variable admixture of peripheral blood with bone marrow; and (3) probably most important, variable degrees of proteolysis of excess newly synthesized α chains (see discussion that follows) that can be influenced by the time of isotopic labeling as well as by the erythroid cell composition of the marrow (that is, the average degree of maturity of the precursors), which, in turn, is influenced by the variable degree of marrow suppression caused by the level of blood transfusion in different patients.

In one study,[27] globin-chain synthesis was studied in early- and late-nucleated erythroid precursor cells that were fractionated from bone marrow of patients with homozygous β⁺ thalassemia and allowed to differentiate for 24 to 48 hours in culture in the presence of erythropoietin. Although globin-chain imbalance was less marked in the purified precursor cells than in total unfractionated marrow (presumably owing to contamination by peripheral blood and marrow reticulocytes), nevertheless, markedly decreased β globin–chain synthesis compared to α globin–chain synthesis was observed in early erythroid precursor cells and during their maturation in culture. These results indicated that imbalanced globin-chain synthesis occurs at all stages of erythroid cell maturation in homozygous β⁺ thalassemia.[27]

Heterozygous β Thalassemia. In heterozygous β thalassemia, an even more interesting and controversial observation was made by Schwartz.[31] In the marrow of such persons, he found that the β/α synthetic ratio was very close to 1.0. This observation was then confirmed in a number of different laboratories.[26, 29, 30, 32, 33] The findings were initially difficult to interpret. It was unlikely that decreased β-chain synthesis occurred only in reticulocytes and not in marrow, because more than 90 per cent of globin-chain synthesis is known to occur in the marrow, and if decreased β-chain synthesis occurred only at the reticulocyte stage, the β-thalassemic heterozygotes should not be anemic and their red cells should not be hypochromic and microcytic. An explanation that was proposed for hypochromia despite relatively equal amounts of α- and β-chain synthesis was that α-chain synthesis as well as β-chain synthesis could be decreased in the marrow cells of patients with heterozygous β thalassemia, whereas in the reticulocytes, the imbalance became manifest as α-chain synthesis returned to normal.[34] There was, however, no experimental evidence to support this type of presumed feedback inhibition of synthesis of the nonaffected globin chain in thalassemia.

Studies by Clegg and Weatherall on globin synthesis in heterozygous β-thalassemia marrow indicated, however, that despite the β/α synthetic ratio of nearly 1.0, there was indeed imbalance between β and α globin-chain synthesis in marrow, evidenced by the finding of a large pool of free α globin chains in such marrow cells,[33] a phenomenon also later observed by Gill and Schwartz.[35] Two mechanisms were postulated for the findings of β/α synthetic ratios close to 1.0: first, in marrow, nonglobin peptides may co-chromatograph with the β chain, thereby falsely increasing the radioactivity in the β-chain region; second, evidence was provided that, *in vitro*, α chains are more unstable in marrow compared with those in peripheral blood and may undergo proteolysis in time, thereby falsely lowering the radioactivity found in the α-chain peak.[33]

Chalevelakis and associates[36, 37] were able to show the presence of a minor nonglobin (? marrow granulocyte) protein contaminating the β-chain peak on carboxymethyl-cellulose columns. More importantly, however, these authors demonstrated clearly, in short pulse-labeling experiments, that the β/α synthetic ratio in heterozygous β-thalassemic marrow changed with time, being abnormal (0.5) after short incubations and nearing unity after longer periods of incubation. Increased α-chain turnover was therefore implicated as the primary cause of the phenomenon. Studies by Wood and Stamatoyannopoulos[38] failed to demonstrate a contaminating nonglobin peptide, but experiments using purified erythroid precursor cells did demonstrate increased free pools of α chains even in the most immature erythroid precursor cells in heterozygous β-thalassemia marrow. These studies provided convincing indirect evidence that turnover (proteolysis) of α chains is the most likely explanation for the unexpected finding of a β/α synthetic ratio of 1.0 in heterozygous β-thalassemic marrow.

A number of subsequent studies have clearly resolved the issue and indicate that proteolysis of excess free α chains does occur in thalassemic erythroid cells and that this proteolytic activity is more active in nucleated erythroid precursor cells than in reticulocytes.[39–42] The process appears to be relatively selective for free α chains and not free β chains, because in some studies, globin-chain synthesis in α-thalassemic marrow cells remained unbalanced without evidence of excessive β-chain turnover.[43, 44] On the other hand, studies in Hb H disease, a doubly heterozygous form of α thalassemia, indicate that proteolysis of excess free β chains occurs in this condition as well,[45] and there are reports of balanced or more nearly balanced bone marrow globin-chain synthesis in heterozygous α thalassemia[46] and Hb H disease.[47,48]

There have been reports of cases of heterozygous β thalassemia of unusual severity in which the marrow β/α synthetic ratio ranges between 0.7 and 0.8 but the peripheral blood ratio remains at the usual level of 0.5.[49,50] It has been proposed that such cases may be associated with diminished or defective proteolysis of excess free α chains.[51]

Summary and Conclusions

Studies of globin synthesis in intact erythroid cells of individuals with α and β thalassemia indicate that there exists in these syndromes imbalance of globin-chain synthesis, with absent or decreased synthesis of β globin chains in β thalassemia and absent or decreased synthesis of α globin chains in α thalassemia. Analysis of globin-chain biosynthesis in marrow cells, in addition, has demonstrated the presence and importance of proteolysis as a mechanism that can modulate the degree of globin-chain imbalance in thalassemic erythroid cells. These studies, however, do not shed any light on the possible molecular mechanisms for the observed imbalance in globin-chain synthesis. A number of other approaches have been used to address this question, and they will be discussed in the following sections.

EARLY MOLECULAR BIOLOGY STUDIES

The details of the normal process of protein and hemoglobin biosynthesis have been reviewed in Chapter 7 (see Fig. 7–1). It is easy to see that in the complex process of protein synthesis, a number of regulatory events could occur that would affect the rate of synthesis of a given protein and result in the presence of decreased amounts of an otherwise structurally normal protein in the cells. Various defects in the process of protein synthesis have been searched for to explain the decreased synthesis of structurally normal globin chains that occurs in thalassemia. Before techniques became available to isolate and directly study the function and amount of globin messenger RNA (mRNA) in thalassemic erythroid cells, a number of studies were performed to analyze in detail the subcellular processes involved in globin-chain assembly in thalassemia. These studies focused on various aspects of the cellular translational apparatus and thereby provided important, although indirect, information concerning globin mRNA translation in thalassemia.

Ribosome Function

The earliest studies on molecular mechanisms in thalassemia involved studies by Marks and coworkers of ribosome function in β-thalassemic reticulocytes compared with that of nonthalassemic reticulocytes.[52-56] These studies revealed that ribosome number[52] and function were similar in β-thalassemic reticulocytes and nonthalassemic reticulocytes. Although specific radioactivity of ribosomes of β-thalassemic reticulocytes incubated with a radioactive amino acid was reduced,[52,53] this reduction could be accounted for by the decreased synthesis of Hb A (and presumably β chains). The radioactive profile of polysomes,[52] the ability to synthesize fetal hemoglobin (Hb F),[52] and the capacity of ribosomes to synthesize polyphenylalanine in response to the artificial mRNA poly(U) were all normal in β-thalassemic ribosomes compared with nonthalassemic ribosomes.[55] The addition of reticulocyte supernatant fraction from nonthalassemic humans or rabbits to β-thalassemic ribosomes in a cell-free system did not stimulate protein synthesis by the thalassemic ribosomes, and thalassemic supernatant fraction did not depress protein synthesis by normal ribosomes.[55] The number of free ribosomal 60S and 40S subunits was found to be increased by 50 per cent in thalassemic reticulocytes compared with normal cells, but the addition of either these thalassemic or other normal ribosomal subunits to a nonthalassemic cell-free system resulted in equal stimulation of protein synthesis, indicating that the ribosomal subunits themselves were not functionally abnormal.[56]

In summary, these studies revealed no significant differences between β-thalassemic and nonthalassemic ribosomes, except for the decreased amount of Hb A and β chains synthesized by the former. The results of these experiments led to the conclusion that the defect in β thalassemia must reside in the globin mRNA or the mRNA ribosome complex.[55]

Rate of Globin-Chain Assembly

One of the early hypotheses for the possible molecular defect in thalassemia postulated that the globin mRNA might contain a base substitution in a codon that results in it coding, not for a different amino acid, but for a different transfer RNA (tRNA) for the normal amino acid. If the specific tRNA were in short supply in the cell, an overall slowing of the rate of synthesis of the affected chain would result. This was the so-called modulation hypothesis to explain thalassemia.[57, 58] There exist, in fact, experimental models for translational control ("modulation") of protein synthesis by tRNA.[59, 60]

This hypothesis was tested by studying the rate of assembly of the β chain in β thalassemia. The technique, originally devised by Dintzis, consists of pulse labeling reticulocytes with a radioactive amino acid for different short periods of time and then examining the appearance of the label in specific peptides at various positions on the globin chain. If there were a slowdown of β-chain synthesis in β thalassemia due to an abnormal codon (or other abnormality), there should be a different pattern or rate of peptide labeling when compared with the pattern obtained from nonthalassemic reticulocytes.

The experiment was first done by Clegg and colleagues,[61] using reticulocytes of Asian patients with β thalassemia. The results indicated normal assembly time of the β chain that was synthesized by these β-thalassemic patients, with no evidence of a slower rate of β-chain mRNA translation compared with that of nonthalassemic controls.

Rieder performed similar studies using peripheral blood from five different patients of Italian ancestry and one black patient with homozygous β thalassemia.[62] Results similar to the previous study were obtained, namely no evidence of abnormally slow assembly time of β globin chains in β thalassemia. In addition, these studies, which utilized radioactive valine as the labeled precursor, indicated that the normal rate of β-chain translation in β thalassemia applied to the earliest measurable amino acid in the β globin chain.

The rate of assembly of globin chains in thalassemia has been also studied in a different manner by the technique of analyzing the distribution of nascent α and β globin chains on polysomes of normal and thalassemic reticulocytes. The number of ribosomes attached to a strand of mRNA at a given time will depend on a number of factors: the rate of initiation, the rate of translation, and the rate of chain termination and release. In normal reticulocytes in man[63, 64] as well as in rabbits,[65] the nascent α and β globin chains are heterogeneously distributed on the polysomes. The larger, more rapidly sedimenting polysomes carry predominantly β chains, whereas the smaller, more slowly sedimenting polysomes carry predominantly α chains. It is generally agreed that the rates of translation (and of termination) of the α and β chains are similar[66]; therefore, the predominance of β chains on larger polysomes is taken to reflect a normally faster rate of initiation of β chains than α chains.[66, 67]

If there were a slowing of the rate of translation (or of initiation or termination) in thalassemia, it should be reflected in the profile of nascent globin chains on thalassemic polysomes. The studies performed with thalassemic cells revealed the same pattern as in nonthalassemic cells: The nascent β chains in β thalassemia are preferentially associated with the same-sized polysomes as in nonthalassemic cells.[63, 68] If the rate of translation of β chains in β thalassemia were abnormally slow (while initiation was normal), the nascent β chains would be associated with larger polysomes than normal. In α thalassemia (Hb H disease), similar studies were performed and also revealed a normal distribution of nascent chains, with α chains predominating on smaller polysomes,[68] indicating normal rates of globin-chain translation and initiation in α thalassemia as well as in β thalassemia.

Initiation of Globin-Chain Synthesis

As described earlier, analysis of the distribution of nascent globin chains on polysomes can provide indirect information about the rate of initiation of α and β globin–chain synthesis, and studies with thalassemic cells suggested normal rates of initiation of the affected globin chain. More direct studies of initiation by Anderson and coworkers, utilizing a totally fractionated cell-free protein synthesizing system,[69-78] also failed to reveal a defect of chain initiation in thalassemia. The initial studies performed involved the incubation of β-thalassemic ribosomes in the cell-free system to study the effect of added normal initiation factors on the translation of endogenous mRNA by the thalassemic ribosomes.[72] These experiments showed that added initiation factors (rabbit or human) did increase total protein synthetic activity by the β-thalassemic ribosomes in the cell-free system, but analysis of the products synthesized revealed that α chains were still synthesized in a great excess over β chains.[72] The decreased β-chain synthesis in β thalassemia therefore did not appear to be associated with a deficiency of initiation factors.

The ability of β-thalassemic ribosomes to initiate and translate exogenously added globin mRNA was also tested in this cell-free system.[73] Thalassemic and nonthalassemic ribosomes were equally effective in translating rabbit globin mRNA, and the relative amounts of rabbit α and β chains synthesized were similar with both types of ribosomes.[73]

In a third set of studies, these workers analyzed the fine details of the initiation process in β thalassemia: the nature of the initial β globin dipeptide synthesized and the function of specific initiator tRNA.[74] The initial dipeptides synthesized in the fractionated cell-free system in the presence of either thalassemic or normal human globin mRNA were found to be identical in both cases: methionine-valine for the α and β chains, and methionine-glycine for the γ chain.[74] In addition, the specific initiator tRNA (methionyl tRNA$_F$) donated the methionine for this initial dipeptide in both the normal and β-thalassemic β chains synthesized in the cell-free system.[74]

All these studies indicated that when some β chain is synthesized in β thalassemia, it is initiated and translated normally. It was concluded that the deficient synthesis of β chains in β$^+$ thalassemia must therefore be due to less frequent initiation of β chains. This could be caused by quantitative deficiency of β-chain mRNA or by a β-chain mRNA that is abnormal in its ability to bind to the ribosome in the process immediately preceding the specific biochemical events of chain initiation.

Chain Termination

In those cases of thalassemia in which some of the affected globin chain is synthesized, no evidence was found for an abnormality of globin-chain termination. If such an abnormality existed, the studies of Clegg and associates[61] and Rieder[62] on the rate of globin-chain assembly in thalassemia would have revealed a slow rate of appearance of completed β chains in lysates and in the postribosomal supernatant fraction of β-thalassemic reticulocytes. Such was not the case.

In those cases of thalassemia in which there is absence of completed globin chains, β^0 thalassemia, one possible explanation could be premature chain termination due to a nonsense mutation of the mRNA: a base substitution changing a normal codon to a chain-termination codon. If this were the case, one might expect to find incomplete fragments of the affected globin chain.[75] One experimental system was devised that suggested that this hypothesis could be tested: In this model system, incomplete globin chains that were initiated at their normal N terminus but prematurely terminated owing to the addition of the antibiotic puromycin were detectable and not immediately degraded in rabbit reticulocytes.[75]

A search for incomplete fragments of β globin chains was performed in reticulocytes of β^0- thalassemic patients from the Ferrara region of Italy, but no such fragments could be identified.[76]

In the severe form of homozygous α thalassemia (hydrops fetalis with Hb Bart's), in which there is total absence of completed α chains, a search was made for N-terminal peptides of α globin chains longer than 11 amino acid residues.[23] None were found, indicating that if a nonsense mutation were present in the α-chain mRNA, it would have to be located within the first 33 nucleotide residues following the initiation codon.[23]

In summary then, no evidence was found in these early studies to support the hypothesis of abnormal chain termination in the thalassemia syndromes. However, as will be discussed in following sections, later structural studies of β globin mRNA and β globin genes in β^0 thalassemia did in fact demonstrate the presence of nonsense mutations in a number of cases of β^0 thalassemia. Nevertheless, in contrast to the model system of Baglioni and colleagues,[75] no abnormal, incomplete β-chain peptides have yet been demonstrated in reticulocytes of such cases, presumably because they are unstable and rapidly degraded and/or because they are synthesized in very low amounts owing to instability and resulting deficiency of the abnormal β globin mRNA itself.

Summary and Conclusions

The large body of work just summarized indicated that in thalassemic erythroid cells, the cytoplasmic translational apparatus appeared to be normal in all of the various components that could be tested. The general conclusion that could be drawn from these studies was that the deficiency of globin-chain synthesis observed in various forms of thalassemia must be due to a defect in the mRNA for the affected globin chain: either a quantitative deficiency of the mRNA or a qualitative abnormality preventing its entry into normal polyribosomes. Further delineation of the molecular basis of thalassemia awaited direct studies of globin mRNA in this disorder.

FUNCTIONAL STUDIES OF THALASSEMIC GLOBIN mRNA IN CELL-FREE PROTEIN SYNTHESIZING SYSTEMS

Direct involvement of mRNA in the thalassemia defect was first demonstrated by translation of mRNA, isolated from thalassemic reticulocytes, in heterologous cell-free protein synthesizing systems capable of translating exogenously added mRNA. The technical developments that allowed these studies included the perfection of techniques for the isolation of biologically functional mRNA from cell extracts, in which it constitutes only a minor component, and the development of efficient cell-free translation systems. The first cell-free systems utilized were the fractionated rabbit reticulocyte system of Anderson and coworkers[69–71] and the Krebs mouse ascites tumor cell system.[77] The wheat germ lysate system,[78] developed somewhat later, also proved quite useful for testing the function of thalassemic globin mRNA.

Reticulocyte mRNA in Homozygous β⁺ Thalassemia

Involvement of globin mRNA in the thalassemia defect was first demonstrated directly by Nienhuis and Anderson[79] and Benz and Forget,[80] who succeeded in isolating functional globin mRNA from β-thalassemic reticulocytes and having it translated in different heterologous cell-free protein synthesizing systems. In both studies, the imbalance of human globin-chain synthesis characteristic of the intact thalassemic reticulocytes was duplicated in the cell-free system in the presence of β-thalassemic globin mRNA, which was the only human or thalassemic reticulocyte component present in the incubation mixture. In control experiments using reticulocyte mRNA from nonthalassemic patients, the cell-free systems synthesized approximately equal amounts of α and β chains. However, in the presence of β-thalassemic mRNA, much more α than β chain was synthesized (Fig. 8–3B) and the β/α synthetic ratio

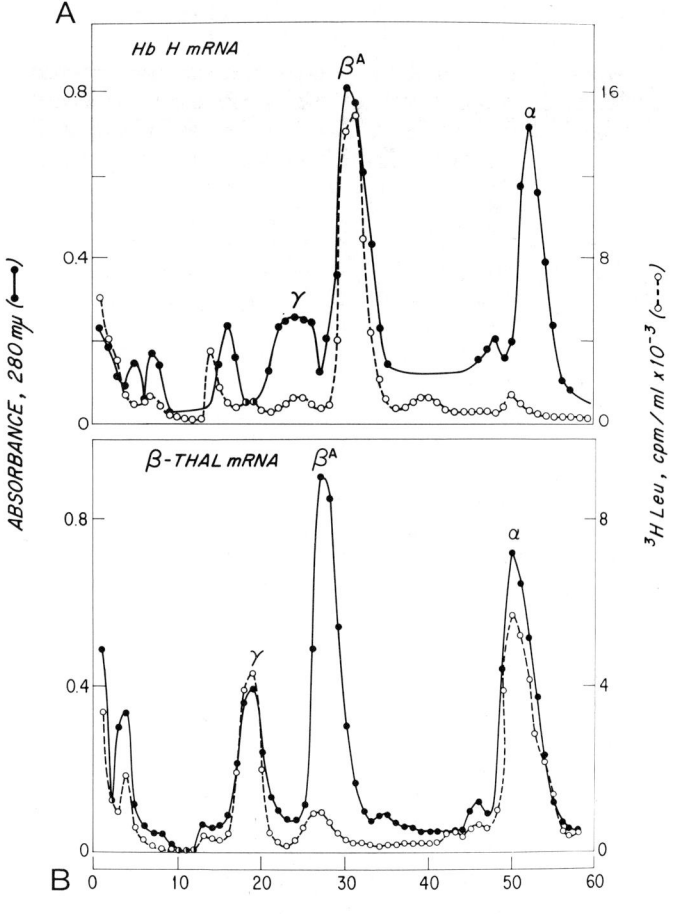

Figure 8–3. Cell-free translation of globin mRNA isolated from a patient with Hb H disease *(A)* and a patient with homozygous β⁺ thalassemia *(B)*. The cell-free protein synthesizing system was derived from Krebs II mouse ascites cells. Deficiency of α and β globin chain synthesis is evident in the respective experiments. (From Forget, B. G.: CRC Crit. Rev. Biochem. 2:311, 1974.)

obtained was similar to that of the patients' intact cells (see Fig. 8–1B).[79, 80]

These experiments conclusively demonstrated that the thalassemic imbalance of globin-chain synthesis was mediated via the cell's globin mRNA. The authors concluded that there must be either true quantitative deficiency of the mRNA for the affected chain or, at least, deficiency of functional mRNA capable of participating in protein synthesis.

These initial experiments were subsequently confirmed by a number of different investigators in many individual patients with homozygous β^+ thalassemia.[26, 30, 74, 81–84] In all cases tested, there was deficiency of functional mRNA for the β globin chain, and the degree of imbalance between α- and β-chain synthesis obtained in the cell-free system was generally similar to that observed in intact reticulocytes of the same patient.

Bone Marrow mRNA in Homozygous β^+ Thalassemia

Because the reticulocyte is an end-stage cell and the thalassemic reticulocyte is metabolically abnormal, it is conceivable (although unlikely) that the deficiency of mRNA in the thalassemic reticulocyte is a "preterminal" event and not representative of the situation in less mature erythroid cells in thalassemia. For this reason, globin mRNA isolated from thalassemic marrow was also tested in cell-free translation systems.[26, 30, 82, 84] In all cases, cell-free translation of the mRNA revealed deficiency of functional mRNA for β globin chains. All of these studies, however, used RNA from total unfractionated marrow, which necessarily contained considerable numbers of reticulocytes. Although the results are convincing and probably valid, the conclusions drawn from the marrow studies would have been more conclusive if the mRNA had been isolated from nucleated marrow cells that had been previously purified of contaminating reticulocytes.

Reticulocyte and Marrow mRNA in Heterozygous β Thalassemia

The function of reticulocyte and marrow globin mRNA was tested in heterozygous β thalassemia in order to study the role of mRNA in the phenomenon of apparently balanced globin-chain synthesis in intact marrow cells of patients with heterozygous β thalassemia.[26, 30] In summary, these studies showed that the mRNA of both reticulocytes and marrow of patients with heterozygous β thalassemia directed the synthesis of less β^A chain than α chain when translated in a cell-free system, even though the intact marrow cells demonstrated balanced globin-chain synthesis. Similar observations were made in three patients doubly heterozygous for β^0 thalassemia and Hb S.[26, 30] The authors concluded that despite the presence of balanced globin-chain synthesis in the marrow cells of these patients with heterozygous β thalassemia, there was evidence for decreased amounts of functional globin mRNA for β chains in these cells.

These studies therefore provided additional support for the conclusions drawn from later studies (see earlier discussion) that the main cause of the balanced globin-chain synthesis observed in intact marrow cells in heterozygous β thalassemia is post-translational proteolysis of excess free α globin chains.

Reticulocyte and Marrow mRNA in β^0 Thalassemia

Study of globin mRNA function in β^0 thalassemia became the focus of particular attention because of observations in β^0 thalassemic patients from Ferrara, Italy (see next section). Studies in these patients were interpreted as showing the presence of substantial amounts of β-chain mRNA that was not translated because of a proposed lack of a specific factor required for its translation or because of the presence of a specific inhibitor of β mRNA translation. Globin mRNA from patients with a number of β^0 thalassemia syndromes (other than Ferrara thalassemia) was studied in various cell-free systems.[26, 30, 81–88] In all cases, there was undetectable cell-free synthesis of β^A globin chains despite use of conditions that favored translation of normal β globin mRNA in the various cell-free systems that were used. These results indicated that in non-Ferrara–type β^0 thalassemia, there was absence of functional mRNA for β globin chains and no evidence for a deficiency or an inhibitor of a factor specifically required for β globin mRNA translation.

Ferrara-Type β^0 Thalassemia

The β^0 thalassemia found in the Ferrara region of northern Italy was once thought to constitute a possible exception to the rule of deficiency of functional β globin mRNA in $β^0$ thalassemia. Intact reticulocytes from these patients synthesize no β chains.[11, 89] However, Conconi and associates[89–91] reported that ribosomes isolated from reticulocytes of patients with homozygous Ferrara $β^0$ thalassemia synthesized $β^A$ globin chains when added to an unusual reconstituted human reticulocyte cell-free system that contained normal or Hb SS reticulocyte supernatant. The phenomenon was abolished by pretreatment of the supernatant by trypsin but not by ribonuclease,[90] suggesting that the permissive factor was protein in nature rather than RNA. Reticulocyte mRNA from Ferrara $β^0$-thalassemic patients was also reported to direct the synthesis of human $β^A$ globin chains in a rabbit reticulocyte cell–free system.[92] The results were interpreted as indicating that in Ferrara thalassemia, substantial amounts of β globin mRNA were present but not translated because of the absence or nonfunction of a specific protein factor required for the translation of β globin mRNA or because of the presence of a specific inhibitor of β globin mRNA translation.

An even more surprising observation was subsequently made by Conconi and colleagues.[90, 93] When patients with Ferrara thalassemia were transfused, it was possible to detect small amounts of β-chain synthesis in their circulating red blood cells approximately 10 to 15 days after the transfusion.

These *in vitro* and *in vivo* observations are difficult to reconcile with the recent conclusive evidence that the Ferrara patients have a nonsense mutation at codon 39.[94] This nonsense mutation is the most common cause of $β^0$ thalassemia in Mediterranean individuals; mRNA-cDNA hybridization assays and gene mapping studies in such $β^0$-thalassemic patients give results similar to those obtained in Ferrara patients[95] (discussed in detail below). It is possible, although unsubstantiated, that the experimental observations described above could have resulted from the action of amber suppressor tRNA, present in reticulocytes,[96] which permitted some full-length translation of the nonsense 39 β mRNA by inserting an amino acid residue at the position of the nonsense termination codon.

Globin mRNA in α Thalassemia

Reticulocyte mRNA from patients with the α-thalassemia syndrome of Hb H disease has also been translated in various cell-free systems,[48, 82, 83, 97, 98] and similar results were obtained in the different studies. The Hb H disease mRNA directed the synthesis of a great excess of β chains over α chains (see Fig. 8–3A), and the imbalance of α- to β-chain synthesis observed in the cell-free systems was much greater than in the intact cells of the same patient (see Fig. 8–1C). This discrepancy was observed both in the Krebs ascites cell and in the wheat germ cell-free systems and indicated that the deficiency of functional α globin mRNA in Hb H disease might be greater than suggested by the degree of imbalance of globin-chain synthesis observed in intact cells. This exaggerated deficiency of α globin mRNA was later confirmed by mRNA-cDNA hybridization studies (see next section). These findings suggest the presence in Hb H disease reticulocytes of a post-translational mechanism—probably proteolysis of nascent β chains—capable of reducing the imbalance of globin-chain accumulation when β globin mRNA is present in a vast excess over α globin mRNA. Kinetic studies of globin-chain synthesis in Hb H disease have in fact demonstrated rapid turnover of newly synthesized excess β globin chains in this condition.[45]

In one study,[48] globin mRNA from bone marrow cells of patients with Hb H disease was also analyzed by cell-free translation. Translation of the bone marrow globin mRNA resulted in roughly the same degree of imbalance of globin-chain synthesis as obtained with reticulocyte globin mRNA from the same patients.[48]

Summary and Conclusions

With the exception of the studies of Ferrara-type $β^0$ thalassemia described above, cell-free translation of thalassemic globin mRNA in all cases tested resulted in the same type of imbalance of globin-chain synthesis as was observed in intact thalassemic cells. These studies provided direct evidence for a deficiency of functional mRNA for α or β globin chain in α and β thalassemia, respectively. The results, however, could be interpreted only as demonstrating deficiency of biological activity but not necessarily true quantitative deficiency, in absolute chemical terms, of the affected globin mRNA species. The studies, therefore, still left open the possibility that there existed in thalassemia substantial amounts of functionally abnormal globin mRNA that was unable to function normally in protein synthesis both in the intact thalassemic cells and in heterologous cell-free systems.

QUANTITATIVE STUDIES OF GLOBIN mRNA AND GENE DNA IN THALASSEMIA BY MOLECULAR HYBRIDIZATION AND OTHER ASSAYS

The next technical advance that allowed substantial progress in thalassemia research was the development of the capacity to assay the relative amounts of α- and β-chain mRNA in thalassemic cells by a direct chemical quantitative assay that did not rely on the ability of the mRNA to function in a cell-free system. Such an assay was essential to definitively settle the issue of whether or not there existed in thalassemia substantial amounts of globin mRNA (for α or β chains) incapable of functioning normally in protein synthesis, either because of a structural abnormality or because of some other abnormality in the cells' protein synthesis "machinery."

Principles of the Hybridization Assay

The technique used for identification and/or quantitation of a specific mRNA present in a mixture of RNAs is molecular hybridization of the RNA mixture with a labeled DNA probe complementary to the specific mRNA in question. Application of this technique to the study of globin mRNA was initially limited by the lack of availability of a suitable DNA probe. However, in the early 1970's, a number of important research contributions made possible the acquisition of separate radioactive DNA probes specific for α and β globin mRNA. The RNA-dependent DNA polymerase of avian myeloblastosis (also referred to as reverse transcriptase and as AMV DNA polymerase) was shown to be capable of synthesizing *in vitro* a radioactive DNA copy (cDNA) of globin mRNA.[99–101] The reaction requires oligo(dT), which acts as a primer and starting point for the cDNA synthesis by binding to the poly(A) sequence situated at the 3' terminus of the globin mRNA. The radioactive cDNA that is synthesized will hybridize almost completely to purified globin mRNA.[99–101]

The cDNA made from total reticulocyte mRNA necessarily consisted of a mixture of α and β chain–specific sequences, but it soon became possible to obtain purified rabbit globin mRNA that was 80 to 90 per cent enriched in α or β chain–specific mRNA. The α-chain mRNA was obtained from a ribonucleoprotein particle found in the postribosomal supernatant fraction of rabbit reticulocytes[102]—a serendipitous observation; the β-chain mRNA was obtained from the largest polysomes of O-methylthreonine–treated reticulocytes.[103] O-methylthreonine is an isoleucine analogue. The rabbit α and β chains contain isoleucine in different positions: In the β chain, isoleucine is first found only at position 112 of the sequence, whereas in the α chain, isoleucine is first encountered at position 10. In the presence of O-methylthreonine, polysomes bearing α and β mRNA will be "blocked" at the site of the first isoleucine codon on the mRNA. In the case of β mRNA, the polysomes will be large because many other ribosomes will have started to translate the mRNA in the time that it takes the first ribosome to reach position 112; on the other hand, the α-chain polysomes will be blocked early in the translation process and will accumulate as small polysomes. This technique also served as a means to obtain relatively purified α-chain mRNA.[103] In the O-methylthreonine procedure, there is an exaggeration of the normal asymmetrical distribution of α and β chain–synthesizing polysomes, with β chains on larger, more rapidly sedimenting polysomes and the α chains on smaller, more slowly sedimenting polysomes.[63–65]

The purified α and β mRNAs were efficient substrates for AMV DNA polymerase, and the resulting cDNAs were found to be specific for α and β chain–specific sequences, as evidenced by cross-hybridization experiments performed between the two types of mRNAs and cDNAs[104–106] (Fig. 8–4). Sufficient homology exists between human and rabbit globin-chain amino acid (and mRNA) sequences that it permitted the use of this type of hybridization assay to detect (and quantitate), with rabbit α and β globin cDNA probes, the relative amounts of human α- and β-chain mRNA sequences in human reticulocyte RNA.[104, 105] An outline of the general procedure is shown in Figure 8–5. The amount of hybridization is detected by digesting the reaction mixture at the end of the hybridization period with the S_1 nuclease of *Aspergillus oryzae* (or another similar enzyme), which specifically degrades single-stranded nucleic acids and leaves intact double-stranded hybrids (Fig. 8–5B). Therefore, even if there is not perfect homology between RNA and cDNA (as in human/rabbit cross-hybridization experiments), the portions of the hybrid complex in which there is good homology will be protected from nuclease digestion, and these nondegraded hybrid complexes will be precipitated by 10 per cent trichloroacetic acid (TCA) and retained on Millipore filters. In such cases, however, 100

Figure 8–4. Model for molecular hybridization assay to quantitate relative amounts of α and β globin mRNA in an RNA sample. Rabbit globin mRNAs were enriched for α- or β-specific sequences, as described in the text, and then radioactive DNA copies (cDNAs) were synthesized from these same mRNAs by means of viral reverse transcriptase. A constant amount of radioactive cDNA was hybridized to progressively increasing amounts of RNA in order to obtain curves showing the range of RNA input required to reach maximum hybridization or full protection of the probe to digestion by single strand-specific S1 nuclease. The hybridization curves reveal marked deficiency of β globin mRNA sequences in the α mRNA preparation *(A)* and marked deficiency of α globin mRNA sequences in the β mRNA preparation *(B)*. (From Housman, D., et al.: Proc. Natl. Acad. Sci. USA 69:1574, 1972.)

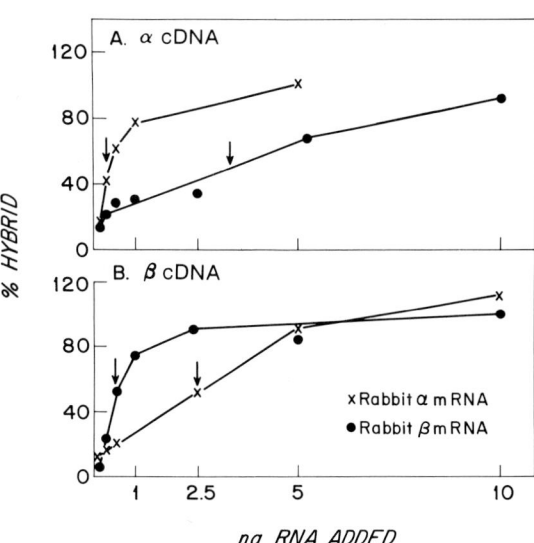

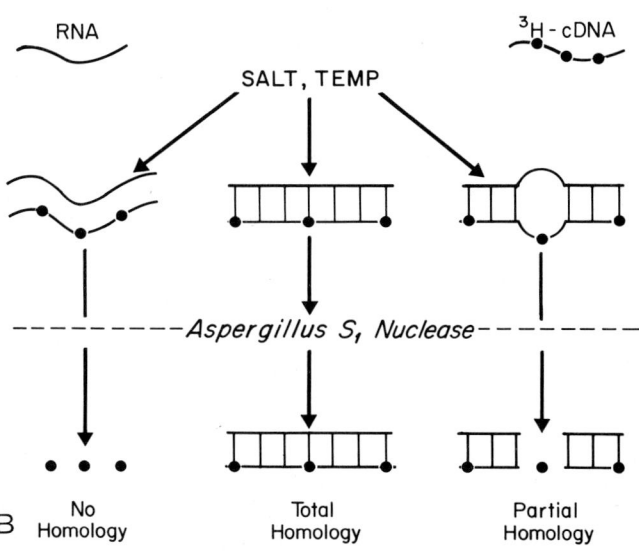

Figure 8–5. Outline of the molecular hybridization procedure initially used to quantitate the ratio of α to β globin mRNA in human reticulocyte RNA. *A,* Partially purified rabbit α and β globin mRNAs, prepared as indicated (see text), were copied into radioactive cDNAs by means of the RNA-dependent DNA polymerase (reverse transcriptase) of avian myeloblastosis virus (AMV). *B,* Two types of hybridization are shown: that in which there is perfect homology beween mRNA and cDNA *(center)*, as in the case of rabbit mRNA/rabbit cDNA hybrids, and that in which there is imperfect homology *(right)*, as in the case of human mRNA/rabbit cDNA hybrids. In the latter case, when maximum hybridization is achieved, less than 100 per cent of the probe is protected after digestion with the single strand-specific S1 nuclease of *Aspergillus oryzae*. (From Forget, B. G.: CRC Crit. Rev. Biochem. 2:311, 1974.)

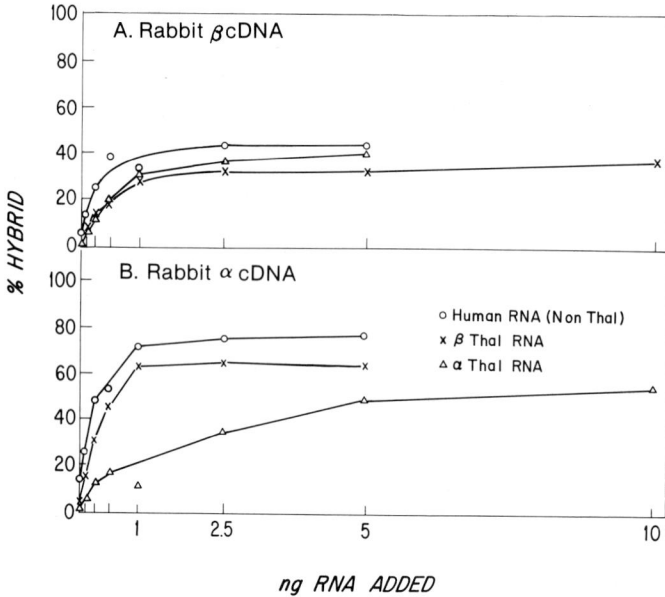

Figure 8-6. Hybridization of human globin mRNAs to rabbit α and β cDNA probes. Hybridization to rabbit α cDNA *(B)* clearly reveals deficiency of α globin mRNA in the case of the mRNA from a patient with α thalassemia (Hb H disease). However, using the rabbit β cDNA probe *(A)*, it is difficult to demonstrate deficiency of β globin mRNA in the RNA from a patient with β thalassemia (homozygous β+ thalassemia). This is probably because of the lower amount of homology between the mRNA and cDNA and also hybridization of γ globin mRNA to the rabbit β cDNA probe under the nonstringent conditions required for the cross-species hybridization. (Modified from Housman, D., et al.: Proc. Natl. Acad. Sci. USA 69:1574, 1972.)

per cent of the counts of the radioactive cDNA probe is never recovered. The nonhomologous (nonhybridized) regions of the cDNA are degraded by the nuclease and therefore remain soluble in the presence of TCA and pass through the filters. The maximum amount or percentage of the probe recovered is proportional to the degree of homology between mRNA and cDNA. When normal (nonthalassemic) human globin mRNA is hybridized to the rabbit α and β globin cDNA probes (Fig. 8-6), it can be seen that there is more homology between human and rabbit α globin mRNA sequences than between the β globin mRNA sequences.

After the initial studies using rabbit α and β globin cDNAs to quantitate human globin mRNAs, various approaches were devised to obtain relatively pure preparations of human α, β, and γ globin cDNAs, which could then be used in more specific hybridization assays. For example, the rabbit β globin cDNA could not be used to differentiate easily between human β and γ globin mRNA sequences; specific cDNAs and highly stringent hybridization conditions are required for such a differentiation. The methods used to obtain relatively pure, chain-specific human globin mRNAs and cDNAs included fractionation of α and β globin mRNAs by acrylamide gel electrophoresis in the presence of the denaturing agent formamide[107]; use of mRNAs from individuals with Hb H disease with marked deficiency of α mRNA as a source of relatively pure β mRNA[104]; and use of differential hybridization and differential elution from hydroxyapatite resin to separate hybridized from nonhybridized cDNAs.[108, 109]

Such hybridization assays were initially used to quantitate the relative amounts of α and β globin mRNA in thalassemic erythroid cells. The assays were then applied to the analysis of globin gene copy number and the search for gene deletions in DNA-cDNA hybridization experiments using total cellular DNA from normal and thalassemic individuals.

Molecular Hybridization Studies of Globin mRNA in Homozygous β+ Thalassemia

Reticulocyte RNA. The first direct demonstration of quantitative deficiency of β globin mRNA in β+ thalassemia was accomplished in 1973 by Housman and coworkers[104] and Kacian and colleagues[105] with the use of RNA-cDNA hybridization assays. These workers demonstrated that reticulocyte RNA from patients with β+ thalassemia, when compared with nonthalassemic reticulocyte RNA, contained substantially less globin mRNA that hybridized to rabbit β globin cDNA than to rabbit α globin cDNA. These initial assays were performed, necessarily, under nonstringent conditions to allow cross-species hybridization; such assays probably also detected γ globin mRNA present in the β+-thalassemic reticulocyte RNA that hybridized to the rabbit β globin cDNA. Consequently, the quantitative results of α to β globin mRNA obtained in these initial hybridization assays did not always correlate closely with the ratio expected on the basis of cell-free translation of the mRNA. In general, although there was a clear deficiency of non-α globin mRNA relative to α globin mRNA, the amount of β globin mRNA was overestimated.

An improvement in the hybridization assay consisted of using a human rather than a rabbit β globin cDNA probe, thus permitting more stringent hybridization conditions to differentiate β from γ globin mRNA. The initial source of human β globin cDNA was the cDNA synthesized from total reticulocyte mRNA isolated from an individual with Hb H disease, which was shown to contain only 10 to 15 per cent as much α globin mRNA as β globin mRNA when hybridized to the rabbit globin cDNA probes.[104] Use of this probe demonstrated more clearly a marked deficiency of β globin mRNA in β+ thalassemia[104] (Fig. 8–7). The β/α mRNA levels obtained by molecular hybridization were approximately 0.1 and corresponded well with the ratio of β to α globin–chain synthesis obtained in intact reticulocytes, or by mRNA-directed cell-free translation in the same individual. Human β globin cDNA was also later prepared by other methods such as differential hybridization[108, 109] and physical separation of β from α globin mRNAs by gel electrophoresis in denaturing conditions[107] and gave results similar to those described earlier. Using these more specific assays, the ratio of β to α globin mRNA was subsequently assayed in a large number of patients with β+ thalassemia. In general, the studies all revealed quantitative deficiency of β chain–specific mRNA sequences that corresponded well with the degree of deficient β-chain synthesis observed in the individual patients' reticulocytes.[82, 110–113]

These early results showing quantitative deficiency of β globin mRNA in reticulocyte RNA of β+ thalassemic patients were interpreted as being consistent with the conclusion that either of two types of general processes could be responsible for the mRNA deficiency: (1) a transcriptional defect in which the mRNA is initially synthesized in reduced amounts at the time of globin gene transcription in the nucleus of the developing erythroid cell, or (2) a post-transcriptional defect in which the mRNA is initially synthesized in normal amounts in the nucleus but the deficiency of cytoplasmic mRNA in reticulocytes (and in marrow cells) results from a defect in processing, transport, or stability of the nascent mRNA in either the nucleus or the cytoplasm of the developing erythroid cells. Studies of nucleated erythroid precursor cells from β+ thalassemic bone marrow were required to help distinguish between the two possibilities.

RNA of Bone Marrow Erythroid Precursor Cells. Nienhuis and coworkers[111] reported the first studies of molecular hybridization analysis of the globin mRNA content in erythroid cells of β+-thalassemic bone marrow. Using labeled α and β globin cDNAs, they studied the relative amounts of α to β globin mRNA in nuclear RNA versus cytoplasmic RNA of three patients with β+ thalassemia. In all three patients, the nuclear RNA contained higher levels of β globin mRNA (relative to α globin mRNA) than the marrow cytoplasmic RNA or reticulocyte RNA of the same patients. In one case, the nuclear RNA actually contained nearly equal amounts of α and β mRNA sequences. In one of the three patients, the bone marrow cytoplasmic RNA had a clearly higher β/α mRNA ratio than the reticulocyte RNA of the same patient. In the other two patients, however, the marrow cytoplasmic β/α mRNA ratio was only slightly higher than that

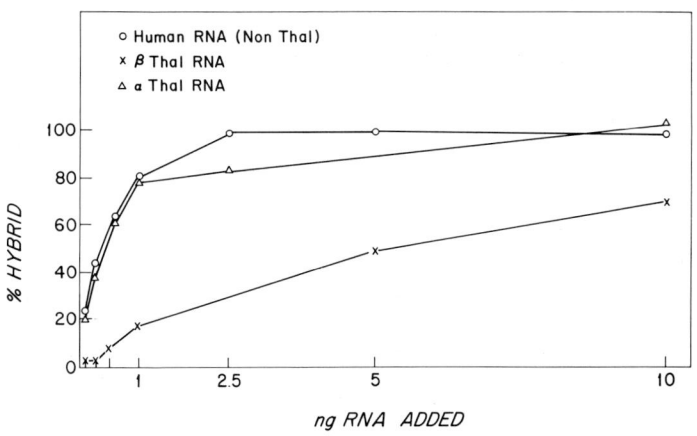

Figure 8–7. Hybridization of human globin mRNAs to a human β-enriched cDNA probe synthesized from the globin mRNA of a patient with Hb H disease. Hybridization was performed under conditions of high stringency, and deficiency of β globin mRNA sequences is now clearly evident in the case of the RNA of an individual with β thalassemia (homozygous β+ thalassemia). (Modified from Housman, D., et al.: Proc. Natl. Acad. Sci. USA 69:1574, 1972.)

of the corresponding reticulocyte RNA. The results of this study clearly demonstrated that in the cases studied, the β+-thalassemic defect was characterized by an intranuclear defect in mRNA processing and/or transport rather than by a primary defect in transcription.

In another study,[47, 114] the technique of velocity sedimentation was used, and nucleated erythroid precursor cells were separated into different fractions containing cells at different stages of maturation and differentiation. The different cell fractions were analyzed for globin-chain synthesis, and total marrow cell RNA was assayed for β/α mRNA content by molecular hybridization. In the one case of β+ thalassemia studied, the results indicated that the degree of deficiency of β-chain synthesis did not vary in different cell fractions and that the β/α mRNA content was similar in all cell fractions: There was less than 10 per cent as much β mRNA as α mRNA in reticulocyte RNA as well as in the total cellular RNA of the most immature erythroid precursor cells. In this study, however, nuclear RNA was not compared with cytoplasmic RNA. The vast majority of the globin mRNA detected by molecular hybridization of total bone marrow cell RNA consists of cytoplasmic globin mRNA. A higher β/α mRNA content in the nucleus than in cytoplasm, such as that observed by Nienhuis and associates in the prior study,[111] would not necessarily have been detected by comparing total bone marrow cell RNA with reticulocyte RNA. Nevertheless, this study clearly did not demonstrate an excess of cytoplasmic β globin mRNA in bone marrow erythroid precursors compared with reticulocytes in the one patient studied.

Later studies using more sensitive and specific molecular hybridization assays provided even more conclusive evidence of a post-transcriptional rather than a transcriptional defect in β globin mRNA biogenesis in the majority of patients with β+ thalassemia. In these studies, the molecular hybridization probes utilized were human globin cDNAs or genomic DNA fragments cloned in bacterial plasmids, which were therefore available in unlimited quantity and in pure form. These cloned probes were used in nonradioactive form and hybridized to radioactive RNA isolated from β+-thalassemic bone marrow cells labeled in short-term cultures with ^{3}H uridine. Alternatively, β globin gene probes, specific for the large intervening sequence of the gene present in precursor but not in mature β globin mRNA molecules, were used as labeled probes for the specific detection of precursor β globin mRNA molecules in β+ thalassemia.

In three different studies,[114–116] analysis of pulse-labeled total bone marrow cell RNA from 11 different patients with β+ thalassemia revealed that in all cases, the β/α mRNA ratio of nascent ^{3}H-labeled RNA was equal or similar to that obtained with labeled nonthalassemic bone marrow RNA and was much higher than the β/α mRNA ratio in the same patient after a 20- to 24-hour "chase" period or in the steady state.[116, 117] In two of the studies,[116, 117] analysis of ^{3}H-labeled nuclear versus cytoplasmic RNA after labeling periods of 30 minutes to 2 hours revealed a much lower ratio of β/α nascent mRNA sequences in the cytoplasm compared with the nucleus in all four cases that were studied. The results of these studies therefore demonstrated that in the cases studied, transcription of the β globin genes appeared to be normal and that the deficit in β mRNA sequences probably occurred at the time of the early post-transcriptional events associated with intranuclear processing and transit of the nascent transcripts from nucleus to cytoplasm.

Direct analysis of precursor β globin mRNA molecules using a variety of techniques demonstrated in three different studies either quantitative[116, 117] or qualitative[115, 116] abnormalities of precursor β mRNA sequences in a number of patients. These abnormalities included excess accumulation (compared with normal) of RNA, containing sequences complementary to the large intervening sequence of the gene,[116, 117] as well as excess accumulation of processing intermediates of the precursor β mRNA molecules.[115, 116] As a result of these studies, it was concluded that in at least some patients with β+ thalassemia, the molecular defect must involve mutations that result in quantitative or qualitative abnormalities in the processing or "splicing out" of intervening sequences present in the precursor β mRNA molecules.

Molecular Hybridization Analysis of Globin mRNA and Globin Gene DNA in Homozygous β⁰ Thalassemia

Reticulocyte and Bone Marrow RNA. Variable results have been obtained in the analysis of reticulocyte globin mRNA from a large number of different patients with β⁰ thalassemia.[110, 118] In some patients (approximately 50 per cent), molecular hybridization assays have revealed a marked deficiency or virtual absence of β mRNA: less than 1 per cent as much β-like mRNA as α mRNA.[87, 110, 118–121, 122–124] The small amount of β-like mRNA seen in these patients was thought, in fact, to represent trace amounts of the mRNA for δ chains.[119, 121] In the other 50 per cent of the patients, however, hybridization assays have revealed a substantial amount of β or β-like mRNA: anywhere from 5 to 30 per cent as much β mRNA as α mRNA.[110, 118, 124–129] The amount of hybridization to β cDNA in these cases was too great to be explained by cross-hybridization of δ-chain mRNA with the β cDNA probe. The β mRNA demonstrable by hybridization assays was always nonfunctional: In heterologous cell-free protein-synthesizing systems, it failed to direct the synthesis of any normal human β globin chains.

The precise nature of the β or β-like globin mRNA detected in β⁰ thalassemia remained unknown for many years. Authentic β chain–specific oligonucleotides were initially demonstrated by RNA fingerprint analysis in one Chinese patient with β⁰ thalassemia who had approximately 15 per cent as much β as α mRNA by hybridization assays.[126] Chang and Kan[130] then successfully determined the structure of the β mRNA in this patient by direct nucleotide sequence analysis of the cDNA synthesized from the mRNA by viral reverse transcriptase and thus established the precedent for the existence of nonsense mutations causing β⁰ thalassemia. They demonstrated a single base substitution in the sequence of the mRNA at codon 17, changing a lysine codon (AAG) to a chain termination codon (UAG). Subsequently, a number of additional nonsense mutations due to base substitutions or frameshifts have been identified by gene cloning and nucleotide sequence analysis as a cause of β⁰ thalassemia in a large number of different patients (see section on Gene Cloning).

The identification of nonsense mutations in patients with β⁰ thalassemia having detectable β mRNA does not in itself explain the marked deficiency of β mRNA relative to α mRNA in these patients. It has been speculated that the low level of the mRNA may be due to accelerated turnover (instability) of the abnormally translated β mRNA. However, such cytoplasmic instability of β globin mRNA in β⁰ thalassemia has not yet been directly demonstrated. Nevertheless, certain results have provided indirect evidence for instability of β mRNA in some cases of β⁰ thalassemia. In a study by Benz and coworkers,[110] three patients

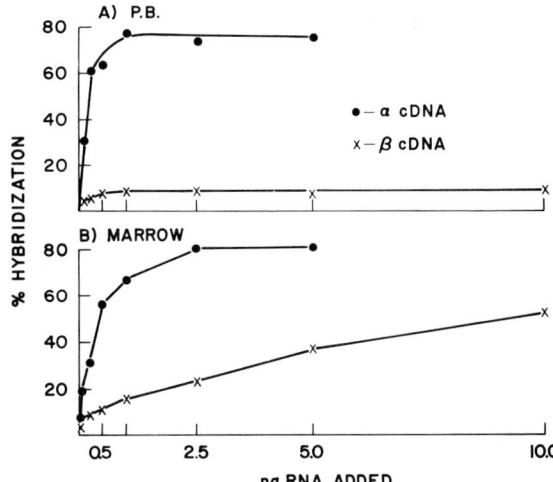

Figure 8–8. Molecular hybridization results in β⁰ thalassemia. RNA from peripheral blood (P.B.) shows virtual absence of β mRNA (A), whereas RNA from marrow of the same patient contains decreased but clearly measurable amounts of β globin mRNA (B). (From Benz, E. J., Jr., et al.: Cell 14:299, 1978.)

demonstrated higher levels of β mRNA (relative to α mRNA) in bone marrow than in peripheral blood (Fig. 8–8). One patient also showed variable levels of reticulocyte β mRNA when tested at different times, with the β/α mRNA ratios ranging from 0.01 to 0.12 (see Fig. 8–9). Nuclear RNA of splenic erythroid cells was studied by Comi and associates[121] in

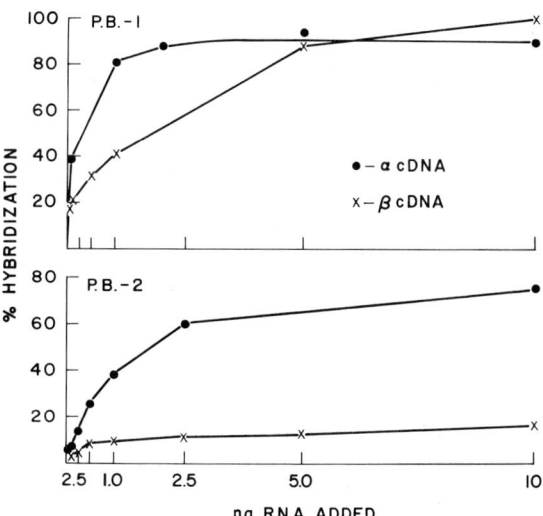

Figure 8–9. Molecular hybridization results in β⁰ thalassemia. Peripheral blood RNA isolated from the same patient at different times (P.B.-1 and P.B.-2) reveals variable amounts of β globin mRNA ranging from virtually absent (P.B.-2) to approximately 10 per cent of α mRNA (P.B.-1). (From Benz, E. J., Jr., et al.: Cell 14:299, 1978.)

two cases of β^0 thalassemia associated with absent cytoplasmic β mRNA: Nuclear β mRNA sequences were found in one case but not in the other, suggesting that post-transcriptional turnover of β mRNA sequences was occurring in one of these cases, whereas a transcriptional defect was suggested in the second patient. Finally, Maquat and colleagues[131] analyzed pulse-labeled bone marrow RNA in Kurdish Jewish patients with β^0 thalassemia and absent reticulocyte β mRNA. Normal electrophoretic profiles of precursor β mRNA and its processing intermediates were detected. The nascent β mRNA transcripts were indistinguishable from normal β mRNA by S1 nuclease mapping (see section on Gene Cloning for methodology). However, following a chase period of 30 minutes, 30 to 75 per cent of the thalassemic β mRNA was degraded.[131] The molecular defect in this type of thalassemia was later found to be a frameshift causing a nonsense mutation[132] (see section on Gene Cloning).

Reticulocyte RNA in Ferrara-Type β^0 Thalassemia. Quantitation of the relative amounts of α and β globin mRNA by molecular hybridization in Ferrara-type β^0 thalassemia has shown the presence of β or β-like mRNA in reticulocyte RNA of these patients in amounts between 5 and 30 per cent of the α mRNA content.[127–129] In one study, Ferrara mRNA failed to totally protect the β cDNA, and the authors concluded that the Ferrara β mRNA might be structurally abnormal.[127] In a second study, however, different results were obtained that indicated that the β mRNA present in Ferrara thalassemia appeared to be substantially similar to normal β mRNA, as judged by the melting temperature of the hybrid formed between the β mRNA and β cDNA.[128] The discrepancies between these two studies may have been due to technical differences such as the state of "intactness" of the mRNA following isolation. In any event, the amounts of β mRNA found in Ferrara β^0 thalassemia did not differ substantially from those found in cases of non-Ferrara β^0 thalassemia with detectable β mRNA.

Globin Gene DNA. Studies of gene quantitation by molecular hybridization in β^0 thalassemia have given uniform results in cases both with and without substantial amounts of detectable β mRNA. DNA-cDNA hybridization studies have shown that the structural genes for β globin chains are in fact present in all cases of β^0 thalassemia studied in a number of different racial groups: Italian, Greek, Pakistani, Chinese, Algerian, and Kurdish Jew.[87, 120, 122, 123, 125–127, 133] Therefore, even cases of β^0 thalassemia with absent β mRNA did not appear to be associated with β globin gene deletions. More sensitive gene mapping studies using restriction endonuclease analysis did, however, later identify a subset of Asian Indian patients and rare black and Dutch patients with partial or total deletions of the β globin gene (see the section on Gene Mapping).

Molecular Hybridization Studies in Heterozygous β Thalassemia

The previously discussed phenomenon of apparently balanced globin-chain synthesis in bone marrow cells of patients with heterozygous β thalassemia prompted a study to analyze the β/α mRNA ratio in partially purified erythroid precursor cells of such patients in order to assess whether or not the expected imbalance of globin mRNA could be directly documented in these cells. Bone marrow erythroid precursor cells were separated from reticulocytes by centrifugation or by velocity sedimentation, and their total cellular RNA was assayed for the relative amounts of α to β globin mRNA by the standard molecular hybridization assays using human α and β globin cDNAs.[114] In all four cases studied, approximately half as much β mRNA as α mRNA was detected in the RNA of bone marrow erythroid cells, levels similar to those detected in peripheral blood reticulocyte RNA of the same individuals. In another report,[113] RNA from total unfractionated bone marrow of an individual with heterozygous β thalassemia yielded an α/β mRNA content of 3.7, a level very similar to that detected in peripheral blood cell RNA of the same individual. These results provided additional support for the role of post-translational turnover of excess α chains as the main cause of apparently balanced globin-chain synthesis in heterozygous β-thalassemic bone marrow cells and ruled out the original hypothesis that equal amounts of α and β globin mRNA might be present in bone marrow precursor cells of β-thalassemia heterozygotes.

Molecular Hybridization Analysis of Globin mRNA and Globin Gene DNA in $\delta\beta$ Thalassemia and Hereditary Persistence of Fetal Hemoglobin (HPFH)

Background and General Considerations. The two syndromes of $\delta\beta$ thalassemia and hereditary persistence of fetal hemoglobin

(HPFH), although relatively rare, are of particular interest because they represent two phenotypically distinct, clinically mild syndromes associated with total absence of β (and δ) globin–chain synthesis. In contrast to $β^0$ thalassemia, both of these syndromes are associated with high levels of γ-chain synthesis that compensates to some degree for the deficient β-chain synthesis (see Chapter 9). It had been hoped that determination of the molecular basis of these syndromes might shed light on factors controlling the fetal to adult hemoglobin switch (see Chapter 7).

Red cells of patients with homozygous δβ thalassemia contain 100 per cent fetal hemoglobin and manifest a thalassemic phenotype with hypochromia and microcytosis because γ-chain synthesis is not equal to α-chain synthesis: There is only approximately one third as much γ-chain synthesis as α-chain synthesis and therefore a net deficit of intracellular hemoglobin. The patients are mildly anemic, and in heterozygotes, the increased amount of Hb F is heterogeneously distributed among the red cells (see Fig. 4–9C). In the usual form of HPFH that occurs in blacks, the red cells of homozygotes also contain 100 per cent Hb F, but because the level of γ-chain synthesis is higher than in δβ thalassemia, the usual phenotypic features of thalassemia are either absent or only minimal. In contrast to the situation in δβ thalassemia, the increased amount of Hb F in heterozygotes with HPFH is relatively uniformly distributed among all of the red cells rather than being heterogeneously distributed among a subpopulation of so-called F cells (see Chapter 4 and Fig. 4–9B). Although the apparent striking qualitative difference in cellular distribution of Hb F between HPFH and δβ thalassemia may be due, in great part, to the quantitative differences in Hb F per cell and the sensitivity of the methods used to detect Hb F cytologically,[5] nevertheless it would appear that the increased amount of Hb F in HPFH is caused by a genetically determined failure to suppress γ globin gene activity postnatally in all erythroid cells rather than by selective survival of the normally occurring subpopulation of F cells such as occurs in sickle cell anemia, $β^+$ thalassemia, $β^0$ thalassemia, and, perhaps to some degree, also δβ thalassemia. These observations constitute the basis

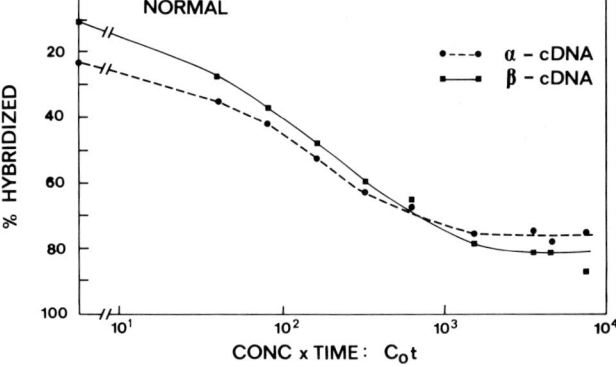

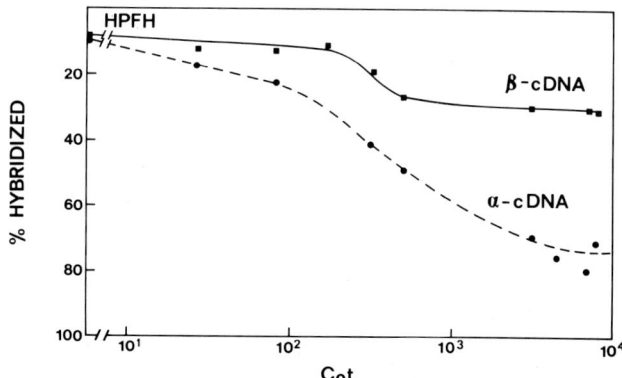

Figure 8–10. Molecular hybridization of globin cDNA to total cellular DNA for quantitation of globin gene number and detection of globin gene deletions. A constant amount of labeled cDNA and total cellular DNA is allowed to hybridize for variable amounts of time in order to generate a curve (C_0t curve) showing the kinetics of hybridization: The amount of probe hybridized is plotted in relation to the C_0t function (concentration × time). The C_0t value at which there is half saturation of hybridization of the probe is an indicator of the number of gene copies in the DNA sample. DNA from an individual homozygous for HPFH *(bottom)* gives no significant hybridization with the β globin cDNA probe consistent with deletion of the β (and δ) globin genes in this individual. (From Forget, B. G., et al.: Cell 7:323, 1976.)

for hoping to find the key to the fetal to adult hemoglobin switch by defining the molecular basis of HPFH.

Molecular Hybridization Results. Almost identical results were obtained in both δβ thalassemia and HPFH when reticulocyte RNA and total cellular DNA were analyzed for β globin mRNA and gene DNA sequences, respectively, by hybridization assays in solution. In the case of reticulocyte RNA, total absence of β or β-like mRNA was observed,[112, 119, 127, 134] and in the case of total cellular DNA, there was marked reduction in hybridization of the DNA to β cDNA (Fig. 8–10), indicating the presence of a substantial deletion of the β (and presumably δ) globin genes in both of these syndromes.[127, 134–137] In one study,[135] the low level of hybridization of DNA to β cDNA was similar in δβ thalassemia and HPFH, but in two other studies,[127, 137] DNA from δβ thalassemia homozygotes hybridized to the β cDNA probe to a significantly greater extent than did DNA from HPFH homozygotes. The latter results were interpreted as indicating that the gene deletion in the β globin gene cluster was more extensive in HPFH than in δβ thalassemia. This conclusion was later verified by gene mapping studies (see the section on Gene Mapping).

In summary, molecular hybridization assays clearly demonstrated the presence of gene deletions as the basis for the absence of β and δ globin gene expression in both δβ thalassemia and HPFH. However, these results left unexplained the molecular basis for the differential effects of these gene deletions on the expression of the neighboring γ globin genes. This topic will be discussed in greater detail in the section on gene mapping.

Molecular Hybridization Studies of Globin mRNA and Gene DNA in α Thalassemia

Background and General Considerations. Alpha thalassemia was first intensively studied in Asian populations, in whom it occurs with a very high frequency[138–140] (see Chapter 9). Four main clinical types of α thalassemia syndromes of progressively increasing severity were defined in this population and were thought to be caused, respectively, by mutation or deletion of one, two, three, or four of the α globin gene loci.[138–140] The four syndromes were called α thalassemia 2, or the silent carrier state (one inactive α globin gene); α thalassemia 1 (two inactive α globin genes); Hb H disease (three inactive α globin genes), caused by double heterozygosity for α thalassemia 2 plus α thalassemia 1; and hydrops fetalis with Hb Bart's (four inactive α globin genes), caused by homozygosity for α thalassemia 1 (Fig. 8–11). An additional common type of α-thalassemia syndrome identified in Asians was associated with the inheritance of Hb Constant Spring (Hb CS), the Hb variant with an elongated α globin chain caused by a chain termination mutation (see Chapters 9 and 10). Heterozygosity for Hb CS was found to interact with α thalassemia 1, in the same manner as did α thalassemia 2, to cause Hb H disease[138–140] (see Fig. 8–11).

On the other hand, the genetic data in blacks with α thalassemia did not fit with the model proposed for the inheritance of α thalassemia in Asians. Although the frequency of apparent heterozygous α thalassemia (that is, α thalassemia 1 phenotype) was quite high in blacks, hydrops fetalis was never observed and Hb H disease was very rare. It was therefore proposed[141] that the α thalassemia 1 phenotype in blacks might be associated with the inactivation or deletion of two α globin genes, but on opposite chromosomes (*in trans*) rather than on the same chromosome (*in cis*) as in Asians (see Fig. 8–11). The advent of molecular hybridization assays, in particular gene quantitation by DNA-cDNA hybridization, led to the first confirmation of some of the genetic theories on the molecular basis of α thalassemia. The refinement of gene mapping technology (see the section on Gene Mapping) provided additional confirmation and further insight into the problem.

Quantitation of α Globin mRNA in the α Thalassemia Syndromes. *Hb H Disease.* The initial molecular hybridization studies of Housman and associates[106] and Kacian and coworkers,[105] demonstrating quantitative deficiency of β globin mRNA in homozygous β thalassemia, also provided evidence for deficiency of α globin mRNA in Hb H disease. In one study,[105] the deficiency of α globin mRNA detected was relatively modest, with an α/β mRNA ratio of approximately 0.6 to 0.7, but in the other study,[106] the deficiency of α globin mRNA (α/β mRNA ratio of approximately 0.1 [see Fig. 8–6]) was much greater than expected on the basis of the relative levels of α and β globin–chain synthesis in reticulocytes of the same patient (α/β globin chain synthetic ratio of 0.3 [see Fig. 8–1C]). As previously noted (see the section on Functional Studies of Thalassemic Globin mRNA in Cell-Free Protein Synthesizing Systems), cell-free translation of globin

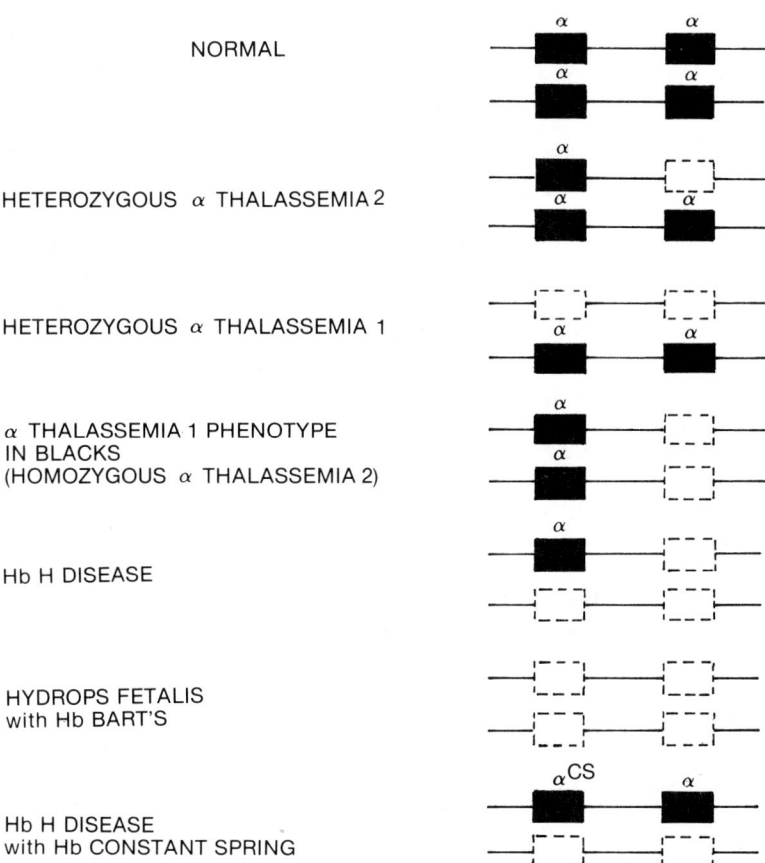

Figure 8–11. Gene deletion model for the molecular basis of the various α-thalassemia syndromes. Gene deletions are represented by the dashed blocks.

mRNA from the same patient also revealed a greater-than-expected deficiency of functional α mRNA relative to β mRNA (see Fig. 8–3A). Marked α globin mRNA deficiency (α/β mRNA ratio of approximately 0.1) was also later noted by molecular hybridization assays in a different case of Hb H disease by Kan and colleagues,[108, 142] but less profound α globin mRNA deficiency, with α/β mRNA ratios of 0.23 to 0.45, has also been observed in a number of additional patients with Hb H disease.[112, 113, 143]

The results of these various studies demonstrated, on the one hand, that all of the cases of Hb H disease analyzed were associated with a quantitative deficiency of α globin mRNA (relative to β globin mRNA), but that in at least some cases, the α globin mRNA deficiency was greater than expected on the basis of α/β globin–chain synthetic ratios in the patients' reticulocytes. These latter results are probably explained by the presence of post-translational turnover of newly synthesized excess β chains in the patients' intact erythroid cells, as discussed previously (see the section on Functional Studies of Thalassemic Globin mRNA in Cell-Free Protein Synthesizing Systems).

Globin mRNA was also quantitated in fractionated bone marrow erythroid cells of the initial Mediterranean patient with Hb H disease studied by Housman and associates.[106] The α/β globin mRNA ratio in total cellular RNA of nucleated erythroid precursor cells was approximately 0.5 at all stages of maturation, a level significantly higher than the ratio of 0.1 obtained with reticulocyte RNA.[47] These results suggested the presence, in the particular patient studied, of unstable α globin mRNA. This Mediterranean patient was subsequently shown to have an unusual form of Hb H disease associated with a partially deleted α globin gene,[144] the *in vivo* transcriptional activity of which is unknown. In the analysis of a different case of Hb H disease, the α/β mRNA ratio was approximately 0.3 in both bone marrow and reticulocytes.[112, 113]

Hydrops Fetalis with Hb Bart's. In the case of the fatal syndrome of hydrops fetalis with Hb Bart's, in which there is total absence of α globin–chain synthesis, hybridization assays in a number of different laboratories have confirmed the expected finding of absence of α globin mRNA.[109, 112, 113, 142, 143]

Heterozygous α Thalassemia. Very sensitive hybridization assays, utilizing purified human α and β globin cDNAs, have been shown to be capable of differentiating the two forms of heterozygous α thalassemia: α thalassemia 1 and α thalassemia 2 (silent carrier state). In a detailed study,[143] Hunt and coworkers obtained α/β mRNA ratios of 0.87 to 1.17 in eight cases of heterozygous α thalassemia 1, and α/β mRNA ratios of 1.34 to 1.75 in five cases of heterozygous α thalassemia 2. In this study, the α/β mRNA ratios obtained with normal reticulocyte RNA ranged between 2.0 and 2.5, a level somewhat higher than that obtained by other investigators[107, 111–114] but consistent with the fact that in normal reticulocytes there probably exists an excess of α globin mRNA relative to β globin mRNA.[67, 145]

Quantitation of α Globin Gene DNA in the α-Thalassemia Syndromes. The quantitation of α globin genes in α thalassemia using cDNA-DNA hybridization assays in solution provided very important early information on the molecular basis of α thalassemia. These assays provided the first direct demonstration of a gene deletion in man and also provided very strong evidence for the presence of normally duplicated α globin genes in the human haploid genome.

Hydrops Fetalis with Hb Bart's. In precedent-setting experiments in 1974, two groups were successful in demonstrating the presence of deletion of the α globin genes in homozygous α thalassemia 1 in Asian subjects. Taylor and colleagues[108] and Ottolenghi and associates,[109] using human α cDNA prepared from total reticulocyte DNA by means of differential hybridization and fractionation techniques, were able to show virtual absence of hybridization of the α cDNA to total DNA isolated from the liver of hydropic infants (Fig. 8–12). Similar results were also subsequently obtained by others[113] and confirmed that deletion of the α globin genes was the basis for absent α globin–chain synthesis in the syndrome of hydrops fetalis with Hb Bart's.

Hb H Disease. In follow-up studies on the question of gene deletion in α thalassemia and the number of α globin genes in normal individuals, Kan and coworkers[142] analyzed the DNA from a Chinese individual with Hb H disease. Hybridization of this DNA to α globin cDNA showed reduced hybridization consistent with deletion of part of the complement of α globin genes. The hybridization profile (see Fig. 8–12) was identical to that obtained with a mixture of hydropic and normal DNA in a 3 to 1 ratio and was definitely different from that obtained with an equal mixture of the two DNAs. These results therefore demonstrated that in Hb H disease, the number of remaining α globin genes is 25 per cent of normal, as expected if each chromosome normally carries two α globin genes rather than one. If there were only one α globin gene per chromosome, one would have expected to see a hybridization profile identical to the 1:1 mixture of normal and hydropic DNA. These experiments provided one of the most conclusive early demonstrations of the normal duplication of the human α globin genes.

Heterozygous α Thalassemia 1. With refinements of the cDNA-DNA hybridization assay, Kan and colleagues subsequently studied a large number of families from different racial groups and were able to reproducibly detect deletion of two out of the four α globin genes in individuals who were obligatory heterozygotes for α thalassemia 1, such as parents of individuals with hydrops fetalis or Hb H disease.[146–149] (Fig. 8–13). A number of additional original observations were made during the course of these studies: (1) The molecular hybridization assays could be accurately ap-

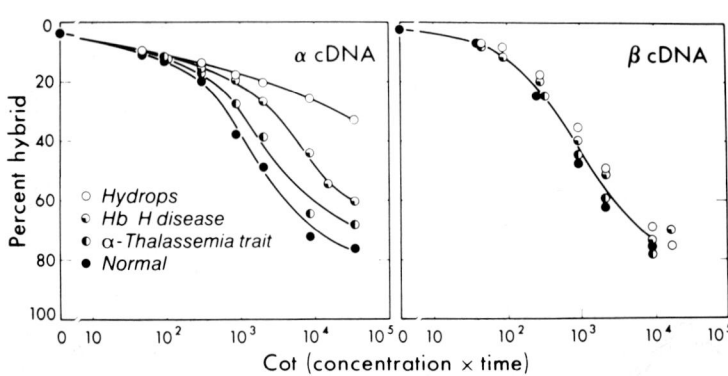

Figure 8–12. Molecular hybridization of DNA from individuals with various α-thalassemia syndromes. The pattern of hybridization to the α globin cDNA is consistent with the deletion of four α globin genes in hydrops fetalis; deletion of three α genes in Hb H disease; and deletion of two α genes in α-thalassemia trait (α thalassemia 1). (From Kan, Y. W.: *In* the Harvey Lectures, Series 76, New York, Academic Press, 1982, p. 75.)

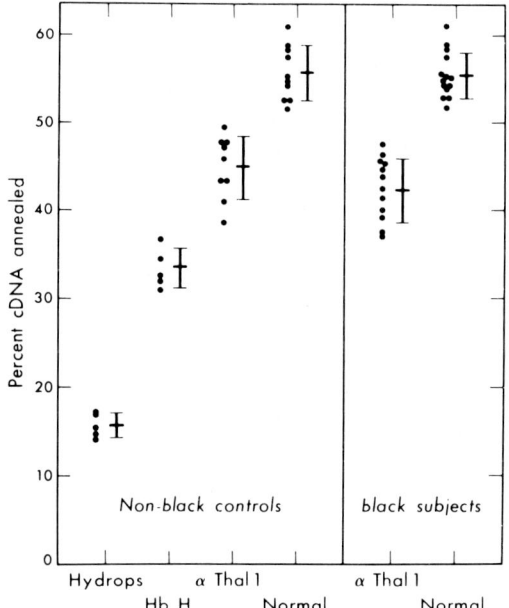

Figure 8–13. Results of DNA/α cDNA hybridization in a series of normal and α-thalassemic individuals. The percentage of cDNA annealed correlates with the number of α globin genes present in the DNA. Black individuals with the α thalassemia 1 phenotype show the same level of hybridization as nonblack individuals with the same phenotype, consistent with the deletion of two α globin genes in these individuals. (From Davis, J. R., Jr., et al.: Am. J. Hum. Genet. 31:569, 1979.)

plied to the prenatal diagnosis of α thalassemia using DNA extracted from amniotic fluid cells.[146] (2) The molecular hybridization patterns of DNA samples from Filipino subjects with α thalassemia were virtually identical to those obtained from Southeast Asian subjects.[147] (3) DNA from black subjects with the phenotype of α thalassemia 1 or with Hb H disease demonstrated the same quantitative deficiency of α globin gene DNA as did Asian patients with the same syndromes.[149]

Nondeletion Forms of α Thalassemia. Although most Asian subjects with α thalassemia could be demonstrated to have α globin gene deletions, Kan and associates[148] identified a Chinese family with two members who had Hb H disease but whose DNA gave a hybridization pattern consistent with the deletion of only two rather than three α globin genes. In addition, a number of family members had the clinical phenotype of α thalassemia 1 without demonstrable evidence of α globin gene deletion by cDNA-DNA hybridization. This report provided the first evidence of a nondeletion type of α thalassemia in Asians (other than Hb Constant Spring) and therefore indicated the presence of heterogeneity in the molecular basis of this disorder.

In a study by Old and colleagues[150] of a case of Hb H disease acquired during the course of a myeloproliferative disorder, it was shown that although the patient had profound deficiency of α globin mRNA, there was no evidence of any α globin gene deletion (see the later section on Gene Mapping in Acquired Hb H Disease).

Summary and Conclusions. Molecular hybridization studies in α thalassemia, particularly the quantitation of α globin gene numbers in the various syndromes, provided a great deal of support and direct confirmation of the model shown in Figure 8–11 for the molecular basis of the different α-thalassemia syndromes in Asian subjects. Although these studies also provided conclusive evidence for α globin gene deletions in blacks with α thalassemia, they left unresolved the issue of gene deletions *in trans* rather than *in cis* to explain the lack of hydrops fetalis and the rarity of Hb H disease in blacks. Finally, evidence of heterogeneity in the molecular basis of α thalassemia, even among Asians, first emerged from the unexpected finding of a nondeletion type of α thalassemia in a Chinese family.

Other Quantitative Assays of Globin mRNA

Two other procedures have been used to demonstrate the presence of quantitative deficiency of chain-specific globin mRNAs in α and β thalassemia: (1) direct visualization of α and β globin mRNAs separated by acrylamide gel electrophoresis in the presence of the denaturing agent formamide; and (2) oligonucleotide fingerprint analysis of RNase digests of thalassemic globin mRNA radioactively labeled by a variety of techniques.

When globin mRNA is analyzed by acrylamide gel electrophoresis under standard conditions, it migrates as a single broad band. However, in the presence of the denaturing agent formamide, which eliminates secondary structure in RNAs, electrophoresis fractionates globin mRNA according to size into two bands: a more rapidly migrating, shorter species, corresponding to α globin mRNA, and a more slowly migrating, longer species, corresponding to β globin mRNA (Fig. 8–14). When globin mRNAs from individuals with α or β thalassemia are analyzed in this manner, one can clearly observe reduced amounts of α globin mRNA in Hb H disease and reduced amounts of β globin mRNA in homozygous β thalassemia[107, 151] (see Fig. 8–14). In the case

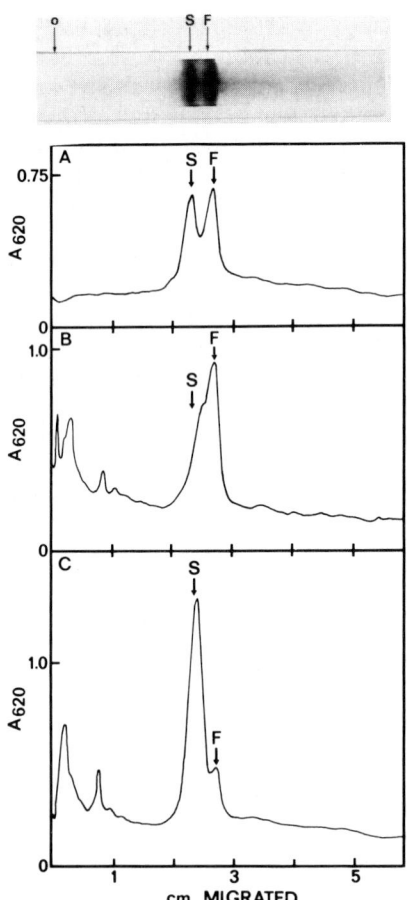

Figure 8–14. Fractionation of human α and β globin mRNAs by polyacrylamide gel electrophoresis in the presence of formamide. Densitometer scans of stained gels containing different RNA samples are shown beneath the photo of a representative gel of a normal RNA sample. *A*, Globin mRNA from a nonthalassemic individual showing roughly equal amounts of RNA in the α (F = fast) and β (S = slow) bands. *B*, Globin mRNA from a patient with homozygous β$^+$ thalassemia showing marked deficiency of β RNA and a moderate amount of RNA in a band (or shoulder) of intermediate mobility, consistent with γ globin mRNA. *C*, Globin mRNA from an individual with Hb H disease showing marked deficiency of α globin mRNA. (From Forget, B. G., et al.: Proc. Natl. Acad. Sci. USA 72:984, 1975.)

of homozygous β thalassemia, actual quantitation of the relative amounts of β to α globin mRNA is difficult by this procedure because γ globin mRNA migrates between the two species and prevents clear separation of the β and α peaks on densitometric scanning of the gels (see Fig. 8–14). Although not as practical as molecular hybridization for the analysis of β globin mRNA in β thalassemia, this procedure has proved to be very useful for the purposes of fractionating normal globin mRNA and isolating relatively pure preparations of α and β globin mRNAs to serve as substrates for the synthesis of cDNAs used in the molecular hybridization assays.[107, 152]

The other procedure that was used for the quantitative estimation of the relative abundance of α and β globin mRNAs was radiolabeling of the mRNA (or of its digestion products) and fractionation of specific nuclease digests of the RNA in two dimensions, followed by autoradiography to obtain oligonucleotide fingerprints of the mRNA. Alpha- and β-specific oligonucleotides, the identities of which were previously determined by nucleotide sequence analysis, were distinguished from one another by this procedure and their relative intensities compared. Three different procedures were used to obtain labeled digests of thalassemic globin mRNA[153, 153a]: (1) radiolabeling of cytosine residues of the mRNA with ^{125}I; (2) 5′-end labeling of oligonucleotides with [γ-^{32}P]-ATP and polynucleotide kinase; and (3) synthesis of globin cDNA from the mRNA by reverse transcriptase and then synthesis of ^{32}P-labeled cRNA from the cDNA by use of RNA polymerase.

Oligonucleotide fingerprinting was used to analyze globin mRNA from various thalassemic individuals and revealed absence of α globin mRNA in hydrops fetalis,[126] marked deficiency of α globin mRNA in a patient with Hb H disease[107] (Fig. 8–15B), virtual absence of β globin mRNA in two unrelated patients with β^0 thalassemia,[110] the presence of authentic β globin mRNA oligonucleotides in yet another patient with β^0 thalassemia,[126] and marked deficiency of β globin mRNA in a case of β$^+$ thalassemia[153a] (see Fig. 8–15C).

GENE MAPPING USING RESTRICTION ENDONUCLEASE DIGESTION OF TOTAL CELLULAR DNA

The introduction by Dr. E. Southern[154] of the technique of gene mapping by analysis of restriction endonuclease digests of total cellular DNA (so-called "Southern gel blotting") rapidly led to the accumulation of a large body of experimental data from numerous laboratories on the nature of various globin gene deletions in the thalassemias. In particular, this technique permitted the elucidation of the fine details of the gene deletions in the different α-thalassemia, δβ-thalassemia, and HPFH syndromes.

Description of the Procedure

The gene mapping procedure of Southern is a very powerful technique, because it allows

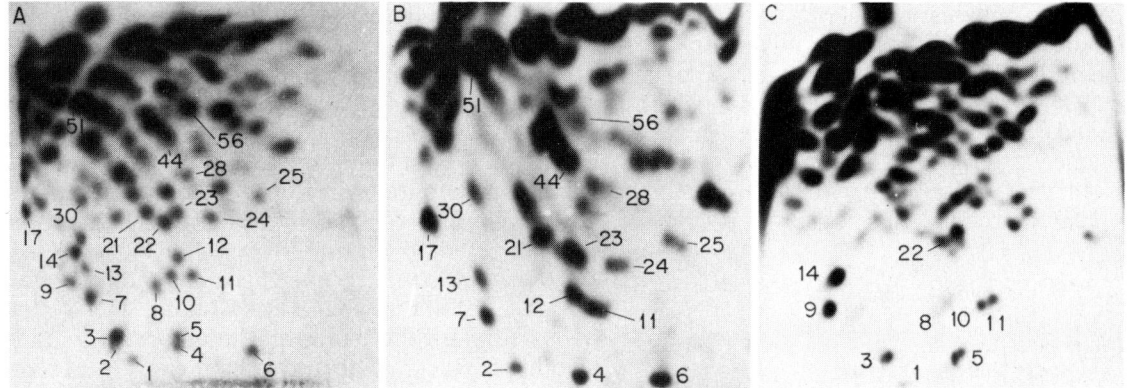

Figure 8–15. Fingerprint patterns of RNAs (cRNAs) complementary to normal and thalassemic globin cDNAs. The different cRNAs, synthesized *in vitro* using DNA-dependent RNA polymerase of *E. coli* and ^{32}P-labeled ribonucleotide triphosphates, were digested with ribonuclease T1 prior to fractionation. Specific oligonucleotides (or spots), present in the fingerprint of normal cRNA *(A)*, are missing or markedly decreased in the cRNA fingerprints of Hb H disease *(B)* and β^+ thalassemia *(C)*, consistent with marked deficiency of sequences corresponding to α and β globin mRNA in the respective thalassemic samples. (From Forget, B. G., et al.: Ann. N.Y. Acad. Sci. *241*:290, 1974.)

one to study the general structure and organization of a gene in total cellular DNA without actually isolating or purifying the gene away from the rest of the cellular DNA. The general principle of the technique is illustrated in Figure 8–16. The procedure relies on the use of restriction endonucleases to digest the DNA under study. These are bacterial enzymes that

Figure 8–16. Outline of the method for gene mapping using the gel blotting procedure of Southern (see text for details). (From Forget, B. G.: Ann. Intern. Med. *91*:605, 1979.)

1) Total Cellular DNA Digested with Restriction Endonuclease

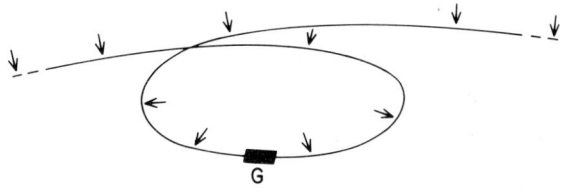

2) Gel Electrophoresis of DNA Fragments

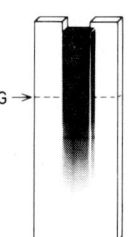

3) Transfer of DNA to Nitrocellulose Filter by Blotting

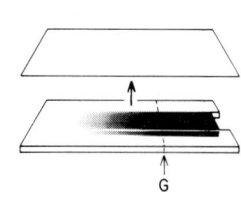

4) Hybridization of Filter with ^{32}P-labeled cDNA (•••)

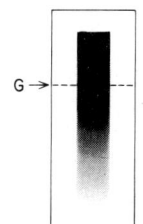

5) Autoradiography

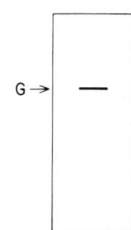

recognize only certain short oligonucleotide sequences in DNA, commonly four to six nucleotides long, and cut the DNA only at those sites. For example, Eco RI, which is isolated from *Escherichia coli*, recognizes the sequence 5'-GAATTC-3'. The substrate for this enzyme is double-stranded DNA, so that the actual structure that it cleaves is

$$\downarrow$$
5'-GAATTC-3'
3'-CTTAAG-5'
$$\uparrow$$

The arrows indicate the bond in each DNA strand that is actually hydrolyzed by this enzyme. This enzyme cuts DNA molecules only at sites that contain this precise sequence, which is expected to occur on a random basis approximately once every 4000 to 16,000 nucleotides. As of early 1984, approximately 475 different restriction endonucleases, with a minimum of 103 different sequence specificities, had been identified.[155]

In the gene mapping procedure (see Fig. 8–16), total cellular DNA is digested with a given restriction endonuclease. The enzyme will cut the DNA, according to its sequence specificity, either within or to either side of a given gene of interest, such as a globin gene, but it will also cut the total DNA in the sample at similar sites, generating probably a million different DNA fragments per genome equivalent. The DNA fragment of interest, however, will have a very discrete size because it is delimited at each end by precise recognition sequences specified by the enzyme used. One then fractionates or separates, according to size, the multitude of fragments in the digested DNA sample by electrophoresis in agarose gels. If one visualizes the DNA after fractionation by staining it with ethidium bromide, only a smear will be seen because the million or so different DNA fragments overlap each other; the single gene of interest is buried in the smear as a fragment of discrete size. To identify it, the DNA in the gel is first denatured to render it susceptible to detection by molecular hybridization and then is transferred to a sheet of nitrocellulose filter paper by simply blotting the gel against the paper. The DNA has a high affinity for the nitrocellulose and therefore becomes transferred. Once the DNA is on this solid support medium, it is ready to be subjected to molecular hybridization. The hybridization probe used is a previously cloned DNA sequence, either a portion of the chromosomal DNA corresponding to the gene of interest or a cloned cDNA copy of the mRNA of that gene rendered radioactive to a high specific activity with ^{32}P by the procedure called "nick translation." When the probe is hybridized to the filter, the radioactive molecules will bind, by complementary (Watson-Crick) base-pairing, only to the DNA fragment(s) containing sequences that are complementary to the probe. The unhybridized radioactivity is washed away and the filter is subjected to autoradiography, which will reveal one or more bands corresponding to the gene of interest and its flanking DNA; the position of the bands on the autoradiograph is directly related to the size of the DNA fragments generated by the restriction endonuclease. This technique allows one to look not only at the gene itself but also at its contiguous flanking DNA contained within the given restriction endonuclease fragment.

A prerequisite to the application and utility of this method in the analysis of mutations causing the thalassemias was the determination of the normal restriction endonuclease map of the α and non-α globin gene clusters in man. Therefore, gene mapping efforts initially focused on normal DNA and led, along with cloning and sequencing of normal human globin genes, to the derivation of detailed maps of the human globin gene clusters, including the determination of the linear chromosomal organization of the linked globin genes as well as their fine structure. In particular, intergene distances were determined as well as the number and size of intervening sequences that interrupt the coding sequences of the globin genes and must be precisely excised (spliced out) from precursor mRNA molecules during the course of normal globin gene expression (see Chapter 7 for details).

Gene Mapping Studies in β⁺ and β⁰ Thalassemia

In the proper circumstances, the gene mapping technique should be capable of detecting deletions or rearrangements of DNA consisting of as little as 100 or so nucleotides. However, with rare exceptions, studies of DNA from a number of individuals with β⁺ or β⁰ thalassemia revealed no evidence of gene deletion or rearrangement[94, 133, 156–159a] and therefore led to the conclusion that in the majority of cases of β⁰ and β⁺ thalassemia, there is no significant disruption in the structure or organization of the β globin gene or its flanking DNA.

Deletion of β Globin Gene Sequences in Some Asian Indian, Black, and Dutch Patients with β⁰ Thalassemia. An early exception to the findings just described was provided by three cases of β⁰ thalassemia in individuals of Asian Indian ancestry.[156, 157] DNA from these individuals, who were homozygous for the β⁰ thalassemia phenotype, yielded gene mapping results consistent with the deletion, in one of the two β globin genes of each patient, of approximately 600 base pairs of DNA at the 3′ extremity of the gene. Subsequent cloning and detailed analysis of this mutant gene revealed that the deletion removed the distal (3′) third of the large intervening sequence (IVS-2) and the entire third exon of the gene, as well as 209 nucleotides of the adjacent 3′-flanking DNA.[160, 161] The nucleotide sequence analysis of the break point of the deletion revealed the presence of a novel heptanucleotide sequence and suggested a complex mechanism for the origin of this mutant gene consisting of a short duplication event prior to the recombination event that generated the deletion.[161]

Analysis of reticulocyte RNA from two patients carrying this partially deleted gene revealed absence of β globin mRNA detectable by molecular hybridization.[156, 157] Although the structure of the abnormal β globin gene explains the absence of normal β globin–chain synthesis, transcription of the gene should be theoretically possible. However, the hypothetical RNA transcript of this gene would be very abnormal: It probably would not be terminated normally owing to the likely absence of normal transcription termination signals in the 3′-flanking DNA of the gene and would lack the processing signal at the 3′ end of IVS-2 as well as the signal for polyadenylation in the 3′-untranslated portion of the mRNA. In all likelihood, such an abnormal mRNA transcript would be rapidly degraded, as occurs in other cases of β⁰ and β⁺ thalassemia associated with abnormal post-transcriptional processing of β globin gene transcripts (see later section on Gene Cloning). Unfortunately, analysis of bone marrow RNA from affected patients or of RNA produced by the abnormal gene in gene transfer/gene expression systems has not been reported. Although this gene was initially thought to be relatively rare, a subsequent survey of Asian Indian subjects has revealed that the gene accounts for approximately 30 per cent of β-thalassemic chromosomes in this population.[162, 162a]

Gene mapping studies in black patients with β thalassemia later detected the presence in rare patients of a deletion of approximately 1.3 kb in length involving the 5′-flanking DNA, exons 1 and 2, and the 5′ end of IVS-2 of the β globin gene.[162b, 162c] A large deletion of 10 kb involving the entire β globin gene but sparing the δ globin gene has also been described in a Dutch family with β⁰ thalassemia.[162d]

Base Substitution in a β⁰-Thalassemic Gene Detected by the Gene Mapping Procedure. Determination of the nucleotide sequence of the normal β globin gene allowed the generation of a detailed map of restriction endonuclease sites present within the gene.[163] In particular, it was found that there existed a site for the enzyme Hph I at the junction between the coding sequence and the 5′ end of the large intervening sequence (IVS-2) of the β globin gene.[163] On the chance that certain forms of β thalassemia might be due to mutations at this site leading to abnormal processing of precursor β mRNA molecules, Baird and associates analyzed Hph I digests of a number of β-thalassemic DNA samples by the gene mapping procedure.[164] DNA from three different β⁰-thalassemic patients (one Italian and two Iranian) yielded results consistent with a mutation that abolished the Hph I site at the 5′ IVS-2 splice junction of the β globin gene. Nucleotide sequence analysis of an independently cloned β⁰-thalassemic gene with presumably the same mutation revealed the abnormality to consist of a single nucleotide base substitution, $\underline{GT} \rightarrow \underline{AT}$,[165] in the consensus dinucleotide (GT) that is required at the 5′ extremity of an intron for proper splicing out of intervening sequences from precursor mRNA molecules[166, 167] (see Chapter 7). This mutation as well as additional mutations that affect restriction endonuclease sites within α or β globin genes will be discussed in greater detail in the section on Gene Cloning.

Gene Mapping in δβ Thalassemia, γδβ Thalassemia, and HPFH

As discussed under Background and General Considerations in the section on Molecular Hybridization of Globin mRNA and Gene DNA in these disorders, the interest in the molecular genetics of δβ thalassemia and HPFH centers on the basis for the different phenotypes of these two syndromes with respect to the quantitative and qualitative aspects of γ globin gene expression. Comparative gene mapping of different deletions causing δβ thalassemia or HPFH has provided a great deal of information concerning the precise extent of these various deletions in the non-α globin gene cluster and has led to the elaboration of a number of theories concerning the possible mechanisms by which these deletions have differential effects on the expression of the γ globin genes in the different syndromes.

δβ Thalassemia. Gene mapping studies were initially performed in the common Mediterranean or Sicilian type of δβ thalassemia, which is associated with the synthesis of both $^G\gamma$ and $^A\gamma$ types of Hb F. The first results confirmed the earlier suggestions—made on the basis of molecular hybridization assays in solution—that less DNA was deleted in δβ thalassemia than in HPFH. Although the normal δ and β globin gene DNA fragments were absent in both syndromes, a new DNA fragment that hybridized to the β globin gene probe was detected in δβ thalassemia but not in HPFH.[168] Detailed mapping studies later showed that this new fragment contained the 5′ end of the δ globin gene,[137, 169] and the precise extent of the gene deletion was subsequently determined. The findings revealed that the entire β globin gene and the 3′-terminal half of the δ gene were deleted, starting near the 3′ end of the large intervening sequence (IVS-2) of the δ gene, as illustrated in Figure 8–17.[137, 169, 169a] Thus, the 5′-terminal (or N-coding) portion of the δ gene up to codon 104 and a portion of IVS-2 are spared from the deletion in this condition. The 3′ end point of the deletion has been variously reported as being located relatively close to[170] or very distant from[171] the 3′ end of the β globin gene. Subsequent studies have indicated that the discrepancy was probably due, in part, to a previously unrecognized restriction fragment length polymorphism in the 3′-flanking DNA of the β gene and that the 3′ end point of the deletion occurs in DNA located approximately 5000 nucleotides (5 kb) to the 3′ side of the β globin gene,[172] as illustrated in Figure 8–17.

A number of additional deletions of different extents have also been found to be associated with δβ thalassemia in different individuals or families of various ethnic origins (see Fig. 8–17). Most of these deletion syndromes involve all or part of the $^A\gamma$ globin gene, so that the phenotype is δβ thalassemia in which the elevated Hb F is exclusively of the $^G\gamma$ type [so-called $^G\gamma(\delta\beta)^0$ or $^G\gamma$ ($^A\gamma \delta\beta)^0$ thalassemia]. These deletions include the following: (1) in a Turkish family, a deletion extending from a point approximately 500 nucleotides 3′ to the

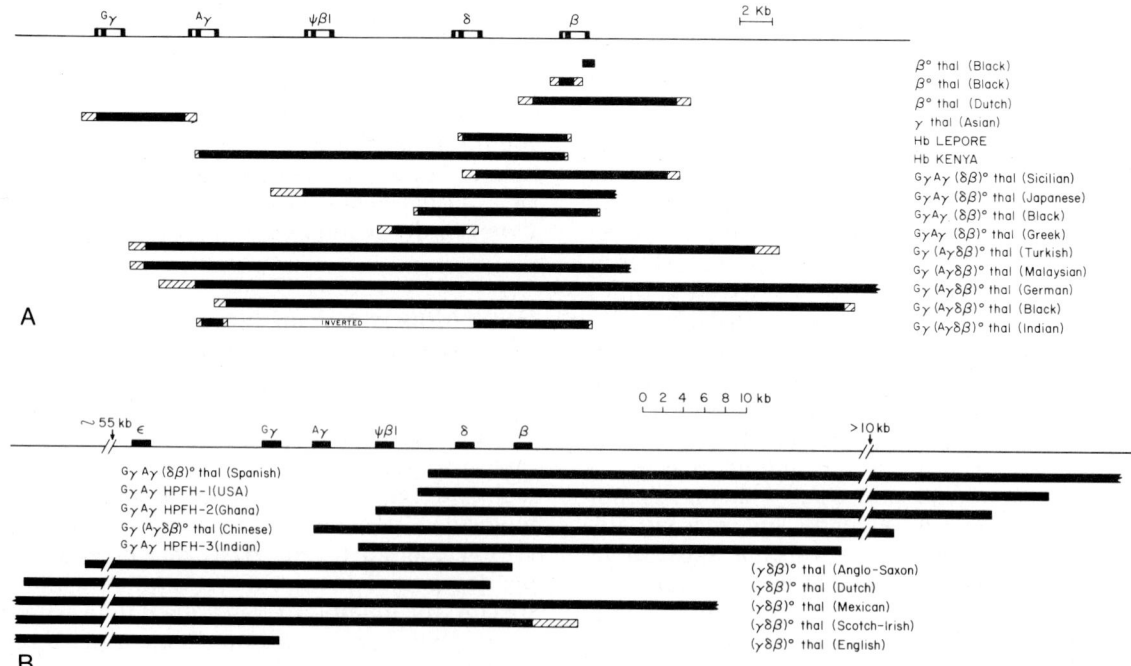

Figure 8–17. Extent of various DNA deletions involving the β globin gene cluster. The cross-hatched bars represent regions where the precise end points of the deletions are indeterminate. *A,* Deletions confined to the cluster or with unknown 3′ end point. *B,* Large deletions extending beyond the cluster.

$^G\gamma$ globin gene to a point approximately 10 kb to the 3′ side of the β globin gene[169, 172–174]; (2) in a Spanish family, a deletion starting at a point 2.75 kb 5′ to the δ globin gene and extending for an unknown distance to a point far beyond the 3′ end of the β globin gene[171, 175]; (3) in a Chinese family, a deletion starting within the large intervening sequence (IVS-2) of the $^A\gamma$ globin gene and extending for an unknown distance to a point far beyond the 3′ end of the β globin gene[176, 176a]; and (4) in families from India and other central Asian countries, a major rearrangement of the β gene cluster, with deletion of portions of the β, δ, and $^A\gamma$ globin genes and an inversion of the preserved intergene DNA between the $^A\gamma$ and δ globin genes.[177–177b]

Nucleotide sequence analysis of the DNA at the junctions of this unusual deletion/inversion event has revealed the presence (or insertion) of foreign DNA sequences that are homologous to sequences involved in recombination events leading to immunoglobulin gene rearrangements during B lymphoid cell differentiation.[177c]

A number of additional deletions have been identified more recently as causes of δβ thalassemia.

$^G\gamma(^A\gamma\delta\beta)^0$ **Thalassemia.** (1) In a Malaysian family, a deletion with a 5′ end point similar to that of the Turkish δβ thalassemia but with a different 3′ end point at an undetermined distance from the β gene.[177a] (2) In a black family, a deletion extending from IVS-2 of the $^A\gamma$ gene to a point approximately 12 kb 3′ to the β gene.[177d] (3) In a German family, a deletion starting at a point between the $^G\gamma$ and $^A\gamma$ genes and extending to a point at least 17 kb 3′ to the β gene but not encompassing DNA detected by HPFH-1 end point probes.[177e]

$^G\gamma^A\gamma(\delta\beta)^0$ **Thalassemia.** (1) In a black individual, a 12-kb deletion extending from a point approximately 2.4 kb 5′ to the δ gene and extending to a point approximately 0.2 kb 3′ to the β gene.[177f] (2) In a Greek family, a 6.5-kb deletion extending from a point approximately 5 kb 5′ to the δ gene and extending into IVS-2 of the δ gene.[177g] The β globin gene is spared by this deletion, but it is inactive for reasons that are not clear, as is the case in certain types of γδβ thalassemia (see below). (3) In a Japanese individual, a deletion starting at a point 3 to 4 kb 3′ to the $^A\gamma$ gene and extending beyond the β gene for an unknown distance.[177h]

Not all patients with δβ thalassemia, however, have deletions within the β gene cluster. One form of δβ thalassemia found in Sardinia and characterized by the synthesis of predominantly $^A\gamma$ globin chains of Hb F is not associated with a demonstrable globin gene deletion.[171] Surprisingly, the β globin gene in such cases has been found to harbor the common Mediterranean nonsense mutation at codon 39.[177i, 177j] Although this finding explains the lack of β-chain synthesis in this condition, it does not shed light on the cause of δ gene silencing or selective $^A\gamma$ gene overexpression. It is possible that multiple mutations coexist on the affected chromosome.

γδβ and γ Thalassemia. The rare syndrome of γδβ thalassemia is characterized clinically, in newborns, by neonatal hemolysis and normoblastemia that are self-limited and, in adults, by the hematological phenotype of heterozygous β thalassemia with normal levels of Hb F and Hb A_2 (see Chapter 9). At the molecular level, extensive deletions have been characterized within the β gene cluster, involving all of the non-α globin genes. Only heterozygotes have been identified; homozygosity would be expected to be lethal very early in gestation. Four different large deletions have been found to be associated with this syndrome (see Fig. 8–17): (1) in a family of Anglo-Saxon ancestry, a deletion of ~100 kb starting at codon 64 of the second exon or coding block of the β globin gene and extending in the 5′ direction to a point ~54 kb to the 5′ side of the ε gene[178, 179]; (2) in a Dutch family, a deletion of approximately the same size starting at a point approximately 2.5 kb 5′ to the β globin gene and extending to a point approximately 6 kb 5′ to the end point of deletion 1 above[179, 180]; (3) in a Mexican-American family, a deletion involving the entire non-α globin gene cluster, the 5′ end of which extends for an unknown distance beyond the 5′ end points of deletions 1 and 2 above and the 3′ end point of which is located at an unknown distance from the 3′ end of the β globin gene: the 3′ end point is at least 17 kb beyond the β globin gene but is proximal to the 3′ end points of the deletions causing HPFH[181] (see below); and (4) in a family of Scottish-Irish ancestry, a deletion involving the entire non-α globin gene cluster, the 5′ end point of which is also located at an unknown distance 5′ to the 5′ end points of deletions 1 and 2, but the 3′ end point of which is located within 6 kb of the 3′ end of the β globin gene.[182]

A most interesting aspect of the γδβ thalassemia in the Dutch family is the fact that the β globin gene on the affected chromosome is intact along with 2.5 kb of its 5′-flanking DNA, but it nevertheless behaves as a β-thalassemic globin gene. The cause of the abnormal function of this β globin gene has been investigated by Grosveld and associates,[183] who found that the cloned β globin gene had a normal structure and functioned normally in a gene transfer/gene expression system using tissue culture cells. However, in fetal liver erythroid cells of an affected individual, the β globin gene from the mutant chromosome was found to be hypermethylated, whereas the β globin gene from the normal chromosome was hypomethylated, as is usually the case in actively transcribing genes. The authors concluded that either the nature of the new DNA sequences juxtaposed to the β globin gene or the disruption of chromosomal and/or chromatin structure caused by the deletion prevents the hypomethylation (usually associated with activity of the β globin gene) from occurring and thereby renders the gene inactive. An analogous and even more striking example of an apparent negative regulatory influence on the β globin gene of a somewhat remote deletion consists of the case in an English family of a large deletion extending from exon 3 of the $^G\gamma$ globin gene to a point beyond the 5′ end point of the Dutch or Anglo-Saxon γδβ-thalassemia deletions.[184] The β gene in this case is not expressed even though approximately 20 kb of its 5′-flanking DNA are intact. The basis for the abnormal β globin gene expression in this syndrome has not yet been established.

A smaller deletion has been identified as a cause of isolated γ thalassemia in individuals found during the course of screening surveys to have unusually high levels of the $^A\gamma$ type of Hb F in cord blood.[185] Gene mapping studies were consistent with a deletion of 5 kb resulting from a nonhomologous crossover between $^G\gamma$ and $^A\gamma$ globin genes, creating a fused γ globin gene having the 5′ end of the $^G\gamma$ globin gene and the 3′ end of the $^A\gamma$ globin gene.[185, 185a] Since the homozygous individual who was studied synthesized chains of the $^A\gamma^T$ type, the crossover in that family must have occurred 5′ to codon 75 in the $^A\gamma$ globin gene, because the polymorphism in which threonine instead of isoleucine is encoded at position 75 of γ globin has been previously identified only in $^A\gamma$ globin chains (see Chapter 7).

Deletion-Type HPFH. Gene mapping studies have revealed the presence of two different forms of gene deletions in the common black type of HPFH, in which both $^G\gamma$ and $^A\gamma$ globin chains of Hb F are actively synthesized ($^G\gamma^A\gamma$ HPFH). In both forms, the δ and β globin genes are totally deleted, but the 5′ and 3′ end points of the deletions differ. In one form, called HPFH-1, the 5′ end point of the deletion is located 3.75 kb to the 5′ side of the δ globin gene,[169, 186, 187] and the 3′ end point is located at a site greater than 60 kb to the 3′ side of the β globin gene.[172, 179] In the second form, called Ghanaian HPFH or HPFH-2, the deletion has a 5′ end point[171, 188, 189] and a 3′ end point[172, 179] that are both displaced by approximately 5 to 6 kb to the 5′ side of the corresponding end points of the HPFH-1 deletion. An individual has also been identified who is doubly heterozygous for both of these forms of HPFH deletions and manifests the same phenotype as individuals who are homozygous for each individual deletion.[172, 179]

These two forms of HPFH constitute two very extensive deletions, involving greater than 70 kb of DNA, that have virtually identical sizes and whose end points are staggered by only 5 to 6 kb. In this regard, it is noteworthy that the first two types of γδβ thalassemia, discussed earlier, also constitute extensive deletions of nearly identical sizes (approximately 100 kb)[179, 180] and with end points that are staggered by only 3 to 6 kb on each side. The implications of these findings with regard to possible molecular mechanisms responsible for the generation of these deletions will be discussed later.

A third deletion is associated with the HPFH phenotype in individuals of Asian Indian ancestry and has been variously referred to as HPFH-3[189a] or Indian (δβ)⁰ thalassemia,[189b] despite pancellular distribution of Hb F. In this case, the 5′ end point of the deletion is slightly 5′ to that of HPFH-2, but the 3′ end point is much more proximal than in the other two HPFH deletions and is located approximately 30 kb 3′ to the β globin gene.[189c]

Nondeletion HPFH. Although the usual variety of HPFH in blacks is associated with deletion of the δ and β globin genes, there are several different rarer subtypes of HPFH, in blacks as well as in other racial groups, that are not associated with β gene deletions and are associated with the synthesis of some β globin chains from the chromosome that bears the HPFH determinant (see Chapter 9 for clinical and hematological aspects). In particular, gene mapping studies have failed to demonstrate the presence of any deletions or rearrangements within the β globin gene cluster in the following syndromes: (1) the Greek type of pancellular HPFH in which $^A\gamma$ chains are predominantly synthesized[186, 189–191]; (2) the black pancellular $^G\gamma\beta^+$ HPFH in which $^G\gamma$ chains are predominantly synthesized[191–193]; (3) the British type of heterocellular HPFH in which $^A\gamma$ chains are predominantly synthesized, but at a much lower level than in Greek-type HPFH[191]; and (4) the Chinese type of HPFH in which $^A\gamma$ chains are predominantly synthesized at a level and in a cellular distribution intermediate between those of the British and Greek types of HPFH.[193]

The precise molecular basis of these nondeletion HPFH syndromes has started to be elucidated through gene cloning and nucleotide sequence analysis of the mutant β gene clusters. In the case of the black $^G\gamma\beta^+$ and Greek types of HPFH, base substitutions have been identified in the 5'-flanking DNA of the genes, which may be responsible for the phenotype (see the section on Gene Cloning).

Gene mapping has also been used to study the linkage of nondeletion forms of heterocellular HPFH to the β gene cluster. This approach analyzes the presence or absence of coinheritance of the HPFH phenotype with a marker for each parental β gene cluster in the form of one or more restriction fragment length polymorphisms such as that created by the polymorphic Hind III sites in the IVS-2 of the γ globin genes (see Chapter 7 and section on Gene Cloning, below). Using this technique, it was shown that the British type of heterocellular HPFH was tightly linked to the β globin gene cluster.[194] In the study of an Asian Indian family with the Swiss type of heterocellular HPFH, in which there is synthesis of relatively low levels of Hb F of both $^G\gamma$ and $^A\gamma$ types, tight linkage of HPFH to the β gene cluster was also demonstrated.[194] However, in this family, in which very good genetic evidence indicated linkage of the heterocellular HPFH trait to a β^S globin gene, a crossover apparently occurred in one individual who inherited the paternal β^S globin gene without the paternal HPFH. Nevertheless, the affected individual inherited the paternal set of polymorphisms corresponding to the chromosome bearing the β^S globin gene, indicating that the heterocellular HPFH determinant in this family was located outside of the immediate β globin gene cluster, that is, either to the 5' side of the ε globin gene or to the 3' side of the β globin gene.[194] In the study of an Italian family with Swiss-type HPFH, different results were obtained that indicated the lack of any linkage, in that particular family, between the heterocellular HPFH determinant and the β globin gene cluster.[195] It would therefore appear that the so-called Swiss type of HPFH is heterogeneous in its molecular basis and in its linkage to the β globin gene cluster. It should also be pointed out that more traditional analyses had previously demonstrated a linkage between Swiss-type HPFH and the β globin gene,[196] but with a recombination rate of approximately 10 per cent in an analysis that probably included mixed genotypes.[197]

Gene mapping studies have also identified a 5' subhaplotype of restriction fragment length polymorphisms in and around the γ genes that is associated with high levels of $^G\gamma$ globin gene expression in patients with sickle cell anemia and β thalassemia.[197a–197d] However, other loci, separate from the β globin gene cluster, also appear to be involved in the regulation of F-cell production in patients with sickle cell anemia.[197e]

A heterocellular type of HPFH, characterized by Hb F levels of 5 to 8 per cent and a $^G\gamma$:$^A\gamma$ ratio of 0.4:0.6, has been found to be associated with a chromosomal translocation involving the short arm of chromosome 11.[197f] However, gene mapping studies have failed to reveal any deletions or rearrangements in the immediate β gene cluster of affected individuals.

Effect of Gene Deletions on γ Globin Gene Expression. The different extents of the gene deletions in δβ thalassemia and HPFH allow one to construct hypothetical models to explain the different effects of the mutations on the levels and patterns of Hb F synthesis that occur in these syndromes and to attempt to understand possible factors that regulate the fetal-to-adult hemoglobin switch in normal individuals. As previously stated, in HPFH, Hb F synthesis occurs at a high level in all erythroid cells, whereas in δβ thalassemia, Hb F synthesis occurs at a lower level and in a heterocellular fashion.

Possible Control Sequences in Inter-γδ Gene DNA at 5' End Point of Deletions. Huisman and associates[198] first proposed the existence of hypothetical control genes situated between the globin genes that might regulate the extent and level of Hb F synthesis in normal persons and in different hemoglobinopathies. One such hypothetical control element is represented by C in Figure 8–18. This neonatal "switch" gene would have two possible functions in the perinatal period: (1) suppression of the activity of the γ globin genes and (2) activation of the β (and δ) globin genes. Deletion of this gene or control element could theoretically lead to the HPFH phenotype because its absence would

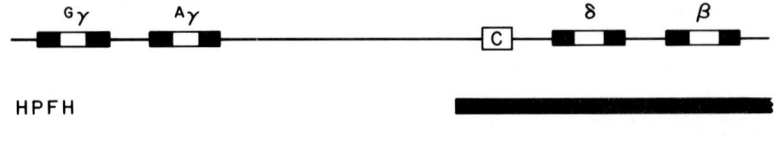

Figure 8–18. Model for putative control region (C) in the inter-γδ globin gene DNA. See text for detailed description of the model.

allow γ globin gene activity to continue uninhibited. In fact, one particular genetic syndrome, Hb Kenya, strongly supports the presence of such a control element between the ^Aγ and δ globin genes. Hb Kenya contains a non-α globin chain that consists of a fused (or hybrid) γβ globin chain. It presumably arose by nonhomologous crossover between the ^Aγ and β globin genes (see Chapter 10 and Fig. 10–7), and thus, all of the normal inter-γδ gene DNA is deleted in this condition, as recently confirmed by gene mapping studies.[199] The fascinating feature about Hb Kenya is that the condition is associated with a HPFH phenotype, thus giving credence to a possible function of the inter-γδ gene DNA in the control of γ globin gene expression.

The results of gene mapping studies summarized in Figure 8–17 provide additional support for the model proposed above, at least in the case of the usual forms of HPFH and the common variety of Mediterranean δβ thalassemia (Sicilian δβ thalassemia) (see Fig. 8–18). In both HPFH-1 and HPFH-2, the deletion of δ and β globin genes is complete and extends into the inter-γδ gene DNA and could thus encompass a hypothetical inter-γδ control element, whereas in Sicilian δβ thalassemia, the deletion stops within the δ gene and leaves the hypothetical control element intact and capable of suppressing γ gene activity.[169, 171, 186–189]

It should be noted that the inter-γδ gene DNA that is deleted in both HPFH-1 and HPFH-2 contains a pair of inverted repetitive DNA sequences of the Alu I family[200] (see Chapter 7). Such sequences are transcribed (at least *in vitro*) by RNA polymerase III to yield low–molecular weight RNA species of as yet unknown function.[200, 201] In HPFH-2 and HPFH-3, both Alu I repetitive DNA sequences are deleted, whereas in HPFH-1, the 5' deletion end point occurs at the midpoint of the 5' (leftward) member of the pair[187] and thereby removes all but one half of one Alu I sequence (Fig. 8–19), which would presumably be rendered inactive by the disruption of its structure. It is difficult to avoid speculating that these repetitive DNA elements may, in some as yet undefined manner, be involved in the control of normal γ globin gene expression and, when deleted or inactivated, contribute to the HPFH phenotype. Certainly, this pair of Alu I repetitive DNA sequences is not deleted in Sicilian δβ thalassemia. In the case of Spanish δβ thalassemia,[171, 175] the deletion does involve a portion of the DNA flanking the 5' end of the δ gene, but its 5' end point occurs within the 3' (rightward) member of the pair of Alu I repetitive DNA sequences, deleting that member almost entirely but leaving the leftward member and all of the inter-Alu DNA completely intact (see Fig. 8–19). If only the 5' end points of these deletions are considered, it must be concluded that the crit-

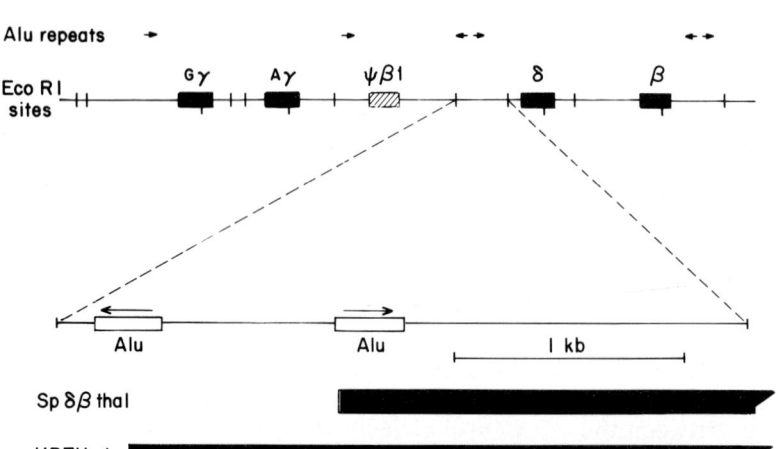

Figure 8–19. Different 5' end points of the HPFH-1 and Spanish (Sp) δβ-thalassemia deletions. (From Collins, F. S., and Weissman, S. M.: Prog. Nucl. Acids Res. Mol. Biol. *31*:315, 1984.)

ical region of DNA perhaps responsible for the difference in HPFH versus δβ-thalassemia phenotype is narrowed down to the 1 kb of DNA, including the leftward Alu sequence and the inter-Alu DNA, that is deleted in HPFH-1 but retained in Spanish δβ thalassemia (see Fig. 8–19).

The findings in the various types of $^G\gamma(^A\gamma\delta\beta)^0$-thalassemia deletions, however, cast doubt on this theory because the presumed control region of DNA is deleted in these syndromes but the phenotype is nevertheless δβ thalassemia and not HPFH, as would be predicted by the model just described. In the case of the Asian Indian $^G\gamma(^A\gamma\delta\beta)^0$-thalassemia (see Fig. 8–17), the DNA of interest is not deleted but is rearranged in an inverted orientation that could be expected to affect the function of those sequences. The various $^G\gamma(^A\gamma\delta\beta)^0$-thalassemia syndromes have in common a complete or partial deletion of the $^A\gamma$ globin gene (hence the $^G\gamma$ phenotype), and the proponents of the inter-γδ control DNA model would propose that two functional γ globin genes are required for the HPFH phenotype to result from deletions or inactivation of the hypothetical control element. This contention is supported somewhat by the findings in the Hb Kenya syndrome. In Hb Kenya, the $^A\gamma$ globin gene is not intact and therefore is not capable of producing normal $^A\gamma$ globin chains, but the $^A\gamma\beta$ fusion gene is functional and its output is approximately equal to that of the linked $^G\gamma$ globin gene. The parameters of γ or γ-like globin gene dosage and output in the Hb Kenya syndrome are therefore more similar to those present in the $^G\gamma^A\gamma$ HPFH syndromes than in the $^G\gamma(^A\gamma\delta\beta)^0$ thalassemias.

The findings in the more recently described Greek type of $^G\gamma^A\gamma(\delta\beta)^0$ thalassemia[177g] are even more difficult to reconcile with the model of inter-γδ control DNA. In this mutation, both γ globin genes are intact and there is a relatively discrete deletion of the hypothetical inter-γδ control region. Nevertheless, the associated phenotype is not that of HPFH, as would be predicted by the model; the heterozygotes in fact manifest little or no increase in Hb F levels.[177g]

In summary, the conclusions with regard to models of γ globin gene control that can be drawn from the comparison of the 5' end points of deletions causing δβ thalassemia and HPFH are as follows:

1. In the situation in which one of the γ globin genes is totally or partially deleted, and therefore nonfunctional, deletion of inter-γδ globin gene sequences is not associated with the HPFH phenotype.

2. In the situation in which two γ (or γ-like) globin genes are intact or functional *in cis* to a deletion, there is no single unifying model that is compatible with all of the deletion syndromes. Although the deletion of 1½ or both of the Alu I repetitive DNA sequences in the 5'-flanking DNA of the δ gene initially appeared to be consistently associated with an HPFH phenotype, the recently reported Greek $^G\gamma^A\gamma\,(\delta\beta)^0$ thalassemia[177g] constitutes a definite exception to the rule.

Therefore, as additional mutations have accumulated, the model for the control of γ globin gene expression by inter-γδ gene DNA sequences, which was supported by some of the initially characterized deletion mutants, has become more and more difficult to rationalize.

Role of Deletion Size and Nature of DNA Sequences at 3' End Point of Deletions. Hypotheses concerning the molecular mechanisms by which deletions in the non-α globin gene cluster cause HPFH rather than δβ thalassemia have more recently focused on differences in the total lengths and 3' end points of the deletions. In many of the δβ thalassemias, the 3' end points of the deletions are located relatively close to the 3' end of the β globin gene in contrast to the two types of HPFH in blacks where the 3' end points are located greater than 60 kb away from the β globin gene. This observation suggests that the overall length of the deletion may be of importance in generating the HPFH phenotype. It is conceivable, as originally suggested by Bernards and Flavell,[189] that very large deletions, such as those associated with HPFH, disrupt chromatin structure in a manner that results in continued expression of the γ globin genes, whereas the shorter deletions associated with many of the δβ thalassemias have no such effect, or a much lesser effect. It is unlikely, however, that deletion size alone is the critical determinant in causing phenotypic differences associated with the various globin gene deletion syndromes because the Chinese and Spanish δβ thalassemias are associated with deletions of at least the same size as those associated with HPFH[176a, 202, 203] (see Fig. 8–17).

Alternatively, it is possible that the DNA that is brought into the vicinity of the γ globin genes from the region of the 3' end point of the deletion may contain sequences, such as enhancer elements or an actively transcribing domain of DNA, that facilitate constitutive expression of the γ globin genes to which they have become juxtaposed. It has been shown in other systems that enhancer-type elements can function at a distance from a target gene in an orientation-independent manner, that is, from a downstream as well as an upstream position.[204] Although enhancer elements were initially characterized in various viruses, they have recently also been identified in cellular DNA, in particular within intervening sequences of immunoglobulin genes.[205-207] Both HPFH-1 and HPFH-2, having 5' and 3' end points that are staggered by approximately the same distance of 5 to 6 kb, bring in, from the remote 3'β–flanking DNA, common DNA sequences to positions located 10 to 11 kb 3' to the $^A\gamma$ gene and 15 to 16 kb 3' to the $^G\gamma$ gene. *In vitro* tests for enhancer activity have, in fact, demonstrated that the DNA sequences adjacent to the 3' end point of the HPFH-1 deletion are active in enhancing the activity of a bacterial gene in a gene transfer system using mammalian tissue culture cells.[208] In addition, these DNA sequences have been found to be hypomethylated[208a] and to contain a DNAse I hypersensitive site[208b] in erythroid but not in nonerythroid cells. It is therefore conceivable that the region of DNA that is translocated to the vicinity of the γ globin genes in HPFH-1 and HPFH-2 contains a gene that is expressed specifically in erythroid cells and is capable of conferring activity to neighboring genes by some position (or other) effect.

In the case of the Spanish δβ thalassemia, the 3' end point is located at least 7 kb further downstream from that of HPFH-1[202, 203] (see Fig. 8–17). Therefore, this deletion removes the DNA sequences that have the unique properties just described, and a δβ thalassemia rather than HPFH phenotype might be explained by the absence of these sequences from the DNA that is brought into the vicinity of the γ globin genes by the deletion.

The deletion in Chinese δβ thalassemia does not appear, at first glance, to be consistent with the model described above. It has a 3' end point that is located approximately 10 kb to the 5' side of that of HPFH-2 and brings in the same remote sequences, as in HPFH-1 and HPFH-2, to a position approximately 20 kb from the 3' end of the $^G\gamma$ globin gene, without causing HPFH[202] (see Fig. 8–17). It is conceivable that both γ globin genes must be functional in order for the hypothetical enhancer elements or other active DNA sequences to generate the HPFH phenotype, and that the partial deletion of the $^A\gamma$ globin gene in the Chinese $^G\gamma(^A\gamma\delta\beta)^0$ thalassemia would prevent this from occurring. Alternatively, the Chinese δβ thalassemia could also be bringing in sequences (absent in the HPFH deletions) that interfere with the action of the hypothetical HPFH-inducing sequences, or there could be some subtle effects of position and distance due to the additional 5 kb of DNA separating the $^G\gamma$ globin gene from these hypothetical sequences. The additional DNA sequences brought in by the Chinese δβ thalassemia do in fact contain a peculiar retrovirus-like structure[176a] that might interfere with the function of any active DNA sequences located downstream to it.

In the Indian type of HPFH (HPFH-3), the 3' end point of the deletion is much more proximal than in HPFH-1 and HPFH-2 (see Fig. 8–17) and thus brings in different downstream sequences to the vicinity of the γ globin genes. The precise molecular basis for the HPFH phenotype in this case is therefore likely to be different from that in HPFH-1 and HPFH-2. It should be pointed out, finally, that the phenotypes of δβ thalassemia and HPFH form a continuum in which there is a certain overlap. Thus, HPFH-3 has been designated by some as a form of δβ thalassemia because of the presence of hypochromia and slight imbalance of globin-chain synthesis in heterozygotes;[177] and also the interaction of one type of δβ thalassemia with the $β^S$ gene results in a phenotype similar to HPFH with pancellular distribution of Hb F.[177]

In conclusion, it is difficult to pick a single hypothesis that convincingly stands out among the others in explaining the molecular mechanisms responsible for the differential effects on γ globin gene expression of the different globin gene deletion syndromes. It is conceivable that different effects caused by the deletions on chromatin structure and configuration are involved, but currently, such phenomena are very difficult to study experimentally.

Gene Mapping Studies in the α-Thalassemia Syndromes

The application of globin gene mapping to the study of the α thalassemias greatly advanced our knowledge of α globin gene structure and organization in these syndromes. In particular, the technique of gene mapping was used to look at questions concerning α globin gene deletions that could not be answered by globin gene analysis using quantitation by molecular hybridization assays in solution. These included (1) identification of individuals with the deletion of only one out of four α globin

THE THALASSEMIAS: MOLECULAR PATHOGENESIS

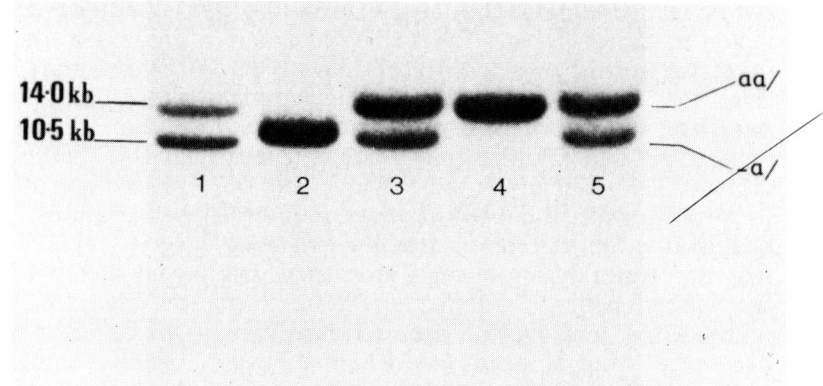

Figure 8–20. Alpha globin gene mapping results in various α-thalassemia syndromes. Total cellular DNA was digested with the restriction endonuclease Bam HI and subjected to the gel blotting procedure of Southern. *1, 3,* and *5,* α Thalassemia 2 heterozygotes. *2,* α Thalassemia 2 homozygote; the same pattern would be observed in a patient with Hb H disease due to double heterozygosity for α thalassemia 2 and the usual variety of α thalassemia 1, although the band would be less intense. *4,* Normal; the same pattern would be observed, although with a less intense band, in patients with Hb H disease due to double heterozygosity for the usual variety of α thalassemia 1 and either Hb Constant Spring or a nondeletion type of α thalassemia 2. (From Weatherall, D. J., and Clegg, J. B.: The Thalassemia Syndromes. 3rd ed. Oxford, Blackwell Scientific Publications, 1981.)

genes; (2) analysis of the extent and end points of α globin gene deletions; (3) differentiation of α globin gene deletions *in trans* from those *in cis;* and (4) reliable identification and characterization of nondeletion types of α thalassemia.

α Thalassemia 2 or α⁺ Thalassemia: One Deleted α Globin Gene Per Chromosome—Designated (– α/). The heterozygous state for deletion of a single α globin gene, or "silent carrier state," can be easily detected by the gene mapping procedure. After digestion with the restriction endonucleases Eco RI or Bam HI and hybridization to an α gene probe, normal DNA with two α globin genes per haploid genome yields a single band of approximately 23 kb with Eco RI and 14 kb with Bam HI (Fig. 8–20). However, DNA from individuals who are obligate carriers for α thalassemia 2 yields, in addition to the normal band, a second shorter band of approximately 19 kb with Eco RI or 10.5 kb with Bam HI (see Fig. 8–20).[209–212] (It should be noted parenthetically that use of Bam HI rather than Eco RI is probably more reliable in detecting the α thalassemia 2 mutation because of the smaller size and greater separation of the fragments and also because a polymorphism creating an Eco RI site has been described[213] that gives a spuriously smaller fragment in the absence of an α-thalassemia deletion.)

Detailed restriction endonuclease mapping of the shorter abnormal α globin gene DNA fragment found in α thalassemia 2 has established that it contains only one of the two α globin genes. By using various restriction endonucleases, two different types of deletions could be defined (Fig. 8–21):

1. A deletion of approximately 3.7 kb, by far the most common, consistent with a deletion created by nonhomologous crossing over between the two α globin gene loci,[210, 214–218] which has been called the "rightward deletion."[214] Gene mapping and mRNA analysis have demonstrated that this mutation is in fact heterogeneous since there are at least three different types of α globin genes associated with it[219]: genes in which the crossover occurred either 5′ to the distal end of IVS-2, within exon 3, or in the distal portion of the

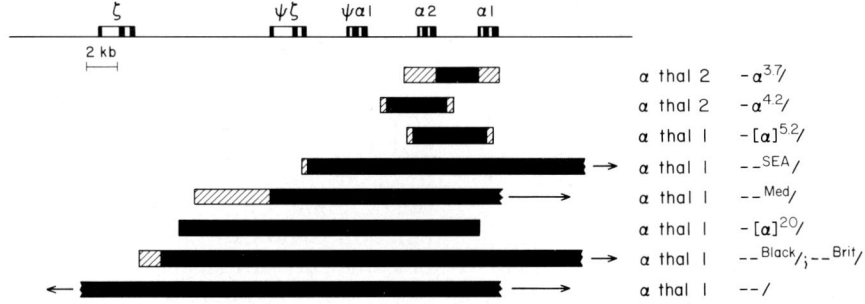

Figure 8–21. Different deletions causing α thalassemia. The cross-hatched bars represent regions where the precise end points of the deletions are indeterminate.

gene corresponding to the far 3'-untranslated region of the α globin mRNA. The first and third types of these α globin genes have been characterized by gene cloning and nucleotide sequence analysis,[219, 219a] as discussed in the section on Gene Cloning that follows. In addition to heterogeneity in the crossover site of the ($-\alpha^{3.7}/$) gene, the locus has been found to be linked to four different restriction fragment length polymorphisms owing either to variation in the length of the hypervariable regions of DNA (V_1 in Fig. 7–9) that is located between the ζ and ψζ genes (see Chapter 7) or to the presence of a single ζ locus.[219b]

2. A deletion of approximately 4.2 kb, consistent with deletion of the 5' or α2 globin gene, which has been called the "leftward deletion."[209, 214]

The rightward deletion was found to constitute a common form of α thalassemia 2 in Asians, those from the Mediterranean area, and blacks,[214–218, 219c, 220] whereas the leftward deletion has been identified essentially only in Asian subjects[214] and very rare black[220a, 220b] individuals.

Homozygosity for α Thalassemia 2 ($-\alpha/-\alpha$) as a Cause of the α Thalassemia 1 Phenotype. When α globin gene mapping was performed using DNA from black individuals with the α thalassemia 1 phenotype (that is, hematologically apparent α-thalassemia "trait"), only a single shorter-than-normal DNA fragment was detected, consistent with the genotype ($-\alpha/-\alpha$). This observation, initially published by Dozy and associates[211] and Higgs and coworkers[212] and subsequently confirmed in a number of different studies,[216, 217, 220–222] confirmed the earlier theories that black individuals with the α thalassemia 1 phenotype carry deletions of two α globin genes in trans ($-\alpha/-\alpha$) (that is, homozygosity for α thalassemia 2), rather than in cis ($--/\alpha\alpha$), as is the case in Asian subjects heterozygous for α thalassemia 1 (see later discussion). These findings therefore provided a definitive explanation for the lack of hydrops fetalis and the rarity of Hb H disease in blacks. Because the α-thalassemic chromosome prevalent in the black population always carries one normal α globin gene ($-\alpha/$), it is impossible for blacks to inherit the genotype found in Asian infants with hydrops fetalis who lack all four α globin genes. The rare cases of Hb H disease in blacks (see later discussion) result from inheritance of the prevalent α-thalassemic chromosome together with a much rarer α-thalassemic chromosome in which both α globin genes are deleted.

Another corollary of the aforementioned findings is that the heterozygous state for α thalassemia 2 must occur extremely frequently in the black population. If the incidence of the α thalassemia 1 phenotype (that is, homozygous α thalassemia 2) is 1 to 2 per cent in the black population, heterozygosity for α thalassemia 2 must approach 30 per cent. In fact, a survey of 211 black American individuals revealed that 27.5 per cent were heterozygous for the α thalassemia 2 genotype ($-\alpha/\alpha\alpha$) and 1.9 per cent were homozygous ($-\alpha/-\alpha$); the overall frequency of the single α globin locus was calculated to be 0.16.[211]

α Thalassemia 1 or α^0 Thalassemia Due to total Deletion of Two α Globin Genes per Chromosome—Designated ($--/$). Gene mapping studies of DNA from hydropic Asian infants with Hb Bart's syndrome have revealed total absence of the 23-kb Eco RI or 14-kb Bam HI DNA fragment that normally hybridizes to α globin gene probes.[173, 209–211, 223–226] DNA from the parents of these hydropic infants and from other Asian individuals with heterozygous α thalassemia 1 yielded a single normal-sized DNA fragment but one of reduced intensity, consistent with the presence of half of the normal α globin gene copy number.[210, 211, 223] These results confirmed that the molecular basis for heterozygous α thalassemia 1 in Asians is the complete deletion of both α globin genes (in cis) on the affected chromosome ($--/$). Results of gene mapping studies in the usual forms of Hb H disease in Asians provided additional confirmation of this conclusion. DNA from individuals with Hb H disease lacking Hb Constant Spring yielded only a single shorter DNA band of the size seen in heterozygous α thalassemia 2, consistent with the genotype ($--/-\alpha$).[209–211, 215] DNA from individuals heterozygous for Hb Constant Spring yielded a qualitatively normal pattern,[227] but with reduced intensity of the normal-sized band. Therefore, individuals with Hb H disease and Hb Constant Spring must have the genotype ($--/\alpha^{CS}\alpha$).

The distance between the 3' end point of the ($--/$) α thalassemia 1 deletion and the α1 gene has not yet been determined, but the 5' end point has been analyzed, and two different deletions have been characterized.[228] The 5' break point of the Southeast Asian (SEA) deletion occurs within a region limited to approximately 450 nucleotides that encompass exon 3 of the ψζ gene[219b] and thereby leaves most of the ψζ gene intact[228] (see Fig. 8–21). The 3' end point of the deletion is separated from the 5' end point by variable amounts of DNA in different individuals. At least seven different variants have been identified. They all share the same precise 5' break point and a common subset of restriction sites in the DNA downstream from the 3' break point. The differences are due to different lengths of intervening hypervariable DNA creating a type of restriction fragment length polymorphism (see Chapter 7). It has not been determined if the hypervariable DNA at the 3' end point of the $(- -^{SEA}/)$ deletion is the same as that normally present 3' to the normal α1 gene (see Fig. 7–9) or if it is derived from DNA normally present further downstream. The seven different subtypes of the mutation could represent polymorphic variants of a single ancestral mutation, or they could conceivably have resulted from separate mutational events. The geographic distribution of the mutation, which is essentially restricted to Southeast Asia, and its conserved 5' break point favor the theory of a single ancestral mutation that subsequently became heterogeneous by recombination events involving a hypervariable region of DNA.

The deletion in one Greek infant[228] and one Cypriot infant[229] with hydrops fetalis was found to have a 5' end point that was located further to the 5' side of that of the Asian deletion, at a point between the ζ and ψζ genes: $(- -^{Med}/)$ (see Fig. 8–21). Because the Mediterranean (Med) deletion completely removes the ψζ gene, without any effect on the production of Hb Portland ($ζ_2γ_2$), the characterization of this deletion provided evidence that the ψζ gene (formerly called ζ1 gene) was nonessential and perhaps nonfunctional before nucleotide sequence analysis demonstrated the presence of a nonsense mutation in the gene.[230]

In rare Asians, the α thalassemia 1 deletion involves the entire α globin gene cluster, including the ζ and ψζ globin genes.[219b, 230a] In the rare black patients with Hb H disease, gene mapping studies have shown the same general pattern as in Asians: a single shorter-than-normal α globin gene DNA fragment consistent with inheritance of the common α thalassemia 2 chromosome from one parent and a rare α thalassemia 1 chromosome, with both α globin genes totally deleted, from the other parent.[215, 231, 232] Gene mapping studies have revealed that the rare α thalassemia 1 deletion (– –/) in blacks is heterogeneous in nature: In some cases the entire α globin gene cluster is deleted, including the ζ and ψζ genes,[233] whereas in others the 5' end point of the deletion is somewhat further to the 5' side of that of the Mediterranean deletion but leaves the ζ gene intact.[234, 234a]

α Thalassemia 1 or $α^0$ Thalassemia Associated with Retention of a Portion of One α Globin Gene—Designated (– [α]/). During the course of gene mapping studies in various Mediterranean patients with Hb H disease, two additional α thalassemia 1 or $α^0$ thalassemia gene deletions were discovered that were characterized by the persistence of a portion of the α1 globin gene on the affected chromosome: (– [α]/) (see Fig. 8–21). In one type of partial deletion, Eco RI digests of DNA from affected individuals yields a new abnormal band of 2.6 kb.[210, 235] Subsequent cloning and sequence analysis of this abnormal α globin gene revealed deletion of the 5' extremity of the α1 globin gene extending up to and including codon 56.[144] The 5' end point of this deletion was initially thought to extend beyond the ζ globin gene,[144] but subsequent studies[236] have indicated that the 5' break point of the deletion occurs between the ζ and ψζ genes and that the overall extent of the deletion is approximately 20 kb $(- [α]^{20}/)$. The overall incidence of this mutation in Mediterranean individuals with Hb H disease is not clear since it was found frequently in one series[210] but infrequently in another series[235] in which the most common genotype in Mediterranean patients with Hb H disease was determined to be the same as in Asians: (– –/– α). The partial deletion associated with the 2.6 kb Eco RI fragment appears to be particularly common in Turkish individuals with Hb H disease.[210, 237]

The other partial deletion of the α globin gene complex leading to α thalassemia 1 was identified in a Greek family.[238] The deletion in this case extended for 5.2 kb and removed the entire α2 globin gene and the 5' end of the α1 globin gene, including the intragenic Hinc II site at codons 96 and 97: $(- [α]^{5.2}/)$ (see Fig. 8–21).

Nondeletion Forms of α Thalassemia: $α^+$ Thalassemia—Designated ($αα^T/$) and ($– α^T/$). Gene mapping studies in patients with Hb H disease from various ethnic groups have identified certain patients in whom α globin gene DNA fragments of normal size are present despite clinical and biochemical evidence of α thalassemia with less α globin–chain production than expected for the number of apparently intact α globin genes present in the affected individuals.

Southeast Asian Nondeletion α Thalassemia. The initial case of Hb H disease with nondeletion α thalassemia, identified by Kan and associates in a Chinese patient by DNA-cDNA hybridization assays in solution,[148] was subsequently shown by gene mapping to have α globin gene DNA fragments of normal size.[209] A nondeletion α thalassemia chromosome was also subsequently identified by gene mapping in a number of additional Asian subjects with Hb H disease[214, 239] associated with the Southeast Asian (SEA) form of α thalassemia 1 ($\alpha\alpha^T/--^{SEA}$).[237] The mutant α globin gene of the original Chinese patient was later cloned and its nucleotide sequence determined[240] (see the section on Gene Cloning). The mutation was shown to consist of a single nucleotide substitution in codon 125 of the α2 globin gene, changing the encoded amino acid from Leu to Pro and resulting in the synthesis of a highly unstable α globin variant[241] that has subsequently been named Hb Quong Sze. The α-thalassemia phenotype in this mutation therefore results from a post-translational phenomenon. Nondeletion forms of α thalassemia have also been detected by gene mapping in individuals from Malaysia[239] and Thailand,[219b] but it is not known if they constitute novel forms of α thalassemia or other examples of the Hb Quong Sze.

Mediterranean Nondeletion α Thalassemia. The analysis of DNA samples from Mediterranean patients with Hb H disease[210, 211, 239] or individuals doubly heterozygous for α thalassemia and the structural variant Hb Hasharon[242] also revealed the unexpected presence of normal-sized, nondeletion, α-thalassemic DNA fragments in a significant number of cases. The nondeletion chromosome in patients with Hb H disease was associated either with the Mediterranean (Med) total-deletion form of α thalassemia 1: ($\alpha\alpha^T/--^{Med}$)[210, 211, 239] or with a partial-deletion form of α thalassemia 1: ($\alpha\alpha^T/-[\alpha]^{20}$).[210]

The molecular basis for one type of Mediterranean nondeletion α thalassemia has been identified by gene cloning and nucleotide sequence analysis.[243] The α2 globin gene from the nondeletion chromosome of an Italian patient was found to have a pentanucleotide deletion involving the 5′ splice junction of IVS-1, thereby preventing normal splicing of α2 globin gene transcripts. This mutation also deletes the recognition site for the restriction endonuclease Hph I and therefore allows detection of the mutation by gene mapping techniques of total cellular DNA. Using this enzyme to analyze DNA from two Turkish patients with nondeletion α thalassemia, it was found that one patient had the same mutation, whereas the other did not.[243] Nondeletion α thalassemia in Mediterranean individuals is therefore heterogeneous in its molecular basis. In fact, most cases of nondeletion α thalassemia in Sardinians have been shown to be due to a base substitution in the initiation codon[243a] (see the section on Gene Cloning).

Saudi Arabian Nondeletion α Thalassemia. Yet another form of nondeletion α thalassemia has been characterized in Saudi Arabia. In this population, Hb H disease results from homozygous inheritance of a nondeletion α-thalassemia chromosome that yields, in gene mapping studies, α globin gene DNA fragments only of normal size: ($\alpha\alpha^T/\alpha\alpha^T$).[239, 244] The α globin genes from affected individuals have been analyzed by gene cloning and nucleotide sequencing[245] (see the section on Gene Cloning). Different mutations were identified in each of the two linked α globin genes: (1) in the α1 globin gene, a single nucleotide deletion at codon 14 results in a frameshift and nonsense mutation, and (2) in the α2 globin gene, a base substitution in the polyadenylation signal of the 3′ untranslated sequence presumably leads to abnormal polyadenylation of the nascent α globin mRNA molecules.[245]

Nondeletion α Thalassemia in Blacks. One case of nondeletion α thalassemia ($\alpha\alpha^T/$) has been identified in a black individual from South Africa,[220] but it is not possible to determine whether it represents a novel form of α thalassemia or one of the mutations also present in one of the other racial groups described previously.

In the analysis of a black family in which the α-chain variant Hb G-Philadelphia and α thalassemia were segregating, gene mapping studies provided evidence for a chromosome bearing a nonfunctional single α globin gene ($-\alpha^T/$) causing α^0 thalassemia.[232, 246] In this family, DNA from a woman with Hb H disease and 100 per cent Hb G yielded a single, shorter-than-normal, α gene DNA fragment consistent with the genotype ($--/-\alpha^G$) or ($-\alpha^T/-\alpha^G$). A half-sibling and an offspring of this individual had the phenotype of α thalassemia 1 without Hb G, and on gene mapping, their DNA yielded both a normal and shorter-than-normal α gene DNA fragment consistent with the genotype ($-\alpha^T/\alpha\alpha$).[232, 246] The child of the proband therefore must have inherited from the mother a chromosome, distinct from the ($-\alpha^G/$) chromosome, bearing a single α gene locus that was nonfunctional.

Other Types of Nondeletion α Thalassemia. Analysis of an Algerian patient with Hb H disease revealed evidence for a ($-\alpha^T/$) genotype causing α^+ thalassemia. The individual with Hb H disease apparently inherited a shorter-than-normal α globin gene DNA fragment of the rightward-deletion type from each parent[218] but had Hb H disease rather than the α thalassemia 1 phenotype, as is the case in black individuals with the genotype ($-\alpha/-\alpha$). The parents, who were first cousins, both manifested a hematologic α-thalassemia phenotype and had a normal offspring who inherited a normal-sized α globin DNA fragment from each parent.[218] The offspring with Hb H disease is therefore presumably homozygous for an α^+ thalassemia of the genotype ($-\alpha^T/-\alpha^T$).

Finally, one should also include in the group of nondeletion α thalassemias the α globin structural variants resulting from chain termination mutations (Hb Constant Spring, Hb Icaria, Hb Koya Dora, and Hb Seal Rock) that are associated with an α-thalassemia phenotype because of markedly decreased synthesis of the variant α chain. Gene mapping studies in affected individuals would also yield α globin gene fragments of normal size. This group of disorders will be discussed later in the section entitled "Structural Variants Associated with Thalassemic Phenotypes."

Molecular Heterogeneity of α-Thalassemia Syndromes. It should be apparent from the previous description of the multiple different molecular defects found to be associated with α thalassemia that the four or so relatively homogeneous clinical α-thalassemia syndromes can result from numerous different interactions between a very large number of different genetic lesions or genotypes. Thus far, there have been identified at least seven different types of α^0 thalassemia (α thalassemia 1) and ten different types of α^+ thalassemia (α thalassemia 2), many of which are genotypically heterogenous (Table 8–1). These multiple different genotypes can theoretically interact to produce more than 100 different genetic combinations, a number of which have in fact already been identified.[219b, 239] For example, Hb H disease can result from the inheritance of any of the five types of α^0 thalassemia together with any of the ten types of α^+ thalassemia, as well as from homozygosity for the Saudi Arabian and Algerian types of α^+ thalassemia. Hydrops fetalis can theoretically result from homozygosity for any of the five types of α^0 thalassemia or from double heterozygosity for any two of the five types of α^0 thalassemia.

The α thalassemias clearly illustrate the well-known genetic phenomenon that a relatively homogeneous clinical entity can result from a wide variety of different genotypes. The same observation applies to the molecular diversity of β^0 thalassemia and β^+ thalassemia uncovered by gene cloning and nucleotide sequence analysis, which will be discussed later (see the section on Gene Cloning).

α Globin Gene Deletions Linked to Genes for α Globin Structural Variants. A number of α globin chain structural variants are found at unexpectedly high levels in red cells of

Table 8–1. DIFFERENT TYPES OF α THALASSEMIA

Phenotype and Mutation	Racial Group	Reference(s)
A. α thalasemia 1 or α^0 thalassemia		
1. ($-\ -^{SEA}/$) (7 polymorphic variants)	Southeast Asian	219b, 228
2. ($-\ -^{Med}/$)	Mediterranean	228, 229
3. ($-\ -^{Black}/$); ($-\ -^{Brit}/$)	Black, British	234, 234a, 460
4. ($-\ -/$)	Southeast Asian, black[1]	219b, 230a
5. ($-[\alpha]^{5.2}/$)	Mediterranean	238
6. ($-[\alpha]^{20}/$)	Mediterranean	144, 236
7. ($-\alpha^T/$)	Black	232, 246
B. α thalasemia-2 or α^+ thalassemia		
1. ($-\alpha^{3.7}/$) (3 types + variants in Table 8–2; 4 polymorphic variants)	Southeast Asian, black, Mediterranean	214–219c
2. ($-\alpha^{4.2}/$) (1 type + variant in Table 8–2)	Southeast Asian (rare black)	209, 214, 219b
3. Hb Constant Spring (3 polymorphic variants)	Southeast Asian	219b, 417
4. Hb Icaria	Mediterranean	418
5. Hb Koya Dora	Asian Indian	419
6. Hb Seal Rock	Black	420
7. Hb Quong Sze	Southeast Asian	240, 241
8. Mediterranean nondeletion (3 types)	Mediterranean	243, 243a, 459
9. Saudi Arabian nondeletion	Saudi Arabian	244, 245
10. Black nondeletion	Black	220

Deletion of the entire α-gene cluster is also associated with some cases of the mental retardation/acquired Hb H disease syndrome in Northern Europeans.[261, 262a]

affected individuals or interact with α thalassemia 1 to produce Hb H disease and, therefore, were long suspected of being associated with a deletion of the linked normal α globin gene on the same chromosome.[5] Gene mapping procedures have provided a definitive method of confirming the presence or absence of α globin gene deletions linked to the various α globin structural variants.[246–255] Table 8–2 lists the various α-chain variants studied in this way and the results of the analysis.

It is apparent from Table 8–2 that a number of α-chain variants occur on α thalassemia 2 chromosomes where the structural variant constitutes the single α globin gene locus. It is impossible to determine if the mutation causing the structural variant occurred on a pre-existing α thalassemia 2 chromosome or if the recombination event generating the α-thalassemic chromosome involved a chromosome that initially carried the variant α locus as well as a normal α locus. In any event, the occurrence of the variant on an α-thalassemic chromosome provided a mechanism for selection by malaria, leading to a high incidence of the variant in appropriate populations.

An unexpected observation was made in the case of an individual with Hb I. Analysis of the individual's globin mRNA indicated that α^I chains were encoded by both α1 and α2 mRNAs, indicating that both α genes on the affected chromosome were mutated.[255b] Because it is extremely unlikely that the same mutation would occur independently in two linked α globin genes, it is assumed that an intrachromosomal gene conversion event occurred that transferred the base substitution of one mutated gene to its linked previously normal partner.

Gene Mapping Studies in Acquired Hb H Disease. There are two distinct syndromes in which Hb H disease occurs as an acquired manifestation in association with a second disorder: in myeloproliferative disorders such as erythroleukemia or acute leukemia and in association with mental retardation.[256]

Hb H Disease Associated with Myeloproliferative Disorders. Hb H disease in association with a myeloproliferative disorder such as erythroleukemia or acute myeloid leukemia usually occurs in elderly men.[257] As noted previously in the section on molecular hybridization assays, this syndrome is associated with markedly reduced amounts of α globin mRNA,[150, 257–259] with levels frequently lower than those in the hereditary form of the disease. In one case,[257] bone marrow RNA had as low a level of α globin mRNA as reticulocyte RNA, suggesting the presence of a transcriptional rather than a post-transcriptional defect. At the level of the α globin genes themselves, hybridization assays revealed a normal copy number of α globin genes in hematopoietic cells of affected individuals.[150, 258] Detailed gene mapping studies have also failed to reveal any abnormality of α globin gene structure or organization in this syndrome.[257, 259] In fact, in one case, there was triplication of one α gene locus,[257] but this phenomenon is known to occur without causing any major effect on α globin gene expression (see later discussion).

The precise cause of the abnormal α globin gene expression in this syndrome is not known. It is possible that the small amount of α globin mRNA is derived exclusively from the small number of residual normal erythroid cells and that the progeny of the neoplastic hematopoietic stem cells have four totally inactive α globin genes. Alternatively, all four affected α globin genes may be markedly hypofunctional.[257, 259]

The α globin mRNA that is present contains the normal ratio of transcripts from the two different (α1 and α2) globin genes, and the α globin genes in affected bone marrow cells appear to be normally hypomethylated when analyzed by the appropriate restriction endonucleases in gene mapping experiments.[259] It is difficult to conceive of the type of acquired mutation that would inactivate or render hypofunctional all four α globin genes on two

Table 8–2. α GLOBIN GENOTYPES ASSOCIATED WITH α-CHAIN STRUCTURAL VARIANTS

Variant		Genotype	Reference(s)
Hb G-Philadelphia:	α 68 Asn→Lys	$(-\alpha^{3.7}/)$ and $(\alpha\alpha/)$	246–248b
Hb Hasharon:	α 47 Asp→His	$(-\alpha^{3.7}/)$	249, 250
Hb Q:	α 74 Asp→His	$(-\alpha^{4.2}/)$	251–253
Hb G:	α 30 Glu→Gln	$(\alpha\alpha/)$	252
Hb J-Tongariki:	α 115 Ala→Asp	$(-\alpha^{3.7}/)$	254
Hb J-Mexico:	α 54 Gln→Glu	$(\alpha\alpha/)$	255
Hb Evanston:	α 14 Trp→Arg	$(-\alpha^{3.7}/)$	255a
HbI:	α 16 Lys→Glu	$(\alpha\alpha/)$	255b

different chromosomes. Any major DNA rearrangements or deletions, if present, must be remote from the α globin gene cluster, because they escaped detection with the α and ζ gene probes. Any acquired *cis*-acting mutations would also need to have occurred independently on both α gene chromosomes or to have been transmitted from one chromosome to the other by some type of mitotic recombination event such as gene conversion.

Hybrid cell lines of mouse erythroleukemia cells containing only one or the other chromosome 16 from affected human hematopoietic cells express normal levels of human α globin mRNA after chemical induction of hemoglobin synthesis,[260] indicating that the α globin genes from hematopoietic cells of affected individuals can function normally in a new environment. These results suggest that the abnormal α globin gene expression in this syndrome is mediated by a mechanism involving a *trans*-acting factor: either lack (or malfunction) of a specific factor required for α globin gene expression or the presence of a factor capable of suppressing α globin gene expression. A similar situation seems to occur in the case of the absent β globin gene expression in K562 erythroleukemia cells, as discussed in Chapter 7.

Hb H Disease in Association with Mental Retardation. In the original report of this syndrome,[261] three unrelated families of Northern European ancestry were described in which a child with Hb H disease and mental retardation had one parent with typical α thalassemia 2 ($α^+$ thalassemia), whereas the second parent was completely normal. Gene mapping studies revealed that the α thalassemia 2 in one family was of the rightward deletion type ($-α/$) whereas in the other two families, it was of a nondeletion type.[261] In the affected patient from the first family, gene mapping confirmed the genotype ($-α/--$), indicating that the patient had inherited the α thalassemia 2 gene from the mother and a spontaneous deletion ($--/$) that must have occurred in the germ cell from the normal father (paternity could not be excluded by the usual means). The deletion chromosome ($--/$) was different from that found in the usual hereditary form of α thalassemia 1; the deletion was more extensive and involved the entire α globin gene cluster, including the ζ globin gene.[261] However, no visible deletion was detected by karyotyping. In the other two families, no abnormalities were noted on gene mapping, and in one of the cases, because of the presence of polymorphisms, it could be shown that both α gene chromosomes were intact in the affected patient.[261] A number of additional cases of this syndrome were subsequently identified,[256, 262] including a case[262a] that by gene mapping was very similar to the one in the first family described previously. In yet another family of Northern European ancestry,[263] a child with multiple congenital abnormalities but no clearcut mental retardation inherited Hb H disease with the genotype ($-α/--$), but the parents were heterozygous for α thalassemia 2 (rightward deletion [$-α/αα$]) and α thalassemia 1 ($--/αα$), respectively. The molecular basis of this unusual syndrome is therefore heterogeneous. Its significance is that near the α globin gene cluster on chromosome 16, there appears to exist a locus or loci that, when spontaneously mutated, or codeleted with the α gene cluster, can lead to mental retardation together with α thalassemia.

Mechanisms Involved in Generation of Globin Gene Deletions

Analysis of the extent and end points of various deletions in the globin gene clusters has permitted the elaboration of theories concerning possible molecular mechanisms involved in the generation of these deletions.

α Globin Gene Deletions. As mentioned previously, the common form of α thalassemia 2 ($-α^{3.7}/$) can be best explained by nonhomologous crossing over between the two α globin gene loci after mispairing of homologous chromosomes during meiosis, as illustrated in Figure 8–22. The gene mapping data are totally consistent with such a phenomenon,[214, 215] and have indicated that at least three different types of crossover events have occurred between the α1 and α2 genes,[219] a conclusion that has been further confirmed by cloning and nucleotide sequence analysis of mutant α-thalassemic genes.[219, 219a] All three crossovers occurred within the homologous segment Z (see Fig. 7–9). If the crossover theory is correct, the reciprocal product of the crossover event, a chromosome bearing three α globin gene loci, should be observed in certain individuals (see Fig. 8–22). Such is indeed the case in a number of different populations.[232, 264–266] The frequency of triplicated α loci is quite low, ranging between 0.004 in Sardinians and American blacks and 0.05 in Greek Cypriots.[264] The frequency of the triplicated α locus would

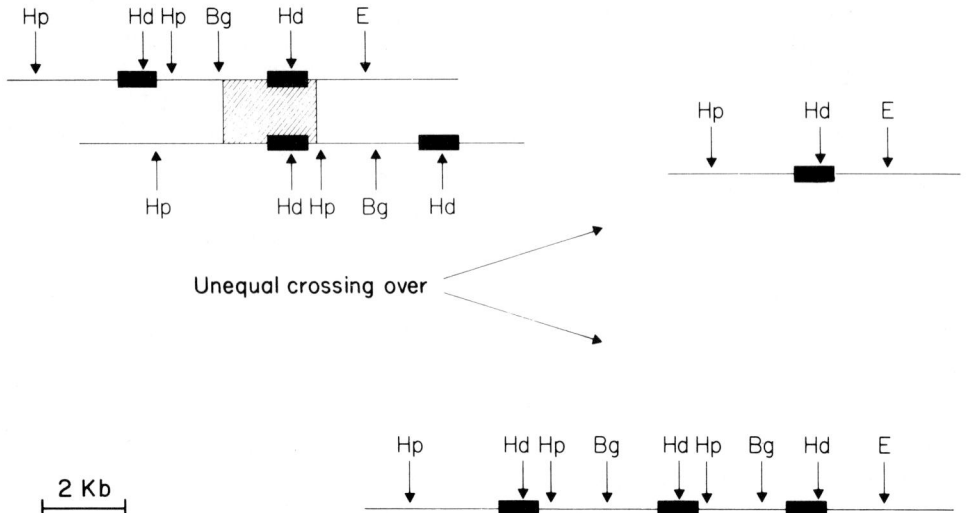

Figure 8–22. Model of unequal crossing over between two normal α globin gene clusters to generate chromosomes bearing the α thalassemia 2 "rightward" deletion ($-\alpha^{3.7}/$) and its reciprocal triple α gene locus. (Modified from Weatherall, D. J., and Clegg, J. B.: The Thalassemia Syndromes. 3rd ed. Oxford, Blackwell Scientific Publications, 1981.)

not be expected to be as high as that of the α thalassemia 2 chromosome because of the usual lack of an α-thalassemic phenotype associated with the former and therefore the lack of selection for it by malaria. The triplicated α locus has also been identified in populations in whom α thalassemia is rare.[265] An interesting feature of the triplicated α locus is the observation that its output of α globin chains usually appears to be equal to that of the normal duplicated α locus,[264, 266] although there seems to be an excess of α globin mRNA in some patients.[265] However, the hematologic phenotype associated with a triplicated locus is variable, suggesting the presence of some genotypic heterogeneity that leads to different levels of α globin gene expression in different individuals; some triplicated loci are associated with levels of α globin–chain synthesis that are clearly above normal,[266a–266d] whereas others are paradoxically associated with decreased α-chain synthesis and an α-thalassemia phenotype.[266e]

Analysis of the α globin gene cluster has revealed, in addition to the structural genes themselves, the presence of homologous stretches of flanking or intergene DNA sequences that could serve as foci for nonhomologous crossing over or recombination[267] (see Fig. 7–9). Indeed, when recombinant DNA bacteriophages containing the cloned normal human α globin gene cluster are grown in culture, recombination frequently occurs, generating deletions of a nature very similar to those observed in the naturally occurring thalassemias.[267] In addition to the expected rightward deletion, the leftward deletion ($-\alpha^{4.2}/$) is also observed.[267] It appears that this deletion occurred by nonhomologous crossing over between misaligned homologous sequences (block X in Fig. 7–9) located in the 3'-flanking DNA of the α2 globin gene and similar sequences located in the 3'-flanking DNA of the ψα1 gene (Fig. 8–23). The reciprocal product of such a crossover would also generate a triplicated α globin gene locus with a distinctive restriction endonuclease map different from that of the previously described triplicated locus (see Fig. 8–22). Such a triplicated locus has in fact been identified in a Chinese individual[268] and a Saudi Arabian individual.[269]

A third crossover event leading to yet another novel triplicated locus has been described in a black individual.[269a] In this case, the crossover event appears to have occurred in the region of the Alu I repetitive sequences located approximately 1 kb 3' to the α2 and α1 genes (see Fig. 7–9). The reciprocal α thalassemia 2 product of this crossover event has not yet been reported.

Deletions in the Non–α Globin Gene Cluster. There is an example of a gene deletion in the non-α gene cluster that probably resulted from nonhomologous crossing over between the two homologous linked γ globin genes, in a fashion similar to that described for α thalassemia 2. This deletion, identified in Asian subjects,[185, 185a] produces a γ thalassemia which, in the homozygous state, is associated with the synthesis of only $^A\gamma$ globin chains (see preceding discussion). The crossover in the two fam-

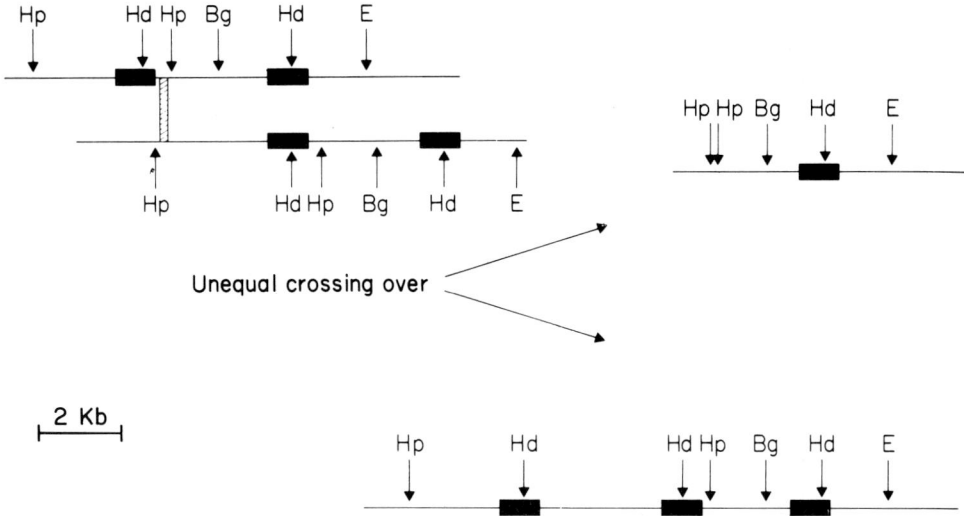

Figure 8–23. Model of unequal crossing over to generate chromosomes bearing the α thalassemia 2 "leftward" deletion (−α$^{4.2}$/) and its reciprocal triple α gene locus. (Modified from Weatherall, D. J., and Clegg, J. B.: The Thalassemia Syndromes. 3rd ed. Oxford, Blackwell Scientific Publications, 1981.)

ilies studied occurred 5′ to codon 75 of the $^Aγ$ globin gene. The reciprocal product of this crossover should consist of a triplicated γ locus with two $^Gγ$ genes and one $^Aγ$ gene. Such a chromosome has in fact been identified in subjects from the New Hebrides Islands.[270]

With regard to the large deletions associated with γδβ thalassemia, HPFH, and some forms of δβ thalassemia, certain observations raise the possibility for the involvement of a different mechanism in the generation of the deletion. The remarkable fact that two different γδβ-thalassemia deletions have respective sizes similar to one another, as do, respectively, the HPFH-1, HPFH-2, and the Chinese $^Gγ$-($^Aγδβ$)^0-thalassemia deletions (see Fig. 8–17), has led Vanin and associates[179] to speculate that these large deletions occurred during the course of a phenomenon thought to take place during normal DNA replication. It is known that chromatin is associated at different points with an intranuclear filamentous structure called the nuclear matrix[271–274] and that loops of chromatin radiate out from these attachment points. Furthermore, it is thought that the loops of chromatin move through the attachment points during replication like a cable through a reel.[274] It is possible that the large deletions in the non–α cluster represent deletions of an entire chromatin loop, with rejoining of the DNA at the attachment points of the DNA to the nuclear matrix, which would constitute the 5′ and 3′ end points of the deletions. Thus, the deletions would be of the same length (equal to one chromatin loop length), but the end points would differ according to what particular region of DNA was attached to the matrix during its movement through the matrix "reel" at the time of the deletion event (Fig. 8–24). This hypothesis is quite attractive but will be difficult to verify experimentally. If it is determined that the two sets of γδβ-thalassemia and HPFH/δβ-thalassemia deletions are of identical overall lengths (which is not yet known), the hypothesis of Vanin and coworkers[179] will be considerably strengthened.

Involvement of Repetitive DNA Sequences in Globin Gene Deletions. The genome of human as well as other mammalian cells contains DNA sequences that are repeated a large number of times throughout the cellular DNA (see Chapter 7). One type of such interspersed repetitive DNA element consists of the Alu I family of repetitive DNA sequences, so called because of the presence at their midpoint of a recognition site for the restriction endonuclease Alu I. These sequences, approximately 300 nucleotides in length, are repeated from 300,000 to 500,000 times in the genome, accounting for approximately 5 per cent of the total cellular DNA.[201] Alu I family repetitive sequences share approximately 80 per cent homology and are frequently found in the vicinity of single copy genes, including the globin genes (see Chapter 7 and Figs. 7–9 and 7–10).

The end points of at least three different globin gene deletion events are found within a repetitive DNA sequence of the Alu I family: (1) the 5′ end point of the HPFH-1 deletion[187] (see Fig. 8–19), (2) the 5′ end point of the

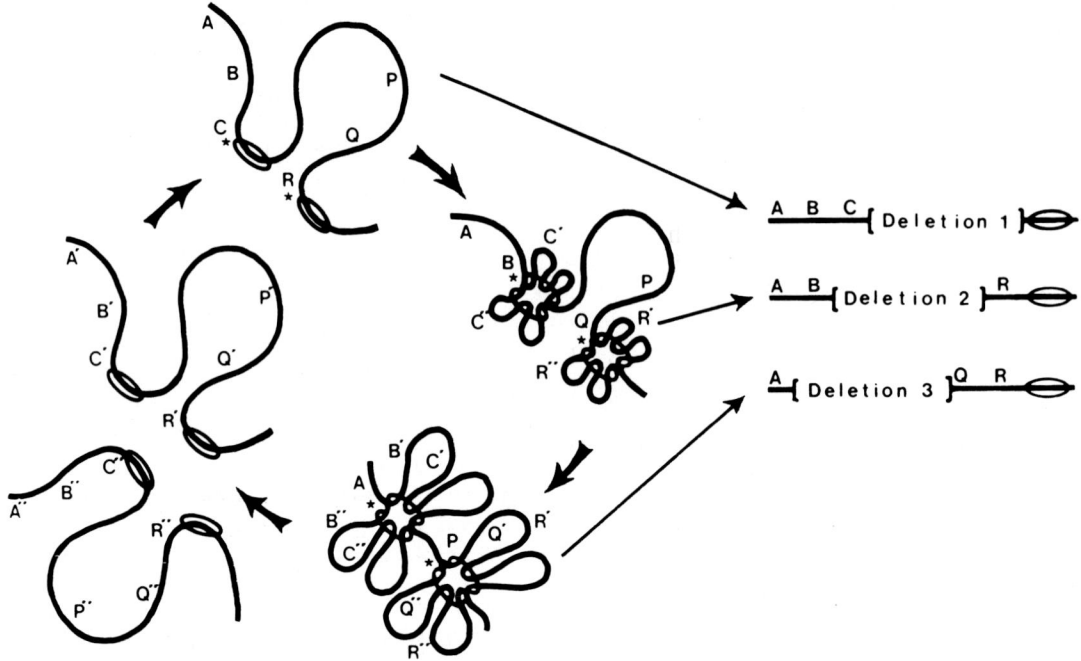

Figure 8–24. Model of possible mechanism for generation of large deletions of approximately the same size but having different staggered end points. The model proposes loss of chromatin loops at different stages of DNA replication as the chromatin moves through attachment sites (ellipses) on the nuclear matrix. Breakage and reunion points are indicated by asterisks. (From Vanin, E. F., et al.: Cell 35:701, 1983.)

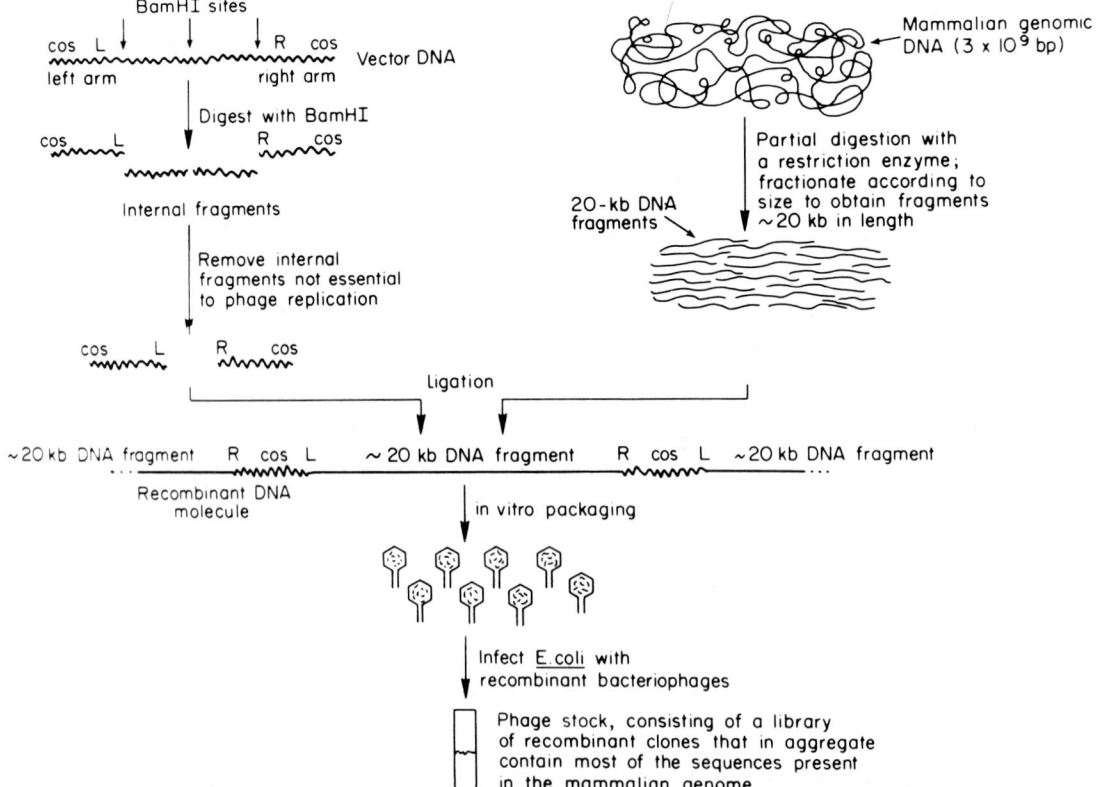

Figure 8–25. Outline of the procedure for constructing recombinant DNA libraries of total cellular DNA in bacteriophage lambda. (From Maniatis, T., et al.: Molecular Cloning. Cold Spring Harbor, New York, Cold Spring Harbor Laboratory, 1983.)

Spanish δβ thalassemia[175] (see Fig. 8–19), and (3) the 5' end point of the partial α1 globin gene deletion $(-[\alpha]^{20}/)$ found in Mediterranean[236] (see Fig. 8–21). Also, as previously noted, one of the three types of triplicated α locus chromosomes presumably arose by recombination between two Alu I family sequences in the α gene cluster.[269a]

It is possible that because of their high degree of homology and ubiquitous interspersion, Alu I repetitive sequences serve as "hot spots" for recombination. However, there is no evidence in the three cases cited earlier that recombination occurred between two different Alu I sequences. On the contrary, in the case of the HPFH-1 and $(-[\alpha]^{20}/)$ deletions, the recombination occurred between an Alu I sequence and nonrepetitive DNA, a so-called illegitimate recombination event.[172] It is more likely that Alu I repetitive DNA sequences occur at the end points of various globin gene deletions by chance alone owing to their abundance in the genome. Nevertheless, there is one example of a deletion involving the gene for the low-density lipoprotein receptor in which Alu-Alu recombination did occur.[274a]

CHARACTERIZATION OF THALASSEMIC GLOBIN GENES BY GENE CLONING, NUCLEOTIDE SEQUENCE ANALYSIS, AND EXPRESSION STUDIES IN GENE TRANSFER SYSTEMS

The definitive identification of the precise molecular defects in nondeletion forms of α and β thalassemia has been made possible in recent years by the advances of recombinant DNA technology that have allowed the isolation of thalassemic globin genes by cloning in *E. coli* bacterial cells. Once the mutant genes were isolated by cloning, their fine structure was determined by DNA sequencing using new rapid sequencing techniques. In some cases, the nucleotide sequence revealed obvious abnormalities to explain the abnormal pattern of expression of the thalassemic gene. However, in other cases, structure-function relationships needed to be established by studying the functional expression of the cloned thalassemic globin genes in an *in vitro* expression system, usually after transfer into tissue culture cells.

Principles of the Technology

Gene Cloning by Recombinant DNA Technology. Recombinant DNA technology consists of the procedures used to construct hybrid or recombinant DNA molecules that contain genetic information derived from different sources, for instance, a hybrid molecule containing both human and bacterial DNA sequences. The vector molecule used is the circular DNA of a bacterial plasmid or bacteriophage that has the ability to replicate independently within bacterial cells. With the use of various restriction endonucleases (see earlier discussion), these DNA molecules can be cleaved at a single site that does not interrupt a vital function, and foreign DNA, digested with the same endonuclease to generate complementary overhanging "sticky ends," can then be inserted and ligated into the vector molecule, as illustrated in Figure 8–25. The recombined DNA molecules can then be introduced into bacterial cells, where the vector molecule will replicate extrachromosomally, generating multiple copies of the vector together with its linked foreign passenger DNA.[275]

In a standard gene cloning experiment, total cellular DNA, digested with the appropriate enzymes, will be ligated to similarly digested bacteriophage DNA. The recombinant bacteriophage DNA is "packaged" *in vitro*, by incubation with extracts containing phage structural proteins, in order to produce infectious bacteriophage particles. *E. coli* bacteria are then infected with the phage and grown on culture plates at a density that will lead to the formation of discrete plaques, each resulting from a single infectious event with lysis of the host bacteria. On the average, one bacterial cell will be infected with only one bacteriophage, so that each plaque contains multiple copies of a single different recombinant bacteriophage with its own particular segment of foreign human DNA. Thus, one to two million bacteriophage plaques, which can be accommodated on a reasonable number of large Petri dishes, can contain DNA fragments spanning the entire human genome. Such a representative collection of recombinant bacteriophages is called a "library."

The one bacteriophage out of several hundred thousand that contains a single copy gene of interest, such as a β globin gene, can be identified by the technique of screening using filter hybridization. A contact imprint of the Petri dish containing the bacteriophage plaques is made onto a disk of nitrocellulose filter paper. The filter paper is then subjected to hybridization, in a manner similar to a Southern gel blot (see earlier discussion), using as a probe a cloned cDNA, complementary to the gene, labeled with ^{32}P by nick translation.

Positive hybridization dots revealed by autoradiography identify candidate plaques from the primary plates (Petri dishes) that can be picked and rescreened at a lower density. A few cycles of rescreening will eventually lead to a pure culture of the recombinant phage of interest.

A prerequisite to the cloning of human globin genes from total cellular DNA using recombinant bacteriophage libraries was the availability of pure cDNA probes for the human globin genes. This was accomplished by synthesizing double-stranded cDNA from globin mRNA by the procedures illustrated in Figure 8–26, ligating it into appropriately treated plasmid DNA, and cloning the separate α, β, and γ recombinant cDNAs in *E. coli* bacteria.[276] After the first genomic β globin gene was cloned,[277] various subclones of this normal gene could be used subsequently to screen new bacteriophage libraries constructed from the DNA of affected individuals to isolate thalassemic β globin genes.

Strategy of Haplotype Analysis for the Identification of Different Thalassemic Globin Genes. The cloning of thalassemic globin genes from different random individuals is likely to lead to the repeated isolation of genes with the same mutation if certain specific forms of thalassemia are particularly prevalent in a given population. In fact, within the period of 1 year, six different groups reported the cloning, from different unrelated Mediterranean individuals, of β⁰-thalassemic globin genes carrying the same mutation consisting of a nonsense codon at position 39 (see discussion that follows). To avoid such fruitless duplication of effort and to assure the efficient characterization of potentially novel β-thalassemic globin genes, Orkin and coworkers devised a strategy to identify different thalassemic β globin genes for cloning and sequence analysis. They reasoned that different types of β-thalassemic globin genes were likely to be associated with different haplotypes or subsets of restriction fragment length polymorphisms present within the non–α globin gene cluster[277a, 277b] (see Chapter 7).

During the course of gene mapping studies in a number of different laboratories, a number of restriction endonuclease sites in and around the non–α globin genes were found to be variably present or absent (that is, polymorphic) among different individuals (see Fig. 7–11). Antonarakis and colleagues[278] observed that these different polymorphisms were not associated with one another in a totally random manner but tended to occur in certain groupings or subsets that were termed "haplotypes." The nine major haplotypes identified are illustrated in Figure 8–27. Orkin and coworkers[279] then demonstrated that in Mediterraneans, different specific β-thalassemic mutations were associated were different haplotypes. The determination of haplotypes by gene mapping therefore provided a relatively simple screening test to identify genes for future study. This strategy was successfully applied to a systematic survey of β-thalassemic mutations in different population groups such as Asian Indians, Chinese, and American blacks[277a, 277b] (see later discussion). Within a given population, a given haplotype will usually be associated with one type of β-thalassemia mutation, but in another population, the same haplotype will usually be associated with a different mutation (see later discussion).

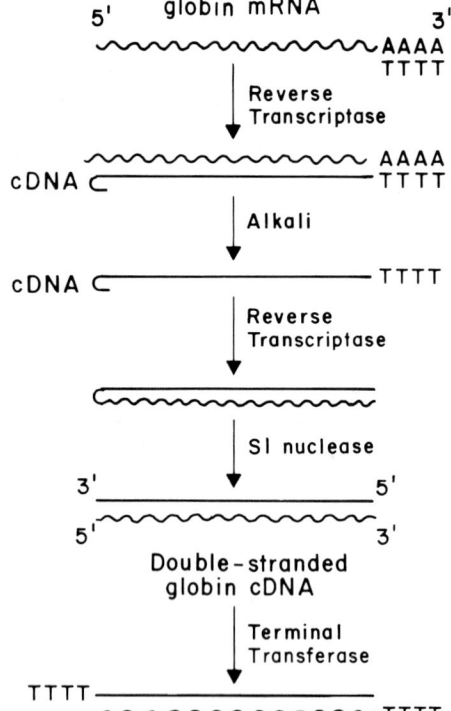

Figure 8–26. Outline of the procedure for synthesizing double-stranded cDNA from mRNA for the purpose of cloning in bacterial plasmids. The cDNA containing T "tails" can be inserted into a plasmid that has been cut at a single site and "tailed" with A residues. If the cDNA is tailed with Cs and the plasmid with Gs at a unique Pst I site, the inserted cDNA can be re-excised by digestion with Pst I. Alternatively, short synthetic oligonucleotide linkers containing sites for various restriction endonucleases can be ligated to the cDNA to allow insertion and re-excision. (From Forget, B. G.: Curr. Top. Hematol. 3:1, 1980.)

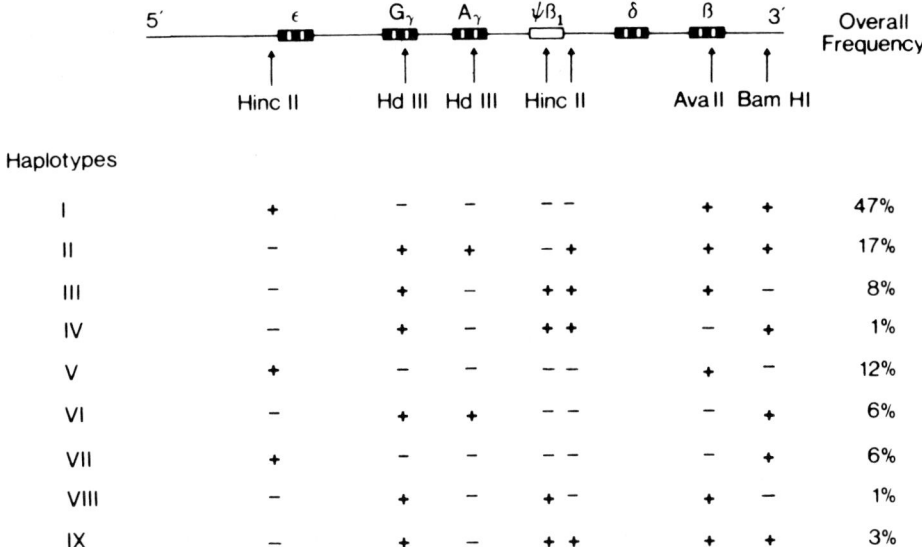

Figure 8–27. Different haplotypes of restriction site polymorphisms in the β gene cluster and their frequency in Mediterranean individuals with β thalassemia. + indicates the presence and − indicates the absence of the particular restriction endonuclease cleavage site. (Modified from Orkin, S. H., et al.: Nature 296:627, 1982.)

DNA Sequencing. A major advance in the study of cloned globin (and other) genes has been the development of rapid DNA sequencing techniques that make feasible the determination of the nucleotide sequence of an entire gene (2000 or so nucleotides long) in a relatively short period of time. Two different techniques have proved to be particularly useful: the technique of Maxam and Gilbert[280] and that of Sanger and associates.[281] In both techniques, the DNA fragment of interest is treated in a manner to generate from it four separate sets of subfragments (one for each nucleotide—C, T, A, or G) that are each truncated in a random fashion at one of the positions where the targeted nucleotide occurs in the DNA sequence. The four different mixtures of ^{32}P-labeled DNA fragments are then fractionated side by side by electrophoresis in polyacrylamide gels, and the gel is subjected to autoradiography, which will reveal a so-called "ladder pattern" from which one can read, going from bottom to top and side to side from one lane to another, the linear sequence of successive nucleotides.[282]

In the technique of Maxam and Gilbert,[280] the DNA fragment is labeled at its 5' ends with polynucleotide kinase and [γ-^{32}P]-ATP, and the generation of subfragments is achieved by various separate, controlled, chemical degradation reactions, each specific for one of the four nucleotides. In the technique of Sanger and colleagues,[281] the DNA fragment is uniformly labeled by primed synthesis using DNA polymerase I and [α-^{32}P]- or ^{35}S-labeled triphosphates. The target DNA is usually initially subcloned in the filamentous bacteriophage M13, which generates single-stranded copies of the recombinant DNA. Appropriate "universal" primers complementary to the vector at the site of insertion of the foreign DNA serve as the starting point for the primed synthesis of the labeled copy of the target DNA. Subfragments are generated by adding to separate synthetic reactions, one of four nucleotide-specific inhibitors of chain elongation (di-deoxynucleotides), present in concentrations that will lead, on a random basis, to chain termination at one of the positions of the target nucleotide in the sequence of the newly synthesized radioactive DNA.

Heterologous Gene Expression Systems. A number of systems have been devised to permit testing of the functional properties of cloned genes. Certain systems consist of cell-free extracts containing RNA polymerase II.[282,283] These systems will generate from added cloned genes RNA transcripts that have faithful 5' termini. However, the transcripts do not terminate accurately or uniformly and are not processed to remove intervening sequences. Furthermore, the relative quantitative level of *in vitro* expression of the added genes does not necessarily accurately reflect their level of expression *in vivo*. For instance, the human δ globin gene is expressed at only a slightly lower level than the β globin gene in such systems.[284] For these various reasons, cell-free systems are not ideal for testing the functional properties of cloned thalassemic globin genes.

More useful systems consist of intact-cell systems in tissue culture, in which transcripts are not only initiated and terminated faithfully but are also spliced accurately and polyadenylated. A number of such systems have been utilized effectively to study normal and thalassemic globin gene function. These systems are of two general types: those in which the transferred gene is expressed transiently for a limited time only and those in which the gene is stably expressed over time. The transient expression systems are as follow: (1) SV40 virus vector systems that cause lytic infection of monkey kidney cells (CV1 cells)[285, 286]; and (2) plasmid vector systems containing the SV40 virus origin of replication and enhancer elements. These vectors are introduced, by DNA-mediated gene transfer, into either HeLa cells[287, 288] or COS cells (monkey kidney cells transformed by the SV40 virus T antigen gene),[289, 290] and the transferred genes are expressed for a day or so 48 hours after transfer. The stable expression systems are as follow: (1) stable transformation of enzyme-deficient mouse fibroblasts[291, 292] or erythroleukemia (MEL) cells[293, 294] by DNA-mediated transfer of the target gene together with the gene for the selectable deficient enzyme, such as thymidine kinase; and (2) bovine papilloma virus (BPV) vector systems in which the recombinant viral DNA transforms mouse fibroblasts and replicates extrachromosomally with high levels of expression of the transferred gene for long periods of time.[295]

In general, studies with thalassemic genes have utilized the transient expression systems, although the BPV system has been used in some studies.[296] Such systems are highly effective not only for the detection of defective processing or splicing of globin mRNA, but also for the identification of quantitative abnormalities in the transcriptional capacity of the transferred gene.

The traditional method used to analyze the globin mRNA produced in such gene expression systems is the S1 nuclease assay originally introduced by Berk and Sharp.[297] In this assay, RNA extracted from the tissue culture cells is hybridized to a ^{32}P-labeled DNA fragment isolated from the gene of interest. The RNA-DNA hybrid is then treated with S1 nuclease, which will digest away the single-stranded portions of the nucleic acids that did not participate in the formation of the double-stranded hybrid. The nuclease-resistant hybrid is then fractionated by electrophoresis in polyacrylamide gels, and the location and size of the labeled, trimmed back DNA fragment are revealed by autoradiography. The principle of the assay is illustrated schematically in Figure 8–28.

The probes used in S1 nuclease assays usually contain intron sequences as well as coding sequences of the gene. Thus, it is possible to assess the presence of abnormal splicing of precursor mRNA molecules in the gene expression system. Normal splicing will result in the protection of only a portion of the labeled genomic DNA probe, resulting in its cleavage at the splice junction and generation of a fragment of a given size. If splicing does not occur normally and intron sequences are retained in the mRNA, a greater portion of the labeled probe will be protected from diges-

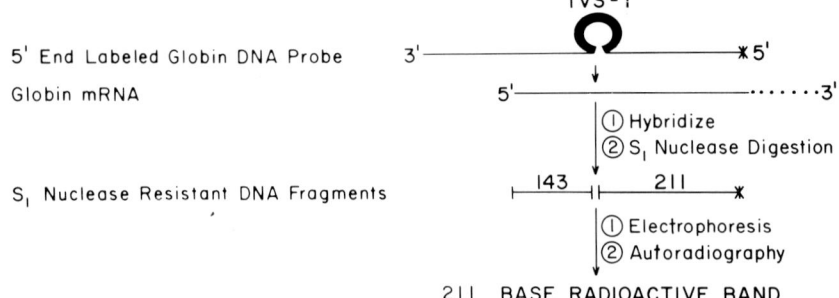

Figure 8–28. Outline of the S1 nuclease assay. In the example shown, the β globin genomic DNA probe is labeled (*) at the Bam HI site at codon 100 and contains the DNA sequences of the first small intervening sequence (IVS-1) that interrupts the gene between codons 30 and 31. The mature processed β globin mRNA will protect the coding sequences of the labeled DNA probe from digestion by the S1 nuclease, but the DNA will be cleaved where the intervening sequence fails to hybridize to the mRNA. In the case where an alternatively spliced β-thalassemic globin mRNA contains sequences from the 3′ end of IVS-1, a longer fragment of the labeled DNA probe will be protected from digestion and detected by autoradiography following acrylamide gel electrophoresis. (From Benz, E. J., Jr., et al.: Trans. Assoc. Am. Phys. 95:325, 1982.)

tion by the S1 nuclease and a larger-than-normal DNA fragment will be detected on the autoradiograph. The length of the abnormal fragment will suggest, by its size, the site in the intron where abnormal splicing occurred. The S1 nuclease assay is also used in a semi-quantitative manner to assess the amount of mRNA accumulation (and thereby, indirectly, the level of transcription from the transferred gene) by inspection of the intensity of hybridization on the autoradiograph in side-by-side comparisons of experiments in which normal and mutant genes were used. The experiments are performed in conditions of excess DNA probe; thus, the relative darkness of the band is proportional to the total amount of RNA available to protect the labeled DNA probe.

Another technique for the analysis of abnormally processed mRNA is the procedure of primer extension,[298] in which a short end-labeled DNA fragment of the gene (the "primer") is hybridized to the RNA and then the enzyme reverse transcriptase is added to synthesize onto the DNA primer a cDNA copy of the mRNA that hybridized to it. This method not only detects abnormally spliced mRNA species by the presence of abnormally sized cDNA fragments (after fractionation of the extension products by polyacrylamide gel electrophoresis) but also allows the isolation and nucleotide sequence analysis of the abnormal cDNA fragments. Thus, it is possible to determine precisely, from the nucleotide sequence of the cDNA, the point at which the precursor mRNA molecules were abnormally spliced.

Cloning and Characterization of β-Thalassemic Globin Genes

β⁺ Thalassemia

The first successful identification of a specific molecular defect causing β⁺ thalassemia was accomplished by Spritz and associates[299] and Westaway and Williamson,[300] who, by cloning and DNA sequence analysis, discovered the same single nucleotide base substitution in the first intron (IVS-1) of the β globin gene of a Greek Cypriot and a Turkish Cypriot individual, respectively. The mutation was subsequently shown to cause β globin mRNA deficiency by a novel process of preferential abnormal alternative splicing of precursor β mRNA molecules[301, 302] (see discussion that follows). A number of additional different mu-

Table 8–3. MUTATIONS CAUSING β⁺ THALASSEMIA

Racial Group and Mutation	Haplotype(s)[1]	Reference(s)
A. Mediterranean		
1. Transcription defects		
−87 from cap site: C→G	VIII	279, 296
−28 from cap site: A→C[2]	N.D.	325, 325a
2. RNA processing defects		
Codon 27: GCC→TCC (Hb Knossos)	I	309
IVS-1 position 5: G→T	V	315a, 315b
IVS-1 position 6: T→C	VI	279, 296
IVS-1 position 110: G→A	I, II, IX	299, 300
IVS-2 position 745: C→G	VII	279, 296
3. Unknown "Silent carrier"	Not linked	327b
B. Black		
1. Transcription defects		
−88 from cap site: C→T	− − − + + +	324
−29 from cap site: A→G	+ − + + + +	327
2. RNA processing defects		
Codon 24: GGT→GGA	+ − − + + +	307
Polyadenylation signal: AATAAA→AACAAA	− − − − + +	327a
C. Asian Indian (AI), Chinese (C), and Southeast Asian (SEA)		
1. Transcription defect		
−28 from cap site: A→G	+ + − + − + (C)	326
2. RNA processing defects		
Codon 26: GAG→AAG (Hb E)	III, IV, V (SEA)	308
IVS-1 position 5: G→C	VII (AI)	162, 296
	− − − − + + (C)	316

[1]The haplotype designations in Roman numerals correspond to those illustrated in Figure 8–27. Haplotypes other than those illustrated in Figure 8–27 are indicated by the convention used in that figure to indicate the presence (+) or absence (−) of the six major polymorphic restriction endonuclease sites in the non–α globin gene cluster (excluding the Hinc II site 5⁺ to the ε gene); additional polymorphic sites have been characterized in the haplotypes associated with those various β-thalassemic genes.[277b, 366b] (N.D. = not determined.)

[2]This mutation was identified in a Kurdish Jewish individual.

tations causing β⁺ thalassemia were later characterized[277a, 277b] (Table 8–3) and can be classified into two groups: (1) those causing abnormal processing or splicing of precursor β mRNA owing to mutations in exon 1, IVS-1, or IVS-2 of the β globin gene and (2) those causing decreased transcription of the β globin gene owing to mutations in the 5'-flanking DNA of the gene.

Mutation Near the 3' End of IVS-1 Causing Preferential Alternative Splicing of Precursor β mRNA Molecules at the Site of the Mutation. The mutation originally identified by Spritz and associates[299] and by Westaway and Williamson[300] consists of a single nucleotide base substitution of G→A at nucleotide 110 of IVS-1 of the β⁺-thalassemic globin gene, 21 nucleotides from the junction between the 3' end of IVS-1 and the adjacent coding sequence at the 5' end of exon 2 of the gene (Fig. 8–29).

Examination of the region of the base substitution in IVS-1 of the β⁺-thalassemic gene revealed a finding that served as the basis for a proposal to explain the molecular basis of this type of β⁺ thalassemia by a post-transcriptional defect in mRNA metabolism. Specifically, the base change creates, within the small intron of the β⁺-thalassemic globin gene, a heptanucleotide sequence that is identical, in all but one nucleotide, to the heptanucleotide sequence situated at the 3' junction between IVS-1 and the adjacent coding region; the one base in the heptanucleotide that differs between the normal and the thalassemic genes has been found to be variable in that position of the normal splicing site in other non–α globin genes in man.[303] More importantly, the specific base substitution of G to A creates an AG dinucleotide, the necessary 3' splicing signal for the excision of intervening sequences[166, 167]; in addition, the AG is preceded by a long stretch of pyrimidines and thus a good 3' or acceptor consensus sequence is generated[167] (see Chapter 7). In Figure 8–29, the heptanucleotide region of sequence homology is shown by the horizontal line underscoring the thalassemic sequence, and the potential splicing sites following AG dinucleotides are shown by arrows.

It was initially suggested by Spritz and coworkers[299] that the base substitution in the β⁺-thalassemic globin gene may create an alternative splicing site for the processing of precursor β mRNA molecules, and a model of the hypothesis is illustrated in Figure 8–30. A given precursor β mRNA molecule could be spliced in one of two ways, either normally, as shown in the lower portion of the figure, or abnormally, as shown in the upper portion of the figure. To explain the 90 per cent deficiency of β mRNA observed in β⁺ thalassemia, the model proposes that the abnormal alternative splicing pathway occurs preferentially, that is, approximately 90 per cent of the time. The abnormally processed mRNA, containing a 19-nucleotide remnant from the 3' end of IVS-1, would then be rapidly turned over, leaving only the 10 per cent or so of the β mRNA, which was normally processed, to accumulate in the steady state in reticulocytes. One possible explanation for the proposed instability of the abnormally processed mRNA is that it would contain an in-phase termination codon derived from the IVS-1 remnant. A number of different β⁰-thalassemic mRNAs with nonsense mutations due to base substitutions or frameshift mutations within the coding sequence are present in markedly reduced amounts in reticulocytes presumably because they are quite unstable (see later discussion).

The postulated mechanism for abnormal processing of precursor globin mRNA as the basis for the deficiency of β mRNA in β⁺ thalassemia was subsequently confirmed by *in vitro* gene transfer and gene expression exper-

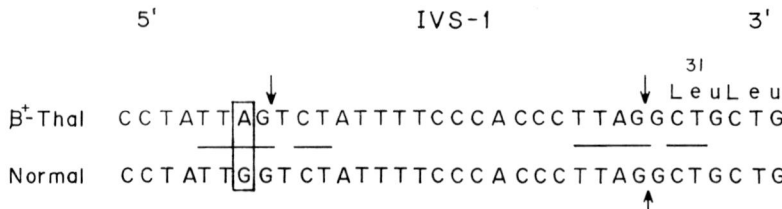

Figure 8–29. Nucleotide sequence of the human β globin gene near the 3' junction between the small intervening sequence (IVS-1) and the adjacent protein encoding sequence. The homologous authentic and alternative internal 3' splice regions are indicated by the interrupted horizontal lines; the potential sites of intron excision are indicated by the arrows. The single nucleotide change in the β⁺-thalassemic DNA sequence at IVS-1 position 110 is indicated by the box. Normal β globin mRNA codon position 31 is numbered. A different mutation has been identified at IVS-1 position 116 of another individual: a T→G base substitution at this nucleotide also creates a new AG dinucleotide that allows alternative splicing at this site.[208] (Modified from Spritz, R. A., et al.: Proc. Natl. Acad. Sci. USA 78:2455, 1981.)

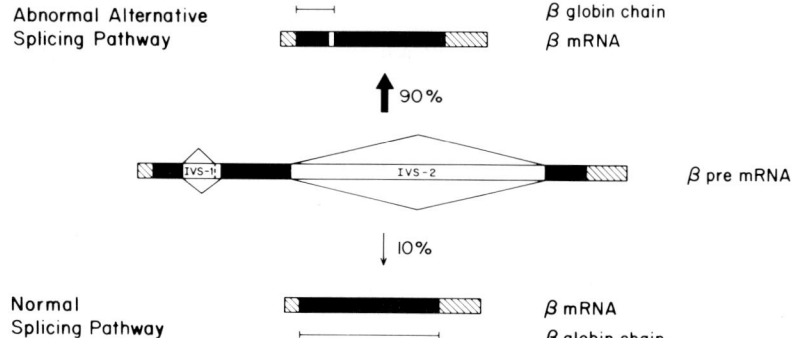

Figure 8–30. Model of alternative splicing in β⁺ thalassemia due to mutation in the β globin gene at IVS-1 position 110, which is indicated by the vertical dashed line.

iments.[301, 302] In summary, the β globin mRNA produced from the transferred β⁺-thalassemic globin gene, in two different transient expression systems, consisted primarily of an abnormally long species containing the predicted 19 additional nucleotides derived from the 3' end of IVS-1,[301, 302] with only approximately 10 per cent as much normally spliced β mRNA. In one study,[302] reticulocyte RNA from two β⁺-thalassemic patients was also examined by the S1 nuclease or primer-extension assays, and small amounts of the same abnormally long β mRNA species in addition to a predominant amount of normally spliced β mRNA were revealed. These results could be best interpreted by the conclusion that approximately 90 per cent of the transcripts originating from the β⁺-thalassemic globin gene were processed abnormally to include the 19 extra nucleotides from the 3' end of IVS-1 but that this abnormal mRNA species was either unstable or abnormally transported, leading to its turnover in developing erythroid cells. As a result, the more mature reticulocytes accumulate and contain essentially only the 10 per cent of the β globin mRNA transcripts that were processed normally and, in addition, a very small amount of the abnormally processed mRNA.

The demonstration that the abnormally processed mRNA species in this form of β⁺ thalassemia could be detected in reticulocyte RNA of affected individuals permitted the establishment of a rapid test for the presence of this mutation by using the S1 nuclease assay. In one study,[304] the reticulocyte RNA of 22 patients of Mediterranean ancestry with the clinical and biochemical phenotype of β⁺ thalassemia was analyzed, and the abnormal β globin mRNA species containing 19 additional nucleotides from IVS-1 was found in 12 of these patients. In another study,[305] 7 of 15 β-thalassemic patients were shown to have the same abnormal mRNA species by S1 nuclease analysis of total bone marrow RNA. Although the assay of reticulocyte or marrow RNA could not distinguish between homozygosity or heterozygosity for the defect, it nevertheless became apparent that this mutation constituted a common cause of β⁺ thalassemia in Mediterraneans.

The studies of restriction fragment length polymorphisms by Orkin and colleagues[279] established that this form of β⁺ thalassemia was associated with haplotype I (see Fig. 8–27) and that this haplotype was found in 47 per cent of Mediterranean patients with β thalassemia. Later studies established that 90 per cent of Mediterranean thalassemic patients with haplotype I carry the IVS-1 position-110 mutation on that chromosome.[277a, 277b, 306] A small proportion of Mediterranean thalassemic patients carry other mutations on chromosomes of haplotype I[306a] (Tables 8–3 and 8–4): a frame shift mutation at codon 6, causing β⁰ thalassemia; a nonsense mutation at codon 39, causing β⁰ thalassemia; a base substitution at IVS-1 position 116, probably causing β⁰ thalassemia[208a]; and Hb Knossos, causing β⁺ thalassemia (see discussions that follow).

Mutations in IVS-1 or Exon 1, Near the 5' End of IVS-1, Causing Alternative Splicing of Precursor β mRNA Molecules at Neighboring Pre-existing Cryptic Splice Sites. A group of mutations have been identified in IVS-1 and in exon 1 that lead to deficiency of authentic β globin mRNA by causing abnormal alternative splicing of precursor β mRNA molecules at one or more sites near the 5' end of IVS-1. All of these mutations leave intact the essential invariant dinucleotide GT sequence at the 5' splice site of IVS-1, thereby allowing some normal processing of precursor β mRNA molecules to occur at that site. However, the base substitutions, all of which occur in the vicinity of the 5' splice site of IVS-1, appear to lead to underutilization of the normal splice site and the abnormal use of one or more pre-existing alternative (or "cryptic") donor splice sites: two located upstream in exon 1 and one located downstream in IVS-1. Figure 8–31 lists

Table 8-4. MUTATIONS CAUSING β⁰ THALASSEMIA

Racial Group and Mutation	Haplotype(s)[1]	Reference(s)
A. Mediterranean		
1. Nonsense and frameshift mutations		
Codon 6: GAG→G-G	I, V. IX	338, 339
Codon 8: AAG→- -G	IV	279, 332
Codon 39: CAG→TAG	I, II, VII, IX	330–335
Codon 44: TCC→TC-[2]	N.D.	132
Codon 121: GAA→TAA[3]	VII	337a
2. RNA processing defects		
IVS-1 position 1: G→A	V	279, 296
IVS-1 position 116: T→G	I	208
IVS-2 position 1: G→A	III, V	165, 279
IVS-2 position 705: T→G	N.D.	317, 318
B. Black		
1. RNA processing defect		
IVS-2 position 849: A→G	- - - + - +	327, 342
C. Chinese		
1. Nonsense and frameshift mutations		
Codon 17: AAG→TAG	N.D.	130
Codons 71/72: TTT AGT→TTTAAGT	VII	316
Codons 41/42: TTC TTT→- - - -TT	N.D.	340
2. RNA processing defect		
IVS-2 position 654: C→T	I	316
D. Asian Indian		
1. Nonsense and frameshift mutations		
Codons 8/9: GAG AAG→GAGGAAG	I	162
Codon 15: TGG→TAG	II	162
Codon 16: GGC→GG-	I	162
Codons 41/42: TTC TTT→- - - -TT	III, V	162
2. RNA processing defects		
IVS-1 position 1: G→T	IX	162
IVS-1 position 108: 25 bp deletion	IX	343
IVS-1 position 117: 17 bp deletion[4]	IX	337a

[1]See Table 8-3.
[2]This mutation was identified in a Kurdish Jewish individual.
[3]This was an apparent spontaneous mutation in a Polish individual.[461]
[4]This mutation was identified in a Kuwaiti individual.[337a]

the normal DNA sequence in this region of the β globin gene, with the normal and cryptic splice sites underlined; all contain the GT dinucleotide sequence required for the 5'-splicing event[166, 168] (see arrows in Fig. 8–31). The figure also illustrates the so-called "consensus" 5'-splicing sequence that usually encompasses the GT, determined from the analysis of a large number of mammalian gene sequences.[166, 167]

Five mutations that occur at the 3' end of exon 1 or the 5' end of IVS-1 (see Fig. 8–31) lead to the activation of one or more of these alternative splice sites by creating a sequence environment that either makes the normal splice site less likely to be used (mutations in IVS-1) or makes one of the alternative splice sites more favorable for selection by the splicing mechanism (mutations in exon 1). None of the mutations create a GT nucleotide (see Fig. 8–31), but they all appear to alter the environment of a pre-existing GT dinucleotide. The use of the alternative splice sites has been confirmed, in the case of the five different mutations, by S1 nuclease analysis of RNA transcribed from the cloned mutant genes after transfer and expression in tissue culture cell systems[296, 307–309] as well as by nucleotide sequence analysis of abnormal cDNA products synthesized from that RNA by the technique of primer extension.[296] However, the abnormally spliced mRNA species, in those cases in which they have been looked for, have not been detected in reticulocyte or bone marrow RNA of affected patients.[307, 308] Therefore, the abnormally spliced RNAs must be highly unstable and rapidly turned over *in vivo*.

The two mutations in IVS-1 that cause alternative splicing are located at positions 5 and 6 of IVS-1 (see Fig. 8–31). The mutation at position 5 occurs in Asian Indian individuals[162] and leads to a moderately severe β⁺-thalassemia syndrome with only low levels of normal β mRNA.[296] The mutation at position 6 occurs in Mediterraneans[277a, 279] and leads to a relatively mild β⁺-thalassemia syndrome,[310, 311] presumably because splicing occurs at the normal site more frequently with this mutation

THE THALASSEMIAS: MOLECULAR PATHOGENESIS

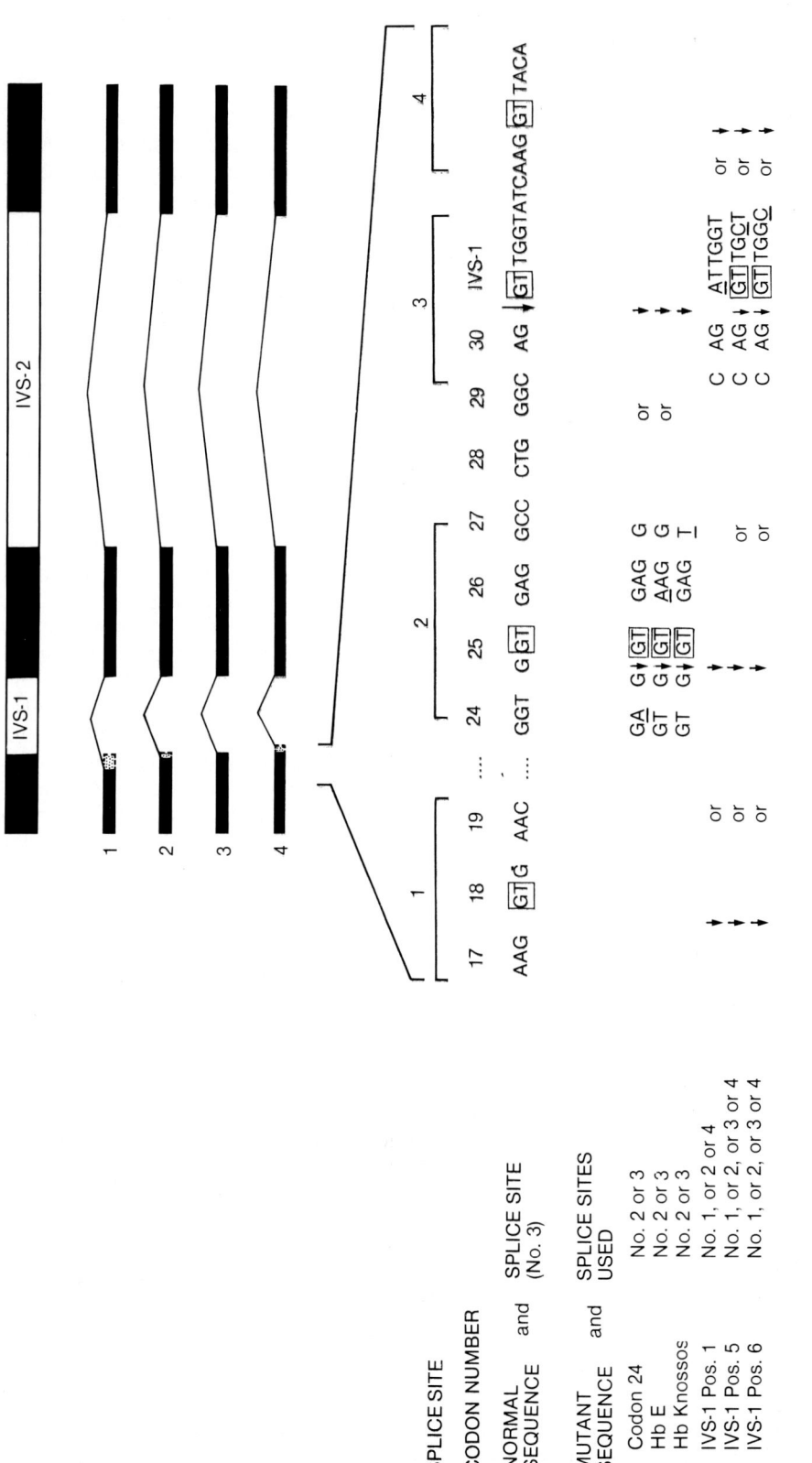

Figure 8–31. Splicing patterns associated with different thalassemic mutations in exon 1 and IVS-1 of the β globin gene. The normal and abnormal 5' or donor splice sites are indicated by the short vertical arrows. The GT dinucleotide sequences required for the splicing events are indicated by the boxes. The nucleotide base substitutions resulting from the mutations are underlined. The stippled boxes indicate the portions of exon 1 that are removed from the processed mRNA by alternative splicing; the open box represents the portion of IVS-1 retained in the processed mRNA.

than with the former,[296] thus resulting in a less severe deficiency of β globin mRNA and less imbalance of globin-chain synthesis. Both of these mutations lead to the activation of all three of the cryptic splicing sites (nos. 1, 2, and 4) shown in Figure 8–31, while still allowing the use (in different relative amounts) of the normal splicing site (no. 3).

The three mutations in exon 1 that cause alternative splicing are located in codons 24, 26, and 27, respectively, within a distance of one to five nucleotides from the alternative splicing signal (GT) in codon 25 (site no. 2 in Fig. 8–31). All three of these mutations lead to the activation of cryptic splicing site no. 2 without the use of sites no. 1 or no. 4; normal splicing in different relative amounts also occurs at the normal 5′ splice site of IVS-1 (site no. 3 in Fig. 8–31). The first of these mutations, which was described in a black patient, consists of a "silent" base substitution in codon 24, GGT→GGA,[307] and therefore does not lead to the synthesis of a structurally abnormal β globin chain from the properly spliced mutant β mRNA. However, the two other mutations at codon 26, GAG→AAG,[308] and codon 27, GCC→TCC,[309] each encode a change in the amino acid sequence of the β globin chain synthesized from translation of the properly spliced mutant β mRNA: β 26 Glu→Lys (Hb E) and β 27 Ala→Ser (Hb Knossos). These two hemoglobin variants were known to be associated with a mild β-thalassemia phenotype[312–315] (see Chapter 10), but the mechanism was not known until gene cloning and expression studies[308, 309] revealed the presence of alternative splicing of precursor β mRNA molecules induced by the base substitutions and, as a result, decreased synthesis of normally spliced β globin mRNA.

With regard to the phenotype of these three mutations, the mutation at codon 24 is associated with a more severe clinical syndrome and with less normal splicing of precursor β mRNA molecules than is the case with Hb E and Hb Knossos.[307–309]

The two syndromes of Hb E and Hb Knossos illustrate the lack of clear-cut distinction between purely qualitative and purely quantitative disorders of hemoglobin synthesis and demonstrate that mutations causing structurally abnormal hemoglobins can have the same or similar effects on globin mRNA metabolism as do mutations that cause quantitative defects in the accumulation of globin mRNA without changing the structure of the encoded globin polypeptide chains. A number of additional structurally abnormal hemoglobin variants that are associated with a thalassemic phenotype will be discussed in a later section of this chapter.

A second mutation involving IVS-1 position 5 has been described more recently: a G → T base substitution in a Greek individual;[315a] the first mutation identified at this site was a G → C base substitution in Asian Indian individuals.[162, 296] Although this second mutation was initially thought to cause β⁰ thalassemia,[315a] more recent studies suggest that it is more likely associated with β⁺ thalassemia.[315b] Studies of globin mRNA expression in gene transfer systems[315b] indicate that the pattern of splicing associated with this mutation is similar, although not identical, to that observed with the other mutation at IVS-1 position 5.

The mutation at position 6 of IVS-1 creates a site, absent in normal DNA, for the restriction endonuclease Sfa NI and is therefore potentially detectable by Southern gel blotting of total cellular DNA.[315c] However, it should be noted that this mutation usually occurs in a β gene that carries the five polymorphisms associated with what has been called a β gene of framework 3[277a, 277b] (see Chapter 7). The polymorphism at codon 2 in such a gene also creates a site for Sfa NI, thus reducing the utility of gene mapping for detection of the mutation: The change in fragment size caused by the thalassemia mutation is from 280 bp to 190 + 90 bp in a gene of framework 3, rather than from ~0.7 kb to ~0.5 kb as was originally suggested, which is a change observed in the nonrelevant 5′-flanking DNA of otherwise normal genes of framework 1 (or 2) and framework 3, respectively.

Mutations in IVS-2 Causing Alternative Splicing of Precursor β mRNA Molecules. A mutation in IVS-2 has been shown to cause β⁺ thalassemia by creating an alternative splicing site while leaving a normal splicing site intact but hypofunctional. This mutation leads to the activation of a second pre-existing cryptic splice site in IVS-2. The defect consists of a base substitution at nucleotide position 745 of IVS-2, which contains a total of 850 nucleotides. The mutation changes a C(T) to a G(T)[279, 296] and thus creates a GT dinucleotide sequence that could potentially serve as a 5′ or donor splice site. Gene transfer and gene expression studies have in fact confirmed that such is the case.[296] A small proportion of precursor β mRNA molecules were processed normally, but the majority were processed abnormally, as illustrated in Figure 8–32. The

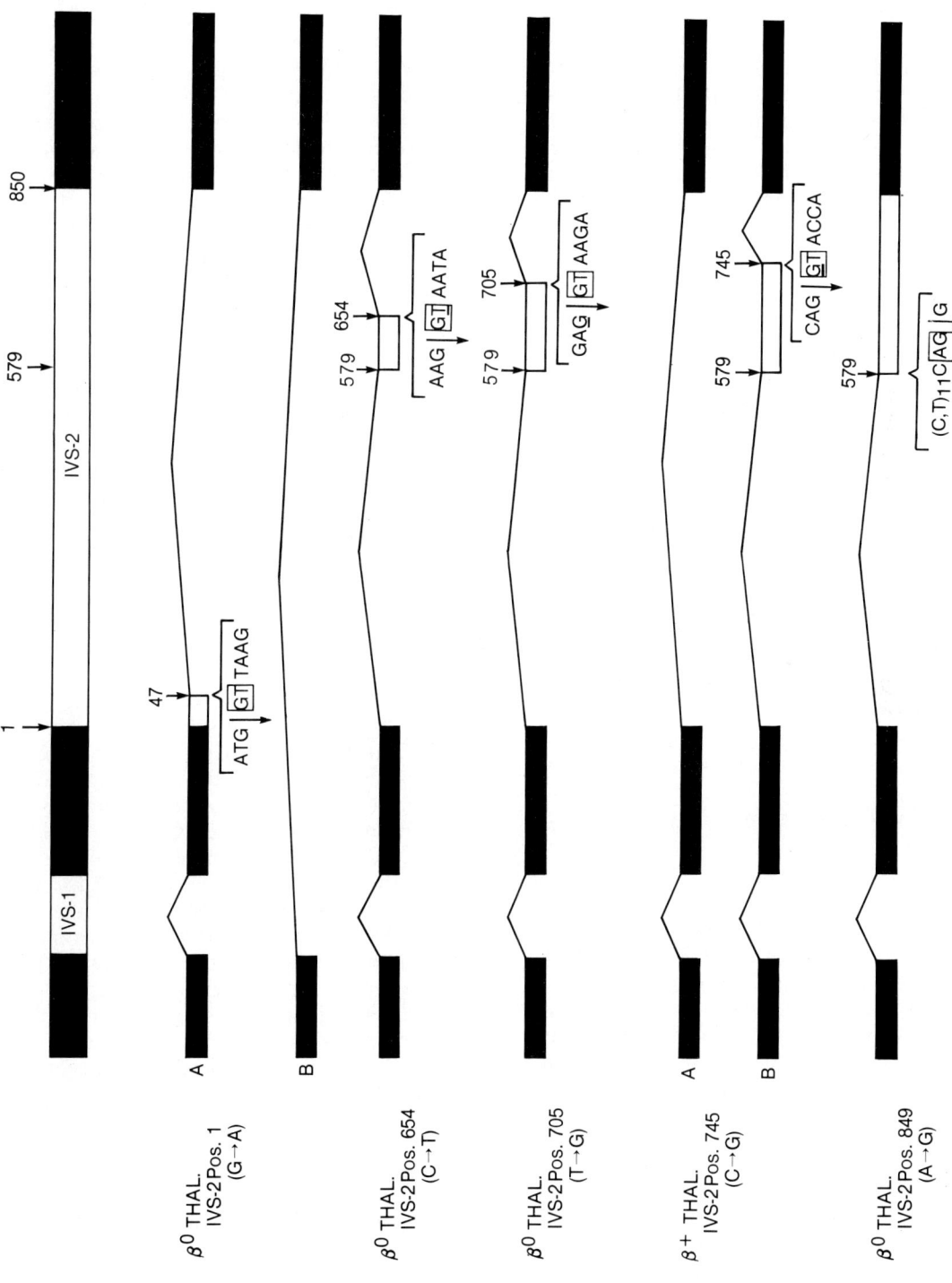

Figure 8–32. Splicing patterns associated with different thalassemic mutations in IVS-2 of the β globin gene. The nucleotide sequences at the cryptic or alternative splicing sites are indicated, with the same conventions as in Figure 8–31. The same cryptic acceptor site at IVS-2 position 579 is utilized in many of the mutations. The portions of IVS-2 retained in the processed mRNAs are indicated by the open boxes. 269

precursor β mRNA molecules are processed in such a way that an internal segment of IVS-2 is retained within the processed mRNA. At the 3' end, the precursor is spliced from the 5' splice site created by the mutation at nucleotide 745 to the normal 3' splice site at the end of IVS-2. However, the size of the abnormal RNA obtained in S1 nuclease assays was not consistent with retention of all of the remainder of IVS-2 upstream from nucleotide 745, and nucleotide sequence analysis of primer-extended cDNA confirmed the presence of an additional abnormal splicing event that had removed the majority of IVS-2 sequences 5' to the mutation. These sequences were spliced from the normal 5' splice site to a pre-existing but normally unused cryptic 3' or acceptor splice site, the AG of which is located at nucleotides 578 and 579 of IVS-2. Thus, the resulting abnormally processed mRNA retains the nucleotides from position 580 to 744 of IVS-2, a total of 164 additional nucleotides. The additional sequence, as in the case of other abnormally spliced mRNAs, contains in-phase nonsense (terminator) codons and therefore would be translated abnormally and presumably would be unstable and rapidly turned over in erythroid cells.

The base substitution at position 745 creates new recognition sites for the restriction endonucleases Rsa I and Kpn I that are not present in normal DNA:

$$\underset{\underset{\text{Kpn I}}{\rule{2cm}{0.4pt}}}{\overset{\overset{\text{Rsa I}}{\rule{2cm}{0.4pt}}}{\text{GCTACC} \rightarrow \text{GGTACC}}}$$

This mutation can therefore be identified by Southern gel blotting of total cellular DNA from affected individuals. Mutant DNA digested with Rsa I reveals a new fragment of 1.9 kb, whereas normal DNA yields a fragment of 2.2 kb.[279] Mutant DNA digested with Kpn I should reveal a new abnormal fragment of approximately 3.7 kb hybridizing to a 3' β globin gene probe, whereas normal DNA yields only a very large fragment of approximately 39 kb.

Two other mutations of IVS-2, at positions 654 and 705,[316, 317] behave in a similar way to the position-745 mutation in that they create or activate an alternative donor splice site near the 3' end of IVS-2 and lead, as well, to activation of the cryptic acceptor splice site at position 579 (see Fig. 8–32). When tested in gene expression systems, however, these mutant genes generate only the abnormally processed β mRNA, with no synthesis of normal β mRNA, even though the normal splicing signals are intact at both ends of IVS-2.[316, 318] These mutations therefore appear to cause β^0 thalassemia rather than β^+ thalassemia (see later discussion and Table 8–4).

Mutations in 5'-Flanking DNA of the β Globin Gene Causing Decreased Transcription of the Gene. Prior to the discovery and realization of the implications of introns, it was commonly assumed that many of the thalassemias, and β^+ thalassemia in particular, might be due to mutations in control regions adjacent to globin genes causing decreased transcription of the affected genes. However, it eventually became apparent that splicing defects accounted for most of the β^+ thalassemias. Nevertheless, certain forms of β^+ thalassemia have subsequently proved to be due to defects in transcription. They are due to mutations in the 5'-flanking DNA of the β globin gene, in the region of promoter sequences thought to be involved in the interactions between RNA polymerase and the gene. Five separate mutations have been identified in the 5'-flanking DNA of the β globin gene (see Table 8–3) in two different regions known to be important for proper transcription of the gene.

The first mutation to be characterized[279, 296] consisted of a C→G base substitution at position −87 in the 5'-flanking DNA of the β gene, that is, 87 nucleotides upstream from, or 5' to, the "cap site" of the gene where transcription is initiated (see Chapter 7). This mutation occurs 10 nucleotides to the 5' side of a conserved sequence CCAAT, the "CCAAT box," that is present in the 5'-flanking DNA of all globin[303] as well as many other mammalian genes and has been shown to be required for efficient transcription of globin genes in gene expression systems utilizing tissue culture cells.[319–321] The sequences 5' to the CCAAT box, in particular the conserved sequence ACACCC, which includes the precise nucleotide substituted in this mutation (underlined), had also been shown to be important for maximum expression of transferred rabbit and mouse β globin genes in tissue culture cell systems.[322, 323] When this thalassemic gene was tested in a transient expression system, the amount of β globin mRNA produced was approximately 10 per cent of the normal amount and was otherwise initiated and processed normally.[296] Although the degree of suppression of β globin gene transcription by this mutation appears to be moderately severe, individuals who are doubly heterozygous for this mutation and the common (severe) form of β⁺ thalassemia due to the IVS-1 position-110 mutation have a milder-than-usual clinical syndrome (in the absence of concomitant α thalassemia) and fall into the category of "thalassemia intermedia."[310] The precise reason for the milder clinical phenotype despite only 10 per cent of normal β globin gene transcription remains unexplained.

A second mutation in this region of DNA, a C to T base substitution at position −88, has been identified as a cause of β⁺ thalassemia in blacks.[324] It presumably has effects similar to those of the −87 mutation and, like it, is associated with a mild form of β thalassemia.

It is noteworthy, and useful for diagnostic purposes, that the −87 mutation eliminates a recognition site, present in normal DNA, for the restriction endonuclease Avr II:

$$\overset{\text{Avr II}}{\underset{}{\text{C}}}\text{CTAGG} \rightarrow \underline{\text{G}}\text{CTAGG}$$

Mutant DNA doubly digested with Avr II and Hind III gives a DNA fragment of approximately 4 kb, whereas normal DNA yields a fragment of 2.3 kb.[279]

The three other β⁺-thalassemic mutations that cause decreased transcription of the β globin gene are base substitutions located at positions −28 or −29 from the cap site in the 5′-flanking DNA of the β globin gene. This region of DNA has been called the TATA or ATA box, because one of these sequences is invariably found approximately 30 nucleotides upstream from the cap site of virtually all mammalian genes and its deletion leads to absent or faulty transcription of cloned genes in various expression systems (see Chapter 7). In the case of the human non–α globin genes, the sequence ATAAAA is found in all members of the family.[303] The thalassemia mutations alter the ATA box sequence of the β globin gene in the following ways:

Normal: ATAAAA[163]
−28 mutation: ATA<u>C</u>AA[325, 325a]
−28 mutation: ATA<u>G</u>AA[326]
−29 mutation: AT<u>G</u>AAA[327]

These mutations, which occur in three different racial groups (see Table 8–3), all lead to decreased transcription of the β globin gene. The decreased amount of β globin mRNA, compared with normal, obtained after expression of the mutant genes in transient expression systems correlates well with the relative degree of β mRNA deficiency in erythroid cells of homozygous individuals.[326, 327] Although experimentally induced deletions or mutations of the ATA box frequently lead to initiation of transcription of the β globin gene at abnormal sites,[319, 320, 323] the β mRNA synthesized from these thalassemic genes *in vivo* and in the gene expression systems has a normal 5′ terminus and is therefore properly initiated.[326, 327]

The A→G mutation at position −29 that occurs in blacks is associated with the production of approximately 25 per cent of the normal amount of β mRNA and constitutes the common form of mild β⁺ thalassemia found in that population.[327] The A→G mutation at position −28 that occurs in Chinese individuals constitutes a more severe form of β⁺ thalassemia, with β mRNA levels that are approximately 10 per cent of the normal level.[326]

Mutation in Polyadenylation Signal. A base substitution of U to C in the conserved hexanucleotide sequence AAUAAA that is thought to constitute the signal for cleavage and polyadenylation at the 3′ end of mRNA transcripts has been found to be associated with β⁺ thalassemia in a black individual with Hb S/β⁺ thalassemia.[327a] Transient expression studies of the cloned mutant gene in HeLa cells revealed the production of only one-tenth the level of stable β mRNA as a normal β gene, and only a portion of the β mRNA was polyadenylated at the normal site. Analysis by S1 nuclease mapping of RNA isolated from the patient's erythroid cells demonstrated the presence of a β mRNA species that was polyadenylated at a point 900 nucleotides downstream from the usual polyadenylation site, at the first AAUAAA hexanucleotide encountered in the 3′-flanking DNA of the β gene.[327a] A small amount of an abnormal β mRNA species 1500 nucleotides in length, consistent with this elongated β mRNA, was also detected by Northern gel analysis. The mutation therefore appears to markedly decrease but not totally abolish the normal cleavage/polyadenylation reaction and leads to the synthesis of an elongated alternatively polyadenylated β mRNA that may be unstable as it accumulates to constitute only a minor portion of the β mRNA in erythroid cells.

Possible Remote Mutation Influencing β Globin Gene Expression. The β globin gene corresponding to a silent carrier allele causing mild β^+ thalassemia (see Chapter 9) has been cloned and subjected to nucleotide sequence analysis.[327b] Surprisingly, no abnormality was detected in the structural gene or its 5′-flanking DNA. It was concluded that the mutation causing β^+ thalassemia in this Albanian family was not linked to the β globin gene. Furthermore, haplotype analysis of restriction fragment length polymorphisms in the β cluster established that the two affected children in the family had inherited different paternal β gene clusters, indicating that the thalassemia allele either was very far removed from the β gene cluster on chromosome 11 or was located on a different chromosome altogether.[327a]

β^0 Thalassemia

Base Substitutions Directly Creating Termination or Nonsense Codons in the β Globin Gene. Mutations at Codons 15 and 17. The first demonstration of the molecular basis of one type of nondeletion β^0 thalassemia was accomplished not by gene cloning, but by direct nucleotide sequence analysis of the mutant β mRNA or, more precisely, by sequence analysis of the cDNA copy of the mutant β mRNA that was present at a level of approximately 15 per cent of normal in reticulocytes of the Chinese individual who was studied.[126] The abnormality that was identified by Chang and Kan[130] consisted of a single nucleotide base substitution at codon 17 of the β mRNA, AAG→UAG, changing a lysine codon to a nonsense codon (Fig. 8–33). This unexpected and precedent-setting observation prompted additional elegant work to demonstrate that the base substitution was not an artifact of the cDNA synthesis. Globin mRNA from the affected patient was translated in a cell-free protein synthesizing system in the presence of added yeast amber suppressor tRNA capable of inserting serine at UAG codons. The cell-free synthesis of full-length β globin chains from the β^0-thalassemic mRNA was obtained in the presence (but not in the absence) of the added suppressor tRNA, thus confirming the presence of the nonsense mutation in the naturally occurring mRNA.[328] In a later study, this same group of workers used site-specific mutagenesis to convert a human lysine tRNA gene to that for an amber suppressor.[329] The gene was microinjected into frog oocytes and was shown to be functional by its ability to produce tRNA capable of suppressing the nonsense mutation of the β^0-thalassemic mRNA that was subsequently microinjected into the oocytes and translated into normal β globin chains.[329] These elegant experiments illustrated one possible approach to gene therapy for this form of β^0 thalassemia (see last section in this chapter).

Subsequently, a nonsense mutation was identified at neighboring codon 15 in an Asian Indian subject: TGG→TAG.[162] The associated phenotype was not reported.

Mutation at Codon 39. Having established the precedent of a nonsense mutation as a cause of β^0 thalassemia, Kan and coworkers proceeded to demonstrate that their initial finding was not a rare isolated example of this phenomenon. They screened various β^0-thalassemic mRNA samples for the presence of nonsense mutations by translation in the presence of suppressor tRNA and observed that the low level (1 to 5 per cent of normal) of β mRNA from Sardinian patients with β^0 thalassemia could direct the synthesis of β globin chains in the presence of amber suppressor tRNA.[330] They subsequently cloned the β globin cDNA from such patients and demonstrated a new nonsense mutation at codon 39 of the β mRNA: CAG→UAG[330] (see Fig. 8–33). Within months, five other groups reported finding the same mutation by cloning and sequence analysis of β globin genes from random, unrelated Mediterranean patients with β^0 thalassemia.[331–335] It was subsequently demonstrated by Orkin and associates that the β 39 nonsense mutation is associated predominantly with two different haplotypes of restric-

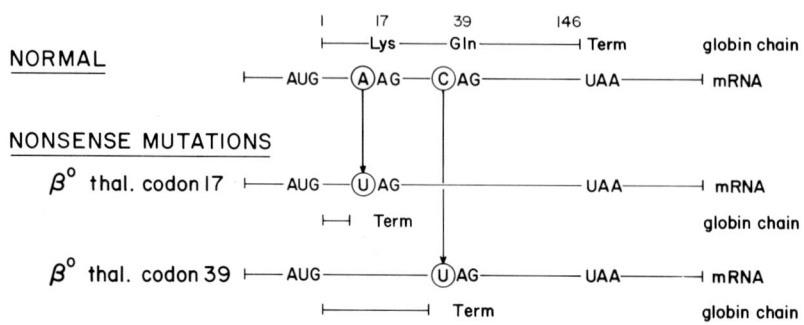

Figure 8–33. Nonsense mutations in cases of β^0 thalassemia. Single nucleotide base substitutions at amino acid codons 17 and 39 lead to premature termination of translation of β globin mRNA and therefore total absence of intact β chains and Hb A. Similar mutations have also been identified at codon 15 and codon 121 in other cases of β^0 thalassemia.

tion enzyme polymorphisms (II and IX [see Fig. 8–27]), which together account for 20 per cent of the β-thalassemic chromosomes in Mediterranean individuals.[332] Thus, in this population, the β 39 nonsense mutation is second in frequency only to the IVS-1 position-110 mutation that causes β$^+$ thalassemia by alternative splicing (see preceding discussion).

Functional studies of the cloned β 39 nonsense thalassemic gene in gene transfer/gene expression systems have produced different results in different laboratories. In the original studies of Moschonas and coworkers,[331] the amount of β mRNA expressed and accumulated after transient expression of the β^0-thalassemic gene in HeLa cells appeared to be normal. The implications of these results were that the marked deficiency of β mRNA observed in erythroid cells of affected individuals must result from different post-transcriptional handling of the mutant β mRNA in the two cell types. There was presumably cytoplasmic instability of the nonsense mRNA in erythroid cells, but not in HeLa cells.

However, in two other laboratories different results have subsequently been obtained in studies of β 39 nonsense thalassemic globin genes isolated from unrelated individuals and analyzed by transient expression in COS cells. In both studies,[336, 337] markedly decreased levels of β globin mRNA (compared with normal) were detected in both nuclei and cytoplasm of COS cells containing the transferred β 39 nonsense thalassemic globin gene. Furthermore, the level of β mRNA did not diminish more rapidly than that of normal β mRNA after inhibition of further gene transcription by the addition of actinomycin D, strongly suggesting that cytoplasmic instability was not the factor responsible for the low level of mutant β globin mRNA.[336, 337] In one study,[337] the amount of unprocessed precursor β mRNA was normal, thereby indicating normal transcription of the mutant gene. No evidence of abnormal processing of precursor β mRNA molecules was detected in either study. In the second study, a rather surprising result was obtained when the gene for a tyrosine amber suppressor tRNA from *Xenopus laevis* was cotransferred into the COS cells with the mutant β globin gene: Normal amounts of β globin mRNA from the β 39 nonsense thalassemic gene were detected in the cytoplasm of the COS cells 48 hours after transfer.[336] Taken together, these various results suggest that the deficiency of the β 39 nonsense thalassemic mRNA is most likely due to early post-transcriptional processes such as intranuclear stability of the mRNA and/or abnormal transport from nucleus to cytoplasm. Furthermore, the abnormality in β globin mRNA metabolism appears to be alleviated by the presence of an amber suppressor tRNA capable of allowing proper full-length translation of the nonsense mRNA. However, the precise molecular mechanisms involved in these phenomena remain to be elucidated.

Both the β 17 and β 39 nonsense mutations create new recognition sites for the restriction endonuclease Mae I that are not present in normal DNA: CAAG and CCAG → CTAG. Therefore, these mutations should be detectable by the Southern gel blotting technique. However, the relatively small size of the fragments, that is, 790 bp → 718 bp for codon 17 mutation and 522 bp for codon 39 mutation, may not provide a practical means for detection of the mutations in total cellular DNA but may limit the application of this assay to the analysis of cloned DNA.

Mutation at Codon 121. A fourth nonsense mutation has been identified more recently in an individual of Polish ancestry: a change in codon 121 from GAA to TAA.[461] This mutation is unusual because it appears to have arisen spontaneously, and in contrast to most other thalassemic mutations, it occurs in exon 3 of the gene. The mutation can be identified easily in genomic DNA by Southern gel blotting because it abolishes the intragenic Eco RI site of the β globin gene.

Frameshift Mutations Due to Base Deletions or Insertions Resulting in the Creation of New In-phase Termination or Nonsense Codons at Points Downstream from the Mutation Itself. Seven additional forms of β^0 thalassemia are caused by frameshift mutations resulting from deletion or insertion of one or more nucleotides in the coding region of the β globin gene (see Table 8–4).[132, 162, 277a, 277b, 332, 338–340] These mutations disrupt the normal reading frame of the mRNA downstream from the mutation. As a result of the new reading frame, a totally anomalous amino acid sequence would be added to the normally initiated nascent globin chain, and almost invariably, a nonsense codon would be encountered, leading to termination of translation of the mutant mRNA at a point preceding the position of the normal termination codon (Fig. 8–34). Although the nucleotide sequence of these β^0-thalassemic genes predicts the synthesis of such abnormal nonsense peptides, they have not been identified in erythroid cells of affected

282 THE THALASSEMIAS: MOLECULAR PATHOGENESIS

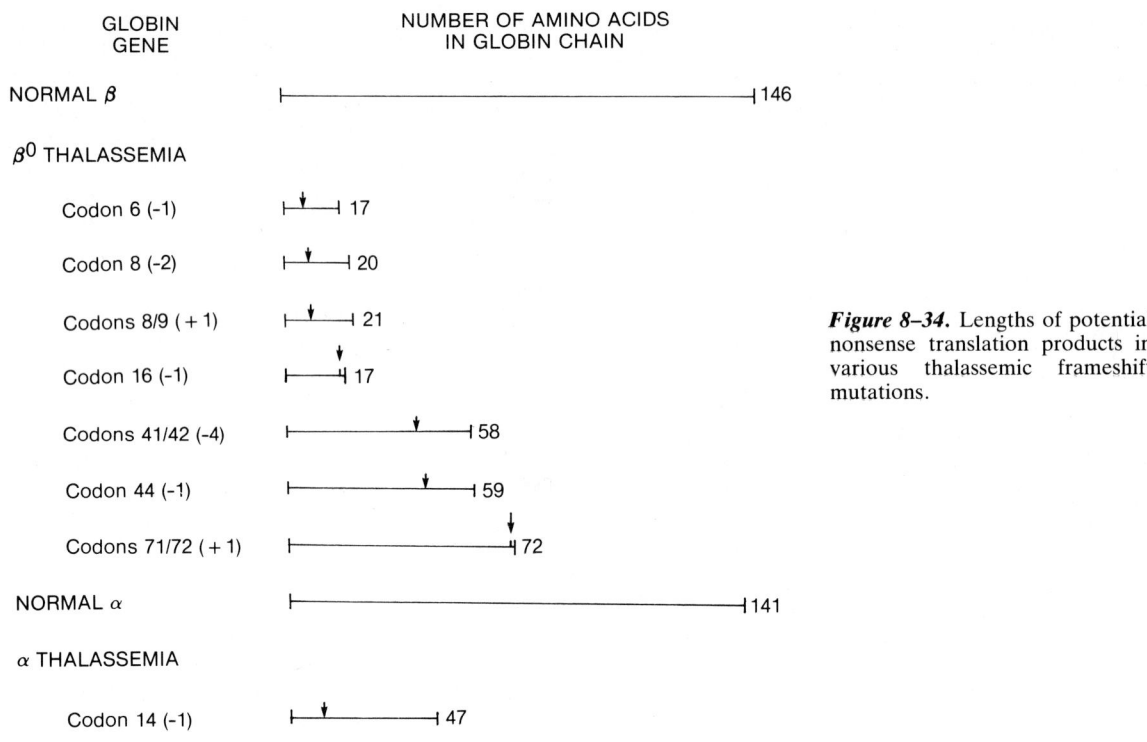

Figure 8–34. Lengths of potential nonsense translation products in various thalassemic frameshift mutations.

patients, presumably because the abnormal proteins are unstable and rapidly turned over. Nevertheless, the basis for the absence of normal β globin chains is clear.

Studies of globin mRNA metabolism have been reported in only one of these mutations[132] and have revealed an extremely short half-life of the mRNA: approximately 30 minutes.[131] It therefore appears that the deletion of a single nucleotide (at codon 44) leads to marked instability and turnover of the mRNA. The basis of this instability is not known; however, the cause of the instability appears to be restricted to erythroid cells, because the abnormal β mRNA is stable in HeLa cells.[340b] Perhaps abnormalities of secondary structure of the mRNA caused by the mutation render it more susceptible to degradation by cellular nucleases. In most cases of frameshift mutations, very low levels of β globin mRNA are detected in erythroid cells of affected individuals.

It is noteworthy that one of these frameshift mutations alters a restriction endonuclease site in the β globin gene and can therefore be detected directly in total cellular DNA by the Southern gel blotting technique (see earlier discussion). The frameshift (−1) at codon 6 abolishes the site for the enzyme Mst II, normally present in the β globin gene.[338, 339] This same site is abolished by the base substitution that causes sickle hemoglobin (Hb S [β 6 Glu→Val]); in fact, the same nucleotide that is deleted in the frameshift mutation is changed from A to T in the sickle mutation. Thus, abolition of the Mst II site, used as a direct test for the prenatal detection of the sickle mutation (see later section), can also be caused by this form of β⁰ thalassemia. Therefore, careful family studies are required to correlate the findings of DNA analysis with the hemoglobin phenotype. The mutation causing the unstable hemoglobin Hb Leiden (β 6 or β 7 deleted) would also be expected to abolish the same Mst II site.[338]

Mutations in Intervening Sequences That Prevent Normal Splicing. A number of mutations have been identified in introns of the β globin gene (see Table 8–4) that totally prevent normal splicing and thus lead to a complete deficiency of normal β globin mRNA. Most of these mutations occur at the junctions between introns and coding sequence, altering the normal splicing signals. However, some mutations that occur within introns, leaving the normal splice junctions intact, nevertheless appear to totally prevent normal splicing of precursor β mRNA molecules.

Base Substitutions at the 5′ Splice Junction of IVS-1 and IVS-2. Two mutations have been identified in β-thalassemic globin genes that consist of single nucleotide base substitutions within the invariant dinucleotide GT that is located at the 5′ ends of introns. The same base substitution, GT→AT, has been identified at the 5' ends of both IVS-1[279] and IVS-2[165] in different β⁰-thalassemic globin genes isolated from Mediterranean individuals. The mutation at the 5' end of IVS-1 leads to the same pattern of abnormal alternative splicing, at three different neighboring cryptic splice sites, as do two other mutations at positions 5 and 6 of IVS-1[296] (see earlier discussion and Fig. 8–31). However, in contrast to the latter two mutations that cause β⁺ thalassemia by allowing some normal splicing to occur, the mutation of position 1 (GT→AT) totally prevents normal splicing[296] and thus leads to β⁰ thalassemia.

The mutation at position 1 of IVS-2 also totally prevents normal splicing of precursor β mRNA molecules. In the HeLa-cell transient expression system, this β⁰-thalassemic gene is transcribed normally and produces a predominant abnormal β globin mRNA species that contains a portion of IVS-2.[165] The precursor β mRNA is spliced from a cryptic 5' splice site, with a GT dinucleotide at positions 48 and 49 of IVS-2, to the normal 3' splice site,[165] thus leaving the first 47 nucleotides of IVS-2 within the abnormally processed β mRNA (see Fig. 8–32). This cryptic site exhibits a low level of homology with the "consensus" 5' splice site[168] and is not utilized in transcripts from normal β globin genes. Another minor abnormal β mRNA species was also detected: It was spliced from the 5' end of IVS-1 to the 3' end of IVS-2, thus completely removing exon 2[165] (see Fig. 8–32). The gene transfer/gene expression studies also demonstrated inefficient processing of precursor β mRNA molecules with increased accumulation of unprocessed precursors in nuclei of transfected cells. In studies of bone marrow cells from an affected individual, pulse labeling of RNA revealed normal transcription,[341] and S1 nuclease analysis of marrow cell RNA demonstrated the presence of the abnormally spliced mRNA species containing a portion of IVS-2.[305] The abnormal mRNA species was also detected in peripheral blood normoblasts of a different affected individual.[341a]

As discussed previously in the section on Gene Mapping, the mutation at position 1 of IVS-2 eliminates a recognition site, present in normal β globin genes, for the restriction endonuclease Hph I:

Hph I

GGTGA → GATGA

This mutation is therefore detectable by Southern gel blotting of total cellular DNA from affected individuals.[164, 279] An abnormal fragment of 1 kb is detected with mutant DNA, whereas normal DNA yields a fragment of 0.9 kb.

Base Substitution at the 3' Splice Junction of IVS-2. Another mutation due to a base substitution in an invariant dinucleotide splicing signal was identified, by two different groups, in β-thalassemic genes isolated from unrelated black individuals. The mutation involved the invariant dinucleotide AG located at the 3' ends of introns and consisted of a change from AG to GG at the 3' end of IVS-2.[327, 342] Gene transfer and expression studies of this mutant gene in tissue culture cells resulted in the synthesis of an abnormal β mRNA containing sequences from the 3' end of IVS-2[327, 342]; no normal splicing was detected. The precursor β mRNA was spliced from the 5' end of IVS-2 to a cryptic acceptor site at position 579 (see Fig. 8–32). The same cryptic acceptor site was utilized in the case of the β⁺ thalassemia due to a base substitution at IVS-2 position 745 (see preceding discussion and Fig. 8–32). However, in this case, there was no further processing of downstream IVS-2 sequences; thus, the 270 nucleotides from positions 580 to 850 were retained in the abnormal β mRNA. The abnormal mRNA species was easily detected, by its abnormal size, in gel fractionated RNA from erythroid cells of an affected individual.[327]

Mutations at the 3' End of IVS-1. Another type of mutation involving a splice junction consists of a 25-nucleotide deletion encompassing the 3' end of IVS-1, identified in the cloned β globin gene of a thalassemic Asian Indian individual.[343] In this case, gene transfer and expression studies revealed the synthesis of an abnormal β mRNA species that retained all of the nondeleted sequences of IVS-1, without evidence of cryptic splicing at other sites within the transcript; IVS-2 sequences were normally spliced.[343] This mutation constitutes the only example thus far described in which a thalassemia mutation in an intron is not associated with an alternative or cryptic splicing event but simply results in the retention of intron sequences without further processing of precursor mRNA molecules in the vicinity of the mutation.

This mutation also removes restriction endonuclease sites, in the deleted DNA, for the enzymes Mst II and Fnu4 HI[277a] and therefore can theoretically be detected by gene mapping procedures.

A different though somewhat similar mutation has been subsequently identified in a Kuwaiti individual. In this case, the deletion involves 17 nucleotides encompassing the 3' end of IVS-1: the terminal 15 nucleotides of the intron and 2 nucleotides of the adjacent 5' end of exon 2.[343a] The same restriction sites are affected as in the case of the 25 base pair deletion discussed previously.

As mentioned previously, a base substitution (T → G) at IVS-1 position 116[208a] is associated with β thalassemia that is probably of the $β^0$ type. As in the case of the mutation at IVS-1 position 110, the mutation creates a potential new AG acceptor dinucleotide in the context of a good consensus sequence. Functional studies of the mutant gene in a transient expression assay resulted in the synthesis of only alternatively spliced β mRNA without any detectable normal β mRNA. Unfortunately, the $β^0$ phenotype could not be ascertained *in vivo* from studies of the affected individual. A $β^0$ phenotype, rather than $β^+$ thalassemia that occurs in the case of the mutation at position 110, could be explained by the observation that the new acceptor dinucleotide created by the mutation at position 116 is separated from the normal acceptor AG by only 12 intervening nucleotides, whereas in a catalogue of normal splice junctions,[167] a second AG was consistently absent between positions −5 and −15 from the normal AG acceptor dinucleotide. It is possible that the proximity to the normal acceptor of the new AG, which is created by the mutation, results in total inactivation of the normal 3' splice site. Thus, the only processed mRNA formed would be abnormally spliced at the site of the mutation and contain 14 additional nucleotides, derived from the 3' end of IVS-1, causing a frameshift leading to an in-phase termination codon in exon 2.

The mutation at IVS-1 position 116 creates a new recognition site, absent in normal DNA, for the enzyme Mae I and should therefore be detectable in total cellular DNA by gene mapping, but fragment sizes are small (Table 8–6):

Mae I
⌐┐
CTA<u>T</u> CTA<u>G</u>

Base Substitutions Within IVS-2 That Cause Alternative Splicing Without the Occurrence of Any Normal Splicing. As previously mentioned in the discussion of $β^+$ thalassemia due to the IVS-2 mutation at position 745, two other mutations have been identified within IVS-2 at positions 654 and 705 that cause a similar pattern of alternative splicing but without the occurrence of any normal splicing of IVS-2, despite the preservation of the normal splicing signals at both of its ends. These mutations therefore cause $β^0$ thalassemia rather than $β^+$ thalassemia, as is the case with the position-745 mutation in which a small amount of normal splicing does occur.

These two mutations consist of a G<u>C</u> to GT change at position 654[316] and a <u>T</u>GT to <u>G</u>GT change at position 705.[318] In gene transfer and expression studies of these mutant genes, no normal splicing of IVS-2 sequences from the precursor β mRNA was observed.[316, 318] All of the transcripts were processed abnormally in a similar fashion to the abnormal pathway (see Fig. 8–32) for the position-745 mutation. Splicing occurs from the 5' end of the IVS-2 to the cryptic acceptor site at position 579 that is used in all of the distal IVS-2 mutations and also from the new cryptic donor sites created (or activated) by the mutations at positions 653 and 706, respectively, to the normal acceptor site at the 3' end of IVS-2 (position 850). Thus, both abnormally spliced mRNAs contain 73 and 126 additional nucleotides, respectively, that are derived from the region of IVS-2 located between the two alternative or cryptic splice sites. The reason for the lack of use of the normal splicing pathway in the case of these two mutations is not known. However, it is noteworthy that abolition of the cryptic acceptor site at position 579 by site-directed mutagenesis results in restoration of normal IVS-2 splicing from RNA transcripts of the β-thalassemic gene still carrying the mutation at position 705.[343b] These results suggest the presence of a certain hierarchy in the preferential use of splice-site pairs.

The mutation at IVS-2 position 654 has been reported by one group to be associated with $β^+$ thalassemia[343c]: There was 15 per cent Hb A in hemolysates of an affected individual where the β gene *in trans* carried the $β^0$-thalassemic nonsense mutation at codons 41 and 42. However, the report did not mention the transfusion status of the patient or provide any results of expression studies using the mutant gene.

Cloning and Sequence Analysis of α-Thalassemic Globin Genes

As previously discussed in the section on Gene Mapping, a few types of α thalassemia are not associated with deletions that are detectable by the Southern gel blotting technique. The elucidation of the molecular basis

Table 8–5. NONDELETION TYPES OF α THALASSEMIA

Phenotype and Mutation	Affected α Gene	Racial Group	Reference(s)
A. α⁺ Thalassemia			
1. Chain termination mutants			
Hb Constant Spring: TAA→CAA	α2	Southeast Asian	417
Hb Icaria: TAA→AAA	α2	Mediterranean	418
Hb Koya Dora: TAA→TCA	α2	Asian Indian	419
Hb Seal Rock: TAA→GAA	α2	Black	420
2. Unstable variants			
Hb Quong Sze; codon 125: CTG→CCG	α2	Southeast Asian	240
3. RNA processing variant			
Polyadenylation signal: AATAAA→AATAAG	α2	Saudi	245
4. Other			
(− α^T/); 2 bp deletion before initiator ATG	(−α$^{3.7}$)	Algerian	218, 459
(αα^T/)	—	Black	220
B. α⁰ Thalassemia			
1. Chain initiation mutant			
AUG→ACG	α2	Mediterranean	243a
2. Frameshift mutant			
Codon 14: TGG→ −GG	α1	Saudi	245
3. RNA processing defect			
5 bp deletion at 5′–IVS-1 splice junction	α2	Mediterranean	243
4. Other			
(− α^T/)	(−α$^{3.7}$)	Black	232, 246

of these nondeletion types of α thalassemia has necessitated the cloning and nucleotide sequence analysis of these mutant genes. The mutations that have been thus identified are listed in Table 8–5.

Short Deletion at the 5′ End of IVS-1 of the α2 Globin Gene That Prevents Normal Splicing. The first mutation identified in a case of "nondeletion" α thalassemia consisted of a short deletion of five nucleotides encompassing the 5′ splice site of IVS-1 of the α2 globin gene in a Mediterranean individual.[243] The deletion involved the T of the invariant GT of the 5′ splice site as well as the adjacent four nucleotides of IVS-1:

    GGTGAGGCT → GGCT
    └──────┘
    Hph I

The mutation eliminates a recognition site, present in normal DNA, for the restriction endonuclease Hph I and can therefore be detected by Southern gel blotting. Mutant DNA yields a fragment of 1.4 kb, whereas normal DNA gives a fragment of 1.1 kb.[243]

Gene transfer and expression studies of this mutant gene were performed in monkey kidney cells using an SV40 viral vector.[344] The level of transcription of the gene was found to be normal, but all of the transcripts were abnormally processed from a cryptic donor site in the middle of exon 1 at codon 15 to the normal acceptor site at the 3′ end of IVS-1[344] (Fig. 8–35); IVS-2 sequences were normally spliced. The mutation therefore has an effect similar to that of the mutations at the 5′ splice site of the β globin gene (see preceding discussion), except that only one rather than three alternative splicing events are observed. The cryptic splice site in exon 1 (GGTAAG) has strong homology with the normal splice site (GGTGAG) as well as with the consensus donor sequence derived from the comparison of many different genes.[166, 167] A small amount of this same alternatively spliced α mRNA was also detected with expression of a normal α globin gene in the tissue culture cells. The abnormally spliced α mRNA species was detected in RNA from bone marrow cells of an affected individual but not in normal bone marrow RNA.[344] This truncated α mRNA is obviously incapable of directing the synthesis of normal α globin. The mutation is therefore associated with an α⁰ thalassemia phenotype.

Base Substitution at Codon 125 of the α2 Globin Gene Causing the Synthesis of a Highly Unstable α-Globin Chain (Hb Quong Sze). The next form of nondeletion α thalassemia to be characterized by gene cloning and sequence analysis was identified in a Chinese individual and consisted of a single nucleotide base substitution in codon 125, CTG→CCG, changing the encoded amino acid from a Leu to a Pro.[240] The hemoglobin variant with the amino acid replacement predicted by this mutation was not detected in hemolysates of the affected individual by hemoglobin electrophoresis, so that the nature of the mutation had been

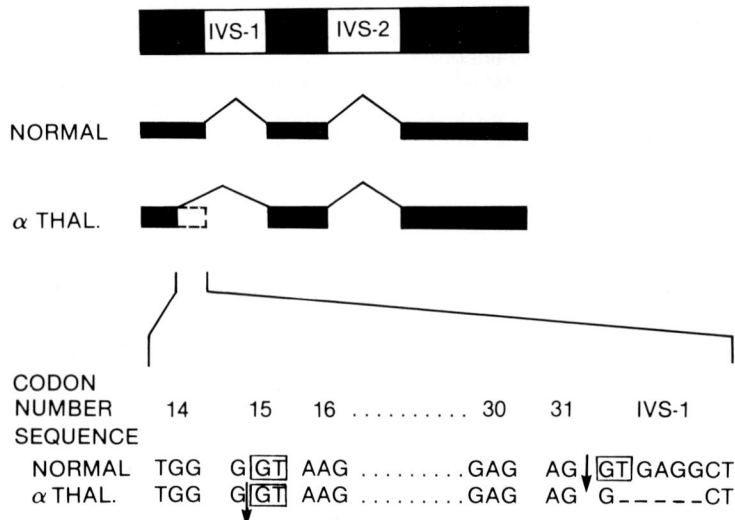

Figure 8–35. Splicing pattern in α thalassemia due to a deletion of five nucleotides at 5'-splice junction of IVS-1. The dashes represent the deleted nucleotides and the open box indicates the portion of exon 1 removed from the processed mRNA by alternative splicing.

totally unexpected prior to gene cloning and sequencing. The α-thalassemia phenotype associated with this mutation results from marked instability of the abnormal α-globin chain that is synthesized. The abnormal α-globin chain could be detected after a short (5- to 20-minute) pulse labeling of reticulocytes with ^{3}H leucine but was not detected after longer periods of labeling, presumably because it was rapidly turned over.[241] The abnormal α-globin chain was in fact more easily detectable and less unstable after translation of reticulocyte globin mRNA from the affected patient in cell-free protein synthesizing systems.[241] This structural variant was subsequently named Hb Quong Sze. The molecular basis of the α-thalassemia phenotype associated with other α globin structural variants, such as Hb Constant Spring, will be discussed in another section.

The relative levels of reticulocyte α globin mRNA derived from the α1 and α2 globin genes can be assayed by a molecular hybridization assay capable of distinguishing transcripts from each α globin gene because of differences in the nucleotide sequences of the 3' untranslated regions of the two genes.[345, 346] The α1/mutant α2 mRNA ratio was assayed in reticulocyte RNA of the affected patient with Hb H disease ($α^Tα/--$) and was found to be normal,[345] indicating that the mutant α globin mRNA was not itself unstable. The results of cell-free translation of the mRNA supported the same conclusion: roughly equal amounts of normal and mutant α globin chains were synthesized after short-term incubation in the cell-free system.[241]

This mutation creates a new restriction endonuclease site for the enzyme Msp I in the affected α globin gene that is not present in normal α globin genes:

$$C\underline{T}GG \rightarrow CC\underline{\,}GG$$
$$\underbrace{}_{Msp\ I}$$

Digestion of mutant DNA with this enzyme will generate fragments of 216 and 121 nucleotide base pairs instead of the normal fragment of 337 base pairs.[240] The mutation is therefore theoretically detectable by Southern gel blotting of total cellular DNA of affected individuals, although the fragment sizes are rather small for detection by this procedure.

Frameshift Due to a Single Base Deletion in the α1 Globin Gene and Base Substitution in the Polyadenylation Signal of the α2 Globin Gene. The nondeletion form of α thalassemia that occurs in Saudis[244] proved to be due to two different mutations in each of the two linked α globin genes: one causing $α^0$ thalassemia, and the other causing a novel form of $α^+$ thalassemia presumably due to a defect in polyadenylation of α globin mRNA. Cloning and nucleotide sequence analysis of the α1 and α2 globin genes from an affected Saudi individual homozygous for the nondeletion α-thalassemia chromosome revealed the following abnormalities[245]:

1. The α1 globin gene had a single nucleotide deletion at codon 14, causing a nonsense mutation due to frameshift: $T\underline{G}G \rightarrow -GG$, resulting in a new in-phase terminator (TGA) at codon 48.

2. The α2 globin gene had a base substitution, AATAA$\underline{A}$→AATAA$\underline{G}$, in the highly conserved hexanucleotide AATAAA that is

located approximately 20 nucleotides from the polyadenylation site of α globin mRNA transcripts and is thought to constitute the mRNA polyadenylation signal in the gene. Alpha globin mRNA is present in reticulocytes of affected individuals at levels of approximately 15 per cent of normal and represents transcripts from the α1 and α2 globin genes in a ratio of approximately 2 to 1. The transcripts from the α2 globin gene that are present in reticulocytes are polyadenylated and are normal in size. However, in a gene transfer/gene expression system in tissue culture cells, abnormally long transcripts of the α2 globin gene were detected, suggesting abnormal 3′-terminal processing and polyadenylation of nascent transcripts.[245] It is conceivable that *in vivo*, only a minor portion of the α2 globin gene transcripts are polyadenylated and that the rest are rapidly turned over because they are unstable. In various experimental systems, it has been shown that mRNA lacking poly(A) is less stable than polyadenylated mRNA (see Chapter 7). Although some modifications of the hexanucleotide polyadenylation signal have been described in different genes, the particular base change associated with the Saudi α2 globin gene has not yet been identified in any other normal genes.

Base Substitution in the Initiation Codon of the α2 Globin Gene. A mutation involving the initiation codon of the α2 globin gene is responsible for the majority of cases of nondeletion α thalassemia in Sardinian individuals.[243a] The base substitution (A$\underline{T}$G → A$\underline{C}$G) prevents the synthesis of normal α globin chains from the mutant mRNA. The steady state level of the mutant α2 mRNA was found to be decreased by approximately twofold: In normal subjects, the α2:α1 mRNA ratio was found to be 3:1, but in an affected individual with Hb H disease (--/α^{T}α) the ratio was 1:1.[243a] It is not clear if the decreased accumulation of the mutant α mRNA is due to decreased transcription of the gene or to decreased stability of the mRNA.

The mutation abolishes a site, present in normal α globin gene DNA, for the restriction endonuclease Nco I:

$$\overset{\text{Nco I}}{\overline{\text{CCA}\underline{\text{T}}\text{GG}}} \longrightarrow \text{CCA}\underline{\text{C}}\text{GG}$$

As a result, this mutation is easily detectable by Southern gel blotting.[243a] Digestion of normal DNA with both Pst I and Nco I yields fragments of 0.6 and 0.9 kb, whereas mutant DNA yields a new fragment of 1.5 kb.

Partial Deletion of the α1 Globin Gene. As noted earlier in the section on Gene Mapping, Southern gel blotting of DNA from certain Mediterranean patients with Hb H disease reveals an abnormally sized Eco RI fragment of 2.6 kb that hybridizes to α globin gene probes.[210] This abnormal fragment has been cloned and the α globin gene region subjected to nucleotide sequence analysis.[144] The restriction endonuclease map of the cloned DNA fragment was consistent with that of the α1 globin gene and its 3′-flanking DNA. However, certain sites normally present at the 5′ end of the α1 globin gene were missing from the cloned DNA. Nucleotide sequence analysis revealed that the 5′ portion of the gene was deleted up to and including codon 56; the first DNA sequence consistent with the α1 globin gene started at codon 57. The published nucleotide sequence[144] of the DNA immediately preceding codon 57 is consistent with that of a repetitive DNA sequence of the Alu I family[200] (see preceding discussion and Chapter 7). Subsequent gene mapping and sequencing studies demonstrated that the Alu I family sequence involved in the recombination event is one of those normally located between the ζ and ψζ globin genes.[236] The break point at the junction between Alu I sequence and α globin gene sequence occurs after nucleotide 93 of the 300 base pair–long Alu I sequence element. Thus, this mutation represents another example of a deletion in a globin gene cluster that involves a repetitive sequence of the Alu I family at its break point. As discussed previously, this phenomenon may have occurred by chance alone and may not be significant with regard to the mechanism(s) that generated these deletions.

The absence of the 5′ end of the α1 globin gene in this mutation would be expected to inactivate its function and thereby constitute a form of α^0 thalassemia. The gene has been studied in an SV40 virus/monkey kidney cell expression system.[347] Transcripts containing α globin mRNA sequences were obtained, but these transcripts also contained sequences complementary to repetitive DNA sequences of the Alu I family. It was not determined if the transcripts originated from promoter sequences in the SV40 virus vector or from the promoter sequences for RNA polymerase III present within the conserved 5′ portion of the

Alu I DNA sequence located immediately upstream from the truncated thalassemic α1 globin gene in the cloned DNA segment. In fact, the highly conserved internal promoter sequences for RNA polymerase III, at nucleotides 75 to 87,[200] are conserved in the Alu I DNA that precedes the mutant α globin gene. There is no information concerning the presence or absence of such transcripts in bone marrow cells of affected patients. It is noteworthy, however, that this mutation was present in a patient with Hb H disease whose α/β mRNA ratio was higher in bone marrow than in peripheral blood, suggesting the presence of an unstable α globin mRNA.[47]

Cloned α Thalassemia 2 ($-\alpha^{3.7}/$) Genes. The single α globin genes from α thalassemia 2 chromosomes of the rightward deletion type ($-\alpha^{3.7}/$) have been cloned from two different Asian individuals and subjected to nucleotide sequence analysis[219, 219a] in order to identify the site at which the recombination event occurred.

As noted previously in the section on Gene Mapping, there are at least three different types of α globin genes associated with the rightward-deletion form of α thalassemia. The most common type involves a crossover between the α1 and α2 genes that occurred 5' to the distal end of IVS-2 in the α1 gene.[219] The nucleotide sequence of such a gene[219a] revealed that the 3' end of the gene, including the distal two thirds of IVS-2, was derived from the α1 gene.

The 5' ends of the normal α1 and α2 genes have identical sequences up to position 54 of IVS-2. Thus, it was impossible to tell precisely where the crossover between the two genes had occurred other than somewhere between positions −869 in the 5'-flanking DNA and position 54 of IVS-2. The DNA 5' to position −869 was clearly derived from 5'-flanking DNA of the α2 gene.[219a] Between positions −869 and −634, the sequence changed from that of α2 to α1 to α2 again, suggesting the occurrence of a gene conversion event.[219a] However, subsequent analysis of other normal and α-thalassemic genes revealed that the apparent interrupted switchover to an α1 sequence could be explained by a polymorphism found in the 5'-flanking DNA of the α2 gene without the need to invoke a gene conversion event.[219] Thus, the area of the crossover can be further narrowed down to between position −634 and the 5' end of IVS-2.

Delta Thalassemia in Man and Nonhuman Primates

Isolated thalassemia affecting the δ globin gene has been identified in individuals who totally lack Hb A_2 and are either homozygous for δ thalassemia or doubly heterozygous for δ thalassemia and δβ thalassemia (see Chapter 9). A form of δ thalassemia has also been described in which there is only partial rather than total suppression of δ-chain synthesis.[348] Thus, there occur both δ^+ and δ^0 forms of δ thalassemia. Gene mapping studies in such individuals do not demonstrate any detectable deletion of the δ globin gene.[169a, 348-350a] A δ globin gene from a Japanese individual with homozygous δ^0 thalassemia has been cloned and its nucleotide sequence determined.[351] No differences in nucleotide sequence were detected between the δ-thalassemic gene and a normal δ gene isolated from a Japanese individual, although two differences were noted in IVS-2 (positions 291 and 292) of both Japanese genes when compared with the δ globin gene sequence of an Anglo-Saxon individual[352]; these differences probably represent polymorphisms. Of note is the fact that the nucleotide sequence analysis included 300 nucleotides of the 5'-flanking DNA of the δ genes upstream from the "cap site" for initiation of mRNA transcription. Thus, the mutation affecting the expression of this δ-thalassemic globin gene must be located outside of the region that was sequenced and is therefore more remote from the gene than the mutations causing the β thalassemias. Functional studies of the cloned δ-thalassemic globin gene in gene transfer/gene expression systems have not yet been reported.

Delta thalassemia also occurs in nonhuman primates, such as the Old World monkeys, who do not synthesize Hb A_2 despite the presence of δ globin genes in their DNA.[353, 354] A number of different mutations have been identified by cloning and nucleotide sequence analysis of δ globin genes from various nonhuman primates, and thus, a picture has emerged on the mechanism of silencing of δ globin gene expression in these animals.[355] The cloned δ globin genes from two evolutionarily distant Old World monkeys (colobus and rhesus) were shown to be transcribed very inefficiently in a cell-free transcription system when compared with a human δ globin gene. The only differences in the nucleotide sequence of the 5'-flanking DNA of these different δ globin genes consisted of three changes (base substitutions) at positions −92, −52, and −23 from the cap site[355]; the base substitution at position −52 was not found in a different Old World species, the baboon.[356] Thus, one (or both) of the other differences between the human and monkey sequences may be the primary cause of the silencing of the δ gene in all of the Old World monkeys by markedly decreasing the transcriptional activity of the gene.[355] Subsequent (? secondary) mutations may have then occurred by evolutionary drift in different monkey species: a 20 nucleotide–long deletion encompassing the cap site in the colobus δ globin gene[355] and a frameshift mutation by insertion of one nucleotide at codon 55 in the δ globin genes of both the rhesus monkey and the baboon,[355, 356] leading to the generation of a termination codon at position 59.

In an evolutionarily more distant prosimian, the brown lemur, a δ pseudogene has resulted from a crossover between the ψβ1 gene (see Chapter 7) and the δ gene, leading to the formation of a Lepore-like fusion gene having the 5' end of the nonfunctional ψβ1 gene and the 3' end (including IVS-2) of the δ globin gene.[357]

Nondeletion HPFH

$^G\gamma\beta^+$ **HPFH.** The molecular basis of the $^G\gamma\beta^+$ type of nondeletion HPFH, which occurs in blacks, has been studied by gene cloning and nucleotide sequence analysis of the γ globin genes from affected individuals. The structure of $^A\gamma$ globin gene has been found to be normal,[357a] but a single nucleotide base substitution has been identified in the 5'-flanking DNA of the $^G\gamma$ globin gene that may explain the persistent expression the $^G\gamma$ globin gene in this syndrome.[357b] The base substitution is a change from C to G at position −202 from the cap site of the $^G\gamma$ gene (Fig. 8–36A). The change occurs in a GC-rich sequence that has homology to elements in the upstream promoter regions of the gene for thymidine kinase (TK) of herpes virus and of the "early region" of SV40 virus (in the 21–base pair repeated sequence). These GC-rich sequences have been shown to be important for the normal function of the viral genes and, in the case of the SV40 promoter, to be involved in the interaction with a specific transcription factor.[357c] It has been proposed that the base change in $^G\gamma\beta^+$ HPFH may represent an "up promoter" mutation leading to enhanced levels of expression of the $^G\gamma$ globin gene even into adult life. However, this theory has not yet been proved by appropriate gene transfer/gene expression studies *in vitro*.

It should be noted that the base change in the $^G\gamma\beta^+$ HPFH eliminates a recognition site, present in normal DNA, for the restriction endonuclease Apa I. The base substitution can therefore be identified by gel blotting of total cellular DNA. The significance of the base change in the pathogenesis of this form of HPFH is underscored by the findings that the Apa I site is missing in 13 other individuals with $^G\gamma\beta^+$ HPFH from 5 different families[357d, 357e] and that it has not been found to be missing (as a random polymorphism) in a large number of black individuals without this form of HPFH.[357c] However, only one of the non-HPFH individuals had a haplotype of restriction site polymorphisms that was closely related, although not identical, to that usually associated with the $^G\gamma\beta^+$ HPFH chromosome. The formal although unlikely possibility therefore exists that the Apa I mutation is not the cause of the HPFH phenotype but consists of a polymorphism found only on this rare chromosome. It is also noteworthy that not all of the individuals lacking the Apa I site carry the HPFH determinant in a β gene cluster that has the same haplotype or subset of restriction site polymorphisms[357f]; the occasional individuals with a different haplotype either carry the same mutation, which may have occurred independently on a different chromosomal background, or may have a different base substitution or mutation in the same region of the 5'-flanking DNA of the $^G\gamma$ globin gene that also abolishes the Apa I site, the recognition sequence of which contains six nucleotides (GGGCCC). Finally, it should be noted that the Apa I site was intact[357d] in an individual from yet another family[192] with the black $^G\gamma\beta^+$ type of nondeletion HPFH, suggesting that different mutations can cause the same phenotype.

There is also a rare heterocellular subtype of $^G\gamma\beta^+$ HPFH that is associated with lower than usual levels of Hb F (3.5 to 9 per cent versus approximately 20 per cent).[357e] The Apa I site 5' to the $^G\gamma$ gene has been found to be normal in such cases, and the high $^G\gamma$ phenotype has been ascribed to the combination of a $^G\gamma$-$^G\gamma$ chromosome and the possible influence of a base change at position −158 that creates a polymorphism for the enzyme Xmn I.[357g]

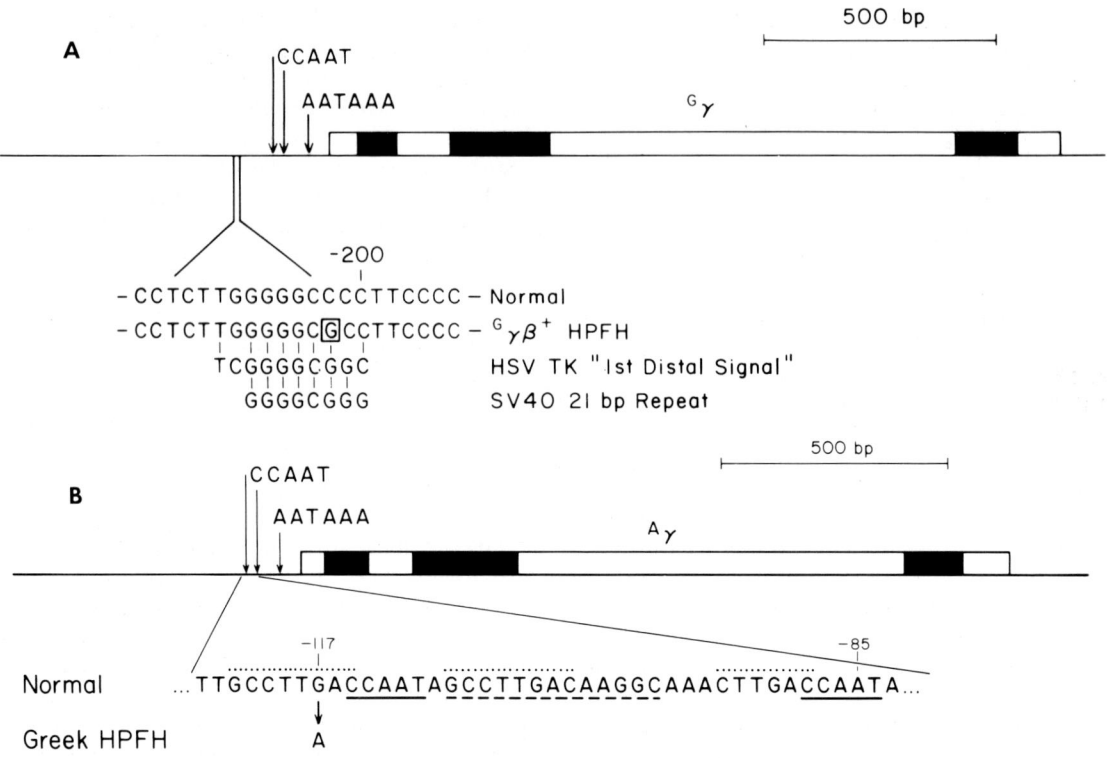

Figure 8–36. *A*, Mutation at position −202 in the 5′-flanking DNA of the $^G\gamma$ globin gene in $^G\gamma\beta^+$ HPFH. The base substitution is indicated by the box. The mutated sequence is compared with that of control elements found in SV40 virus and in the promoter region of the thymidine kinase (TK) gene of herpes simplex virus (HSV). (From Collins, F. S., et al.: Proc. Natl. Acad. Sci. USA *81*:4894, 1984.) *B*, Mutation at position −117 in the 5′-flanking DNA of the $^A\gamma$ globin gene in Greek HPFH. The peculiar structure of the duplicated CCAAT box of the γ gene promotor is shown: The dotted line above the sequence indicates a directly repeated sequence around the CCAAT sequences and the dashed line under the sequence indicates a 13-bp palindrome. (From Collins, F. S., et al.: Nature *313*:325, 1985.)

Greek ($^A\gamma$) Type of HPFH. In the case of nondeletion Greek or $^A\gamma$ type of HPFH, a different point mutation has been identified in the 5′-flanking DNA of the $^A\gamma$ globin gene: a base substitution of G→A at position −117 from the cap site of the $^A\gamma$ gene[357h, 357i] (Fig. 8–36B). This mutation is particularly noteworthy because it is the first naturally occurring mutation to be found in close proximity to the CCAAT "box" of a eukaryotic promoter element. The base change involves the nucleotide located two base pairs to the 5′ side of the upstream CCAAT box (which is duplicated in the case of the γ globin genes [see Chapter 7 and Fig. 8–36B]): GACCAAT → AACCAAT. A survey of published nucleotide sequences of mammalian embryonic and fetal globin genes reveals that the sequence TTGA precedes the CCAAT in all cases, implying a functional role for these nucleotides. Furthermore, studies of site-directed mutagenesis of the mouse β^{major} globin gene promoter region have demonstrated that a G → A mutation in the same position relative to the CCAAT box resulted in an approximately twofold increase in the expression of that gene following transfer and transient expression in HeLa cells.[357j] It is remarkable therefore that a mutation in a highly conserved sequence within a promoter element leads to increased rather than decreased expression of the involved gene. Although a direct cause-and-effect relationship between the mutations and the HPFH phenotype has not yet been established, the indirect evidence for such a relationship is compelling.

In an Italian individual with the phenotype of $^A\gamma$ HPFH, a different mutation was found: a C to T base change at position −196 from the cap site of the $^A\gamma$ gene.[357k] This mutation may have similar effects on γ gene expression as the −202 mutation in the black $^G\gamma\beta^+$ type of HPFH.

General Conclusions

Cloning and nucleotide sequence analysis of thalassemic globin genes together with functional studies of the cloned genes in expression systems have provided, in the majority of cases, the key to the discovery of the precise molecular basis of different forms of α and β thalassemia. What has emerged from this large body of recent information is a picture of thalassemia as a disorder with a previously unexpected diversity of etiologies that nevertheless has, within a certain range, a relatively homogeneous phenotype from the point of view of biochemical and clinical manifestations. Particularly remarkable has been the identification of multiple defects, at virtually each of the defined stages or steps of gene expression, that have as their end result the synthesis or accumulation of reduced amounts of the mRNA and/or polypeptide chains for one of the globin chain subunits. Thus, the following have been characterized: defects in globin gene transcription; post-transcriptional processing of precursor mRNA molecules, including splicing and polyadenylation; intranuclear stability and/or nucleus-to-cytoplasm transport of nascent mRNA molecules; possibly cytoplasmic stability of mutant globin mRNA; abnormal translation of globin mRNAs with nonsense mutations leading to premature termination of translation and synthesis of nonsense peptides; and finally, the synthesis of highly unstable globin chains that are so rapidly degraded that they are not normally detected in hemolysates of affected erythroid cells. It would have been difficult to anticipate or predict the existence of such an all-encompassing array of naturally occurring mutations in a genetic disorder that has a relatively limited amount of biochemical and clinical heterogeneity. More significantly, the precise characterization of the basis of thalassemia mutations has permitted the development of more precise methods to make the diagnosis of specific forms of thalassemia prenatally, as well as in the course of population surveys, as will be discussed in the following section.

IMPLICATIONS FOR PRENATAL DIAGNOSIS OF THALASSEMIA

The characterization of thalassemia mutations at the DNA level has led to the application of various molecular biology techniques for the prenatal detection of thalassemia. As discussed in Chapter 9, prenatal diagnosis of thalassemia was initially achieved by fetal blood aspiration and analysis of the globin-chain synthesis in the fetal blood cells. Although quite accurate, this technique has the drawbacks that fetal blood sampling can only be performed in a small number of centers by experienced individuals and is associated, even in the best of hands, with a significant risk of mortality (approximately 5 per cent) or of morbidity to the fetus. Amniocentesis is a much safer procedure and can provide fetal cells as a source of DNA for the molecular diagnosis of thalassemia. The procedure of chorionic villus biopsy in the first trimester is currently being investigated as an alternative procedure for obtaining DNA for prenatal detection of abnormal globin (and other) genes.[358–362]

Prenatal Detection of Globin Gene Deletions

The earliest applications of molecular biology to prenatal detection of thalassemia consisted of molecular hybridization assays[146, 361, 362] or gene mapping studies[173, 224] to detect thalassemia syndromes due to gene deletions, such as the common forms of α thalassemia and δβ thalassemia. Theoretically, any thalassemia defect that is associated with an abnormal globin gene pattern on Southern gel blotting can be detected in this way. Simpler hybridization assays have subsequently been devised for the prenatal demonstration of total absence of α globin gene DNA in hydrops fetalis with Hb Bart's. These assays utilize the technique of direct "dot blotting"[362a, 462] or "slot blotting"[362b] of DNA, and they have the advantage that they can give a definitive diagnosis with only a small amount of DNA and without the need to perform restriction endonuclease digestion or the gel electrophoresis and transfer steps of the Southern gel blotting procedure.

However, most of the demand for prenatal diagnosis concerns pregnancies in which the fetus is at risk for homozygous β thalassemia in which the molecular defects are of the nondeletion type, and different strategies had to be devised for the prenatal diagnosis of these disorders, as will be discussed in the following sections.

Prenatal Detection of Thalassemia by Gene Mapping Using Restriction Fragment Length Polymorphisms

A widely applicable procedure for prenatal diagnosis of thalassemia in the absence of gene deletion or of a direct assay for the mutant gene was gradually developed with the identification of relatively frequent polymorphisms for a number of different restriction endonuclease sites within the non–α globin gene cluster. Thus, it became possible by Southern gel blotting to identify and track, in a given family, linkage of polymorphisms for Hind III sites in IVS-2 of the γ globin genes,[363] or for a Bam HI site in the 3'-flanking DNA of the β globin gene,[364] or both,[365] to β-thalassemic genes that were coinherited with the marker polymorphism(s) in the family. This procedure was initially used for the prenatal detection of sickle cell anemia at the DNA level after it was discovered that a polymorphism for a Hpa I site in the 3'-flanking DNA of the β globin gene was linked to the sickle cell mutation in a high proportion of the cases[226] (see Chapter 7). In the case of thalassemia, this procedure is relatively tedious, as it requires the study of a large number of family members to establish the pattern of inheritance of a given polymorphism with the particular thalassemic globin genes in the family. It also has limited applicability, not being feasible in the cases of first pregnancies and families in which parents do not display heterozygosity for the polymorphic marker, although it is estimated that with the combined use of the Bam HI with the Hind III polymorphisms, prenatal diagnosis of β thalassemia can be accomplished in approximately 75 per cent of cases.[365]

The observation that the polymorphisms at seven different sites in the non–α globin gene cluster were associated with one another in a nonrandom fashion,[278] forming nine general haplotypes or chromosome subsets, led to the subsequent demonstration that specific molecular forms of thalassemia were associated, in a given population group, with one particular haplotype or subset of polymorphisms[279] (see Tables 8–3 and 8–4). The prenatal diagnosis of thalassemia by full haplotype analysis of restriction endonuclease polymorphisms in amniocyte DNA thus became more generally applicable and quite precise. In a large study of 32 pregnancies in which the fetus was at risk for β thalassemia, prenatal diagnosis was achieved solely by analysis of DNA polymorphisms in 86 per cent of the cases, without any diagnostic errors.[366] In another study of 20 Cypriot and 42 Asian families, the prenatal diagnosis of homozygous β thalassemia by haplotype analysis of multiple restriction fragment length polymorphisms was possible in 76 per cent of the Asian and 35 per cent of the Cypriot families.[366a] The low feasibility rate in Cypriots is due to the fact that haplotype I (see Fig. 8–27) is the preponderant haplotype in this population and that the most common type of β thalassemia in Cypriots is the mutation of IVS-1 position 110, which is also linked to haplotype I. However, a polymorphism of an Ava II site in the ψβ gene has subsequently been identified that is in linkage disequilibrium with this type of β-thalassemia gene and increases the feasibility of successful prenatal diagnosis in the same Cypriot population from 35 per cent to 90 per cent.[366b]

Although quite accurate, haplotype analysis remains a labor-intensive procedure requiring multiple analyses with different enzymes. A moderate amount of amniocyte DNA is needed, and this usually requires the time-consuming and expensive procedure of culturing the amniotic fluid to obtain more cells. In addition, the test may not provide a definitive answer in approximately 10 to 15 per cent of cases. Ideally, one would prefer a procedure that has 100 per cent applicability and can directly, rather than indirectly, identify the mutation by a single analysis requiring a small amount of DNA such as can be isolated directly from aspirated amniotic fluid cells rather than a culture of these cells. Such procedures have in fact been devised and fall into two categories, as discussed in the sections that follow.

Direct Identification of Mutations by Differences in Restriction Endonuclease Cleavage Pattern Due to the Mutation Itself

A number of the base substitutions (or other subtle mutations) causing α or β thalassemia abolish or create cleavage sites for different restriction endonucleases at the precise point of the mutation and are therefore directly detectable by Southern gel blotting of total cellular DNA from affected individuals. Table 8–6 lists the various types of thalassemia that can be detected directly at the DNA level by changes in restriction endonuclease cleavage sites. This approach was first used for the successful prenatal diagnosis[367] of Hb O-Arab (β 121 Glu→Lys), in which the base substitution abolishes the intragenic Eco RI site of the β globin gene[367, 368] and has subsequently been applied to the detection of a number of other hemoglobin variants.[369–370a] A particularly useful application of this type of analysis was developed when restriction endonucleases were identified, initially Dde I[371, 372] and then

Table 8–6. THALASSEMIC MUTATIONS THAT AFFECT RESTRICTION ENDONUCLEASE RECOGNITION SITES

Mutation	Recognition Site[1]	Fragment Size	
		Normal	Thalassemic
A. α Thalassemias			
1. Initiation codon mutations	Nco I (−)	0.6 + 0.9 kb[2]	1.5 kb[2]
2. Codon 14 frameshift	Msp I (+)	162 bp	79 + 82 bp
3. IVS-1 5′ splice junction (5 bp deletion)	Hph I (−)	1.1 kb	1.4 kb
4. Hb Quong Sze	Msp I (+)	337 bp	216 bp
B. β Thalassemias			
1. −87 from cap site	Avr II (−)	2.3 kb[3]	4 kb[3]
2. Codon 6 frameshift	Mst II (−)	1.15 kb	1.35 kb
3. Codon 17 nonsense	Mae I (+)	790 bp	72 + 718 bp
4. IVS-1 position 6	Sfa NI (+)	280 bp[4]	90 + 190 bp
5. IVS-1 position 116	Mae I (+)	790 bp	226 + 564 bp
6. Deletions of 25 bp and 17 bp at 3′ end of IVS-I	Mst II (−)	202 bp	291 bp
7. Codon 39 nonsense	Mae I (+)	790 bp	268 + 522 bp
8. IVS-2 position 1	Hph I (−)	0.9 kb	1.0 kb
9. IVS-2 position 745	Rsa I (+)	2.2 kb	1.9 kb
	Kpn I (+)	~39 kb	~35 + 3.7 kb
10. IVS-2 position 849	Alu I (−)	130 bp	180 bp

[1](+) indicates that the site is created by the thalassemic mutation, and (−) indicates that the site is abolished by the mutation.
[2]The sizes are for DNA doubly digested with Pst I + Nco I.[243a]
[3]The sizes are for DNA doubly digested with Avr II + Hind III.[279]
[4]The size is for a framework 3 gene in which the polymorphism at codon 2 creates a new Sfa NI site; the fragment size in genes of framework 1 or 2 is ~700 bp.

Mst II,[373–375] that have recognition sites encompassing β globin codon 6 that are abolished by the base substitution causing the sickle cell mutation (β 6 Glu→Val). Successful prenatal diagnosis of Hb S has been accomplished by this procedure,[375, 376] and direct DNA diagnosis using the enzyme Mst II now constitutes the method of choice for prenatal diagnosis of sickle cell anemia (see Chapter 12 and Fig. 12–22).

In the case of β thalassemia, although there are a number of mutations that affect restriction endonuclease sites (see Table 8–6), these constitute, in general, relatively rare forms of the disease, and actual attempts at prenatal diagnosis of these mutations have not yet been reported. In some cases, such as the IVS-2 acceptor site mutation, the small size of the affected DNA fragments would make direct prenatal detection using amniocyte DNA difficult and perhaps impractical. Furthermore, it is particularly unfortunate that the most common forms of β thalassemia in Mediterraneans, such as the mutation at IVS-1 position 110, do not affect restriction endonuclease sites and are therefore not directly detectable at the DNA level by restriction endonuclease analysis. Although the common β 39 nonsense mutation creates a new cleavage site for the enzyme Mae I[463] (see Table 8–6), fragment sizes and other factors generated may not allow a practical prenatal detection test. A different strategy has therefore been devised for the direct DNA diagnosis of these and other thalassemic mutations, as described in the next section.

Direct Identification of Single Base Substitutions by the Use of Synthetic Oligonucleotide Probes

The precedent-setting work of Wallace and associates[377] established the feasibility of direct detection of single nucleotide base substitutions in globin gene DNA by the use of labeled synthetic oligonucleotide probes 19 nucleotides long, in which the central nucleotide was either identical or different from that in the target DNA being analyzed. Hybridization conditions were established that would allow annealing of the synthetic probe to its target only if all 19 nucleotides were perfectly complementary. If the one central nucleotide was different, no hybridization was observed. Thus, it was possible to distinguish $β^A$ globin DNA from $β^S$ globin DNA with such oligonucleotide probes, initially in cloned DNA samples[377] and then in total cellular DNA,[378] thereby establishing the basis for using this procedure to detect base substitutions in β globin gene DNA of amniocytes or placental villi.

The general strategy of this approach consists of using two oligonucleotide probes, one complementary to the normal sequence and the other complementary to the mutant sequence with the single nucleotide substitution. With two probes, one can have positive and negative controls for the detection of both the normal and the mutant sequence, thereby allowing the detection of heterozygotes as well as homozygotes for the target sequences. Because, on a random basis, total cellular DNA contains multiple regions that can hybridize to a given 19 base oligonucleotide, it is not possible to perform the analysis directly on dots or spots of total unfractionated DNA. However, if the DNA is digested with a restriction endonuclease and then fractionated by gel electrophoresis and processed according to regular Southern gel blotting procedures, it is possible to separate the specific target fragment (containing globin gene sequences) away from the nonspecifically hybridizing fragments located elsewhere in the genome. In the case of the human β globin gene, a convenient enzyme for this purpose is Bam HI; it yields a 1.8-kb fragment containing the 5' end of the β globin gene that is well separated from higher–molecular weight fragments that hybridize to oligonucleotide probes directed at sequences in exon 1 or IVS-1 of the β globin gene. An example of such an analysis is shown in Figure 8–37.

This technique has been applied to the direct detection in DNA of the two most common forms of β thalassemia: the mutation at IVS-1 position 110 causing β$^+$ thalassemia by alternative splicing, and the nonsense mutation at codon 39 causing β^0 thalassemia by premature chain termination. Both mutations are caused by single nucleotide base substitutions. Synthetic oligonucleotide probes were prepared corresponding to the normal and mutant sequences in both regions and were shown to be capable of directly detecting the target mutations in total cellular DNA of affected individuals.[379, 380] This approach has been used successfully for the prenatal diagnosis of β^0 thalassemia due to the codon 39 nonsense mutation in a large number of pregnancies in which the fetus was at risk and was found to be quite accurate and reliable[380, 464] (see Fig. 8–37).

It should therefore be feasible, with a battery of oligonucleotide probes, to directly identify specific β-thalassemia mutations in parents heterozygous for β thalassemia and then use

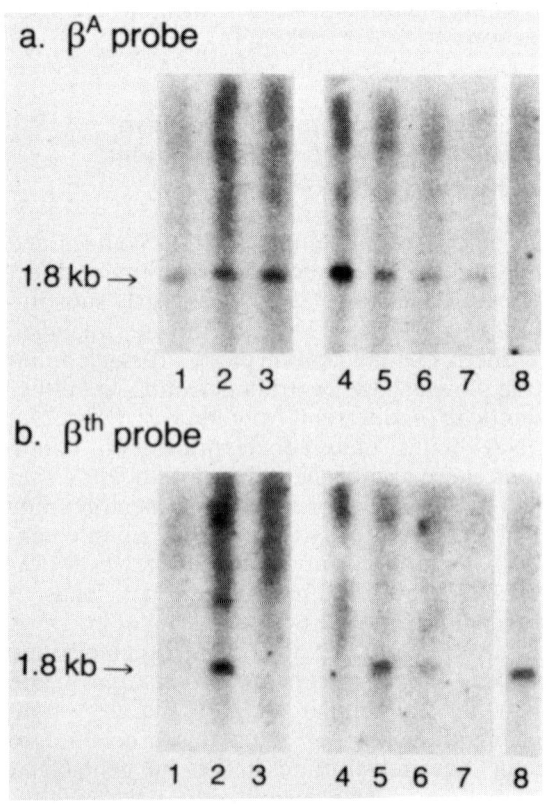

Figure 8–37. Detection of β^0 thalassemia due to the β 39 nonsense mutation by hybridization of synthetic oligonucleotide probes to restriction endonuclease digests of total cellular DNA. The filter from the Southern gel blot was hybridized initially to an oligonucleotide complementary to the normal β globin gene (β^A probe) and then later washed and rehybridized to an oligonucleotide complementary to the sequence with the single base substitution causing the β 39 nonsense mutation (βth probe). The target band derived from DNA digested with Bam HI is 1.8 kb in length. Normal DNA samples (lanes 1, 3, 4, and 7) show hybridization only to the β^A probes; DNA sample from an individual homozygous for the mutation (lane 8) shows hybridization only to the βth probe, whereas DNA samples from individuals heterozygous for the mutation (lanes 2, 5, and 6) show hybridization to both probes. (From Pirastu, M., et al.: N. Engl. J. Med. *309*:284, 1983.)

the appropriate probes for detection of the presence or absence of these mutations in DNA samples from pregnancies in which the fetus is at risk. Such studies could utilize DNA either from amniocytes or eventually, after the safety of the procedure is demonstrated, from chorionic villi. In addition to the oligonucleotide probes for the two common mutations discussed earlier, probes are currently available that have been shown to be effective for the detection of three β-thalassemic mutations due to base substitutions at positions 1, 5, and 6 of IVS-1.[310, 311, 381] In the future, this approach will no doubt constitute the method of choice for direct prenatal detection of thalassemia at the DNA level.

Detection of Base Substitutions by Differential Mobility of Restriction Fragments in Denaturing Gradient Gels

A novel technique has been devised that allows the identification of different single base substitutions in a fragment of DNA by its differential mobility in a specialized acrylamide gel system that subjects the migrating DNA fragments to a gradient of denaturing forces.[381a] Thus, fragments with different types of base substitutions at a given position or with substitutions at different positions (and therefore in different sequence environments) will denature and acquire altered mobility at different positions in the gel because different DNA sequences will usually require somewhat different conditions of denaturation in order for the two strands to separate or "melt." The differential mobility between mutant and normal fragments can be further enhanced by mixing them together and then subjecting them to denaturation and renaturation, thus allowing the formation of heteroduplexes or hybrid DNA fragments in which one strand is normal and the complementary strand contains the base substitution. The heteroduplexes will be substantially more unstable than the parent molecules and thus will be more widely separated from the latter after gel electrophoresis. The technique, which was initially applied to the study of cloned globin genes, has also been used successfully to detect single base substitutions in thalassemic globin genes by analysis of total cellular DNA digested with appropriate restriction enzymes. This technique therefore constitutes another screening procedure for the identification of individuals carrying novel or specific mutations in a given region of a globin (or other) gene.

APPLICATIONS TO POPULATION SURVEYS AND ANALYSIS OF GENETIC MECHANISMS

A number of the observations and results obtained during the course of molecular genetic studies of thalassemia have made possible an in-depth genetic analysis of the incidence and distribution of specific thalassemia mutations in different population groups. Haplotyping of restriction fragment length polymorphisms, on the one hand, followed by direct detection of suspected mutations using restriction endonuclease digestion or hybridization to synthetic oligonucleotide probes (see preceding discussion), can provide a very precise picture of the incidence and distribution of thalassemia subtypes in a given population.

The Mediterranean population has been studied most extensively thus far. The prevalence of different haplotypes in Mediterranean β-thalassemic patients is shown in Figure 8–27. Follow-up studies of this population[381] using synthetic oligonucleotides (or restriction endonuclease digestion) for direct identification of thalassemic mutations have led to some interesting observations. In general, a given haplotype within this population is usually associated with one specific type of thalassemia.[277a, 277b, 279, 306] Thus, by haplotype analysis, one can predict, with approximately 90 per cent accuracy, the specific molecular type(s) of β thalassemia present in a given individual. However, there are exceptions: more than one type of thalassemia can be found within a given haplotype, and a specific thalassemia mutation may be associated with two or more haplotypes in the same population.[277a, 277b, 279, 381, 382] With haplotype I, which is the most common haplotype in Mediterranean β-thalassemic patients (see Fig. 8–27), approximately 90 per cent of cases are associated with the mutation at IVS-1 position 110.[277a, 277b, 306, 381, 382] However, other β-thalassemic mutations are also associated with haplotype I in Mediterraneans: the frameshift mutation at codon 6,[338] Hb Knossos,[309] the mutation at IVS-1 position 116,[208] and even the β 39 nonsense mutation.[381, 383] Thus, it cannot be assumed that all Mediterranean β-thalassemic individuals with haplotype I have the IVS-1 position 110 mutation. This result is not totally surprising; it would be expected that multiple different independent mutations might occur on the same chromosomal background if the latter is particularly common in a given normal population, as is haplotype I.

Although a number of examples exist of the association of a given specific β-thalassemic mutation with more than one different haplotype,[279, 381, 382] the most interesting cases consist of the β 39 nonsense and $β^E$ globin genes. In the case of the β 39 nonsense mutation, the defect has been shown, by hybridization studies using synthetic oligonucleotide probes, to be associated with at least seven different haplotypes.[381, 382–383a] In the case of five of the haplotypes, the differences in restriction fragment length polymorphisms are located in the block of sites 5' to the δ gene; the polymorphic sites within (or very close to) the β globin gene itself are uniform. Thus, the observation could be explained by a single mutation in an ancestral β globin gene that then "spread" to other chromosomes by recombination, with the crossover site being located between the two blocks of restriction fragment length polymorphisms (indicated by the brackets labeled I and II in Fig. 7–11). Such a crossover event between these two regions of the non-α globin gene cluster has in fact been documented in one family.[384]

However, the β 39 nonsense mutation has also been identified in β globin genes with different intragenic polymorphic sites (see Fig. 7–11) or, in the terminology of Kazazian and colleagues,[382] in different β globin gene "frameworks." There are three (or four) basic β globin gene frameworks that differ by two to five intragenic nucleotide base substitutions.[277a, 277b, 279, 382] The occurrence of the same mutation in two different β gene frameworks, especially the two differing by five nucleotides (one in exon 1 and four in IVS-2) implies that the identical mutation must have arisen spontaneously at least twice, once in each framework.[382] Alternatively, if one holds to the theory of a single ancestral mutation, the findings can only be explained by a rare localized interchromosomal recombination event called gene conversion.[385] Such short, discrete, recombination or gene conversion events appear to have occurred in the case of IVS-2 of the γ globin genes[386, 387] as well as in the histocompatibility and immunoglobulin genes.[388–390] In the case of the Hb E mutation in Asian populations, it also has been identified in two different β globin gene frameworks, differing by four nucleotides.[382, 391] The same explanations must also apply in this case: separate identical mutations or gene conversion.

As noted previously in the introduction to the section on Gene Cloning, the occurrence of different haplotypes of restriction fragment length polymorphisms provided a strategy for the rapid screening of individuals likely to be carrying different β-thalassemic genes and thus facilitated the efficient cloning and characterization of many different forms of β thalassemia.[277a, 277b, 279] The theory, subsequently proved in practice, states that in a given population, different molecular forms of thalassemia are likely to be associated with different haplotypes. Thus, when surveying a particular racial group for the presence of different thalassemic mutations, one should choose for cloning and sequence analysis, β-thalassemic genes that are linked to different haplotypes. This strategy has proved fruitful for the identification of new β-thalassemic mutations in Mediterranean,[279, 381, 392, 392a] Asian Indian,[162, 382] American black,[327] and Chinese[316] populations.

An interesting observation that has emerged from the comparison of haplotypes and β-thalassemic mutations in different populations is that a given haplotype is usually associated with different forms of β thalassemia in different populations (see Tables 8–3 and 8–4).[277b, 382, 393] In fact, a given molecular form of β thalassemia appears to be generally restricted to a particular population, because the same mutation is not usually found in two different racial groups.[277b, 393] Thus far, there are only two examples of the same mutation occurring in two different populations.[277b] The G to C mutation at position 5 of IVS-1 has been identified in one Chinese family as well as in many Asian Indians.[316, 392] The mutation in the Chinese family was in a different globin gene framework than that in Asian Indians, suggesting that it had an independent origin. The second biracial mutation is the frameshift mutation due to a four base pair deletion at codons 41 and 42 that has been identified in both Asian Indian and Chinese individuals[340, 392] (see Table 8–4). The haplotype of the affected Chinese chromosome has not been reported, but in Asian Indians, the mutant gene is associated with two different haplotypes sharing the same β gene framework.

Finally, the availability of oligonucleotide probes allows the definitive identification of specific β-thalassemic mutations that are suspected to exist in various patients or subpopulations on the basis of their associated clinical phenotype or haplotype, as illustrated by the following examples: (1) the IVS-1 mutation at position 6 was shown to be responsible for the mild form of thalassemia (thalassemia intermedia) found in certain Cypriot[310] and Portuguese[311] individuals; (2) despite its association with seven different haplotypes, the β^0 thalassemia in Sardinia was shown to consist almost exclusively of the β 39 nonsense mutation[382]; (3) the β^0 thalassemia in the Po river valley, in Rovigo and in Ferrara, was shown to consist of the β 39 nonsense mutation.[95]

THALASSEMIA-LIKE DISORDERS ASSOCIATED WITH STRUCTURALLY ABNORMAL GLOBIN CHAINS

In the usual forms of thalassemia, the affected globin chain, which is synthesized in decreased amounts, is structurally normal, that is, it shows no evidence of an amino acid substitution. There are a number of thalassemia-like disorders, however, in which an abnormal globin chain is in fact synthesized, and these will be discussed individually in the following sections.

The Hemoglobin Lepore and Anti-Lepore Syndromes

Hb Lepore is a structurally abnormal hemoglobin in which the abnormal globin chain is a hybrid or fused globin chain, having the N-terminal amino acid sequence of the normal δ chain and the C-terminal amino acid sequence of the normal β chain. The different molecular types of the Lepore and anti-Lepore hemoglobins and their origin by nonhomologous crossing over between δ and β globin genes are discussed in Chapter 10 (see Fig. 10–7 and Table 10–2E). The Hb Lepore gene behaves as a β-thalassemic gene because there is only a low level of synthesis of its gene product (the $\delta\beta$ Lepore globin chain) and absence of a normal β-chain locus on the affected chromosome: homozygotes produce no Hb A.[5] Gene mapping studies have confirmed the deletion, predicted by a δ-β crossover event, of the 5' end of the β globin gene as well as the 3' end of the δ gene and adjacent inter–$\delta\beta$ globin gene DNA.[368, 394] In the most common form, Hb Lepore-Boston (also called Hb Lepore-Washington), the recombination event occurred at or to the 5' side of the 5' end of IVS-2 of the β globin gene, because gene mapping studies have shown the presence of the β IVS-2 and its specific restriction endonuclease sites in the Lepore gene DNA.[395–397b]

The reasons for the low level of synthesis of Hb Lepore are not definitively known. There may be decreased synthesis because of relative instability of the mRNA for the Lepore chain: Globin-chain synthetic studies reveal that synthesis of the Lepore $\delta\beta$ chain, like that of the δ chain of Hb A_2,[8, 398–401] occurs primarily in bone marrow cells and is virtually absent or much lower in peripheral blood reticulocytes.[399–402] Molecular hybridization assays have in fact revealed virtual absence or markedly decreased levels of β-like ($\delta\beta$) globin mRNA in peripheral blood RNA of affected patients.[110, 396, 403–405] In one study,[405] RNA isolated from nuclei of spleen cells of homozygous patients contained somewhat higher levels of β-like mRNA than did RNA isolated from spleen cell cytoplasm or reticulocytes. The latter results are consistent with some instability of the Lepore $\delta\beta$ mRNA.

Alternatively, transcription of the Lepore $\delta\beta$ gene may be reduced because it shares the same 5'-flanking (promoter) sequences as the δ globin gene, and these sequences, which differ from the corresponding sequences of the β gene,[352] are very likely to be responsible for the normally low level of δ globin gene expression (see Chapter 7). Hybridization studies of pulse-labeled RNA or steady-state levels of precursor δ mRNA from bone marrow cells have revealed that the low level of δ globin gene expression is due at least in part to decreased transcription.[116, 117] Studies of cloned δ and "synthetic" Lepore $\delta\beta$ globin genes in a gene transfer/gene expression system are also consistent with decreased transcriptional ability of these genes: 50-fold lower levels of δ and $\delta\beta$ globin mRNA, compared with β mRNA, accumulate during transient expression of these genes over 48 hours in tissue culture cells.[290]

Whatever the relative contributions of mRNA instability and decreased gene transcription, it is difficult to understand why Hb Lepore accumulates to a level of 10 to 15 per cent of the total hemoglobin, whereas Hb A_2 is rarely increased to levels much greater than 5 per cent. The 5'-flanking δ gene DNA cannot be the only factor influencing the level of expression of the Lepore $\delta\beta$ gene, otherwise Hb Lepore would accumulate only to a level similar to that of Hb A_2. The possible role of intervening sequences in the generation of the Lepore phenotype will be noted in the discussion that follows on the molecular phenomena associated with the anti-Lepore syndromes.

Finally, it should be noted that the role of

post-translational processes, such as those influencing α:non-α dimer formation, has not been thoroughly investigated as a factor in the pathogenesis of the Lepore phenotype.

The anti-Lepore syndromes are not associated with a β thalassemia phenotype because the affected chromosome carries, in addition to the mutant gene, normal β and δ genes (see Fig. 10–7). Gene mapping studies in the case of Hb Miyada have confirmed this expected chromosomal organization as well as the structure of the βδ fusion gene.[405a] The anti-Lepore hemoglobins accumulate in the red cell to approximately the same levels as do the Lepore hemoglobins. As in the case of Hb Lepore, their synthesis is virtually absent in reticulocytes and is limited essentially to bone marrow cells.[406–408] This phenomenon was interpreted as evidence for instability of the anti-Lepore globin mRNA and evidence that both the 5′- and 3′-terminal sequences of globin mRNA are important in maintaining its stability.[406, 408a] An in vitro test of this hypothesis consisted of gene expression studies of a "synthetic" anti-Lepore gene in tissue culture cells, using a hybrid gene that contained the 3′ end of a cloned δ gene linked at the intragenic Eco RI site at codon 121 to the 5′ end of β gene.[290] The levels of globin mRNA obtained with the synthetic anti-Lepore gene were similar to those obtained with a normal β globin gene.[290] Therefore, these studies did not provide evidence for a negative effect of the δ 3′-untranslated sequences on mRNA accumulation, at least during transient expression experiments lasting 48 hours.

Some new information on the possible mechanisms involved in the pathogenesis of the Lepore and anti-Lepore phenotypes has been obtained from the study of chimeric genes constructed to contain one or both of the δ gene introns in an otherwise unmodified β globin gene.[408b] The β gene containing δ IVS-1 was expressed normally after transfer and transient expression in HeLa cells, but the β genes containing δ IVS-2 or δ IVS-1 + δ IVS-2 were expressed at levels intermediate between those of the unmodified δ and β genes, respectively. These results were interpreted as indicating the presence of negative regulatory sequences in IVS-2 of the δ gene that could decrease the level of expression of a gene, such as the anti-Lepore gene, that is transcribed from a normal β gene promoter. As a corollary, it was suggested that β IVS-2 might contain positive regulatory sequences capable of increasing the level of expression of a gene, such as the Lepore gene, that is transcribed from the δ gene promoter.[408b]

One final noteworthy observation on the phenotype of anti-Lepore hemoglobins is the finding that despite the presence of two structurally normal β globin genes, biosynthesis studies reveal a deficit of β globin chain synthesis and α/β globin chain synthetic ratios suggestive of mild β thalassemia.[407, 408] It is possible that the globin gene rearrangement on the abnormal chromosome bearing the anti-Lepore gene impairs, in some yet-to-be-determined fashion, the expression of the structurally normal β globin gene located downstream from the anti-Lepore globin gene.[407]

Beta Globin Chain Structural Variants

Hb E and Hb Knossos. As noted previously in the section describing β-thalassemic mutations involving the 5′ end of IVS-1, two structurally abnormal hemoglobins, Hb E (β 26 Glu→Lys) and Hb Knossos (β 27 Ala→Ser), are associated with a β-thalassemic phenotype because the base substitutions causing the amino acid replacements also cause alternative splicing of precursor β mRNA molecules by the activation of a cryptic "donor" or 5′ splice site that is located at nearby codon 25[308, 309] (see Fig. 8–31). A "silent" base substitution at the third position of codon 24 has a similar effect on splicing and causes β thalassemia without the association of a structurally abnormal hemoglobin.[307] Prior to the gene cloning and expression studies that established the aforementioned mechanism as a cause for β thalassemia, a number of studies had explored the pathogenesis of the Hb E syndromes at the level of globin mRNA metabolism, as described in the following section.

Abnormal Globin mRNA Metabolism Associated with Hb E. The clinical and hematological aspects of Hb E are discussed in Chapter 10. It was initially shown that the hematologic phenotype of β thalassemia (hypochromia and microcytosis) associated with Hb E could be correlated with a decreased β/α globin chain synthetic ratio[312, 313, 409, 410] and a parallel decrease in reticulocyte β globin mRNA, as assayed by molecular hybridization assays.[312, 313]

In a subsequent study by Traeger and colleagues,[411] α/β mRNA ratios were measured in bone marrow RNA preparations from four Hb E homozygotes and compared with those in normal individuals. The mean α/β mRNA ratio in the Hb E individuals was 1.59 in bone marrow nuclei, 2.59 in bone marrow cytoplasm, and 4.36 in reticulocytes, whereas in normal individuals, the values were 1.29, 1.84, and 1.79, respectively. It was concluded from these data that the β^E globin mRNA must be unstable and progressively degraded in the cytoplasm during erythroid cell maturation.

These results are somewhat difficult to reconcile with the subsequent findings, based on gene cloning and gene expression studies in tissue culture cells,[308] that alternative splicing is responsible for the β-thalassemia phenotype associated with Hb E. It is not unreasonable to expect that the abnormal alternatively spliced β^E mRNA might be unstable, at least in nuclei. Orkin and coworkers[308] examined bone marrow RNA from one Hb E homozygote by S1 nuclease analysis and found little or no abnormally spliced β mRNA. Thus, it was concluded that the abnormally spliced β^E mRNA must be turned over very rapidly in erythroid cells. It is therefore unlikely that the decline of β^E mRNA observed by Traeger and associates[411] during erythroid maturation represented gradual loss of the abnormally spliced β^E mRNA. It is conceivable, however, that the normally spliced β^E mRNA could be somewhat less stable than β^A mRNA owing to differences in secondary structure and that this phenomenon could provide an additional contribution to the β mRNA deficiency in this syndrome.

Other β-Chain Structural Variants. A number of additional β-chain structural variants are associated with a β-thalassemic phenotype that is caused by different molecular mechanisms. Hb Indianapolis (β 112 Cys→Arg) is a highly unstable variant that is detectable as a radioactive globin gene product in short-term labeling experiments but does not accumulate to any substantial degree in red cells and thus is not visible on hemoglobin electrophoresis of unlabeled hemolysates.[412, 413] Heterozygotes manifest thalassemic hematologic features, with a moderate hemolytic anemia presumably due to membrane damage caused by precipitation of the unstable hemoglobin. The β^A/α globin chain synthetic ratio was found to be 0.5 in reticulocytes and 1.0 in bone marrow cells, results similar to those found in heterozygous β thalassemia. The labeled $\beta^{Indianapolis}/\alpha$ ratio was 0.28 after a 1.25-minute labeling but decreased to 0.16 after 20 minutes. The half-life of the mutant globin chain was calculated to be approximately 7 minutes, and labeled $\beta^{Indianapolis}$ chains were shown to become rapidly associated with red cell membranes.[412] The mechanism of production of the thalassemic phenotype in this condition is analogous to that which was later identified in the case of the α globin chain variant Hb Quong Sze (see preceding discussion), but in the latter case, a hemolytic component was not observed, presumably because the turnover of the mutant α globin chain or hemoglobin is not associated with membrane damage.

Hb Leiden (β 6 or 7→0) is another unstable hemoglobin variant that is associated with a thalassemia phenotype because of accelerated turnover of the mutant globin chain with resulting hypochromia, microcytosis, and a thalassemic β/α globin chain synthetic ratio.[414] However, in this case, the mutant hemoglobin does accumulate within red cells to a level of approximately 25 per cent of the total hemoglobin. A mild degree of globin chain synthetic imbalance, with excess accumulation of α globin chains, has also been observed in a number of additional unstable hemoglobin syndromes.[415]

Two other β-chain variants are associated with a thalassemic phenotype that does not appear to be related to instability of the mutant globin chain: Hb Vicksburg (β 75→0)[413] and Hb North Shore (β 134 Val→Glu).[416] In these cases, there appears to be an inappropriately low level of production of the abnormal globin chain. In the case of Hb Vicksburg, the defect in synthesis of the mutant β globin chain is more severe and is associated with very low levels of β globin mRNA.[413] It has not yet been determined if the β-thalassemia phenotype in these syndromes is due to the mutation causing the structural abnormality itself or to the possible coexistence of this mutation within a β-thalassemic globin gene with another defect such as one of those described previously. Gene cloning and expression studies will be required to answer this question.

Structural Variants Associated With α-Thalassemia Phenotype

Hb Constant Spring and Related Disorders. As discussed earlier in this chapter (see Fig. 8–21) as well as in Chapter 10, α thalassemia can result from the inheritance of the α-chain structural variant Hb Constant Spring as well as the related variants Hb Icaria, Hb Koya Dora, and Hb Seal Rock. Structural studies of these variants (see Chapter 10) are totally consistent with the notion that they are all due to different base substitutions in the normal α-chain termination codon changing it to an amino acid codon and resulting in readthrough of the 3' unstranslated sequence of the α mRNA until a new in-phase termination codon is encountered 31 codons later (see Fig. 7–7A). The striking feature of these variants with elongated α chains is that they are present in only very low amounts in red cells of heterozygotes (1 to 2 per cent of the total hemoglobin), hence the α-thalassemia phenotype. What is not clear, however, is the precise molecular basis for the uniformly very low level of expression of these chain termination mutants. Most of the studies of this issue have been performed in patients with Hb Constant Spring, either simple heterozygotes or individuals doubly heterozygous for the variant and α thalassemia 1 ($\alpha^{CS}\alpha/--$), a very common cause of Hb H disease in Southeast Asia (see Chapter 9).

It is clear that the low level of Hb Constant Spring is not due primarily to instability of the mutant globin chain itself, because biosynthetic studies reveal that the variant globin chain does not have a high specific activity and is therefore not rapidly turning over in reticulocytes or marrow cells.[417, 421] The rate of globin chain elongation, or translation time, was also measured and was found to be the same for α^{CS} globin chains as for normal α^{A} globin chains.[417] However, similar to the situation in the Hb Lepore syndromes, the mutant α globin chain is synthesized virtually exclusively in bone marrow erythroid cells, with little or no synthesis in peripheral blood,[421, 422] suggesting the possibility of instability of the α^{CS} mRNA as a basis for the low level of synthesis of the mutant globin chain.

The ratio of reticulocyte α to β globin mRNA has been measured by molecular hybridization assays in individuals heterozygous for Hb Constant Spring ($\alpha^{CS}\alpha/\alpha\alpha$) and doubly heterozygous for Hb Constant Spring and α thalassemia 1 ($\alpha^{CS}\alpha/--$). The α/β mRNA levels were found to be very similar to the α/β mRNA levels found in heterozygotes for deletion-type α thalassemia 2 ($-\alpha/\alpha\alpha$) and in double heterozygotes for α thalassemia 2 plus α thalassemia 1 ($-\alpha/--$), respectively.[143] These results therefore confirmed the expected absence or marked deficiency of α^{CS} mRNA in reticulocytes of affected individuals.

As noted previously, it is possible to differentiate the two individual α1 and α2 globin genes and their respective mRNA transcripts because of nucleotide sequence differences in the portions of the genes corresponding to the 3' untranslated sequence of the α mRNA[345, 346] (see Chapter 7). Thus, it has been possible to establish that the Constant Spring mutation affects the α2 globin gene because the amino acid sequence of the elongated portion of the α^{CS} globin chain corresponds to the expected readthrough product of the α2 (see Fig. 7–7A) but not to the α1 globin mRNA. Reticulocyte RNA and bone marrow RNA were analyzed by the S1 nuclease assay that differentiates α1 from α2 globin mRNA in a patient with Hb H disease due to double heterozygosity for Hb Constant Spring and deletion-type α thalassemia 1 ($\alpha^{CS}\alpha/--$).[243] In reticulocyte RNA, the only detectable α globin mRNA was derived from the normal α1 globin gene, whereas in bone marrow RNA, transcripts from both the α1 and α2 (α^{CS}) globin genes could be detected, although the relative amounts of each could not be accurately measured because of technical difficulties.[243] These studies provided the most direct evidence to date for instability of the α^{CS} globin mRNA.

The cause of the instability of α^{CS} mRNA remains unknown. It is difficult to theorize how a single base substitution in the termination codon could destabilize the mRNA. It has been suggested[5] that the process of translation of the normally untranslated 3' portion of the α mRNA alters its conformation or disturbs the interaction between the poly(A) tail and mRNA-associated proteins that may contribute to the stability of the mRNA, thus rendering the mRNA more susceptible to degradation by intracellular nucleases. The precise sequences in the 3' untranslated region of the mRNA that might be important for the stability of the mRNA have not yet been determined. However, it is likely that they are situated distally, because of the findings in the Hb Wayne syndrome.

Hb Wayne is a different type of α globin readthrough product that results from a single nucleotide deletion at codon 138 or 139, causing a frameshift and readthrough of the first 15 nucleotides of the normally untranslated portion of the α mRNA (see Table 10–8). Although the total amount of Hb Wayne in reticulocytes is rather low (7 to 11 per cent of total α chains), this is probably due to instability of Hb Wayne itself rather than to instability of its mRNA. Synthesis of α^{Wayne} globin chains is quite active in reticulocytes[423] (see Chapter 10). Because of the apparent stability of α^{Wayne} mRNA, readthrough of sequences located more distally to the termination point of α^{Wayne} globin chains may be responsible for the instability of the α^{CS} mRNA.

It is noteworthy that the readthrough of the α^{CS} mRNA proceeds into the hexanucleotide sequence AATAAA that is highly conserved in most if not all eukaryotic mRNAs, approximately 20 nucleotides from the site of poly(A) addition, and is thought to constitute a polyadenylation signal[424] (see Chapter 7). In fact, the termination codon UAA for the α^{CS} chain is located within this hexanucleotide (see Fig. 7–7A). It is conceivable that this hexanucleotide sequence, or the region of the mRNA in which it is located, is responsible in some yet-to-be-defined manner for the stability of mRNAs and that its invasion by the translation process renders the mRNA unstable. In this regard, it should be noted that the two β globin readthrough products, Hb Cranston and Hb Tak, that result from frameshift mutations near the normal β globin mRNA termination codon (see Chapter 10) accumulate at high levels in red cells and are actively synthesized in reticulocytes. In the case of these β-chain variants, the readthrough of the β mRNA extends for 28 nucleotides beyond the normal termination codon but stops well short of the region of the polyadenylation signal, which is located 76 nucleotides further downstream. However, possibly contradicting the theory of the importance of noninvasion of the polyadenylation signal for mRNA stability is the fact that the gene for the β subunit of human chorionic gonadotropin (HCG) has evolved in such a way that its mRNA uses the UAA within the polyadenylation signal (AA<u>UAA</u>A) as its normal termination codon.[425] The mRNA for β HCG therefore constitutes an example of a stable mRNA that is normally translated up to its polyadenylation signal. It is possible, nevertheless, that the gene for β HCG is an exception to the rule and has developed other features during evolution to ensure the stability of its mRNA.

Other Structural Variants Associated with α-Thalassemia Phenotypes. As in the case of β-chain structural variants, certain α-chain variants are highly unstable and are associated with an α-thalassemia phenotype because of rapid turnover of the mutant chain, leading to overall α globin chain deficiency in the cell. As discussed previously (see the section on Gene Cloning), Hb Quong Sze (α 125 Leu→Pro)[240, 241] constitutes the classic example of this phenomenon: the variant globin chain is so highly unstable that it can be detected only as a radioactive product in short-term labeling experiments. In this regard, it behaves in a manner analogous to the β-chain structural variant Hb Indianapolis (see preceding discussion). Hb Quong Sze, however, is probably even more unstable than Hb Indianapolis, and it is not associated with a hemolytic component due to membrane damage caused by precipitation of the mutant hemoglobin.

Two other unstable α-chain structural variants, detectable in unlabeled hemolysates of affected individuals, have been found to be associated with an α-thalassemia phenotype: Hb Suan-Dok (α 109 Leu→Arg)[426] and Hb Petah Tikva (α 110 Ala→Asp).[427] In both instances, the mutant hemoglobins were detected in individuals with Hb H disease resulting from the inheritance of α thalassemia 1 from one parent and the mutant hemoglobin from the other parent. In the case of Hb Suan-Dok, the variant accounted for approximately 9 per cent of the total hemoglobin in the patient with Hb H disease and approximately 2 per cent in a simple heterozygote (the patient's aunt).[426] In the case of Hb Petah Tikva, the variant α chains represented approximately 32 per cent of the total amount of α chains synthesized by bone marrow cells of the affected patients with Hb H disease and present in their unlabeled peripheral blood; synthesis in peripheral blood, however, was reduced to 13 to 17 per cent of the total α-chain synthesis,[427] suggesting some instability of the mutant α globin mRNA in a manner analogous to other variants such as Hb Lepore and Hb Constant Spring.

It is not clear that the α-thalassemia phenotype associated with these two variants is due entirely to the instability of the mutant α chains and/or mRNAs. Other factors may be involved, such as the coexistence of another thalassemic mutation in the affected α globin gene or alternative splicing caused by the primary mutation itself. It is interesting to note, with regard to the latter possibility, that the two mutants affect neighboring codons—109 and 110. However, the mutations themselves do not create new donor (GT) or acceptor (AG) dinucleotides. The nearest potential splicing signal in the neighboring normal sequence is a GT located at codon 107, six and nine nucleotides away from the two mutations. The GT is not encompassed within a particularly convincing consensus sequence. Nevertheless, the possibility of alternative splicing at this site cannot be excluded because not all of the sequence requirements for normal and alternative splicing are known. Gene cloning and expression studies will ultimately be required to definitively establish the presence or absence of additional molecular mechanisms associated with these mutations.

Finally, a rather surprising result was the finding of an α-thalassemia phenotype associated with a β-chain structural variant: Hb New York (β 113 Val→Glu) was shown to produce an apparent decrease in α-chain synthesis by a unique pathophysiologic mechanism. $β^{NY}$ globin chains are synthesized at an accelerated rate compared with $β^A$ globin chains, and they compete more efficiently than $β^A$ chains in binding to newly synthesized α chains. However, Hb New York is unstable, and its degradation results secondarily in relative α-chain deficiency, producing a syndrome similar to heterozygous α thalassemia 1.[428]

ANIMAL MODELS OF THALASSEMIA

It is only recently that animal models of thalassemia have been identified and characterized. The availability of such animal models should greatly accelerate and facilitate attempts to perform gene therapy of thalassemia by transfer of normal globin genes into hematopoietic stem cells of affected animals. In fact, somewhat premature attempts at gene therapy in thalassemic patients[429] were criticized, among other reasons, for failure to await the availability of animal model systems for testing the feasibility of the experimental procedures prior to proceeding with actual human experimentation.[430]

The Belgrade Rat

A radiation-induced, recessively inherited, hypochromic microcytic anemia in Belgrade laboratory rats was thought for many years to constitute an animal model for thalassemia because of the striking similarity of the morphology of the red blood cells in these anemic animals when compared with that of patients with homozygous β thalassemia.[431] However, subsequent studies demonstrated that the abnormality in the animals was a defect in iron transport and heme synthesis and not a primary defect in the ratio of α to β globin chain synthesis.[432–434] However, despite the lack of imbalance of α to β globin chain synthesis, overall globin chain synthesis is decreased,[432, 433] and abnormalities of reticulocyte globin mRNA have been demonstrated in these animals by cell-free translation and molecular hybridization assays.[435, 436]

Cell-free translation assays revealed that total reticulocyte RNA of Belgrade rats was less effective than RNA from control rats in stimulating globin chain synthesis, and RNA-cDNA hybridization assays revealed that the number of globin mRNA molecules per unit of total reticulocyte RNA in mutant rats was approximately 45 per cent of that in normal rats.[436] However, the ratio of α to β globin chain synthesis directed by polysomal mRNA in the wheat germ cell-free system was the same for mutant and normal rats.[435, 436] It is likely that the abnormalities of globin mRNA and globin synthesis in these mutant rats are secondary to the defect in heme synthesis that results from the abnormality in iron transport.

Mouse Models of α Thalassemia

Three different mouse strains have been identified that have hematologic features consistent with heterozygous α thalassemia: two were induced by x-irradition[437, 438] and one by exposure to the chemical triethylene-melamine.[439] Studies of globin chain synthesis and globin mRNA quantitation by RNA-cDNA hybridization assays revealed a reduced α/β globin chain synthetic ratio and a parallel decrease of the α/β globin mRNA ratio.[440] Gene mapping studies in all three strains demonstrated the deletion from the affected chromosome of both α globin genes as well as the linked gene for the α-like embryonic x chain.[441, 442]

Matings of heterozygous mice from all three strains have not produced mice with homozygous α thalassemia. A number of presumably homozygous embryos became necrotic and died, starting at approximately 5 to 5.5 days of gestation, a time several days before the activation of the globin genes.[442, 443] It is thought that the deletion event in these mice probably involves an additional linked gene, the activity of which is required for normal embryonic development.[442, 443] Unfortunately, these findings seriously limit the usefulness of these mice as models for gene therapy of homozygous α thalassemia.

Mouse Model of β Thalassemia

More recently, a spontaneously occurring mutation in the mouse has been identified that is a very good model for β thalassemia[444] and probably constitutes the best animal model system thus far characterized for the study of gene transfer modalities in the therapy of thalassemic defects of globin gene expression. In reticulocytes of homozygous animals, there is total absence of synthesis of the $β^{major}$ chain of mouse adult hemoglobin. The non-α chains synthesized by these homozygous animals consisted exclusively of $β^{minor}$ globin chains, the gene for which is closely linked to the 3′ side of the $β^{major}$ gene and probably arose from it by a gene duplication event (see Chapter 7). The $β^{minor}/α$ synthetic ratio is 0.78 in homozygotes and 0.95 in heterozygotes, indicating a high level of compensation by the $β^{minor}$ gene for the deficient output of the $β^{major}$ gene. Nevertheless, homozygous animals manifest a moderate hypochromic microcytic anemia with severe anisocytosis, poikilocytosis, and reticulocytosis, as well as the presence of inclusion bodies in many of the red cells and increased numbers of circulating nucleated red blood cells.[444]

Globin gene mapping studies have revealed that the basis for the absence of $β^{major}$ globin chain synthesis in these mice is a 3.3-kb deletion that encompasses the entire $β^{major}$ globin gene and approximately 1.5 kb of its 5′-flanking DNA.[444] Other interesting features of this mutation include the following[444a]: (1) the increased level of synthesis of $β^{minor}$ globin chains is associated with a parallel increase in $β^{minor}$ globin mRNA; (2) the level of synthesis of $β^{minor}$ globin chains can be further increased by treatment of the mice with 5-azacytidine; (3) the $β^{minor}$ globin gene of the mutant mice contains in its 5′-flanking DNA a DNase I hypersensitive site that is absent in normal mice; and (4) nucleotide sequence analysis of the break point of the deletion revealed the insertion at this site of a 68 bp–long sequence of foreign DNA with structural homology to certain transposable DNA elements as well as to the myc oncogene.

CONCLUSIONS AND FUTURE PROSPECTS FOR GENE THERAPY

The progressive unraveling of what was once the mystery of the molecular basis of thalassemia has been a fascinating phenomenon to observe. There have been many surprises, such as the unexpected degree of heterogeneity of molecular defects that have been uncovered as well as the dramatic effects shown to be exerted on globin gene expression by simple and seemingly insignificant changes in globin gene structure, such as a "silent" base substitution in an amino acid codon, or base substitutions in regions of intervening sequences not normally encompassed in traditional "splicing" signals. As impressive an accomplishment as the acquisition of this large body of new knowledge represents, it is nevertheless sobering to realize that the promise of the anticipated molecular cure or therapy for thalassemia, hoped for on the basis of such knowledge, remains essentially unfulfilled.

Putting aside considerations of γ globin gene activation such as by 5-azacytidine (see Chapter 9), it is clear from the heterogeneity and nature of the molecular defects that cause thalassemia that any practical attempts at gene therapy for thalassemia should be directed at substituting, by various gene transfer technologies, normal globin genes for the defective thalassemic genes, rather than attempting direct correction of the specific defect associated with the mutant gene. One possible exception to the preceding statement is the potential for correcting the effect of nonsense mutations in thalassemic globin genes and mRNAs by the transfer of suppressor tRNA genes into hematopoietic stem cells, thus providing erythroid progenitor cells with a means to translate the mutant globin mRNA into a full-length, functional globin chain. As discussed previously, the mutant β globin mRNA associated with the nonsense mutation at β globin codon 17 has been successfully translated into normal β globin chains in frog oocytes after transfer into these cells of genes for a lysine suppressor tRNA.[329] The amount of mutant β mRNA associated with the nonsense mutation at codon 39 has also been shown to be increased in monkey kidney (COS) tissue culture cells by cotransfer of a gene for an amber suppressor tRNA.[336] However, for such a strategy to be effective in an affected patient, the suppressor tRNA genes must be stably introduced into the individual's pluripotential (or committed erythroid) stem cells and the transfected cells must repopulate the bone marrow and indefinitely maintain their capacity for self-renewal. The purely technical difficulties of this approach at the hematopoietic stem cell level will be discussed later in relation to globin gene transfer experiments. However, a particular concern regarding gene therapy using amber suppressor tRNA genes resides in the nonspecificity of the approach. In addition to allowing full-length translation of the mutant β globin mRNAs, the amber suppressor tRNAs will allow the readthrough of all normal cellular mRNAs that have a UAG termination codon and therefore lead to the synthesis of abnormal proteins analogous to Hb Constant Spring. The potential harmful effects on hematopoietic cells of such readthrough proteins remain unknown, although in prokaryotic systems, amber suppressor tRNAs do not have a notably harmful or lethal effect. In this regard, short-term viability of frog oocytes was not appreciably affected by the presence of amber suppressor tRNA in the experiments of Temple and colleagues on the translation of $β^0$-thalassemic globin mRNA.[329]

With regard to gene therapy by transfer of normal globin genes into hematopoietic cells, two major categories of obstacles must be overcome: (1) those related to the pattern of expression of globin genes after transfer into a foreign chromosomal environment and (2) those related to the cell biology of hematopoietic cells. Great progress has been made in the technical ability to transfer cloned globin gene DNA into a variety of tissue culture cells as well as into living animals. However, it has become apparent during the course of these experiments that the transferred genes do not function normally in their new chromosomal environment. It would be expected that the most likely experiments to be successful would be those in which the transferred gene was in an erythroid cell environment or subjected to the changes that accompany hematopoietic cell development and differentiation. However, the results of such experiments have been disappointing. When stably introduced into mouse erythroleukemia (MEL) cells, human β globin genes can be "induced" to produce human β globin mRNA after exposure of the cells to DMSO or other inducing agents, but the level of expression is very low: at best only 1/100 of the level of the endogenous mouse β globin genes, even though as many as 50 to 100 copies of human β globin genes are integrated into the mouse chromosome.[293, 294] The level of expression also varies greatly from cell line to cell line, suggesting that the site of integration can influence the function and quantitative output of the transferred genes.

A similar conclusion was drawn from the results of experiments in which rabbit β globin genes were microinjected into mouse oocytes and the embryos allowed to develop into adult animals.[445] Although multiple copies of the rabbit globin genes were successfully incorporated into the chromosomal DNA of the test mice, the site of integration was in different chromosomes in different mice. In none of the mice was there expression of rabbit globin mRNA in erythroid cells of the animals, although, in some mice, very low levels of expression of globin mRNA was observed in ectopic sites such as the testis and muscle.[445] Analogous results have been obtained in a number of different studies.[445a–445d] However, more promising results were subsequently obtained by two groups using different β globin genes[445c, 445e, 445f]; mice from a number of transgenic lines expressed the transferred genes predominantly in erythroid cells. In most cases, the level of expression was quite low,[445e] but in one animal it was nearly equal to that of the endogenous β genes.[445c] In a subsequent study, the transferred β globin genes were shown to be developmentally regulated, being inactive in embryonic but active in fetal liver cells.[445g]

It is possible that in order for transferred globin genes to be reproducibly expressed at high levels and in a tissue-specific manner, they may have to become integrated at or near the normal chromosomal site of the endogenous globin gene. Unfortunately, the technology does not yet exist to target the integration of transferred genes to specific chromosomal sites.

The obstacles for globin gene therapy related to the cell biology of hematopoietic stem cells center on the difficulties of obtaining such cells in sufficient numbers to successfully perform *in vitro* globin gene transfer, which is currently a highly inefficient process. A large number of cells must be treated to allow selection of the few successfully transfected cells *in vitro* or *in vivo* and permit their subsequent engraftment to significantly populate the marrow in test animals. The rationale and technical aspects of this aspect of globin gene therapy have been extensively discussed[446–448] following the first unsuccessful globin gene transfer attempts in thalassemic patients.[429, 430] There have, however, been reports of the successful transfer of genes for the selectable enzymes dihydrofolate reductase (DHFR) and thymidine kinase into murine bone marrow cells.[449–452] The transfected marrow cells were able to proliferate after transplantation into irradiated mice, and the transferred DHFR genes were expressed in the transplanted animals. With more efficient transfer systems, such as retroviral-based or other viral vectors, this approach may be successful one day in the case of human hematopoietic stem cells. In fact, highly efficient transfer of foreign genes into hematopoietic cells has been achieved using such vectors,[453-455] and it is likely that gene therapy for certain inborn errors of metabolism will soon be attempted in humans using transfer of cloned genes into bone marrow cells.[456-458] The problems of tissue-specificity and levels of expression in the case of these contemplated attempts do not constitute obstacles such as those faced in the case of globin gene therapy.

In conclusion, much progress in gene manipulation and gene transfer has been achieved in the last few years, but much more is required before globin gene therapy is a reality for the management of thalassemia. However, if advances in this field over the coming years occur with the same explosive rapidity as they recently have in the case of studies on the molecular basis of thalassemia, one can anticipate numerous breakthroughs and perhaps the realization, sooner than one can now imagine, of what is for many the "impossible dream."

REFERENCES

1. Guidotti, G.: Thalassemia. In Conference on Hemoglobin. Arden House, Columbia University, New York, 1962.
2. Baglioni, C.: Correlations between genetics and chemistry of human hemoglobins. In Taylor, J. H. (ed.): Molecular Genetics. Part I. New York, Academic Press, 1963, p. 452.
3. Jones, R. T., and Schroeder, W. A.: Chemical characterization and subunit hybridization of human hemoglobin H and associated compounds. Biochemistry 2:1357, 1963.
4. Schroeder, W. A., Huisman, T. H. J., Shelton, J. R., Apell, G., Shelton, J. B., Brodie, A. R., Lutcher, C. L., Blunt, M. H., and Miller, A.: On the structure of the hemoglobins A, A_2 and F in a Negro with homozygous β-thalassemia. Biochem. Med. 10:276, 1974.
5. Weatherall, D. J., and Clegg, J. B.: The Thalassemia Syndromes. 3rd ed. Oxford, Blackwell Scientific Publications, 1981.
6. Heywood, J. D., Karon, M., and Weissman, S.: Amino acids: Incorporation into α and β chains of hemoglobin by normal and thalassemic reticulocytes. Science 146:530, 1964.
7. Heywood, D., Karon, M., and Weissman, S.: Asymmetrical incorporation of amino acids into the α and β chains of hemoglobin synthesized in thalassemic reticulocytes. J. Lab. Clin. Med. 66:476, 1965.
8. Weatherall, D. J., Clegg, J. B., and Naughton, M. A.: Globin synthesis in thalassemia: An in vitro study. Nature 208:1061, 1965.
9. Bank, A., and Marks, P. A.: Excess α chain synthesis relative to β chain synthesis in thalassemia major and minor. Nature 212:1198, 1966.
10. Clegg, J. B., Naughton, M. A., and Weatherall, D. J.: An improved method for the characterization of human hemoglobin mutants: Identification of $\alpha_2\beta_2$ 95 Glu hemoglobin N (Baltimore). Nature 207:945, 1965.
11. Bargellesi, A., Pontremoli, S., and Conconi, F.: Absence of β globin synthesis and excess of α globin synthesis in homozygous β-thalassemia. Eur. J. Biochem. 1:73, 1967.
12. Modell, C. B., Lotter, A., Steadman, J. H., and Huehns, E. R.: Hemoglobin synthesis in β-thalassemia. Br. J. Haematol. 17:485, 1969.
13. Weatherall, D. J., Clegg, J. B., Na-Nakorn, S., and Wasi, P.: The pattern of disordered hemoglobin synthesis in homozygous and heterozygous β-thalassemia. Br. J. Haematol. 16:251, 1969.
14. Conconi, F., Bargellesi, A., Del Senno, L., Menegatti, E., Pontremoli, S., and Russo, G.: Globin chain synthesis in Sicilian thalassemic subjects. Br. J. Haematol. 19:469, 1970.
15. Ramot, B., Ben-Bassat, I., Mozel, M., and Shacked, N.: Globin synthesis in α- and β-thalassemia. Isr. J. Med. Sci. 9:1469, 1973.
16. Friedman, S., Oski, F. A., and Schwartz, E.: Bone marrow and peripheral blood globin synthesis in an American black family with β-thalassemia. Blood 39:785, 1972.
17. Friedman, S., Hamilton, R. W., and Schwartz, E.: β-Thalassemia in the American Negro. J. Clin. Invest. 52:1453, 1973.
18. Braverman, A. S., McCurdy, P. R., Manos, O., and Sherman, A.: Homozygous β-thalassemia in American blacks: The problem of mild thalassemia. J. Lab. Clin. Med. 81:857, 1973.
19. Friedman, S., Schwartz, E., Ahern, V., and Ahern, E.: Globin synthesis in the Jamaican Negro with β-thalassemia. Br. J. Haematol. 28:505, 1974.
20. Bank, A., Braverman, S., O'Donnell, J. V., and Marks, P. A.: Absolute rates of globin chain synthesis in thalassemia. Blood 31:226, 1968.
21. Clegg, J. B., and Weatherall, D. J.: Hemoglobin synthesis in α-thalassemia (hemoglobin H disease). Nature 215:1241, 1967.
22. Kan, Y. W., Schwartz, E., and Nathan, D. G.: Globin chain synthesis in α-thalassemia syndromes. J. Clin. Invest. 47:2515, 1968.
23. Weatherall, D. J., Clegg, J. B., and Wong, H. B.: The hemoglobin constitution of infants with the hemoglobin Bart's hydrops fetalis syndrome. Br. J. Haematol. 18:357, 1970.
24. Schwartz, E., and Atwater, J.: α-Thalassemia in the American Negro. J. Clin. Invest. 51:412, 1972.
25. Braverman, A. S., and Bank, A.: Changing rates of globin chain synthesis during erythroid cell maturation in thalassemia. J. Mol. Biol. 42:57, 1969.
26. Natta, C., Banks, J., Niazi, G., Marks, P. A., and Bank, A.: Decreased β globin mRNA activity in bone marrow cells in homozygous and heterozygous β-thalassemia. Nature (New Biol.) 244:280, 1973.
27. Kim, H. C., Marks, P. A., Rifkind, R. A., Maniatis, G. M., and Bank, A.: Isolation and in vitro differentiation of human erythroid precursor cells. Blood 47:767, 1976.
28. Musumeci, S., Schiliro, G., Romeo, M. A., Pizzarelli, G., Fischer, A., and Russo, G.: Haemoglobin synthesis in bone marrow of patients with β^0 and β^+ thalassemia. Acta Haematol. 65:170, 1981.
28a. Saglio, G., Camaschella, C., Guerrasio, A., Cambrin, G. R., Capaldi, A., Pich, P. G., Trento, M., and Mazza, U.: $^G\gamma$ and $^A\gamma$ globin chain synthesis in bone marrow and peripheral blood of β-thalassaemia homozygotes. Br. J. Haematol. 52:225, 1982.
29. Shchory, M., and Ramot, B.: Globin chain synthesis in the marrow and reticulocytes of β-thalassemia,

hemoglobin H disease, and βδ-thalassemia. Blood 40:105, 1972.
30. Nienhuis, A. W., Canfield, P. H., and Anderson, W. F.: Hemoglobin messenger RNA from human bone marrow: Isolation and translation in homozygous and heterozygous β-thalassemia. J. Clin. Invest. 52:1735, 1973.
31. Schwartz, E.: Heterozygous β-thalassemia: Balanced globin synthesis in bone marrow cells. Science 167:1513, 1970.
32. Kan, Y. W., Nathan, D. G., and Lodish, H. F.: Equal synthesis of α and β globin chains in erythroid precursors in heterozygous β-thalassemia. J. Clin. Invest. 51:1906, 1972.
33. Clegg, J. B., and Weatherall, D. J.: Hemoglobin synthesis during erythroid maturation in β-thalassemia. Nature (New Biol.) 240:190, 1972.
34. Nathan, D. G.: Thalassemia. N Engl J Med 286:586, 1972.
35. Gill, F., and Schwartz, E.: Free α globin pool in human bone marrow. J. Clin. Invest. 52:3057, 1973.
36. Chalevelakis, G., Clegg, J. B., and Weatherall, D. J.: Imbalanced globin chain synthesis in heterozygous β-thalassemic bone marrow. Proc. Natl. Acad. Sci. USA 72:3853, 1975.
37. Chalevelakis, G., Clegg, J. B., and Weatherall, D. J.: Globin synthesis in normal human bone marrow. Br. J. Haematol. 34:535, 1976.
38. Wood, W. G., and Stamatoyannopoulos, G.: Globin synthesis in fractionated normoblasts of β-thalassemia heterozygotes. J. Clin. Invest. 55:567, 1975.
39. Hanash, S. M., and Rucknagel, D. L.: Proteolytic activity in erythrocyte precursors. Proc. Natl. Acad. Sci. USA 75:3427, 1978.
40. Ballas, S. K., and Burka, E. R.: Catabolism of hemoglobin by human erythrocyte membranes. J. Lab. Clin. Med. 92:387, 1978.
41. Testa, U., Hinard, N., Beuzard, Y., Tsapis, A., Galacteros, F., Thomopoulos, P., and Rosa, J.: Excess α chains are lost from β-thalassemic reticulocytes by proteolysis. J. Lab. Clin. Med. 98:352, 1981.
42. Braverman, A. S., and Lester, D.: Evidence for increased proteolysis in intact β-thalassemia erythroid cells. Hemoglobin 5:549, 1981.
43. Steinberg, M. H., Coleman, M., and Dreiling, B.: Unbalanced globin chain synthesis in erythroid precursor cells of heterozygous α-thalassemia. Br. J. Haematol. 34:55, 1976.
44. Wood, W. G., and Stamatoyannopoulos, G.: Globin synthesis during erythroid cell maturation in α-thalassemia. Hemoglobin 1:135, 1976–1977.
45. Sancar, G. B., Cedeno, M. M., and Rieder, R. F.: Rapid destruction of newly synthesized excess β globin chains in Hb H disease. Blood 57:967, 1981.
46. Zaizov, R., Steinherz, M., Wollach, B., and Kirschmann, C.: Balanced bone marrow globin synthesis in Mideastern α-thalassemia. Acta Haematol. 64:136, 1980.
47. Benz, E. J., Glass, J., Tsistrakis, G. A., Hillman, D. G., Cavallesco, C., Coupal, E., Forget, B. G., Turner, P. A., Kantor, J. A., and Nienhuis, A. W.: Heterogeneity of messenger RNA defects in the thalassemia syndromes. Ann. N. Y. Acad. Sci. 344:101, 1980.
48. Kirschmann, C., Lupovitz, Z., Steinherz, M., and Zaizov, R.: Globin chain synthesis in Hb H disease: The activity of red cell precursors and their mRNA. Isr. J. Med. Sci. 14:1102, 1978.

49. Friedman, S., Ozsoylu, S., Luddy, R., and Schwartz, E.: A new form of β-thalassemia trait of unusual severity. Blood 42:990, 1973.
50. Stamatoyannopoulos, G., Woodson, R., Papayannopoulou, T. H., Heywood, D., and Kurachi, S.: Inclusion body β-thalassemia trait: A new form of β-thalassemia producing clinical manifestations in simple heterozygotes. N. Engl. J. Med. 290:939, 1974.
51. Ballas, S. K., Burka, E. R., and Gill, F. M.: Abnormal red cell membrane proteolytic activity in severe heterozygous β-thalassemia. J. Lab. Clin. Med. 99:263, 1982.
52. Burka, E. R., and Marks, P. A.: Ribosomes active in protein synthesis in human reticulocytes: A defect in thalassemia major. Nature 199:706, 1963.
53. Marks, P. A., and Burka, E. R.: Hemoglobins A and F: Formation in thalassemia and other hemolytic anemias. Science 144:552, 1964.
54. Marks, P. A., Burka, E. R., and Rifkind, R. A.: Control of protein synthesis in reticulocytes and the formation of hemoglobins A and F in thalassemia syndromes and other hemolytic anemias. Medicine 43:769, 1964.
55. Bank, A., and Marks, P. A.: Protein synthesis in a cell-free human reticulocyte system: Ribosome function in thalassemia. J. Clin. Invest. 45:330, 1966.
56. Fuhr, J., Natta, C., Marks, P. A., and Bank, A.: Protein synthesis in cell-free systems from reticulocytes of thalassemic patients. Nature 224:1305, 1969.
57. Ingram, V. M.: A molecular model for thalassemia. Ann. N. Y. Acad. Sci. 119:485, 1964.
58. Itano, H. A.: The synthesis and structure of normal and abnormal hemoglobins. In Jonxis, J. H. P. (ed.): Abnormal Hemoglobins in Africa. Oxford, Blackwell Scientific Publications, 1965, p. 3.
59. Anderson, W. F., and Gilbert, J. M.: tRNA dependent translational control of in vitro hemoglobin synthesis. Biochem. Biophys. Res. Commun. 36:456, 1969.
60. Weiss, G. B.: Translational control of protein synthesis by tRNA unrelated to changes in tRNA concentration. J. Mol. Evol. 2:199, 1973.
61. Clegg, J. B., Weatherall, D. J., Na-Nakorn, S., and Wasi, P.: Hemoglobin synthesis in β-thalassemia. Nature 220:664, 1968.
62. Rieder, R. F.: Translation of β globin mRNA in β-thalassemia and the S and C hemoglobinopathies. J. Clin. Invest. 51:364, 1972.
63. Nathan, D. G., Lodish, H., Kan, Y. W., and Housman, D.: β-Thalassemia and translation of globin messenger RNA. Proc. Natl. Acad. Sci. USA 68:2514, 1971.
64. Clegg, J. B., Weatherall, D. J., and Eunson, C. E.: The distribution of nascent globin chains on human reticulocyte polysomes. Biochem. Biophys. Acta 247:109, 1971.
65. Hunt, R. T., Munro, A. J., and Hunter, A. R.: Control of hemoglobin synthesis: A difference in the size of polysomes making α and β chains. Nature 220:481, 1968.
66. Lodish, H. F., and Jacobsen, M.: Regulation of hemoglobin synthesis: Equal rates of translation and termination of α and β globin chains. J. Biol. Chem. 247:3622, 1972.
67. Lodish, H. F.: α and β globin messenger ribonucleic acid: Different amounts and rates of initiation of translation. J. Biol. Chem. 246:7131, 1971.

68. Cividalli, G., Nathan, D. G., and Lodish, H. F.: Translational control of hemoglobin synthesis in thalassemic marrow. J. Clin. Invest. 53:955, 1974.
69. Gilbert, J. M., and Anderson, W. F.: Cell-free hemoglobin synthesis. II. Characteristics of the transfer ribonucleic acid–dependent assay system. J. Biol. Chem. 245:2342, 1970.
70. Crystal, R. G., Nienhuis, A. W., Elson, N. A., and Anderson, W. F.: Initiation of globin synthesis: Preparation and use of reticulocyte ribosomes retaining initiation region messenger ribonucleic acid fragments. J. Biol. Chem. 247:5357, 1972.
71. Crystal, R. G., and Anderson, W. F.: Initiation of hemoglobin synthesis: Comparison of model reactions that use artificial templates, with those using natural messenger RNA. Proc. Natl. Acad. Sci. USA 69:706, 1972.
72. Gilbert, J. M., Thornton, A. G., Nienhuis, A., and Anderson, W. F.: Cell-free hemoglobin synthesis in β-thalassemia. Proc. Natl. Acad. Sci. USA 67:1854, 1970.
73. Nienhuis, A. W., Laycock, D. G., and Anderson, W. F.: Translation of rabbit hemoglobin messenger RNA by thalassemic and nonthalassemic ribosomes. Nature (New Biol.) 231:205, 1971.
74. Crystal, R. G., Elson, N. A., Nienhuis, A., Thornton, A. C., and Anderson, W. F.: Initiation of globin synthesis in β-thalassemia. N. Engl. J. Med. 288:1091, 1973.
75. Baglioni, C., Colombo, B., and Jacobs-Lorena, M.: Chain termination: A test for a possible explanation of thalassemia. Ann. N. Y. Acad. Sci. 165:212, 1969.
76. Dreyfus, J. C., Labie, D., Vibert, M., and Conconi, F.: An attempt at demonstrating the existence of a nonsense mutation in β-thalassemia. Eur. J. Biochem. 27:291, 1972.
77. Mathews, M. B., and Korner, A.: Mammalian cell-free protein synthesis directed by viral ribonucleic acid. Eur. J. Biochem. 17:328, 1970.
78. Roberts, B. E., and Paterson, B. M.: Efficient translation of tobacco mosaic virus RNA and rabbit globin 9S RNA in a cell-free system from commercial wheat germ. Proc. Natl. Acad. Sci. USA 70:2330, 1973.
79. Nienhuis, A. W., and Anderson, W. F.: Isolation and translation of hemoglobin messenger RNA from thalassemia, sickle cell anemia and normal human reticulocytes. J. Clin. Invest. 50:2458, 1971.
80. Benz, E. J., Jr., and Forget, B. G.: Defect in messenger RNA for human hemoglobin synthesis in β-thalassemia. J. Clin. Invest. 50:2755, 1971.
81. Dow, L. W., Terada, M., Natta, C., Metafora, S., Grossbard, E., Marks, P. A., and Bank, A.: Globin synthesis of intact cells and activity of isolated mRNA in β-thalassemia. Nature (New Biol.) 243:114, 1973.
82. Forget, B. G., Baltimore, D., Benz, E. J., Jr., Housman, D., Lebowitz, P., Marotta, C. A., McCaffrey, R. P., Skoultchi, A., Swerdlow, P. S., Verma, I. M., and Weissman, S. M.: Globin messenger RNA in the thalassemia syndromes. Ann. N. Y. Acad. Sci. 232:76, 1974.
83. Pritchard, J., Longley, J., Clegg, J. B., and Weatherall, D. J.: Assay of thalassemic messenger RNA in the wheat germ system. Br. J. Haematol. 32:473, 1976.
84. Gambino, R., Kacian, D. L., Ramirez, F., Dow, L. W., Grossbard, E., Natta, C., Spiegelman, S., Marks, P. A., and Bank, A.: Decreased globin messenger RNA in thalassemia by hybridization and biologic activity assays. Ann. N. Y. Acad. Sci. 232:6, 1974.
85. Kan, Y. W., Dozy, A. M., and Holland, J. P.: Absence of functional β globin mRNA in homozygous β^0-thalassemia. Blood 42:991, 1973.
86. Benz, E. J., Jr., Swerdlow, P. S., and Forget, B. G.: Absence of functional messenger RNA activity for β globin chain synthesis in β^0-thalassemia. Blood 45:1, 1975.
87. Ramirez, F., Starkman, D., Bank, A., Kerem, H., Cividalli, G., and Rachmilewitz, E. A.: Absence of β mRNA in β^0-thalassemia in Kurdish Jews. Blood 52:735, 1978.
88. DiSegni, G., Kerem, H., Cividalli, G., Rachmilewitz, A., and Kaempfer, R.: Absence of functional β globin messenger RNA in Kurdish Jews with β^0-thalassemia. Isr. J. Med. Sci. 14:1116, 1978.
89. Conconi, F., Rowley, P. T., Del Senno, L., Pontremoli, S., and Volpato, S.: Induction of β globin synthesis in the β-thalassemia of Ferrara. Nature (New Biol.) 238:83, 1972.
90. Conconi, F., and Del Senno, L.: The molecular defect of the Ferrara β-thalassemia. Ann. N. Y. Acad. Sci. 232:54, 1974.
91. Rowley, P. T., and Kosciolek, B.: Distinction between two types of β-thalassemia by inducibility of the cell-free synthesis of β chains by nonthalassemic soluble fraction. Nature (New Biol.) 239:234, 1972.
92. Conconi, F., Bernardi, F., Buzzoni, D., Casoni, I., Del Senno, L., Marchetti, G., and Perrotta, C. M.: β-Globin messenger RNA in Ferrara β^0 thalassemia. Ann. N. Y. Acad. Sci. 344:120, 1980.
93. Conconi, F., Del Senno, L., Ferrarese, P., Menini, C., Borgatti, F., Vullo, C., and Labie, D.: Appearance of β globin synthesis in erythroid cells of Ferrara β^0-thalassemic patients following blood transfusion. Nature 254:256, 1975.
94. Pirastu, M., del Senno, L., Conconi, F., Vullo, C., and Kan, Y. W.: Ferrara β^0 thalassemia caused by the β^{39} nonsense mutation. Nature 307:76, 1984.
95. Del Senno, L., Conconi, F., Little, P. F. R., and Williamson, R.: Restriction enzyme analysis of the β globin gene in DNA from β^0-thalassemic subjects from Ferrara. Biochem. Biophys. Res. Commun. 91:548, 1979.
96. Geller, A. I., Rich, A.: A UGA termination suppression $tRNA^{Trp}$ active in rabbit reticulocytes. Nature 283:41, 1980.
97. Grossbard, E., Terada, M., Dow, L. W., and Bank, A.: Decreased α globin messenger RNA activity associated with polyribosomes in α-thalassemia. Nature (New Biol.) 241:209, 1973.
98. Benz, E. J., Jr., Swerdlow, P. S., and Forget, B. G.: Globin messenger RNA in hemoglobin H disease. Blood 42:825, 1973.
99. Verma, I. M., Temple, G. F., Fan, H., and Baltimore, D.: In vitro synthesis of DNA complementary to rabbit reticulocyte 10S RNA. Nature 235:163, 1972.
100. Kacian, D. L., Spiegelman, S., Bank, A., Terada, M., P. A.: In vitro synthesis of DNA components of human genes for globin. Nature 235:167, 1972
101. Ross, J., Aviv, H., Scolnick, E., and Leder, P.: In vitro synthesis of DNA complementary to purified rabbit globin mRNA. Proc. Natl. Acad. Sci. USA 69:264, 1972.
102. Jacobs-Lorena, M., and Baglioni, C.: Messenger RNA for globin in the postribosomal supernatant

of rabbit reticulocytes. Proc. Natl. Acad. Sci. USA 69:1425, 1972.
103. Temple, G., and Housman, D.: Separation and translation of the mRNA's coding for α and β chains of rabbit globin. Proc. Natl. Acad. Sci. USA 69:1574, 1972.
104. Housman, D., Forget, B. G., Skoultchi, A., and Benz, E. J., Jr.: Quantitative deficiency of chain-specific globin mRNA in the thalassemia syndromes. Proc. Natl. Acad. Sci. USA 70:1809, 1973.
105. Kacian, D. L., Gambino, R., Dow, L. W., Grossbard, E., Natta, C., Ramirez, F., Spiegelman, S., Marks, P. A., and Bank, A.: Decreased globin messenger RNA in thalassemia detected by molecular hybridization. Proc. Natl. Acad. Sci. USA 70:1886, 1973.
106. Housman, D., Skoultchi, A., Forget, B. G., and Benz, E. J., Jr.: Use of globin cDNA as a hybridization probe for globin mRNA. Ann. N. Y. Acad. Sci. 241:280, 1974.
107. Forget, B. G., Housman, D., Benz, E. J., Jr., and McCaffrey, R. P.: Synthesis of DNA complementary to separated human alpha and beta globin messenger RNAs. Proc. Natl. Acad. Sci. USA 72:984, 1975.
108. Taylor, J. M., Dozy, A., Kan, Y. W., Varmus, H. E., Lie-Ingo, L. E., Ganeson, J., and Todd, D.: Genetic lesion in homozygous α thalassaemia (hydrops fetalis). Nature 251:392, 1974.
109. Ottolenghi, S., Lanyon, W., Paul, J., Williamson, R. W., Weatherall, D. J., Clegg, J., Pritchard, J., Pootrakul, S., and Wong, H.: The severe form of α thalassaemia is caused by a haemoglobin gene deletion. Nature 251:389, 1974.
110. Benz, E. J., Jr., Forget, B. G., Hillman, D. G., Cohen-Solal, M., Pritchard, J., Cavallesco, C., Prensky, W., and Housman, D.: Variability in the amount of β globin mRNA in $β^0$-thalassemia. Cell 14:299, 1978.
111. Nienhuis, A. W., Turner, P., and Benz, E. J., Jr.: Relative stability of α and β globin messenger RNAs in homozygous $β^+$-thalassemia. Proc. Natl. Acad. Sci. USA 74:3960, 1977.
112. Ramirez, F., O'Donnell, J. V., Natta, C., and Bank, A.: Quantitation of human gamma globin genes and gamma globin mRNA with purified gamma globin complementary DNA. J. Clin. Invest. 58:1475, 1976.
113. Ramirez, F., Clayton, N., O'Donnell, J. V., Canale, V., Bailey, G., Sanguensermsri, T., Maniatis, G. M., Marks, P. A., and Bank, A.: Relative numbers of human globin genes assayed with purified α and β complementary human DNA (thalassemia). Proc. Natl. Acad. Sci. USA 72:1150, 1975.
114. Benz, E. J., Jr., Pritchard, J., Hillman, D., Glass, J., and Forget, B. G.: β Globin messenger RNA content of bone marrow erythroblasts in heterozygous β-thalassemia. Am. J. Hematol. 16:33, 1984.
115. Maquat, L. E., Kinniburgh, A. J., Beach, L. R., Honig, G. R., Lazerson, J., Ershler, W. B., and Ross, J.: Processing of the human β globin mRNA precursor to mRNA is defective in three patients with $β^+$-thalassemia. Proc. Natl. Acad. Sci. USA 77:4287, 1980.
116. Kantor, J. A., Turner, P. H., and Nienhuis, A. W.: β-Thalassemia: Mutations which affect processing of the β globin mRNA precursor. Cell 21:149, 1980.
117. Benz, E. J., Jr., Scarpa, A. L., Tonkonow, B. L., Pearson, H. A., and Ritchey, A. K.: Post-transcriptional defects in β globin mRNA metabolism in β-thalassemia: Abnormal accumulation of β mRNA precursor sequences. J. Clin. Invest. 68:1526, 1981.
118. Old, J. M., Proudfoot, N. J., Wood, W. G., Longley, J. I., Clegg, J. B., and Weatherall, D. J.: Characterization of β globin mRNA in the $β^0$-thalassemias. Cell 14:289, 1978.
119. Forget, B. G., Benz, E. J., Jr., Skoultchi, A., Baglioni, C., and Housman, D.: Absence of messenger RNA for β globin chain in $β^0$-thalassemia. Nature 247:279, 1974.
120. Tolstoshev, P., Mitchell, J., Lanyon, G., Williamson, R., Ottolenghi, S., Comi, P., Giglioni, B., Masera, G., Modell, B., Weatherall, D. J., and Clegg, J. B.: Presence of gene for β globin in homozygous $β^0$-thalassemia. Nature 259:95, 1976.
121. Comi, P., Giglioni, B., Barbarano, L., Ottolenghi, S., Williamson, R., Novakova, M., and Masera, G.: Transcriptional and post-transcriptional defects in $β^0$-thalassemia. Eur. J. Biochem. 79:617, 1977.
122. Ottolenghi, S., Lanyon, W. G., Williamson, R., Weatherall, D. J., Clegg, J. B., and Pitcher, C. S.: Human globin gene analysis for a patient with $β^0/δβ^0$-thalassemia. Proc. Natl. Acad. Sci. USA 72:2294, 1975.
123. Godet, J., Verdier, G., Nigon, V., Belhani, M., Richard, F., Colonna, P., Mitchell, J., Williamson, R., and Tolstoshev, P.: $β^0$-Thalassemia from Algeria: Genetic and molecular characterization. Blood 50:463, 1977.
124. Belhani, M., Morle, F., Colonna, P., and Godet, J.: Heterogeneity in $β^0$ thalassemia from Algeria: Genetic, clinical and molecular studies. Hum. Genet. 54:251, 1980.
125. Kan, Y. W., Holland, J. P., Dozy, A. M., and Varmus, H. E.: Demonstration of nonfunctional β globin mRNA in homozygous $β^0$-thalassemia. Proc. Natl. Acad. Sci. USA 72:5140, 1975.
126. Temple, G. F., Chang, J. C., and Kan, Y. W.: Authentic β globin mRNA sequences in homozygous $β^0$-thalassemia. Proc. Natl. Acad. Sci. USA 74:3047, 1977.
127. Ramirez, F., O'Donnell, J. V., Marks, P. A., Bank, A., Musumeci, S., Schiliro, G., Pizzarelli, G., Russo, G., Luppis, B., and Gambino, R.: Abnormal or absent β mRNA in $β^0$-Ferrara and gene deletion in δβ-thalassemia. Nature 263:471, 1976.
128. Ottolenghi, S., Comi, P., Giglioni, B., Williamson, R., Vullo, G., and Conconi, F.: Direct demonstration of β globin mRNA in homozygous Ferrara $β^0$-thalassemia patients. Nature 266:231, 1977.
129. Forget, B. G., and Hillman, D. G.: β Globin mRNA in Ferrara $β^0$-thalassaemia. Nature 269:355, 1977.
130. Chang, J. C., and Kan, Y. W.: $β^0$-thalassemia, a nonsense mutation in man. Proc. Natl. Acad. Sci. USA 76:2886, 1979.
131. Maquat, L. E., Kinniburgh, A. J., Rachmilewitz, E. A., and Ross, J.: Unstable β-globin mRNA in mRNA-deficient $β^0$ thalassemia. Cell 27:543, 1981.
132. Kinniburgh, A. J., Maquat, L. E., Schedl, T., Rachmilewitz, E., and Ross, J.: mRNA deficient $β^+$-thalassemia results from a single nucleotide deletion. Nucleic Acids Res. 10:5421, 1982.
133. Tuan, D., Biro, P. A., deRiel, J. K., and Forget, B. G.: Analysis of β globin genes in $β^0$-thalassemia. Ann. N. Y. Acad. Sci. 344:12, 1980.
134. Forget, B. G., Hillman, D. G., Lazarus, H., Barell,

E. F., Benz, E. J., Jr., Caskey, C. T., Huisman, T. H. J., Schroeder, W. A., and Housman, D.: Absence of messenger RNA and gene DNA for beta globin chains in hereditary persistence of fetal hemoglobin. Cell 7:323, 1976.
135. Ottolenghi, S., Comi, P., Giglioni, B., Tolstoshev, P., Lanyon, W. G., Mitchell, G. H., Williamson, R., Russo, G., Musumeci, S., Schiliro, G., Tsistrakis, G., Charache, S., Wood, W. G., Clegg, J. B., and Weatherall, D. J.: δβ-Thalassemia is due to a gene deletion. Cell 9:71, 1976.
136. Kan, Y. W., Holland, J. P., Dozy, A. M., Charache, S., and Kazazian, H. H.: Deletion of the β globin structure gene in hereditary persistence of fetal hemoglobin. Nature 258:162, 1975.
137. Ottolenghi, S., Giglioni, B., Comi, P., Gianni, A. M., Polli, E., Acquaye, C. T. A., Oldham, J. H., and Masera, G.: Globin gene deletion in HPFH, $\delta^0\beta^0$ thalassemia and Hb Lepore disease. Nature 278:654, 1979.
138. Wise, P.: The alpha thalassemia genes. J. Med. Assoc. Thai. 53:677, 1970.
139. Wasi, P., Na-Nakorn, S., and Pootrakul, S.: The α thalassaemias. Clin. Haematol. 3:2, 1974.
140. Wasi, P.: Is the human globin α-chain locus duplicated? Br. J. Haematol. 24:267, 1973.
141. Lehmann, H.: Different types of alpha-thalassemia and significance of haemoglobin Bart's in neonates. Lancet 2:73, 1970.
142. Kan, Y. W., Dozy, A. M., Varmus, H. E., Taylor, J. M., Holland, J. P., Lie-Injo, L. E., Ganesan, J., and Todd, D.: Deletion of α globin genes in haemoglobin H disease demonstrates multiple α globin structural loci. Nature 255:255, 1975.
143. Hunt, D. M., Higgs, D. R., Old, J. M., Clegg, J. B., Weatherall, D. J., and Marsh, G. W.: Determination of alpha thalassaemia phenotypes by messenger RNA analysis. Br. J. Haematol. 45:53, 1980.
144. Orkin, S. H., and Michelson, A.: Partial deletion of the α globin structural gene in human α-thalassaemia. Nature 286:538, 1980.
145. Lodish, H. F.: Model for the regulation of mRNA translation applied to haemoglobin synthesis. Nature 251:385, 1974.
146. Kan, Y. W., Golbus, M. S., and Dozy, A. M.: Prenatal diagnosis of α-thalassemia: Clinical application of molecular hybridization. N. Engl. J. Med. 295:1165, 1976.
147. Dozy, A. M., Kabisch, H., Baker, J., Koenig, H. M., Kurachi, S., Stamatoyannopoulos, G., Todd, D., and Kan, Y. W.: The molecular defects of α-thalassemia in the Filipino. Hemoglobin 1(6):539, 1977.
148. Kan, Y. W., Dozy, A. M., Trecartin, R., and Todd, D.: Identification of a nondeletion defect in α-thalassemia. N. Engl. J. Med. 291:1081, 1977.
149. Davis, J. R., Jr., Dozy, A. M., Lubin, B., Koenig, H. M., Pierce, H. I., Stamatoyannopoulos, G., and Kan, Y. W.: α-Thalassemia in blacks is due to gene deletion. Am. J. Hum. Genet. 31:569, 1979.
150. Old, J., Longley, J., Wood, W. G., Clegg, J. B., and Weatherall, D. J.: Molecular basis for acquired haemoglobin H disease. Nature 269:524, 1977.
151. Kazazian, H. H., Jr., Ginder, G. D., Snyder, P. G., van Beneden, R. J., and Woodhead, A. P.: Further evidence of a quantitative deficiency of chain-specific globin mRNA in the thalassemia syndromes. Proc. Natl. Acad. Sci. USA 72:567, 1975.
152. Nudel, U., Ramirez, F., Marks, P. A., and Bank, A.: Preparative polyacrylamide gel electrophoretic purification of human α- and β-globin messenger RNAs. J. Biol. Chem. 252:2182, 1977.
153. Forget, B. G.: The structure of human globin messenger RNA. Functional, genetic and evolutionary implications. In Piomelli, S., and Yachnin, S. (eds.): Current Topics in Hematology. Vol. 3. New York, Alan R. Liss, Inc., 1980, pp. 1–74.
153a. Forget, B. G., Marotta, C. A., Weissman, S. M., Verma, I. M., McCaffrey, R. P., and Baltimore, D.: Nucleotide sequences of human globin messenger RNA. Ann. N.Y. Acad. Sci. 241:290, 1974.
154. Southern, E. M.: Detection of specific sequences among DNA fragments separated by gel electrophoresis. J. Mol. Biol. 98:503, 1975.
155. Roberts, R. J.: Restriction and modification enzymes and their recognition sequences. Nucleic Acids Res. 13(Suppl.):r 165, 1985.
156. Flavell, R. A., Bernards, R., Kooter, J. M., deBoer, E., Little, P. F. R., Annison, G., and Williamson, R.: The structure of the human β globin gene in β-thalassemia. Nucleic Acids Res. 6:2749, 1979.
157. Orkin, S. H., Old, J. M., Weatherall, D. J., and Nathan, D. G.: Partial deletion of β-globin gene DNA in certain patients with β^0-thalassemia. Proc. Natl. Acad. Sci. USA 76:2400, 1979.
158. Tam, J. W. O., Kaufman, R. E., and Nienhuis, A. W.: Analysis of globin gene structure in patients with β-thalassemia by restriction endonuclease mapping. Hemoglobin 5:209, 1981.
159. Kanavakis, E., Metaxotou-Mavromati, A., Kattamis, C., Aksoy, M., Weatherall, D. J., and Wood, W. G.: Globin gene mapping in normal Hb A_2 types of β-thalassemia. Br. J. Haematol. 51:59, 1982.
159a. Mathew, C. G. P., Rousseau, J., Berman, P., and Harley, E. H.: Restriction endonuclease mapping of globin genes in beta-thalassaemia. S. Afr. Med. J. 64:394, 1983.
160. Orkin, S. H., Kolodner, R., Michelson, A., and Husson, R.: Cloning and direct examination of a structurally abnormal human β^0-thalassemia globin gene. Proc. Natl. Acad. Sci. USA 77:3558, 1980.
161. Spritz, R. A., and Orkin, S. H.: Duplication followed by deletion accounts for the structure of an Indian deletion β^0-thalassemia gene. Nucleic Acids Res. 10:8025, 1982.
162. Kazazian, H. H., Jr., Orkin, S. H., Antonarakis, S. E., Sexton, J. P., Boehm, C. D., Goff, S. C., and Waber, P. G.: Molecular characterization of seven β-thalassemia mutations in Asian Indians. EMBO J. 3:593, 1984.
162a. Thein, S. L., Old, J. M., Wainscoat, J. S., Petrou, M., Modell, B., and Weatherall, D. J.: Population and genetic studies suggest a single origin for the Indian deletion β^0 thalassaemia. Br. J. Haematol. 57:271, 1984.
162b. Padanilam, B. J., Felice, A. E., and Huisman, T. H. J.: Partial deletion of the 5′ β-globin gene region causes β^0-thalassemia in members of an American black family. Blood 64:941, 1984.
162c. Boehm, C. D., Dowling, C. E., and Kazazian, H. H., Jr.: β-thalassemia due to a rare deletion involving the β-globin gene in an American Black. Am. J. Hum. Genet. 36(Suppl.):133S, 1984.
162d. Gilman, J. G., Huisman, T. H. J., and Abels, J.:

Dutch β⁰-thalassaemia: A 10 kilobase DNA deletion associated with significant γ-chain production. Br. J. Haematol. 56:339, 1984.
163. Lawn, R. M., Efstratiadis, A., O'Connell, C., and Maniatis, T.: The nucleotide sequence of the human β globin gene. Cell 21:647, 1980.
164. Baird, M., Driscoll, C., Schreiner, H., Sciaratta, G. V., Sansone, G., Niazi, G., Ramirez, F., and Bank, A.: A nucleotide change at a splice junction in the human β-globin gene is associated with β⁰-thalassemia. Proc. Natl. Acad. Sci. 78:4218, 1981.
165. Treisman, R., Proudfoot, N. J., Shander, M., and Maniatis, T.: A single base change at a splice site in a β⁰-thalassemic gene causes abnormal RNA splicing. Cell 29:903, 1982.
166. Brethnach, R., Benoist, C., O'Hare, K., Gannon, F., and Chambon, P.: Ovalbumin gene: Evidence for a leader sequence in mRNA and DNA sequences at the exon-intron boundaries. Proc. Natl. Acad. Sci. USA 75:4853, 1978.
167. Mount, S. M.: A catalogue of splice junction sequences. Nucleic Acids Res. 10:459, 1982.
168. Mears, J. G., Ramirez, F., Leibowitz, D., Nakamura, F., Bloom, A., Konotey-Ahulu, F., and Bank, A.: Changes in restricted human cellular DNA fragments containing globin gene sequences in thalassemias and related disorders. Proc. Natl. Acad. Sci. USA 75:1222, 1978.
169. Fritsch, E. F., Lawn, R. M., and Maniatis, T.: Characterization of deletions which affect the expression of fetal globin genes in man. Nature 279:598, 1979.
169a. Baird, M., Driscoll, M. C., Ben-Bassat, I., Ohta, Y., Nakamura, F., Bloom, A., and Bank, A.: Gene analysis in δβ and δ⁰ thalassemia. J. Biol. Chem. 259:512, 1984.
170. Bernards, R., Kotter, J. M., and Flavell, R. A.: Physical mapping of the globin gene deletion in (δβ)⁰-thalassemia. Gene 6:265, 1979.
171. Ottolenghi, S., Giglioni, B., Taramelli, R., Comi, P., Mazza, U., Saglio, G., Camaschella, C., Izzo, P., Cao, A., Galanello, R., Gimferrer, E., Baiget, M., and Gianni, A. M.: Molecular comparison of δβ-thalassemia and hereditary persistence of fetal hemoglobin DNAs: Evidence of a regulatory area? Proc. Natl. Acad. Sci. USA 79:2347, 1982.
172. Tuan, D., Feingold, E., Newman, M., Weissman, S. M., and Forget, B. G.: Different 3'-end-points of deletions causing δβ-thalassemia and hereditary persistence of fetal hemoglobin: Implications for the control of γ-globin gene expression in man. Proc. Natl. Acad. Sci. USA 80:6937, 1983.
173. Orkin, S. H., Alter, B. P., Altay, C., Mahoney, M. J., Lazarus, H., Hobbins, J. C., and Nathan, D. G.: Application of endonuclease mapping to the analysis and prenatal diagnosis of thalassemias caused by globin-gene deletion. N. Engl. J. Med. 299:166, 1978.
174. Orkin, S. H., Alter, B. P., and Altay, C.: Deletion of the ᴬγ-globin gene in ᴳγ-δβ-thalassemia. J. Clin. Invest. 64:886, 1979.
175. Ottolenghi, S., and Giglioni, B.: The deletion in a type of δ⁰-β⁰-thalassemia begins in an inverted Alu I repeat. Nature 300:770, 1982.
176. Jones, R. W., Old, J. M., Trent, R. J., Clegg, J. B., and Weatherall, D. J.: Restriction mapping of a new deletion responsible for ᴳγ(δβ)⁰-thalassemia. Nucleic Acids Res. 9:6813, 1981.
176a. Mager, D. L., and Henthorn, P. S.: Identification of a retrovirus-like repetitive element in human DNA. Proc. Natl. Acad. Sci. USA 81:7510, 1984.
177. Jones, R. W., Old, J. M., Trent, R. J., Clegg, J. B., and Weatherall, D. J.: Major rearrangement in the human β globin gene cluster. Nature 291:39, 1981.
177a. Trent, R. J., Jones, R. W., Clegg, J. B., et al.: (ᴬγδβ)⁰ Thalassemia: Similarity of phenotype in four different molecular defects, including one newly described. Br. J. Haematol. 57:279, 1984.
177b. Nakatsuji, T., Gilman, J. G., Sukumaran, P. K., Huisman, T. H. J.: Restriction endonuclease gene mapping studies of an Indian (ᴬγδβ)⁰-thalassemia, previously identified as ᴳγ-HPFH. Br. J. Haematol. 57:663, 1984.
177c. Jennings, M. W., et al.: Analysis of an inversion within the human beta globin gene cluster. Nucleic Acids Res. 13:2897, 1985.
177d. Henthorn, P. S., Smithies, O., Nakatsuji, T., Felice, A. E., Gardiner, M. B., Reese, A. L., and Huisman, T. H. J.: (ᴬγδβ)⁰-Thalassemia in Blacks is due to a deletion of 34 kbp of DNA. Br. J. Haematol. 59:343, 1985.
177e. Anagnou, N. P., Papayannopoulou, T., Stamatoyannopoulos, G., and Nienhuis, A. W.: In vitro modulation of γ-gene expression by fetal sheep "switching factor" in two types of (ᴬγδβ)⁰ thalassemia. Blood 64(Suppl. 1):61A, 1984.
177f. Anagnou, N. P., Papayannopoulou, T., Stamatoyannopoulos, G., and Nienhuis, A. W.: Structurally diverse molecular deletions in the β-globin gene cluster exhibit an identical phenotype on interaction with the β^S gene. Blood 65:1245, 1985.
177g. Wainscoat, J. S., et al.: A novel deletion in the β globin gene complex. Ann. N. Y. Acad. Sci. 445:20, 1985.
177h. Motsunaga, E., Kimura, A., Yamada, H., Fukumaki, Y., and Takaji, Y.: A novel deletion in δβ-thalassemia found in Japan. Biochem. Biophys. Res. Commun. 126:185, 1985.
177i. Pirastu, M., Kan, Y. W., Galanello, R., and Cao, A.: Multiple mutations produce δβ⁰ thalassemia in Sardinia. Science 223:929, 1984.
177j. Guida, S., Gigioni, B., Comi, P., Ottolenghi, S., Camaschella, C., and Saglio, G.: The β-globin gene in Sardinian δβ⁰-thalassemia carries a C → T nonsense mutation at codon 39. EMBO J. 3:785, 1984.
178. Orkin, S. H., Goff, S. C., and Nathan, D. G.: Heterogeneity of DNA deletion in γδβ-thalassemia. J. Clin. Invest. 67:878, 1981.
179. Vanin, E. F., Henthorn, P. S., Kioussis, D., Grosveld, F., and Smithies, O.: Unexpected relationships between four large deletions in the human β-globin gene cluster. Cell 35:701, 1983.
180. Van der Ploeg, L. H. T., Konings, A., Oort, M., Roos, D., Bernini, L., and Flavell, R. A.: γβ-Thalassemia studies showing that deletion of the γ and δ genes influences β globin gene expression in man. Nature 283:637, 1980.
181. Fearon, E. R., et al.: The entire β-globin gene cluster is deleted in a form of γδβ-thalassemia. Blood 61:1273, 1983.
182. Pirastu, M., Kan, Y. W., Lin, C. C., Baine, R. M., and Holbrook, C. T.: Hemolytic disease of the newborn caused by a new deletion of the entire β-globin cluster. J. Clin. Invest. 72:602, 1983.
183. Kioussis, D., Vanin, E., deLange, T., Flavell, R. A., and Grosveld, F. G.: β-Globin gene inactivation by DNA translocation in γβ-thalassaemia. Nature 306:662, 1983.
184. Curtin, P., Kan, Y. W., Gobert-Jones, J. A., Stephens, A. D., and Lehmann, H.: Gene deletion distant from the β-globin locus inactivates the β-globin gene. Clin. Res. 32:493A, 1984.

185. Sukumaran, P. K., Nakatsuji, T., Gardiner, M. B., Reese, A. L., Gilman, J. G., and Huisman, T. H. J.: Gamma thalassemia from the deletion of a γ-globin gene. Nucleic Acids Res. *11*:4635, 1983.

185a. Nakatsuji, T., Ohba, Y., and Huisman, T. H. J.: Hb F-Yamaguchi (γ 75 Thr, γ 80 Asn, γ 136 Ala) is associated with ^{G}γ-thalassemia. Am. J. Hematol. *16*:189, 1984.

186. Tuan, D., Biro, P. A., deRiel, J. K., Lazarus, H., and Forget, B. G.: Restriction endonuclease mapping of the human γ globin gene loci. Nucleic Acids Res. *6*:2519, 1979.

187. Jagadeeswaran, P., Tuan, D., Forget, B. G., and Weissman, S. M.: A gene deletion ending at the midpoint of a repetitive DNA sequence in one form of hereditary persistence of fetal haemoglobin. Nature *296*:469, 1982.

188. Tuan, D., Murnane, M. J., deRiel, J. K., and Forget, B. G.: Heterogeneity in the molecular basis of hereditary persistence of fetal haemoglobin. Nature *285*:335, 1980.

189. Bernards, R., and Flavell, R. A.: Physical mapping of the globin gene deletion in hereditary persistence of fetal hemoglobin (HPFH). Nucleic Acids Res. *8*:1521, 1980.

189a. Kutlar, A., Gardiner, M. B., Headlee, M. G., Reese, A. L., Cleek, M. P., Nagle, S., Sukumaran, P. K., and Huisman, T. H. J.: Heterogeneity in the molecular basis of three types of hereditary persistence of fetal hemoglobin and the relative synthesis of the ^{G}γ and ^{A}γ types of γ chain. Biochem. Genet. *22*:21, 1984.

189b. Wainscoat, J. S., Old, J. M., Wood, W. G., Trent, R. J., and Weatherall, D. J.: Characterization of an Indian (δβ)^0 thalassaemia. Br. J. Haematol. *58*:353–360, 1984.

189c. Mager, D. L., and Henthorn, P. S.: Personal communication.

190. Papayannopoulou, T., Lawn, R. M., Stamatoyannopoulos, G., and Maniatis, T.: Greek (^{A}γ) variant of hereditary persistence of fetal haemoglobin: Globin gene organization and studies of expression of fetal haemoglobins in clonal erythroid cultures. Br. J. Haematol. *50*:387, 1982.

191. Jones, R. W., Old, J. M., Wood, W. G., Clegg, J. B., and Weatherall, D. J.: Restriction endonuclease maps of the β-like globin gene cluster in the British and Greek forms of HPFH, and for one example of ^{G}γβ$^+$ HPFH. Br. J. Haematol. *50*:415, 1982.

192. Balsley, J. F., Rappaport, E., Schwartz, E., and Surrey, S.: The γ-δ-β-globin gene region in ^{G}γ-β$^+$-hereditary persistence of fetal hemoglobin. Blood *59*:828, 1982.

193. Farquhar, M., Gelinas, R., Tatsis, B., Murray, J., Yagi, M., Mueller, R., and Stamatoyannopoulos, G.: Restriction endonuclease mapping of γ-δ-β-globin region in ^{G}γ(β)$^+$ HPFH and a Chinese ^{A}γ HPFH variant. Am. J. Hum. Genet. *35*:611, 1983.

194. Old, J. M., Ayyub, H., Wood, W. G., Clegg, J. B., and Weatherall, D. J.: Linkage analysis of nondeletion hereditary persistence of fetal hemoglobin. Science *215*:981, 1983.

195. Gianni, A. M., Bregni, M., Cappellini, M. D., Fiorelli, G., Taramelli, R., Giglioni, B., Comi, P., and Ottolenghi, S.: A gene controlling fetal hemoglobin expression in adults is not linked to the non-α globin cluster. EMBO J. *2*:921, 1983.

196. Dover, G. J., and Boyer, S. H.: F-cell production in sickle cell anemia: Regulation by genes linked to β-hemoglobin locus. Science *211*:1441, 1981.

197. Wood, W. G., Weatherall, D. J., and Clegg, J. B.: Interaction of heterocellular hereditary persistence of foetal haemoglobin with β thalassemia and sickle cell anaemia. Nature *264*:247, 1976.

197a. Gilman, J. G., and Huisman, T. H. J.: Two independent genetic factors in the β-globin gene cluster are associated with high ^{G}γ levels in the Hb F of SS patients. Blood *64*:452, 1984.

197b. Labie, D., Pagnier, J., Lapoumeroulie, C., Rouabhi, F., et al.: Common haplotype dependency of high ^{G}γ gene expression and high Hb F levels in β-thalassemia and sickle cell anemia patients. Proc. Natl. Acad. Sci. USA *82*:2111, 1985.

197c. Harano, T., et al.: Five haplotypes in black β-thalassaemia heterozygotes: Three are associated with high and two with low ^{G}γ values in fetal haemoglobin. Br. J. Haematol. *59*:333, 1985.

197d. Wainscoat, J. S., et al.: A genetic marker for elevated levels of haemoglobin F in homozygous sickle cell disease? Br. J. Haematol. *60*:261, 1985.

197e. Boyer, S. H., Dover, G. J., Serjeant, G. R., Smith, K. D., Antonarakis, S. E., Embury, S. H., Margolet, L., Noyes, A. N., Boyer, M. L., and Bias, W. B.: Production of F cells in sickle cell anemia: Regulation by a genetic locus or loci separate from the β-globin gene cluster. Blood *64*:1053, 1984.

197f. Jensen, M., Wirtz, W., Walther, J.-U., Schemken, E. M., Laryea, M. D., and Driesel, A. J.: Hereditary persistence of fetal haemoglobin (HPFH) in conjunction with a chromosomal translocation involving the haemoglobin β locus. Br. J. Haematol. *56*:87, 1984.

198. Huisman, T. H. J., et al.: The present status of the heterogeneity of fetal hemoglobin in β-thalassemia: An attempt to unify some observations in thalassemia and related conditions. Ann. N. Y. Acad. Sci. *232*:107, 1974.

199. Ojwang, P. J., Nakatsuji, T., Gardiner, M. B., Reese, A. L., Gilman, J. G., and Huisman, T. H. J.: Gene deletion as the molecular basis for the Kenya-^{G}γ-HPFH condition. Hemoglobin *7(2)*:115, 1983.

200. Schmid, C. W., and Jelinek, W. R.: The structure and organization of the major interspersed repetitious sequence in mammalian DNA: The Alu sequence. Science *216*:1065, 1982.

201. Duncan, C., Biro, P. A., Choudary, P. V., Elder, J. T., Wang, R. R. C., Forget, B. G., deRiel, J. K., and Weissman, S. M.: RNA polymerase III transcriptional units are interspersed among human non-α globin genes. Proc. Natl. Acad. Sci. USA *76*:5095, 1979.

202. Ottolenghi, S., Giglioni, B., Comi, P., Taramelli, R., Guida, S., Mantovani, R., Crema, A. L., Cappellini, M. D., and Gianni, A. M.: Regulation of fetal hemoglobin synthesis. In Bertazzoni, U., Bollum, F. J., and Ghione, M. (eds.): Contributions of Modern Biology to Medicine. New York, Raven Press, 1985, pp. 125–130.

203. Ottolenghi, S.: Personal communication.

204. Yaniv, M.: Enhancing elements for activation of eukaryotic promoters. Nature *297*:17, 1982.

205. Boss, M. A.: Enhancer elements in immunoglobulin genes. Nature *303*:281, 1983.

206. Khoury, G., and Gruss, P.: Enhancer elements. Cell *33*:313, 1983.

207. Marx, J. L.: Immunoglobulin genes have enhancers. Science *221*:735, 1983.

208. Feingold, E. A., Collins, F. S., Metherall, J. E.,

Stoeckert, C. J., Jr., Weissman, S. M., and Forget, B. G.: Molecular analysis of deletion and nondeletion hereditary persistence of fetal hemoglobin and identification of a new mutation causing β-thalassemia. Ann. N.Y. Acad. Sci. 445:159, 1985.
208a. Feingold, E. A., and Forget, B. G.: Erythroid-specific hypomethylation and potential enhancer element in the DNA juxtaposed to the γ-globin genes in hereditary persistence of fetal hemoglobin (HPFH). Clin. Res. 33:541A, 1985.
208b. Elder, J. T., and Groudine, M.: Personal communication.
209. Embury, S. H., Lebo, R. V., Dozy, A. M., and Kan, Y. W.: Organization of the α-globin genes in the Chinese α-thalassemia syndromes. J. Clin. Invest. 63:1307, 1979.
210. Orkin, S. H., Old, J., Lazarus, H., Altay, C., Gurgey, A., Weatherall, D. J., and Nathan, D. G.: The molecular basis of α-thalassemias: Frequent occurrence of dysfunctional α loci among non-Asians with Hb H disease. Cell 17:33, 1979.
211. Dozy, A. M., Kan, Y. W., Embury, S. H., Mentzer, W., C., Lubin, B., Davis, J. R., Jr., and Koenig, H. M.: α-Globin gene organization in blacks precludes the severe form of α-thalassemia. Nature 280:605, 1979.
212. Higgs, D. R., Old, J. M., Clegg, J. B., Pressley, L., Hunt, D. M., Weatherall, D. J., and Serjeant, G. R.: Negro α-thalassaemia is caused by deletion of a single α-globin gene. Lancet 2:272, 1979.
213. Beutler, E., Kuhl, W., and Johnson, C.: A common mutant Eco RI restriction endonuclease site in the 5' flanking portion of the human α-globin gene. Proc. Natl. Acad. Sci. USA 78:7056, 1981.
214. Embury, S. H., Miller, J. A., Dozy, A. M., Kan, Y. W., Chan, V., and Todd, D.: Two different molecular organizations account for the single α-globin gene of the α-thalassemia-2 genotype. J. Clin. Invest. 66:1319, 1980.
215. Phillips, J. A., III, Vik, T. A., Scott, A. F., Young, K. E., Kazazian, H. H., Jr., Smith, K. D., Fairbanks, V. F., and Koenig, H. M.: Unequal crossing-over: A common basis of single α-globin genes in Asians and American blacks with hemoglobin-H disease. Blood 55:1066, 1980.
216. Higgs, D. R., Pressley, L., Serjeant, G. R., Clegg, J. B., and Weatherall, D. J.: The genetics and molecular basis of alpha thalassaemia in association with Hb S in Jamaican Negroes. Br. J. Haematol. 47:43, 1981.
217. Higgs, D. R., Pressley, L., Clegg, J. B., Weatherall, D. J., and Serjeant, G. R.: α Thalassemia in black populations. Johns Hopkins Med. J. 146:300, 1980.
218. Whitelaw, E., Pagnier, J., Verdier, G., Henni, T., Godet, J., and Williamson, R.: Mapping the α-globin genes in an Algerian Hb H patient and his family. Blood 55:511, 1980.
219. Higgs, D. R., Hill, A. V. S., Bowden, D. K., Weatherall, D. J., and Clegg, J. B.: Independent recombination events between the duplicated human α globin genes; implications for their concerted evolution. Nucleic Acids Res. 12:6965, 1984.
219a. Michelson, A. M., and Orkin, S. H.: Boundaries of gene conversion within the duplicated human α-globin genes: Concerted evolution by segmental recombination. J. Biol. Chem. 258:15245, 1983.
219b. Winichagoon, P., Higgs, D. R., Goodbourn, S. E. Y., Clegg, J. B., Weatherall, D. J., and Wasi, P.: The molecular basis of α-thalassaemia in Thailand. EMBO J. 3:1813, 1984.
219c. Hill, A. V. S., et al.: Melanesians and Polynesians share a unique α-thalassemia mutation. Am. J. Hum. Genet. 37:571, 1985.
220. Mathew, C. G. P., Rousseau, J., Rees, J. S., and Harley, E. H.: The molecular basis of alpha thalassaemia in a South African population. Br. J. Haematol. 55:103, 1983.
220a. Embury, S. H., Gholson, M. A., Gillette, P., and Rieder, R. F.: The leftward deletion α-thalassemia-2 in a black subject with Hb SS. Blood 65:769, 1985.
220b. Wong, S. C., et al.: Double heterozygosity for two genotypes of α-thalassemia 2: Hematological, biosynthetic and DNA studies. Hemoglobin 9:111, 1985.
221. Ohene-Frempong, K., Rappaport, E., Atwater, J., Schwartz, E., and Surrey, S.: Alpha-gene deletions in black newborn infants with Hb Bart's. Blood 56:931, 1980.
222. Higgs, D. R., Pressley, L., Clegg, J. B., Weatherall, D. J., Higgs, S., Carey, P., and Serjeant, G. R.: Detection of alpha thalassaemia in Negro infants. Br. J. Haematol. 46:39, 1980.
223. Orkin, S. H.: The duplicated human α globin genes lie close together in cellular DNA. Proc. Natl. Acad. Sci. USA 75:5950, 1978.
224. Dozy, A. M., Kan, Y. W., Forman, E. N., Abuelo, D. N., Barsel-Bowers, G., Mahoney, M. J., and Forget, B. J.: Antenatal diagnosis of homozygous α-thalassemia. J. A. M. A. 241:1610, 1979.
225. Surrey, S., Chambers, J. S., Muni, D., and Schwartz, E.: Restriction endonuclease analysis of human globin genes in cellular DNA. Biochem. Biophys. Res. Commun. 83:1125, 1978.
226. Kan, Y. W., and Dozy, A. M.: Polymorphism of DNA sequence adjacent to human β-globin structural gene: Relationship to sickle mutation. Proc. Natl. Acad. Sci. USA 75:5631, 1978.
227. Lie-Injo, L. E., Solai, A., Herrera, A. R., Nicolaisen, L., Kan, Y. W., Wan, W. P., and Hasan, K.: Hb Bart's level in cord blood and deletions of α-globin genes. Blood 59:370, 1982.
228. Pressley, L., Higgs, D. R., Clegg, J. B., and Weatherall, D. J.: Gene deletions in α-thalassemia prove that the 5'-ζ locus is functional. Proc. Natl. Acad. Sci. USA 77:3586, 1980.
229. Sophocleous, T., Higgs, D. R., Aldridge, B., Trent, R. J., Pressley, L., Clegg, J. B., and Weatherall, D. J.: The molecular basis for the haemoglobin Bart's hydrops fetalis syndrome in Cyprus. Br. J. Haematol. 47:153, 1981.
230. Proudfoot, N. J., Gil, A., and Maniatis, T.: The structure of the human ζ globin gene and a closely linked, nearly identical pseudogene. Cell 31:553, 1982.
230a. Chang, J. C., and Kan, Y. W.: Deletion of the entire human α-globin gene cluster. Clin. Res. 32:549A, 1984.
231. Phillips, J. A., III, Scott, A. F., Smith, K. D., Young, K. E., Lightbody, K. L., Jiji, R. M., and Kazazian, H. H., Jr.: A molecular basis for hemoglobin-H disease in American blacks. Blood 54:1439, 1979.
232. Sancar, G. B., Cedeno, M. M., and Riedler, R. F.: The varied arrangement of the α globin genes in α thalassemia and Hb H disease in American blacks. Johns Hopkins Med. J. 146:264, 1980.
233. Felice, A. E., Cleek, M. P., McKie, K., McKie, V., and Huisman, T. H. J.: The rare α-thalassemia-1 of Blacks is a ζα-thalassemia-1 associated with deletion of all α- and ζ-globin genes. Blood 63:1253, 1984.
234. Embury, S. H., Monroy, G. C., and Kark, J. A.:

Identification of the rare α-thalassemia-1 deletion in the black population. Blood 62(Suppl. 1):66a, 1983.
234a. Steinberg, M. H., Coleman, M. B., Adams, J. G., Hartmann, R. C., Saba, H., and Anagnou, N. P.: A new gene deletion in the α-like globin gene cluster as the molecular basis for the rare α-thalassemia-1 in blacks: Hb H disease in sickle cell trait. Blood 64(Suppl. 1):60a, 1984.
235. Molecular basis of hemoglobin-H disease in the Mediterranean population. Blood 54:1434, 1979.
236. Nicholls, R. D., Higgs, D. R., Clegg, J. B., and Weatherall, D. J.: α^0-Thalassemia due to recombination between the α1-globin gene and an Alu I repeat. Blood 65:1434, 1985.
237. Altay, C., Gurgey, A., and Tuncbilek, E.: Hematological evaluation of patients with various combinations of α-thalassemia. Am. J. Hematol. 9:261, 1980.
238. Pressley, L., Higgs, D. R., Aldridge, B., Metaxatou-Mavromati, A., Clegg, J. B., and Weatherall, D. J.: Characterisation of a new α thalassemia 1 defect due to a partial deletion of the α globin gene complex. Nucleic Acids Res. 8:4889, 1980.
239. Higgs, D. R., Pressley, L., Aldridge, B., Clegg, J. B., Weatherall, D. J., Cao, A., Hadjiminas, M. G., Kattamis, C., Metaxatou-Mavromati, A., Rachmilewitz, E. A., and Sophocleous, T.: Genetic and molecular diversity in nondeletion Hb H disease. Proc. Natl. Acad. Sci. USA 78:5833, 1981.
240. Goossens, M., Lee, K. Y., Liebhaber, S. A., and Kan, Y. W.: Globin structural mutant α is a novel cause of α-thalassemia. Nature 296:864, 1982.
241. Liebhaber, S. A., and Kan, Y. W.: α-Thalassemia caused by an unstable α-globin mutant. J. Clin. Invest. 71:461, 1983.
242. Del Senno, L., Bernardi, F., Buzzoni, D., Marchetti, G., Perrotta, C., and Conconi, F.: Molecular characteristics of a non-deletion α-thalassaemia of the Po River delta. Eur. J. Biochem. 116:127, 1981.
243. Orkin, S. H., Goff, S. C., and Hechtman, R. L.: Mutation in an intervening sequence splice junction in man. Proc. Natl. Acad. Sci. USA 78:5041, 1981.
243a. Pirastu, M., Saglio, G., Chang, J. C., Cao, A., and Kan, Y. W.: Initiation codon mutation as a cause of α thalassemia. J. Biol. Chem. 259:12315, 1984.
244. Pressley, L., Higgs, R. D., Clegg, J. B., Perrine, R. P., Pembrey, M. E., and Weatherall, D. J.: A new genetic basis for hemoglobin-H disease. N. Engl. J. Med. 303:1381, 1980.
245. Higgs, D. R., Goodbourn, S. E. Y., Lamb, J., Clegg, J. B., and Weatherall, D. J.: α-Thalassaemia caused by a polyadenylation signal mutation. Nature 306:398, 1983.
246. Sancar, G. B., Tatsis, B., Cedeno, M. M., and Rieder, R. F.: Proportion of hemoglobin G Philadelphia ($\alpha_2^{68Asn-Lys}\beta_2$) in heterozygotes is determined by α-globin gene deletions. Proc. Natl. Acad. Sci. USA 77:6874, 1980.
247. Surrey, S., Ohene-Frempong, K., Rappaport, E., Atwater, J., and Schwartz, E.: Linkage of $\alpha^{G-Philadelphia}$ to α-thalassemia in African-Americans. Proc. Natl. Acad. Sci. USA 77:4885, 1980.
248. Felice, A. E., Ozdonmez, R., Headlee, M. E., and Huisman, T. H. J.: Organization of α-chain genes among Hb G-Philadelphia heterozygotes in association with Hb S, β-thalassemia, and α-thalassemia-2. Biochem. Genet. 20:689, 1982.
248a. Bruzdzinski, C. J., Sisco, K. L., Ferrucci, S. J., and Rucknagel, D. L.: The occurrence of the $\alpha^{G-Philadelphia}$-globin allele on a double-locus chromosome. Am. J. Hum. Genet. 36:101, 1984.
248b. Sciarratta, G. V., Sansone, G., Ivaldi, G., Felice, A. E., and Huisman, T. H. J.: Alternate organization of α G-Philadelphia globin genes among U.S. black and Italian Caucasian heterozygotes. Hemoglobin 8:537, 1984.
249. Del Senno, L., Bernardi, F., Marchetti, G., Perrotta, C., Conconi, F., Vullo, C., Salsini, G., Cristofori, G., Cappellozza, G., Bellinello, F., Bedendo, B., and Mercuriati, M.: Organization of α-globin genes and mRNA translation in subjects carrying haemoglobin Hasharon (α47 Asp-His) from the Ferrara region (northern Italy). Eur. J. Biochem. 111:125, 1980.
250. Giglioni, B., Comi, P., Taramelli, R., Ottolenghi, S., Ciocca-Vasino, M. A., Ane, C., Cappellini, M. D., and Gianni, A. M.: Organization of α-globin genes in Hb Hasharon (α 47Asp-His) carriers. Blood 56:1145, 1980.
251. Higgs, D. R., Hunt, D. M., Drysdale, H. C., Clegg, J. B., Pressley, L., and Weatherall, D. J.: The genetic basis of Hb Q-H disease. Br. J. Haematol. 46:387, 1980.
252. Lie-Injo, L. E., Dozy, A. M., Kan, Y. W., Lopes, M., and Todd, D.: The α-globin gene adjacent to the gene for Hb Q–α74Asp-His is deleted, but not that adjacent to the gene for Hb G–α30 Glu-Gln: three-fourths of the α-globin genes are deleted in Hb Q–α thalassemia. Blood 54:1416, 1979.
253. Pagnier, J., Elion, J., Lapoumeroulie, C., Vigneron, C., and Labie, D.: Homozygous deletional α^+-thalassemia associated with unequal expression of the two remaining α_1 genes (α_1^A and α_1^Q). Br. J. Haematol. 52:115, 1982.
254. Bowden, D. K., Pressley, L., Higgs, D. R., Clegg, J. B., and Weatherall, D. J.: α-Globin gene deletions associated with Hb J Tongariki. Br. J. Haematol. 51:243, 1982.
255. Trabuchet, G., Morle, F., Verdier, G., Godet, J., Benabadji, M., and Nigon, V. M.: Mapping the α-globin genes in Hb J Mexico carriers. Hum. Genet. 62:164, 1982.
255a. Honig, G. R., Shamsuddin, M., Vida, L. N., Mompoint, M., Valcourt, E., Bowie, L. J., Jones, E. C., Powers, P. A., Spritz, R. A., Guis, M., Embury, S. H., Conboy, J., Kan, Y. W., Mentzer, W. C., Weil, S. C., Hirata, R. K., Waloch, J., O'Riordan, J. F., and Goldstick, T. K.: Hemoglobin Evanston (α14 Trp→Arg): An unstable α-chain variant expressed as α-thalassemia. J. Clin. Invest. 73:1740, 1984.
255b. Liebhaber, S. A., Rappaport, E. F., Cash, F. E., Ballas, S. K., Schwartz, E., and Surrey, S.: Hemoglobin I mutation encoded at both α-globin loci on the same chromosome: Concerted evolution in the human genome. Science 226:1449, 1984.
256. Weatherall, D. J., Higgs, D. R., Clegg, J. B., and Wood, W. G.: The significance of haemoglobin H in patients with mental retardation or myeloproliferative disease. Br. J. Haematol. 52:351, 1982.
257. Higgs, D. R., Wood, W. G., Barton, C., and Weatherall, D. J.: Clinical features and molecular analysis of acquired hemoglobin H disease. Am. J. Med. 75:181, 1983.
258. Weatherall, D. J., Old, J., Longley, J., Wood, W. G., Clegg, J. B., Pollock, A., and Lewis, M. J.: Acquired haemoglobin H disease in leukemia:

Pathophysiology and molecular basis. Br. J. Haematol. 38:305, 1978.
259. Anagnou, N. P., Ley, T. J., Chesbro, B., Wright, G., Kitchens, C., Liebhaber, S., Nienhuis, A. W., and Deisseroth, A. B.: Acquired α-thalassemia in preleukemia is due to decreased expression of all four α-globin genes. Proc. Natl. Acad. Sci. USA 80:6051, 1983.
260. Deisseroth, A., Helder, J. C., Higgs, D., and Weatherall, D.: Trans inactivation of alpha globin gene expression in leukemic patients with hemoglobin H disease. Blood 64(Suppl. 1):56a, 1984.
261. Weatherall, D. J., Higgs, D. R., Bunch, C., et al: Hemoglobin H disease and mental retardation: A new syndrome or a remarkable coincidence? N. Engl. J. Med. 305:607, 1981.
262. Vives Corrons, J. L. L., Aquilar, J. L. L., and Mateo, M.: Haemoglobin H (Hb H) disease and severe glutathione peroxidase deficiency: An undescribed association in a mentally retarded child. Br. J. Haematol. 54:160, 1983.
262a. Bowcock, A. M., Van Tonder, S., and Jenkins, T.: The haemoglobin H disease mental retardation syndrome: Molecular studies on the South African case. Br. J. Haematol. 56:69, 1984.
263. Hjelle, B., Charache, S., and Phillips, J. A., III: Hemoglobin H disease and multiple congenital anomalies in a child of northern European origin. Am. J. Hematol. 13:319, 1982.
264. Goossens, M., Dozy, A. M., Embury, S. H., Zachariades, Z., Hadjiminas, M. G., Stamatoyannopoulos, G., and Kan, Y. W.: Triplicated α-globin loci in humans. Proc. Natl. Acad. Sci. USA 77:518, 1980.
265. Higgs, D. R., Old, J. M., Pressley, L., Clegg, J. B., and Weatherall, D. J.: A novel α-globin gene arrangement in man. Nature 284:632, 1980.
266. Sancar, G. B., Cedeno, M. M., Bellevue, R., and Rieder, R. F.: Interaction of chromosomes bearing 1, 2 or 3 α-globin genes in an American black family with α-thalassemia. Hemoglobin 6:99, 1982.
266a. Sampietro, M., Cazzola, M., Cappellini, M. D., and Fiorelli, G.: The triplicated alpha-gene locus and heterozygous beta thalassaemia: A case of thalassaemia intermedia. Br. J. Haematol. 55:709, 1983.
266b. Galanello, R., Ruggeri, R., Paglietti, E., Addis, M., Melis, M. A., and Cao, A.: A family with segregating triplicated alpha globin loci and beta thalassemia. Blood 62:1035, 1983.
266c. Thein, S. L., Al-Hakim, I., and Hoffbrand, A. V.: Thalassemia intermedia: A new molecular basis. Br. J. Haematol. 56:333, 1984.
266d. Higgs, D. R., Clegg, J. B., Weatherall, D. J., Serjeant, B. E., and Serjeant, G. R.: Interaction of the αααα globin gene haplotype and sickle haemoglobin. Br. J. Haematol. 58:671, 1984.
266e. Kanavakis, E., Metaxotou-Mavromati, A., Kattamis, C., Wainscoat, J. S., and Wood, W. G.: The triplicated α gene locus and β thalassemia. Br. J. Haematol. 54:201, 1983.
267. Lauer, J., Shen, C. K. J., and Maniatis, T.: The chromosomal arrangement of human α-like globin genes: Sequence homology and α-globin gene deletions. Cell 20:119, 1980.
268. Lie-Injo, L. E., Herrera, A. R., and Kan, Y. W.: Two types of triplicated α-globin loci in humans. Nucleic Acids Res. 9:3707, 1981.
269. Trent, R. J., Higgs, D. R., Clegg, J. B., and Weatherall, D. J.: A new triplicated α-globin gene arrangement in man. Br. J. Haematol. 49:149, 1981.
269a. Platica, O., Cedeno, M., and Rieder, R. F.: A novel chromosome bearing three alpha-globin genes. Blood 62(Suppl. 1):69a, 1983.
270. Trent, R. J., Bowden, D. K., Old, J. M., Wainscoat, J. S., Clegg, J. B., and Weatherall, D. J.: A novel rearrangement of the human β-like globin gene cluster. Nucleic Acids Res. 9:6723, 1981.
271. Paulson, J. R., and Laemmli, U. K.: The structure of histone-depleted metaphase chromosomes. Cell 12:817, 1977.
272. Marsden, M. P. F., and Laemmli, U. K.: Metaphase chromosome structure: Evidence for a radial loop model. Cell 17:849, 1979.
273. Vogelstein, B., Pardoll, D. M., and Coffey, D. S.: Supercoiled loops and eucaryotic replication. Cell 22:79, 1980.
274. Pardoll, D. M., Vogelstein, B., and Coffey, D. S.: A fixed site of DNA replication in eucaryotic DNA cells. Cell 19:527, 1980.
274a. Lehrman, M. A., Schneider, W. J., Sudhof, T. C., Brown, M. S., Goldstein, J. L., and Russell, D. W.: Mutation in LDL receptor: Alu-Alu recombination deletes exons encoding transmembrane and cytoplasmic domains. Science 227:140, 1985.
275. Cohen, S. N.: Gene manipulation. N. Engl. J. Med. 294:883, 1976.
276. Wilson, J. T., Wilson, L. B., deRiel, J. K., Villa-Komaroff, L., Efstratiadis, A., Forget, B. G., and Weissman, S. M.: Insertion of synthetic copies of human globin genes into bacterial plasmids. Nucleic Acids Res. 5:563, 1978.
277. Lawn, R. M., Fritsch, E. F., Parker, R. C., Blake, G., and Maniatis, T.: The isolation and characterization of linked δ- and β-globin genes from a cloned library of human DNA. Cell 15:1157, 1978.
277a. Orkin, S. H., Antonarakis, S. E., and Kazazian, H. H., Jr.: Polymorphism and molecular pathology of the human beta-globin gene. Prog. Hematol. 13:49, 1983.
277b. Orkin, S. H., and Kazazian, H. H., Jr.: The mutation and polymorphism of the human β-globin gene and its surrounding DNA. Ann. Rev. Genet. 18:131, 1984.
278. Antonarakis, S. E., Boehm, C. D., Giardina, P. J. V., and Kazazian, H. H., Jr.: Nonrandom association of polymorphic restriction sites in the β-globin gene cluster. Proc. Natl. Acad. Sci. USA 79:137, 1982.
279. Orkin, S. H. Kazazian, H. H., Jr., Antonarakis, S. E., Goff, S. C., Boehm, C. D., Sexton, J. P., Waber, P. G., and Giardina, P. J. V.: Linkage of β-thalassemia mutations and β globin gene polymorphisms with DNA polymorphisms in human β globin gene cluster. Nature 296:627, 1982.
280. Maxam, A. M., and Gilbert, W.: A new method for sequencing DNA. Proc. Natl. Acad. Sci. USA 74:560, 1977.
281. Sanger, F., Nicklen, S., and Coulson, A. R.: DNA sequencing with chain-terminating inhibitors. Proc. Natl. Acad. Sci. USA 74:5463, 1977.
282. Manley, J. L., Fire, A., Cano, A., Sharp, P. A., and Gefter, M. L.: DNA-dependent transcription of adenovirus genes in a soluble whole-cell extract. Proc. Natl. Acad. Sci. USA 77:3855, 1980.
283. Weil, P. A., Luse, D. S., Segall, J., and Roeder, R. G.: Selective and accurate initiation of transcription at the Ad 2 major late promoter in a soluble

system dependent on purified RNA polymerase II and DNA. Cell 18:469, 1979.
284. Proudfoot, N. J., Shander, M. H. M., Manley, J. L., Gefter, M. L., and Maniatis, T.: Structure and in vitro transcription of human globin genes. Science 209:1329, 1980.
285. Mulligan, R. C., Howard, B. H., and Berg, P.: Synthesis of rabbit β-globin in cultured monkey kidney cells following infection with a SV40 β-globin recombinant genome. Nature 277:108, 1979.
286. Hamer, D. H., and Leder, P.: Expression of the chromosomal mouse β^{maj}-globin gene cloned in SV40. Nature 281:35, 1979.
287. Banerji, J., Rusconi, S., and Schaffner, W.: Expression of a β-globin gene is enhanced by remote SV40 DNA sequences. Cell 27:299, 1981.
288. de Villiers, J., and Schaffner, W.: A small segment of polyoma virus DNA enhances the expression of a cloned β-globin gene over a distance of 1400 base pairs. Nucleic Acids Res. 9:6251, 1981.
289. Mellon, P., Parker, V., Gluzman, Y., and Maniatis, T.: Identification of DNA sequences required for transcription of the human αl-globin gene in a new SV40 host-vector system. Cell 27:279, 1981.
290. Humphries, R. K., Ley, T., Turner, P., Moulton, A. D., and Nienhuis, A. W.: Differences in human α-, β- and δ-globin gene expression in monkey kidney cells. Cell 30:173, 1982.
291. Mantei, N., Boll, W., and Weissmann, C.: Rabbit β-globin mRNA production in mouse L cells transformed with cloned rabbit β-globin chromosomal DNA. Nature 281:40, 1979.
292. Wold, B., Wigler, M., Lacy, E., Maniatis, T., Silverstein, S., and Axel, R.: Introduction and expression of a rabbit β-globin gene in mouse fibroblasts. Proc. Natl. Acad. Sci. USA 76:5684, 1979.
293. Chao, M. V., Mellon, P., Charnay, P., Maniatis, T., and Axel, R.: The regulated expression of β-globin genes introduced into mouse erythroleukemia cells. Cell 32:483, 1983.
294. Wright, S., deBoer, E., Grosveld, F. G., and Flavell, R. A.: Regulated expression of the human β-globin gene family in murine erythroleukaemia cells. Nature 305:333, 1983.
295. DiMaio, D., Treisman, R., and Maniatis, T.: Bovine papillomavirus vector that propagates as a plasmid in both mouse and bacterial cells. Proc. Natl. Acad. Sci. USA 79:4030, 1982.
296. Treisman, R., Orkin, S. H., and Maniatis, T.: Specific transcription and RNA splicing defects in five cloned β-thalassaemia genes. Nature 302:591, 1983.
297. Berk, A. J., and Sharp, P. A.: Sizing and mapping of early adenovirus mRNAs by gel electrophoresis of S$_1$ endonuclease digested hybrids. Cell 12:721, 1977.
298. Ghosh, P. K., Reddy, V. B., Piatak, M., Lebowitz, P., and Weissman, S. M.: Determination of RNA sequences by primer directed synthesis and sequencing of their cDNA transcripts. Methods Enzymol. 65:580, 1980.
299. Spritz, R. A., Jagadeeswaran, P., Choudary, P. V., Biro, P. A., Elder, J. T., deRiel, J. K., Manley, J. L., Gefter, M. L., Forget, B. G., and Weissman, S. M.: Base substitution in an intervening sequence of a β$^+$-thalassemic human globin gene. Proc. Natl. Acad. Sci. USA 78:2455, 1981.
300. Westaway, D., and Williamson, R.: An intron nucleotide sequence variant in a cloned β$^+$-thalassemia globin gene. Nucleic Acids Res. 9:1777, 1981.
301. Busslinger, M., Moschonas, N., and Flavell, R. A.: β$^+$-Thalassemia: Aberrant splicing results from a single point mutation in an intron. Cell 27:289, 1981.
302. Fukumaki, Y., Ghosh, P. K., Benz, E. J., Jr., Reddy, V. B., Lebowitz, P., Forget, B. G., and Weissman, S. M.: Abnormally spliced messenger RNA in erythroid cells from patients with β$^+$-thalassemia and monkey cells expressing a cloned β$^+$-thalassemic gene. Cell 28:585, 1982.
303. Efstratiadis, A., Posakony, J. W., Maniatis, T., Lawn, R. M., O'Connell, C., Spritz, R. A., deRiel, J. K., Forget, B. G., Weissman, S. M., Slightom, J. L., Blechl, A. E., Smithies, O., Baralle, F. E., Shoulders, C. C., and Proudfoot, N. J.: The structure and evolution of the human β globin gene family. Cell 21:653, 1980.
304. Benz, E. J., Jr., Scarpa, A. L., and Forget, B. G.: Defective processing of β mRNA in different forms of β$^+$-thalassemia. Trans. Assoc. Am. Physicians 95:325, 1982.
305. Ley, T., Anagnou, N. P., Pepe, G., and Nienhuis, A. W.: RNA processing errors in patients with β-thalassemia. Proc. Natl. Acad. Sci. USA 79:4775, 1982.
306. Kazazian, H. H., Jr., Chakravarti, A., and Orkin, S. H.: Identity of different mutations for deleterious genes. Nature 301:176, 1983.
307. Goldsmith, M. E., Humphries, R. K., Ley, T., Cline, A., Kantor, J. A., and Nienhuis, A.: "Silent" nucleotide substitution in a β$^+$-thalassemia globin gene activates splice site in coding sequence RNA. Proc. Natl. Acad. Sci. USA 88:2318, 1983.
308. Orkin, S. H., Kazazian, H. H., Jr., Antonarakis, S. E., Ostrer, H., Goff, S. C., and Sexton, J. P.: Abnormal RNA processing due to the exon mutation of β^E globin gene. Nature 300:768, 1982.
309. Orkin, S. H., Antonarakis, S. E., and Loukopoulos, D.: Abnormal processing of β^{Knossos} RNA. Blood 64:311, 1984.
310. Wainscoat, J. S., Old, J. M., Weatherall, D. J., and Orkin, S. H.: The molecular basis for the clinical diversity of β thalassaemia in Cypriots. Lancet 1:1235, 1983.
311. Tamagnini, G. P., Lopes, M. C., Castanheira, M. E., Wainscoat, J. S., and Wood, W. G.: β$^+$ Thalassaemia-Portuguese type: Clinical haematological and molecular studies of a newly defined form of β thalassaemia. Br. J. Haematol. 54:189, 1983.
312. Traeger, J., Wood, W. G., Clegg, J. B., Weatherall, D. J., and Wasi, P.: Defective synthesis of Hb E is due to reduced levels of β^E mRNA. Nature 288:497, 1980.
313. Benz, E. J., Jr., Berman, B. W., Tonkonow, B. L., Coupal, E., Coates, T., Boxer, L. A., Altman, A., and Adams, J. G., III: Molecular analysis of the β-thalassemia phenotype associated with inheritance of hemoglobin E($α_2β_2^{26}$Glu-Lys). J. Clin. Invest. 68:118, 1981.
314. Fessas, P., Loukopoulos, D., Loutradi-Anagnostou, A., and Komes, G.: "Silent" β-thalassaemia caused by a "silent" β-chain mutant: The pathogenesis of a syndrome of thalassaemia intermedia. Br. J. Haematol. 51:577, 1982.
315. Arous, N., Galacteros, F., Fessas, P. H., Loukopoulos, D., Blouquit, Y., Komes, G., Sellaye, M.,

Boussiou, M., and Rosa, J.: Structural study of hemoglobin Knossos, β27 (B9) Ala-Ser. FEBS Lett. *147*:247, 1982.

315a. Atweh, G. F., Hsu, H., and Forget, B. G.: A new IVS-1 position 5 mutation resulting in β⁰-thalassemia in Mediterraneans. Blood *64*(Suppl. 1):55a, 1984.

315b. Atweh, G. F., and Forget, B. G.: Unpublished observations.

315c. Gilman, J. G., Huisman, T. H. J., Stojanovski, N., and Efremov, G. D.: Characterization of the β⁺-thalassemia mutation in a homozygous Yugoslavian patient. Hemoglobin *8*:529, 1984.

316. Cheng, T.-C., Orkin, S. H., Antonarakis, S. E., Potter, M. J., Sexton, J. P., Giardina, P. J. V., Li, A., and Kazazian, H. H., Jr.: β-Thalassemia in Chinese: Use of in vivo RNA analysis and oligonucleotide hybridization in systematic characterization of molecular defects. Proc. Natl. Acad. Sci. USA *81*:2821, 1984.

317. Spence, S. E., et al.: Five nucleotide changes in the large intervening sequence of an α globin gene in a β⁺-thalassemia patient. Nucleic Acids Res. *10*:1283, 1982.

318. Dobkin, C., Pergolizzi, R. G., Bahre, P., and Bank, A.: Abnormal splice in a mutant human β globin gene not at the site of a mutation. Proc. Natl. Acad. Sci. USA *80*:1184, 1983.

319. Dierks, P., van Ooyen, A., Mantei, N., and Weissmann, C.: DNA sequences preceding the rabbit β-globin gene are required for formation in mouse L cells of β-globin RNA with the correct 5′ terminus. Proc. Natl. Acad. Sci. USA *78*:1411, 1981.

320. Grosveld, G. C., de Boer, E., Shewmaker, C. K., and Flavell, R. A.: DNA sequences necessary for transcription of the rabbit β-globin gene in vivo. Nature *295*:120, 1982.

321. Charnay, P., Mellon, P., and Mariatis, T.: Linker scanning mutagenesis of the 5′ flanking region of the mouse β-major globin gene: Sequence requirements for transcription in erythroid and non-erythroid cells. Mol. Cell. Biol. *5*:1498, 1985.

322. Grosveld, G. C., Rosenthal, A., and Flavell, R. A.: Sequence requirements for the transcription of the rabbit β-globin gene in vivo: The −80 region. Nucleic Acids Res. *10*:4951, 1982.

323. Dierks, P., van Ooyen, A., Cochran, M. D., Dobkin, C., Reiser, J., and Weissmann, C.: Three regions upstream from the cap site are required for efficient and accurate transcription of the rabbit β-globin gene in mouse 3T6 cells. Cell *32*:695, 1983.

324. Orkin, S. H., Antonarakis, S. E., and Kazazian, H. H., Jr.: Base substitution at position −88 in a β-thalassemic globin gene: Further evidence for the role of distal promoter element ACACCC. J. Biol. Chem. *259*:8679, 1984.

325. Poncz, M., et al.: β-Thalassemia in a Kurdish Jew. Single base changes in the T-A-T-A box. J. Biol. Chem. *257*:5994, 1982.

325a. Surrey, S., Delgrosso, K., Malladi, P., and Schwartz, E.: Functional analysis of a β-globin gene containing a TATA box mutation from a Kurdish Jew with β thalassemia. J. Biol. Chem. *260*:6507, 1985.

326. Orkin, S. H., et al.: ATA box transcription mutation in β-thalassemia. Nucleic Acids Res. *11*:4727, 1983.

327. Antonarakis, S. E., Orkin, S. H., Cheng, T.-C., Scott, A. F., Sexton, J. P., Trusko, S., Charache, S., and Kazazian, H. H., Jr.: β Thalassemia in American blacks: Novel mutations in the "TATA" box and an acceptor splice site. Proc. Natl. Acad. Sci. USA *81*:1154, 1984.

327a. Orkin, S. H., Cheng, T.-C., Antonarakis, S. E., and Kazazian, H. H., Jr.: Thalassemia due to a mutation in the cleavage-polyadenylation signal of the human β-globin gene. EMBO J. *4*:453, 1985.

327b. Semenza, G. L., Delgrosso, K., Poncz, M., Malladi, P., Schwartz, E., and Surrey, S.: The silent carrier allele: β thalassemia without a mutation in the β-globin gene or its immediate flanking regions. Cell *39*:123, 1984.

328. Chang, J. C., Temple, G. F., Trecartin, R. F., and Kan, Y. W.: Suppression of the nonsense mutation in homozygous β⁰-thalassaemia. Nature *281*:602, 1979.

329. Temple, G. F., Dozy, A. M., Roy, K. L., and Kan, Y. W.: Construction of a functional human suppressor tRNA gene: An approach to gene therapy for β-thalassaemia. Nature *296*:537, 1982.

330. Trecartin, R. F., Liebhaber, S. A., Chang, J. C., Lee, K. Y., Kan, Y. W., Furbetta, M., Angius, A., and Cao, A.: β-Thalassemia in Sardinia is caused by a nonsense mutation. J. Clin. Invest. *68*:1012, 1981.

331. Moschonas, N., deBoer, E., Grosveld, F. G., Dahl, H. H. M., Wright, S., Shewmaker, C. K., and Flavell, R. A.: Structure and expression of a cloned β⁰-thalassemic globin gene. Nucleic Acids Res. *9*:4391, 1981.

332. Orkin, S. H., and Goff, S. C.: Nonsense and frameshift mutations in β⁰-thalassemia detected in cloned β globin genes. J. Biol. Chem. *256*:9782, 1981.

333. Pergolizzi, R., Spritz, R. A., Spence, S., Goossens, M., Kan, Y. W., and Bank, A.: Two cloned β-thalassemia genes are associated with amber mutations at codon 39. Nucleic Acids Res. *9*:7065, 1981.

334. Jackson, I. J., Freund, R. M., Wasylyk, B., Malcolm, A. D. B., and Williamson, R.: The isolation, mapping and transcription in vitro of a β⁰-thalassaemia globin gene. Eur. J. Biochem. *121*:27, 1981.

335. Gorski, J., Fiori, M., and Mach, B.: A new nonsense mutation as the molecular basis for β⁰-thalassemia. J. Mol. Biol. *154*:537, 1982.

336. Takeshita, K., Forget, B. G., Scarpa, A., and Benz, E. J., Jr.: Intranuclear defect in β globin mRNA accumulation due to a premature translation termination codon. Blood *64*:13, 1984.

337. Humphries, R. K., Ley, T. J., Anagnou, N. P., Baur, A. W., and Nienhuis, A. W.: β⁰-39-thalassemia gene: A premature termination codon causes β mRNA deficiency without changing cytoplasmic β mRNA stability. Blood *64*:23, 1984.

337a. Orkin, S. H., and Kazazian, H. H., Jr.: Personal communication.

338. Kazazian, H. H., Jr., Orkin, S. H., Boehm, C. D., Secton, J. P., and Antonarakis, S. E.: β-Thalassemia due to a deletion of the nucleotide which is substituted in the βˢ-globin gene. Am. J. Hum. Genet. *35*:1028, 1983.

339. Chang, J. C., Alberti, A., and Kan, Y. W.: A β-thalassemia lesion abolishes the same Mst II site as the sickle mutation. Nucleic Acids Res. *11*:7789, 1983.

340. Kimura, A., Matsunaga, E., Takihara, Y., Nakamura, T., Takagi, Y., Lin, S., and Lee, H.: Structural analysis of a β-thalassemia gene found in Taiwan. J. Biol. Chem. *258*:2748, 1983.

340a. Maquat, L. E., and Kinniburgh, A. J.: A β⁰-

thalassemic β-globin RNA that is labile in bone marrow cells is relatively stable in HeLa cells. Nucleic Acids Res. *13*:2855, 1985.
341. Benz, E. J., Jr., et al.: Analysis of specific abnormalities of β-globin messenger RNA processing in different forms of β-thalassemia. Blood *58*:52a, 1981.
341a. Oppenheim, A., et al.: Expression of a mutant globin gene defective in splicing in peripheral blood normoblasts from β-thalassemia. Blood *64*(Suppl. 1):59a, 1984.
342. Atweh, G. F., et al.: β-thalassemia resulting from a single nucleotide substitution in an acceptor slice site. Nucleic Acids Res. *13*:777, 1985.
343. Orkin, S. H., Sexton, J. P., Goff, S. C., and Kazazian, H. H., Jr.: inactivation of an acceptor RNA splice site by a short deletion in β-thalassemia. J. Biol. Chem. *258*:7249, 1983.
343a. Orkin, S. H., and Kazazian, H. H., Jr.: Personal communication.
343b. Dobkin, C., and Bank, A.: Mutagenesis of a cryptic splice site abolishes abnormal splicing in a β thalassemia gene. Blood *64*(Suppl. 1):56a, 1984.
343c. Takihara, Y., Matsunaga, E., Nakamura, T., Lin, S-t., Lee, H.-t., Fukumaki, Y., and Takagi, Y.: One base substitution in IVS-2 causes a β$^+$-thalassemia phenotype in a Chinese patient. Biochem. Biophys. Res. Commun. *121*:324, 1984.
344. Felber, B. K., Orkin, S. H., and Hamer, D. H.: Abnormal RNA splicing causes one form of α-thalassemia. Cell *29*:895, 1982.
345. Liebhaber, S. A., and Kan, Y. W.: Differentiation of the mRNA transcripts originating from the α1 and α2 globin loci in normals and α-thalassemics. J. Clin. Invest. *68*:439, 1981.
346. Orkin, S. H., and Goff, S. C.: The duplicated human α globin genes: Their relative expression as measured by RNA analysis. Cell *24*:345, 1981.
347. Orkin, S., and Hamer, D.: Personal communication.
348. Pirastu, M., Galanello, R., Melis, M. A., Brancati, C., Tagarelli, A., Cao, A., and Kan, Y. W.: δ$^+$-Thalassemia in Sardinia. Blood *62*:341, 1983.
349. Wilson, J. T., Wilson, L. B., and Ohta, Y.: A case of homozygous δ thalassemia not due to a deletion of the δ globin structural gene. Biochem. Biophys. Res. Commun. *99*:1035, 1981.
350. Taramelli, R., Giglioni, B., Comi, P., Ottolenghi, S., Brancati, C., Tagarelli, A., Polli, E., and Gianni, A. M.: Delta thalassemia: A non-deletion defect. Eur. J. Biochem. *129*:589, 1983.
350a. Morlé, M., Morlé, F., Dorléac, E., Baklouti, F., Baudonnet, C., Godet, J., and Delaunay, J.: The association of hemoglobin Knossos and hemoglobin Lepore in an Algerian patient. Hemoglobin *8*:229, 1984.
351. Kimura, A., Matsunaga, E., Ohta, Y., Fujjyoshi, T., Matsuo, Y., Nakamura, T., Imamura, T., Yanase, T., and Takagi, Y.: Structure of cloned δ-globin gene region of Japanese individuals. Nucleic Acids Res. *10*:5725, 1982.
352. Spritz, R. A., deRiel, J. K., Forget, B. G., and Weissman, S. M.: Complete nucleotide sequence of the human δ-globin gene. Cell *21*:639, 1980.
353. Martin, S. L., Zimmer, E. A., Kan, Y. W., and Wilson, A. C.: Silent δ-globin gene in Old World monkeys. Proc. Natl. Acad. Sci. USA *77*:3563, 1980.
354. Barrie, P. A., Jeffreys, A. J., and Scott, A. F.: Evolution of the β globin gene cluster in man and the primates. J. Mol. Biol. *149*:319, 1981.
355. Martin, S. L., Vincent, K. A., and Wilson, A. C.: Rise and fall of the delta globin gene. J. Mol. Biol. *164*:513, 1983.
356. Kimura, A., and Takagi, Y.: A frameshift addition causes silencing of the δ-globin gene in an Old World monkey, an anubis (*Papio doguera*). Nucleic Acids Res. *11*:2541, 1983.
357. Jeffreys, A. J., Barrie, P. A., Harris, S., Fawcett, D. H., Nugent, Z. J., and Boyd, A. C.: Isolation and sequence analysis of a hybrid δ-globin pseudogene from the brown lemur. J. Mol. Biol. *156*:487, 1982.
357a. Jones, R. W., Goodbourn, S. E. Y., Old, J. M., and Weatherall, D. J.: The sequence of the $^A\gamma$ globin gene in a $^G\gamma\beta^+$ type of hereditary persistence of fetal haemoglobin. Br. J. Haematol. *59*:357, 1985.
357b. Collins, F. S., Stoeckert, C. J., Jr., Serjeant, G. R., Forget, B. G., and Weissman, S. M.: $^G\gamma\beta^+$ hereditary persistence of fetal hemoglobin: Cosmid cloning and identification of a specific mutation 5' to the $^G\gamma$ gene. Proc. Natl. Acad. Sci. USA *81*:4894, 1984.
357c. Gidoni, D., Dynan, W. S., and Tjian, R.: Multiple specific contacts between a mammalian transcription factor and its cognate promoters. Nature *312*:409, 1984.
357d. Collins, F. S., Boehm, C. D., Waber, P. G., Stoeckert, C. J., Jr., Weissman, S. M., Forget, B. G., and Kazazian, H. H., Jr.: Concordance of a point mutation 5' to the $^G\gamma$-globin gene with $^G\gamma\beta^+$ hereditary persistence of fetal hemoglobin in the black population. Blood *64*:6, 1984.
357e. Gilman, J. G., Harano, T., Nakatsuji, T., Bakioglu, I., Reese, A. L., Gardiner, M. B., and Huisman, T. H. J.: The ratio of the $^G\gamma$ and $^A\gamma$ chains: Variations due to anomalies at the molecular level. Ann. N.Y. Acad. Sci. *445*:235, 1985.
357f. Gilman, J. G., and Huisman, T. H. J.: Personal communication.
357g. Gilman, J. G., and Huisman, T. H. J.: A mutation 158 base pairs 5' to the $^G\gamma$ gene is associated with elevated $^G\gamma$ production. Blood *64*(Suppl. 1):62a, 1984.
357h. Collins, F. S., Metherall, J. E., Yamakawa, M., Pan, J., Weissman, S. M., and Forget, B. G.: A point mutation in the $^A\gamma$-globin gene promoter in Greek hereditary persistence of fetal haemoglobin. Nature *313*:325, 1985.
357i. Gelinas, R., Endlich, B., Pfeiffer, C., Yagi, M., and Stamatoyannopoulos, G.: G to A substitution at the distal CCAAT box of the $^A\gamma$-globin gene in Greek hereditary persistence of fetal haemoglobin. Nature *313*:323, 1985.
357j. Myers, R. M., and Maniatis, T.: Personal communication.
357k. Giglioni, B., Casini, C., Mantovani, R., Merli, S., Comi, P., Ottolenghi, S., Saglio, G., Camaschella, C., and Mazza, U.: A molecular study of a family with Greek hereditary persistence of fetal hemoglobin and β-thalassemia. EMBO J. *3*:2641, 1984.
358. Williamson, R., Eskdale, J., Coleman, D. V., Niazi, M., Loeffler, F. E., and Modell, B. F.: Direct gene analysis of chorionic villi: A possible technique for first-trimester antenatal diagnosis of haemoglobinopathies. Lancet *2*:1125, 1981.
359. Old, J. M., Ward, R. H. T., Karagozlu, F., Petrou, M., Modell, B., and Weatherall, D. J.: First-trimester fetal diagnosis for haemoglobinopathies: Three cases. Lancet *2*:1413, 1982.

360. Goossens, M., Dumez, Y., Kaplan, L., Lupker, M., Chabret, C., Henrion, R., and Rosa, J.: Prenatal diagnosis of sickle-cell anemia in the first trimester of pregnancy. N. Engl. J. Med. *309*:831, 1983.
361. Koenig, H. M., Vedvick, T. S., Dozy, A. M., et al.: Prenatal diagnosis of hemoglobin H disease. J. Pediatr. *92*:278, 1978.
362. Wong, V., Ma, H. K., Todd, D., et al.: Diagnosis of homozygous α-thalassemia in cultured amniotic fluid fibroblasts. N. Engl. J. Med. *298*:669, 1978.
362a. Huang, S., Zeng, Y., Cheng, G., Cong, J., Huang, Y., Zhou, X., and Shen, M.: The prenatal diagnosis method of α-thalassemia. II: Rapid micro DNA hybridization. Shanghai Med. *7*:36, 1984.
362b. Rubin, E. M., and Kan, Y. W.: A simple sensitive prenatal test for hydrops fetalis caused by α-thalassaemia. Lancet *1*:75, 1985.
363. Little, P. F. R., Annison, G., Darling, S., and Williamson, R.: Model for antenatal diagnosis of β-thalassemia and other monogenic disorders by molecular analysis of linked DNA polymorphisms. Nature *285*:144, 1980.
364. Kan, Y. W., Lee, K. Y., Furbetta, M., Angus, A., and Cao, A.: Polymorphism of DNA sequence in the β globin gene region: Application to prenatal diagnosis of $β^0$-thalassemia in Sardinia. N. Engl. J. Med. *302*:185, 1980.
365. Kazazian, H. H., Phillips, J. A., Boehm, C. D., Wik, T. A., Mahoney, M. J., and Ritchey, A. K.: Prenatal diagnosis of β-thalassemias by amniocentesis: Linkage analysis using multiple polymorphic restriction endonuclease sites. Blood *56*:926, 1980.
366. Boehm, C. D., Antonarakis, S. E., Phillips, J. A., III, Stetten, G., and Kazazian, H. H., Jr.: Prenatal diagnosis using DNA polymorphisms. N. Engl. J. Med. *308*:1054, 1983.
366a. Old, J. M., Petrou, M., Modell, B., and Weatherall, D. J.: Feasibility of antenatal diagnosis of β thalassaemia by DNA polymorphisms in Asian Indian and Cypriot populations. Br. J. Haematol. *57*:255, 1984.
366b. Wainscoat, J. S., Old, J. M., Thein, S. L., and Weatherall, D. J.: A new DNA polymorphism for prenatal diagnosis of β-thalassemia in Mediterranean populations. Lancet *2*:1299, 1984.
367. Phillips, J. A., III, Scott, A. F., Kazazian, H. H., Jr., Smith, K. D., Stetten, G., and Thomas, G. H.: Prenatal diagnosis of hemoglobinopathies by restriction endonuclease analysis: Pregnancies at risk for sickle cell anemia and S-O[Arab] disease. Johns Hopkins Med. J. *145*:57, 1979.
368. Flavell, R. A., Kooter, J., deBoer, E., Little, P. F. R., and Williamson, R.: Analysis of the βδ-globin gene loci in normal and Hb Lepore DNA: Direct determination of gene linkage and intergene distance. Cell *15*:25, 1978.
369. Little, P. F. R., Whitelaw, E., Annison, G., Williamson, R., Kooter, J. M., Flavell, R. A., Goossens, M., Serjeant, G. R., and Montgomery, D.: The detection and use of hemoglobin mutants in the direct analysis of human globin genes. Blood *55*:1060, 1980.
370. Horst, J., Schafer, R., Kleihauer, E., and Kohne, E.: Analysis of the Hb M Milwaukee mutation at the DNA level. Br. J. Haematol. *54*:643, 1983.
370a. Trent, R. J., Davis, B., Wilkinson, R., and Kronenberg, H.: Identification of β variant hemoglobins by DNA restriction endonuclease mapping. Hemoglobin *8*:443, 1984.
371. Geever, R. F., Wilson, L. B., Nallaseth, F. S., Milner, P. F., Bittner, M., and Wilson, J. T.: Direct identification of sickle cell anemia by blot hybridization. Proc. Natl. Acad. Sci. USA *78*:5801, 1981.
372. Chang, J. C., and Kan, Y. W.: Antenatal diagnosis of sickle cell anaemia by direct analysis of the sickle mutation. Lancet *2*:1127, 1981.
373. Wilson, J. T., Milner, P. F., Summer, M. E., Nallaseth, F. S., Fadel, H. E., Reindollar, R. H., McDonough, P. G., and Wilson, L. B.: Use of restriction endonucleases for mapping the allele for $β^S$-globin. Proc. Natl. Acad. Sci. USA *79*:3628, 1982.
374. Chang, J. C., and Kan, Y. W.: A sensitive new prenatal test for sickle-cell anemia. N. Engl. J. Med. *307*:30, 1982.
375. Orkin, S. H., Little, P. F. R., Kazazian, H. H., Jr., and Boehm, C. D.: Improved detection of the sickle mutation by DNA analysis. N. Engl. J. Med. *307*:32, 1982.
376. Chang, J. C., Golbus, M. S., and Kan, Y. W.: Antenatal diagnosis of sickle cell anaemia by sensitive DNA assay. Lancet *1*:1463, 1982.
377. Wallace, R. B., Schold, M., Johnson, M. J., Dembek, P., and Itakura, K.: Oligonucleotide directed mutagenesis of the human β-globin gene: A general method for producing specific point mutations in cloned DNA. Nucleic Acids Res. *9*:3647, 1981.
378. Conner, B. J., Reys, A. A., Morin, C., Itakura, K., Teplitz, R. L., and Wallace, R. B.: Detection of sickle cell $β^S$-globin allele by hybridization with synthetic oligonucleotides. Proc. Natl. Acad. Sci. USA *80*:278, 1983.
379. Orkin, S. H., Markham, A. F., and Kazazian, H. H., Jr.: Direct detection of the common Mediterranean β-thalassemia gene with synthetic DNA probes: An alternative approach for prenatal diagnosis. J. Clin. Invest. *71*:775, 1983.
380. Pirastu, M., Kan, Y. W., Cao, A., Conner, B. J., Teplitz, R. L., and Wallace, R. B.: Prenatal diagnosis of β-thalassemia: Detection of a single nucleotide mutation in DNA. N. Engl. J. Med. *309*:284, 1983.
381. Kazazian, H. H., Jr., Orkin, S. H., Markham, A. F., Chapman, C. R., Youssoufian, H., and Waber, P. G.: Quantification of the close association between DNA haplotypes and specific β-thalassaemia mutations in Mediterraneans. Nature *310*:152, 1984.
381a. Myers, R. M., Lumelsky, N., Lerman, L. S., and Maniatis, T.: Detection of single base substitutions in total genomic DNA. Nature *313*:495, 1985.
382. Kazazian, H. H., Jr., Antonarakis, S. E., Cheng, T., Boehm, C. D., and Waber, P. G.: DNA polymorphisms in the β-globin gene cluster: Use in discovery of mutations and prenatal diagnosis. *In* Caskey, C. T., and White, R. L., (eds.): Recombinant DNA Applications to Human Disease. New York, Cold Spring Harbor Laboratory, 1983, p. 29.
383. Pirastu, M., Doherty, M., Galanello, R., Cao, A., and Kan, Y. W.: Frequent crossing over in human DNA generates multiple chromosomes containing the sickle and β-thalassemia genes and increases Hb F production. Blood *62*(Suppl. 1):75a, 1983.
383a. Wainscoat, J. S., Bell, J. I., Old, J. M., Weatherall, D. J., Furbetta, M., Galanello, R., and Cao, A.: Globin gene mapping studies in Sardinian patients

homozygous for β⁰ thalassemia. Mol. Biol. Med. *1*:1, 1983.
384. Gerhard, D. S., Kidd, K. K., Kidd, J. R., Egeland, J. A., and Housman, D. E.: Identification of a recent recombination event within the human β-globin gene cluster. Proc. Natl. Acad. Sci. USA *81*:7875, 1984.
385. Szostak, J. W., Orr-Weaver, T. L., Rothstein, R. J., and Stahl, F. W.: The double-strand-break repair model for recombination. Cell *33*:25, 1983.
386. Slightom, J. L., Blechl, A. E., and Smithies, O.: Human fetal $^G\gamma$ and $^A\epsilon$ globin genes: Complete nucleotide sequences suggest that DNA can be exchanged between these duplicate genes. Cell *21*:627, 1980.
387. Shen, S., Slightom, J. L., and Smithies, O.: A history of the human fetal globin gene duplication. Cell *26*:191, 1981.
388. Weiss, E. H., Mellor, A., Golden, L., Fahrner, K., Simpson, E., Hurst, J., and Flavell, R. A.: The structure of a mutant H-2 gene suggests that the generation of polymorphism in H-2 genes may occur by gene conversion-like events. Nature *301*:671, 1983.
389. Pease, L. R., Schulze, D. H., Pfaffenbach, G. M., and Nathenson, S. G.: Spontaneous H-2 mutants provide evidence that a copy mechanism analogous to gene conversion generates polymorphism in the MHC. Proc. Natl. Acad. Sci. USA *80*:242, 1983.
390. Ollo, R., and Rougeon, F.: Gene conversion and polymorphism: Generation of mouse immunoglobulin γ2a chain alleles by differential gene conversion by γ2b chain gene. Cell *32*:515, 1983.
391. Antonarakis, S. E., Orkin, S. H., Kazazian, H. H., Jr., Goff, S. C., Boehm, C. D., Waber, P. G., Sexton, J. P., Ostrer, H., Fairbanks, V. F., and Chakravarti, A.: Evidence for multiple origins of the β^E globin gene in Southeast Asia. Proc. Natl. Acad. Sci. USA *79*:6608, 1982.
392. Chehab, F., Deeb, S., Pirastu, M., and Kan, Y. W.: Molecular heterogeneity of β-thalassemia in Lebanon: Application to prenatal diagnosis. Blood *64*(Suppl. 1):55a, 1984.
392a. Giampaolo, A., Mavilio, F., Massa, A., Gabbianelli, M., Guerriero, R., Sposi, N. M., Caré, A., Cianciulli, P., Tentori, L., and Marinucci, M.: Molecular heterogeneity of beta thalassaemia in the Italian population. Br. J. Haematol. *56*:79, 1984.
393. Kazazian, H. H., Jr., Orkin, S. H., Antonarakis, S. E., Cheng, T.-C., and Sexton, J. P.: β-thalassemia mutations differ among various ethnic groups. Blood *62*:68a, 1983.
394. Mears, J. G., Ramirez, F., Leibowitz, D., and Bank, A.: Organization of human δ- and β-globin genes in cellular DNA and the presence of intragenic inserts. Cell *15*:15, 1978.
395. Baird, M., Schreiner, H., Driscoll, C., and Bank, A.: Localization of the site of recombination in formation of the Lepore Boston globin gene. J. Clin. Invest. *68*:560, 1981.
396. Mavilio, F., Giampaolo, A., Care, A., Sposi, N. M., and Marinucci, M.: The δβ crossover region in Lepore Boston hemoglobinopathy is restricted to a 59 base pairs region around the 5′ splice junction of the large globin gene intervening sequence. Blood *62*:230, 1983.
397. Chebloune, Y., and Verdier, G.: The delta-beta–crossing-over site in the fusion gene of the Lepore-Boston disease might be localized in a preferential recombination region. Acta Haematol. *69*:294, 1983.
397a. Chebloune, Y., Poncet, D., and Verdier, G.: S₁-nuclease mapping of the genomic Lepore-Boston DNA demonstrates that the entire large intervening sequence of the fusion gene is of β-type. Biochem. Biophys. Res. Commun. *120*:116, 1984.
397b. Chebloune, Y., Trabuchet, G., Poncet, D., Cohen-Solal, M., Faure, C., Verdier, G., and Nigon, V.: A new method for detection of small modifications in genomic DNA, applied to the human δ-β globin gene cluster. Eur. J. Biochem. *142*:473, 1984.
398. Rieder, R. F., and Weatherall, D. J.: Studies on hemoglobin biosynthesis: Asynchronous synthesis of hemoglobin A and A₂ by human erythrocyte precursors. J. Clin. Invest. *44*:42, 1965.
399. Wood, W. G., Old, J. M., Roberts, A. V. S., Clegg, J. B., Weatherall, D. J., and Quattrin, N.: Human globin gene expression: Control of β, δ and δβ chain production. Cell *15*:437, 1978.
400. White, J. M., Lang, A., Lorkin, P. A., and Lehmann, H.: Synthesis of haemoglobin Lepore. Nature *235*:208, 1972.
401. Roberts, A. V., Weatherall, D. J., and Clegg, J. B.: The synthesis of human haemoglobin A₂ during erythroid maturation. Biochem. Biophys. Res. Commun. *47*:81, 1972.
402. Gill, F., Atwater, J., and Schwartz, E.: Hemoglobin Lepore trait: Globin synthesis in bone marrow and peripheral blood. Science *178*:623, 1972.
403. Forget, B. G., Cavallesco, C., Benz, E. J., Jr., McClure, P. D., Hillman, D. G., Krieger, H., Clarke, B., and Housman, D.: Studies of globin chain synthesis and globin mRNA content in a patient homozygous for hemoglobin Lepore. Hemoglobin *2*:117, 1978.
404. Ramirez, F., Mears, J. G., Nudel, U., et al.: Defects in DNA and globin mRNA in homozygotes for hemoglobin Lepore. J. Clin. Invest. *63*:736, 1979.
405. Giglioni, B., Comi, P., Taramelli, R., Pozzoli, M., Zanollo, A., Ottolenghi, S., and Gianni, A. M.: β-Like globin RNA sequences in hemoglobin Lepore disease. Eur. J. Biochem. *95*:1979.
405a. Driscoll, M. C., Ohta, Y., Nakamura, F., Bloom, A., and Bank, A.: Hemoglobin Miyada: DNA analysis of the anti-Lepore δβ fusion gene. Am. J. Hematol. *17*:355, 1984.
406. Roberts, A. V., Clegg, J. B., Weatherall, D. J., and Ohta, Y.: Synthesis *in vitro* of anti-Lepore haemoglobin. Nature *245*:23, 1973.
407. Abu-Sin, A., Felice, A. E., Gravely, M. E., et al.: Hb P Nilotic in association with β⁰-thalassemia: cis-mutation of a hemoglobin β^A chain regulatory determinant. J. Lab. Clin. Med. *93*:973, 1979.
408. Honig, G. R., Shamsuddin, M., Mason, R. G., and Vida, L. N.: Hemoglobin Lincoln Park: A βδ fusion (anti-Lepore) variant with an amino acid deletion in the δ chain–derived segment. Proc. Natl. Acad. Sci. USA *75*:1745, 1978.
408a. Modiano, G., and Pepe, G.: The quantitative expression of δ and β human globin genes is controlled by both 5′ and 3′ untranslated regions. Mol. Biol. Med. *1*:157, 1983.
408b. Kosche, K., Dobkin, C., and Bank, A.: The role of intervening sequences (IVS) in human β globin gene expression. Blood *64*(Suppl. 1):58a, 1984.
409. Fairbanks, V. G., Rhaiza, O., Brandabur, J. H., Willis, R. R., and Fiester, R. F.: Homozygous

hemoglobin E mimics β-thalassemia minor without anemia or hemolysis: Hematologic, functional, and biosynthetic studies of first North American cases. Am. J. Hematol. 8:109, 1980.
410. Wong, S. C., and Ali, M. A. M.: Hemoglobin E diseases: Hematological, analytical, and biosynthetic studies in homozygotes and double heterozygotes for α-thalassemia. Am. J. Hematol. 13:15, 1982.
411. Traeger, J., Winichagoon, P., and Wood, W. G.: Instability of β^E–messenger RNA during erythroid cell maturation in hemoglobin E homozygotes. J. Clin. Invest. 69:1050, 1982.
412. Adams, J. G., III, Boxer, L. A., Baehner, R. L., Forget, B. G., Tsistrakis, G. A., and Steinberg, M. H.: Hemoglobin Indianapolis (β112[G14] arginine): An unstable β-chain variant producing the phenotype of severe β-thalassemia. J. Clin. Invest. 63:931, 1979.
413. Adams, J. G., III, Steinberg, M. H., Newman, M. V., Morrison, W. T., Benz, E. J., Jr., and Iyer, R.: β-Thalassemia present in cis to a new β chain structural variant, Hb Vicksburg [β75 (E19) Leu→0]. Proc. Natl. Acad. Sci. USA 78:469, 1981.
414. Rieder, R. F., and James, G. W., III: Imbalance in α and β globin synthesis associated with a hemoglobinopathy. J. Clin. Invest. 54:948, 1974.
415. Honig, G. R., Mason, R. G., Vida, L. N., and Shamsuddin, M.: Synthesis of hemoglobin Abraham Lincoln (β32 Leu-Pro). Blood 43:657, 1974.
416. Smith, C. M., II, Hedlund, B., Cich, J. A., Tukey, D. P., Olson, M., Steinberg, M. H., and Adams, J. G., III: Hemoglobin North Shore: A variant hemoglobin associated with the phenotype of β-thalassemia. Blood 61:378, 1983.
417. Clegg, J. B., Weatherall, D. J., and Milner, P. F.: Haemoglobin Constant Spring—a chain termination mutant? Nature 234:337, 1971.
418. Clegg, J. B., Weatherall, D. J., Contopolou-Griva, I., Caroutsos, K., Poungouras, P., and Tsevrenis, H.: Haemoglobin Icaria, a new chain-termination mutant which causes α thalassemia. Nature 251:245, 1974.
419. DeJong, W. W., Khan, P. M., and Bernini, L. F.: Hemoglobin Koya Dora: High frequency of a chain termination mutant. Am. J. Hum. Genet. 27:81, 1975.
420. Bradley, T. B., Wohl, R. C., and Smith, G. J.: Elongation of the α-globin chain in a black family: Interaction with Hb G-Philadelphia. Clin. Res. 23:131A, 1975.
421. Weatherall, D. J., and Clegg, J. B.: The α-chain termination mutants and their relation to the α-thalassaemais. Philos Trans. R. Soc. Lond. [Biol.] 271:411, 1975.
422. Kan, Y. W., Todd, D., and Dozy, A. M.: Haemoglobin Constant Spring synthesis in red cell precursors. Br. J. Haematol. 28:103, 1974.
423. Hanash, S. M., Winter, W. P., and Rucknagel, D. L.: Synthesis of haemoglobin Wayne in erythroid cells. Nature 269:717, 1977.
424. Proudfoot, N. J., and Brownlee, G. G.: 3' Noncoding region sequences in eukaryotic messenger RNA. Nature 263:211, 1976.
425. Fiddes, J. C., and Goodman, H. M.: The cDNA for the β-subunit of human chorionic gonadotropin suggests evolution of a gene by readthrough into the 3'-untranslated region. Nature 286:684, 1980.
426. Sanguansermsri, T., Matragoon, S., Changloah, L., and Flatz, G.: Hemoglobin Suan-Dok ($\alpha_2^{109(G16)Leu\rightarrow Arg}\beta_2$): An unstable variant associated with α-thalassemia. Hemoglobin 3:161, 1979.
427. Honig, C. R., Shamsuddin, M., Zaizov, R., Steinherz, M., Solar, I., and Kirschmann, C.: Hemoglobin Petah Tikva (α110Ala→Asp): A new unstable variant with α-thalassemia–like expression. Blood 57:705, 1981.
428. Todd, D., Chan, V., Schneider, R. G., Dozy, A. M., Kan, Y. W., and Chan, T. K.: Globin chain synthesis in haemoglobin New York ($\beta^{113Valine\rightarrow Glutamic Acid}$). Br. J. Haematol. 46:557, 1980.
429. Kolata, G. B., and Wade, N.: Human gene treatment stirs new debate. Science 210:407, 1980.
430. Wade, N.: UCLA gene therapy racked by friendly fire. Science 210:509, 1980.
431. Sladic-Simic, D., Martinovitch, P. N., Zivkovic, N., Pavic, D., Martinovic, J., Kahn, M., and Ranney, H. M.: A thalassemia-like disorder in Belgrade laboratory rats. Ann. N.Y. Acad. Sci. 165:93, 1969.
432. Edwards, J. A., Garrick, L. M., and Hoke, J. E.: Defective iron uptake and globin synthesis by erythroid cells in the anemia of the Belgrade laboratory rat. Blood 51:347, 1978.
433. Garrick, L. M., Edwards, J. A., and Hoke, J. E.: The effect of hemin on globin synthesis and iron uptake by reticulocytes of the Belgrade rat. FEBS Lett. 93:109, 1978.
434. Edwards, J. A., Sullivan, A. L., and Hoke, J. E.: Defective delivery of iron to the developing red cell of the Belgrade laboratory rat. Blood 55:645, 1980.
435. Crkvenjakov, R., Cusic, S., Ivanovic, I., and Glisin, V.: Rat b/b anemia: Translation of normal and anemic globin mRNA in wheat-germ cell-free system. Eur. J. Biochem. 71:85, 1976.
436. Chu, M.-L., Garrick, L. M., and Garrick, M. D.: Deficiency of globin messenger RNA in reticulocytes of the Belgrade rat. Biochemistry 17:5128, 1978.
437. Russell, L. B., Russell, W. L., Popp, R. A., Vaughan, C., and Jacobson, K. B.: Radiation-induced mutations at mouse hemoglobin loci. Proc. Natl. Acad. Sci. USA 73:2843, 1976.
438. Popp, R. A., and Enlow, M. K.: Radiation-induced α-thalassemia in mice. Am. J. Vet. Res. 38:569, 1977.
439. Whitney, J. B., III, and Russell, E. S.: Linkage of genes for adult α-globin and embryonic α-like globin chains. Proc. Natl. Acad. Sci. USA 77:1087, 1980.
440. Martinell, J., Whitney, J. B., III, Popp, R. A., Russell, L. B., and Anderson, W. F.: Three mouse models of human thalassemia. Proc. Natl. Acad. Sci. USA 78:5056, 1981.
441. Whitney, J. B., III, Martinell, J., Popp, R. A., Russell, L. B., and Anderson, W. F.: Deletions in the α-globin gene complex in α-thalassemic mice. Proc. Natl. Acad. Sci. USA 78:7644, 1981.
442. Anderson, W. F., Martinell, J., Whitney, J. B., III, and Popp, R. A.: Mouse models of human thalassemia. In Desnick, R. J. (ed.): Animal Models of Inherited Metabolic Diseases. New York, Alan R. Liss Inc., 1982, pp. 11–26.
443. Popp, R. A., Bradshaw, B. S., and Skow, L. C.: Effects of alpha thalassemia on mouse development. Differentiation 17:205, 1980.
444. Skow, L. C., Burkhart, B. A., Johnson, F. M., Popp, R. A., Popp, D. M., Goldberg, S. Z., Anderson, W. F., Barnett, L. B., and Lewis, S.

E.: A mouse model for β-thalassemia. Cell 34:1043, 1983.
444a. Goldberg, S. Z., Kantoff, P. W., Kuebbing, D., Trauber, D. R., Lewis, S., Popp, R., and Anderson, W. F.: Molecular characterization of β-thalassemic mice. Blood 64(Suppl. 1):57a, 1984.
445. Lacy, E., Roberts, S., Evans, E. P., Burtenshaw, M. D., and Constantini, F. D.: A foreign β-globin gene in transgenic mice: Integration at abnormal chromosomal positions and expression in inappropriate tissues. Cell 34:343, 1983.
445a. Stewart, T. A., Wagner, E. F., and Mintz, B.: Human β-globin gene sequences injected into mouse eggs, retained in adults, and transmitted to progeny. Science 217:1046, 1982.
445b. Humphries, R. K., Berg, P., DiPietro, J., Bernstein, S., Bauer, A., Nienhuis, A., and Anderson, W. F.: Transfer of human and murine globin gene sequences into transgenic mice. Am. J. Hum. Genet. 37:295, 1985.
445c. Townes, T. M., Chen, H. Y., Lingrel, J. B., Palmiter, R. D., and Brinster, R. L.: Expression of human β globin genes in transgenic mice: Effects of a flanking metallothionein/human growth hormone fusion gene. Mol. Cell Biol., in press.
445d. Lau, Y. F., Dozy, A. M., Chen, H. E., Brinster, R. L., and Kan, Y. W.: Retrieval of the human α-globin genes from transgenic mice. Blood 62(Suppl. 1):68a, 1983.
445e. Chada, K., Magram, J., Raphael, K., Radice, G., Lacy, E., and Costantini, F.: A foreign β-globin gene expressed specifically in erythroid cells of transgenic mice. Nature 314:377, 1985.
445f. Townes, T. M., Chen, H. Y., Lingrel, J. B., Brinster, R. L., and Palmiter, R. D.: Erythroid specific expression of human β globin genes in transgenic mice. EMBO J., in press.
445g. Magram, J., Chada, K., and Costantini, F.: Developmental regulation of a cloned adult β-globin gene in transgenic mice. Nature 315:338, 1985.
446. Anderson, W. F., and Fletcher, J. C.: Gene therapy in human beings: When is it ethical to begin? N. Engl. J. Med. 303:1293, 1980.
447. Mercola, K. E., and Cline, M. J.: The potentials of inserting new genetic information. N. Engl. J. Med. 303:1297, 1980.
448. Cline, M. J.: Genetic engineering of mammalian cells: Its application to genetic diseases of man. J. Lab. Clin. Med. 99:299, 1982.
449. Cline, M. J., Stang, H., Mercola, K., Morse, L., Ruprecht, R., Browne, J., and Salser, W.: Gene transfer in intact animals. Nature 284:422, 1980.
450. Mercola, K. C., Stang, H. D., Browne, J., Salser, W., and Cline, M. J.: Insertion of a new gene of viral origin into bone marrow cells of mice. Science 208:1033, 1980.
451. Bar-Eli, M., Stang, H. D., Mercola, K. E., and Cline, M. J.: Expression of a methotrexate-resistant dihydrofolate reductase gene by transformed hematopoietic cells of mice. Somatic Cell Genet. 9:55, 1983.
452. Carr, F., Medina, W. D., Dube, S., and Bertino, J. R.: Genetic transformation of murine bone marrow cells to methotrexate resistance. Blood 62:180, 1983.
453. Joyner, A., Keller, G., Phillips, R. A., and Bernstein, A.: Retrovirus transfer of a bacterial gene into mouse haematopoietic progenitor cells. Nature 305:556, 1983.
454. Williams, D. A., Lemischka, I. R., Nathan, D. G., and Mulligan, R. C.: Introduction of new genetic material into pluripotent haematopoietic stem cells of the mouse. Nature 310:476, 1984.
455. Karlsson, S., Humphries, R. K., Gluzman, Y., and Nienhuis, A. W.: Transfer of genes into hematopoietic cells using recombinant DNA viruses. Proc. Natl. Acad. Sci. USA 82:158, 1985.
456. Weatherall, D.: A step nearer gene therapy? Nature 310:452, 1984.
457. Anderson, W. F.: Prospects for human gene therapy. Science 226:401, 1984.
458. Culliton, B. J.: Gene therapy: Research in public. Science 227:493, 1985.
459. Morlé, F., Lopez, B., Henni, T., and Godet, J.: α-Thalassemia associated with the deletion of two nucleotides at the position -2 and -3 preceding the AUG codon. EMBO J., in press.
460. Higgs, D. R., Ayyub, H., Clegg, J. B., Hill, A. V. S., Nicholls, R. D., Teal, H., Wainscoat, J. S., and Weatherall, D. J.: α Thalassaemia in British people. Br. Med. J. 290:1303, 1985.
461. Kazazian, H. H., Jr., Orkin, S. H., Boehm, C. D., Goff, S. C., Wang, C., Dowling, C. E., Newburger, P. E., Knowlton, R. G., Brown, V., and Donis-Keller, H.: Spontaneous mutation to a β thalassemia allele in a Polish American. Am. J. Hum. Genet., in press.
462. Zeng, Y.-T. and Huang, S.-Z.: α-Globin gene organisation and prenatal diagnosis of α-thalassaemia in Chinese. Lancet 1:304, 1985.
463. Thein, S. L., Wainscoat, J. S., Lynch, J. R., Weatherall, D. J., Sampietro, M., and Fiorelli, G.: Direct detection of β⁰ 39 thalassaemic mutation with Mae I. Lancet 1:1095, 1985.
464. Rosatelli, C., Falchi, A. M., Tuveri, T., Scalas, M. T., DiTucci, A., Monni, G., and Cao, A.: Prenatal diagnosis of beta-thalassemia with the synthetic-oligomer technique. Lancet 1:241, 1985.

THE THALASSEMIAS—CLINICAL MANIFESTATIONS

9

As discussed in the preceding chapter, the thalassemia syndromes are a group of hereditary disorders in which there is a defect in the synthesis of one or more of the globin polypeptide chains of hemoglobin. This defect causes absent or decreased synthesis of the affected chain. As a result, the erythrocytes have a low intracellular hemoglobin content (hypochromia) and are smaller than normal (microcytosis). In addition, the continued normal synthesis of the unaffected globin chain leads to the accumulation of unstable aggregates of these unmatched chains. These aggregates precipitate within the erythroid cell, damage its membrane, and cause its premature destruction in the peripheral circulation as well as at earlier stages of maturation in the bone marrow. In α thalassemia, synthesis of the α chain of normal adult hemoglobin is impaired, whereas in β thalassemia, it is the synthesis of β chains that is reduced or absent. In this chapter, we will describe the clinical and hematologic aspects of thalassemia. A more extensive and detailed discussion of this topic can be found in the excellent monograph by Weatherall and Clegg.[1]

HISTORICAL BACKGROUND

The first description of the clinical features of homozygous β thalassemia was provided by Dr. Thomas B. Cooley and colleagues in Detroit in 1925 and 1927.[2,3] They reported a number of patients with anemia, splenomegaly, a peculiar mongoloid facial appearance, and red blood cells with increased resistance to osmotic lysis. Over the following years, a number of additional reports of Cooley's anemia were published, and it became apparent that the disorder affected primarily individuals of Mediterranean ancestry. The term "thalassemia," derived from the Greek θαλασσα (the sea), was first coined by Whipple and Bradford in 1932[4] to indicate the association of the disease with the Mediterranean area.

Between 1925 and 1935, a number of Italian workers described a disorder characterized by mild anemia and increased osmotic resistance of red cells.[5-7] The condition was named, after the workers who described it, "la malattia di Rietti-Greppi-Micheli" and almost certainly consisted of different forms of heterozygous β thalassemia.[8]

Despite the virtually simultaneous descriptions, in different countries, of the homozygous and heterozygous forms of β thalassemia, almost 15 years passed before it was realized that Cooley's anemia or thalassemia resulted from the homozygous inheritance of the Rietti-Greppi-Micheli syndrome. This conclusion was drawn initially by Caminopetros in Greece in 1936 and 1938[9, 10] and by Angelini in Italy in 1937.[11] In the early to mid 1940's a number of workers in Europe and the United States independently characterized the genetic basis of thalassemia; these included Sivestroni and Bianco, Wintrobe and coworkers, Dameshek, Strauss and coworkers, Valentine and Neel, Gatto, and Smith.[1, 8, 12]

Over the ensuing years, the manifestations and patterns of inheritance of thalassemia were further characterized by a large number of workers, and it became apparent that the disorder was genetically and hematologically quite heterogeneous. In the mid 1960's, the establishment of techniques to quantitate the synthesis of α and β globin chains of hemoglobin (see Chapter 8) and the identification and characterization of inclusion bodies in the erythroid cells of β-thalassemic patients[13] further extended our understanding of the basis and pathophysiology of the thalassemia syndromes.

INCIDENCE AND POPULATION GENETICS

Thalassemia primarily affects people of Mediterranean, African, and Asian ancestry (Fig. 9-1). However, sporadic cases have been reported in many varied ethnic groups. It is believed that malaria has exerted selective pressure for the propagation of the thalassemia genes,[1] although the precise scientific basis for the proposed protection of the thalassemia heterozygote against malaria is unknown. It has been proposed that in the case of β-thalassemia heterozygotes, the main protection may be against cerebral malaria in the first 1 to 1½ years of life because of a slower-than-normal decline of neonatal Hb F levels and a demonstrated disadvantage for malarial growth in red cells containing Hb F.[1, 14] An alternative explanation proposes that the red cell membrane in heterozygous thalassemia is

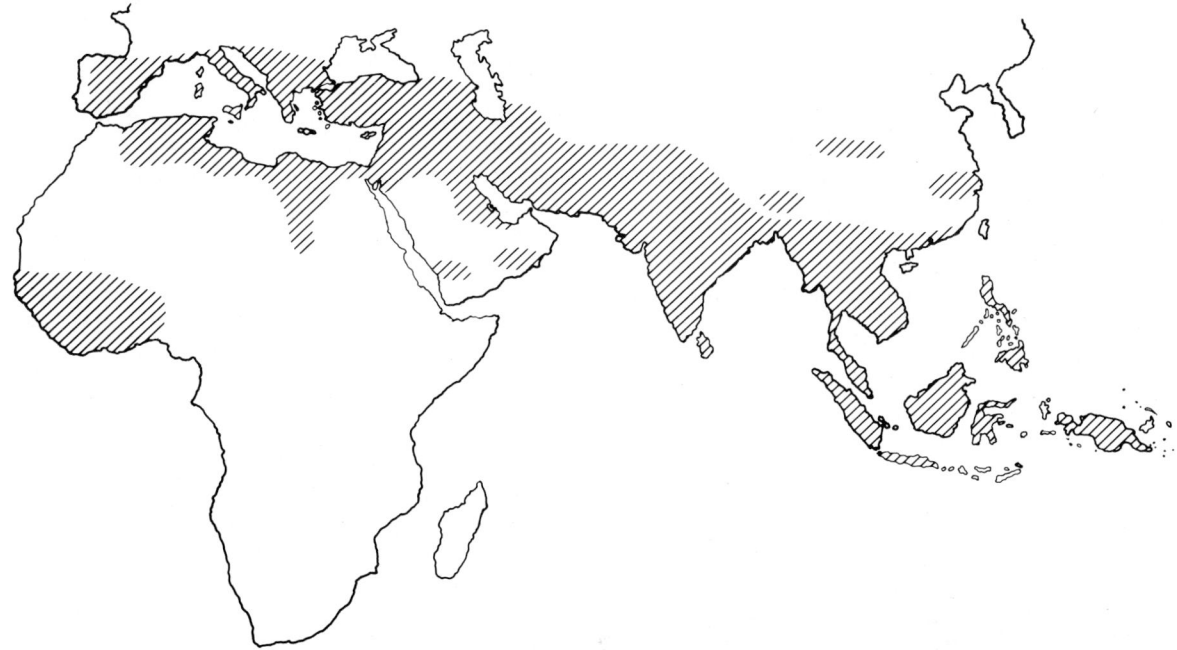

Figure 9-1. Worldwide distribution of β thalassemia. The map is a composite of the information of D. J. Weatherall and J. B. Clegg (The Thalassemia Syndromes. 3rd ed. Oxford, Blackwell Scientific Publications, 1981) and of M. J. Friedman and W. Trager (Scientific American, *244*:154, 1981.)

particularly susceptible to damage by oxidation and that infection with the malaria parasite gives rise to sufficient oxidative stress to perturb intracellular metabolism in a manner that leads to premature death of the parasite.[14a] This latter hypothesis provides a unifying theory for the selective survival of heterozygotes for α thalassemia[14b] as well as for β thalassemia, glucose 6 phosphate dehydrogenase (G6PD) deficiency, and Hb S.[14a]

The prevalence of thalassemia in various populations has been estimated in a number of different surveys.[1] In southern Italian, Sicilian, and Greek populations, approximately 10 per cent of individuals are heterozygous for β thalassemia. In certain Greek islands and some villages in Sardinia, the incidence reaches 20 to 30 per cent. In Southeast Asian populations, the prevalence of heterozygous β thalassemia is approximately 5 per cent, although a higher incidence is encountered in certain regions. In African and American blacks, the incidence of heterozygous β thalassemia is approximately 1.5 per cent.

In the case of heterozygous α thalassemia, the highest incidence occurs in blacks and Southeast Asians. Approximately 3 per cent of blacks have phenotypic α-thalassemia "trait" (α thalassemia 1 phenotype), but as discussed in Chapter 8, this phenotype results from homozygosity for the deletion of a single α globin gene on each chromosome (α thalassemia 2 genotype). Thus, approximately 25 to 30 per cent of blacks are heterozygous for the α thalassemia 2 gene deletion.[15] The cause of this extraordinarily high gene frequency is poorly understood. It is difficult to explain a selective advantage against malaria when the red blood cells in heterozygous α thalassemia 2 are difficult to distinguish hematologically from normal red blood cells. In Thailand, where the α-thalassemia phenotype is due to the deletion of two α globin genes on the same chromosome (*in cis*), the prevalence of this form of heterozygous α thalassemia is approximately 10 per cent; an additional 10 per cent or so of Thais are heterozygous for α thalassemia 2. Thus, the combined prevalence of heterozygous α thalassemia in Thailand is approximately 20 per cent, although in northern Thailand it is higher and approaches 30 per cent. In certain regions of new Guinea, the combined incidence of heterozygous and homozygous α thalassemia 2 is greater than 80 per cent.[14b] In other Southeast Asian populations, the prevalence of heterozygous α thalassemia approaches approximately 5 per cent.

In Mediterranean populations, α thalassemia is less common than β thalassemia, with an incidence of approximately 5 per cent in Sardinia and Greece. In Cyprus, the incidence is somewhat higher and approaches 10 per cent.

PATHOPHYSIOLOGY OF THE ANEMIA IN THALASSEMIA

There are many primary and secondary causes for the anemia observed in thalassemia. It is easy to understand how reduced synthesis of one or another of the globin chains of Hb A will result in an overall deficit of Hb A accumulation in red cells and cause a hypochromic, microcytic anemia with a low mean corpuscular hemoglobin concentration in affected erythrocytes. This is true in both the heterozygous and homozygous states. In the homozygous state, however, another pathophysiologic process worsens the anemia and is responsible for the major clinical manifestations of Cooley's anemia. The continued synthesis in normal amounts of the nonaffected globin chain results in the accumulation, within the erythroid cells, of excessive amounts of these normal chains. Not finding complementary globin chains with which to bind, these chains form aggregates and precipitate within the cell.[13, 16–18] These precipitates lead to membrane damage and premature destruction of the red cells.[19, 20] In β thalassemia, the resulting α-chain aggregates are called inclusion bodies or, perhaps improperly, Heinz bodies. In contrast to true Heinz bodies, which are made up of total precipitated hemoglobin ($\alpha_2\beta_2$), these inclusion bodies have been shown, convincingly, to consist of only α globin chains,[21] which do have some attached heme in the form of hemichromes.[22] The process of inclusion body formation occurs extensively in the erythroid precursor cells of the marrow and is responsible for the marked ineffective erythropoiesis that characterizes homozygous β thalassemia. In α thalassemia, the resulting β_4 tetramers constitute Hb H, which is less insoluble than α-chain aggregates. In the neonatal and fetal periods, γ_4 tetramers are formed and constitute Hb Bart's. Hemoglobin Bart's is also seen in occasional adults with Hb H disease, particularly those with Hb Constant Spring.

In β thalassemia, the role of thalassemic inclusions in the pathophysiology of the hemolytic anemia provides an explanation for the genesis of a heterogeneous red cell population in this disorder. Hb F is very heterogeneously distributed among β-thalassemic red cells. Those cells that have the most Hb F are those that will have the least relative excess of α chains, since the γ chains combine with α chains to form Hb F. It has been demonstrated in β thalassemia that Hb A has a more rapid turnover (shorter half-life) than Hb F.[23] This finding is consistent with the presence of different populations of red cells: Those containing mainly Hb A are short-lived, and those containing much more Hb F have a longer survival.[23] Indeed, differential centrifugation of red cells in β thalassemia reveals that the older, more rapidly sedimenting red cells contain much Hb F and have relatively few α-chain inclusions, whereas the younger, more slowly sedimenting cells are relatively deficient in Hb F and contain many α-chain inclusions.[16, 20, 24] The severity of the disease in β thalassemia also correlates well with the size of the free α-chain pool and the degree of α to non–α globin chain imbalance.[25, 26] In addition, the co-inheritance of α thalassemia together with homozygous β thalassemia reduces the degree of α to non–α globin chain imbalance and leads to a milder clinical course (discussed later). These findings serve to emphasize the relationship of the α-chain inclusions to the hemolytic process and ineffective erythropoiesis, as well as the beneficial role of γ-chain synthesis in lessening the imbalance of globin-chain synthesis, decreasing the formation of α-chain inclusions and thus increasing the effective production of red cells as well as prolonging their survival in the circulation.

In β thalassemia, the α-chain inclusions are found in large quantities in the bone marrow erythroid precursor cells,[13, 17, 18] a phenomenon that is probably the cause of the marked ineffective erythropoiesis or intramedullary destruction of erythroid cells that is observed in homozygous β thalassemia.[27] Prior to splenectomy, these inclusion bodies are practically never seen in peripheral red blood cells, but following splenectomy, they appear in large numbers.[13] This observation correlates well with the demonstrated role of the spleen (and reticuloendothelial system) in removing inclusion bodies of the Heinz-body type from red cells, thereby damaging and/or destroying these cells.[28–30] This phenomenon can be dramatically observed under phase microscopy in fresh wet preparations obtained from scrapings of β-thalassemic spleens removed at surgery (Fig. 9–2).

Although the major cause of red cell injury

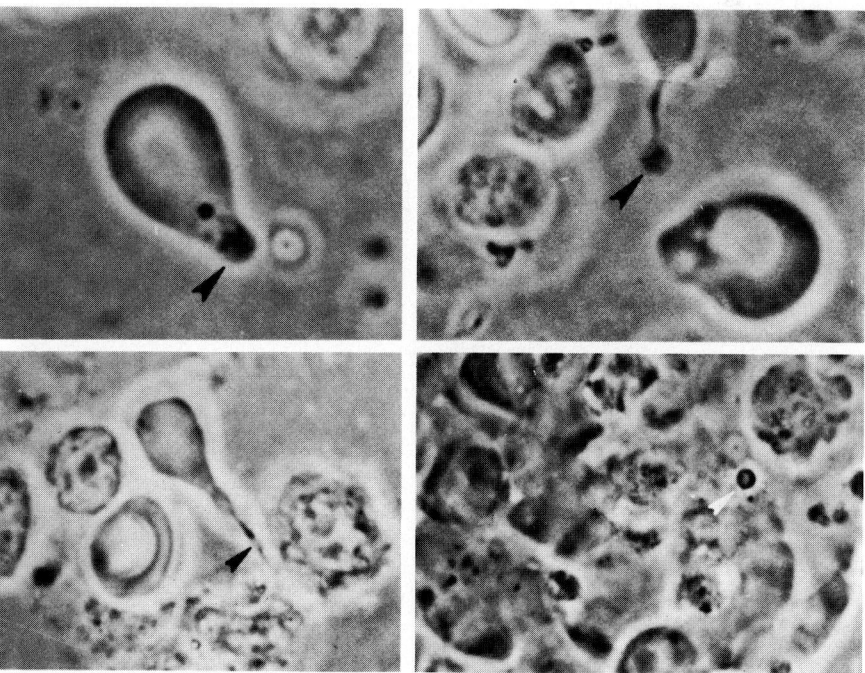

Figure 9–2. Phase microscopy of a wet preparation of scrapings from the spleen of a patient with homozygous β thalassemia. Note α-chain inclusion bodies (arrows) within teardrop-shaped red cells, inclusions being pulled out or "pitted" from the red cell by reticuloendothelial cell action (lower left), and inclusions free in the splenic pulp (white arrow). (From Nathan, D. G.: N. Engl. J. Med. *286*:586, 1972.)

and destruction in homozygous β thalassemia is probably the physical trauma due to the presence of the rigid α-chain inclusions and the mechanical injury resulting from the interactions between the abnormal red cells and the reticuloendothelial cells, there are other abnormalities of red cell metabolism that may further damage the cells.[1, 342] These include oxidant damage to the membrane (lipid peroxidation) resulting from generation of superoxide and formation of hemichrome by the excess of α chains.[31, 32] These abnormalities may be enhanced by vitamin E deficiency and iron overload resulting from transfusions.[33]

In the α-thalassemia syndrome of Hb H disease, the resulting β_4 tetramers (Hb H) are more stable than α-chain aggregates and precipitate more slowly. Therefore, one does not observe the marked ineffective erythropoiesis and intramedullary destruction of erythroid cells that is seen in β thalassemia, although some Hb H inclusions are occasionally seen in marrow normoblasts.[34, 35] The precipitation of β_4 tetramers to form inclusions proceeds more gradually and occurs mainly in mature red cells rather than erythroid precursor cells. The spleen removes these inclusions and thus damages the red blood cells,[16, 20, 29, 36] resulting in their premature destruction. Prior to splenectomy, no preformed Hb H inclusions are seen in the peripheral red blood cells, although soluble Hb H is present and can be induced to precipitate in the form of small, stippled inclusions after *in vitro* incubation of the blood with the oxidant compound brilliant cresyl blue (Fig. 9–3A; also see Color Plate 2L). After splenectomy, large, usually single, round preformed inclusions are seen in the red cells after staining with methyl violet or by phase and electron microscopy[16, 35, 36] (Fig. 9–3B) and occasionally on routine blood smear (see Color Plate 2K).

In addition to the primary pathophysiologic processes operative in thalassemia, a number of secondary abnormalities occur that can worsen the anemia or its effects on the affected patients. In thalassemia intermedia or in patients on low transfusion programs, the anemia may be aggravated by folic acid deficiency, which can easily develop because of the high folic acid requirement resulting from the massive marrow erythroid hyperplasia and cellular turnover.[37–39] Such patients may also experience sudden worsening of their anemia during aplastic crises induced by infection with the recently characterized parvovirus that causes similar crises in patients with sickle cell anemia (see Chapter 12) and other chronic hemolytic anemias.[39a–39c] The splenomegaly invariably associated with homozygous β thalassemia also contributes to the anemia either by simply acting as a third space, increasing intravascular volume and causing hemodilution,[40] or by causing true hypersplenic destruction of red blood cells. After splenectomy, the liver may act in a similar fashion but less effectively. Finally, since red cells containing fetal hemoglobin have high oxygen affinity (see Chapter 4), there may exist actual tissue hypoxia at hemoglobin levels that would otherwise seem adequate to provide proper tissue oxygenation if the hemoglobin were all normal adult Hb A.[41, 42] In fact, thalassemic red cells appear to adapt poorly to anemia, as reflected by inappropriately low levels of red cell 2,3-DPG and relatively increased oxygen affinity.[1, 42, 43]

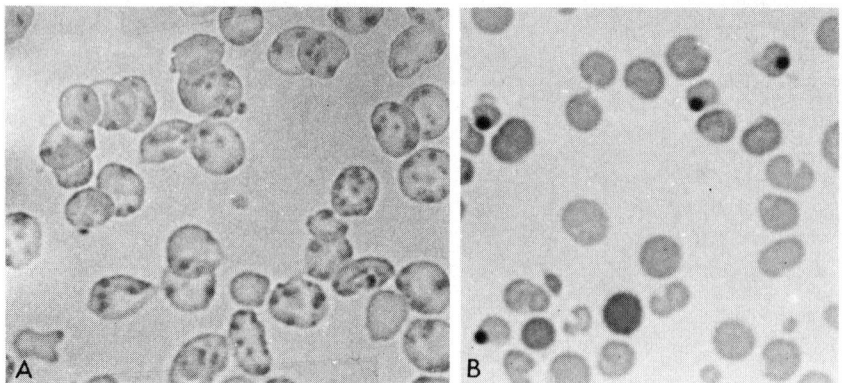

Figure 9–3. Red cell inclusions in Hb H disease. *A*, Inclusions induced by incubating peripheral blood in 1 per cent brilliant cresyl blue (BCB) and 0.4 per cent citrate for 30 minutes at 37°C (patient not splenectomized). *B*, Preformed inclusions, in peripheral blood of a splenectomized patient, stained by new methylene blue reticulocyte stain. (*From* Bunn, H. F., Forget, B. G., and Ranney, H. M.: Human Hemoglobins. Philadelphia, W. B. Saunders Company, 1977.)

CLASSIFICATION OF THE THALASSEMIA SYNDROMES

The thalassemia syndromes are usually classified according to the type of globin chain that is absent or present in decreased amount. The different types of thalassemia syndromes are listed in Table 9–1. The two major categories consist of the α and the β thalassemias, each of which can be subdivided into a number of different subtypes that may be inherited in the heterozygous state, the homozygous state, or in various doubly heterozygous states to generate a large number of diverse clinical and hematologic syndromes.

In the α-thalassemia syndromes, heterozygous α thalassemia can occur in two forms: a phenotypically apparent form, referred to as α thalassemia 1, and a very mild defect, with little or no hematologic abnormalities, called α thalassemia 2 or the "silent carrier" state. The α thalassemia 1 phenotype can also result from homozygosity for α thalassemia 2. The heterozygous state for Hb Constant Spring is phenotypically similar to α thalassemia 2, except that small amounts (1 to 2 per cent) of

Table 9–1. **CLINICAL AND HEMATOLOGICAL CLASSIFICATION OF THE THALASSEMIA AND THALASSEMIA-LIKE SYNDROMES**

α-Thalassemia Syndromes
1. Heterozygous α thalassemia 2 or "silent carrier" state
2. Heterozygous α thalassemia 1 or α-thalassemia trait
3. Hb H disease: double heterozygosity for α thalassemia 1 + α thalassemia 2
4. Hydrops fetalis with Hb Bart's: homozygous α thalassemia 1
5. Hb Constant Spring syndromes
6. α + β thalassemia
7. Hb S or Hb SS/α thalassemia

β-Thalassemia Syndromes
1. Heterozygous β thalassemia, β-thalassemia trait, or β thalassemia minor
   a. With elevated Hb A_2 ± elevated Hb F
   b. With normal Hb A_2 and elevated Hb F: δβ thalassemia, or F thalassemia
      i. $^G\gamma^A\gamma(\delta\beta)^0$ thalassemia
      ii. $^G\gamma(^A\gamma\delta\beta)^0$ thalassemia
   c. With normal Hb A_2 and Hb F
      i. "Silent carrier," including Hb Knossos
      ii. Concomitant δ + β thalassemia, *in cis* or *in trans*
      iii. γδβ thalassemia
      iv. Other: atypical δβ thalassemia; concomitant iron deficiency
   d. Hb Lepore trait
2. Homozygous β thalassemia, Cooley's anemia, or β thalassemia major
   a. True homozygosity for one or another β-thalassemia gene
   b. Double heterozygosity for any two different β-thalassemia genes
3. β thalassemia intermedia (see Table 9–3)

Rare Forms of Thalassemia
1. γ thalassemia
2. δ thalassemia
3. γδβ thalassemia

Interacting Thalassemia
1. α thalassemia + α-chain variant
   a. Hb Q/α thalassemia
   b. Hb G/α thalassemia
2. β thalassemia + β-chain variant
   a. Sickle/β thalassemia
   b. Hb C/β thalassemia
   c. Hb E/β thalassemia

Hereditary Persistence of Fetal Hemoglobin (HPFH)
1. Pancellular
   a. $^G\gamma^A\gamma(\delta\beta)^0$ HPFH
   b. Hb Kenya ($^G\gamma$ HPFH)
   c. Black $^G\gamma\beta^+$ HPFH with high Hb F
   d. Greek $^A\gamma$ HPFH
   e. Chinese $^A\gamma$ HPFH
2. Heterocellular
   a. Swiss-type $^G\gamma^A\gamma$ HPFH
   b. British-type $^A\gamma$ HPFH
   c. Other: Seattle-type $^G\gamma^A\gamma$ HPFH; Atlanta type—black $^G\gamma\beta^+$ HPFH with low Hb F; Saudi high Hb F determinant

the abnormal hemoglobin are detectable. The homozygous state for α thalassemia 1 is the syndrome of hydrops fetalis with Hb Bart's. The doubly heterozygous state for α thalassemia 1 and α thalassemia 2 (or Hb Constant Spring) results in the less severe syndrome of Hb H disease.

In the β-thalassemia syndromes, the heterozygous state for β thalassemia (thalassemia minor) is quite heterogeneous, as indicated by the variations in the amounts of the minor components of hemoglobin present in red cells of affected individuals. The various heterozygous states include (1) β thalassemia with high Hb A_2; (2) δβ thalassemia, or F thalassemia, characterized by normal Hb A_2 but elevated Hb F; (3) β-thalassemia trait with normal amounts of Hb F and Hb A_2; and (4) Hb Lepore trait, which is phenotypically similar to heterozygous β thalassemia but characterized by normal levels of Hb A_2, the presence of small amounts (10 to 15 per cent) of the abnormal hemoglobin (Hb Lepore), and some elevation of Hb F. Thalassemia major or Cooley's anemia may result from the combination of any two of these genes. Occasionally, an individual will inherit a combination of thalassemic genes that results in a syndrome that is clinically less severe than in the usual cases of homozygous β thalassemia and is called "β thalassemia intermedia." A number of different genotypes can be associated with β thalassemia intermedia (as discussed later).

THE ALPHA-THALASSEMIA SYNDROMES

Alpha thalassemia is associated with four general clinical syndromes (see Fig. 8–11 for genotypes):
 1. Mild or inapparent heterozygous α thalassemia: α thalassemia 2, or the "silent carrier" state (with or without associated Hb Constant Spring).
 2. Phenotypically apparent α-thalassemia "trait": α thalassemia 1.
 3. Hemoglobin H disease: double heterozygosity for α thalassemia 1 + α thalassemia 2.
 4. Hydrops fetalis with Hb Bart's: homozygosity for α thalassemia 1.

As discussed in Chapter 8, α thalassemia 2 is caused by deletion (or inactivation) of one of the four α globin genes (– α/αα), whereas α thalassemia 1 results from the deletion (or inactivation) of two α globin genes. In Asians (and many Mediterraneans), the α thalassemia 1 phenotype is associated with the deletion of two α globin genes on the same chromosome (*in cis*) (– –/αα), whereas in blacks, the same phenotype also results from the deletion of two α globin genes but on opposite chromosomes (*in trans*) (– α/– α) and therefore constitutes homozygosity for α thalassemia 2. Because of this difference in gene organization, Hb H disease is very rare in blacks and hydrops fetalis with Hb Bart's has thus far not been reported. The infrequent cases of Hb H disease in blacks are due to the inheritance of a rare α thalassemia 1 gene of the (– –/) genotype (see Chapter 8) together with the common α thalassemia 2 gene.

α Thalassemia 1 Phenotype

This condition is clinically benign. The hematologic features are essentially indistinguishable in the two distinct genotypes found in different racial groups: (– –/αα) or (– α/– α). Affected individuals are usually detected on routine hematologic examination or during family studies of patients with the more symptomatic α-thalassemic disorders. Alpha thalassemia 1 is characterized by microcytosis and hypochromia of the red blood cells, with a mild degree of anisocytosis and poikilocytosis (see Color Plate 2G). The hemoglobin level may be slightly depressed (10 to 12 g/dl) or near normal as a result of an elevated red cell count (greater than 5 million/mm^3). Alpha thalassemia 1 can be distinguished from β-thalassemia trait by the presence of normal levels of Hb F and normal or decreased levels of Hb A_2 (see Chapter 4). Beyond the neonatal period, the clinical diagnosis is often difficult; iron deficiency and other causes of hypochromia and microcytosis must be ruled out before the diagnosis can be accepted. Although it is possible to confirm the suspected diagnosis by studies of globin chain synthesis (see Chapter 8 and Fig. 8–2), the most definitive method to unequivocally establish the diagnosis is to perform gene mapping studies of the patient's DNA (see Chapter 8 and Fig. 8–20).

Heterozygous α Thalassemia 2

The hematologic findings in patients heterozygous for α thalassemia 2 are essentially normal or only very minimally abnormal with a slightly lower than normal MCV and MCH and an unremarkable blood smear. Globin-chain synthetic studies may show a small deficit of α globin chain synthesis, but there is a great deal of overlap with the normal range of α/β synthetic ratios (see Fig. 8–2). The diagnosis is usually inferred from the study of parents of individuals with Hb H disease and can be established definitively, in family studies as well as in population surveys, by gene mapping studies demonstrating the deletion of one α globin gene (– α/αα) (see Fig. 8–20).

During the neonatal period, α thalassemia 1 and α thalassemia 2 can be diagnosed by the level of Hb Bart's (γ_4) present in cord blood. This association has been studied most thoroughly in Thailand.[1, 44, 45] Cord blood of normal infants has no detectable Hb Bart's, but that of infants with heterozygous α thalassemia 2 has levels of 1 to 2 per cent Hb Bart's and that of infants with α thalassemia 1 has levels of approximately 5 to 6 per cent Hb Bart's. By the age of approximately 6 months, Hb Bart's is usually no longer detectable in α thalassemia 1 or α thalassemia 2. In Sardinia, somewhat similar results were obtained in infants with the α thalassemia 1 phenotype, but only approximately 40 per cent of infants with heterozygous α thalassemia 2 were found to have elevations of Hb Bart's in cord blood.[45a]

Hemoglobin H Disease

This condition is characterized by a chronic hemolytic anemia of variable severity.[1, 36] Most patients have a hemoglobin level of approximately 8 to 10 g/dl, with moderate reticulocytosis (5 to 10 per cent). However, the variation is wide, and one can see patients with either severe anemia or very mild anemia. Patients with mongoloid facies similar to that associated with homozygous β thalassemia have occasionally been described. Splenomegaly is usually present, and hepatomegaly is not uncommon. Anemia may become more severe during pregnancy or infection, or after ingestion of oxidant drugs, which accelerate the oxidation and precipitation of the Hb H (β_4). The peripheral blood smear typically shows hypochromia, microcytosis, poikilocytosis, polychromasia, and targeting of the red cells (see Color Plate 2J). Incubation of blood with 1 per cent brilliant cresyl blue (BCB) causes *in vitro* precipitation of Hb H, which is seen in the form of multiple speckled bodies (see Color Plate 2L and Fig. 9–3A). After splenectomy, large Hb H inclusion bodies, formed *in vivo* during red blood cell aging, can be seen by supravital staining and occasionally on routine blood smear. They are usually single and round[16, 35] (see Color Plate 2K and Fig. 9–3B). The bone marrow typically shows erythroid hyperplasia. Punctate hemoglobin H inclusions can be demonstrated by BCB incubation in nucleated erythroid precursor cells in the marrow, but large, single, round preformed inclusion bodies, although present in some normoblasts,[34, 35] are much less abundant than the numerous α-chain inclusion bodies found in cells of patients with homozygous β thalassemia.

The diagnosis can be established by hemoglobin electrophoresis (Fig. 9–4A). In the newborn, approximately 20 to 40 per cent Hb Bart's (γ_4) is found. This is gradually replaced in older children and adults by Hb H (β_4), the level of which varies between 5 and 30 per cent. Both Hb H and Hb Bart's migrate more rapidly than Hb A when electrophoresis is performed at pH 8.6, with Hb H being the faster of the two components. Hb A_2 is reduced to about 1 to 1.5 per cent. Biosynthetic studies have shown that in peripheral blood reticulocytes, there is approximately a 50 to 75 per cent reduction in α-chain synthesis compared to β-chain synthesis (see Chapter 8 and Fig. 8–1C). Gene mapping studies usually reveal the deletion of three α globin genes in affected individuals (– –/– α), although cases associated with nondeletion forms of α thalassemia are occasionally observed (see Chapter 8).

Study of the families of patients with Hb H disease usually reveals that one parent has hematologic findings characteristic of α thalassemia 1, whereas the other is hematologically normal and therefore a presumptive "silent carrier" of an α thalassemia 2 gene. Gene mapping studies will usually confirm the deletion of two (– –/αα) and one (– α/αα) α globin genes in the respective parents except in cases of nondeletion α thalassemia, in which many different patterns can be observed (see Chapter 8). A significant proportion of Asians with Hb H disease have Hb Constant Spring, as will be discussed in one of the sections that follow.

Acquired Hb H Disease

Hb H has been described as an acquired defect, usually during the course of erythroleukemia or other myeloproliferative disorders, including "preleukemic" syndromes, such as myelofibrosis and refractory anemia, that eventually progress to acute nonlymphocytic

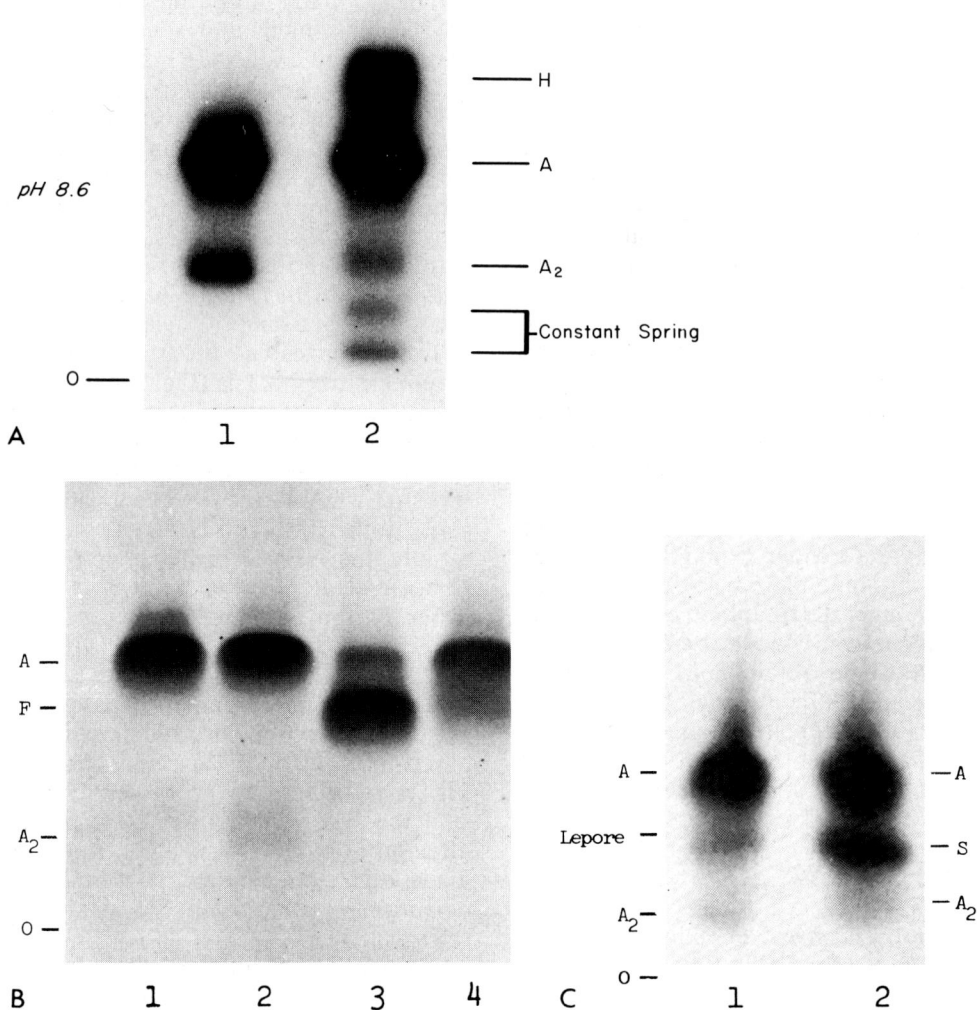

Figure 9–4. Hemoglobin electrophoresis. *A*, Starch-gel electrophoresis at pH 8.6; 1, Normal; 2, Hb H disease with Hb Constant Spring. *B*, Agarose electrophoresis at pH 8.6; 1, Normal; 2, β-thalassemia trait with increased Hb A_2; 3 and 4, homozygous β thalassemia with different relative amounts of Hb A and Hb F. *C*, Starch-gel electrophoresis at pH 8.6; 1, Hb lepore trait; 2, sickle cell trait. (O indicates the origin and the anode is at the top.) (*From* Bunn, H. F., Forget, B. G., and Ranney, H. M.: Human Hemoglobins. Philadelphia, W. B. Saunders Company, 1977.)

leukemia.[1, 46, 47] The disorder usually affects males over the age of 60 and is characterized by a dimorphic blood smear containing both normal red cells and hypochromic cells from the leukemic clone that contain numerous inclusion bodies after incubation with brilliant cresyl blue. As the disease progresses, the abnormal clone becomes increasingly predominant. The degree of imbalance of globin-chain synthesis and of α globin mRNA deficiency is greater than in hereditary Hb H disease. It is even conceivable that cells of the abnormal "leukemic" clone of erythroid cells synthesize no α globin chains at all, but this phenomenon is difficult to document in total blood as long as some normal erythroid cells are being produced. The general clinical manifestations of this disorder are those associated with the primary myeloproliferative disorder, although symptoms of anemia may appear to be inappropriately severe in relation to the total hemoglobin level owing to the very high oxygen affinity of Hb H, resulting in the lack of physiological oxygen delivery (see the section that follows on the pathophysiology of Hb H disease). The molecular basis of this fascinating disorder remains obscure (see Chapter 8). It is clear, however, that the marked deficiency of α globin chain synthesis is not due to the deletion of any of the α globin genes and that the defect, in all likelihood, involves the suppression or silencing of all four α globin genes (see Chapter 8).

A second syndrome that is associated with Hb H on an acquired basis is the disorder of mental deficiency with Hb H, first described by Weatherall and coworkers.[48] In this disorder, the affected individuals of northern European ancestry have mental retardation (with I.Q.s in the range of 50 to 70) and Hb H disease that was inherited in a nontraditional manner: Although one parent had α thalassemia 2 by various criteria, the other parent was completely normal. It is presumed that a mutation occurred on the chromosome 16 inherited from the "normal" parent that resulted in both mental retardation and reduced globin gene expression. In one case, this mutation was documented to consist of a large deletion encompassing the entire α globin gene complex, including the ζ globin gene, but in two other cases, no deletion could be demonstrated.[48] Following the initial report, a number of additional cases were subsequently identified and studied (see Chapter 8). The hematologic and biochemical abnormalities in this disorder are similar in severity to those in the traditional hereditary form of Hb H disease. The significance of this syndrome is that certain acquired mutations of chromosome 16 can cause both mental retardation and defective α globin gene expression, perhaps by affecting neighboring genetic loci on the chromosome.

Pathophysiology of Hb H Disease

Deficiency of α-chain synthesis results in overall decreased synthesis of Hb A and, hence, hypochromia and microcytosis. The excess β chains that accumulate form the $β_4$ tetramers of Hb H. Hb H has a very high oxygen affinity and lacks the Bohr effect as well as subunit cooperativity (see Chapter 3). Hence, it is a useless pigment for oxygen delivery under physiologic conditions. In addition, Hb H is an unstable tetramer. It is easily oxidized and tends to precipitate as the red cells age. These precipitates, which form gradually *in vivo*, are normally removed by the spleen and can be demonstrated most abundantly in peripheral blood cells after splenectomy. They cause disturbances in red cell metabolism and interfere with normal membrane function and deformability.[16, 20] All of these factors lead to shortened red cell survival and the hemolytic component of the disease.

Hemoglobin Constant Spring Syndromes

In as many as 50 per cent of Asian subjects with Hb H disease, hemoglobin electrophoresis shows, in addition to the usual findings, one or two more slowly migrating hemoglobin components, derived from Hb Constant Spring (Hb CS), which account for 3 to 5 per cent of the total hemoglobin[49, 50] (Fig. 9–4A). Hb CS is made up of two normal β chains and two elongated α chains, which have either 28 or 31 additional amino acid residues at their C-terminal end, resulting from readthrough of the normally untranslated 3′ portion of the α globin mRNA due to a base substitution in the chain termination codon converting it to a codon for glutamine (see Chapters 8 and 10). The shorter $α^{CS}$ chain presumably results from proteolytic digestion of the longer $α^{CS}$ chain. Typically, one of the parents of a patient with Hb H/CS disease has α thalassemia 1 trait, whereas the other appears to be hematologically normal except that hemoglobin electrophoresis shows the presence of approximately 1 per cent Hb CS. Therefore, heterozygotes for Hb CS are phenotypically similar to individuals with heterozygous α thalassemia 2. An α thalassemia 2 phenotype is also associated with heterozygosity for three other elongated α-chain variants[1] resulting from different base substitutions in the normal α globin mRNA termination codon: Hb Icaria,[51] Hb Koya Dora,[52] and Hb Seal Rock[53] (see Chapters 8 and 10).

The homozygous state for Hb CS is an interesting syndrome that has some unusual and unexpected clinical and hematologic features. One would expect this condition to have a phenotype similar to that of homozygous α thalassemia 2, i.e., the phenotype of apparent α-thalassemia "trait" or α thalassemia 1 but with increased levels of Hb CS. On the contrary, such individuals in fact present a picture of a mild hemolytic anemia with splenomegaly and reticulocytosis. Hemolysates contain approximately 5 to 7 per cent Hb CS and even small amounts of Hb Bart's, but there is no significant hypochromia and microcytosis.[54–58] It is also noteworthy that patients with Hb H disease and Hb CS ($- -/α^{CS}α$) have a somewhat more severe degree of anemia with higher levels of Hb H and Hb Bart's than patients with ordinary Hb H disease ($- -/- α$).[59, 60] Even more unexpected has been the observation, in both heterozygotes and homozygotes for Hb CS, of excess β to α globin chain synthesis in biosynthetic studies[56, 57] rather than the expected deficit of α globin chain synthesis. These puzzling findings have been greatly clarified by the recent studies of Derry and co-workers.[61] These workers found that in short-term pulse-labeling studies there was in fact the expected deficit of α globin chain synthesis but that this deficit was masked at longer time points owing to unusually rapid degradation of excess newly synthesized β globin chains. Analysis of free β globin chain pools and of intracellular Hb H inclusion bodies revealed that the homozygous state for Hb CS was hematologically and pathophysiologically more similar to Hb H disease than to α thalassemia 1.[61] What is unexplained in these detailed and well-executed studies is the basis for the difference in handling of the excess β globin chain subunits in homozygous Hb CS when the degree of imbalance of α to β globin chain synthesis is quite similar to that in α thalassemia 1, in which there is no accumulation of free β globin chains, no inclusion body formation, and, therefore, no hemolytic anemia.

Hydrops Fetalis Associated with Hb Bart's

The homozygous state for α thalassemia 1 results in the syndrome of hydrops fetalis with Hb Bart's.[1] The affected fetus is usually delivered prematurely and is either stillborn or dies within an hour after birth; it is grossly hydropic (Fig. 9–5) with marked anemia and hepatosplenomegaly.[62–65] This syndrome occurs almost exclusively in individuals from Southeast Asia, although rare cases have been described in Greek and Cypriot infants.[66–69] No cases have thus far been described in people of black ancestry.

The peripheral blood smear is characterized by large hypochromic red cells, reticulocytosis, and large numbers of nucleated red blood cells (see Color Plates 2H and I). On hemoglobin electrophoresis, the predominant hemoglobin is Hb Bart's (γ_4).[62] In addition, there is found a small amount of Hb H and 10 to 20 per cent of another component with an electrophoretic mobility similar to Hb A, Hb Portland ($\zeta_2\gamma_2$).[70–72] Although the embryonic ζ globin chain is usually synthesized exclusively in yolk sac–derived erythroid cells,[72a] the gene deletion causing α thalassemia 1 is associated with persistent expression of the ζ globin gene *in cis,* in the heterozygous as well as the homozygous state.[72b, 72c] Studies of globin chain syn-

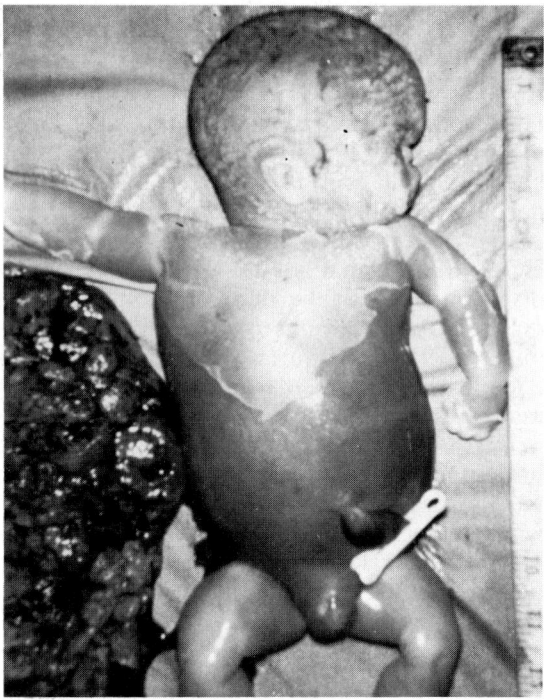

Figure 9–5. Hydropic infant and markedly enlarged placenta caused by homozygous α thalassemia 1. (Courtesy of Dr. R. Osathanondh.)

thesis in cases of Hb Bart's syndrome reveal total absence of α-chain synthesis,[70] and gene mapping studies have demonstrated the deletion of all four α globin genes (– –/– –) (see Chapter 8). Family studies in such cases invariably reveal the presence of deletion-type α thalassemia 1 (– –/αα) in both parents.

Hb Bart's has a very high oxygen affinity similar to that of Hb H. Thus, the bulk of the hemoglobin present in these infants cannot deliver oxygen effectively to the tissues. The cause of the hydropic changes and death is severe hypoxia. Delivery by cesarean section and exchange transfusion were attempted in one case but were not successful in prolonging life for more than a few hours,[70] and it is doubtful that this approach would be successful in salvaging such infants in view of the probable damage to brain and other organs caused by the prolonged hypoxia during gestation. However there is one instance in which a hydropic infant not initially suspected of having Hb Bart's syndrome was successfully resuscitated and subsequently maintained on transfusions.[72d] The neurological status of the child remains uncertain. In view of the oxygen affinity properties of Hb Bart's, it is somewhat astounding that the infants survive to the age of 30 to 40 weeks of gestation. In all likelihood, they obtain their oxygenation through the function of Hb Portland, which has a physiological oxygen dissociation curve.[73]

The cause of the hemolytic anemia in this syndrome remains unknown. Hb Bart's, in contrast to Hb H, is not particularly unstable and does not tend to form inclusion bodies.

THE BETA THALASSEMIAS

Heterozygous Beta Thalassemia

The hallmark of heterozygous β thalassemia is microcytosis and hypochromia. With the widespread use of electronic cell counting equipment, the diagnosis is frequently first suspected by the discovery of a low MCV and MCH on routine blood counts.[74] β-Thalassemia heterozygotes are usually asymptomatic. Mild anemia is present in most individuals, although there is a wide range of Hb levels,[1] and some individuals have normal Hb and Hct levels owing to elevated red cell counts. Anemia may be more pronounced in infancy and during pregnancy. The MCV and MCH are usually decreased well below normal, with typical values of 55 to 70 μ^3 and 16 to 20 pg, respectively. Despite the microcytosis, the MCHC is not usually as low as in iron deficiency. The peripheral blood smear typically shows microcytosis, hypochromia, and anisocytosis and poikilocytosis with targeting and basophilic stippling of the red cells (see Color Plate 2B). The bone marrow shows mild erythroid hyperplasia, with many of the normoblasts showing poor hemoglobinization. Mild to moderate splenomegaly may occur in a minority of cases. A more detailed review of the clinical and hematologic features of heterozygous β thalassemia is provided in Weatherall and Clegg's monograph.[1]

The differential diagnosis between iron deficiency and β- (or α-) thalassemia trait can be difficult in practice. Table 9–2 lists the differentiating features. In thalassemic heterozygotes, the MCV tends to be lower when related to the red cell count than in iron deficiency. This observation has led to the derivation of various formulas to differentiate thalassemia trait from iron deficiency on the basis of the red cell indices[75–77] (see Table 9–2). Although such findings are helpful, they do not provide conclusive evidence of the diagnosis. Precise diagnosis requires hemoglobin electrophoresis and measurement of the serum iron and iron binding capacity. Demonstration of absent stainable iron in bone marrow aspirates may be necessary to identify individuals with combined thalassemia trait and iron deficiency. This combination is quite common in early childhood and during pregnancy. Medicinal iron should not be withheld when iron deficiency complicates thalassemia trait.

It is noteworthy that the presence of iron deficiency may obscure the diagnosis of concomitant β-thalassemia trait. Iron deficiency causes a decrease in Hb A_2 levels in normal individuals as well as in those with β-thalassemia trait: With iron deficiency, the usually elevated Hb A_2 levels in a β-thalassemic heterozygote may fall into the normal range.[78, 79] β-thalassemia trait should therefore be suspected in cases in which anemia responds only partially and in which hypochromia and microcytosis persist after therapy for iron deficiency.

Table 9–2. DIFFERENTIATION OF β-THALASSEMIA TRAIT FROM IRON DEFICIENCY ANEMIA (Hb 9 to 11 g/100 ml)

	β-Thal Trait	Iron Deficiency Anemia
I. Definitive Tests		
A. Serum iron	Normal	Decreased
B. TIBC	Normal	Increased
C. % saturation	Nomal	Decreased
D. Hb electrophoresis		
HB A_2	Increased	Decreased
Hb F	± Increased	Normal
II. Associated Findings		
MCV/RBC*	< 13	> 13
RBC protoporphyrin	Normal	Increased
RBC morphology	3 to 4+ Abnormal	Tr-1+ Abnormal
Serum ferritin	Normal	Low
Dominant inheritance	+	0
Color of plasma	Straw-colored	Colorless

*See Mentzer, W. C.: Lancet 1:449, 1973.

The Hb A_2 levels will return to their normally elevated values in such patients after replenishment of iron stores.

Moderately severe anemia has been described occasionally in apparent heterozygous thalassemia.[80-84] However, severe anemia is unusual, and when it occurs, one should look for associated secondary causes such as concomitant iron or folic acid deficiency. Such cases should also be distinguished by family studies from the milder forms of homozygous β thalassemia or double heterozygosity for β-thalassemia genes of different types and severity. The term "thalassemia intermedia" has been used to refer to either severe heterozygous β thalassemia or mild homozygous β thalassemia.

There are at least four different clinical types of heterozygous β thalassemia, which can be distinguished on the basis of hemoglobin electrophoresis:

1. *High Hb A_2 β thalassemia.* By far the most common variety, it is characterized by an increased Hb A_2 level of 4 to 6 per cent (see Fig. 9–4B) and a normal level of Hb F, although in approximately half of the cases a slightly elevated level of Hb F (2 to 3 per cent) may be present.[85-86a]

2. *δβ Thalassemia (or F thalassemia).* In this type of heterozygous β thalassemia, the Hb A_2 level is normal or slightly decreased, and the Hb F level is increased, with levels between 5 and 20 per cent.

3. *β Thalassemia with normal levels of Hb A_2 and Hb F.* This type of heterozygous β thalassemia is difficult to distinguish clinically from heterozygous α thalassemia. It is usually suspected by the finding of a clinically significant β-thalassemia syndrome in an offspring. Studies of globin chain biosynthesis in peripheral blood reticulocytes may be the only laboratory means to make this diagnosis in an affected heterozygote. This disorder is quite heterogeneous in its phenotype, as discussed later.

4. *Hb Lepore trait.* This condition is characterized by normal Hb A_2, slight elevation of Hb F, and the finding of 6 to 15 per cent Hb Lepore, which has an electrophoretic mobility similar to that of Hb S (see Fig. 9–4C).

The clinical picture in all four types of heterozygous β thalassemia is rather similar, although there are certain exceptions to this general rule. In δβ thalassemia[87] and in a subset of black patients with high Hb A_2 β-thalassemia trait,[88] anemia, microcytosis, and morphologic abnormalities of the red cells are less pronounced than in other types of heterozygous β thalassemia. In some cases of β thalassemia with normal levels of Hb A_2 and Hb F, the hematologic findings may be virtually normal, and the term "silent carrier" state has been applied to such cases. Finally, as discussed in the section on thalassemia intermedia, α thalassemia can interact with heterozygous β thalassemia to produce red cells with virtually normal morphology and indices but increased levels of Hb A_2.

The presence or absence of elevated Hb F in heterozygous high Hb A_2 β thalassemia is usually of no prognostic significance with regard to the severity of disease in a homozygous offspring. One exception to this rule is a rare variety of high Hb A_2 β thalassemia, found in Dutch and black individuals, that is characterized by an unexpectedly high Hb F level, ranging between 5 and 15 per cent.[89, 90] The homozygous state for this rare disorder is much milder than homozygosity for the usual type of high Hb A_2 β thalassemia.[90] These cases have subsequently been shown to be associated with deletions of different lengths in the β gene cluster[90a, 90b] (see Chapter 8). They are therefore somewhat analogous, with regard to molecular basis and possible cause of increased Hb F production, to cases of δβ thalassemia, but with intact δ genes and therefore the capacity to accumulate increased amounts of Hb A_2. Other cases of high Hb A_2 β thalassemia with increased increased levels of Hb F may be due to co-inheritance of a gene for heterocellular HPFH (discussed later) that is linked *in cis* to an ordinary β-thalassemia gene. It is known that a heterocellular HPFH determinant can have a favorable modifying effect on the clinical severity of homozygous β thalassemia,[86, 91-92b] of Hb S/β thalassemia,[92c] and of sickle cell anemia (see Chapter 12). Heterozygous β thalassemia with increased levels of Hb F can also result from the inheritance of heterocellular HPFH *in trans,* but in this situation there is lack of co-inheritance of the high Hb F determinant together with β-thalassemia trait in siblings or offspring.[92c, 92d]

The results of globin-chain biosynthetic studies in heterozygous β thalassemia have been discussed in Chapter 8. The β/α synthetic ratio is approximately 0.5 in peripheral blood reticulocytes. In contrast, the ratio in bone marrow cells is close to 1. As discussed in Chapter 8, this finding of apparently balanced globin-chain synthesis in the bone marrow appears to be due to accelerated turnover and degradation of newly synthesized excess α chains.

The study of β-thalassemia homozygotes and of individuals doubly heterozygous for β thalassemia and a β-chain structural variant such as Hb S makes it possible to evaluate the amount of $β^A$-chain synthesis directed by a given β-thalassemia gene. In high Hb A_2 β thalassemia, it is possible to distinguish two general categories or phenotypes: one in which the synthesis of β globin chains is present but diminished ($β^+$ thalassemia), and the other in which it is totally absent ($β^0$ thalassemia). In various populations or geographic regions, one type tends to predominate over the other. $β^0$ thalassemia is by far the predominant form of thalassemia in northern Italy (Ferrara and Po Valley),[93] Sardinia,[94, 95] and Thailand[96] and probably the rest of Southeast Asia. $β^+$ thalassemia, on the other hand, is by far the most common form of β thalassemia in blacks[88] and Cypriots.[97] In Greece, southern Italy, and Sicily both forms exist, but $β^+$ thalassemia accounts for the majority of cases.[1, 98, 99] It should be pointed out, however, that in these regions, homozygous patients with a $β^+$-thalassemia phenotype are frequently doubly heterozygous for $β^0$ and $β^+$ thalassemia. In Mediterraneans, it is nearly impossible to distinguish $β^0$- from $β^+$-thalassemia heterozygotes on the basis of hematologic criteria alone.[1]

Homozygous High Hb A_2 β Thalassemia

Clinical Manifestations

The clinical course in most cases of homozygous β thalassemia is severe. At birth, anemia is not evident, and examination of the peripheral blood smear shows only occasional hypochromic red cells. Diagnosis, however, can be established by study of globin chain synthesis in the cord blood.[100] Within a year or so, severe hypochromic, microcytic, hemolytic anemia develops, and a regular transfusion program must be undertaken to maintain an adequate hemoglobin level.

The clinical manifestations of homozygous β thalassemia in childhood have changed considerably over the last decade or two owing to changes in the philosophy and practice of transfusion therapy (see the section that follows on management). With modern transfusion therapy, most children will develop normally, with little or no skeletal abnormalities, and will have a reasonably good quality of life until the onset of cardiac complications due to iron overload, which usually develop in the mid to late teens or early twenties.

However, with less adequate transfusion therapy, a different clinical picture emerges.[1] The spleen and liver become progressively enlarged. A typical facies develops (Fig. 9–6), with prominent frontal bossing, prominent cheek bones, and protruding upper jaw due to expansion of the marrow in the skull and facial bones. Radiography of the skull demonstrates the typical "hair on end" appearance (Fig. 9–7A). The long bones may also become rarefied from the marrow expansion (Fig. 9–7B) and may become subject to repeated pathological fractures. Occasionally, the expanding marrow extrudes from ribs or vertebrae and forms large intrathoracic masses. Gallstones and leg ulcers are frequent complications, as they are in other severe hemolytic anemias. Intercurrent infection is extremely common, and along with neglected anemia, it is the most common cause of death in early childhood. A benign form of pericarditis with pericardial effusion frequently occurs and is usually self-limited. Secondary hypersplenism may develop and cause thrombocytopenia, leukopenia, and rapid destruction of transfused red cells. This complication may pose a severe management problem, and splenectomy may be required to control it. The incidence of overwhelming infection (septicemia) following splenectomy is very high in thalassemic patients,[101, 102] and such patients should be observed carefully and treated aggressively during febrile episodes. The administration of antipneumococcal vaccines prior to splenectomy may decrease the incidence of this complication (see the section that follows on management).

Physical growth and development are usually impaired. Menarche and secondary sexual characteristics are usually absent, and the final stature of affected patients tends to be short. This problem has been well reviewed.[103] Growth retardation becomes most significant and noticeable at 9 to 10 years of age. Even in well-transfused patients, there is a decrease in growth rate in late childhood and an absent or greatly diminished pubertal growth spurt.[104, 105] The basis for this growth retardation is not known. There is no evidence of growth hormone deficiency,[106–108] and it has been speculated that somatomedin deficiency may play a role.[105, 109] Decreased levels of somatomedin have in fact been detected in some patients.[109a]

Delay or failure of puberty is probably caused by end-organ damage of ovaries and

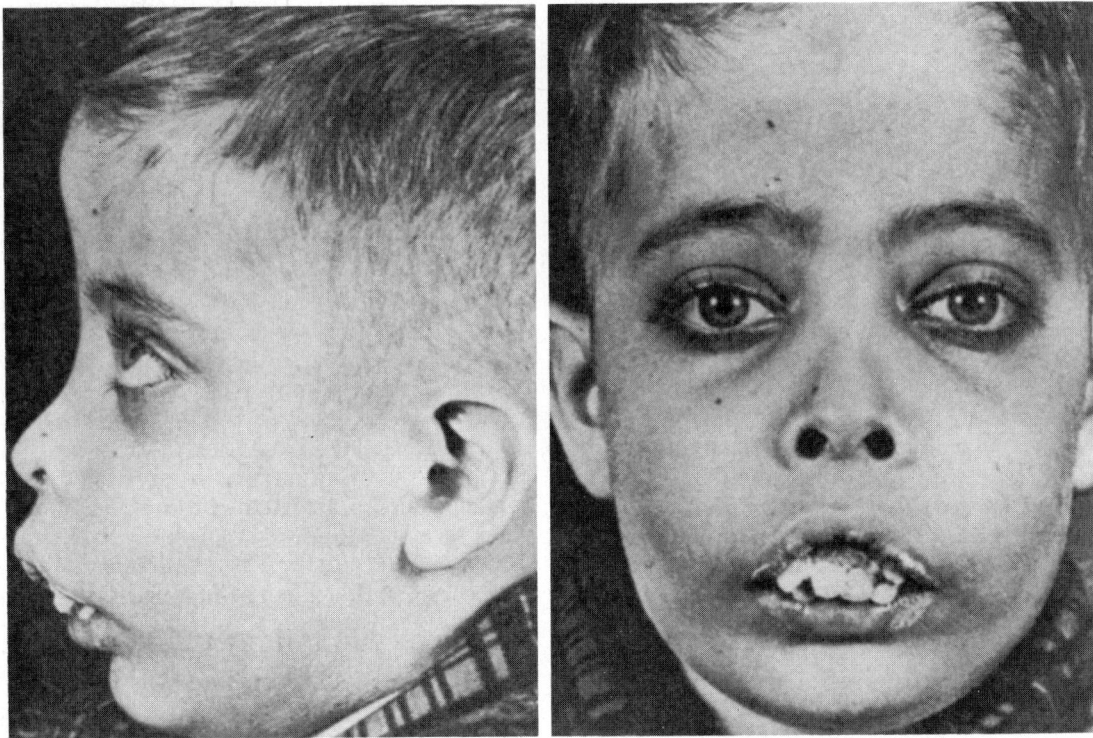

Figure 9–6. Typical facial appearance of a child with homozygous β thalassemia not treated by a high transfusion program. (From Jurkiewicz, M. J., et al.: Ann. N.Y. Acad. Sci. *165*:437, 1969.)

testes as a consequence of iron overload.[104, 106, 108, 110] Although aggressive iron chelation from an early age may prevent or ameliorate this complication in some patients, such successful results are not universal.

Iron overload due to repeated blood transfusions is the major cause of morbidity and mortality in the second decade of life and is responsible for damage to the heart, liver, pancreas, endocrine and other organs. Cardiac failure and arrhythmias due to cardiac siderosis are the most common causes of death as these patients survive to their twenties.[111] Diabetes mellitus and hepatic insufficiency may also pose difficult management problems. Increased iron absorption may contribute substantially to iron overload in homozygous β thalassemia. This phenomenon is probably related to ineffective erythropoiesis, which can be suppressed by adequate blood transfusions. It is hoped that treatment with vigorous iron chelation starting early in childhood will prevent or greatly delay the complications of iron overload and prolong the life of transfusion-dependent individuals with β thalassemia. However, long-term follow-up studies are not yet available to document that this will in fact be the case. Initiation of such therapy in mid to late childhood once transfusional hemosiderosis is already established may not significantly prolong the life span of the patients (see the section that follows on management).

Although the preceding clinical descriptions apply to most patients with homozygous β thalassemia, a small number of patients have a much milder clinical course (so-called thalassemia intermedia) and may require few or no blood transfusions. This is especially true of homozygous β^+ thalassemia in blacks, which is a much milder disease (discussed later).

Laboratory Findings

In the absence of blood transfusions, anemia is severe, and the findings on peripheral blood smear are striking (see Color Plate 2*D*). The red cells show severe hypochromia and microcytosis, marked anisocytosis and poikilocytosis with teardrop-shaped red cells, polychromasia, and basophilic stippling. Poorly hemoglobinized normoblasts are frequently found in the peripheral blood, and their number increases markedly following splenectomy (see Color Plate 2*E*). Even when anemia is severe, the

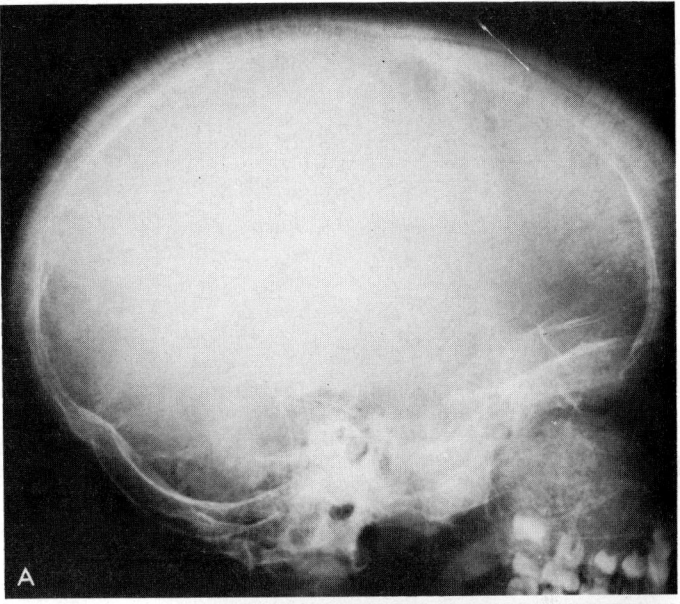
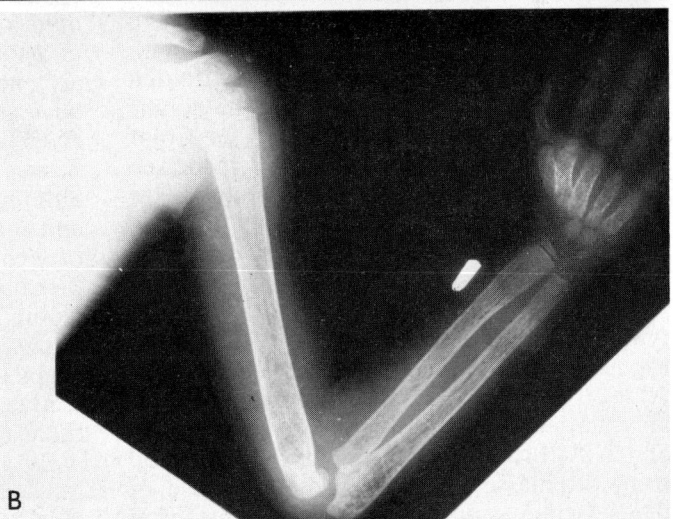

Figure 9–7. Bone changes in severe homozygous β thalassemia. *A,* Skull radiograph. (From Beck, W. S. [ed.]: Hematology. 2nd ed. Boston, MIT Press, 1976.) *B,* Radiograph of forearm and hand. (From Nathan, D. G.: N. Engl. J. Med. *286*:586, 1972.)

reticulocyte count is usually not very high because of massive destruction of erythroid precursor cells in the bone marrow, i.e, ineffective erythropoiesis.

The red cell osmotic fragility is decreased, a phenomenon explained by the marked hypochromia and thus the increased ability of the red cells to adapt to an increase in intracellular volume. The bone marrow is very hypercellular, with marked erythroid hyperplasia characterized by normoblasts that are poorly hemoglobinized (micronormoblastic). Storage cells resembling Gaucher cells are frequently found in the marrow (and spleen).[112, 113] Examination of the marrow under phase microscopy or after supravital staining reveals the presence of many inclusion bodies (α-chain aggregates) in the normoblasts. This finding can be used as a diagnostic test for homozygous β thalassemia.[13, 17] The α-chain inclusions are also seen in peripheral blood red cells after splenectomy (Fig. 9–8).

Elevated nonconjugated bilirubin levels and other biochemical evidence of hemolysis are usually observed. Dipyrroles resulting from increased heme catabolism give the urine a dark brown color.[114, 115] The findings on Hb electrophoresis vary from patient to patient and with the type of thalassemia (see Fig. 9–3B); they are primarily informative if the patient has not been previously transfused. In homozygous β⁺ thalassemia, a variable

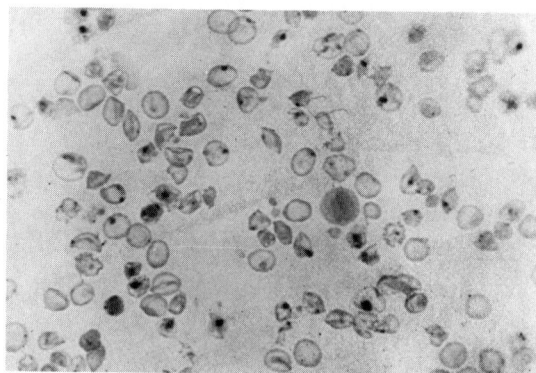

Figure 9–8. Supervital stain (methyl violet) of the peripheral blood cells from a patient with homozygous β thalassemia following splenectomy. (From Nathan, D. G., and Oski, F. A.: Hematology of Infancy and Childhood. 2nd ed. Philadelphia, W. B. Saunders Company, 1981.)

amount of Hb A is present. The Hb F is usually elevated and may represent from 10 to 90 per cent of the patient's total hemoglobin. The Hb F is heterogeneously distributed among the red cells as in other hemolytic anemias, such as sickle cell anemia (see Color Plate 3C), that are associated with increased production and selective survival of F cells (see Chapter 7). The Hb A_2 level may be low, normal, or increased, but the ratio of Hb A_2 to Hb A is usually higher than the normal ratio of 1 to 40, suggesting more efficient synthesis of Hb A_2 relative to Hb A in homozygous β thalassemia even if the absolute Hb A_2 level is below normal. Cell selection probably plays a role in lowering the total amount of Hb A_2 in hemolysates of peripheral blood from β-thalassemia homozygotes because of the selective survival in these patients of F cells, which synthesize decreased amounts of Hb A_2 (see Chapter 4). Free α chains may also be seen occasionally in trace amounts as a slow-moving component on hemoglobin electrophoresis.[116] Hb A is totally absent in untransfused patients with homozygous $β^0$ thalassemia. In general, patients doubly heterozygous for the high Hb A_2 β thalassemia and δβ thalassemia have a higher level of Hb F and a lower level of Hb A_2 than homozygotes for high Hb A_2 β thalassemia.

δβ Thalassemia or F Thalassemia

Heterozygous δβ thalassemia is a condition characterized by mild hypochromia and microcytosis. Red cell indices and morphological changes are generally less abnormal than in the usual form of heterozygous β thalassemia found in Mediterraneans. The changes may be barely noticeable. Hemoglobin electrophoresis reveals low or normal Hb A_2 and elevation of Hb F (5 to 20 per cent). When analyzed by acid elution or immunofluorescent staining of blood smears, the Hb F is heterogeneously distributed among the red cells (see Fig. 4–9C). The condition has been especially studied in Greeks,[87] but it has also been found in a number of other populations and racial groups. In association with the usual variety of high Hb A_2 β thalassemia, a thalassemia intermedia syndrome usually results, characterized by high levels of Hb F and only mild to moderate anemia that does not require treatment with regular transfusions of red cells.[117]

Homozygous δβ thalassemia is also a relatively mild disorder and may be barely symptomatic. The affected individuals usually have mild to moderate anemia (a hemoglobin level of 9 to 10 g/dl), mild or moderate splenomegaly, and no transfusion requirement. They have 100 per cent Hb F, with no Hb A or Hb A_2. The relatively benign nature of δβ thalassemia seems to be related to the fact that although it is associated with totally absent β- and δ-chain synthesis, there is a higher level of γ-chain synthesis than in the usual forms of β thalassemia: The overall degree of α/non–α globin chain imbalance is not as pronounced,[1, 118–120] and therefore, there is less α-chain inclusion body formation and less ineffective erythropoiesis and hemolysis than in the usual forms of homozygous β thalassemia.

By the analysis of Hb F subtypes in δβ-thalassemic individuals, it is possible to subdivide δβ thalassemia into two different types: that associated with synthesis of both ^{G}γ and ^{A}γ globin chains of Hb F [^{G}γ^{A}γ (δβ) thalassemia] and that associated with synthesis of only the ^{G}γ globin chain [^{G}γ (^{A}γδβ)^0 thalassemia].[1] The ^{G}γ^{A}γ type of δβ thalassemia occurs primarily in Mediterraneans and is itself heterogeneous. In most patients, ^{G}γ and ^{A}γ chains are usually present in a ratio of roughly 1:1 or 2:3, as in the Hb F of normal adults. However, in the δβ thalassemia found in Sardinia,[121] ^{G}γ and ^{A}γ chains are present in a ratio of roughly 1:10. The ^{G}γ variety of δβ thalassemia has been found in blacks, Asian Indians, Southeast Asians, Arabs, and Turks. Aside from these qualitative differences in Hb F, the two subtypes of δβ thalassemia are quite similar clinically and hematologically. The heterogeneity of the molecular basis of δβ thalassemia has been discussed in Chapter 8.

β Thalassemia with Normal Levels of Hb A_2 and Hb F

In the study of parents of children with apparent homozygous β thalassemia, one occasionally encounters a parent in whom both Hb A_2 and Hb F levels are normal. Some of these individuals may be atypical heterozygotes for δβ thalassemia in which, for unexplained reasons, the Hb F level is only at the upper limits of normal instead of constituting over 5 per cent of the total hemoglobin. Cases of δβ thalassemia have been documented in which there is a low level of Hb F that is not constant within the family: Other members in the family with thalassemia trait usually have the expected elevated Hb F levels.[87] Also, as noted previously, iron deficiency can result in a lowering of the Hb A_2 level in typical β-thalassemia trait.

Nevertheless, there are other well-characterized β-thalassemic disorders, distinct from those mentioned earlier, that are associated with normal levels of Hb A_2 and Hb F. These fall into two general categories: (1) the "silent carrier" state for β thalassemia, in which hematologic abnormalities of the red cells are not apparent; and (2) phenotypically apparent heterozygous β thalassemia with the usual degree of microcytosis, hypochromia, and morphologic abnormalities.

The silent carrier state for β thalassemia was first described by Schwartz.[122] He reported an Albanian family in which two children had β thalassemia of intermediate severity. The mother had typical high Hb A_2 β-thalassemia trait, whereas the father was essentially hematologically normal, having normal red blood cell indices and morphology and normal levels of Hb A_2 and Hb F. However, an abnormal β/α synthetic ratio of 0.6, characteristic of mild heterozygous β thalassemia, was observed in globin-chain biosynthetic studies of peripheral blood from the father and a number of his relatives. Subsequently, a number of additional cases of this condition have been reported.[123–125] The diagnosis relies on the demonstration of decreased production of β globin chains by studies of globin-chain synthesis. As discussed in Chapter 8, the molecular defect in the family initially reported by Schwartz does not appear to be linked to the β globin gene.

The phenotype of silent β thalassemia has also been found to be associated with a β-chain variant, Hb Knossos (β 27 Ala → Ser), that can be detected by isoelectric focusing but not by standard hemoglobin electrophoresis.[125a] Heterozygotes have low (or normal) levels of Hb A_2, normal levels of Hb F, and little or no microcytosis or morphological abnormalities of the red cells, but a decreased β/α synthetic ratio is observed after isotopic labeling of peripheral blood cells.[125b] Co-inheritance of Hb Knossos together with high Hb A_2 β thalassemia or Hb Lepore results in the clinical picture of β thalassemia intermedia.[125b–125e] As discussed in Chapter 8, Hb Knossos (like Hb E) causes β thalassemia by abnormal processing of precursor β mRNA molecules.

Phenotypically apparent β-thalassemia trait with normal levels of Hb A_2 and Hb F has also been described in at least two additional distinct syndromes: δ + β thalassemia and γδβ thalassemia. In contrast to the less severe thalassemic syndrome associated with double heterozygosity for high Hb A_2 β thalassemia together with the silent carrier state or the usual type of δβ thalassemia, a severe, transfusion-dependent thalassemia major syndrome can result from the interaction of high Hb A_2 β thalassemia with phenotypically apparent β-thalassemia trait associated with normal levels of Hb A_2 and Hb F.[123–125, 126] The hematologic features of this disorder are the same as those of typical high Hb A_2 β thalassemia. Both $β^0$ and $β^+$ forms have been described.[125] The most likely explanation for this disorder is the coexistence of separate thalassemias of the δ and β globin gene, i.e., δ + β thalassemia. In fact, it was clearly shown in one study[126] that the δ and β thalassemias were situated *in trans* to one another and segregated independently in different families. This was not the case, however, in other studies.[123–125] It was once postulated that β thalassemia with normal levels of Hb A_2 might be theoretically caused by a Lepore-like δβ crossover event resulting in a fusion product that was indistinguishable structurally from a normal β globin chain because the crossover occurred at a point before the first amino acid difference between δ and β globin chains.[127] However, recent gene mapping studies have ruled out such a process in a series of patients with normal Hb A_2 β thalassemia.[128]

The last disorder in the category of normal Hb A_2 β thalassemia is γδβ thalassemia, which was first described by Kan and coworkers[129] in a newborn infant with a self-limited hemolytic anemia associated with hypochromia and microcytosis (discussed later). A number of family members were found to have typical thalassemic red cell indices, abnormal morphology, normal levels of Hb A_2 and Hb F, and a β/α synthetic ratio of 0.5 characteristic of heterozygous β thalassemia. The findings suggested that the thalassemia defect in this family involved the γ-, δ-, and β-chain genes on the same chromosome, a theory that was later confirmed when gene mapping studies revealed the presence of an extensive deletion of the non–α globin gene cluster in affected family members[130] (see Chapter 8). The basis for normal levels of Hb A_2 and Hb F is the deletion of the δ and γ globin genes *in cis* to the β-thalassemic globin gene. A number of additional cases of γδβ thalassemia have subsequently been described, associated with different types of large deletions in the γδβ globin gene cluster (see Chapter 8).

Hb Lepore Syndromes

Hb Lepore is composed of two α chains and two abnormal non–α chains, which are δβ fusion chains having the amino acid sequence of the δ chain at their N terminus and that of the β chain at their C terminus.[131] The Lepore globin gene resulted from nonhomologous crossing over between the δ and β globin gene loci (see Chapter 10 and Fig. 10–7). Three different Lepore hemoglobins have been described, which differ by the point at which the crossing over occurred between the δ- and β-chain structural genes (see Table 10–2E).

Hb Lepore is produced at a markedly reduced rate, and in the heterozygote it accounts for only approximately 6 to 15 per cent of the total hemoglobin. Hb Lepore is easily detected by standard hemoglobin electrophoresis, having approximately the same mobility as Hb S (see Fig. 9–4C). Hemoglobin electrophoresis, in addition to the abnormal hemoglobin, reveals low or normal Hb A_2 and, in most cases, slight elevation of Hb F in the range of 2 to 3 per cent. The peripheral blood findings are similar to those of heterozygous high Hb A_2 β thalassemia, with microcytosis, hypochromia, and the usual morphological changes. Homozygosity for Hb Lepore and double heterozygosity for high Hb A_2 β thalassemia and Hb Lepore may be clinically indistinguishable from homozygous high Hb A_2 β thalassemia or may be associated with a milder clinical syndrome analogous to β thalassemia intermedia.[1] The milder clinical course in the latter situation may be related to the fact that Hb Lepore trait is usually associated with a higher level of Hb F than that which is ordinarily seen in high Hb A_2 β-thalassemia trait.[1] In homozygous Hb Lepore, there is no Hb A or Hb A_2, only Hb F (approximately 75 per cent) and Hb Lepore (10 to 20 per cent), because the chromosome bearing the Lepore gene carries no normal δ or β globin genes (see Fig. 10–7).

β Thalassemia Intermedia

A number of different genetic interactions can result in a milder-than-usual clinical course in a patient with homozygous β thalassemia. In general, the term "thalassemia intermedia" is used to describe cases of homozygous (or doubly heterozygous) β thalassemia in which the anemia is not severe enough to require treatment with regular transfusions of red cells. However, the term has also been used to describe severe heterozygous β thalassemia in which there is evidence of inclusion body formation and hemolysis. Table 9–3 lists the various syndromes that have been associated with the clinical picture of β thalassemia intermedia. In general, such a clinical picture is due either to the inheritance of mild β-thalassemia genes or to the co-inheritance of genes for α thalassemia or heterocellular HPFH.

Certain forms of β thalassemia are milder and produce a less severe clinical syndrome in the homozygous (or doubly heterozygous) state than is the case with the usual forms of β thalassemia.[131a] This is especially true of homozygous β$^+$ thalassemia in blacks, which is usually a mild disease.[1] Two different base substitutions in the 5′-flanking DNA of the β globin gene have been found to be associated with mild β$^+$ thalassemia in blacks: one at position −28, by far the most common,[131b] and the other at position −88[131c] (see Chapter 8). Mild β-thalassemia genes have also been characterized in Mediterraneans. These include the "silent carrier" states, including Hb Knossos, described earlier and the β thalassemia associated with two specific mutations of the β globin gene—the base substitution at position 6 of IVS-1[132, 133] and that at position −87 in the 5′-flanking DNA of the gene[132] (see Chapter 8). These β thalassemias are associated, *in vivo* or in various *in vitro* assay systems,[133a] with less reduction of β globin chain synthesis than that observed with the usual forms of β thalassemia. Thus, homozygotes or double heterozygotes presumably manifest less β to α globin chain imbalance, and hence, less inclusion body formation and less hemolysis.

Homozygous δβ thalassemia tends to be

Table 9–3. β THALASSEMIA INTERMEDIA

I. Homozygosity for Two Mild β-Thalassemia Genes or Double Heterozygosity for One Mild Gene and a Gene of Usual Severity
   A. Mild genes associated with less-than-usual impairment of β-chain synthesis
      1. β$^+$ thalassemia in blacks due to mutations at either position -28 or position -88 of 5′-flanking DNA
      2. "Silent carrier" gene
      3. Hb Knossos in Mediterraneans and blacks
      4. β$^+$ thalassemia in Mediterraneans due to mutation at IVS-1 position 6
      5. β$^+$ thalassemia in Mediterraneans due to mutation at position -87 of 5′-flanking DNA
   B. Genes associated wih high levels of Hb F production
      1. δβ thalassemia
      2. Hb Lepore
      3. β^0 thalassemia due to gene deletions in Dutch and black patients
      4. Pancellular HPFH
II. Homozygosity or Double Heterozygosity for β-Thalassemia Genes of Usual Severity but with Co-inheritance of a Modifying Factor
   A. Co-inheritance of α thalassemia
      1. α thalassemia 1
      2. α thalassemia 2
      3. Some cases of the triplicated α locus
      4. Some cases of concomitant Hb H disease
   B. Co-inheritance of heterocellular HPFH
III. Heterozygous β Thalassemia of Unusual Severity
   A. Concomitant heterozygosity or homozygosity for some cases of the triplicated α locus
   B. Hb Indianapolis, a highly unstable β-chain variant
   C. Unknown etiology: syndrome of inclusion body formation and dyserythropoiesis in northern Europeans

relatively mild because the high level of Hb F synthesis associated with this disorder results in less imbalance between α and non–α globin chains. Double heterozygosity for δβ thalassemia and high Hb A$_2$ β thalassemia also produces a disease of intermediate severity[87, 117] for the same reason. As mentioned previously, homozygous or doubly heterozygous Hb Lepore syndromes may also be associated with a clinical course of intermediate severity, perhaps owing to increased Hb F production. The Dutch and black cases of β^0 thalassemia due to deletions in the β globin gene cluster[89–90b] are also associated with increased production of Hb F and a mild clinical phenotype. It appears from these various examples that perturbations caused by even small deletions in the β gene cluster can result in enhanced Hb F production with beneficial clinical consequences. Another cause for increased Hb F synthesis and a milder than usual course in homozygous β thalassemia is the co-inheritance of a gene for the heterocellular type of HPFH,[86, 91–92b] which will be discussed later. Co-inheritance of β thalassemia with pancellular HPFH also results in a mild disorder.[1]

The co-inheritance of α thalassemia together with homozygous β thalassemia will usually result in a clinical picture of β thalassemia intermedia because of the overall decrease in α to non–α globin chain imbalance and the resulting beneficial effect on reducing inclusion body formation. This association was first described by Kan and Nathan[134] in a Mediterranean family in which α thalassemia 1 coexisted with β thalassemia. Double heterozygotes for α thalassemia 1 and β thalassemia had increased Hb A$_2$ levels but β/α synthetic ratios of approximately 1.0, indicating the corrective influence of concomitant α thalassemia on the globin chain imbalance usually observed in heterozygous β thalassemia. The β-thalassemia homozygote who also inherited α thalassemia 1 had a hemoglobin level of 10.0 g/dl with 40 per cent Hb F and did not require regular transfusions. A number of similar cases were subsequently described by others.[91, 135]

With the ease of detection of both α thalassemia 2 and α thalassemia 1 by gene mapping techniques, it has been possible to screen the DNA of large numbers of individuals with β thalassemia intermedia and to show the high frequency of co-inheritance of α thalassemia in this syndrome.[132, 136–139] A somewhat surprising finding has been the association not only of α thalassemia 1 but also of α thalassemia 2 with homozygous β thalassemia intermedia.[132, 136–137, 139] It therefore appears that even a very small decrease in α globin chain synthesis can have a beneficial effect on the clinical course of homozygous β thalassemia. In a study from Sardinia,[140] it was found that the incidence of heterozygosity and especially homozygosity for α thalassemia 2 was much higher in β-thalassemia homozygotes than in the general population, suggesting a beneficial effect of the co-inheritance of α thalassemia on the clinical course and survival of patients with homozygous β thalassemia. However, the patients were not characterized from the point of view of transfusion dependence or other clinical criteria of β thalassemia intermedia.

The co-inheritance of homozygous β thalassemia with a chromosome bearing three α globin genes instead of the usual two loci has also been found to be associated in some cases with a milder-than-usual clinical course consistent with β thalassemia intermedia.[140a] This surprising result, which is the opposite of what one would have expected, strongly suggests that, at least in some cases, the triplicated α globin gene complex may be defective in its overall output of α globin mRNA and may constitute a form of mild α thalassemia. Most individuals who co-inherit a triplicated α locus together with β-thalassemia trait are phenotypically indistinguishable from simple β-thalassemia heterozygotes.[140a, 140b] However, there are reports of β-thalassemia heterozygotes who co-inherited either one[140c] or two[140b, 140d] triplicated α loci and manifested a more severe clinical syndrome consistent with β thalassemia intermedia. In these cases, α globin chain production directed by the triplicated α gene complex must be actually increased above normal.[140b]

The doubly heterozygous state for β thalassemia and α thalassemia is also worthy of further comment. Studies utilizing gene mapping techniques for the identification of α-thalassemia genotypes have revealed that patients who co-inherit heterozygous β thalassemia and α thalassemia 2 in either the heterozygous (−α/αα) or homozygous (−α/−α) state have much milder hematologic abnormalties than patients with simple heterozygous β thalassemia: There is less anemia, less hypochromia, and less microcytosis, together with a more balanced β/α globin chain synthetic ratio.[141–142a] In some cases, the red blood cells can actually have normal indices, but an elevated Hb A_2 level will still allow the diagnosis of heterozygous β thalassemia to be made.[141–142a] These findings point out the difficulty of relying on the MCV alone as a screening test for heterozygous β thalassemia and may explain the basis for some of the "mild" or "silent" β-thalassemia alleles that have been reported in the literature.

Conversely, patients with the α-thalassemia syndrome of Hb H disease who also inherit a β-thalassemia gene have less Hb H formation and less anemia than patients with simple Hb H disease.[1, 134] The co-inheritance of homozygous β thalassemia together with the genotype for Hb H disease has also been reported.[143, 144] The condition was characterized by markedly hypochromic red cells, nearly balanced α/β globin chain synthesis, and a clinical picture that could be characterized as β thalassemia intermedia in some cases[143] but as β thalassemia major in others.[144]

Finally, in a discussion of thalassemia intermedia, one should include cases of heterozygous β thalassemia of unusual severity associated with inclusion body formation and hemolysis or with features of dyserythropoietic anemia. Such cases are rare and have usually been identified in northern Europeans and individuals of other racial groups in which thalassemia is generally rare.[81–84, 145–147] In most cases, the basis for the disorder is not known. Although β/α globin chain synthetic ratios in peripheral blood cells have been found to be similar to those observed in the usual form of heterozygous β thalassemia, the ratios measured in bone marrow cells were 0.7 to 0.8 instead of the usual 1.0,[82, 83, 145, 146] perhaps indicating a greater degree of globin-chain synthetic imbalance or impaired proteolysis of excess α chains. In the family described by Weatherall and coworkers,[145] it was proposed, on the basis of the lack of hypochromia, that the disorder might have resulted from a primary increase in α-chain synthesis in the presence of normal levels of β-chain production. In one family,[84] it was clearly shown that the heterozygous β-thalassemia phenotype with hemolysis was due to a highly unstable hemoglobin variant, Hb Indianapolis, that was degraded so rapidly that it did not accumulate to any appreciable degree within red cells, thus leading to hypochromia and a thalassemia phenotype (see Chapter 8).

Interaction of Thalassemia with Abnormal Hemoglobins

When a patient acquires a thalassemia gene for a given globin chain on one chromosome and a gene for a structural variant of the same type of globin chain on the other chromosome, the percentage of the structurally abnormal hemoglobin observed is increased over the level found in a simple heterozygote for the structural variant, and the clinical severity of the condition approaches that of homozygosity for the abnormal hemoglobin (so-called interacting thalassemia). On the other hand, when a patient inherits the combination of thalassemia for one type of globin chain (i.e., β) and a gene for a structural variant of the other type of globin chain (i.e., α), no increase in the abnormal hemoglobin is observed, and the clinical manifestations of the condition are similar to those of the heterozygous state for the structural variant (non-interacting thalassemia). In fact, when α thalassemia is co-inherited with a gene for a β-chain structural variant (and vice versa), the amount of the abnormal hemoglobin observed is usually less than in the simple heterozygous state for the variant. Post-translational assembly of globin-chain subunits is responsible for the latter phenomenon (see Chapter 10): In the face of limiting amounts of the opposite globin chain, the mutant subunits cannot compete as effectively as usual with the normal subunits for the reduced numbers of the complementing globin chains. In addition to the finding of the abnormal hemoglobin, the common feature in all of these syndromes is hypochromia and microcytosis of the red cells, as in thalassemia trait. Only the clinically or genetically important combinations will be briefly described here.

β Thalassemia in Association with β-Chain Structural Variants

Sickle Cell/β Thalassemia. This disorder is described in more detail in Chapter 12. Hb S/β thalassemia primarily affects people of African and Mediterranean ancestry. The clinical picture resembles that of sickle cell anemia, but the disease in general tends to run a milder course. Splenomegaly is a common feature and is helpful in differentiating Hb S/β thalassemia from sickle cell anemia in older children and adults. Occasionally, the disease can be extremely mild, and the diagnosis may be discovered as an incidental finding. Hb S/β$^+$ thalassemia is generaly a much milder disorder than Hb S/β^0 thalassemia (see Table 12–5).

Laboratory findings include a variable degree of anemia accompanied by targeting, hypochromia, and microcytosis of the red cells as well as occasional irreversibly sickled forms in the blood smear of the more severely affected patients (see Color Plate 2F). Hemoglobin electrophoresis reveals 60 to 90 per cent Hb S, 0 to 30 per cent Hb A, increased levels of Hb A_2, and 1 to 15 per cent Hb F (see Table 12–4 and Fig. 12–18).

Hb C/β Thalassemia. This condition occurs mainly in blacks and is associated with a mild anemia. The blood smear is characterized by hypochromia and pronounced targeting of the red cells (see Color Plate 3H). Hemoglobin electrophoresis reveals 65 to 80 per cent Hb C, with the remainder being made up of Hb A (in Hb C/β$^+$ thalassemia) and a low level of Hb F (2 to 5 per cent). Hb C/β^0 thalassemia is less common and is associated with a more severe anemia and splenomegaly; Hb A is totally absent on hemoglobin electrophoresis.

Hb E/β Thalassemia. This is a common disease in Thailand and Southeast Asia. For reasons that are poorly understood, it is almost as severe as homozygous β thalassemia. As discussed in Chapter 8, Hb E is itself associated with a β-thalassemia phenotype because of decreased β^E-chain synthesis due to decreased functional β^E mRNA formation secondary to abnormal processing of the β^E precursor globin mRNA. However, the overall deficit in globin synthesis in homozygous Hb E is about equivalent to that in heterozygous β thalassemia, and homozygous Hb E is a benign disorder. It is therefore difficult to understand why double heterozygosity for Hb E and β thalassemia should be so severe a condition. One would expect instead a thalassemia intermedia syndrome as occurs in double heterozygosity for a mild β-thalassemia gene and a β-thalassemia gene of standard severity. It has been suggested[1] that since Hb E is oxidatively unstable, the greater excess of α chains generated in the doubly heterozygous state (compared with homozygous Hb E) might provide a sufficient oxidative stress to cause accelerated denaturation and precipitation of Hb E and increased hemolysis on that basis.

The hematological findings are similar to those in homozygous β thalassemia (see Color Plate 3E). Hemoglobin electrophoresis shows Hb E, a high percentage of Hb F (approximately 50 per cent), and usually no Hb A, since most cases are associated with β^0 thalassemia.

α Thalassemia in Association with α- and β-Chain Structural Variants

Hb Q/α Thalassemia. This condition is also found mainly in Thailand and Southeast Asia. The clinical picture is similar to that of Hb H disease. This syndrome is of interest mainly because of the associated hemoglobin electrophoresis findings. The affected individuals display a total absence of Hb A, a finding that was initially interpreted (and later proved by gene mapping studies [see Chapter 8]) to indicate that the α gene *in cis* to the α^Q gene is deleted ($-\alpha^Q/$) and that the α^Q gene behaves as an α thalassemia 2 determinant. Thus, affected individuals with Hb H disease have the genotype ($- -/- \alpha^Q$).

Hb G[Philadelphia]**/α Thalassemia.** Hb G[Philadelphia] is an α-chain variant that occurs predominantly in blacks and, like Hb Q, is usually associated with deletion of the linked α globin gene *in cis* ($- \alpha^G/$) (see Chapter 8), which accounts for the different amounts of Hb G observed in heterozygotes.[148–150a] Since the α thalassemia 1 chromosome ($- -/$) is rare in blacks, Hb H disease with Hb G has been described in only two families[1]; in both cases, there was total absence of Hb A, consistent with the genotype ($- -/- \alpha^G$). On the other hand, double heterozygosity for Hb G[Philadelphia] and α thalassemia 2 ($- \alpha^G/- \alpha$) is much more common and accounts for the differences in the percentage of Hb G[Philadelphia] observed in affected individuals: Double heterozygotes ($- \alpha^G/- \alpha$) have levels of approximately 40 per cent Hb G, whereas simple heterozygotes ($- \alpha^G/\alpha\alpha$) have levels of approximately 30 per cent Hb G.[149–150a] Rare individuals have been identified in whom the α^G gene is not associated with a deletion of the linked α gene *in cis*.[150b, 150c] Such individuals, with the genotype ($\alpha\alpha^G/\alpha\alpha$), have even lower levels of Hb G, in the range of 20 per cent.

Hb S/α Thalassemia. This combination of hemoglobinopathies is of interest because of the effects that associated α thalassemia has on the amount of Hb S that accumulates in SA heterozygotes and on the clinical features of Hb SS disease.

It was initially recognized by a number of workers[151–153] that individuals who inherited a phenotype of α thalassemia 1 as well as heterozygosity for Hb S had levels of Hb S that were lower than in simple SA heterozygotes: 25 to 35 per cent versus 40 to 45 per cent. It was subsequently shown that the low level of Hb S is due to post-translational turnover of β^S chains that cannot compete as efficiently as β^A chains for the limited pool of available α chains (see Chapter 10). The use of gene mapping studies for the identification of α thalassemia has confirmed the correlation between the percentage of Hb S and α globin gene number in Hb S heterozygotes: Individuals with four α globin genes generally have >36 per cent Hb S; those with three α genes have 30 to 36 per cent Hb S; and those with two α genes have <30 per cent Hb S.[154–156]

There is some controversy concerning the role of concomitant α thalassemia as a modifier of the clinical severity of homozygous Hb S disease (see Chapter 12). Although it is generally agreed that the degree of anemia, hemolysis, and other red cell abnormalities are less in SS or SC patients with concomitant homozygous α thalassemia 2 than in patients without α thalassemia,[157–159c] there is conflicting evidence concerning the issue of whether or not the association leads to a milder clinical course from the point of view of vaso-occlusive phenomena. In one study,[157] patients with associated homozygous α thalassemia 2 had fewer episodes of acute chest syndrome and chronic leg ulceration, but in another study,[159] α thalassemia did not appear to provide any protection from the vaso-occlusive complications of Hb SS disease. It has been proposed that the decreased hemolysis and increased number of circulating red cells that are associated with co-inheritance of homozygous α thalassemia 2 can have a deleterious effect on the rheology of the red cells in homozygous SS disease,[159] although in one study[160] the rheological properties of the red cells *in vitro* were actually improved in the presence of concomitant homozygous α thalassemia 2. In a population survey in Africa and the United States, it was found that patients with SS disease had a higher incidence of heterozygous and homozygous α thalassemia 2 than in the general population and that the frequency of this association was higher in the older age groups.[161] These findings suggested an association between concomitant α thalassemia and a longer life expectancy in homozygous SS disease.

γδβ AND γ THALASSEMIA

As mentioned earlier, γδβ thalassemia was first described in an infant with hemolytic disease of the newborn associated with hypochromic microcytic red cells.[129] Heterozygous β thalassemia, with normal levels of Hb A_2 and Hb F, was found in the father and many of his relatives. Globin-chain synthesis studies revealed a decrease in γ- and β-chain synthesis in the reticulocytes of this infant. The disease was self-limited: As the baby grew older, the hemolytic anemia resolved, and the child developed the phenotype of simple heterozygous β thalassemia. It was believed that this child represented an example of heterozygous γδβ thalassemia, and this hypothesis was later confirmed by gene mapping studies[130] (see Chapter 8). The disease should be suspected in cases of hypochromic hemolytic disease in the newborn. A number of clinically similar cases have been subsequently described,[162–164] associated with deletions of different extents in the non–α globin gene cluster (see Fig. 8–17B).

Cases of isolated γ thalassemia have also been described. These have usually been identified by an abnormal ratio of $^G\gamma$ to $^A\gamma$ globin chains detected during the course of cord blood screening surveys. Thus, infants from various racial groups have been identified who have unexpectedly low or absent levels of $^G\gamma$ globin chains.[165] Two infants, one Chinese and one Asian Indian, were found to have total absence of $^G\gamma$ globin chains; the Indian case was found to be associated with a gene deletion resulting from nonhomologous crossing over between the $^G\gamma$ and $^A\gamma$ globin loci (see Chapter 8). Infants with total absence of $^G\gamma$ globin chains, resulting from homozygosity for this form of $^G\gamma$ thalassemia, are clinically asymptomatic: they have lower-than-normal levels of Hb F in cord blood, but no significant anemia,[165] even though $^G\gamma$ globin chains are the predominant γ chains synthesized in newborns. These infants in fact synthesize a fused γ globin chain having the C-terminal end of the $^A\gamma$ chain but the N-terminal end of the $^G\gamma$ chain, presumably under the control of the $^G\gamma$ globin gene promoter and thus programmed to be expressed at higher levels than the authentic $^A\gamma$ globin gene.

Not all individuals with abnormal ratios of $^G\gamma$ to $^A\gamma$ chains have γ thalassemia. In some instances, abnormal ratios result from the inheritance of unusual $^G\gamma$-$^G\gamma$ or $^A\gamma$-$^A\gamma$ alleles caused either by point mutations or limited gene conversion events[166] (see Chapter 7).

Homozygosity for a form of γ thalassemia affecting both γ globin genes (such as γδβ thalassemia) would be expected to be fatal *in utero* and has not yet been documented.

δ THALASSEMIA

Isolated δ thalassemia has been described as an incidental finding in both the heterozygous[167] and homozygous forms.[168–169] The latter condition is especially prevalent in Japan. In the heterozygote, there is decreased Hb A_2; in the homozygote, total absence of Hb A_2 is noted. In neither situation are hypochromia, anemia, or red cell morphological changes observed. The doubly heterozygous state for δ thalassemia plus δβ thalassemia[170] and δ thalassemia plus HPFH[171] has also been described and is clinically similar to simple heterozygosity for δβ thalassemia or HPFH except that there is total absence of Hb A_2. Although these various reports indicate that δ thalassemia is frequently of the δ^0 type, a form of δ^+ with reduced rather than absent Hb A_2 in homozygotes has been described in Sardinians.[172] As mentioned previously, the concomitant inheritance of heterozygous δ + β thalassemia results in a β-thalassemia trait phenotype with normal levels of Hb A_2.[123–126] It is noteworthy in this regard that low or normal levels of Hb A_2, caused by the presence of a linked δ^0 thalassemia, have been found to be associated with the gene for Hb Knossos, a β-chain variant that behaves as a mild β-thalassemia allele.[125a–125c] The linked δ^0 thalassemia is found in Mediterranean patients but not black patients with Hb Knossos,[125d, 125e] indicating probable separate origins of the mutations in these two populations.

HEREDITARY PERSISTENCE OF FETAL HEMOGLOBIN (HPFH) AND RELATED DISORDERS

The term "hereditary persistence of fetal hemoglobin" or HPFH, is used to describe a heterogeneous group of inherited disorders characterized by increased levels of Hb F in the absence of the usual clinical and hematological features of thalassemia. The disorder can be broadly classified into two categories: (1) pancellular HPFH, in which all of the red cells of affected individuals contain increased levels of Hb F; and (2) heterocellular HPFH, in which only a subpopulation of red cells contains Hb F.

The strict classification of HPFH disorders into one category or the other is sometimes difficult and depends on some degree on the technique used to determine the distribution of Hb F among red cells, i.e., the acid elution procedure of Betke and Kleihauer or immunofluorescence using anti–Hb F antibodies. In some cases, what may appear to be heterocellular distribution of Hb F by the acid elution technique could be interpreted as pancellular by immunofluorescence because of the increased sensitivity of the latter technique. Nevertheless, a number of relatively well-defined syndromes have been characterized within the traditional classification.

Pancellular HPFH in Blacks

$^G\gamma^A\gamma(\delta\beta)^0$ HPFH

The most common variety of HPFH in blacks is associated with the synthesis of both

$^G\gamma$ and $^A\gamma$ globin chains of Hb F, in the usual "adult" ratio of approximately 2:3 and with total absence of δ and β globin gene expression *in cis* to the HPFH gene, thus the designation $^G\gamma^A\gamma(\delta\beta)^0$ HPFH. Heterozygotes are characterized by the presence of approximately 30 per cent Hb F, which is relatively uniformly distributed among the red cells, although after acid elution there is some variability from cell to cell in the intensity of staining of the residual Hb F (see Fig. 9–4*B*). Hemoglobin levels, red cell indices, red cell morphology, and α/non–α globin chain synthetic ratios are all essentially within normal limits.[173–176] In homozygotes, there is 100 per cent Hb F without detectable Hb A or Hb A_2. In contrast to homozygous δβ thalassemia, however, there is no anemia, and there may even be a slight degree of polycythemia, presumably because of the hypoxic stress resulting from the increased oxygen affinity of the red cells. Although, by definition, HPFH is not supposed to be associated with thalassemic characteristics, it must be pointed out that homozygosity for this form of HPFH does share some features in common with mild β thalassemia: In HPFH homozygotes, the γ/α globin chain synthetic ratio is approximately 0.5,[177, 178] a value similar to the β/α ratio in heterozygous β thalassemia; the red cells of HPFH homozygotes are also slightly microcytic and hypochromic. Despite the presence of 100 per cent Hb F, the red cells of homozygotes do not have the other characteristics of fetal red cells such as "i" antigen expression and low carbonic anhydrase levels.[178] It is therefore inaccurate to consider this condition as a failure of the physiologic fetal to adult "switch." If this were the case, the overall fetal erythroid cell pattern of protein synthesis should persist and the $^G\gamma$ and $^A\gamma$ genes should be expressed in the "fetal" ratio of 3:2 rather than the "adult" ratio of 2:3. As discussed in Chapter 8, this condition is caused by at least three different extensive deletions of DNA in the non–α globin gene cluster. The pattern of γ gene expression varies somewhat in the three different deletion syndromes with regard to the ratio of $^G\gamma$ to $^A\gamma$ globin gene expression: The percentage of $^G\gamma$ chains averages 69, 51, and 32 per cent, respectively, in the three different syndromes.[179] Even in homozygotes, this condition is essentially asymptomatic and is usually discovered by chance during the course of family studies or population surveys.

In association with Hb S, this type of HPFH gives hemoglobin electrophoresis findings similar to those found in Hb S/$β^0$ thalassemia or homozygous sickle cell anemia but with an unusually high level of Hb F: absent Hb A, decreased Hb A_2, 70 to 80 per cent Hb S, and 20 to 30 per cent Hb F (see Table 12–4). Clinically, however, this disorder is benign, with no anemia, hemolysis, hypochromia, or painful crises. The benign nature of this disorder is no doubt related to the fact that the Hb F is relatively evenly distributed among the red cells and thus is present in all cells in sufficient amounts to inhibit or reduce the polymerization of Hb S within the usual physiologic range of oxygen desaturation experienced by affected individuals (see Chapter 12).

$^G\gamma\beta^+$ HPFH

A less common form of pancellular HPFH found in blacks is associated with increased synthesis of essentially only the $^G\gamma$ globin chain of Hb F without total loss of activity of the linked β globin gene *in cis*, as evidenced by the synthesis of both Hb A and Hb S or Hb C in double heterozygotes who inherit this form of HPFH together with the gene for those β-chain variants *in trans*.[180–184] The amount of Hb F in heterozygotes is somewhat less than in $^G\gamma^A\gamma(\delta\beta)^0$ HPFH and ranges between 15 and 20 per cent. In double heterozygotes for $^G\gamma\beta^+$ HPFH and Hb S, there is approximately 45 per cent Hb S and 35 per cent Hb A in addition to the 20 per cent Hb F. Thus, in contrast to patients with Hb S trait, there is more Hb S than Hb A. It has been calculated that Hb A accumulation is approximately half of normal.[181] Therefore, it appears that the $β^A$ gene *in cis* to the $^G\gamma\beta^+$ HPFH determinant is hypoactive or negatively regulated in a manner to ensure that the total output of the non–α (γ + β) globin genes on the affected chromosome does not exceed that of the normal $β^A$ globin gene in adults. However, it has not yet been determined whether the linked $β^A$ globin gene is totally normal structurally or possibly affected by a mild $β^+$-thalassemia mutation. In contrast to $^G\gamma^A\gamma(\delta\beta)^0$ HPFH, there are no deletions within the non–α globin gene cluster in this syndrome, and its molecular basis appears to be a single nucleotide base substitution in the 5′-flanking of the $^G\gamma$ gene that allows increased expression of the gene (see Chapter 8). As in the case of $^G\gamma^A\gamma$ HPFH, this condition is clinically benign and is not associated with hematological abnormalities of the red cells. Homozygotes have not yet been identified.

Hb Kenya

Hb Kenya is an abnormal hemoglobin found in blacks that is associated with an HPFH phenotype[185–189] and that has provided the basis for certain models on the regulation of γ globin gene expression (see Chapter 8). The non–α chain of Hb Kenya consists of a fusion product containing the N terminus of the γ chain and the C terminus of the β chain, the result of nonhomologous crossing over between the $^A\gamma$ globin gene and the β globin gene (see Fig. 10–7). The crossover from γ to β sequence occurred between residues 81 and 86 of the γ chain, i.e, before position 136 that distinguishes $^A\gamma$ from $^G\gamma$ globin chains. Thus, it was not possible to tell from the structure of Hb Kenya alone whether the $^A\gamma$ or $^G\gamma$ gene was involved in the crossover event. However, individuals with Hb Kenya had increased levels of Hb F in their red cells that was all of the $^G\gamma$ type, and it was assumed that this Hb F was in all likelihood derived from the $^G\gamma$ globin gene *in cis* to the Kenya gene. Therefore, the 5' end of the Kenya γδ globin gene was thought to be derived from the $^A\gamma$ gene. Gene mapping studies subsequently confirmed the postulated crossover and demonstrated deletion of the inter–$^A\gamma\beta$ globin gene DNA.[190]

Hb Kenya, unlike Hb Lepore, is not associated with a β-thalassemic phenotype but rather a phenotype of pancellular HPFH. Hb Kenya has been found in the simple heterozygous state as well as in association with Hb S; homozygotes have not yet been identified. In the simple heterozygote, Hb Kenya usually composes approximately 7 to 12 per cent of the total hemoglobin,[186, 187] although in some cases it can account for 20 to 23 per cent of the total.[187, 188] Double heterozygotes for Hb S and Hb Kenya have 62 to 69 per cent Hb S and 17 to 19 per cent Hb Kenya.[186] All of the affected individuals are essentially asymptomatic. There is no hypochromia, microcytosis, or morphological abnormalities of the red cells. In all cases, Hb F is elevated in the range of 5 to 10 percent, and is uniformly distributed among the red cells.[186–188] As noted previously, it is exclusively of the $^G\gamma$ type.[186, 187] Unlike the situation in the Hb Lepore and anti–Lepore syndromes, the synthesis of the fused Kenya globin chain is active in reticulocytes, and there is balanced α/non–α globin chain synthesis.[189]

As discussed in Chapter 8, the phenotype of HPFH associated with the Hb Kenya crossover and its resulting DNA deletion has been used to support the theory for the presence of regulatory sequences in the inter–γβ globin gene region, the deletion of which would prevent the normal postnatal suppression of γ globin gene expression.

Greek HPFH: $^A\gamma$ HPFH

A form of pancellular HPFH has been identified in Greek individuals that is characterized by increased levels of Hb F in the range of 10 to 20 per cent, approximately 90 per cent of which is of the $^A\gamma$ type.[191–194] As in other types of HPFH, individuals are asymptomatic, and the red cells manifest normal hematological features[191, 193, 194] and balanced or nearly balanced α/non–α globin chain synthesis.[193–195] This condition has not yet been identified in the homozygous state or in association with β-chain structural variants *in trans*; thus, it was not possible to definitely ascertain whether the β^A globin gene *in cis* to the HPFH determinant was active or inactive. However, a number of individuals have been described who are doubly heterozygous for β thalassemia and this type of HPFH.[191, 193, 194] Such individuals have mild anemia (a hemoglobin level of 9 to 11 g/dl) with hypochromia and microcytosis. Hemoglobin electrophoresis reveals 25 to 45 per cent Hb F, 4 to 5 per cent Hb A_2, and the remainder Hb A. Globin-chain synthesis studies reveal somewhat more α/non–α globin chain synthesis imbalance than observed in simple β-thalassemia heterozygotes, indicating that the HPFH chromosome does not have a totally normal output of non–α globin chains. By calculating the total amount of Hb A per cell in such double heterozygotes, it is possible to ascertain that the Hb A content is too high to be derived solely from a β^+-thalassemia allele *in trans* to the $^A\gamma$ HPFH allele.[1] It is also likely that some of these double heterozygotes carry a gene for β^0 thalassemia, a conclusion that has been subsequently confirmed by molecular analyses in some cases (see Chapter 8). Thus, the Hb A in such double heterozygotes must be derived from the β gene *in cis* to the HPFH determinant. Hemoglobin synthesis in erythroid colonies grown *in vitro* from affected individuals reveals a substantial amount of $^G\gamma$ globin chain production, indicating that the $^G\gamma$ gene *in cis*, like that *in trans* to the HPFH determinant, is probably capable of normal function.[196] As discussed in Chapter 8, gene mapping studies have failed to reveal any evidence of gene deletions in this disorder, but gene cloning and sequence analysis have revealed a base substitution in the 5'-flanking

DNA of the $^A\gamma$ gene that is probably responsible for the disorder.

A similar disorder has been identified in a Chinese family,[184] but in this family, the Hb F was somewhat less elevated than in the Greek cases, with levels of only 10 to 14 per cent. Nevertheless, the Hb F was distributed in a pancellular (or quasi-pancellular) fashion and was predominantly of the $^A\gamma$ globin type. As in the Greek cases, gene mapping studies failed to reveal the presence of any gene deletion or rearrangement.[184]

Heterocellular HPFH

In contrast to the disorders just described, a number of conditions have been characterized in which there is an elevated level of Hb F that is distributed in only a subpopulation of the red cells. This group of conditions has been called heterocellular HPFH.[197] In general, the levels of Hb F are lower than in the pancellular disorders, ranging between 2 and 10 per cent of the total hemoglobin. This condition is rather heterogeneous from the point of view of the overall Hb F levels as well as the relative amounts of the $^G\gamma$ and $^A\gamma$ subtypes of Hb F present in red cells of affected individuals. In some cases, Hb F levels are only slightly elevated and could simply represent normal variation of Hb F and F-cell numbers at the high end of the bell-shaped curve of distribution of normal values in the general population. In other cases, however, the Hb F is clearly elevated and consists predominantly of only one subtype of Hb F, so that it is difficult to escape the conclusion that one is dealing with a clear-cut genetic abnormality.

Genetics of Normal Hb F Levels in Adults

In normal adults, Hb F rarely exceeds 1 per cent of the total Hb, and rather than being distributed uniformly among all red cells, it is found only in a minor subpopulation of red cells, called F cells, that make up approximately 1 to 7 per cent of the total red cell population.[197–200] It is clear, however, that the level of Hb F and F cells in a given individual is relatively constant and under genetic control, being transmissible as an autosomal trait within a given family.[197–200b] Therefore, the number of F cells and hence the Hb F levels in normal adults appear to be under genetic control. Abnormalities of these genes may be responsible for some if not all types of heterocellular HPFH.

Swiss-Type Heterocellular HPFH

This condition is characterized by only slightly elevated levels of Hb F, usually in the range of 2 to 3 per cent or slightly higher. It was first described by Marti[201] in a survey of Swiss army personnel and has been identified subsequently in a number of racial groups, including blacks and Mediterraneans.[1] The Hb F contains both $^G\gamma$ and $^A\gamma$ subtypes of γ globin chains, and the increased levels of Hb F are inherited in an autosomal dominant fashion. Individuals are asymptomatic, and there are no other hematological abnormalities. The condition appears to represent a continuum within the normal pattern of Hb F and F-cell inheritance, with the only difference being the quantitative levels of Hb F and F cells that are significantly above "normal."

This condition is of particular interest because it may be found linked *in cis* on chromosome 11 to a gene for β thalassemia or sickle hemoglobin.[1] In such cases, the inheritance *in trans* of a second gene for β thalassemia[86, 91, 92c] or sickle hemoglobin[202, 203] is associated with a clinical syndrome of less severity than in the usual cases of homozygous β thalassemia, Hb S/β thalassemia, or sickle cell anemia because of the synthesis of increased levels of Hb F (in the range of 19 to 30 per cent for patients with SS/heterocellular HPFH)[202–204] that can modulate the severity of the pathophysiology of the homozygous disorder.

Studies of families in which this form of heterocellular HPFH occurs in association with Hb S or β thalassemia have allowed an assessment of the closeness of the linkage between the heterocellular HPFH gene and the β globin gene locus.[1] Three crossover or recombination events between the two loci were observed in 27 opportunities, indicating that the two loci are not as tightly linked to one another as are the non-α globin genes to each other. Gene mapping studies in a family with one such recombination event indicated that the heterocellular HPFH determinant was located outside of the immediate non-α globin gene cluster.[205] However, not all heterocellular HPFH determinants are linked, even remotely, to the β gene cluster on chromsome 11, as illustrated by gene mapping studies in another family[206] that showed no linkage whatsoever of the heterocellular HPFH determinant to the non–α globin gene complex. In another family demonstrating lack of linkage of the HPFH determinant to the β gene cluster, the presence of a polymorphic variant of the $^A\gamma$ chain (the $^A\gamma^T$ chain [see Chapter 4]) allowed the demonstration that the increased γ-chain synthesis caused by the HPFH determinant was directed by both chromosomes.[92b]

Other Forms of Heterocellular HPFH in Blacks

Somewhat different forms of heterocellular HPFH have also been described in individual black families and are referred to in the literature according to the city or state of origin of the cases: Georgia-type,[207] Atlanta-type,[208] and Seattle-type[209] heterocellular HPFH. In general, the Hb F levels are somewhat higher than in Swiss-type heterocellular HPFH, reaching 6 to 8 per cent in some cases. In the Georgia and Atlanta families, the Hb F was predominantly or exclusively of the $^G\gamma$ type, whereas in the Seattle family, there were roughly equal amounts of the $^G\gamma$ and $^A\gamma$ subtypes of Hb F, in a fashion analogous to Swiss-type heterocellular HPFH but with somewhat higher levels of Hb F.

In the case of the Atlanta-type HPFH, also called $^G\gamma\beta^+$ HPFH with low levels of Hb F, the probable cause of the disorder is the inheritance of a $^G\gamma$-$^G\gamma$ chromosome with a haplotype of restriction fragment length polymorphisms that is associated with high levels of $^G\gamma$ gene expression[209a] (see Chapter 8).

British-Type Heterocellular HPFH

This disorder, originally described by Weatherall and coworkers in a large family of Anglo-Saxon ancestry,[210] is characterized in heterozygotes by the presence of 3.5 to 10 per cent Hb F, approximately 90 per cent of which is of the $^A\gamma$ type, clearly distinguishing this type of heterocellular HPFH from the other varieties described previously. Three individuals apparently homozygous for the disorder had Hb F levels of 18 to 21 per cent, with the high level of Hb A indicating good activity of the β^A globin gene linked *in cis* to the HPFH determinant; Hb A_2, although present, was significantly reduced (<2 per cent). The condition is clinically benign, and the red blood cells manifest no hematological abnormalities or imbalance in α/non–α globin chain synthesis. Globin gene mapping studies of restriction fragment length polymorphisms within the non–α globin gene cluster (see Chapters 7 and 8) clearly demonstrated linkage of this disorder to the β globin gene complex.[205] This disorder is clearly distinguished from the Greek type of $^A\gamma$ HPFH by the lower levels and more uneven distribution of Hb F.

Wood and coworkers[211] studied the postnatal changes in Hb F in two heterozygotes as well as the pattern of hemoglobin synthesis in erythroid colonies grown *in vitro* from affected individuals. They observed normal levels of Hb F and normal ratios of $^G\gamma/^A\gamma$ globin chain synthesis at birth with a delayed decline in Hb F levels with age as well as a parallel decline in the proportion of $^G\gamma$ chains. Hemoglobin synthesis in erythroid colonies of both heterozygotes and homozygotes showed the normal pattern of asynchrony between γ- and β-chain synthesis but with an overall increase in γ-chain production compared with normal. It was concluded from these studies that the defect in the British type of heterocellular HPFH must involve an abnormality in the regulatory mechanisms for postnatal repression of γ-chain synthesis.[211]

The Saudi High Hb F Determinant

Population surveys in Saudi Arabia have revealed a group of homozygous sickle cell anemia patients with an unusually mild clinical course[212, 213] associated with high levels of Hb F, in the range of 25 to 40 per cent[204, 212–215] (see Chapter 12). A similar syndrome has also been described in certain Asian Indian individuals with sickle cell anemia.[216, 217] However, in contrast to American or Jamaican blacks with SS disease and high levels of Hb F, one cannot usually identify in the Saudi or Indian families a parent with slight elevation of Hb F consistent with the Swiss type of heterocellular HPFH.[214, 217] The nature of this high Hb F determinant is obscure. Since there is no definite phenotypic expression in heterozygotes, the condition cannot be properly called a form of hereditary persistence of fetal hemoglobin. Nevertheless, it is clear that the Saudi SS patients synthesize more γ globin chains than patients of African origin.[215]

The same phenomenon of unexpectedly high levels of Hb F occurs in Saudi patients with Hb S/β^0 thalassemia[218] and thus is not restricted to homozygous Hb SS disease. Although Saudi heterozygotes for Hb S do not have increased levels of Hb F, they do have, on average, slightly elevated numbers of F cells.[214] Thus, during the course of cell selection that occurs with the hemolysis in Hb SS disease and in Hb S/β thalassemia, higher-than-usual levels of Hb F may accumulate in affected Saudis as a result of cell selection acting on a larger than usual pool of F cells, which may be expanded even further in response to the anemic stress of the sickling disorder[1] (see Chapter 11). It has also been demonstrated that the erythroid progenitor cells of affected individuals have a program for the production of higher-than-normal levels of Hb F in their progeny erythroblasts, as evidenced by quantitative measurements of Hb F in BFU-E–derived colonies grown in culture.[218a]

MANAGEMENT OF THE THALASSEMIA SYNDROMES

Prevention

An important step in the prevention of the occurrence of severely affected children with homozygous α or β thalassemia is the detection of the heterozygous state in adults of reproductive age. Physicians should be aware of the possibility of thalassemia trait occurring in individuals with hypochromic anemias that are refractory to iron therapy and should perform the necessary diagnostic studies to confirm the diagnosis. In areas where there is a high incidence of thalassemia trait, general population screening surveys can be established. Once identified, the affected individuals can be educated and counseled with respect to the disease process and its genetics. Two affected heterozygotes contemplating marriage and planning to have a family should be aware of the one-in-four chance of having a severely affected homozygous child. Although such information will rarely alter the reproductive behavior of couples at risk of having homozygous infants, the counseling and education of such couples should include information concerning the availability of prenatal diagnosis for homozygous β thalassemia.

Prenatal diagnosis of hemoglobinopathies has undergone many changes over the last decade. Recent advances have elucidated the molecular basis of the thalassemias and led to the application of this newly gained knowledge to prenatal diagnosis of thalassemia at the DNA level (see Chapter 8).

Before the availability of DNA-based diagnosis, prenatal diagnosis of thalassemia required fetal blood sampling at 18 to 20 weeks of gestation and analysis of globin-chain synthesis by isotopic labeling and globin-chain separation to identify the abnormality of globin-chain synthesis. A fetal blood sample can be obtained in one of two ways: (1) "blind" needle aspiration of the placenta after localizing its position by ultrasound[219]; or (2) needle aspiration of a placental blood vessel (when the placenta is in a posterior or fundal position) under direct visualization using an amnioscope or fetoscope.[220, 221] The procedure is not totally safe. In a few cases, fetal loss has occurred owing to infection, hemorrhage, premature labor, or undetermined causes.[222, 223] It is estimated from large surveys of the worldwide experience with this procedure that even in the best of hands, there exists a risk of death or serious injury to the fetus on the order of approximately 5 to 10 per cent,[224–227a] a much higher risk than that associated with amniocentesis.

In the early years, it was often difficult to obtain a pure or relatively pure fetal blood sample: There was frequently variable contamination of the fetal blood with maternal placental blood. The contamination problem was overcome by various techniques that concentrated or purified the fetal red cells either by differential agglutination with anti-"i" antibody[228] or by differential lysis of maternal cells[229, 230] by the so-called Orskov phenomenon, which relies on differences in the carbonic anhydrase content of fetal versus adult red cells, allowing much more rapid lysis of adult cells in the face of a hypotonic challenge induced by ammonium bicarbonate and ammonium chloride.[231] Methods were also devised to correct for the maternal contamination by calculations based on differences in specific activity between fetal and maternal samples or by determining globin-chain synthesis in various known mixtures of fetal plus maternal red blood cells.[232, 233] Finally, another approach to the problem of maternal blood contamination has been to transfuse the mother prior to the procedure in order to suppress her erythropoiesis and thereby reduce the proportion of synthetically active reticulocytes in the maternal peripheral blood.[222, 234] However, with increased experience in performing fetoscopies, significantly contaminated samples are obtained relatively infrequently, especially in centers where the procedure is done with some frequency and by experienced personnel. The purity of the sample can be monitored rapidly in the fetoscopy suite by an electronic cell counter and particle size analyzer equipped with a screen to display the size distribution of the aspirated red cells. Since fetal red cells are much larger than adult red cells, contamination is readily detected and quantitated by the position and size of the peaks on the display screen and its printout chart.[228]

From the biochemical and technical points of view, prenatal diagnosis of α and β thalassemia and structural hemoglobinopathies poses no major obstacles. In the case of α thalassemia and α-chain structural variants, the detection of a quantitative or qualitative abnormality in α-chain synthesis is easily detectable, since the α chain is normally fully expressed in the first trimester. With respect to β thalassemia and β-chain structural variants, the β gene is normally expressed at only a very low level in the first and second trimesters, but there is still sufficient β-chain synthesis in utero to allow detection of an abnormal β chain and to determine, from the study of a large number of cases, the range of normal fetal β-chain synthesis, below which β thalassemia should fall.[222, 232, 233, 235] Although a number of different procedures have been used to analyze hemoglobin and globin-chain synthesis in fetal red blood cells,[1] the technique most commonly used and found to be most useful is globin-chain separation by carboxymethyl-cellulose column chromatography (see Fig. 8–1). The procedure has been widely used for the prenatal diagnosis of sickle cell anemia and homozygous β thalassemia. A number of summaries of the results obtained in large numbers of cases have been published[224–227a] and indicate that the procedure is quite accurate and reliable.

With the availability of DNA-based prenatal diagnosis, the demand for prenatal diagnosis by fetoscopy and analysis of globin-chain synthesis has decreased markedly, at least in the United States, and will probably progressively decline in those countries where fetoscopy is still commonly used, once the technology of DNA-based diagnosis becomes more widely established. Use of fetoscopy will ultimately be limited to cases in which DNA diagnosis is not possible, because of lack of knowledge of the genotype of the parents or lack of sufficient information concerning linkage of restriction fragment length polymorphisms (see Chapter 8) or because the case presents itself too late in the course of the pregnancy to obtain the necessary baseline DNA information from parents and other family members.

The technology and principles of DNA-based prenatal diagnosis of hemoglobinopathies are discussed in detail in Chapter 8. In summary, the procedure relies on the ability to detect, in fetal cell DNA from any tissue, the presence or absence of a mutant globin gene either directly, by gene mapping or hybridization to synthetic oligonucleotides, or indirectly, through the analysis of linked restriction fragment length polymorphisms (see Chapter 8). The big advantage of this procedure is its safety, since fetal blood sampling by fetoscopy is not required. Sufficient fetal DNA can be isolated from amniotic fluid cells obtained by amniocentesis after 14 weeks of gestation, with or without subsequent tissue culture. In the future, the source of DNA will in all likelihood be chorionic villi obtained by biopsy in the first trimester.[236–237a] This procedure not only provides an ample amount of DNA for the necessary studies but also allows the studies to be done much earlier in pregnancy and thus is much less traumatic emotionally to the parents.

It is not certain that prenatal diagnosis will significantly reduce the worldwide incidence of homozygous thalassemic individuals, especially since many of the regions with a very high gene frequency are in Third World countries that have limited access to proper genetic education and counseling as well as to the sophisticated technology required for all forms of prenatal diagnosis. In addition, many cases will still arise in instances in which the parents are unaware, before the birth of their first affected child, that they have thalassemia trait. Furthermore, some parents may object to abortion yet wish to attempt to have unaffected children. In many countries and individual families, however, the availability of precise prenatal diagnosis has been greatly welcomed and will no doubt play an important role in reducing the incidence and public health impact of this serious disorder.[237b, 237c]

Supportive Therapy

Transfusion Regimens

There is currently no definitive therapy for the correction of the pathophysiologic abnormalities in the severely affected homozygous thalassemic patient. Treatment is mainly supportive and consists of a regular transfusion program to control the anemia. In the past, a standard program consisted of transfusing the patient only as frequently as required to maintain a "safe" hemoglobin level. This usually meant transfusing the patient when the hemoglobin dropped to a level of 6 or 8 g/dl, hopefully before the patient became symptomatic.

A second type of transfusion program, the so-called high transfusion or hypertransfusion regimen, originally devised by Wolman in 1964,[238] is now the program of choice whenever and wherever it is feasible. This approach consists of transfusing the patients as frequently as necessary to maintain a "normal" hemoglobin level, which is not allowed to drop below a minimum of 10 g/dl (Hct 30 per cent). A modification of this approach is "supertransfusion," in which the Hct is not allowed to drop below 35 per cent.[239] Such programs usually entail the transfusion of 2 to 3 units of packed red cells at intervals of every 2 to 4 weeks. The hypertransfusion regimens have the apparent disadvantage that the patient may receive a much larger total body burden of iron than in a low-transfusion program. Early calculations of this excess infusion of iron, in comparison with the previously more standard transfusion regimen, gave minimum values in the range of 1 to 4 g of elemental iron per year for the net increment of additional iron accumulated.[240-242] Since the major cause of death in these children is related to the effects of iron overload in the second or third decade, many physicians were initially reluctant to adopt such hypertransfusion programs. However, good evidence rapidly accumulated that children who were maintained on hypertransfusion did very well and probably better than children maintained on the older regimen of more limited transfusions. In general, the children in the hypertransfusion group had fewer intercurrent illnesses, in particular fewer infections, were more active, and led more normal and happy lives.[238, 243] There was less cardiomegaly and hepatosplenomegaly as well as fewer bone changes and orthodontic problems.[241, 242] There was initially some dispute as to whether hypertransfusion actually improved the growth and development of these children. Some studies claimed that hypertransfusion did improve growth,[238, 241, 242, 244] whereas other studies did not find improved growth,[103, 243, 245, 246] and one study even found some decrease in growth in the hypertransfusion group.[247] It is now generally agreed that even in patients well transfused from an early age, there is an absent or reduced pubertal growth spurt.[104, 105]

The question concerning the additional iron burden imposed on the patient by hypertransfusion compared with low-transfusion programs is generally addressed by the reasoning that the increment of excess iron received in the additional blood is probably balanced by the decrease in the excess absorption of food iron that is known to occur in thalassemic patients[248] owing to marked ineffective erythropoiesis. Iron absorption should be reduced to normal following the suppression of the ineffective erythropoiesis by hypertransfusion.[239, 249] In the case of the supertransfusion programs, after an initial short period of equilibration, the overall blood requirements of the patients are no greater than those in the more standard hypertransfusion programs[239, 250]; this is probably due to the reduction in blood volume that occurs in these patients as a result of the marked suppression of erythropoiesis and thus reduced blood flow to marrow and reticuloendothelial organs.[239] Although life may not be prolonged by hypertransfusion alone, the results of various series indicate that it is probably not shortened. The general improvement in the quality of life that results from hypertransfusion[244, 251-257] has led to its acceptance as the preferred form of transfusion therapy for patients with thalassemia major, in conjunction with a program of iron chelation therapy (discussed later). It is important to institute such a program from an early age if one wishes to lessen the development of severe facial deformities, bony changes, cardiomegaly, and hepatosplenomegaly in these patients.

Because of the issue of iron overload resulting from transfusions, an approach has been devised to reduce the overall blood requirements in hypertransfusion programs by selectively transfusing young red cells (so-called "neocytes") that have a longer survival than total unfractionated red cells. This technique was initially devised and tested in animals by Piomelli and coworkers,[258] and its effectiveness in the transfusion of thalassemic patients was subsequently studied by a number of additional investigators.[239, 259-261] The procedure is based on the fact that younger red cells are larger and more buoyant (less dense) than older red cells and thus, after centrifugation, are located in the top layer of the packed red cells. In practice, such cell separation may be achieved by simple centrifugation of blood bags in blood bank centrifuges or by apheresis of a donor using a cell separator to remove only the top layer of red cells for transfusion. Because this top layer also contains many leukocytes, it is necessary to treat the cells by freezing in glycerol followed by extensive washing after thawing in order to eliminate the leukocytes, which can cause troublesome febrile reactions. Red cells prepared in this manner have been shown by isotopic labeling with ^{51}Cr to have a significantly longer half-life after transfusion than total unfractionated red cells—42 to 47 days compared with 28 to 29 days, respectively.[239, 259, 260] However, in two studies,[261, 261a] the use of neocyte transfusions in thalassemic patients did not result in a lowering of the total blood requirement or any improvement in the pretransfusion hemoglobin level. This procedure is generally considered to have limited applicability because it is time-consuming and costly, is associated with inefficient use of donated blood, and requires a high degree of donor motivation in the case of apheresis.

Any chronic transfusion regimen is associated with a certain incidence of transfusion-related complications. Hepatitis and other viral diseases such as cytomegalovirus infections are always a risk and are treated symptomatically. One case of transfusion-related acquired immune deficiency syndrome (AIDS) has been confirmed in a thalassemic patient.[345] Also, two cases of the pre-AIDS lymphadenopathy syndrome have been described in thalassemic patients who received blood from an initially healthy donor who subsequently developed AIDS many months after the blood donation.[261b] It is hoped that the availability of screening tests for the detection of anti–HTLV III antibodies in potential donors will reduce the risk of such occurrences in the future. Isoimmunization to minor blood group antigens (Kell, Duffy, C, K, E), although relatively rare, may cause difficulties in cross-matching and in survival time of the transfused red cells. This complication may be avoided by careful, full minor blood typing of the patient before the institution of transfusions and by careful selection of blood donors in appropriate cases. Urticarial reactions usually respond to epinephrine or antihistamines and may be prevented in some cases by treatment with antihistamines prior to the transfusion. A more difficult problem is the febrile reaction due to prior sensitization of the patient to white blood cell or plasma protein antigens. These may be prevented by use of white cell–free blood, i.e., washed or frozen and washed red cells or blood passed through various filters to remove leukocytes. Antipyretics and, occasionally, corticosteroids are necessary to treat severe febrile reactions.

Splenectomy

Splenectomy has an important place in the management of patients with homozygous β thalassemia. If a child is maintained on a good hypertransfusion regimen from an early age, marked splenomegaly may not develop[241, 242] because of decreased turnover of abnormal red cells and therefore less stimulus for hyperplasia of the reticuloendothelial system. Even established splenomegaly may be reversible to some degree following institution of hypertransfusion.[262] However, most patients, despite adequate transfusions, will eventually develop significant splenomegaly with increasing age, and this may cause problems. Progressive splenomegaly usually aggravates the anemia and increases the transfusion requirement by causing a dilutional type of anemia due to the sequestration of transfused red cells in the large third space provided by the spleen's size. Thalassemic children with splenomegaly have a greatly increased intravascular blood volume, which can be reversed by splenectomy.[262] In addition, patients may develop hypersplenism, with evidence of sequestration and destruction of white cells and platelets as well as red cells. More frequently, however, hypersplenism is manifested primarily by an increasing or inordinate transfusion requirement. Modell[256] has stressed the importance of maintaining accurate transfusion records and calculating, for the achievement of a given mean hemoglobin level, the ratio of the actual over the expected transfusion requirement (in ml of rbc/kg/yr) by reference to standard curves obtained from a group of splenectomized patients. A ratio greater than 2 usually indicates the likelihood that splenectomy will be beneficial. Rapid onset of splenomegaly and splenic destruction of transfused red cells may be triggered by isoimmunization to minor blood group antigens. Such an occurrence is usually associated with difficulty in cross-matching the blood as well as with the development of a positive Coombs' test.

Splenomegaly, on the other hand, may be symptomatic simply by the sheer size of the spleen, causing discomfort from pressure in the abdomen or pain from splenic infarcts. In such cases, splenectomy is usually recommended.

Splenectomy will usually result in a lessening of the transfusion requirement[256, 264, 265] and, in combination with a good transfusion program, will usually make it possible to maintain the patient's hemoglobin at a near normal level much more easily than before splenectomy and thus achieve the benefits of hypertransfusion. Although the decision to perform splenectomy may be aided by doing various isotopic studies and scans to assess red cell survival and splenic sequestration,[266] clinical criteria such as the transfusion requirement[256] are generally more helpful in reaching the decision to recommend splenectomy.

Splenectomy is rarely necessary before the child reaches 5 or 6 years of age and is generally avoided before the age of 3 or 4 years because of the demonstration of increased instances of rapidly fatal septicemia in children who have undergone splenectomy, for whatever reason, before that age.[267] Thalassemic children of all ages are particularly susceptible to fatal gram-positive septicemia following splenectomy,[101,102] although the overall incidence has been somewhat lower in more recent series[264,265] than in the past. The offending organisms are usually pneumococci or streptococci, although other organisms have been implicated, including penicillin-resistant staphylococci.[264] The reasons for the high incidence of postsplenectomy sepsis are unclear.[268] The spleen and the reticuloendothelial (RE) system in general probably function as bacterial filters of the circulation. In the asplenic thalassemic individual, the loss of splenic filter function is probably further aggravated by some degree of RE system blockade throughout the body. The spleen probably also has a function in antibody synthesis, the absence of which may put the thalassemic patient at an additional disadvantage in handling infections. Indeed, immunoglobulin levels have been found to be low in some splenectomized thalassemic individuals,[269] but not all.[265,270] Because of the increased risk of postsplenectomy sepsis, it is probably advisable after splenectomy to maintain thalassemic children on prophylactic doses of penicillin for at least 2 years (the time of peak incidence of postsplenectomy septicemia), if not indefinitely. The administration of anti-pneumococcal vaccines prior to splenectomy is also advisable, although such vaccines do not confer absolute protection against infection.

There is some controversy in the literature concerning whether or not splenectomy enhances the development of iron overload in the liver and heart, owing to the removal of a large storage depot for reticuloendothelial iron. In some series,[271–274] splenectomized patients appeared to have evidence of greater iron loading than nonsplenectomized patients, but this was not the case in another series of patients.[275] One possible explanation for the apparent harmful effect of splenectomy on iron loading is that splenectomized patients in general may have more severe disease than nonsplenectomized patients. The question is definitely not yet settled, but in general, it would be unwise to defer splenectomy in a patient with definite hypersplenism, because the excess iron resulting from the increased transfusion requirement is likely to be more harmful in the long run than the loss of the spleen as a storage site for iron. It has been observed that in nonsplenectomized patients maintained on a hypertransfusion program, red cell transfusion requirements tend to eventually exceed 250 ml/kg/yr by the time the child reaches 6 to 8 years of age. At such a transfusion level, it is difficult to maintain iron balance by iron chelation therapy,[276] and thus, it has been suggested that splenectomy be seriously considered when transfusion requirements reach or exceed the level of 200 to 250 ml of rbc/kg/yr.[264]

Use of Iron-Chelating Agents

Because of the marked iron overload that occurs in β thalassemia as a result of repeated blood transfusions, it should be clinically advantageous to remove the excess iron stores by the long-term administration of iron-chelating agents. There is essentially only one such agent currently in clinical use—desferrioxamine, which was introduced in 1963 and which must be given parenterally in order to be effective.[277] It is a derivative of hydroxamic acid and a member of a family of compounds produced by microorganisms as part of their iron transport system. The initial clinical experience with desferrioxamine, administered as a single daily intramuscular injection, was disappointing, and use of the drug waned because the amount of iron chelated from thalassemic patients, as monitored by urinary excretion of the chelate, was observed to decrease in time.[242,277] In retrospect, this phenomenon was probably not due to tachyphylaxis, as was initially concluded, but was more likely caused by variations in the distribution of the chelated iron between the urinary and biliary routes of excretion, as was later observed to occur with the drug. Excretion via the biliary route is proportionally greater when higher doses of the drug are used and when ineffective erythropoiesis is suppressed by hypertransfusions.[278] It was also observed that higher levels of urinary excretion of iron could be achieved by giving higher doses of the drug, including intravenous infusions at the time of transfusion, and by concomitant administration of oral vitamin C.[279–282] Targeted delivery of desferrioxamine to the RE system, by packaging it into resealed, hemoglobin-free red cell membrane "ghosts," was also attempted,[283] but this approach has not been widely used.

Interest in the drug was revived in 1974, when a study of transfused thalassemic patients treated with intramuscular desferrioxamine revealed that these patients had less liver iron deposition and fibrosis than a control group of patients who had not received the drug.[284] A later retrospective study of similar patients treated with intramuscular desferrioxamine revealed that they had a small but significant increase in life expectancy compared with untreated control patients.[285]

However, widespread interest in the use of desferrioxamine did not occur until 1976, when it was shown by Propper and coworkers[286] that the drug was much more effective in enhancing urinary excretion of iron when it was given as a slow continuous infusion rather than as a bolus. This observation led to the establishment of the technique of subcutaneous infusion of desferrioxamine[287–290] by means of a battery-operated syringe or "pump" attached to a narrow-gauge "butterfly" needle inserted under the skin of the anterior abdominal wall (Fig. 9–9). In practice, the infusions are done overnight to minimize inconvenience to the patient. The dose of the drug given varies with the age of the patient and the degree of iron overload: In children below the age of 6 years, the dose ranges between 0.25 and 1.0 g/12 hr; in older children, the dose is usually 2 g/12 hr; and in heavily iron-overloaded patients, up to 4.0 g/12 hr are commonly administered.[291]

There has been some controversy concerning the role of vitamin C as an adjunct in iron chelation therapy. Thalassemic patients are frequently deficient in vitamin C and vitamin E, presumably because of increased requirements of these nonspecific anti-oxidant substances due to the oxidant stress of iron overload. It was shown early on that the administration of vitamin C to thalassemic patients greatly enhanced urinary excretion of iron in response to desferrioxamine.[279, 282] However, there were concerns, on theoretical grounds, that vitamin C might increase the labile, potentially toxic pool of iron within tissues or facilitate the transfer of iron from RE cells to parenchymal cells, where it is more likely to be toxic.[292] This concern increased with the report of cardiac decompensation coincident with the administration of large doses of vitamin C (500 mg/day) during iron

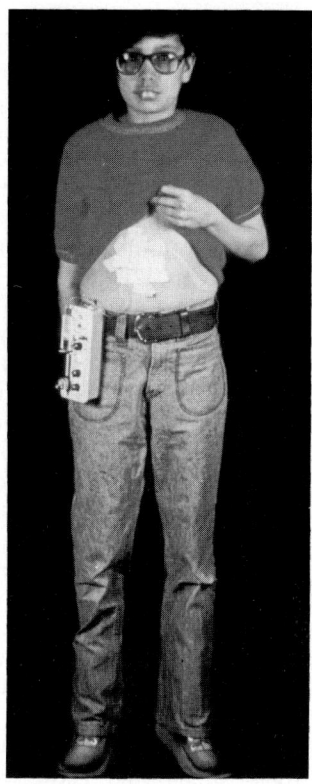

Figure 9–9. Thalessemic patient with portable battery-operated pump for the subcutaneous administration of desferrioxamine. (Courtesy of Dr. R. Propper.)

chelation therapy.[293, 294] It is generally considered safe, however, to administer lower doses of vitamin C, in the range of 100 to 200 mg/day, that are sufficient to correct any actual ascorbate deficiency in the patient.[291]

The results of intensive iron chelation therapy using subcutaneous desferrioxamine are thus far encouraging from the point of view of the total amount of iron chelated, but the long-term effect on the life span of treated patients must await many more years of follow-up of patients who were started on the therapy at a young age. The hope is that institution of an intensive iron chelation program starting at an early age will prevent (or greatly delay) the occurrence of fatal iron overload. In this regard, the early results are rather promising: Even young patients can be maintained in negative iron balance,[295, 296] and slightly older patients have been put into negative iron balance and have manifested objective evidence of reversal of iron overload such as a fall in serum ferritin levels, sometimes to normal,[297–301] and improvement in abnormal liver function tests, together with biopsy-proven reduction or complete removal of excess iron stores.[300, 301a] Even older patients with no preexisting cardiac disease can be protected from developing cardiac complications by compliant use of subcutaneous desferrioxamine.[302] Finally, patients with established cardiac disease can also benefit from the use of desferrioxamine, administered either in high doses intravenously or in conventional doses taken on a compliant basis.[302–302c]

This type of therapy, however, is not without certain disadvantages and shortcomings. It is extremely expensive and therefore not widely applicable to developing countries where thalassemia is a major public health problem. The cost of the "pump" is approximately $1000 and that of the desferrioxamine, $2.50/g or $3650/yr for a patient requiring 4 g/day of the drug. Because of the inconvenience of the route of administration, compliance can also be a problem in some patients, especially as they reach adolescence. The known toxicity of the drug is minimal, although the long-term consequences of intensive chelation therapy have not yet been established. Some dose-related ocular complications have been described, including cataracts in animals (although rarely in man) and retinal abnormalities such as reversible night blindness and field defects.[303] Rare anaphylactic drug reactions have also been described, but in one case, it was possible to desensitize the patient and reuse the drug.[304]

With regard to other iron-chelating agents, the search continues for an orally absorbable agent as a substitute for desferrioxamine. One oral compound, 2,3-dihydroxybenzoic acid, unfortunately proved to be relatively inefficient with regard to the amount of iron that it could chelate in transfused patients.[305] Another orally effective compound, cholylhydroxamic acid, is still under study, as are more effective parenteral agents such as rhodotorulic acid and others.[306, 307]

The role of iron chelation in non–transfusion-dependent thalassemia intermedia is not clear. Patients with thalassemia intermedia do develop progressive iron overload as they grow older,[308] presumably because of increased gastrointestinal absorption of food iron due to ineffective erythropoiesis. It has been calculated that by the time such patients reach the third or fourth decade, the level of their iron stores may approach that of transfusion-dependent thalassemics. Obviously, it should be advantageous to decrease gastrointestinal iron absorption in such patients, and it has been suggested that tea may be effective in this role,[249, 309] although the long-term efficiency of tea in preventing or decreasing iron overload in thalassemia intermedia remains to be established.

Other General Measures

The management of a child with homozygous β thalassemia otherwise involves good general medical care, which includes a close relationship among physician, patient, and parents and education of parents and child with regard to seeking early medical attention for any illness, especially febrile episodes. Because of the increased predisposition of these children to life-threatening septicemia, especially after splenectomy, it is probably wise to treat any febrile illness, after the taking of appropriate cultures, with systemic broad-spectrum antibiotics until a specific diagnosis becomes apparent.

Because of marked marrow hyperplasia due to ineffective erythropoiesis and hemolysis, patients with thalassemia intermedia in whom erythropoiesis is not suppressed by blood transfusions should be maintained on folic acid replacement (1 mg daily) to prevent the development of folic acid deficiency and a megaloblastic crisis, which may aggravate the anemia.

The consequences of iron overload must be treated as they develop—diabetes with appropriate diet and insulin therapy and hepatic dysfunction by dietary and other supportive means. Frequently, thalassemic children may have a bleeding diathesis associated with a prolonged prothrombin time that, despite its probable hepatocellular basis, may respond to vitamin K therapy. Some malabsorption of vitamin K may occur because of chronic pancreatic insufficiency due to pancreatic siderosis and fibrosis.

The most serious and life-threatening complication is that of cardiac siderosis, resulting in arrhythmias and/or chronic congestive heart failure. When these complications develop, the patients must be treated vigorously with low-salt diet, digitalis, diuretics, anti-arrhythmic medications, and other symptomatic measures. The monitoring of cardiac function is important as the patients grow older in order to detect the first signs of cardiac dysfunction and to determine as early as possible the need to institute effective therapeutic measures. One of the more sensitive tests of early cardiac dysfunction has been found to be radionuclide cineangiography during exercise.[310] This procedure should also prove useful to monitor the effect of iron chelation programs on cardiac function.

As noted previously, deficiencies of vitamin C[279, 282, 311-313] and vitamin E[31, 311, 314-316] occur not infrequently in thalassemic patients, presumably owing to increased requirements resulting from the oxidant stress of iron overload. Correction of these deficiencies by vitamin supplementation therapy is recommended. Proper supplementation of vitamin C can be very important to achieve the maximum effects of iron chelation therapy (discussed previously). In the case of vitamin E, it was thought that its deficiency might aggravate the anemia in thalassemic patients because of the increased propensity of vitamin E–deficient red cells to lyse when subjected to an oxidant stress.[31] However, there is no evidence that vitamin E supplementation will prolong red cell survival in thalassemic patients.[316]

Hormonal replacement therapy has been used in certain patients in an attempt to treat various endocrine deficiencies presumably due to transfusional hemosiderosis and thus to improve development of secondary sexual characteristics. The therapy is not usually effective because sexual underdevelopment is probably due in great part to target organ unresponsiveness (related to siderotic or hypoxic damage) rather than to hormonal deficiency. Hormonal therapy, however, may have a role, on a temporary basis, in the treatment of delayed puberty in certain cases of thalassemia intermedia.

Future Treatment

The future may offer more definitive forms of therapy for thalassemia. Two means of therapy now considered experimental may one day be routinely available to the child with thalassemia major: (1) bone marrow transplantation and (2) correction of, or compensation for, the biochemical defect by gene therapy or manipulation of gene expression.

Bone Marrow Transplantation

The art of bone marrow transplantation has been developed in a number of medical centers. Transplants have been successfully performed in the treatment of a large number of patients with aplastic anemia and acute leukemia, with the source of bone marrow being an unaffected sibling who is histocompatible with the patient.[317] Bone marrow transplantation has also been used recently in the treatment of a number of patients with homozygous β thalassemia.[318-319a] In one series,[318, 319] five patients underwent the transplant in the first 2 years of life, before receiving multiple transfusions that could have led to their sensitization and graft rejection. The patients were pretreated with dimethyl busulfan and cyclophosphamide to essentially eradicate the thalassemic hematopoietic cells in the endogenous marrow prior to the transplant. Three of the patients are now hematologically normal, growing normally, and apparently cured of the disease, but two patients died from transplantation-related complications. In another series,[319a] the patients received bone marrow transplants at an older age after prolonged transfusion support; the transplantations were successful in only 2 of 13 patients. However, in a subsequent study by the same investigators,[344] sustained engraftment was obtained in 22 of 30 patients aged 6 months to 7 years; actuarial disease-free survival was 73 per cent.

Bone marrow transplantation is therefore not a benign procedure, and its use in the treatment of homozygous β thalassemia poses a number of ethical questions. Even in the best centers, there is a failure and/or mortality rate of approximately 20 per cent owing to various complications such as hemorrhage or infection, during the stage of pancytopenia, and graft-versus-host disease. One is therefore faced with a serious ethical dilemma: Is the 20 per cent risk of failure worth taking in a young child when, by current conventional therapy, the patient can be reasonably well assured of a good quality of life for approximately 20 years and perhaps even longer if intensive iron chelation therapy started at a young age proves to be effective in prolonging survival of transfusion-dependent thalassemics? There is also always the possibility that new and safer forms of effective therapy could be developed in the next decade. This dilemma must obviously be resolved on an individual basis by thorough discussions between the patient's parents and the responsible physician. It should also be pointed out that bone marrow transplantation can usually be performed only if there is a histocompatible sibling to act as the donor; the chances of this occurring are one in four for each sibling. Methods are being developed to allow marrow transplantation across the histocompatibility barrier, but these techniques are still in the experimental stages and are not yet in general use. In conclusion, bone marrow transplantation, despite its risks, may provide a definitive form of therapy for selected patients with homozygous β thalassemia. The long-term results of the recent successful transplants will be awaited with great interest.

Gene Therapy and Manipulation of Gene Expression

As discussed in Chapter 8, gene therapy for thalassemia by means of transfer of normal globin genes into hematopoietic cells will not be a realistic option until some time in the future. A number of scientific breakthroughs must first occur to overcome a number of technical difficulties such as the low efficiency of gene transfer and lack of regulated expression, as well as low level of expression, of transferred globin genes. However, pharmacologic manipulation of γ globin gene expression has been recently accomplished and has been shown in short-term studies to have a favorable influence on the pathophysiological abnormalities in homozygous β thalassemia as well as in sickle cell anemia.

As discussed previously, increased synthesis of Hb F can have a modulating effect on the severity of homozygous β thalassemia and sickle cell anemia. In adult bone marrow cells, the DNA of the inactive γ globin genes is in a state of hypermethylation,[320, 321] as is usually the case for inactive genes in animal cells[323] (see Chapter 7). In contrast, the DNA of active γ globin genes in fetal liver erythroid cells is hypomethylated,[320, 321] as expected for any active gene.[322, 323] The importance of DNA methylation in γ globin gene expression is also illustrated by the finding that methylated γ globin genes are not expressed normally after gene transfer into tissue culture cells.[324] The chemotherapeutic agent 5-azacytidine prevents the methylation of DNA during DNA replication by inhibiting the enzyme DNA methyltransferase.[325] On the basis of the aforementioned information, DeSimone and coworkers[326] reasoned that the administration of 5-azacytidine might result in enhanced γ globin gene expression, and this was in fact the result they obtained after infusion of the drug into baboons.[326, 326a]

Based on these animal studies, clinical trials of 5-azacytidine therapy were then performed in patients with homozygous β thalassemia and sickle cell anemia.[327-329] The initial results were very encouraging: Following administration of the drug, there was a fourfold to eightfold increase in the level of Hb F, which was accompanied by evidence of decreased hemolysis and decreased ineffective erythropoiesis as well as by a sustained increase in the total hemoglobin level for up to 40 days.[327-329] Studies of DNA methylation showed a decrease in methylation of the γ (and ε) globin genes in bone marrow cells starting as early as 2 days after the drug was given and lasting for up to 21 days.[327-329] 5-Azacytidine has also been shown to be capable of activating human γ globin genes in mouse erythroleukemia cells containing human chromosome 11.[329a]

As exciting as these results may be, they have been greeted with some caution regarding the general applicability and long-term safety of the therapy.[330] One concern has been that with generalized demethylation of genes, aberrant and potentially harmful gene expression might occur in various tissues, including the activation of latent viruses. Such inappropriate gene expression has thus far not been observed. In particular, levels of alpha-fetoprotein and carcinoembryonic antigen did not change significantly in treated patients.[328] Long-term therapy may also be complicated by neutropenia due to the myelosuppressive effects of the drug. The biggest concern, however, is the strong possibility that the drug is a mutagen and carcinogenic[330-332] and that long-term therapy might lead to the development of tumors. In summary then, although this therapy provides an important precedent and will stimulate the search for other less toxic agents that might have similar effects, the use of 5-azacytidine to stimulate Hb F synthesis in patients with homozygous β thalassemia should still be considered highly experimental and, for the time being, should be limited in its application to patients with advanced disease until more information accumulates regarding long-term side effects.

Parenthetically, there is currently further controversy concerning the actual mechanism of action of 5-azacytidine. Although the increase in Hb F production is associated with decreased methylation of the γ globin genes, it is not yet clear whether the primary action of the drug responsible for increased Hb F production is, in fact, inhibition of DNA methylation. It has been proposed that the drug induces cell selection and preferential accumulation in the marrow of F-committed erythroid precursor cells (i.e., F-cell precursors) that would naturally be expected to already have their γ globin genes in an active, hypomethylated state. Since 5-azacytidine is a cell cycle–specific agent that is toxic primarily to dividing cells, it is argued that the rapidly dividing late erythroid progenitor cells (CFU-Es) might be selectively killed by the drug, sparing the noncycling early erythroid progenitor cells (BFU-Es) that have a greater commitment and potential for giving rise to F-cell progeny than do CFU-Es[333, 334] (see Chapter 7). Studies of erythroid progenitor cells from baboons treated with 5-azacytidine have in fact demonstrated perturbations in progenitor cell pools that are consistent with such a model.[335] Assays of erythroid progenitor cells in bone marrow of leukemic patients recovering from chemotherapy with high doses of 5-azacytidine also demonstrated a profound deficiency of CFU-E– compared with BFU-E–derived erythroid colonies,[336] but analogous findings were not observed in patients with sickle cell anemia and thalassemia treated with lower doses of the drug for enhancement of Hb F production.[337]

Additional evidence for the possible role of cell selection in this phenomenon has been provided by studies in which the administration of other cell cycle–specific agents such as hydroxyurea and cytosine arabinoside to nonhuman primates resulted in increased Hb F accumulation but to levels somewhat lower than those observed with 5-azacytidine.[338, 339] Hydroxyurea has also been shown to be effective in increasing Hb F levels in patients with sickle cell anemia.[340, 341]

A third possible mechanism for the effect of 5-azacytidine and other cell cycle–specific agents on Hb F synthesis is the reprogramming of the pattern of globin gene expression of erythroid progenitor and precursor cells through perturbations unrelated to effects of methylation on the globin genes.[343] The main evidence in favor of such reprogramming is the rapidity of onset of the effect. The first evidence of increased Hb F production, provided by a rise in the percentage of F reticulocytes, is observed within 2 days after administration of the drug,[329, 337] and this phenomenon occurs too rapidly to be explained by cell selection at the level of progenitor cells such as BFU-Es and CFU-Es but suggests a direct effect of the drug on dividing erythroblasts. There is also evidence for reprogramming of late erythroid progenitor cells by the drug. CFU-E–derived colonies, grown from bone marrow aspirated from patients treated with the drug for 2 days, contain increased amounts of Hb F compared with normal colonies in the absence of any evidence of cytotoxicity.[337] Exposure of normal bone marrow cells to 5-azacytidine in tissue culture for 24 hours leads to similar effects in subsequently formed CFU-E–derived colonies.[337] These various findings all strongly suggest that the increase in Hb F synthesis results from a direct effect of 5-azacytidine on both erythroid precursor and progenitor cells.

This topic will no doubt be the subject of much future experimentation. It is likely that multiple factors play a role in the enhanced accumulation of Hb F that occurs after the administration of 5-azacytidine and other cell cycle–specific agents.

In summary, the future holds the promise of effective and definitive forms of therapy for thalassemia such as bone marrow transplantation and perhaps even gene therapy or gene manipulation, but at present, the use of these modalities is still very much in the experimental and developmental stages. Technical and ethical issues as well as issues of long-term safety and effectiveness need to be resolved before these approaches can be accepted as standard practice. In the meantime, the cornerstones of the treatment of thalassemia must remain good general medical care and proper supportive management of the patient with diligent use of blood transfusions and iron chelation therapy.

References

1. Weatherall, D. J., and Clegg, J. B.: The Thalassemia Syndromes. 3rd ed. Oxford, Blackwell Scientific Publications, 1981.
2. Cooley, T. B., and Lee, P.: A series of cases of splenomegaly in children with anemia and peculiar bone changes. Trans. Amer. Pediat. Soc. 37:29, 1925.
3. Cooley, T. B., Witwer, E. R., and Lee, P.: Anemia in children with splenomegaly and peculiar changes in bones; report of cases. Am. J. Dis. Child. 34:347, 1927.
4. Whipple, G. H., and Bradford, W. L.: Mediterranean disease—thalassemia (erythroblastic anemia of Cooley). J. Pediatr. 9:279, 1936.
5. Rietti, F.: Ittero emolitico primitivo. Atti Accad Scient Med Nat Ferrara 2:14, 1961.
6. Greppi, E.: Ittero emolitico familiare con aumento della resistenza dei globuli. Min. Med., 8:1, 1928.
7. Micheli, F., Penati, F., and Momigliano, L. G.: Ulteriori ricerche sulla anemia ipocromica splenomegalica con poichilocitosi. Atti Soc. It. Emat. Haematologica 16(Suppl.):10, 1935.
8. Chini, V., and Valeri, C. M.: Mediterranean hemopathic syndromes. Blood 4:989, 1949.
9. Caminopetros, J.: Kliniki 12, 1936.
10. Caminopetros, J.: Recherches sur l'anémiérythroblastique infantile des peuples de la Méditerranée

10. orientale, édute anthropologique, étiologique et pathogénique; la transmission héréditaire de la maladie. Ann. Med. 43:104, 1938.
11. Angelini, V.: Primi risultati di ricerche ematologiche nei familiari di ammalati di anemia di Cooley. Minerva Med. 28:331, 1937.
12. Marmont, A., and Bianchi, V.: Mediterranean anaemia. Acta Haematol. 1:4, 1948.
13. Fessas, P.: Inclusions of hemoglobin in erythroblasts and erythrocytes of thalassemia. Blood 21:21, 1963.
14. Pasvol, G., Weatherall, D. J., and Wilson, R. J. M.: Effects of foetal haemoglobin on susceptibility of red cells to *Plasmodium falciparum*. Nature 270:171, 1977.
14a. Friedman, M. J., and Traeger, W.: The biochemistry of resistance to malaria. Sci. Am. 244:154, 1981.
14b. Oppenheimer, S. J., Higgs, D. R., Weatherall, D. J., Barker, J., and Spark, R. A.: α Thalassemia in Papua New Guinea. Lancet 2:424, 1984.
15. Dozy, A. M., Kan, Y. W., Embury, S. H., Mentzer, W. C., Wang, W. C., Lubin, B., Davis, J. R., Jr., and Koenig, H. M.: α-globin gene organization in blacks precludes the severe form of α-thalassemia. Nature 280:605, 1979.
16. Nathan, D. G., and Gunn, R. B.: Thalassemia: The consequences of unbalanced hemoglobin synthesis. Am. J. Med. 41:815, 1966.
17. Yataganas, X., and Fessas, P.: The pattern of hemoglobin precipitation in thalassemia and its significance. Ann. N. Y. Acad. Sci. 165:270, 1969.
18. Wickramasinghe, S. N., Letsky, E., and Moffatt, B.: Effect of α-chain precipitates on bone marrow function in homozygous β-thalassaemia. Br. J. Haematol. 25:123, 1973.
19. Gunn, R. B., Silvers, D. N., and Rosse, W. F.: Potassium permeability in β-thalassemia minor red blood cells. J. Clin. Invest. 51:1043, 1972.
20. Nathan, D. G., Stossel, T. B., Gunn, R. B., Zarkowsky, H. S., and Laforet, M. T.: Influence of hemoglobin precipitation on erythrocyte metabolism in alpha and beta thalassemia. J. Clin. Invest. 48:33, 1969.
21. Fessas, P., Loukopoulos, D., and Kaltsoya, A.: Peptide analysis of the inclusions of erythroid cells in β-thalassemia. Biochim. Biophys. Acta 124:430, 1966.
22. Rachmilewitz, E. A., and Thorell, B.: Hemichromes in single inclusion bodies in red cells of beta thalassemia. Blood 39:794, 1972.
23. Gabuzda, T. G., Nathan, D. G., and Gardner, F. H.: The turnover of hemoglobins A, F, and A_2 in the peripheral blood of three patients with thalassemia. J. Clin. Invest. 42:1678, 1963.
24. Loukopoulos, D., and Fessas, P.: The distribution of hemoglobin types in thalassemic erythrocytes. J. Clin. Invest. 44:231, 1965.
25. Weatherall, D. J., Clegg, J. B., Na-Nakorn, S., and Wasi, P.: The pattern of disordered haemoglobin synthesis in homozygous and heterozygous β-thalassaemia. Br. J. Haematol. 16:251, 1969.
26. Bargellesi, A., Pontremoli, S., Menini, C., and Conconi, F.: Excess of alpha globin synthesis in homozygous beta-thalassemia and its removal from the red blood cell cytoplasm. Eur. J. Biochem. 3:364, 1968.
27. Finch, C. A., Deubelbeiss, K., Cook, J. D., Eschbach, K., Harker, L. A. Funk, D. D., Marsaglia, G., Hillman, R. S., Slichter, S., Adamson, J. W., Ganzoni, A., and Giblet, E. G.: Ferrokinetics in man. Medicine 49:17, 1970.
28. Rifkind, R. A., and Danon, D.: Heinz body anemia—an ultrastructural study: I. Heinz body formation. Blood 25:885, 1965.
29. Wennberg, E., and Weiss, L.: Splenic erythroclasia: An electronic microscopic study of hemoglobin H disease. Blood 31:778, 1968.
30. Slater, L. M., Muir, W. A., and Weed, R. I.: Influence of splenectomy on insoluble hemoglobin inclusion bodies in β-thalassemic erythrocytes. Blood 31:766, 1968.
31. Rachmilewitz, E. A., Lubin, B. H., and Shohet, S. B.: Lipid membrane peroxidation in beta thalassaemia major. Blood 47:495, 1976.
32. Kahane, I., Shifter, A., and Rachmilewitz, E. A.: Cross-linking of red blood cell membrane proteins induced by oxidative stress in β thalassemia. FEBS Lett. 85:267, 1978.
33. Rachmilewitz, E. A., and Kahane, I.: The red blood cell membrane in thalassaemia. Br. J. Haematol. 46:1, 1980.
34. Fessas, P., and Yataganas, X.: Intraerythroblastic instability of hemoglobin $β_4$ (Hgb H). Blood 31:323, 1968.
35. Wickramasinghe, S. N., Hughes, M., Hollan, S. R., Horanyi, M., and Szelenya, J.: Electron microscope and high resolution autoradiographic studies of the erythroblasts in haemoglobin H disease. Br. J. Haematol. 45:401, 1980.
35a. Wickramasinghe, S. N., Hughes, M., Fucharoen, S., and Wasi, P.: The fate of excess β globin chains within erythropoietic cells in α-thalassaemia 2 trait, α-thalassaemia 1 trait, haemoglobin-H disease and haemoglobin Q-H disease: An electron microscope study. Br. J. Haematol. 56:473, 1984.
36. Rigas, D. A., and Koler, R. D.: Decreased erythrocyte survival in hemoglobin H disease as a result of the abnormal properties of hemoglobin H: The benefit of splenectomy. Blood 18:1, 1961.
37. Jandl, J. H., and Greenberg, M. S.: Bone marrow failure due to relative nutritional deficiency in Cooley's hemolytic anemia. N. Engl. J. Med 280:461, 1959.
38. Luhby, A. L., and Cooperman, J. M.: Folic acid deficiency in thalassaemia major. Lancet 2:490, 1961.
39. Luhby, A. L., Cooperman, J. M., Feldman, R., Ceraolo, J., Herrero, J., and Marley, J. F.: Folic acid deficiency as a limiting factor in the anemias of thalassemia major. Blood 18:786, 1961.
39a. Davis, L. R.: Aplastic crisis in haemolytic anemias: The role of a parvovirus-like agent. Br. J. Haematol. 55:391, 1983.
39b. Young, N. S., Mortimer, P. P., Moore, J. G., and Humphries, R. K.: Characterization of a virus that causes transient aplastic crisis. J. Clin. Invest. 73:224, 1984.
39c. Young, N., and Mortimer, P.: Viruses and bone marrow failure. Blood 63:729, 1984.
40. Prankerd, T. A. J.: The spleen and anaemia. Br. Med. J. 2:517, 1963.
41. Maurer, H. S., Behrman, R. E., and Honig, G. R.: Dependence of the oxygen affinity of blood on the presence of foetal or adult hemoglobin. Nature 227:388, 1970.
42. DeFuria, F. G., Miller, D. R., and Canale, V. C.: Red blood cell metabolism and function in transfused β-thalassemia. Ann. N. Y. Acad. Sci. 232:323, 1974.
43. Pearson, H. A., Motoyama, E., Genel, M., Kramer, M., and Zigas, C. J.: Intraerythrocytic adaptation (2,3-DPG, P_{50}) in thalassemia minor. Blood 49:463, 1977.

44. Pootrakul, S., Wasi, P., Pornpatkul, M., and Na-Nakorn, S.: Incidence of alpha thalassemia in Bangkok. J. Med. Assoc. Thai. 53:250, 1970.
45. Na-Nakorn, S., and Wasi, P.: Alpha-thalassemia in Northern Thailand. Am. J. Hum. Genet. 22:645, 1970.
45a. Galanello, R., Maccioni, L., Ruggeri, R., Perseu, L., and Cao, A.: Alpha thalassemia in Sardinian newborns. Br. J. Haematol. 58:361, 1984.
46. Weatherall, D. J., Higgs, D. R., Clegg, J. B., and Wood, W. G.: The significance of haemoglobin H in patients with mental retardation or myeloproliferative disease. Br. J. Haemat. 52:351, 1982.
47. Higgs, D. R., Wood, W. G., Barton, C., and Weatherall, D. J.: Clinical features and molecular analysis of acquired hemoglobin H disease. Am. J. Med. 75:181, 1983.
48. Weatherall, D. J., Higgs, D. R., Bunch, C., et al.: Hemoglobin H disease and mental retardation; a new syndrome or a remarkable coincidence? N. Engl. J. Med. 305:607, 1981.
49. Milner, P. F., Clegg, J. B., and Weatherall, D. J.: Haemoglobin H disease due to a unique haemoglobin variant with an elongated α-chain. Lancet 1:729, 1971.
50. Clegg, J.B., Weatherall, D. J., and Milner, P. F.: Haemoglobin Constant Spring—a chain-termination mutant? Nature 234:337, 1971.
51. Clegg, J. B., Weatherall, D. J., Contopolou-Griva, I., Caroutsos, K., Poungouras, P., and Tsevrenis, H.: Haemoglobin Icaria, a new chain-termination mutant which causes α thalassemia. Nature 251:245, 1974.
52. DeJong, W. W., Khan, P. M., and Bernini, L. F.: Hemoglobin Koya Dora: High frequency of a chain termination mutant. Am. J. Hum. Genet. 27:81, 1975.
53. Bradley, T. B., Wohl, R. C., and Smith, G. J.: Elongation of the α-globin chain in a black family: Interaction with Hb G-Philadelphia. Clin. Res. 23:131A, 1975.
54. Lie-Injo, L. E., Ganesan, J., Clegg, J. B., and Weatherall, D. J.: Homozygous state for Hb Constant Spring (slow-moving Hb X components). Blood 43:251, 1974.
55. Lie-Injo, L. E., Ganesan, J., and Lopez, C. G.: The clinical haematological and biochemical expression of hemoglobin Constant Spring and its distribution. In Schmidt, R. M. (ed.): Abnormal Hemoglobins and Thalassemia. New York, Academic Press, 1975, p. 75.
56. Pongsamart, S., Pootrakul, S., Wasi, P., and Na-Nakorn, S.: Hemoglobin Constant Spring: Hemoglobin synthesis in heterozygous and homozygous states. Biochem. Biophys. Res. Comm. 64:681, 1975.
57. Pootrakul, P., Winichagoon, P., Fucharoean, S., Pravatmuang, P., Piankijagum, A., and Wasi, P.: Homozygous haemoglobin Constant Spring: A need for revision of concept. Hum. Genet. 59:250, 1981.
58. Winichagoon, P., Adirojnanon, P., and Wasi, P.: Levels of haemoglobin H and proportions of red cells with inclusion bodies in the two types of haemoglobin H disease. Br. J. Haematol. 46:507, 1980.
59. Wasi, P., Pootrakul, S., Pootrakul, P., Pravatmuang, P., Winichagoon, P., and Fucharoon, S.: Thalassemia in Thailand. N. Y. Acad. Sci. 344:352, 1981.
60. Higgs, D. R., Hunt, D. M., Drysdale, H. C., Clegg, J. B., Pressley, L., and Weatherall, D. J.: The genetic basis of Hb Q-H disease. Br. J. Haematol. 46:387, 1980.
61. Derry, S., Wood, W. G., Pippard, M., Clegg, J. B., Weatherall, D. J., Wickramasinghe, S., Darley, J., Winichagoon, P., and Wasi, P.: Hematologic and biosynthetic studies in homozygous Hemoglobin Constant Spring. J. Clin. Invest. 73:1673, 1984.
62. Lie-Injo, L. E., and Jo, B. H.: A fast-moving haemoglobin in hydrops fetalis. Nature 185:698, 1960.
63. Lie-Injo, L. E.: Alpha-chain thalassemia and hydrops fetalis in Malaya: Report of five cases. Blood 20:581, 1962.
64. Todd, D., Lai, M. C. S., and Braga, C. A.: Thalassaemia and hydrops foetalis—family studies. Br. Med. J. 3:347, 1967.
65. Kan, Y. W., Allen, A., and Loewnstein, L.: Hydrops fetalis with alpha thalassemia. N. Engl. J. Med. 276:18, 1967.
65a. Pootrakul, S., Wasi, P., and Na-Nakorn, S.: Haemoglobin Bart's hydrops foetalis in Thailand. Ann. Hum. Genet. 30:203, 1967.
66. Diamond, M. P., Cotgrove, I., and Parker, A.: Case of intrauterine death due to α-thalassemia. Br. Med. J. 2:278, 1965.
67. Sophocleous, T., Higgs, D. R., Aldridge, B., Trent, R. J., Pressley, L., Clegg, J. B., and Weatherall, D. J.: The molecular basis for the Haemoglobin Bart's hydrops fetalis syndrome in Cyprus. Br. J. Haematol. 47:153, 1981.
68. Kattamis, C., Metaxotou-Mavromati, A., Tsiarta, E., Metaxotou, C., Wasi, P., Wood, W. G., Pressley, L., Higgs, D. R., Clegg, J. B., and Weatherall, D. J.: Haemoglobin Bart's hydrops syndrome in Greece. Br. Med. J. 2:268, 1980.
69. Pressley, L., Higgs, D. R., Clegg, J. B., and Weatherall, D. J.: Gene deletions in α-thalassemia prove that the $5'$-ζ locus is functional. Proc. Natl. Acad. Sci. USA 77:3586, 1980.
70. Weatherall, D. J., Clegg, J. B., and Wong, H. B.: The haemoglobin constitution of infants with the haemoglobin Bart's hydrops foetalis syndrome. Br. J. Haematol. 18:357, 1970.
71. Todd, D., Lai, M. C. S., Beaven, G. H., and Huehns, E. R.: The abnormal haemoglobins in homozygous α-thalassaemia. Br. J. Haematol. 19:27, 1970.
72. Capp, G. L., Rigas, D. A., and Jones, R. T.: Evidence for a new haemoglobin chain (ζ-chain). Nature 228:278, 1970.
72a. Peschle, C., Mavilio, F., Carè, A., Migliaccio, G., Migliaccio, A. R., Salvo, G., Samoggia, P., Petti, S., Guerriero, R., Marinucci, M., Lazzaro, D., Russo, G., and Mastroberardino, G.: Haemoglobin switching in human embryos: Asynchrony of ζ → α and ε → γ globin switches in primitive and definitive erythropoietic lineage. Nature 313:235, 1985.
72b. Chung, S. W., Wong, S. C., Clarke, B. J., Patterson, M., Walker, W. H. C., and Chui, D. H. K.: Human embryonic ζ-globin chains in adult patients with α-thalassemias. Proc. Natl. Acad. Sci. USA 81:6188, 1984.
72c. Chui, D. H. K., Wong, S. C., Chung, S.-W., and Poon, M.-C.: Expression of human embryonic ζ globin genes in adult individuals. Blood 64(Suppl. 1):55a, 1984.
72d. Yanofsky, R. A., Beaudry, M. A., Ferguson, D. J., Pearse, K., Rubin, E. M., and Kan, Y. W.: Survival of a hydropic infant with α thalassemia. Blood 64(Suppl. 1):60a, 1984.

73. Tuchinda, S., Nagai, K., and Lehmann, H.: Oxygen dissociation curve of haemoglobin Portland. FEBS Lett. *49*:390, 1975.
74. Pearson, H. A., O'Brien, R. T., and McIntosh, S.: Screening for thalassemia trait by electronic measurement of mean corpuscular volume (MCV). N. Engl. J. Med. *288*:351, 1973.
75. England, J. M., and Fraser, P. M.: Differentiation of iron deficiency from thalassaemia trait by routine blood-count. Lancet *1*:449, 1973.
76. Mentzer, W. C.: Differentiation of iron deficiency from thalassemia trait. Lancet *1*:882, 1973.
77. Torlontano, G., Tata, A., and Camagna, A.: A rapid screening test for thalassaemic trait. Acta Haematol. *48*:234, 1972.
78. Wasi, P., Disthasongchan, P., and Na-Nakorn, S.: The effect of iron deficiency on the levels of hemoglobins A_2 and E. J. Lab. Clin. Med. *71*:85, 1983.
79. Kattamis, C., Lagos, P., Metaxotou-Mavromati, A., and Matsaniotis, N.: Serum iron and unsaturated iron-binding capacity in the β-thalassemia trait: Their relation to the levels of haemoglobins A, A_2, and F. J. Med. Genet. *9*:154, 1972.
80. Askoy, M.: Thalassemia intermedia: A genetic study of 11 patients. J. Med. Genet. *7*:47, 1970.
81. McCarthy, G. M., Temperley, I. J., Clegg, J. B., and Weatherall, D. J.: Thalassemia in an Irish family. Ir. J. Med. Sci. *1*:303, 1968.
82. Stamatoyannopoulos, G., Woodson, R., Papayannopoulou, T., Heywood, D., and Kurachi, S.: Inclusion-body β-thalassemia trait: A form of β thalassemia producing clinical manifestations in simple heterozygotes. N. Engl. J. Med. *290*:939, 1974.
83. Friedman, S., Ozsoylu, S., Luddy, R., and Schwartz, E.: Heterozygous beta thalassaemia of unusual severity. Br. J. Haematol. *32*:65, 1976.
84. Adams, J. G. III, Boxer, L. A., Baehner, R. L., Forget, B. G., Tsistrakis, G. A., and Steinberg, M. H.: Hemoglobin Indianapolis (β112[G14] arginine): An unstable β-chain variant producing the phenotype of severe β-thalassemia. J. Clin. Invest. *63*:931, 1979.
85. Pootrakul, P., Wasi, P., and Na-Nakorn, S.: Haematological data in 312 cases of β-thalassaemia trait in Thailand. Br. J. Haematol. *24*:703, 1973.
86. Knox-Macaulay, H. H. M., Weatherall, D. J., Clegg, J. B., and Pembrey, M. E.: Thalassemia in the British. Br. J. Med. *3*:150, 1973.
86a. Mazza, U., Saglio, G., Cappio, F. C., Camaschella, C., Neretto, G., and Gallo, E.: Clinical and haematological data in 254 cases of beta-thalassaemia trait in Italy. Br. J. Haematol. *33*:91, 1976.
87. Stamatoyannopoulos, G., Fessas, P., and Papayannopoulou, T.: F-thalassemia: A study of thirty-one families with simple heterozygotes and combinations of F-thalassemia with A_2-thalassemia. Am. J. Med. *47*:194, 1969.
88. Millard, D. P., Mason, K., Serjeant, B. E., and Serjeant, G. R.: Comparison of haematological features of the $β^0$ and $β^+$ thalassaemia traits in Jamaican negroes. Br. J. Haematol. *36*:161, 1977.
89. Weatherall, D. J.: Biochemical phenotypes of thalassemia in the American negro population. Ann. N. Y. Acad. Sci. *119*:450, 1964.
90. Schokker, R. C., Went, L. N., and Bok, J.: A new genetic variant of beta-thalassemia. Nature *209*:44, 1966.
90a. Gilman, J. G., Huisman, T. H. J., and Abels, J.: Dutch $β^0$-thalassemia: A 10 kilobase DNA deletion associated with significant γ-chain production. Br. J. Haematol. *56*:339, 1984.
90b. Padanilam, B. J., Felice, A. E., and Huisman, T. H. J.: Partial deletion of the 5' β-globin gene region causes $β^0$-thalassemia in members of an American black family. Blood *64*:941, 1984.
91. Weatherall, D. J., Clegg, J. B., Wood, W. G., Old, J. M., Higgs, D. R., Pressley, L., and Darbre, P. D.: The clinical and molecular heterogeneity of the thalassaemia syndromes. Ann. N. Y. Acad. Sci. *344*:83, 1980.
92. Cappellini, G., Fiorelli, G., and Bernini, L. F.: Interaction between homozygous $β^0$ thalassaemia and the Swiss type of hereditary persistence of fetal haemoglobin. Br. J. Haematol. *48*:561, 1981.
92a. Marinucci, M., Mavilio, F., Giuliani, A., Gabbianelli, M., Tentori, L., Jr., and Tentori, L.: β thalassemia associated with increased Hb F production. Evidence for the existence of a heterocellular hereditary persistence of fetal hemoglobin (HPFH) determinant linked to β thalassemia in a Southern Italian population. Hemoglobin *5*:1, 1981.
92b. Giampaolo, A., Mavilio, F., Sposi, N. M., Carè, A., Massa, A., Cianetti, L., Petrini, M., Russo, R., Cappellini, M. D., and Marinucci, M.: Heterocellular abnormal γ-gene expression in association with β thalassemia and linkage relationship with the β-globin gene cluster. Hum. Genet. *66*:151, 1984.
92c. Wood, W. G., Weatherall, D. J., Clegg, J. B., Hamblin, T. J., Edwards, J. H., and Barlow, A. M.: Heterocellular hereditary persistence of fetal haemoglobin (heterocellular HPFH) and its interaction with β thalassemia. Br. J. Haematol. *36*:461, 1977.
92d. Soummer, A. M., Testa, U., Dujardin, P., Guerrasio, A., Henri, A., Gazaix, M., Riou, J., Rochant, H., Beuzard, Y., and Rosa, J.: Genetic regulation of γ gene expression: Study of the interaction of β-thalassemia with heterocellular HPFH. Hum. Genet. *57*:371, 1981.
93. Bargellesi, A., Pontrennoli, S., and Conconi, F.: Absence of beta-globin synthesis and excess of alpha-globin synthesis in homozygous beta-thalassemia. Eur. J. Biochem. *1*:73, 1967.
94. Cao, A., Galanello, R., Furbetta, M., Muroni, P. P., Garbato, L., Rosatelli, C., Scalas, M. T., Ruggeri, R. R., Laccione, L., and Melis, M. A.: Thalassemia types and their incidence in Sardinia. J. Med. Genet. *15*:443, 1978.
95. Gallanello, R., Melis, M. A., Ruggeri, R., Addis, M., Scalas, M. T., Maccioni, L., Furbetta, M., Angius, A., Tuveri, T., and Cao, A.: $β^0$ thalassaemia trait in Sardinia. Hemoglobin *3*:33, 1979.
96. Wasi, P., Na-Nakorn, S., and Pootrakul, S.: Alpha- and beta-thalassemia in Thailand. Ann. N. Y. Acad. Sci. *165*:60, 1969.
97. Modell, C. B., and Berdoukas, V. A.: The Clinical Approach to Thalassemia. New York, Grune and Stratton, 1981.
98. Conconi, F., Bargellesi, A., Del Senno, L., Menegatti, E., Pontremoli, S., and Russo, G.: Globin chain synthesis in Sicilian thalassemic subjects. Br. J. Haematol. *19*:469, 1970.
99. Schiliro, G., Musumeci, S., Pizzarelli, G., di Gregorio, L., Fischer, A., and Russo, G.: β-thalassemia in Sicily: Hematological and biosynthetic studies. Acta Haematol. *60*:193, 1978.

374 THE THALASSEMIAS—CLINICAL MANIFESTATIONS

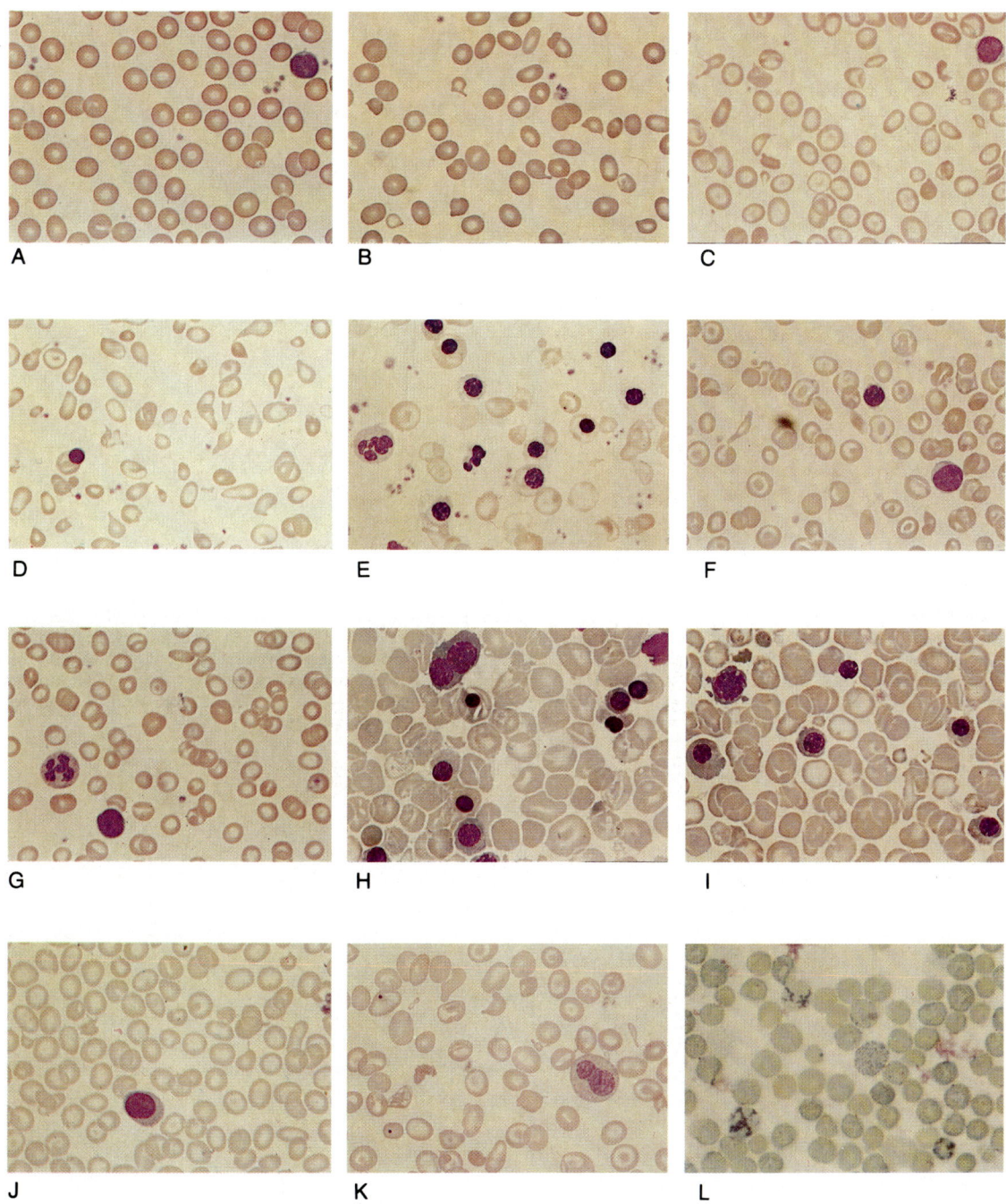

Color Plate I. *A*, Deoxy Hb (α_1—yellow; β_1—blue; α_2—green; β_2—turquoise; heme—red). *B*, Carboxy Hb. (See *A* for color Key.) *C*, Deoxy Hb, showing hydrogen atoms. (See *A* for color key.) *D*, Carboxy Hb, showing hydrogen atoms. (See *A* for color key.) *E*, Sickle polymer, double strand, showing lateral contacts between light blue and dark blue molecules (heme—red; β 6 Val—yellow). (Courtesy of Dr. Eduardo Padlan, Johns Hopkins University.) *F*, Perutz and student. *G*, Human carboxy Hb (heme—red; arginine and lysine residues—blue; glutamic and aspartic acid residues—yellow). (*A–D* and *G*, Prepared by Richard Feldman, National Institutes of Health.)

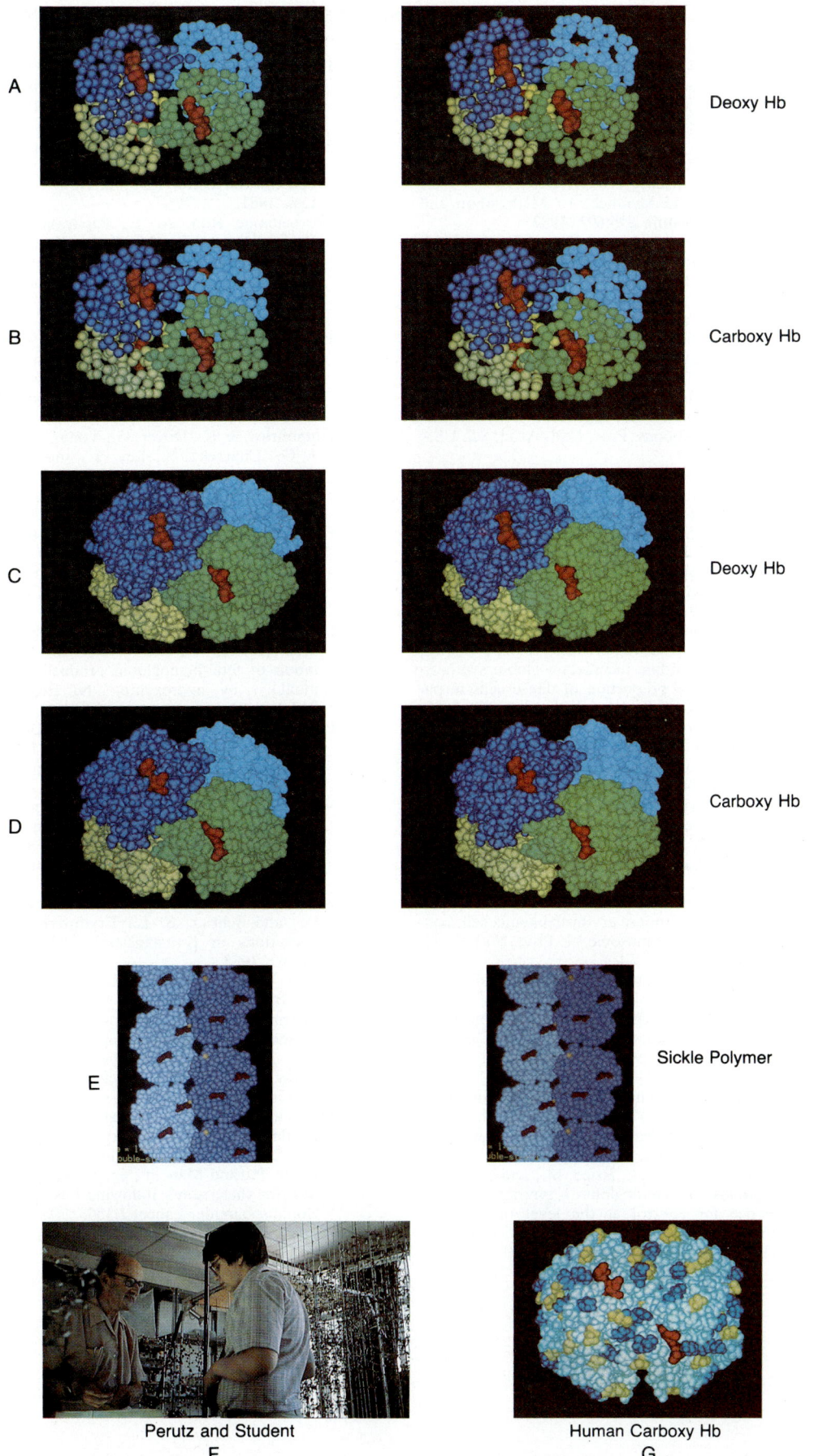

A — Deoxy Hb
B — Carboxy Hb
C — Deoxy Hb
D — Carboxy Hb
E — Sickle Polymer
F — Perutz and Student
G — Human Carboxy Hb

C.: Molecular mechanisms of human hemoglobin switching: Selective undermethylation and expression of globin genes in embryonic, fetal, and adult erythroblasts. Proc. Natl. Acad. Sci. USA 80:6907, 1983.
322. Razin, A., and Riggs, A. D.: DNA methylation and gene function. Science 210:604, 1980.
323. Felsenfeld, G., and McGhee, J.: Methylation and gene control. Nature 296:602, 1982.
324. Busslinger, M., Hurst, J., and Flavell, R. A.: DNA methylation and the regulation of globin gene expression. Cell 34:197, 1983.
325. Creusot, F., Acs, G., and Christman, J. K.: Inhibition of DNA methyltransferase and induction of Friend erythroleukemia cell differentiation by 5-Azacytidine and 5-Aza-2'-deoxycytidine. J. Biol. Chem. 257:2041, 1982.
326. DeSimone, J., Heller, P., Hall, L., and Zwiers, D.: 5-Azacytidine stimulates fetal hemoglobin synthesis in anemic baboons. Proc. Natl. Acad. Sci. USA 79:4428, 1982.
326a. Heller, P., and DeSimone, J.: 5-Azacytidine and fetal hemoglobin. Am. J. Hematol. 17:439, 1984.
327. Ley, T. J., DeSimone, J., Anagnou, N. P., Keller, G. H., Humphries, R. K., Turner, P. H., Young, N. S., Heller, P., and Nienhuis, A. W.: 5-Azacytidine selectively increases gamma-globin synthesis in a patient with beta+ thalassemia. N. Engl. J. Med. 307:1469, 1982.
328. Ley, T. J., DeSimone, J., Noguchi, C. T., Turner, P. H., Schechter, A. N., Heller, P., and Nienhuis, A. W.: 5-azacytidine increases γ-globin synthesis and reduces the proportion of dense cells in patients with sickle cell anemia. Blood 62:370, 1983.
329. Charache, S., Dover, G., Smith, K., Talbot, C. C., Jr., Moyer, M., and Boyer, S.: Treatment of sickle cell anemia with 5-azacytidine results in increased fetal hemoglobin production and is associated with nonrandom hypomethylation of DNA around the γ-δ-β-globin gene complex. Proc. Natl. Acad. Sci. USA 80:4842, 1983.
329a. Ley, T. J., Chiang, Y. L., Haidaris, D., Anagnou, N. P., Wilson, V. L., and Anderson, W. F.: DNA methylation and regulation of the human β-globin–like genes in mouse erythroleukemia cells containing human chromosome 11. Proc. Natl. Acad. Sci. USA 81:6618, 1984.
330. 5-Azacytidine for beta-thalassaemia? (Editorial.) Lancet 1:36, 1983.
331. Landolph, J. R., and Jones, D. A.: Mutagenicity of 5-azacytidine and related nucleosides in C3H/10 T 1/2 clone 8 and V79 cells. Cancer Res. 42:817, 1982.
332. Bioassay of 5-azacytidine for possible carcinogenicity, CAS no. 320-67-2: NCI-CG-TR-42: DHN/PUB/NIH-78-842, National Cancer Institute, Carcinogenesis Program.
333. Papayannopoulou, T. H., Brice, M., and Stamatoyannopoulos, G.: Hemoglobin F synthesis in vitro: Evidence for control at the level of primitive erythroid stem cells. Proc. Natl. Acad. Sci. USA 74:2923, 1977.
334. Papayannopoulou, T. H., Nakamoto, B., Kurachi, S., Kurnit, D., and Stamatoyannopoulos, G.: Cell biology of hemoglobin switching. II. Studies on the regulation of fetal hemoglobin synthesis in human adults. In Stamatoyannopoulos, G., and Nienhuis, A. W. (eds.): Hemoglobins in Development and Differentiation. New York, Alan R. Liss, 1981.
335. Torrealba-de Ron, A. T., Papayannopoulou, T., Knapp, M. S., Fu, M. F.-R., Knitter, G., and Stamatoyannopoulos, G.: Perturbations in the erythroid marrow progenitor cell pools may play a role in the augmentation of HbF by 5-Azacytidine. Blood 63:201, 1984.
336. Perrine, S., Rubin, E., Shatsky, M., Faller, D. V., and Kan, Y. W.: Increased γ-globin synthesis in AML patients on 5-azacytidine is associated with selective destruction of CFUE. Blood 62(Suppl. 1):75a, 1983.
337. Humphries, R. K., Dover, G., Young, N. S., Moore, J. G., Charache, S., Ley, T., and Nienhuis, A. W.: 5-Azacytidine acts directly on both erythroid precursors and progenitors to increase production of Hb F. J. Clin. Invest. 75:547, 1985.
338. Papayannopoulou, T., Torrealba de Ron, A. T., Veith, R., Knitter, G., and Stamatoyannopoulos, G.: Arabinosylcytosine induces fetal hemoglobin in baboons by perturbing erythroid cell differentiation kinetics. Science 224:617, 1984.
339. Letvin, N. L., Linch, D. C., Beardsley, G. P., McIntyre, K. W., and Nathan, D. G.: Augmentation of fetal-hemoglobin production in anemic monkeys by hydroxyurea. N. Engl. J. Med. 310:869, 1984.
340. Platt, O. S., Orkin, S. H., Dover, G., Beardsley, G. P., Miller, B., and Nathan, D. G.: Hydroxyurea enhances fetal hemoglobin production in sickle cell anemia. J. Clin. Invest. 74:652, 1984.
341. Veith, R., Galanello, R., Fu, M., Kurachi, S., Papayannopoulou, T., and Stamatoyannopoulos, G.: Stimulation of Hb F synthesis in Hb S homozygotes treated wtih ARA-C. Blood 64(Suppl. 1):64a, 1984.
342. Rachmilewitz, E. A., Shinar, E., Shalev, O., Galili, U., and Schrier, S. L.: Erythrocyte membrane alterations in β-thalassaemia. Clin. Haematol. 14:163, 1985.
343. Dover, G. J., Humphries, R. K., Young, N., Ley, T., Boyer, S., Charache, S., and Nienhuis, A.: Pharmacologic manipulation of fetal hemoglobin synthesis. In Stamatoyannopoulos, G., and Nienhuis, A. W. (eds.): Experimental Approaches for Study of Hemoglobin Switching. New York, Alan R. Liss, Inc., in press.
344. Lucarelli, G., Polchi, P., Galimberti, M., Izzi, T., Delfini, C., Manna, M., Agostinelli, F., Baronciani, D., Giorgi, C., Angelucci, E., Giardini, C., Politi, P., and Manenti, F.: Marrow Transplantation for thalassemia following busulphan and cyclophosphamide. Lancet 1:1355, 1985.
345. Hilgartner, M., and Giardina, P.: Personal communication.

Wapnick, A. A., and Charlton, R. W.: The role of ascorbic acid in the metabolism of storage iron. Br. J. Haematol. 20:155, 1971.
293. Nienhuis, A. W.: Vitamin C and iron. N. Engl. J. Med. 304:170, 1981.
294. Henry, W.: Echocardiographic evaluation of the heart in thalassemia major. In Nienhuis, A. W. (moderator): Thalassemia major: Molecular and clinical aspects. Ann. Intern. Med. 91:892, 1979.
295. Pippard, M. J., Letsky, E. A., Callender, S. T., and Weatherall, D. J.: Prevention of iron loading in transfusion-dependent thalassaemia. Lancet 1:1178, 1978.
296. Russo, G., Romeo, M. A., Musumeci, S., Schiliro, G., and Di Gregorio, F.: Early iron chelation therapy in thalassemia major. Haematologica 68:69, 1983.
297. Weiner, M., Karpatkin, M., Hart, D., Seaman, C., Vora, S. K., Henry, W. L., and Piomelli, S.: Cooley anemia: High transfusion regimen and chelation therapy, results, and perspective. J. Pediatr. 92:653, 1978.
298. Silvestroni, E., Bianco, I., Graziani, B., Carboni, C., and Constantini, S.: Subcutaneous desferrioxamine in homozygous β-thalassaemia. Lancet 1:1178, 1978.
299. Graziano, J. H., Markenson, A., Miller, D. R., Chang, H., Bestak, M., Meyers, P., Pisciotto, P., and Rifkind, A.: Chelation therapy in β-thalassemia major. I. Intravenous and subcutaneous deferoxamine. J. Pediatr. 92:648, 1978.
300. Hoffbrand, A. V., Gorman, A., Laulicht, M., Garidi, M., Economidou, J., Georgipoulou, P., Hussain, M. A. M., and Flynn, D. M.: Improvement in iron status and liver function in patients with transfusional iron overload with long-term subcutaneous desferrioxamine. Lancet i:947, 1979.
301. Cohen, A., and Schwartz, E.: Decreasing iron stores during intensive chelation therapy. Ann. N. Y. Acad. Sci. 344:405, 1980.
301a. Cohen, A., Martin, M., and Schwartz, E.: Depletion of excessive liver iron stores with desferrioxamine. Br. J. Haematol. 58:369, 1984.
302. Wolfe, L. C., Olivieri, N., Sallan, D., et al.: Prevention of cardiac disease by subcutaneous desferoxamine in patients with thalassemia major. N. Engl. J. Med. 312:1600, 1985.
302a. Marcus, R. E., Davies, S. C., Bantock, H. M., Underwood, S. R., Walton, S., and Huehns, E. R.: Desferrioxamine to improve cardiac function in iron-overloaded patients with thalassemia major. Lancet 1:392, 1984.
302b. High-dose chelation therapy in thalassaemia. (Editorial.) Lancet 1:373, 1984.
302c. Freeman, A. P., Giles, R. W., Berdoukas, V., Walsh, W., Choy, D., and Murray, P. C.: Early left ventricular dysfunction and chelation therapy in thalassemia. Ann. Intern. Med. 99:450, 1983.
303. Davies, S. C., Marcus, R. E., Hungerford, J. L., Miller, M. H., Arden, G. B., and Huehns, E. R.: Ocular toxicity of high-dose intravenous desferrioxamine. Lancet 2:181, 1983.
304. Miller, K. B., Rosenwasser, L. J., Bessette, J. A. M., Deer, D. J., and Rocklin, R. E.: Rapid desensitisation for desferrioxamine anaphylactic reaction. Lancet 1:1069, 1981.
305. Peterson, C. M., Grady, R. W., Jones, R. L., Cerami, A., Graziano, J. H., Markenson, A. L., Lavi, U., Canale, V., Gray, G. F., and Miller, D. R.: 2,3-DHB ineffective in treatment of iron overload. N. Engl. J. Med. 297:1404, 1977.
306. Hershko, C., Grady, R. W., and Link, G.: Evaluation of iron-chelating agents in an in vivo system: Potential usefulness of EHPG, a powerful iron-chelating drug. Br. J. Haematol. 51:251, 1982.
307. Jacobs, A.: Iron chelation therapy for iron loaded patients. Br. J. Haematol. 43:1, 1979.
308. Pippard, M. J., Callender, S. T., Warner, G. T., and Weatherall, D. J.: Iron absorption and loading of β-thalassaemia intermedia. Lancet 2:819, 1979.
309. Disler, P. B., Lynch, S. R., Charlton, R. W., Torrance, J. D., Bothwell, T. H., Walker, R. B., and Mayet, F.: The effect of tea on iron absorption. Gut 16:193, 1975.
310. Leon, M. B., Borer, J. S., Bacharach, S. L., Green, M. V., Benz, E. J., Griffith, P., and Nienhuis, A. W.: Detection of early cardiac dysfunction in patients with severe beta-thalassemia and chronic iron overload. N. Engl. J. Med. 301:1143, 1979.
311. Modell, C. B., and Beck, J.: Long-term desferrioxamine therapy in thalassemia. Ann. N. Y. Acad. Sci. 232:201, 1974.
312. Cohen, A., Cohen, I. J., and Schwartz, E.: Scurvy and altered iron stores in thalassemia major. N. Engl. J. Med. 304:158, 1981.
313. Charlton, R. W., and Bothwell, T. H.: Iron ascorbic acid and thalassemia. Iron metabolism and thalassemia. Birth Defects: Original Article Series, XII. Bergsma, D., Cerami, A., Peterson, C. M., and Graziano, J. H. (eds.). New York, Alan R. Liss, 1976.
314. Hyman, C. B., Landing, B., Alfin-Slater, R., Kozak, L., Weitzman, J., and Ortega, J. A.: D1-alpha-tocopherol, iron and lipofuscin in thalassemia. Ann. N. Y. Acad. Sci. 232:211, 1974.
315. Zannos-Mariolea, L., Tzortzatou, F., Dendaki-Svolaki, K., Katerellos, C., Kavallari, M., and Matsaniotis, N.: Serum vitamin E levels with beta-thalassemia major: Preliminary report. Br. J. Haematol. 26:193, 1974.
316. Rachmilewitz, E. A., Shifter, A., and Kahane, I.: Vitamin E deficiency in β thalassemia major. Changes in hematological and biochemical parameters following a therapeutic trial with alpha-tocopherol. Am. J. Clin. Nutr. 32:1850, 1980.
317. Storb, R., and Santos, G. W.: Application of bone marrow transplantation in leukemia and aplastic anemia. Clin. Haematol. 12:721, 1983.
318. Thomas, E. D., Buckner, C. D., Sanders, J. E., Papayannopoulou, T., Borgna-Pignatti, C., DeStefano, P., Sullivan, K. M., Clift, R. A., and Storb, R.: Marrow transplantation for thalassaemia. Lancet 2:227, 1982.
319. Thomas, E. D.: Marrow transplantation for nonmalignant disorders. N. Engl. J. Med. 312:46, 1985.
319a. Lucarelli, G., Polchi, P., Izzi, T., Manna, M., Agostinelli, F., Delfini, C., Porcellini, A., Galimberti, M., Moretti, L., Manna, A., Sparaventi, G., Baronciani, D., Proietti, A., and Buckner, C. D.: Allogeneic marrow transplantation for thalassemia. Exp. Hematol. 12:676, 1984.
320. van der Ploeg, L. H. T., and Flavell, R. A.: DNA methylation in the human γδβ-globin locus in erythroid and nonerythroid tissues. Cell 19:947, 1980.
321. Mavilio, F., Biampaolo, A., Care, A., Migliaccio, G., Calandrini, M., Russo, G., Pagliardi, G. L., Mastroberardino, G., Marinucci, M., and Peschle,

sion therapy. Proc. Natl. Acad. Sci. USA 75:3474, 1978.
259. Corash, L., Klein, H., Deisseroth, A., Shafer, B., Rosen, S., Beman, J., Griffith, P., and Nienhuis, A.: Selective isolation of young erythrocytes for transfusion support of thalassemia major patients. Blood 57:599, 1981.
260. Graziano, J. H., Piomelli, S., Seaman, C., Wang, T., Cohen, A. R., Kelleher, J. F., Jr., and Schwartz, E.: A simple technique for preparation of young red cells for transfusion from ordinary blood units. Blood 59:865, 1982.
261. Anderson, J., and Lay, H.: Neocyte transfusions for thalassemia major. Transfusion 22:539, 1982.
261a. Marcus, R. E., Wonke, B., Bantock, H. M., Thomas, M. J. G., Parry, E. S., Taite, H., and Huehns, E. R.: A prospective trial of young red cells in 48 patients with transfusion-dependent thalassemia. Br. J. Haematol. 60:153, 1985.
261b. Boiteux, F., Vilmer, E., Girot, R., Muller, J.-Y., Rouzioux, C., Chamaret, S., and Montagnier, L.: Lymphadenopathy syndrome in two thalassemic patients after LAV contamination by blood transfusion. N. Engl. J. Med. 312:648, 1985.
262. O'Brien, R. T., Pearson, H. A., and Spencer, R. P.: Transfusion induced decrease in spleen size in thalassemia major: Documentation by radioisotope scan. J. Pediatr. 81:105, 1972.
263. Blendis, L. M., Modell, C. B., Bowdler, A. J., and Williams, R.: Some effects of splenectomy in thalassaemia major. Br. J. Haematol. 28:77, 1974.
264. Cohen, A., Markenson, A. L., and Schwartz, E.: Transfusion requirements and splenectomy in thalassemia major. J. Pediatr. 97:100, 1980.
265. Engelhard, D., Cividalli, G., and Rachmilewitz, E. A.: Splenectomy in homozygous beta thalassaemia: A retrospective study of 30 patients. Br. J. Haematol. 31:391, 1975.
266. Lewis, S. M.: Newer methods of assessment for splenectomy. In Weatherall, D. J. (ed.): Pitman Medical, 1978, p. 200.
267. Eraklis, A. J., Kevy, S. V., Diamond, L. K., and Gross, R. E.: Hazard of overwhelming infection after splenectomy in childhood. N. Engl. J. Med. 276:1225, 1967.
268. Bullen, A. W., and Losowsky, M. S.: Consequences of impaired splenic function. Clin. Sci. 57:129, 1979.
269. Wasi, P.: Streptococcal infection leading to cardiac and renal involvement in thalassaemia. Lancet 1:949, 1971.
270. Valassi-Adam, H., Nassika, E., Kattamis, C., and Matsaniotis, N.: Immunoglobulin levels in children with homozygous beta-thalassemia. Acta Paediatr. Scand. 65:23, 1976.
271. Witzleben, C. L., and Wyatt, J. P.: The effect of long survival on the pathology of thalassaemia major. J. Path. Bact. 87:1, 1961.
272. Berry, C. L., and Marshall, W. C.: Iron distribution in the liver of patients with thalassaemia major. Lancet 1:1031, 1967.
273. Okon, E., Levij, I. S., and Rachmilewitz, E. A.: Splenectomy, iron overload and liver cirrhosis in beta-thalassemia major. Acta Haematol. 56:142, 1976.
274. Pootrakul, P., Rugkiatsakul, R., and Wasi, P.: Increased transferrin iron saturation in splenectomized thalassaemic patients. Br. J. Haematol. 46:143, 1980.
275. Risdon, A. R., Barry, M., and Flynn, D. M.: Transfusional iron overload: The relationship between tissue iron concentration and hepatic fibrosis in thalassaemia. J. Pathol. 116:83, 1975.
276. Graziano, J. H., Piomelli, S., Hilgartner, M., Giardina, P., Karpatkin, M., Andrew, M., Loiacono, N., and Seaman, C.: Chelation therapy in β-thalassemia major. III. The role of splenectomy in achieving iron balance. J. Pediatr. 99:695, 1981.
277. Smith, R. S.: Chelating agents in the diagnosis and treatment of iron overload in thalassemia. Ann. N. Y. Acad. Sci. 119:776, 1964.
278. Pippard, M. J., Callender, S. T., and Finch, C. A.: Ferrioxamine excreted in iron-loaded man. Blood 60:288, 1982.
279. Wapnick, A. A., Lynch, S. R., Charlton, R. W., Seftel, H. C., and Bothwell, T. H.: The effect of ascorbic acid deficiency on desferrioxamine-induced urinary iron excretion. Br. J. Haematol. 17:563, 1969.
280. Modell, C. B., and Beck, J.: Long-term desferrioxamine therapy in thalassemia. Ann. N. Y. Acad. Sci. 232:201, 1974.
281. Constantoulakis, M., Economidou, J., Karagiorga, M., Katsantoni, A., and Gyftaki, E.: Combined long term treatment of hemosiderosis with desferrioxamine and DTPA in homozygous β-thalassemia. Ann. N. Y. Acad. Sci. 232:193, 1974.
282. O'Brien, R. T.: Ascorbic acid enhancement of desferrioxamine-induced urinary iron excretion in thalassemia major. Ann. N. Y. Acad. Sci. 232:221, 1974.
283. Green, R., Lamon, J., and Curran, D.: Clinical trial of desferrioxamine entrapped in red cell ghosts. Lancet 2:327, 1980.
284. Barry, M., Flynn, D. M., Letsky, E. A., and Risdon, R. A.: Long-term chelation therapy in thalassemia major: Effect on liver iron concentration, liver histology and clinical progress. Br. Med. J. 2:16, 1974.
285. Modell, B., Letsky, E. A., Flynn, D. M., Peto, R., and Weatherall, D. J.: Survival and desferrioxamine in thalassaemia major. Br. Med. J. 284:1081, 1982.
286. Propper, R. D., Shurin, S. B., and Nathan, D. G.: Reassessment of the use of desferrioxamine B in iron overload. N. Engl. J. Med. 294:1421, 1976.
287. Propper, R. D., Cooper, B., Rufo, R. R., Nienhuis, A. W., Anderson, W. F., Bunn, F., Rosenthal, A., and Nathan, D. G.: Continuous subcutaneous administration of deferoxamine in patients with iron overload. N. Engl. J. Med. 297:418, 1977.
288. Pippard, M. J., Callendar, S. T., and Weatherall, D. J.: Intensive iron-chelating therapy with desferrioxamine in iron-loading anaemias. Clin. Sci. 54:99, 1978.
289. Hussain, M. A. M., Flynn, D. M., Green, N., Hussein, S., and Hoffbrand, A. V.: Subcutaneous infusion and intramuscular injection of desferrioxamine in patients with transfusional iron overload. Lancet 2:1278, 1976.
290. Hussain, M. A. M., Flynn, D. M., Green, N., and Hoffbrand, A. V.: Effect of dose, time, and ascorbate on iron excretion after subcutaneous desferrioxamine. Lancet 1:977, 1977.
291. Pippard, M. J., and Callender, S. T.: The management of iron chelation therapy. Br. J. Haematol. 54:503, 1983.
292. Lipschitz, D. A., Bothwell, T. H., Seftel, H. C.,

Rosatelli, C., Scalas, M. T., Fais, R., Cao, A., Angioni, G., and Caminiti, F.: Prenatal diagnosis of β thalassaemia by fetal red cell enrichment with NH_4Cl-NH_4HCO_3 differential lysis of maternal cells. Br. J. Haematol. 44:441, 1980.
231. Boyer, S. H., Noyes, A. N., and Boyer, M. L.: Enrichment of erythrocytes of fetal origin from adult-fetal blood mixtures via selective hemolysis of adult blood cells: An aid to antenatal diagnosis of hemoglobinopathies. Blood 47:883, 1976.
232. Cividalli, G., Nathan, D. G., Kan, W. Y., Santamarina, B., and Frigoletto, F.: Relation of beta to gamma synthesis during the first trimester: An approach to prenatal diagnosis of thalassemia. Pediatr. Res. 8:553, 1974.
233. Chang, H., Modell, C. B., Alter, B. P., Dickinson, M. J., Frigoletto, F. D., Huehns, E. R., and Nathan, D. G.: Expression of the β-thalassemia gene in the first trimester fetus. Proc. Natl. Acad. Sci. USA 72:3633, 1975.
234. Nathan, D. G., and Alter, B. P.: Antenatal diagnosis of the haemoglobinopathies. Br. J. Haematol. (Suppl.) 31:143, 1975.
235. Kazazian, H. H., and Woodhead, A. P.: Adult hemoglobin synthesis in the human fetus. Ann. N.Y. Acad. Sci. 241:691, 1974.
236. Williamson, R., Eskdale, J., Coleman, D. V., Niazi, M., Loeffler, F. E., and Modell, B. F.: Direct gene analysis of chorionic villi: A possible technique for first-trimester antenatal diagnosis of haemoglobinopathies. Lancet 2:1125, 1981.
237. Old, J. M., Ward, R. H. T., Petrou, M., Karagozlu, F., Modell, B., and Weatherall, D. J.: First-trimester fetal diagnosis for haemoglobinopathies: Three cases. Lancet 2:1413, 1982.
237a. Goossens, M., Dumez, Y., Kaplan, L., Lupker, M., Chabret, C., Henrion, R., and Rosa, J.: Prenatal diagnosis of sickle-cell anemia in the first trimester of pregnancy. N. Engl. J. Med. 309:831, 1983.
237b. Modell, B., Petrou, M., Ward, R. H. T., Fairweather, D. V. I., Rodeck, C., Varnavides, L. A., and White, J. M.: Effect of fetal diagnostic testing on birth-rate of thalassemia major in Britain. Lancet 2:1383, 1984.
237c. Scriver, C. R., Bardanis, M., Cartier, L., Clow, C. L., Lancaster, G. A., and Ostrowsky, J. T.: β-Thalassemia disease prevention: Genetic medicine applied. Am. J. Hum. Genet. 36:1024, 1984.
238. Wolman, I. J.: Transfusion therapy in Cooley's anemia: Growth and health as related to long-range hemoglobin levels, a progress report. Ann. N. Y. Acad. Sci. 119:736, 1964.
239. Propper, R. D., Button, L. N., and Nathan, D. G.: New approaches to the transfusion management of thalassemia. Blood 55:55, 1980.
240. Necheles, T. F., Allen, D. M., and Finkel, H. E.: Clinical disorders of hemoglobin structure and synthesis. New York, Appleton-Century-Crofts, 1969.
241. Piomelli, S., Danoff, S. J., Becker, M. H., Lipera, M. J., and Travis, S. F.: Prevention of bone malformations and cardiomegaly in Cooley's anemia by early hypertransfusion regimen. Ann. N.Y. Acad. Sci. 165:427, 1969.
242. Beard, M. E. J., Necheles, T. F., and Allen, D. M.: Clinical experience with intensive transfusion therapy in Cooley's anemia. Ann. N. Y. Acad. Sci. 165:415, 1969.
243. Wolman, I. J., and Ortolani, M.: Some clinical features of Cooley's anemia patients as related to transfusion schedules. Ann. N. Y. Acad. Sci. 165:407, 1969.
244. Kattamis, C., Touliatos, N., Haidas, S., and Matsaniotis, N.: Growth of children with thalassemia: Effect of different transfusion regimens. Arch. Dis. Child. 45:502, 1970.
245. Johnston, F. E., Hertzog, K. P., and Malina, R. M.: Longitudinal growth in thalassemia major: Relationship to hemoglobin level. Am. J. Dis. Child. 112:396, 1966.
246. Wolff, J. A., and Luke, K. H.: Management of thalassemia: A comparative program. Ann. N. Y. Acad. Sci. 165:423, 1969.
247. Brook, C. G., Thompson, E. N., Marshall, W. C., and Whitehouse, R. H.: Growth in children with thalassemia major and effect of two different transfusion regimens. Arch. Dis. Child. 44:612, 1969.
248. Erlandson, M. E., Walden, B., Stern, G., Hilgartner, M. W., Wehman, J., and Smith, C. H.: Studies on congenital hemolytic syndromes. IV. Gastrointestinal absorption of iron. Blood 19:359, 1962.
249. De Alarcon, P. A., Donovan, M. E., Forbes, G. B., Landaw, S. A., and Stockman, J. A.: Iron absorption in the thalassemia syndromes and its inhibition by tea. N. Engl. J. Med. 300:5, 1979.
250. Masera, G., Terzoli, S., Avanzini, A., Fontanelli, G., Mauri, R. A., Placentini, G., and Ferrari, M.: Evaluation of the supertransfusion regimen in homozygous beta-thalassaemia children. Br. J. Haematol. 52:111, 1982.
251. Necheles, T. F., Chung, S., Sabbah, R., and Whitten, D.: Intensive transfusion therapy in thalassemia major: An eight year follow-up. Ann. N. Y. Acad. Sci. 232:179, 1974.
252. Piomelli, S., Karpatkin, M. H., Arzanian, M., Zamani, M., Becker, M. H., Geneiser, N., Danoff, S. J., and Kuhns, W. J.: Hypertransfusion regimen in patients with Cooley's anemia. Ann. N. Y. Acad. Sci. 232:186, 1974.
253. Rotoli, B.: Thalassemia in Italy: Treatment of Cooley's disease and iron kinetics in heterozygotes. Birth Defects: Original Article Series, XII. Bergsma, D., Cerami, A., Peterson, C. M., and Graziani, J. H. (eds.). New York, Alan R. Liss, 1976, p. 53.
254. Loukopoulos, D.: Present status of treatment of thalassemia in Greece. Birth Defects: Original Article Series, XII. Bergsma, D., Cerami, A., Peterson, C. N., and Graziano, J. H. (eds.). New York, Alan R. Liss, 1976, p. 1.
255. Esposito, L., Ferrara, M., and Ponte, G.: Blood transfusion therapy in thalassemia major. Experience of a 5-year period of activity in the Center for Hemoglobinopathies of the Pediatric Clinic of Naples. Pediatria 86:537, 1978.
256. Modell, C. B.: Total management in thalassaemia major. Arch. Dis. Child. 52:489, 1977.
257. Weiner, M., Karpatkin, M., Hart, D., Seaman, C., Vora, S. K., Henry, W. L., and Piomelli, S.: Cooley anemia: High transfusion regimen and chelation therapy, results, and perspective. J. Pediatr. 92:653, 1978.
258. Piomelli, S., Seaman, C., Reibman, J., Tytun, A., Graziano, J. H., Tabachnik, N., and Corash, L.: Separation of younger red cells with improved survival in vivo: An approach to chronic transfu-

B. P., Grenett, H. E., and Garver, F. A.: Increased HbF in sickle cell anemia is determined by a factor linked to the β^s gene from one parent. Blood 63:64, 1984.
201. Marti, H. R.: Normale und anormale menschliche Hamoglobine. Berlin, Springer Verlag, 1963, p. 81.
202. Wood, W. G., Weatherall, D. J., and Clegg, J. B.: Interaction of heterocellular hereditary persistence of foetal haemoglobin with β thalassemia and sickle cell anaemia. Nature 264:247, 1976.
203. Serjeant, G. R., Serjeant, B. E., and Mason, K.: Heterocellular hereditary persistence of fetal haemoglobin and homozygous sickle-cell disease. Lancet 1:795, 1977.
204. Dover, G. J., and Boyer, S. H.: F-cell production in sickle cell anemia: Regulation by genes linked to β-hemoglobin locus. Science 211:1441, 1981.
205. Old, J. M., Ayyub, H., Wood, W. G., Clegg, J. B., and Weatherall, D. J.: Linkage analysis of nondeletion hereditary persistence of fetal hemoglobin. Science 215:981, 1983.
206. Gianni, A. M., Bregni, M., Cappellini, M. D., Fiorelli, G., Taramelli, R., Giglioni, B., Comi, P., and Ottolenghi, S.: A gene controlling fetal hemoglobin expression in adults is not linked to the non-α globin cluster. EMBO J 2:921, 1983.
207. Sukumaran, P. K., Huisman, T. H. J., Schroeder, W. A., McCurdy, P. R., Freehafer, J. T., Bouver, N., Shelton, J. R., Shelton, J. B., and Apell, G.: A homozygote for the Hb$_{G\gamma}$ type of foetal haemoglobin in India: A study of two Indian and four Negro families. Br. J. Haematol. 23:403, 1972.
208. Altay, C., Huisman, T. H. J., and Schroeder, W. A.: Another form of hereditary persistence of fetal hemoglobin (the Atlanta type)? Hemoglobin 1:125, 1976–77.
209. Stamatoyannopoulos, G., Wood, W. G., Papayannopoulou, T., and Nute, P. E.: A new form of hereditary persistence of fetal hemoglobin in blacks and its association with sickle cell trait. Blood 46:683, 1975.
209a. Gilman, J. G., and Huisman, T. H. J.: A mutation 158 base pairs 5′ to the $^G\gamma$ gene is associated with elevated $^G\gamma$ production. Blood 64(Suppl. 1):62a, 1984.
210. Weatherall, D. J., Cartner, R., Clegg, J. B., Wood, W. G., MacRae, I. A., and Mackenzie, A.: A form of hereditary persistence of fetal hemoglobin characterized by uneven cellular distribution of haemoglobin F and the production of haemoglobins A and A$_2$ in homozygotes. Br. J. Haematol. 29:205, 1975.
211. Wood, W. G., MacRae, I. A., Darbre, P. D., Clegg, J. B., and Weatherall, D. J.: The British type of non-deletion HPFH: Characterization of developmental changes in vivo and erythroid growth in vitro. Br. J. Haematol. 50:401, 1982.
212. Perrine, R. P., Brown, M. J., Clegg, J. B., Weatherall, D. J., and May, A.: Benign sickle-cell anaemia. Lancet 2:1163, 1972.
213. Perrine, R. P., Pembrey, M. E., John, P., Perrine, S., and Shoup, F.: Natural history of sickle-cell anaemia in Saudi Arabs: A study of 270 subjects. Ann. Intern. Med. 88:1, 1978.
214. Pembrey, M. E., Wood, W. G., Weatherall, D. J., and Perrine, R. P.: Fetal haemoglobin production and the sickle gene in the oases of eastern Saudi Arabia. Br. J. Haematol. 40:415, 1978.
215. Wood, W. G., Pembrey, M. E., Serjeant, G. R., Perrine, R. P., and Weatherall, D. J.: Hb F synthesis in sickle cell anaemia: A comparison of Saudi Arab cases with those of African origin. Br. J. Haematol. 45:431, 1980.
216. Brittenham, G., Lozoff, B., Harris, J. W., Sharma, V. S., and Marasimhan, S.: Sickle cell anemia and trait in a population of southern India. Am. J. Hematol. 2:25, 1977.
217. Brittenham, G., Lozoff, B., Harris, J. W., Mayson, S. M., Miller, A., and Huisman, T. H. J.: Sickle cell anemia and trait in Southern India: Further studies. Am. J. Hematol. 6:107, 1979.
218. Pembrey, M. E., Perrine, R. P., Wood, W. G., and Weatherall, D. J.: Sickle-β^0 thalassemia in eastern Saudi Arabia. Am. J. Hum. Genet. 32:26, 1980.
218a. Miller, B. A., Salameh, M., Ahmed, M., Antognetti, G., Weatherall, D. J., and Nathan, D. G.: High fetal hemoglobin production in sickle cell anemia patients from the oases of Saudi Arabia is genetically determined. Blood 64(Suppl. 1):51a, 1984.
219. Kan, Y. W., Valenti, C., Carnazza, V., Guidotti, R., and Rieder, R. F.: Fetal blood-sampling in utero. Lancet 1:79, 1974.
220. Hobbins, J. C., and Mahoney, M. J.: In utero diagnosis of hemoglobinopathies. Technic for obtaining fetal blood. N. Engl. J. Med. 290:1065, 1974.
221. Hobbins, J. C., and Mahoney, M. J.: Fetal blood drawing. Lancet 2:107, 1975.
222. Alter, B. P., Modell, C. B., Fairweather, D., Hobbins, J. C., Mahoney, M. J., Frigoletto, F. D., Sherman, A. S., and Nathan, D. G.: Prenatal diagnosis of hemoglobinopathies. A review of 15 cases. N. Engl. J. Med. 295:1437, 1976.
223. Kan, Y. W., Golbus, M. S., Trecartin, R. F., Filly, R. A., Valenti, C., Furbetta, M., and Cao, A.: Prenatal diagnosis of β-thalassaemia and sickle-cell anaemia: Experience with 24 cases. Lancet 1:269, 1977.
224. Alter, B. P.: Antenatal diagnosis of thalassemia: A review. Ann. N.Y. Acad. Sci. 445:393, 1985.
225. Cao, A., Cossu, P., Falchi, A. M., Monni, G., Pirastu, M., Rosatelli, C., Scalas, M. T., and Tuveri, T.: Antenatal diagnosis of thalassemia major in Sardinia. Ann. N.Y. Acad. Sci. 445:380, 1985.
226. Loukopoulos, D., Karababa, P., Antsaklis, A., et al.: Prenatal diagnosis of thalassemia and Hb S syndromes in Greece: An evaluation of 1500 cases. Ann. N.Y. Acad. Sci. 445:357, 1985.
227. Matsakis, M., Berdoukas, V. A., Angastiniotis, M., Mouzouras, M., Ioannou, P., Ferrari, M., Modell, B., Fairweather, D. V. I., Ward, R. H. T., Loukopoulos, D., and Sakarellou, N.: Haematological aspects of antenatal diagnosis for thalassaemia in Britain. Br. J. Haematol. 46:185, 1980.
227a. Alter, B. P.: Advances in the prenatal diagnosis of hematologic diseases. Blood 64:329, 1984.
228. Kan, Y. W., Nathan, D. G., Cividalli, G., and Crookston, M. C.: Concentration of fetal red blood cells from a mixture of maternal and fetal blood by anti-i serum: An aid to prenatal diagnosis of hemoglobinopathies. Blood 43:411, 1974.
229. Alter, B. P., Metzger, J. B., Yock, P. G., Rothchild, S. B., and Dover, G. J.: Selective hemolysis of adult red blood cells: An aid to prenatal diagnosis of hemoglobinopathies. Blood 53:279, 1979.
230. Furbetta, M., Angius, A., Ximenes, A., Tuveri, T.,

174. Natta, C. L., Niazi, G. A., Ford, S., and Bank, A.: Balanced globin chain synthesis in hereditary persistence of fetal hemoglobin. J. Clin. Invest. 54:433, 1974.
175. Friedman, S., Schwartz, E., Ahern, E., and Ahern, V.: Variations in globin chain synthesis in hereditary persistence of fetal haemoglobin. Br. J. Haematol. 32:357, 1976.
176. Huisman, T. H. J., Miller, A., Cook, L., Gordon, S., and Schroeder, W. A.: The molecular heterogeneity of some types of hereditary persistence of fetal hemoglobin (HPFH). Proceedings of the International Istanbul Symposium on Abnormal Hemoglobins and Thalassemia. Aksoy, M. (ed.) Ankara, 1975, p. 95.
177. Forget, B. G., Hillman, D. G., Lazarus, H., Barell, E. F., Benz, E. J., Jr., Caskey, C. T., Huisman, T. H. J., Schroeder, W. A., and Housman, D.: Absence of messenger RNA and gene DNA for beta globin chains in hereditary persistence of fetal hemoglobin. Cell 7:323, 1976.
178. Charache, S., Clegg, J. B., and Weatherall, D. J.: The Negro variety of hereditary persistence of fetal hemoblogin is a mild form of thalassemia. Br. J. Haematol. 34:527, 1976.
179. Kutlar, A., Gardiner, M. B., Headlee, M. G., Reese, A. L., Cleek, M. P., Nagle, S., Sukumaran, P. K., and Huisman, T. H. J.: Heterogeneity in the molecular basis of three types of hereditary persistence of fetal hemoglobin and the relative synthesis of the $^G\gamma$ and $^A\gamma$ types of γ chain. Biochem. Genet. 22:21, 1984.
180. Huisman, T. H. J., Miller, A., and Schroeder, W. A.: A $^G\gamma$ type of the hereditary persistence of fetal hemoglobin with β chain production in cis. Am. J. Hum. Genet. 27:765, 1975.
181. Friedman, S., and Schwartz, E.: Hereditary pesistence of foetal haemoglobin with β chain synthesis in cis position ($^G\gamma$-β^+-HPFH) in a negro family. Nature 259:138, 1976.
182. Tatsis, B.: Hereditary persistence of fetal hemoglobin (HPFH) with β-chain production in cis: A new case in interaction with α-thalassemia. Blood 52:119, 1978.
183. Higgs, D. R., Clegg, J. B., Wood, W. G., and Weatherall, D. J.: $^G\gamma\beta^+$ type of hereditary persistence of fetal haemoglobin in association with Hb C. J. Med. Genet. 16:288, 1979.
184. Farquhar, M., Gelinas, R., Tatsis, B., Murray, J., Yagi, M., Mueller, R., and Stamatoyannopoulos, G.: Restriction endonuclease mapping of γ-δ-β-globin region in $^G\gamma(\beta)^+$ HPFH and a Chinese $^A\gamma$ HPFH variant. Am. J. Hum. Genet. 35:611, 1983.
185. Huisman, T. H. J., Wrightstone, R. N., Wilson, J. B., Schroeder, W. A., and Kendall, A. G.: Hemoglobin Kenya, the product of fusion of γ and β polypeptide chains. Arch. Biochem. Biophys. 153:850, 1972.
186. Kendall, A. G., Ojwang, P. J., Schroeder, W. A., and Huisman, T. H. J.: Hemoglobin Kenya, the project of a γ-β fusion gene: Studies of the family. Am. J. Hum. Genet. 25:548, 1973.
187. Smith, D. H., Clegg, J. B., Weatherall, D. J., and Gilles, H. M.: Hereditary persistence of foetal haemoglobin associated with a $\gamma\beta$ fusion variant, haemoglobin Kenya. Nature 246:184, 1973.
188. Nute, P. E., Wood, W. G., Stamatoyannopoulos, G., Olweny, C., and Fialkow, P. J.: The Kenya form of hereditary persistence of fetal haemoglobin: Structural studies and evidence for homogeneous distribution of haemoglobin F using fluorescent anti-haemoglobin F antibodies. Br. J. Haematol. 32:55, 1976.
189. Wood, W. G., Clegg, J. B., Weatherall, D. J., Gyde, O. H. B., Obeid, D. A., Tarlow, M. J., Brown, M. J., and Hewitt, S.: $^G\gamma$ $\delta\beta$ thalassaemia and $^G\gamma$ HPFH (Hb Kenya type) comparison of two new cases. J. Med. Genet. 14:237, 1977.
190. Ojwang, P. J., Nakatsuji, T., Gardiner, M. B., Reese, A. L., Gilman, J. G., and Huisman, T. H. J.: Gene deletion as the molecular basis for the Kenya-$^G\gamma$-HPFH condition. Hemoglobin 7:115, 1983.
191. Fessas, P., and Stamatoyannopoulos, G.: Hereditary persistence of fetal hemoglobin in Greece. A study and a comparison. Blood 24:223, 1964.
192. Huisman, T. H. J., Schroeder, W. A., Stamatoyannopoulos, G., Bouver, N., Shelton, J. R., Shelton, J. B., and Apell, G.: Nature of fetal hemoglobin in the Greek type of hereditary persistence of fetal hemoglobin with and without concurrent β-thalassemia. J. Clin. Invest. 49:1035, 1970.
193. Sofroniadou, K., Wood, W. G., Nute, P. E., and Stamatoyannopoulos, G.: Globin chain synthesis in the Greek type ($^A\gamma$) of hereditary persistence of fetal haemoglobin. Br. J. Haematol. 29:137, 1975.
194. Clegg, J. B., Metaxatou-Mavromati, A., Kattamis, C., Sofroniadou, K., Wood, W. G., and Weatherall, D. J.: Occurrence of $^G\gamma$ Hb F in Greek HPHF: Analysis of heterozygotes and compound heterozygotes with β thalassaemia. Br. J. Haematol. 43:521, 1979.
195. Camaschella, C., Ciocca-Vasino, M. A., Guerrasio, A., Balegno, G., Barberis, E., Delponte, D., and Saglio, G.: Biosynthetic studies and γ-chain composition in the Greek type of hereditary persistence of fetal hemoglobin and in its association with β-thalassemia. Acta Haematol. 61:272, 1979.
196. Papayannopoulou, T., Lawn, R. M., Stamatoyannopoulos, G., and Maniatis, T.: Greek ($^A\gamma$) variant of hereditary persistence of fetal haemoglobin: Globin gene organization and studies of expression of fetal haemoglobins in clonal erythroid cultures. Br. J. Haematol. 50:387, 1982.
197. Boyer, S. H., Margolet, L., Boyer, M. L., Huisman, T. H. J., Schroeder, W. A., Wood, W. G., Weatherall, D. J., Clegg, J. B., and Cartner, R.: Inheritance of F cell frequency in heterocellular hereditary persistence of fetal hemoglobin. An example of allelic exclusion. Am. J. Hum. Genet. 29:256, 1977.
198. Boyer, S. H., Belding, T. K., Margolet, L., and Noyes, A. N.: Fetal hemoglobin restriction to a few erythrocytes (F cells) in normal human adults. Science 188:361, 1975.
199. Wood, W. G., Stamatoyannopoulos, G., Lim, G., and Nute, P. E.: F-cells in the adult: Normal values and levels in individuals with hereditary and acquired elevations of Hb F. Blood 46:671, 1975.
200. Zago, M. A., Wood, W. G., Clegg, J. B., Weatherall, D. J., O'Sullivan, M., and Gunson, H.: Genetic control of F cells in human adults. Blood 53:977, 1979.
200a. Mason, K. P., Grandison, Y., Hayes, R. J., Serjeant, B. E., Serjeant, G. R., Vaidya, S., and Wood, W. G.: Post-natal decline of fetal haemoglobin in homozygous sickle cell disease: Relationship to parental Hb F levels. Br. J. Haematol. 52:455, 1982.
200b. Milner, P. F., Leibfarth, J. D., Ford, J., Barton,

150b. Bruzdzinski, C. J., Sisco, K. L., Ferrucci, S. J., and Rucknagel, D. L.: The occurrence of the $\alpha^{\text{G-Philadelphia}}$-globin allele on a double-locus chromosome. Am. J. Hum. Genet. 36:101, 1984.

150c. Sciarratta, G. V., Sansone, G., Ivaldi, G., Felice, A. E., and Huisman, T. H. J.: Alternate organization of α G-Philadelphia globin genes among U.S. black and Italian Caucasian heterozygotes. Hemoglobin 8:537, 1984.

151. DeSimone, J., Kleve, L., Longley, M. A., and Shaeffer, J.: Unbalanced globin chain synthesis in reticulocytes of sickle cell trait individual with low concentrations of hemoglobin S. Biochem. Biophys. Res. Comm. 59:564, 1974.

152. Steinberg, M. H., Adams, J. G. III, and Dreiling, B. J.: Alpha thalassaemia in adults with sickle-cell trait. Br. J. Haematol. 30:31, 1975.

153. Felice, A. E., Webber, B., Miller, A., Mayson, S. M., Harris, H. F., Henson, J. B., Gravely, M. E., and Huisman, T. H. J.: The association of sickle cell anemia with heterozygous and homozygous α-thalassemia-2: In vitro HB chain synthesis. Am. J. Hematol. 6:91, 1979.

154. Higgs, D. R., Old, J. M., Clegg, J. B., Pressley, L., Hunt, D. M., and Weatherall, D. J.: Negro α-thalassaemia is caused by deletion of a single α-globin gene. Lancet 2:272, 1979.

155. Brittenham, G., Lozoff, B., Harris, J. W., Kan, Y. W., Dozy, A. M., and Nayudu, N. V. S.: Alpha globin gene number: Population and restriction endonuclease studies. Blood 55:706, 1980.

156. Higgs, D. R., Pressley, L., Serjeant, G. R., Clegg, J. B., and Weatherall, D. J.: The genetics and molecular basis of alpha thalassaemia in association with Hb S in Jamaican Negroes. Br. J. Haematol. 47:43, 1981.

157. Higgs, D. R., Aldridge, B. E., Lamb, J., Clegg, J. B., Weatherall, D. J., Hayes, R. J., Grandison, Y., Lowrie, Y., Mason, K. P., Serjeant, B. E., and Serjeant, G. R.: The interaction of alpha-thalassemia and homozygous sickle-cell disease. N. Engl. J. Med. 306:1441, 1982.

158. Embury, S. H., Dozy, A. M., Miller, J., Davis, J. R., Jr., Kleman, K. M., Preisler, H., Vichinsky, E., Lande, W. N., Lubin, B. H., Kan, Y. W., and Mentzer, W. C.: Concurrent sickle-cell anemia and α-thalassemia: Effect on severity of anemia. N. Engl. J. Med. 306:270, 1982.

159. Steinberg, M. H., Rosenstock, W., Coleman, M. B., Adams, J. G., Platica, O., Cedeno, M., Rieder, R. F., Wilson, J. T., Milner, P., West, S., and the Cooperative Study of Sickle Cell Disease: Effects of thalassemia and microcytosis on the hematologic and vasoocclusive severity of the sickle cell anemia. Blood 63:1353, 1984.

159a. Steinberg, M. H., Coleman, M. B., Adams, J. G., Platica, O., Gillette, P., and Rieder, R. F.: The effects of alpha-thalassaemia in HbSC disease. Br. J. Haematol. 55:487, 1983.

159b. Serjeant, G. R., Foster, K., and Serjeant, B. E.: Red cell size and the clinical and haematological features of homozygous sickle cell disease. Br. J. Haematol. 48:445, 1981.

159c. Embury, S. H., Clark, M. R., Monroy, G., and Mohandas, N.: Concurrent sickle cell anemia and α-thalassemia: Effect on pathological properties of sickle erythrocytes. J. Clin. Invest. 73:116, 1984.

160. Serjeant, B. E., Mason, K. P., Kenny, M. W., Stuart, J., Higgs, D. R., Weatherall, D. J., Hayes, R. J., and Serjeant, G. R.: Effect of alpha thalassaemia on the rheology of homozygous sickle cell disease. Br. J. Haematol. 55:479, 1983.

161. Mears, J. G., Lachman, H. M., Labie, D., and Nagel, R. L.: Alpha-thalassemia is related to prolonged survival in sickle cell anemia. Blood 62:286, 1983.

162. Oort, M., Heerspink, W., Roos, D., Flavell, R. A., and Bernini, L. F.: Haemolytic disease of the newborn and chronic anaemia induced by γδβ thalassaemia in a Dutch family. Br. J. Haematol. 48:251, 1981.

163. Fearon, E. R., Kazazian, H. H., Jr., Waber, P. G., Lee, J. I., Antonarakis, S. E., Orkin, S. H., Vanin, E. F., Henthorn, P. S., Grosveld, F. G., Scott, A. F., and Buchanan, G. R.: The entire β-globin gene cluster is deleted in a form of γδβ-thalassemia. Blood 61:1273, 1983.

164. Pirastu, M., Kan, W. Y., Lin, C. C., Baine, R. M., and Holbrook, C. T.: Hemolytic disease of the newborn caused by a new deletion of the entire β-globin cluster. J. Clin. Invest. 72:602, 1983.

165. Huisman, T. H. J., Reese, M. B., Gardiner, M. B., Wilson, J. B., Lam, H., Reynolds, A., Nagle, S., Trowell, P., Yi-tao, Z., Shu-zheng, H., Sukumaran, P. K., Miwa, S., Efremov, G. D., Petkov, G., Sciaratta, G. V., and Sansone, G.: The occurrence of different levels of $^G\gamma$ chain and of the $^A\gamma^T$ variant of fetal hemoglobin in newborn babies from several countries. Am. J. Hematol. 14:133, 1983.

166. Powers, P. A., Altay, C., Huisman, T. H. J., and Smithies, O.: Two novel arrangements of the human fetal globin genes: $^G\gamma$-$^G\gamma$ and $^A\gamma$-$^A\gamma$. Nucleic Acids Res. 12:7023, 1984.

167. Fraser, G. R., Stamatoyannopoulos, G., Kattamis, C., Loukopoulos, D., Deteranas, B., Kitsos, C., Zannos-Mariolea, L., Choremis, C., Fessas, P., and Motulsky, A. G.: Thalassemias, abnormal hemoglobins, and glucose-6-phosphate dehydrogenase deficiency in the Arta area of Greece: Diagnostic and genetic aspects of complete village studies. Ann. N. Y. Acad. Sci. 119:415, 1964.

168. Ohta, Y., Yamaoka, K., Sumida, I., Fujita, S., Fujimura, T., and Yanse, T.: Homozygous delta-thalassemia first discovered in Japanese family with hereditary persistence of fetal hemoglobin. Blood 376:706, 1971.

168a. Ohta, Y., Yasukawa, M., Saito, S., Fujita, S., and Kobayashi, Y.: Homozygous delta thalassemia in Japan. Hemoglobin 4:417, 1980.

169. Yasukawa, M., Saito, S., Fujita, S., Ohta, Y., Ikeda, K., Matsumoto, I., and Kobayashir, Y.: Five families with homozygous δ-thalassemia in Japan. Br. J. Haematol. 46:199, 1980.

170. Fessas, P., and Stamatoyannopoulos, G.: Absence of hemoglobin A_2 in an adult. Nature 195:1215, 1962.

171. Thompson, R. B., Warrington, R., Odom, J., and Bell, W. N.: Interaction between genes for delta thalassemia and hereditary persistence of foetal hemoglobin. Acta Genet. 15:190, 1965.

172. Pirastu, M., Galanello, R., Melis, M. A., Brancati, C., Tagarelli, A., Cao, A., and Kan, Y. W.: δ^+-thalassemia in Sardinia. Blood 62:341, 1983.

173. Conley, C. L., Weatherall, D. J., Richardson, S. N., Shepard, M. D., and Charache, S.: Hereditary persistence of fetal hemoglobin: A study of 79 affected persons in 15 Negro families in Baltimore. Blood 21:261, 1963.

Gamma-beta thalassemia: A cause of hemolytic disease of newborns. N. Engl. J. Med. *286*:129, 1972.
130. Orkin, S. H., Goff, S. C., and Nathan, D. G.: Heterogeneity of DNA deletion in γδβ-thalassemia. J. Clin. Invest. *67*:878, 1981.
131. Baglioni, C.: The fusion of two peptide chains in hemoglobin Lepore and its interpretation as a genetic deletion. Proc. Natl. Acad. Sci. USA *48*:1880, 1962.
131a. Kattamis, C., Metaxotou-Mavromati, A., Ladis, V., Tsiarta, H., Laskari, S., and Kanavakis, E.: The clinical phenotype of β and δβ thalassemias in Greece. Eur. J. Pediat. *139*:135, 1982.
131b. Antonarakis, S. E., Irkin, S. H., Cheng T.-C., Scott, A. F., Sexton, J. P., Trusko, S. P., Charache, S., and Kazazian, H. H., Jr.: β-thalassemia in American blacks: Novel mutations in the "TATA" box and an acceptor splice site. Proc. Natl. Acad. Sci. USA *81*:1154, 1984.
131c. Orkin, S. H., Antonarakis, S. E., and Kazazian H. H., Jr.: Base substitution at position −88 in a β-thalassemic globin gene: Further evidence for the role of distal promoter element ACACCC. J. Biol. Chem. *259*:8679, 1984.
132. Wainscoat, J. S., Old, J. M., Weatherall, D. J., and Orkin, S. H.: The molecular basis for the clinical diversity of β thalassaemia in Cypriots. Lancet *1*:1235, 1983.
133. Tamagnini, G. P., Lopes, M. C., Castanheira, M. E., Wainscoat, J. S., and Wood, W. G.: β$^+$ thalassaemia—Portuguese type: Clinical, haematological and molecular studies of a newly defined form of β thalassaemia. Br. J. Haematol. *54*:189, 83.
133a. Treisman, R., Orkin, S. H., and Maniatis, T.: Specific transcription and RNA splicing defects in five cloned β-thalassemia genes. Nature *302*:591, 1983.
134. Kan, Y. W., and Nathan, D. G.: Mild thalassemia: The result of interaction of alpha and beta thalassemia genes. J. Clin. Invest. *49*:635, 1970.
135. Musumeci, S., Schiliro, G., Pizzarelli, G., Fischer, A., and Russo, G.: Thalassaemia of intermediate severity resulting from the interaction between α- and β-thalassaemia. J. Med. Genet. *15*:448, 1978.
136. Weatherall, D. J., Wood, W. G., Pressley, L., Higgs, D. R., and Clegg, J. B.: Molecular basis for mild forms of homozygous beta-thalassaemia. Lancet *1*:527, 1981.
137. Trent, E. J., Wainscoat, J. S., Huehns, E. R., Clegg, J. B., and Weatherall, D. J.: The molecular basis for β^0 thalassaemia intermedia in an Iranian individual. Br. J. Haematol. *52*:511, 1982.
138. Lie-Injo, L. E., Duraisamy, G., and Vasudevan, S.: Influence of two α-globin gene deletions on homozygous β^0-thalassaemia. Hemoglobin *6*:115, 1982.
139. Wainscoat, J. S., Kanavakis, E., Wood, W. G., Letsky, E. A., Huehns, E. R., Marsh, G. W., Higgs, D. R., Clegg, J. B., and Weatherall, D. J.: Thalassaemia intermedia in Cyprus: The interaction of α and β thalassaemia. Br. J. Haematol. *53*:411, 1983.
140. Pirastu, M., Lee, K. Y., Dozy, A.M., Kan, Y. W., Stamatoyannopoulos, G., Hadjiminas, M. G., Zachariades, Z., Angius, A., Furbetta, M., Rosatelli, C., and Cao, A.: Alpha-thalassemia in two Mediterranean populations. Blood *60*:509, 1982.
140a. Kanavakis, E., Metaxotou-Mavromati, A., Kattamis, C., Wainscoat, J. S., and Wood, W. G.: The triplicated α gene locus and β thalassaemia. Br. J. Haematol. *54*:201, 1983.
140b. Galanello, R., Ruggeri, R., Paglietti, E., Addis, M., Melis, M. A., and Cao, A.: A family with segregating triplicated alpha globin loci and beta thalassemia. Blood *62*:1035, 1983.
140c. Sampietro, M., Cazzola, M., Cappellini, M. D., and Fiorelli, G.: The triplicated alpha-gene locus and heterozygous beta thalassaemia: A case of thalassaemia intermedia. Br. J. Haematol. *55*:709, 1983.
140d. Thein, S. L., Al-Hakim, I., and Hoffbrand, A. V.: Thalassemia intermedia: A new molecular basis. Br. J. Haematol. *56*:333, 1984.
141. Kanavakis, E., Wainscoat, J. S., Wood, W. G., Weatherall, D. J., Cao, A., Furbetta, M., Galanello, R., Georgiou, D., and Sophocleous, T.: The interaction of α thalassaemia with heterozygous β thalassaemia. Br. J. Haematol. *52*:465, 1982.
142. Melis, M. A., Pirastu, M., Galanello, R., Furbetta, M., Tuveri, T., and Cao, A.: Phenotypic effect of heterozygous α and β^0-thalassemia interaction. Blood *62*:226, 1983.
142a. Rosatelli, C., Falchi, A. M., Scalas, M. T., Tuveri, T., Furbetta, M., and Cao, A.: Hematological phenotype of the double heterozygous state for alpha and beta thalassemia. Hemoglobin *8*:25, 1984.
143. Loukopoulos, D., Loutradi, A., and Fessas, P.: A unique thalassaemic syndrome: Homozygous α-thalassaemia + homozygous β-thalassaemia. Br. J. Haematol. *39*:377, 1978.
144. Furbetta, M., Galanello, R., Ximenes, A., Angius, A., Melis, M. A., Serra, P., and Cao, A.: Interaction of alpha and beta thalassaemia genes in two Sardinian families. Br. J. Haematol. *41*:203, 1979.
145. Weatherall, D. J., Clegg, J. B., Knox-Macaulay, H. H. M., Bunch, C., Hopkins, C. R., and Temperley, I. J.: A genetically determined disorder with features both of thalassaemia and congenital dyserythropoietic anaemia. Br. J. Haematol. *24*:681, 1973.
146. Hruby, M. A., Mason, R. G., and Honig, G. R.: Unbalanced globin chain synthesis in congenital dyserythropoietic anemia. Blood *42*:843, 1973.
147. Berrebi, A., and Nir, E.: An unusual type of congenital dyserythropoietic anemia with thalassemia features. Isr. J. Med. Sci. *14*:1135, 1978.
148. Baine, R. M., Rucknagel, D. L., Dublin, P. A., Jr., and Adams, J. G. III: Trimodality in the proportion of hemoglobin G Philadelphia in heterozygotes: Evidence for heterogeneity in the number of human alpha chain loci. Proc. Natl. Acad. Sci. USA *73*:3633, 1976.
149. Sancar, G. B., Tatsis, B., Cedeno, M. M., and Rieder, R. F.: Proportion of hemoglobin G Philadelphia ($\alpha_2^{68Asn\ Lys}\beta_2$) in heterozygotes is determined by α-globin gene deletions. Proc. Natl. Acad. Sci. USA *77*:6874, 1980.
150. Surrey, S., Ohene-Frempong, K., Rappaport, E., Atwater, J., and Schwartz, E.: Linkage of $\alpha^{G-Philadelphia}$ to α-thalassemia in African-Americans. Proc. Natl. Acad. Sci. USA *77*:4885, 1980.
150a. Felice, A. E., Ozdonmez, R., Headlee, M. E., and Huisman, T. H. J.: Organization of α-chain genes among Hb G-Philadelphia heterozygotes in association with Hb S, β-thalassemia, and α-thalassemia-2. Biochem. Genet. *20*:689, 1982.

100. Gaburro, D., Volpato, S., and Vigi, V.: Diagnosis of beta thalassemia in the newborn by means of hemoglobin synthesis. Acta Pediatr. Scand. 59:523, 1970.
101. Smith, C. H., Erlandson, M. E., Stern, G., and Hilgartner, M. W.: Postsplenectomy infection in Cooley's anemia. N. Engl. J. Med. 266:737, 1962.
102. Smith, C. H., Erlandson, M. E., Stern, G., and Hilgartner, M. W.: Postsplenectomy infection in Cooley's anemia. Ann. N. Y. Acad. Sci. 119:748, 1964.
103. Logothetis, J., Loewenson, R. B., Augoustaki, O., Economidou, J., and Constantoulakis, M.: Body growth in Cooley's anemia (homozygous beta-thalassemia) with a correlative study as to other aspects of the illness in 138 cases. Pediatrics 50:92, 1972.
104. Modell, C. B.: Management of thalassaemia major. Br. Med. Bull. 32:270, 1976.
105. Costin, G., Kogut, M. D., Hyman, C. B., and Orega, J. A.: Endocrine abnormalities in thalassemia major. Am. J. Dis. Child. 133:497, 1979.
106. Zaino, E. C., Juo, B., and Roginsky, M. S.: Growth retardation in thalassemia major. Ann. N. Y. Acad. Sci. 232:238, 1974.
107. Canale, V. C., Steinherz, P., New, M., and Erlandson, M.: Endocrine function in thalassemia major. Ann. N.Y. Acad. Sci. 232:333, 1974.
108. Lassman, M. N., Genel, M., Wise, J. K., Hendler, R., and Felig, P.: Carbohydrate homeostasis and pancreatic islet cell function in thalassemia. Blood 80:65, 1974.
109. Lassman, M. N., O'Brien, R. T., Pearson, H. A., Wise, J. K., Donabedian, R. K., Felig, P., and Genel, M.: Endocrine evaluation in thalassemia major. Ann. N. Y. Acad. Sci. 232:226, 1974.
109a. Saenger, P., Schwartz, E., Markenson, A. L., Graziano, J. H., Levine, L. S., New, M. I., and Hilgartner, M. W.: Depressed serum somatomedin activity in β-thalassemia. J. Pediatr. 96:214, 1980.
110. Flynn, D. M., Fairney, A., Jackson, D., and Clayton, B. E.: Hormonal changes in thalassaemia major. Arch. Dis. Child. 51:828, 1976.
111. Engle, M. A.: Cardiac involvement in Cooley's anemia. Ann. N. Y. Acad. Sci. 119:694, 1964.
112. Beltrami, C. A., Bearzi, I., and Fabris, G.: Storage cells of spleen and bone marrow in thalassemia: An ultrastructural study. Blood 41:901, 1973.
113. Resegotti, L., Dalforno, S., Infelise, V., and Rossi, M.: Gaugher-like cells in the spleen of an adult with Cooley's anaemia. Panminerva Med. 16:261, 1974.
114. Kreimer-Birnbaum, M., Pinkerton, P. H., Bannerman, R. M., and Hutchinson, H. E.: Dipyrrolic urinary pigments in congenital Heinz body anaemia due to Hb Köln and in thalassaemia. Br. Med. J. 2:396, 1966.
115. Kreimer-Birnbaum, M., Pinkerton, P. H., Bannerman, R. M., and Hutchinson, H. E.: Urinary "dipyrroles"; their occurrence and significance in thalassemia and other disorders. Blood 28:993, 1966.
116. Fessas, P., and Loukopoulos, D.: Alpha-chain of human hemoglobin: Occurrence in vivo. Science 143:590, 1964.
117. Kattamis, C., Metaxotou-Mavromati, A., Karamboula, K., Nasika, E., and Lehmann, H.: The clinical and haematological findings in children inheriting two types of thalassaemia: High-A$_2$ type β-thalassemia, and high-F type or δβ-thalassaemia. Br. J. Haematol. 25:375, 1973.
118. Russo, G., Musumeci, S., Schiliro, G., D'Agate, A., and Pizzarelli, G.: Hemoglobin synthesis in δβ-thalassemia. Atti del V Congresso sulle Microcitemia, Cozenza, Arte Della Stampa, Roma, 1973.
119. Shchory, M., and Ramot, B.: Globin chain synthesis in the marrow and reticulocytes of beta thalassemia, hemoglobin H disease and beta delta thalassemia. Blood 40:105, 1970.
120. Gimferrer, E., Baiget, M., and Rutllant, M. I.: Homozygous δβ-thalassaemia in a Spanish woman. Acta Haematol. 61:226, 1979.
121. Cao, A., Melis, M. A., Galanello, R., Angius, A., Furbetta, M., Giordano, P., and Bernini, L. F.: δβ(F)-thalassaemia in Sardinia. J. Med. Genet. 19:184, 1982.
122. Schwartz, E.: The silent carrier of beta-thalassemia. N. Engl. J. Med. 281:1327, 1969.
123. Askoy, M., Erdem, S., and Dincol, G.: β-thalassemia with normal levels of hemoglobins F and A$_2$. Simple heterozygous and homozygous forms and doubly heterozygous state with β-thalassemia with increased hemoglobin A$_2$. Study in seven families. Proceedings of the International Istanbul Symposium on Abnormal Hemoglobins and Thalassemia. Ankara, 1975, p. 289.
124. Aksoy, M., Dincol, G., and Erdem, S.: Different types of beta-thalassaemia intermedia. Acta Haematol. 59:178, 1978.
125. Kattamis, C., Metaxotou-Mavromati, A., Wood, W. G., Nash, J. R., and Weatherall, D. J.: The heterogeneity of normal Hb A$_2$-β thalassaemia in Greece. Br. J. Haematol. 42:109, 1979.
125a. Arous, N., Galacteros, F., Fessas, P., Loukopoulos, D., Blouquit, Y., Komis, G., Sellaye, M., Boussiou, M., and Rosa, J.: Structural study of hemoglobin Knossos, β27 (B9) Ala → Ser. A new abnormal hemoglobin present as a silent β-thalassemia. FEBS Lett. 147:247, 1982.
125b. Fessas, P., Loukopoulos, D., Loutradi-Anagnostou, A., and Komis, G.: "Silent" β-chain mutant: The pathogenesis of a syndrome of thalassemia intermedia. Br. J. Haematol. 51:577, 1982.
125c. Rouabhi, F., Chardin, P., Boissel, J. P., Beghoul, F., Labie, D., and Benabadji, M.: Silent β-thalassemia associated with Hb Knossos β27 (B9) Ala → Ser in Algeria. Hemoglobin 7:555, 1983.
125d. Galacteros, F., Garin, J. D., Monplaisir, N., Namoune, S., Arous, N., Blouquit, Y., Mamalaki, A., Tulliez, M., Ouka, M., Goossens, M., and Rosa, J.: Two new cases of heterozygosity for hemoglobin Knossos $\alpha_2\beta_2^{27\ Ala\ \rightarrow Ser}$ detected in the French West Indies and Algeria. Hemoglobin 8:215, 1984.
125e. Morlé, L., Morlé, B., Dorléac, E., Baklouti, F., Baudonnet, C., Godet, J., and Delaunay, J.: The association of hemoglobin Knossos and hemoglobin Lepore in an Algerian patient. Hemoglobin 8:229, 1984.
126. Silvestroni, E., Bianco, I., Graziani, B., and Carboni, C.: Heterozygous β-thalassaemia with normal haemoglobin pattern. Acta Haematol. 59:332, 1978.
127. Stamatoyannopoulos, G., Papayannopoulou, T., Fessas, P., and Motulsky, A. G.: The beta-delta thalassemias. Ann. N. Y. Acad. Sci. 165:25, 1969.
128. Kanavakis, E., Metaxotou-Mavromati, A., Kattamis, C., Aksoy, M., Weatherall, D. J., and Wood, W. G.: Globin gene mapping in normal Hb A$_2$ types of β-thalassaemia. Br. J. Haematol. 51:59, 1982.
129. Kan, Y. W., Forget, B. G., and Nathan, D. G.:

Color Plate II. *A*, Normal. *B*, β-thalassemia trait. *C*, β thalassemia intermedia. *D*, β thalassemia major. *E*, β thalassemia major, after splenectomy. *F*, Sickle/β thalassemia. *G*, α-thalassemia trait. *H* and *I*, Hydrops fetalis. *J*, Hemoglobin H disease. *K*, Hemoglobin H disease, after splenectomy. *L*, Hemoglobin H disease—Heinz body preparation. (Prepared by Carola Von Kapff, Harvard Medical School. Some of the blood films were loaned by Dr. Virgil Fairbanks and Dr. David Todd.)

THE THALASSEMIAS—CLINICAL MANIFESTATIONS

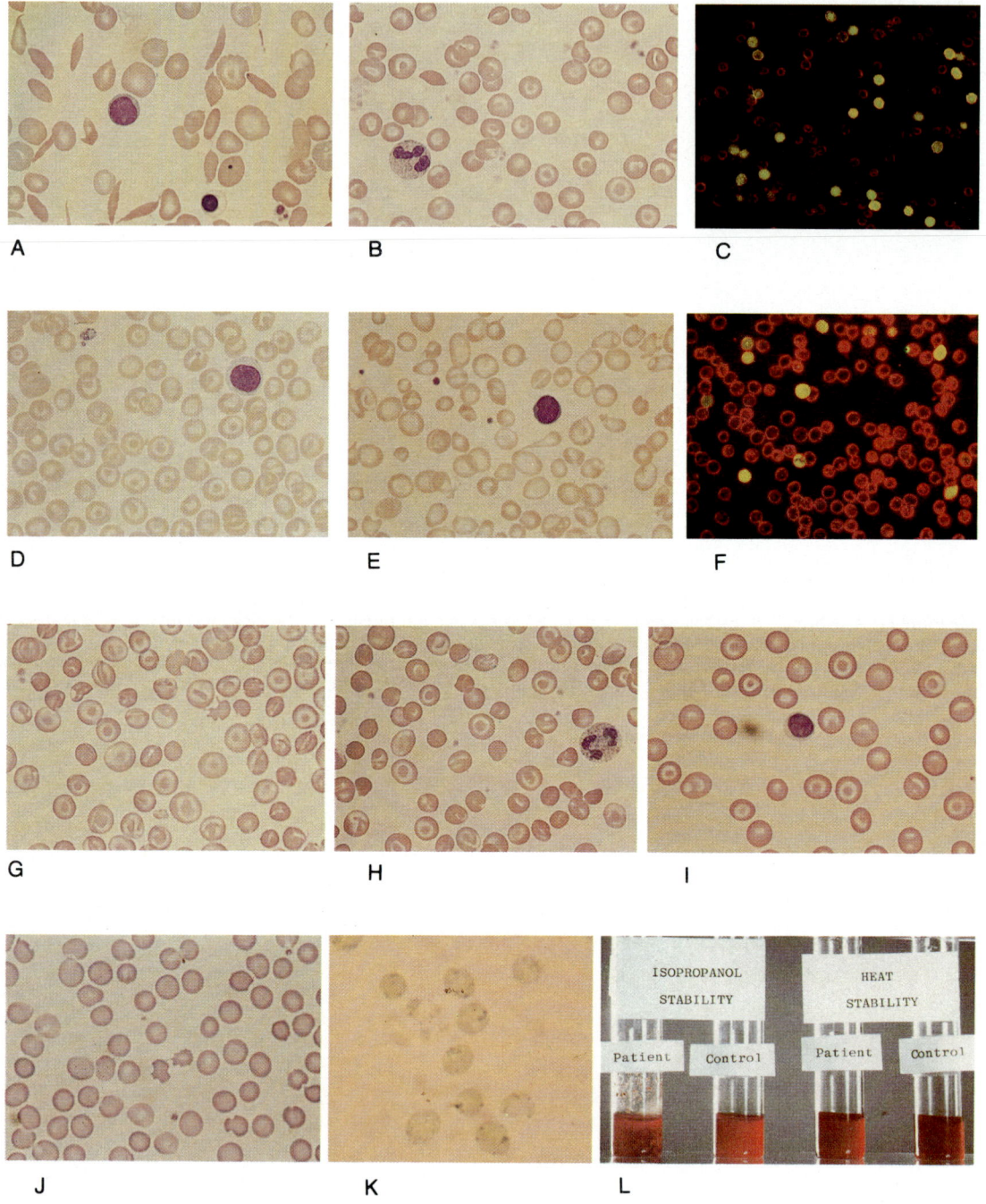

Color Plate III. *A,* SS disease. *B,* SC disease. *C,* SS—30% F cells. *D,* EE. *E,* E-β thalassemia. *F,* AS—6% F cells. *G,* CC. *H,* C-β thalassemia. *I,* AC. *J,* CHBA. *K,* CHBA—Heinz body preparation. *L,* CHBA—heat and isopropanol stability. (Prepared by Carola Von Kapff, Harvard Medical School. Some of the blood films were loaned by Dr. Virgil Fairbanks and Dr. David Todd.)

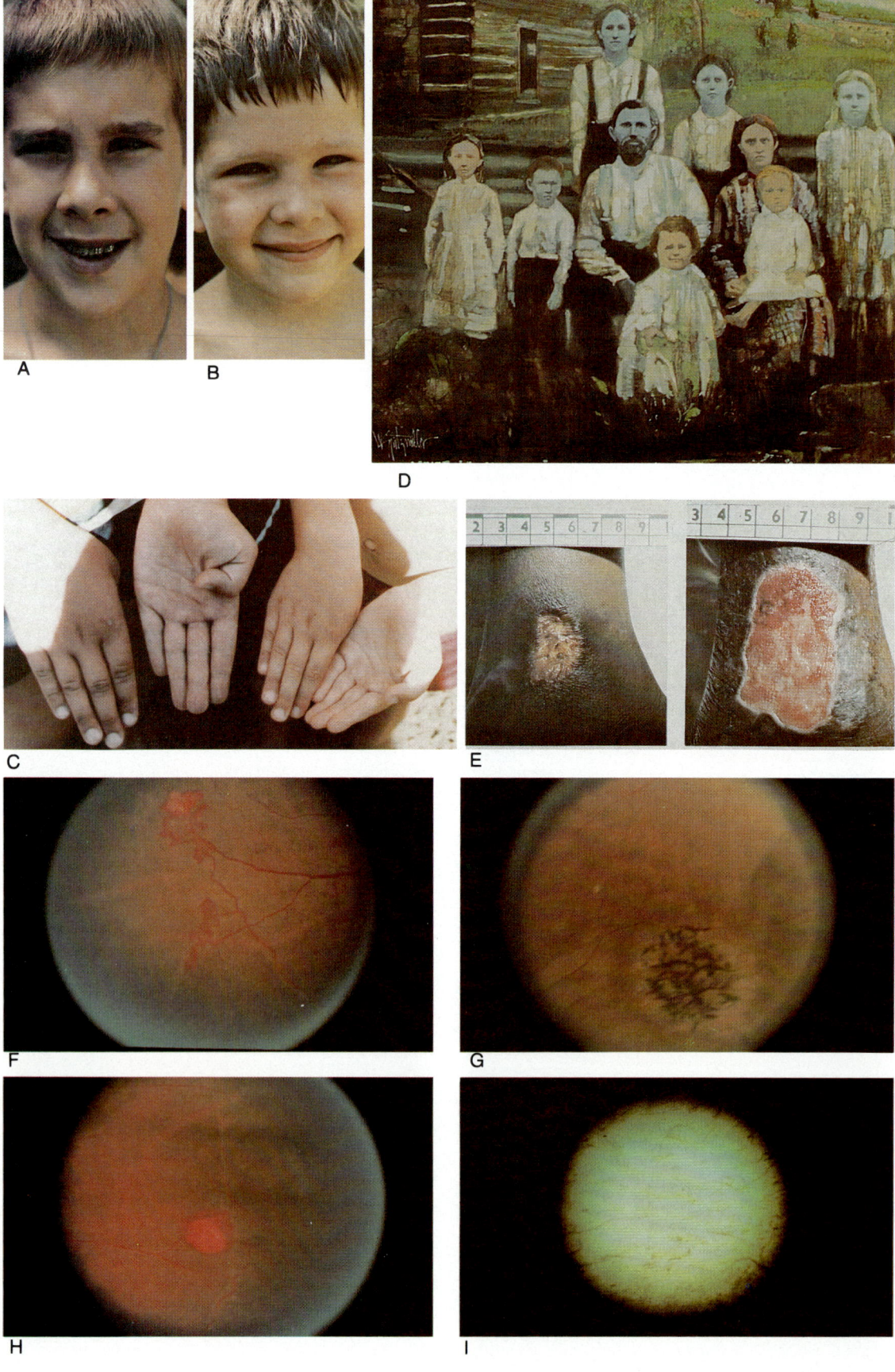

Color Plate IV. *A,* Boy with Hb M-Boston. *B,* Normal brother of boy shown in *A. C,* Hands of boy shown in *A* (left) and of his brother shown in *B* (right). (*A–C,* Courtesy of Dr. Carol Crowley.) *D,* Family with congenital methemoglobinemia (deficiency of cytochrome b_5 reductase). (Courtesy of Walt Spitzmiller and Science '81.) *E,* Ankle ulcers in patients with homozygous sickle cell anemia. (From Sergeant, G. R.: Arch. Intern. Med. *133*:6;90, 1974.) *F,* Sea fan SC disease. *G,* Black sunburst, SS disease. *H,* Salmon patch, SS disease. *I,* SS Conjuntival "corkscrews." (*F–I,* Courtesy of Dr. Lee Jampol, Northwestern University Medical Center.)

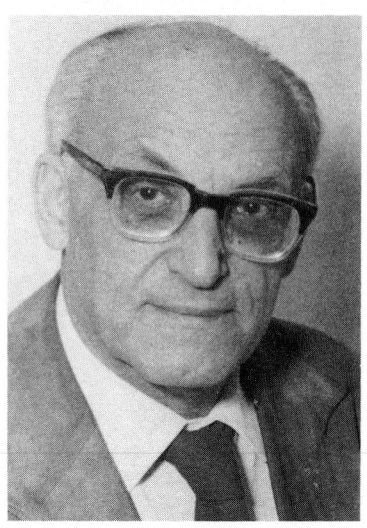

HERMANN LEHMANN

Hermann Lehmann shares his birthplace, Halle, in Saxony, with George Frederick Handel. Both men had long careers, producing large volumes of work of great vitality and originality.

Lehmann received his medical training at the universities in Basel and Heidelberg. While working in the famous biochemistry laboratory of Otto Meyerhof, he showed that ATP can phosphorylate creatine. This work attracted the attention of Professor Sir Frederic Gowland Hopkins, who invited Lehmann to Cambridge University for a visit in 1934 and for good in 1936. Except for a few important interruptions, he has remained there since.

Despite his nationality, Lehmann served in the British Army in India during World War II. There, he developed the copper sulfate drop screening test for anemia that is still used in many blood banks around the world. Immediately after the war, he worked with starved victims from Japanese prisoner-of-war camps. He then went to Uganda to investigate the dimorphic anemia of Central Africa. He showed that it arose from a combination of iron therapy and continued blood loss due to hookworm infestation. In Uganda, his attention was drawn to sickle cell anemia. Thereafter, he became, and remained, the leading investigator of human hemoglobin variants.

During the 1950's, Lehmann served as chemical pathologist at St. Bartholomew's Hospital, the oldest hospital in London and best known to readers of this book for Hb Bart's. During this time, he completed exhaustive population surveys demonstrating the origin and distribution of the sickle cell gene as well as initial studies on other prevalent hemoglobin variants, particularly Hbs, C, D, and E. He built the first laboratory devoted to the systematic study of protein variation in man and other animals. An impressive proportion of the nearly 400 human hemoglobin variants mentioned in Chapter 10 were discovered and characterized by a combination of Lehmann's indefatigable field studies, which have taken him to all corners of the world, and his expertise in analysis of protein structure. This cumulative information provided powerful proof of the universality of the genetic code. Lehmann's studies on Hb Q and Hb Bart's led to an understanding of the genetic basis and pathogenesis of the α thalassemias. The explosion of information on the human hemoglobin variants allowed Lehmann and Perutz to propose coherent stereochemical explanations of those with abnormal oxygen binding or instability (see Chapters 13, 14, and 15). This information has contributed greatly to current understanding of structure-function relationships in hemoglobin.

Lehmann's scientific pursuits extend far beyond hemoglobin. He has an abiding interest in protein polymorphisms and molecular evolution. At present, he and his laboratory staff are completing a comprehensive characterization of animal myoglobins.

Like George Frederick Handel, Lehmann became a bona fide Englishman. He delights in British institutions, particularly Christ College, Cambridge, where he has made a strong impact. In the larger sense, he is a citizen of the world. No one has done more to make hemoglobin research an international enterprise.

HUMAN HEMOGLOBIN VARIANTS

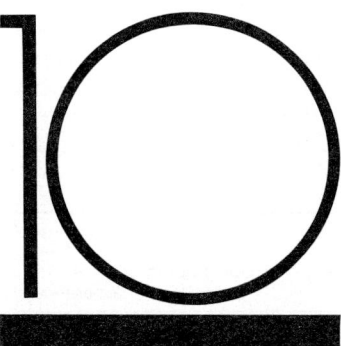

To the nonspecialist, perhaps the most bewildering aspect of "hemoglobinology" is the number and variety of human hemoglobin variants. At present, there are nearly 400 variants of known structure (Tables 10–1 and 10–2). It is not surprising that the first human hemoglobin variants to be recognized were those that attracted clinical attention. In 1948, Hörlein and Weber[263] reported the first hemoglobinopathy. They studied a family with congenital cyanosis and demonstrated that affected family members had hemoglobin with abnormal spectral properties. Later, it was shown that they had one of the M hemoglobins (M-Saskatoon).

In the early 1950's, sickle cell anemia was found to be due to an electrophoretically abnormal hemoglobin having a single amino acid substitution in the β chain (β 6 Glu→Val). Thereafter, electrophoresis became widely employed in the search for other human hemoglobin variants. Those having relatively high gene frequencies were discovered quite readily. Hemoglobins C, D, and E were identified within two years following the structural identification of hemoglobin S. Large-scale screening programs were initiated to find other abnormal hemoglobins. Initally, new variants were named by successive letters of the alphabet. By the time hemoglobin Q was encountered, it became apparent that the letters of the alphabet would soon be exhausted. To add to the confusion, some hemoglobins with identical electrophoretic properties were shown to have different structures. Gradually, investigators agreed to give new hemoglobins a specific name, most often reflecting the origin of the patient. Many colorful and provocative names have appeared in the literature, some exotic (Hb Aida), others chauvinistic (Hb Brigham), parochial (Hb Riverdale-Bronx), or patriotic (Hb Abraham Lincoln). For a while, the naming of hemoglobin variants was treated somewhat lightly because many believed the hemoglobin would be remembered more often by its structure rather than by its eponym. However, just as people naturally tend to call

Table 10-1. HUMAN HEMOGLOBIN VARIANTS: 1984*

	Total	Unstable	Abnormal O_2 Affinity†	Hbs M	No Clinical Manifestations
α Chain	126	16	6	2	102
β Chain	232	68	39	3	122
γ Chain	38	1		1	
δ Chain	15				
Fusion	9				
	420				

*Compiled from Table 12–2.
†Does not include variants with abnormal oxygen affinity but no clinical manifestations.

their friends by name rather than by social security number, the names of the variants have stuck. As Table 10–2 shows, the same variant (with specific structural abnormality) is often rediscovered in different laboratories all over the world: α 47 Asp→Gly has nine interesting names.

DETECTION OF HEMOGLOBIN VARIANTS

The majority of hemoglobin variants listed in Table 10–2 were detected because of abnormal electrophoretic behavior. The screening of variants usually employs electrophoresis on cellulose acetate or starch gel at a slightly alkaline pH (8.3 to 8.8). Of the 200-odd variants associated with no clinical manifestations, 95 per cent have an amino acid substitution involving a change of charge, allowing their separation from Hb A by routine electrophoresis. In contrast, a significant proportion (45 per cent) of the clinically significant variants have substitutions that do not alter the overall charge of the protein. In order to identify these variants as well as to distinguish among

Text continued on page 399

Table 10-2. HUMAN HEMOGLOBIN VARIANTS†

A. Variants of the Alpha Chain

Structure	Name	% of Total Hb	Hb (g/dl)	Reticulocytes (%)	Properties	Geographic Origin‡	Reference(s)
2 (NA2) Leu→Arg	Chongqing				↑ O_2 affinity, unstable	A	1
5 (A3) Ala→Asp	J-Toronto	25	14.2		Neg HB; neg heat	WE	1a, 2
6 (A4) Asp→Ala	Sawara				↑ O_2 affinity	EA	3, 4, C14
Asp→Asn	Dunn				↑ O_2 affinity	Af	5, C14
Asp→Val	Ferndown				↑ O_2 affinity		5a
Asp→Tyr	Woodville				↑ O_2 affinity		5b
11 (A9) Lys→Glu	Anantharaj	44	14.2			SEA	6
Lys→Gln	J-Wenchang Wuming						6a
Lys→Asn	Albany-Suma	19	14.8		↑ O_2 affinity	A	6b, 6c
12 (A10) Ala→Asp	J-Paris-I, J-Aljezur	22–26			Neg HB; neg heat	SE	7
14 (A12) Trp→Arg	Evanston	15–17			Thalassemic phenotype	Af	8a
15 (A13) Gly→Asp	I-Interlaken	20	13.5		Neg HB; neg heat	E	9
	J-Oxford	23				E	10, 11
Gly→Arg	Ottawa	25			Neg heat	EE	12
	Siam	15				SEA	13
16 (A14) Lys→Glu	I	15–28	13.1	1.7	Neg HB; nl O_2 affinity	Af	14–19
Lys→Asn	Beijing	19	15.4	0.3	Neg HB; neg Iso	A	19a
Lys→Met	Harbin				↑ O_2 affinity, unstable	A	1

†This Table was prepared from the list of hemoglobin variants compiled by Dr. Ruth Wrightstone at the International Hemoglobin Information Center, Augusta, Georgia. Relevant laboratory data were obtained from primary sources (References 1 to 477) and added to this table. Variants with a substitution at the $α_1β_1$ interface are denoted by one asterisk (*), and those with a substitution at the $α_1β_2$ interface are denoted by two asterisks (**). Further information on the unstable variants, those with abnormal oxygen affinity, and the M hemoglobins can be obtained from more complete tables in Chapters 13 to 15.
‡Geographic information was obtained from Dr. William Winter.[634] This reference contains more detail. *Key:* Prefixes: N = North; S = South; E = East; W = West; C = Central; M = Middle. Suffixes: A = Asia; Am = America; Af = Africa; *Af* = Afro-American; C = Caucasian; E = Europe; I = India. Exception: ME = Middle East.
Abbreviations: Hb = hemoglobin; HB = Heinz body; Iso = isopropanol test; Nl = normal; Sl = slight. C13, C14, and C15 refer to Chapters 13, 14, and 15.

Table 10–2. HUMAN HEMOGLOBIN VARIANTS† Continued

A. Variants of the Alpha Chain

Structure	Name	% of Total Hb	Hb (g/dl)	Reticulocytes (%)	Properties	Geographic Origin‡	Reference(s)
18 (A16) Gly→Arg	Handsworth	11	11.6		Neg heat; neg Iso	CA	20
19 (AB1) Ala→Asp	J-Kurosh	25				ME	21
Ala→Glu	J-Tashikuergan	21	13			A	21a
20 (B1) His→Tyr	Necker Enfants-Malades	30	12–14	0.3	Neg HB; nl O_2 affinity	CAm	22
His→Gln	LeLamentin	20			Nl O_2 affinity; neg Iso	Af	22a
21 (B2) Ala→Asp	J-Nyanza	35			Variant/α thal	Af	23
22 (B3) Gly→Asp	J-Medellin	20				Af	24
23 (B4) Glu→Gln	Memphis				Variant/Hb S	Af	25
Glu→Lys	Chad	16	14			Af	26
Glu→Val	G-Audhali	25				ME	27
26 (B7) Ala→Glu	Shenyang	22	Nl		Sl + Iso; Sl + HB	A	27a
27 (B8) Glu→Gly	Fort Worth	5	11–12	2	Sl + heat; sl + HB	Af	28
Glu→Lys	Shuangfeng						28a
Glu→Val	Spanish Town	11–12	13.4	1.7	Neg heat	Af	29
30 (B11) Glu→Lys	O-Padova	25			Nl O_2 affinity; neg heat	SE	30
Glu→Gln	G-Honolulu	35	12–14				31
	G-Singapore					SEA	32
	G-Chinese					EA	33
	G-Hong Kong					EA	34
31 (B12) Arg→Ser*	Prato					SE	34, 35
34 (B15) Leu→Arg*	Queens	13	15		Nl O_2 affinity; neg Iso		36, 36a
40 (C5) Lys→Glu	Kariya	15	15		↑ O_2 affinity	A	36b
43 (CE1) Phe→Val	Torino				Unstable	SE	37, C13
Phe→Leu	Hirosaki				Unstable	EA	38
44 (CE2) Pro→Leu**	Milledgeville				↑ O_2 affinity		39, C14
Pro→Arg**	Kawachi				↑ O_2 affinity	A	39a, C14
45 (CE3) His→Arg	Fort de France				↑ O_2 affinity		40, C14
His→Gln	Bari	20	13.6		Nl O_2 affinity; neg heat; neg Iso		41
47 (CE5) Asp→Gly	Umi	12	Nl	2–4	Unstable		42, 43, 43a C13
	Kokura						
	Michigan-I						
	Michigan-II						
	Yukuhashi-II						
	L-Gaslini						
	Tagawa-II						
	Beilinson						
	Mugino						
Asp→His	Hasharon	18			Unstable	ME	44, C13
	Sinai						45
	Sealy						46
	L-Ferrara					SE	47, 48
Asp→Asn	Arya	22			Sl unstable; neg HB	ME	49
Asp→Ala	Cordele				Sl unstable		49a
48 (CE6) Leu→Arg	Montgomery	20				Af	50
49 (CE7) Ser→Arg	Savaria	30	9.8	7	Neg heat; nl O_2 affinity; hemoly unrel to var	EA	51
50 (CE8) His→Asp	J-Sardegna	16–20					52
His→Arg	Aichi	21			Sl + Iso; nl O_2 affinity	A	52a
51 (CE9) Gly→Asp	J-Abidjan	23				Af	53
Gly→Arg	Russ	11–12				C	54
53 (E2) Ala→Asp	J-Rovigo	23–30	13–15	1–5	Unstable	SE	55, 56, C13
54 (E3) Gln→Arg	Shimonoseki Hikoshima	13			Nl O_2 affinity	EA	57, 58

Table continued on following page

Table 10–2. HUMAN HEMOGLOBIN VARIANTS† Continued

A. Variants of the Alpha Chain

Structure	Name	% of Total Hb	Hb (g/dl)	Reticulocytes (%)	Properties	Geographic Origin‡	Reference(s)
Gln→Glu	Mexico	20–55	10–15	1	Variant/α thal	CAm	59
	J						59
	J-Paris-II					SE	60, 62
	Uppsala						61
56 (E5) Lys→Thr	Thailand	28	12.1	0.4%	Nl O$_2$ affinity	SEA	63
Lys→Glu	Shaare Zedek	10–20	11.5		Variant/α thal		64
57 (E6) Gly→Arg	L-Persian Gulf	18				ME	65
Gly→Asp	J-Norfolk	28				E	66
	Kagoshima	20					67
	Nishik-I, II, III						68
58 (E7) His→Tyr	M-Boston				↓ O$_2$ affinity	NE	69–72, C15
59 (E8) Gly-Val	Tottori				Unstable		73, C13
60 (E9) Lys→Asn	Zambia					Af	74
Lys→Glu	Dagestan	30					75
61 (E10) Lys→Asn	J-Buda	16–21			Neg HB; neg heat	EE	76
63 (E12) Ala→Asp	Pontoise	12			Unstable	WE	77
64 (E13) Asp→Asn	G-Waimanalo	19, 27			Nl O$_2$ affinity	EA	78
	Aida						79
Asp→His	Q-India	8–20	11–12	1		I	80
Asp→Tyr	Perspolis	20				I	21
68 (E17) Asn→Asp	Ube-2				Sl ↑ O$_2$ affinity	EA	58, 81
Asn→Lys	G-Philadelphia	33–45			Variant/α thal	Af	82
	G-Knoxville-I						83
	Stanleyville-I					Af	84
	D-Washington						83
	D-St. Louis						85
	G-Bristol						86
	G-Azakuoli						
	D-Baltimore						
71 (E20) Ala→Glu	J-Habana	38				CAm	87
72 (EF1) His→Arg	Daneskgah-Tehran	25			Neg HB	ME	88
74 (EF3) Asp→His	G-Taichung	35			Variant/α thal	EA	89
	Mahidol						90
	Q-Thailand					EA	91
	Kurashiki						
	Asabara						
Asp→Asn	G-Pest	23				EE	76
Asp→Gly	Chapel Hill	24	15.5		Sl ↑ O$_2$ affinity		92
Asp→Ala	Lille						93
75 (EF4) Asp→His	Q-Iran	25				ME	91
Asp→Ala	Duan	25	12.5		Neg HB		94
Asp→Tyr	Winnipeg	20	14.4	1.7	Neg heat	WE	95
Asp→Asn	Matsue-Oki	12–14				EA	96
Asp→Gly	Mizshi	14	13.7		Neg Iso; nl O$_2$ affinity	EA	97
76 (EF5) Met→Lys	Noko						98
77 (EF6) Pro→Arg	GuiZhou	25	10	1	Neg Iso; neg heat	A	98a
78 (EF7) Asn→Lys	Stanleyville-II	24			Variant/Hb S	Af	99
Asn→Asp	J-Singa						99a
80 (F1) Leu→Arg	Ann Arbor				Unstable	C	100, 101
81 (F2) Ser→Cys	Nigeria				Variant/Hb S/α thal; nl O$_2$ affinity	Af	102

Table 10–2. HUMAN HEMOGLOBIN VARIANTS† Continued

A. Variants of the Alpha Chain

Structure	Name	% of Total Hb	Hb (g/dl)	Reticulocytes (%)	Properties	Geographic Origin‡	Reference(s)
82 (F3) Ala→Asp	Garden State					Af	103
84 (F5) Ser→Arg	Etobicoke				Unstable	WE	104, 105, C13
85 (F6) Asp→Asn	G-Norfolk	18–23			↑ O_2 affinity	WE	106, 107, C14
Asp→Tyr	Atago	23				EA	108
Asp→Val	Inkster	22	14		Variant/β thal	C	109
86 (F7) Leu→Arg	Moabit				Unstable		110
87 (F8) His→Tyr	M-Iwate				Ferri-Hb	EA	111–113, C15
His→Arg	Iwata				Unstable	EA	114
90 (FG2) Lys→Asn	J-Broussais Tagawa-I	20	10.7	1.5	Nl O_2 affinity	WE	115–117 68
Lys→Met	Handa	18	14	2.4	Sl ↑ O_2 affinity	A	117a
Lys→Thr	J-Rajappen	26–28	13–15	1	Neg HB; neg heat	I	118
91 (FG3) Leu→Pro**	Port Phillip				Unstable		119
92 (FG4) Arg→Gln**	J-Cape Town	10–50			↑ O_2 affinity	Af	120, 121
Arg→Leu	Chesapeake	25–30			↑ O_2 affinity	C	122, 123
94 (G1) Asp→Tyr**	Setif				Unstable	NAf	124, C13
Asp→Asn	Titusville				↓ O_2 affinity	Af	125
Asp→His	Sunshine Seth	16–19	13–15		Neg Iso	C	126
95 (G2) Pro→Leu**	G-Georgia	23			↑ O_2 affinity	Af	127, 128, C14
Pro→Ser	Rampa	15–48			↑ O_2 affinity	I	129, C14
Pro→Ala	Denmark Hill	19			↑ O_2 affinity	CAm	130, C14
Pro→Arg	St. Luke's	10			↑ O_2 affinity		131
97 (G4) Asn→Lys	Dallas	23			↑ O_2 affinity		131a
102 (G9) Ser→Arg	Manitoba	5	10.4	0.6	Sl unstable	WE	132
103 (G10) His→Arg	Contaldo	18	13		S1 unstable	SE	132a
109 (G16) Leu→Arg	Suan-Dok				Unstable	SEA	133, C13
110 (G17) Ala→Asp*	Petah Tikva				Unstable		134, C13
112 (G19) His→Asp	Hopkins-II	17–27			Unstable		135, 136, C13
His→Arg	Strumica	16	13–15	1		EE	137
	Serbia	27				EE	138
113 (GH1) Leu→His	Twin Peaks						138a
114 (GH2) Pro→Arg*	Chiapas	25			Neg HB; neg heat	CAm	59
115 (GH3) Ala→Asp	J-Tongariki	50, 97			Variant/α thal	SEA	139–141
116 (GH4) Glu→Lys	O-Indonesia Buginese-X Oliviere	20	13			SEA	142 143 144
Glu→Ala	Ube-4	10–12	15		Neg heat; neg Iso; nl O_2 affinity	EA	145
Glu→Gln	Oleander				Nl O_2 affinity		146
120 (H3) Ala→Glu	J-Meerut	24				I	147
	J-Birmingham	20	13.6	1.4		I	148
122 (H5) His→Gln*	Westmead	50	14.4		Variant/α thal; neg Iso; neg heat; + HB		149
125 (H8) Leu→Pro	Quong Sze	0			Variant/HB H disease		149a, 149b
126 (H9) Asp→Asn*	Tarrant				↑ O_2 affinity		150, C14

Table continued on following page

Table 10–2. HUMAN HEMOGLOBIN VARIANTS† Continued

A. Variants of the Alpha Chain

Structure	Name	% of Total Hb	Hb (g/dl)	Reticulocytes (%)	Properties	Geographic Origin‡	Reference(s)
127 (H10) Lys→Thr	St. Claude	27–29	15.6		Neg heat	WE	151
Lys→Asn	Jackson	25			Neg heat; neg Iso	Af	152
136 (H19) Leu→Pro	Bibba				Unstable	C	153, C13
139 (HC1) Lys→Thr	Tokoname				Sl ↑ O_2 affinity	A	153a
141 (HC3) Arg→Pro**	Singapore	25				SEA	154
Arg→His**	Suresnes				↑ O_2 affinity	WE	155, C14
Arg→Ser**	J-Cubujuqui	37	15		↑ O_2 affinity		156
Arg→Leu**	Legnano				↑ O_2 affinity	SE	157, C14
Arg→Gly**	J-Camagüey	28	14–16	0.6	Neg heat; neg Iso	CAm	158

B. Variants of the Beta Chain

Structure	Name	% of Total Hb	Hb (g/dl)	Reticulocytes (%)	Properties	Geographic Origin‡	Reference(s)
1 (NA1) Val→AcAla	Raleigh				↓ O_2 affinity	C	159, C14
Val→Met	South Florida	50	14	1	Elongation at β-NH_2	C	160d
2 (NA2) His→Arg	Deer Lodge				↑ O_2 affinity	WE, Af	160, C14
His→Gln	Okayama	47	13.9	1	↑ O_2 affinity	EA	160a
His→Pro	Marseille, Long Island				Elongated at β-NH_2		160b, 636
5 (A2) Pro→Arg	Warwickshire						160c
6 (A3) Glu→Val	S	25–40			Sickling	Af, ME	161, C11–C12
Glu→Lys	C	35–40			Variant/S	Af	162, C10
Glu→Ala	G-Makassar				Sl hemolysis in homozyg	SEA	163
Glu→Gln	Machida		13.6		Neg sickling; neg Iso; Nl O_2 affinity	A	163a
7 (A4) Glu→Gly	G-San Jose		12.7		Nl O_2 affinity; sl unstable	SE	164
Glu→Lys	Siriraj	33–40	15		Var/β thal; homozyg	SEA	165, 166
8 (A5) Lys→Thr	Rio Grande						166a
Lys→Gln	J-Luhe					A	166b
9 (A6) Ser→Cys	Porto Alegre				↑ O_2 affinity; polymerization	SAm	167, 168
10 (A7) Ala→Asp	Ankara	42			Subj had iron def	ME	169
11 (A8) Val→Ile	Hamilton	38					169a
13 (A10) Ala→Asp	J-Lens	53	14		Neg heat; neg Iso		169b
14 (A11) Leu→Arg	Sögn	30–32			Sl unstable; neg HB; nl O_2 affinity	NE	170
Leu→Pro	Saki				Unstable	A	171, 172
15 (A12) Trp→Arg	Belfast				Unstable	C	173, 174
16 (A13) Gly→Asp	J-Baltimore	52–55 40–60	11–17	1	Variant/S; Var/C; Variant/β thal	Af	175–179
Gly→Arg	D-Bushman	34–39	11–13			Af	180
17 (A14) Lys→Glu	Nagasaki	43				EA	181
Lys→Asn	Amiens						181a
19 (B1) Asn→Lys	D-Ouled Rabah	47				ME	182, 183
Asn→Asp	Alamo	53	14			Af	184
20 (B2) Val→Met	Olympia				↑ O_2 affinity		185
21 (B3) Asp→Tyr	Yusa	40	14		Nl O_2 affinity		186
Asp→Asn	Cocody						186a
Asp→Gly	Connecticut				↓ O_2 affinity		187, C14
22 (B4) Glu→Lys	E-Saskatoon	35–40	14.5			WE	188–190
Glu→Gly	G-Taipei					EA	191

Table 10–2. HUMAN HEMOGLOBIN VARIANTS† Continued

B. Variants of the Beta Chain

Structure	Name	% of Total Hb	Hb (g/dl)	Reticulocytes (%)	Properties	Geographic Origin‡	Reference(s)
Glu→Ala	G-Saskatoon				Nl O$_2$ affinity	NAm	192,193
	G-Coushatta					NAm	194,195
Glu→Gln	D-Iran	40	14		Nl O$_2$ affinity; neg HB	ME	196
23 (B5) Val→Asp	Strasbourg				↑O$_2$ affinity	WE	197, 198, C14
Val→Gly	Miyashiro				↑O$_2$ affinity; unstable		198a
Val→Phe	Palmerston North				↑O$_2$ affinity		198b, C14
24 (B6) Gly→Arg	Riverdale-Bronx				Unstable	CE	199, C13
Gly→Val	Savannah				Unstable	C	200, C13
Gly→Asp	Moscva				Unstable	EE	201
25 (B7) Gly→Arg	G-Taiwan Ami					EA	202
26 (B8) Glu→Lys	E	35			Thalassemic phenotype		203, C10
Glu→Val	Henri Mondor		7.5	2	Subj had iron def; sl unstable		204
27 (B9) Ala→Asp	Volga				Unstable	EE	205, 206, C13
Ala→Ser	Knossos	33			Variant/β thal	EE	206a 206b
28 (B10) Leu→Gln	St. Louis				Unstable	WE	207, 208, C13
Leu→Pro	Genova				Unstable	Af, SE	209, 210, C13
29 (B11) Gly→Asp	Lufkin				Unstable	Af	211, C13
30 (B12) Arg→Ser*	Tacoma				Unstable	E	212, C13
31 (B13) Leu→Pro	Yokohama				Unstable		212a
32 (B14) Leu→Pro	Perth				Unstable		213, C13
	Abraham Lincoln					Af	214
Leu→Arg	Castilla				Unstable	SE	215, C13
34 (B16) Val→Phe**	Pitie-Salpetriere				↑O$_2$ affinity		216, C14
35 (C1) Tyr→Phe*	Philly				Unstable	E, WE	217
36 (C2) Pro→Thr	Linkoping		18		↑O$_2$ affinity	E	217a
37 (C3) Trp→Ser**	Hirose				↑O$_2$ affinity	EA	218
Trp→Arg**	Rothschild				↓O$_2$ affinity		219
38 (C4) Thr→Pro	Hazebrouck	31	10.8	9	↓O$_2$ affinity; +HB	E	219a, C13
39 (C5) Gln→Lys	Alabama	38	10.8	1.5		Af	220
Gln→Glu	Vaasa		12	2.4	Sl unstable (+Iso)	NE	221
40 (C6) Arg→Lys**	Athens-Ga				↑O$_2$ affinity	C	222, C14
Arg→Ser**	Austin				↑O$_2$ affinity	CAm	223, C14
41 (C7) Phe→Tyr**	Mequon				Unstable	WE	224, C13
42 (CD1) Phe→Ser	Hammersmith				Unstable		225, 226, C13
Phe→Leu	Louisville, Bucuresti				Unstable	NAm EE	227, C13, 228
43 (CD2) Glu→Ala**	G-Galveston					Af	229
Glu→Gln**	Hoshida	42	13.6		Nl O$_2$ affinity	EA	230
44 (CD3) Ser→Cys	Mississippi				Forms disulfide bonds with other globin subunits	A	230a
45 (CD4) Phe→Ser	Cheverly				Unstable		230b, C13
46 (CD5) Gly→Glu	K-Ibadan	50				Af	231
Gly→Arg	Gainesville-Ga						231a
47 (CD6) Asp→Asn	G-Copenhagen					NE	232
Asp→Gly	Gavello	42			Nl O$_2$ affinity; neg HB	SE	233

Table continued on following page

Table 10–2. HUMAN HEMOGLOBIN VARIANTS† Continued

B. Variants of the Beta Chain

Structure	Name	% of Total Hb	Hb (g/dl)	Reticulocytes (%)	Properties	Geographic Origin‡	Reference(s)
Asp→Ala	Avicenna	40			Neg heat		234
Asp→Tyr	Maputo						234a
48 (CD7) Leu→Arg	Okaloosa				Unstable	C	235, C13
50 (D1) Thr→Lys	Edmonton	20				EE	236
51 (D2) Pro→Arg	Willamette				↑ O$_2$ affinity	Af	237, C14
52 (D3) Asp→Asn	Osu-Christiansborg	36			Variant/S	Af, ME	238
Asp→Ala	Ocho Rios					Af	239
Asp→His	Summer Hill	44	13.1		Nl O$_2$ affinity	ME	240
56 (D7) Gly→Asp	J-Bangkok J-Meinung J-Korat	57–65					241, 242, 243
Gly→Arg	Hamadan	40			Neg HB	ME	244
57 (E1) Asn→Lys	G-Ferrara				Unstable	SE	245, C13
Asn→Asp	J-Daloa	37	14			Af	245a
58 (E2) Pro→Arg	Yukuhashi, Dhofar	15				A, ME	68, 246
59 (E3) Lys→Glu	I-High Wycombe					WE	247
Lys→Thr	J-Kaohsiung	47				EA	248, 249
Lys→Asn	J-Lome	50	16.7		Nl O$_2$ affinity; ↑ auto-oxidation	Af	250
60 (E4) Val→Leu	Yatsushiro	45					251
Val→Ala	Collingwood				Unstable		251a
61 (E5) Lys→Glu	N-Seattle	50				Af	252
Lys→Asn	Hikari	54–69			Nl O$_2$ affinity	EA	253
Lys→Met	Bologna				↓ O$_2$ affinity		254, C14
62 (E6) Ala→Pro	Duarte				Unstable	CE	255, C13
63 (E7) His→Arg	Zürich				Unstable	CE	256, C13
His→Tyr	M-Saskatoon				Ferri-Hb	NAm	257–265, C15
His→Pro	Bicetre				Unstable		266, C13
64 (E8) Gly→Asp	J-Calabria				Unstable	SE	267, C13
65 (E9) Lys→Asn	J-Sicilia	40	11.6	1.8		SE	268
Lys→Gln	J-Cairo				↓ O$_2$ affinity	NAf	269, C14
66 (E10) Lys→Glu	I-Toulouse				Unstable	WE	270, C13
67 (E11) Val→Asp	Bristol				Unstable		271, C13
Val→Glu	M-Milwaukee-I				Ferri-Hb	E	257, C15
Val→Ala	Sydney				Unstable	C	272, C13
68 (E12) Leu→Pro	Mizuho				Unstable	EA	273, C13
Leu→His	Brisbane Great Lakes				↑ O$_2$ affinity		274, C13 275
69 (E13) Gly→Asp	J-Cambridge J-Rambam	11–15	1–2			WE	232 276
Gly→Ser	City of Hope	45	16		Nl O$_2$ affinity		276a
Gly→Arg	Kenitra						276b
70 (E14) Ala→Asp	Seattle				Unstable		277, C13
71 (E15) Phe→Ser	Christchurch				Unstable		278, C13
73 (E17) Asp→Tyr	Vancouver				↓ O$_2$ affinity	EA	279, C14
Asp→Asn	Korle-Bu G-Accra					Af	280, 281
Asp→Val	Mobile				↓ O$_2$ affinity	Af	282, 279, C14
74 (E18) Gly→Val	Bushwick				Unstable	SE	283, C13
Gly→Asp	Shepherds Bush				Unstable	WE	284, C13

Table 10-2. HUMAN HEMOGLOBIN VARIANTS† Continued

B. Variants of the Beta Chain

Structure	Name	% of Total Hb	Hb (g/dl)	Reticulocytes (%)	Properties	Geographic Origin‡	Reference(s)
75 (E19) Leu→Pro	Atlanta				Unstable	C	285, C13
Leu→Arg	Pasadena				Unstable		286, C13
76 (E20) Ala→Asp	J-Chicago	53	12.4	0.6		Af	287
77 (EF1) His→Asp	J-Iran		14.2			ME	288
78 (EF2) Leu→Arg	Quin-Hai	21	12.2		Neg Iso	EA	288a
79 (EF3) Asp→Gly	G-Hsi-Tsou				↑ O_2 affinity	EA	289–290, C14
Asp→Tyr	Tampa	33			Homozygote; neg HB; neg Iso		291
80 (EF4) Asn→Lys	G-Szuhu	40			Homozygote; n1 O_2 affinity	EA	292, 293
81 (EF5) Leu→Arg	Baylor				Unstable	E	294, C13
82 (EF6) Lys→Asn, Lys→Asp	Providence				↓ O_2 affinity	Af	295, 296, C14
Lys→Thr	Rahere				↑ O_2 affinity	WE	297, C14
Lys→Met	Helsinki				↑ O_2 affinity		298, C14
83 (EF7) Gly→Cys	Ta-Li	40	15	0.4	Sl + heat; polymerization	EA	299
Gly→Asp	Pyrgos	52	12.5	1	Variant/S; neg HB; neg heat; s1 ↓ O_2 affinity	SE, EA	300, 301
85 (F1) Phe→Ser	Bryn Mawr / Buenos Aires				Unstable	SAm, C	302, C13 / 303
87 (F3) Thr→Lys	D-Ibadan				Variant/S	WA	304
88 (F4) Leu→Arg	Borås				Unstable	NE	305, C13
Leu→Pro	Santa Ana				Unstable	C	306, C13
89 (F5) Ser→Asn	Creteil				↑ O_2 affinity		307, C14
Ser→Arg	Vanderbilt				↑ O_2 affinity		308, C14
90 (F6) Glu→Lys	Agenogi				↓ O_2 affinity	EA, Af	309, C14
91 (F7) Leu→Pro	Sabine				Unstable	WE, CE	310, C13
Leu→Arg	Caribbean				Unstable	CAm	311, C13
92 (F8) His→Tyr	M-Hyde Park				Ferri-Hb	Af	312, 313, C15
His→Gln	St. Etienne / Istanbul				Unstable		314, C13 / 315
His→Asp	J-Altgeld Gardens				Nl O_2 affinity	Af	316
His→Arg	Mozhaisk				Unstable		316a, C13
His→Pro	Newcastle				Unstable	WE	317, C13
93 (F9) Cys→Arg	Okazaki	40	13.5	1.4	↑ O_2 affinity; +Iso	A	317a
94 (FG1) Asp→His	Barcelona				↑ O_2 affinity		C14
Asp→Asn	Bunbury				↑ O_2 affinity		317b
95 (FG2) Lys→Glu	N-Baltimore	50–60			Nl O_2 affinity	Af	318–322
Lys→Asn	Detroit	48	13.7		Nl O_2 affinity; neg HB; neg Iso		323
96 (FG3) Leu→Val	Regina				↑ O_2 affinity		323a
97 (FG4) His→Gln**	Malmö				↑ O_2 affinity	NE	324, C14
His→Leu**	Wood				↑ O_2 affinity	NE	325, 326, C14
His→Pro**	Nagoya				Unstable		326a
98 (FG5) Val→Met**	Köln				Unstable	CE	327–329, C13
Val→Gly**	Nottingham				Unstable	C	330, C13
Val→Ala**	Djelfa				Unstable		331, C13
99 (G1) Asp→Asn**	Kempsey				↑ O_2 affinity	WE	332, C14
Asp→His**	Yakima				↑ O_2 affinity	NE	333, C14
Asp→Ala**	Radcliffe				↑ O_2 affinity	WE	334, C14

Table continued on following page

Table 10–2. **HUMAN HEMOGLOBIN VARIANTS**† Continued

B. Variants of the Beta Chain

Structure	Name	% of Total Hb	Hb (g/dl)	Reticulocytes (%)	Properties	Geographic Origin‡	Reference(s)
Asp→Tyr**	Ypsilanti				↑ O_2 affinity	Af	335, C14
Asp→Gly**	Hotel-Dieu				↑ O_2 affinity		336, C14
Asp→Val**	Chemilly	40	18.7		↑ O_2 affinity	E	336a, C14
100 (G2) Pro→Leu**	Brigham				↑ O_2 affinity	C	337, C14
101 (G3) Glu→Lys**	British Columbia				↑ O_2 affinity	SEA	338, C14
Glu→Gln**	Rush				Unstable	Af	339, C13
Glu→Gly**	Alberta				↑ O_2 affinity	C	340, C14
Glu→Asp**	Potomac				↑ O_2 affinity	NE	341, C14
102 (G4) Asn→Lys**	Richmond				Asymmetric hybrids	Af	342
Asn→Thr**	Kansas				↓ O_2 affinity	WE	343, C14
Asn→Ser**	Beth Israel				↓ O_2 affinity	SE, EE	344, C14
Asn→Tyr**	Saint Mande				↓ O_2 affinity	WE	345, C14
103 (G5) Phe→Leu	Heathrow				↑ O_2 affinity	WE	346, C14
104 (G6) Arg→Ser	Camperdown	50	11–19		Sl +heat; +Iso; nl O_2 affinity	SE	347
Arg→Thr	Sherwood Forest	50	12.5		Neg heat; neg Iso	ME	348
106 (G8) Leu→Pro	Southampton Casper				Unstable	WE C	349, C13 350
Leu→Gln	Tübingen				Unstable	CE	351, 352, C13
107 (G9) Gly→Arg	Burke				Unstable		353, C13
108 (G10) Asn→Asp*	Yoshizuka				↓ O_2 affinity	EA	354, C14
Asn→Lys*	Presbyterian				↓ O_2 affinity	CE	355, C14
109 (G11) Val→Met	San Diego				↑ O_2 affinity		356, C14
111 (G13) Val→Phe	Peterborough				Unstable	SE	357, C13
112 (G14) Cys→Arg*	Indianapolis				Very unstable	NE	358, C13
113 (G15) Val→Glu	New York	40–45			Variant/β thal	EA	359, 360
115 (G17) Ala→Pro*	Madrid				Unstable	WE	361, C13
117 (G19) His→Arg	P-Galveston	45	13.1	1	Abn RBC morphology	Af	362
His→Pro	Saitama				Unstable		362a
118 (GH1) Phe→Tyr	Minneapolis-Laos						362b
119 (GH2) Gly→Asp	Fannin-Lubbock	41–45	12–14	1.5	Sl +heat; +HB; nl O_2 affinity		363, 364
Gly→Val*	Bougardirey-Mali	35	15	1.5	Sl unstable; nl O_2 affinity	SEA	365
120 (GH3) Lys→Glu	Hijiyama	58				EA	366
Lys→Asn	Riyadh	55	10.8	1.5	Neg heat; neg Iso	ME, CAm	367, 368
Lys→Gln	Takamatsu	49	12.1	1.0	Nl O_2 affinity	EA	369
Lys→Ile	Jianghua	50	12		+Iso; +HB	EA	369a
121 (GH4) Glu→Gln	D-Los Angeles D-Punjab D-Chicago	30–40			↑ O_2 affinity		370–377, C10
Glu→Lys	O-Arab				Variant/β thal	Af EE, NAf, Af, ME	378
Glu→Val	Beograd				Variant/β thal	EE	379
124 (H2) Pro→Arg*	Khartoum				Unstable	Af	380, C13
Pro→Gln*	Ty Gard				↑ O_2 affinity		381, C14
126 (H4) Val→Glu	Hofu	51	11	1.3		EA, WE, ME Af	382
Val→Ala	Beirut	44	Nl		Neg Iso; nl O_2 affinity		383

Table 10–2. **HUMAN HEMOGLOBIN VARIANTS**† Continued

B. Variants of the Beta Chain

Structure	Name	% of Total Hb	Hb (g/dl)	Reticulocytes (%)	Properties	Geographic Origin‡	Reference(s)
127 (H5) Gln→Glu*	Hacettepe	45	14.6		Neg heat		384
128 (H6) Ala→Asp*	J-Guantanamo				Unstable	CAm	385, C13
129 (H7) Ala→Asp	J-Taichung	41				EA	386
Ala→Glu or Asp	K-Cameroon						231
Ala→Pro	Crete				↑ O_2 affinity		387
130 (H8) Tyr→Asp	Wien				Unstable	CE	388, C13
131 (H9) Gln→Glu*	Camden	45	11.1	0.1	Nl O_2 affinity	Af	389, 391
Gln→Lys*	Shelby	34	13	1–3	Nl O_2 affinity; +heat	Af	389a, 467–469
132 (H10) Lys→Gln	K-Woolwich	40			Variant/S; Var/C	CAm	231, 390
134 (H12) Val→Glu	North Shore				Unstable	WE	392, 393, C13
135 (H13) Ala→Pro	Altdorf				Unstable	CE	394, C13
136 (H14) Gly→Asp	Hope				Unstable; ↓ O_2 affinity	Af	395, C13
138 (H16) Ala→Pro	Brockton				Unstable		396, C13
139 (H17) Asn→Asp	Geelong						396a
140 (H18) Ala→Thr	St.-Jacques				↑ O_2 affinity		396b, C14
141 (H19) Leu→Arg	Olmsted				Unstable	C	324, C13
142 (H20) Ala→Asp	Ohio				↑ O_2 affinity		397, C14
Ala→Pro	Toyoake				Unstable		398, C13
143 (H21) His→Arg	Abruzzo				↑ O_2 affinity	SE	399, C14
His→Gln	Little Rock				↑ O_2 affinity		400, C14
His→Pro	Syracuse				↑ O_2 affinity	C	401, C14
144 (HC1) Lys→Asn	Andrew-Minneapolis				↑ O_2 affinity		402, C14
145 (HC2) Tyr→His**	Bethesda				↑ O_2 affinity		403, C14
Tyr→Cys**	Rainier				↑ O_2 affinity	SE	403, C14
Tyr→Asp**	Fort Gordon				↑ O_2 affinity		404, C14
	Osler					Af	405
	Nancy					Af	406
Tyr→Term**	McKees Rocks				↑ O_2 affinity	C	407
146 (HC3) His→Asp**	Hiroshima				↑ O_2 affinity	EA	408, C14
His→Pro**	York				↑ O_2 affinity	C	409, C14
His→Arg**	Cochin-Port Royal	48	13.3	1.5	Nl O_2 affinity		410
His→Leu**	Cowtown				↑ O_2 affinity		411, C14

Table continued on following page

Table 10-2. **HUMAN HEMOGLOBIN VARIANTS†** Continued

C. Variants of the Delta Chain

Residue	Substitution	Name	Reference
2 (NA2)	His→Arg	A₂-Sphakiá	412
12 (A9)	Asn→Lys	A₂-NYU	413
16 (A13)	Gly→Arg	A₂' (B₂)	414
20 (B2)	Val→Glu	A₂-Roosevelt	415
22 (B4)	Ala→Glu	A₂-Flatbush	416
24 (B6)	Gly→Asp	A₂-Victoria	416a
43 (CD2)	Glu→Lys	A₂-Melbourne	417
51 (D2)	Pro→Arg	A₂-Adria	418
69 (E13)	Gly→Arg	A₂-Indonesia	419
99 (G1)	Asp→Asn*	A₂-Canada	419a
116 (G18)	Arg→His	A₂-Coburg	420
121 (GH4)	Glu→Val	A₂-Manzonares	420a
125 (H3)	Gln→Glu	A₂-Zagreb	420b
136 (H14)	Gly→Asp	A₂-Babinga	421
142 (H20)	Ala→Asp	A₂-Fitzroy	421a

*Increased O_2 affinity.

D. Variants of the Gamma Chain

Residue	Substitution		Name	Reference(s)
1 (NA1)	Gly→Cys	(ᴳγ)*	F-Malaysia	422
5 (A2)	Glu→Lys	(ᴬγᴵ)	F-Texas-I	423
	Glu→Gly	(ᴳγᴵ)	F-Meinohama	423a
6 (A3)	Glu→Lys	?	F-Texas-II	424
	Glu→Gly	(ᴬγᴵ)	F-Kotobuki	424a
	Glu→Gln	(ᴬγᴵ)	F-Pordenone	424b
7 (A4)	Asp→Asn	(ᴳγ)	F-Auckland	425
12 (A9)	Thr→Lys	?	Alexandra	426
	Thr→Arg	(ᴳγᴵ)	Heather	426a
	Thr→Arg	(ᴬγᴵ)	F-Calluna	426b
16 (A13)	Gly→Arg	(ᴳγ)	F-Melbourne	427
22 (B4)	Asp→Gly	(ᴬγ)	F-Kuala Lumpur	428
34 (B16)	Val→Ile	(ᴳγ)	F-Tokyo	428a
36 (B18)	Pro→Arg	(ᴬγᴵ)	F-Pendergrass	428b
39 (C5)	Gln→Arg	(ᴬγᴵ)	F-Bonaire-Ga	428c
44 (CD3)	Ser→Arg	(ᴳγᴵ)	F-Lòdz	428d
55 (D6)	Met→Arg	(ᴳγ)	F-Kingston	428e
61 (E5)	Lys→Glu	(ᴳγ)	F-Jamaica	429
63 (E7)	His→Tyr	(ᴬγ)	F-M-Osaka	430
66 (E10)	Lys→Arg	(ᴳγᴵ)	F-Shanghai	430a
72 (E16)	Gly→Arg	(ᴬγᴵ)	F-Iwata	431
75 (E19)	Ile→Thr		F-Sardinia	C4
77 (EF1)	His→Arg	(ᴳγᴵ)	F-Kennestone	431a
79 (EF3)	Asp→Asn	(ᴬγ)	F-Dammon	431b
80 (EF4)	Asp→Tyr	(ᴬγ)	F-Victoria Jubilee	432
	Asp→Asn	(ᴳγᴵ)	F-Marietta	432a
	Asp→Asn	(ᴬγᵀ)	F-Yamaguchi	431
94 (FG1)	Asp→Asn	(ᴳγᴵ)	F-Columbus-Ga	432b
97 (FG4)	His→Arg	(ᴬγ)	F-Dickinson	433
101 (G3)	Glu→Lys	(ᴳγ)	F-La Grange	433a
108 (G10)	Asn→Lys	?	F-Ube	434
117 (G19)	His→Arg	(ᴳγ)	F-Malta-I**	435,435a
120 (GH3)	Lys→Gln	(ᴳγ)	F-Caltech	435b
121 (GH4)	Glu→Lys	(ᴬγᴵ)	F-Hull	436
	Glu→Lys	(ᴬγᵀ)	F-Siena	436a
	Glu→Lys	(ᴳγ)	F-Carlton	427
125 (H3)	Glu→Ala	(ᴳγ)	F-Port Royal	437
130 (H8)	Trp→Gly	(ᴳγ)	F-Poole†	438,C13

*ᴳγ:γ subunit has glycine at position 136
ᴬγ:γ subunit has alanine at position 136
γᴵ:γ subunit has isoleucine at position 75
γᵀ:γ subunit has threonine at position 75
**Increased oxygen affinity
†Unstable

Table 10–2. HUMAN HEMOGLOBIN VARIANTS† Continued

E. Fusion Hemoglobins

	A6	A9	B4	D1	F2	F3	G18	G19	H2	H4	H15	Reference
	9	12	22	50	86	87	116	117	124	126	137	
δ Chain	Thr	Asn	Ala	Ser	Ser	Gln	Arg	Asn	Gln	Met	Val	
β Chain	Ser	Thr	Glu	Thr	Ala	Thr	His	His	Pro	Val	Val	
Lepore-Hollandia	———— δ — — β ————————————————											439
Lepore-Baltimore	———————— δ — — β ————————————											440
Lepore-Washington-Boston	———————————————— δ — — β ————											441
Parchman	———— δ — — β — β — — δ ————————											442
Miyada	———— β — — δ ————————————————											443
P-Congo	———— β — — — — — — — — δ ————											444
P-Nilotic	———— β — — δ ————————————————											445
Lincoln Park	———— β — — δ ———————————— δ 137 Val→0											446

	NA1	EF4	EF5	F2	F3		HC3	
	1	80	81	86	87		146	
γ Chain	Gly	Asp	Leu	Ala	Gln		His	
β Chain	Val	Asn	Leu	Ala	Thr		His	
Kenya	———— γ — — β ————————————————							447

F. Extended Chains

	Residues	Name	Major Abnormal Property	Reference(s)
α 141	140 Tyr-Arg-Gln- Ala-Gly-Ala-Ser-Val-Ala-Val-Pro-Pro- 150 160 Ala-Arg-Trp-Ala-Ser-Gln-Arg-Ala-Leu- Leu-Pro-Ser-Leu-His-Arg-Pro-Phe-Leu- 170 Val-Phe-Glu	Constant Spring		448, 449
α 141	31 additional residues—identical to Hb Constant Spring except for residue 142, which is lysine instead of glutamine	Icaria		450
α 141	140 (16 or 17 additional residues) Tyr-Arg (Ser,Ala,Gly,Ala,Ser,Val,Ala, 150 Val,Pro,Pro,Ala)-Arg(?,Ala,Ser,Gln)-Arg-COOH	Koya Dora		451
α 139–141	140 Thr-Ser-Asn-Thr-Val-Lys-Leu-Glu-Pro-Arg-COOH	Wayne		455
α 115–118	115 116 117 118 119 Ala-Glu-Phe-Thr-*Glu-Phe-Thr*-Pro (insertion)	Grady, Dakar		457, 458
β 146	146 His-Thr-Lys-Leu- 150 Ala-Phe-Leu-Leu-Ser-Asn-Phe-Tyr-COOH	Tak	↑ O_2 affinity	452–454

Table continued on following page

Table 10–2. HUMAN HEMOGLOBIN VARIANTS† Continued

F. Extended Chains

	Residues	Name	Major Abnormal Property	Reference(s)
β 145	144 150 Lys-Ser-Ile-Thr-Lys-Leu-Ala-Phe-Leu- 155 Leu-Ser-Asn-Phe-Tyr-COOH	Cranston	Unstable	456
β 143	142 145 150 Ala-Pro-Ser-Ile-Thr-Lys-Leu-Ala-Phe- 155 Leu-Leu-Ser-Asn-Phe-Tyr-COOH	Saverne	Unstable	456a
β NH$_2$	1 H$_2$N-*Met*-Val-*Pro*-Leu- H$_2$N-*Met*-*Met*-His-Leu-	Marseille South Florida		160b 160d

G. Deletions

Residue	Substitution	Name	Major Abnormal Property	Reference
α 6	Asp→0	Boyle Heights	Unstable	458a
β 6 or 7	Glu→0	Leiden	Unstable; sl ↑ O$_2$ affinity	459
β 17–18	(Lys-Val)→0	Lyon	↑ O$_2$ affinity; sl unstable	460
β 23	Val→0	Freiburg	Unstable, ↑ O$_2$ affinity	461
β 43–45	(Phe-Glu-Ser)→0 or (Glu-Ser-Phe)→0	Niteroi	Unstable, ↓ O$_2$ affinity	462
β 56–59	(Gly-Asn-Pro-Lys)→0	Tochigi	Unstable; O$_2$ affinity not known	463
β 74–75	(Gly-Leu)→0	St. Antoine	Unstable; Nl O$_2$ affinity	464
β 75	Leu→0	Vicksburg	Stable	465
β 87	Thr→0	Tours	Unstable; ↑ O$_2$ affinity	464
β 91–95	(Leu-His-Cys Asp-Lys)→0	Gun Hill	Unstable; ↑ O$_2$ affinity	466
β 141	Leu→0	Coventry	Unstable; Nl O$_2$ affinity	470
β 145	(Tyr-His)→0	McKees Rocks	Stable; ↑ O$_2$ affinity	Table 10–2—Section B, C14

H. More Than One Point Mutation in the Same Polypeptide Chain

Residue	Substitution	% of Total	Name	Major Abnormal Property	Reference
β 6 (A3)	Glu→Val 73 Asp→Asn	40	C-Harlem, C-Georgetown	Nl O$_2$ affinity	471 472
	Glu→Val 58 Pro→Arg	35, 43	C-Ziguinchor	Nl O$_2$ affinity; ↑ autoxidation	475
	Glu→Val 142 Ala→Val		S-Travis	↑ O$_2$ affinity	476
	Glu→Lys 95 Lys→Glu		Arlington Park		473
α 78–79	Asn→Asp Ala→Gly	22–24	J-Singapore		474

Table 10–2. HUMAN HEMOGLOBIN VARIANTS† Continued

I. Alphabetical List of the Variants*

A_2-Adria	δ 51	Bunbury	β 94
$A_2'(B_2)$	δ 16	Burke	β 107
A_2-Babinga	δ 136	Bushwick	β 74
A_2-Canada	δ 99	B_2	δ 16
A_2-Coburg	δ 116	C	β 6
A_2-Fitzroy	δ 142	C-Georgetown	β 6, β 73
A_2-Flatbush	δ 22	C-Harlem	β 6, β 73
A_2-Indonesia	δ 69	C-Ziguinchor	β 6, β 58
A_2-Manzonares	δ 121	Camden	β 131
A_2-Melbourne	δ 43	Camperdown	β 104
A_2-NYU	δ 12	Caribbean	β 91
A_2-Roosevelt	δ 20	Casper	β 106
A_2-Sphakiá	δ 2	Castilla	β 32
A_2-Victoria	δ 24	Chad	α 23
A_2-Zagreb	δ 125	Chapel Hill	α 74
Abraham Lincoln	β 32	Chaya	β 43 Gln
Abruzzo	β 143	Chemilly	β 99
Agenogi	β 90	Chesapeake	α 92
Aichi	α 50	Cheverly	β 45
Aida	α 64	Chiapas	α 114
Alabama	β 39	Chiba	β 42 Ser
Alamo	β 19	Chongqing	α 2
Albany-Suma	α 11	Christchurch	β 71
Alberta	β 101	City of Hope	β 69
Alexandra	γ 12	Cochin–Port Royal	β 146
Altdorf	β 135	Cocody	β 21
Amiens	β 17	Collingwood	β 60
Anantharaj	α 11	Connecticut	β 21
Andrew-Minneapolis	β 144	Constant Spring	α 141 Extended chain
Ankara	β 10	Contaldo	α 103
Ann Arbor	α 80	Cordele	α 47
Arlington Park	β 6, β 95	Coventry	β 141 Deletion
Arya	α 47	Cowtown	β 146
Asabara	α 74	Cranston	β 145 Extended chain
Atago	α 85	Crete	β 129
Athens-Ga	β 40	Creteil	β 89
Atlanta	β 75	D-Baltimore	α 68
Austin	β 40	D-Bushman	β 16
Avicenna	β 47	D-Camperdown	β 121 Val
Barcelona	β 94	D-Chicago	β 121
Bari	α 45	D-Ibadan	β 87
Baylor	β 81	D-Iran	β 22
Beijing	α 16	D-Los Angeles	β 121
Beilinson	α 47	D-North Carolina	β 121 Gln
Beirut	β 126	D-Ouled Rabah	β 19
Belfast	β 15	D-Portugal	β 121 Gln
Beograd	β 121	D-Punjab	β 121
Bethesda	β 145	D-St. Louis	α 68
Beth Israel	β 102	D-Washington	α 68
Bibba	α 136	Dagestan	α 60
Bicetre	β 63	Dakar	α 115–118 Extended chain
Bologna	β 61	Dallas	α 97
Borås	β 88	Daneskgab-Tehran	α 72
Bougardirey-Mali	β 119	Deer Lodge	β 2
Boyle Heights	α 6 Deletion	Denmark Hill	α 95
Brigham	β 100	Detroit	β 95
Brisbane	β 68	Dhofar	β 58
Bristol	β 67	Djelfa	β 98
British Columbia	β 101	Drenthe	β 27 Asp
Brockton	β 138	Duan	α 75
Bryn Mawr	β 85	Duarte	β 62
Bucuresti	β 42	Dunn	α 6
Buenos Aires	β 85	E	β 26
Buginese-X	α 116	E-Saskatoon	β 22

*The most common names for each variant are listed in Table 10–2, *A* to *H*. This part of the table also includes other names that are designated with the substituted residue. Thus, Hb Chaya is β 43 Glu→Gln.

Table continued on following page

Table 10-2. HUMAN HEMOGLOBIN VARIANTS† Continued

I. Alphabetical List of the Variants*

Edmonton	β 50	G-Port Arthur	β 43 Ala
Egypt	β 121 Lys	G-San Jose	β 7
Etobicoke	α 84	G-Saskatoon	β 22
Evanston	α 14	G-Singapore	α 30
F-Alexandra	γ 12	G-Szuhu	β 80
F-Auckland	γ 7	G-Taegu	β 22 Ala
F-Bonaire	γ 39	G-Taichung	α 74
F-Calluna	γ 12	G-Taipei	β 22
F-CalTech	γ 120	G-Taiwan Ami	β 25
F-Carlton	γ 121	G-Texas	β 43 Ala
F-Columbus-Ga	γ 94	G-Waimanalo	α 64
F-Damman	γ 79	Gainesville	β 46
F-Dickinson	γ 97	Garden State	α 82
F-Heather	γ 12	Gavello	β 47
F-Hull	γ 121	Genova	β 28
F-Iwata	γ 72	Gifu	β 80 Lys
F-Jamaica	γ 61	Gothenburg	α 58 Tyr
F-Kennestone	γ 77	Grady	α 115–118 Extended chain
F-Kingston	γ 55	Great Lakes	β 68
F-Kotobuki	γ 6	GuiZhou	α 77
F-Kuala Lumpur	γ 22	Gun Hill	β 91–95 Deletion
F-La Grange	γ 101	Hacettepe	β 127
F-Lódz	γ 44	Hamadan	β 56
F-Malaysia	γ 1	Hamilton	β 11
F-Malta-I	γ 117	Hammersmith	β 42
F-Marietta	γ 80	Handa	α 90
F-Meinohama	γ 5	Handsworth	α 18
F-Melbourne	γ 16	Harbin	α 16
F-M-Osaka	γ 63	Hasharon	α 47
F-Pendergrass	γ 36	Hazebrouck	β 38
F-Poole	γ 130	Heather	γ 12
F-Pordenone	γ 6	Heathrow	β 103
F-Port Royal	γ 125	Helsinki	β 82
F-Sardinia	γ 75	Henri Mondor	β 26
F-Shanghai	γ 66	Hijiyama	β 120
F-Siena	γ 121	Hikari	β 61
F-Texas-I	γ 5	Hikoshima	α 54
F-Texas-II	γ 6	Hirosaki	α 43
F-Tokyo	γ 34	Hirose	β 37
F-Ube	γ 108	Hiroshima	β 146
F-Victoria Jubilee	γ 80	Hofu	β 126
F-Yamaguichi	γ 80	Hope	β 136
Fannin-Lubbock	β 119	Hopkins-I	β 95 Glu
Ferndown	α 6	Hopkins-II	α 112
Ferrara	α 47	Horlein-Weber	β 63 Tyr
Fort de France	α 45	Hoshida	β 43
Fort Gordon	β 145	Hotel-Dieu	β 99
Fort Worth	α 27	Hsin Chu	β 22 Ala
Freiburg	β 23 Deletion	Hyogo	β 28 Pro
G-Accra	β 73	I	α 16
G-Audhali	α 23	I-Burlington	α 16 Glu
G-Azakuoli	α 68	I-High Wycombe	β 59
G-Bristol	α 68	I-Interlaken	α 15
G-Chinese	α 30	I-Philadelphia	α 16 Glu
G-Copenhagen	β 47	I-Skamania	α 16 Glu
G-Coushatta	β 22	I-Tagawa	α 90
G-Ferrara	β 57	I-Texas	α 16 Glu
G-Galveston	β 43	I-Toulouse	β 66
G-Georgia	α 95	Icaria	α 141 Extended chain
G-Hong Kong	α 30	Indianapolis	β 112
G-Honolulu	α 30	Inkster	α 85
G-Hsi-Tsou	β 79	Istanbul	β 92
G-Knoxville-I	α 68	Iwata	α 87
G-Makassar	β 6	J	α 54
G-Norfolk	α 85	J-Abidjan	α 51
G-Pest	α 74	J-Aljezur	α 12
G-Philadelphia	α 68	J-Altgeld Gardens	β 92

Table 10–2. HUMAN HEMOGLOBIN VARIANTS† Continued

I. Alphabetical List of the Variants*

J-Baltimore	β 16	Knossos	β 27
J-Bangkok	β 56	Kobe	β 32 Pro
J-Bari	β 64 Asp	Kokura	α 47
J-Birmingham	α 120	Köln	β 98
J-Broussais	α 90	Korle-Bu	β 73
J-Buda	α 61	Kotobuki	γ 6
J-Cairo	β 65	Koya Dora	α 141 Extended chain
J-Calabria	β 64	Kurashiki	α 74
J-Camaguey	α 141	L-Ferrara	α 47
J-Cambridge	β 69	L-Gaslini	α 47
J-Cape Town	α 92	L-Persian Gulf	α 57
J-Chicago	β 76	Legnano	α 141
J-Cosenza	β 64 Asp	Leiden	β 6 or 7 Deletion
J-Cubujuqui	α 141	Leipzig	β 63 Tyr
J-Daloa	β 57	LeLamentin	α 20
J-Georgia	β 16 Asp	Lepore-Baltimore	Fusion hemoglobin
J-Guantanamo	β 128	Lepore-Hollandia	Fusion hemoglobin
J-Habana	α 71	Lepore-Washington-Boston	Fusion hemoglobin
J-Honolulu	β 59		
J-Iran	β 77	Lille	α 74
J-Ireland	β 16 Asp	Lincoln Park	Fusion hemoglobin
J-Kaohsiung	β 59	Little Rock	β 143
J-Korat	β 56	Linkoping	β 36
J-Kurosh	α 19	Louisville	β 42
J-Lens	β 13	Lufkin	β 29
J-Lome	β 59	Lyon	β 17–18 Deletion
J-Luhe	β 8	M-Akita	β 92
J-Manado	β 56 Asp	M-Arhus	β 63
J-Medellin	α 22	M-Boston	α 58
J-Meerut	α 120	M-Chicago	β 63
J-Meinung	β 56	M-Emory	β 63
J-Norfolk	α 57	M-Erlangen	β 63
J-Nyanza	α 21	M-Hida	β 63
J-Oxford	α 15	M-Hyde Park	β 92
J-Paris-I	α 12	M-Iwate	α 87
J-Paris-II	α 54	M-Kankakee	α 87
J-Rajappen	α 90	M-Kiskunhalas	α 58
J-Rambam	β 69	M-Kurume	β 63
J-Rovigo	α 53	M-Milwaukee-I	β 67
J-Sardegna	α 50	M-Oldenburg	α 87
J-Sicilia	β 65	M-Osaka	α 58
J-Singa	α 78	M-Radom	β 63
J-Singapore	α 78–79	M-Saskatoon	β 63
J-Taichung	β 129	M-Sendai	α 87
J-Tashikuergan	α 19	Machida	β 6
J-Tongariki	α 115	Madrid	β 115
J-Toronto	α 5	Mahidol	α 74
J-Trinidad	β 16	Malmö	β 97
J-Wenchang	α 11	Manitoba	α 102
Jackson	α 127	Maputo	β 47
Jenkins	β 95 Glu	Marseille	β 2
Jianghua	β 120	Matsue-Oki	α 75
Jinan	β 139	McKees Rocks	β 145–146 Deletion
K-Cameroon	β 129	Memphis	α 23
K-Ibadan	β 46	Mequon	β 41
K-Woolwich	β 132	Mexico	α 54
Kagoshima	α 57	Michigan-I	α 47
Kansas	β 102	Michigan-II	α 47
Kaohsiang	β 113 Glu	Milledgeville	α 44
Karatsu	β 120 Asn	Minneapolis-Laos	β 118
Kariya	α 40	Mississippi	β 44
Kawachi	α 44	Miyada	Fusion hemoglobin
Kempsey	β 99	Miyashiro	β 23
Kenitra	β 69	Mizuho	β 68
Kenwood	β 95 Glu	Mizunami	β 83 Asp
Kenya	Fusion hemoglobin	Mizushi	α 75
Khartoum	β 124	Moabit	α 86

Table continued on following page

Table 10–2. HUMAN HEMOGLOBIN VARIANTS† Continued

I. Alphabetical List of the Variants*

Name	Position	Name	Position
Mobile	β 73	Quin-Hai	β 78
Montgomery	α 48	Quong Sze	α 125
Moscva	β 24	Radcliffe	β 99
Motown	β 131 Glu	Rahere	β 82
Mozhaisk	β 92	Rainier	β 145
Mugino	α 47	Rajappen	α 90
Munakata	α 90 Met	Raleigh	β 1
N-Baltimore	β 95	Regina	β 96
N-Cosenza	α 15 Asp	Rampa	α 95
N-Memphis	β 95 Glu	Richmond	β 102
N-New Haven	β 16 Asp	Rio Grande	β 8
N-Seattle	β 61	Riverdale-Bronx	β 24
Nagasaki	β 17	Riyadh	β 120
Nagoya	β 97	Rothschild	β 37
Nancy	β 145	Rush	β 101
Necker Enfants-Malades	α 20	Russ	α 51
Newcastle	β 92	S	β 6
New York	β 113	S-Travis	β 6, β 142
Nigeria	α 81	Sabine	β 91
Nishik-I, II, III	α 57	Saitama	β 117
Niteroi	β 43–45 Deletion	Saki	β 14
Noko	α 76	San Diego	β 109
North Shore	β 134	San Francisco (Pacific)	β 98 Met
North Shore–Caracas	β 134	Santa Ana	β 88
Nottingham	β 98	Savannah	β 24
Novi Sad	β 63 Tyr	Savaria	α 49
O-Arab	β 121	Saverne	β 143 Extended chain
O-Indonesia	α 116	Sawara	α 6
O-Padova	α 30	Sealy	α 47
Oak Ridge	β 121 Gln	Seattle	β 70
Ocho Rios	β 52	Serbia	α 112
Ogi	α 34 Arg	Setif	α 94
Ohio	β 142	Shaare Zedek	α 56
Okaloosa	β 48	Shelby	β 131
Okayama	β 2	Shenyang	α 26
Okazaki	β 93	Shepherds Bush	β 74
Oleander	α 116	Sherwood Forest	β 104
Oliviere	α 116	Shimonoseki	α 54
Olmsted	β 141	Shuangfeng	α 27
Olympia	β 20	Siam	α 15
Osler	β 145	Sinai	α 47
Osu-Christiansborg	β 52	Singapore	α 141
Ottawa	α 15	Siriraj	β 7
P-Congo	Fusion hemoglobin	Sögn	β 14
P-Galveston	β 117	Southampton	β 106
P-Nilotic	Fusion hemoglobin	South Florida	β 1
Palmerston-North	β 23	Spanish Town	α 27
Parchman	Fusion hemoglobin	Stanleyville-I	α 68
Pasadena	β 75	Stanleyville-II	α 78
Perspolis	α 64	St. Antoine	β 74–75 Deletion
Perth	β 32	St. Claude	α 127
Petah Tikva	α 110	St. Etienne	β 92
Peterborough	β 111	St.-Jacques	β 140
Philly	β 35	St. Louis	β 28
Pitie-Salpetriere	β 34	St. Luke's	α 95
Pontoise	α 63	St. Mandé	β 102
Port Phillip	α 91	Strasbourg	β 23
Porto Alegre	β 9	Strumica	α 112
Potomac	β 101	Suan-Dok	α 109
Prato	α 31	Summer Hill	β 52
Presbyterian	β 108	Sunshine Seth	α 94
Providence	β 82	Suresnes	α 141
Pyrgos	β 83	Sydney	β 67
Q-India	α 64	Syracuse	β 143
Q-Iran	α 75	Tacoma	β 30
Q-Thailand	α 74	Tagawa-I	α 90
Queens	α 34	Tagawa-II	α 47

Table 10–2. HUMAN HEMOGLOBIN VARIANTS† Continued

I. Alphabetical List of the Variants*

Tak	β 146 Extended chain	Vanderbilt	β 89
Takamatsu	β 120	Vicksburg	β 75 Deletion
Ta-Li	β 83	Volga	β 27
Tampa	β 79	Waco	β 40 Lys
Tarrant	α 126	Warwickshire	β 5
Thailand	α 56	Wayne	α 139–141 Extended chain
Titusville	α 94	Westmead	α 122
Tochigi	β 56–59 Deletion	Wien	β 130
Tokoname	α 139	Willamette	β 51
Tokuchi	β 131 Glu	Winnipeg	α 75
Torino	α 43	Wood	β 97
Tottori	α 59	Woodville	α 6
Tours	β 87 Deletion	Yakima	β 99
Toyoake	β 142	Yatsushiro	β 60
Tübingen	β 106	Yokohama	β 31
Twin Peaks	α 113	York	β 146
Ty Gard	β 124	Yoshizuka	β 108
Ube-1	β 98 Met	Ypsilanti	β 99
Ube-2	α 68	Yukuhashi	β 58
Ube-4	α 116	Yukuhashi-II	α 47
Umi	α 47	Yusa	β 21
Uppsala	α 54	Zambia	α 60
Vaasa	β 39	Zürich	β 63
Vancouver	β 73		

the electrophoretically abnormal variants, other techniques must be employed. In many laboratories, electrophoresis on citrate agar at pH 6.0 to 6.5 is used. Schneider[478] has shown that this technique can be very informative in the initial detection and identification of variants. Figure 10–1 shows the comparative electrophoretic separations on cellulose acetate and citrate agar for 102 variants. Most variants, irrespective of charge, behave like Hb A when analyzed by electrophoresis on citrate agar. Those variants that have abnormal migration on citrate agar generally have structural alterations at sites that bind polyanions such as 2,3-DPG.[479, 479a] When electrophoresis on cellulose acetate (pH 8.6) and on citrate agar (pH 6.0 to 6.5) is coupled with electrophoresis of globin chains in 6 M urea, presumptive identification of most variants can be made (Fig. 10–1[480, 481]). Alternatively, a higher-resolution electrophoretic method can be used for identification of variants. Rosa and colleagues in Paris[482, 483] have shown that the vast majority of variants can be separated by isoelectric focusing on thin slabs of polyacrylamide gel. Figure 10–2 shows a representative pattern as well as the relative focusing positions of many of the variants that have been studied. High-performance liquid chromatography has also proved useful for isolating variants that escape detection by other methods.[383] More specialized techniques required for separation of a few of the functionally abnormal variants are described in Chapters 13 to 15.

Recently, immunologic techniques have been developed for the detection and identification of hemoglobin variants. Garver and colleagues[484] have prepared monospecific antibodies that recognize 40 specific hemoglobin variants and do not cross react with Hb A or other variants. Thus, these antibodies can be used for definitive identification. The most "antigenic" variants are those that have a structural alteration on the surface of the molecule.[485] Fortunately, these include nearly all of the frequently encountered variants. Immunologic detection has many advantages: It can be performed with very small amounts of sample and does not require purification of the variant. The assay can be partially automated and can provide results in 24 to 48 hours. The most extensive experience has involved the radioimmune assay.[486] An enzyme-linked assay may be more suitable for clinical applications.[487] In laboratories that have immunologic capability, this approach can be utilized to screen and identify the relatively commonly encountered variants, reserving time-consuming and costly structural analyses for the few that remain.

Methods used in the structural analysis of hemoglobin variants are outlined in Chapter 2. Recent advances in high-performance liquid chromatography, automated microsequencing,

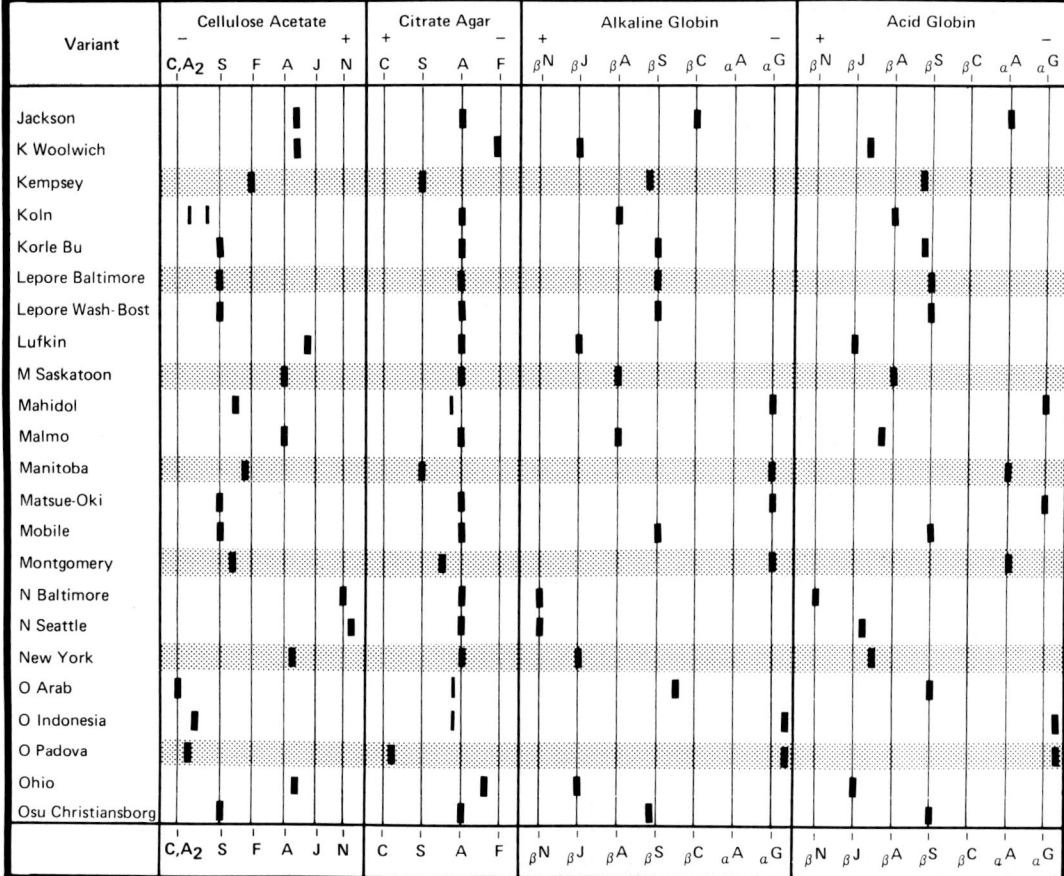

Figure 10-1. Comparative electrophoretic mobilities of 102 mutant hemoglobins and their chains. (Courtesy of Drs. Winston Moo-Penn and Danny Jue.)

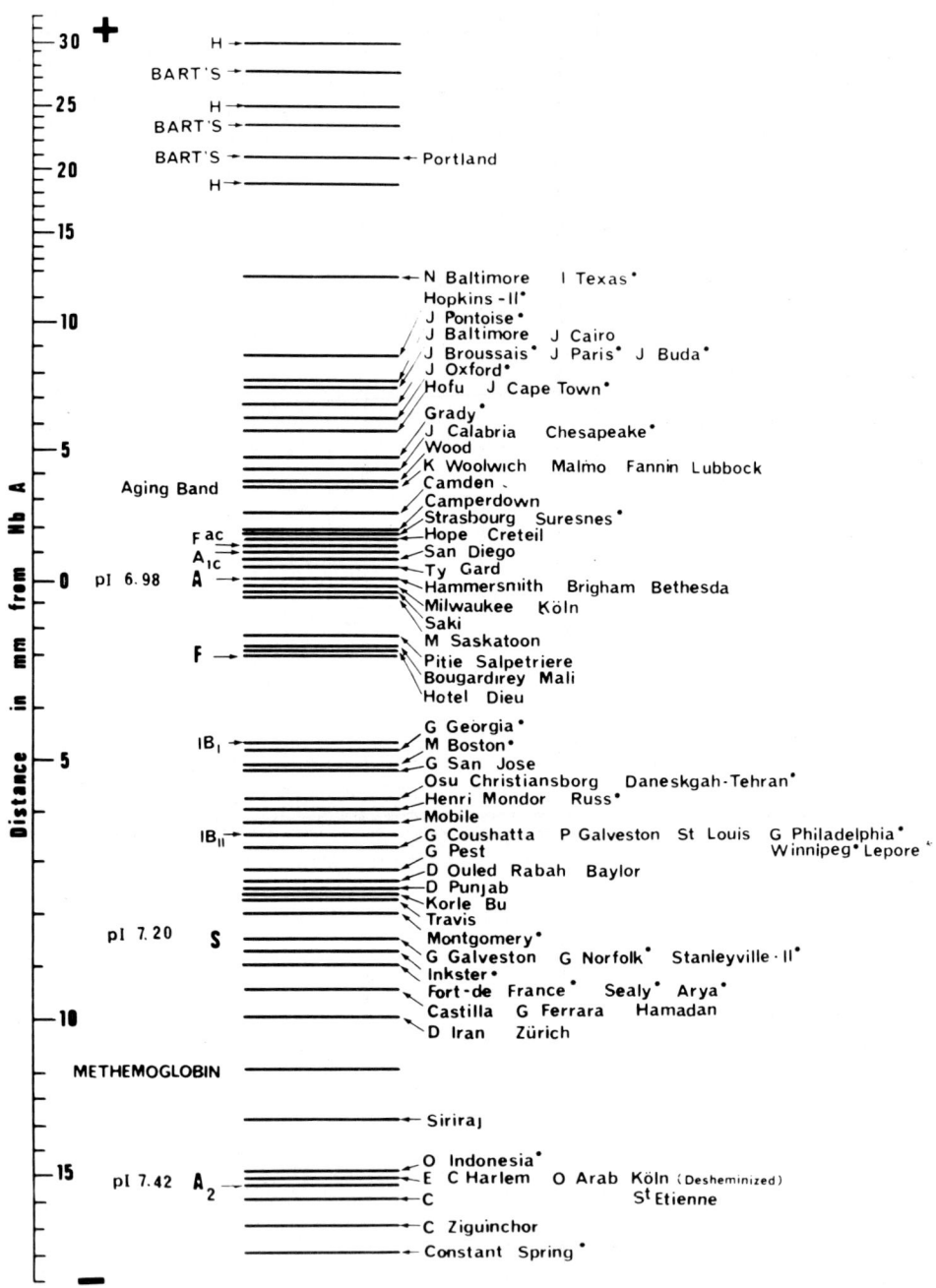

Figure 10–2. Comparison of 57 human hemoglobin variants by electrofocusing on polyacrylamide slabs. Asterisk (*) denotes alpha-chain variants. IB_I and IB_{II} are partially oxidized hemoglobin A ($\alpha_2\beta_2^{\frac{1}{2}}$ and $\alpha_2^{\frac{1}{2}}\beta_2$, respectively) (see Chapter 16). (From Basset, P., et al.: J. Chromatogr. Biomed. Appl. 227:267, 1982.)

and mass spectrometry[487a] have facilitated the identification of structural abnormalities.

CLINICAL CLASSIFICATION

The large list of human hemoglobin variants presented in Table 10–2 is more readily comprehended if the variants are classified according to their clinical manifestations (see Table 10–3). The majority of known variants are unassociated with any apparent clinical sequelae. Many of these were discovered accidentally or during the survey of large populations. Harris[488] has estimated that in populations lacking commonly encountered variants such as S, E, or C, one individual in 800 has a hemoglobin variant that can be detected by electrophoresis. Certain variants have provided insights on population genetics and the migration of peoples.

Functional studies were seldom included in the analysis of hemoglobin variants that were discovered prior to 1975. However, recent reports often include stability and oxygenation measurements, even when there are no associated clinical or hematological abnormalities. Thus, the hemoglobin variants compose a spectrum ranging from those with normal properties to those that produce clinical manifestations such as hemolysis or erythrocytosis.

The clinically significant human hemoglobin variants are classified in Table 10–3. Disorders due to the presence of sickle hemoglobin constitute the most important group both in the United States and worldwide. The sickle syndromes are discussed in detail in Chapters 11 and 12. Hb E is the next most commonly encountered variant worldwide. It is associated with a thalassemic phenotype and is discussed in detail at the end of this chapter. In the United States, Hb C is the second most prevalent variant. Like Hb S, Hb C has decreased solubility within the red cell. The pathogenesis of homozygous Hb C disease is also discussed at the end of this chapter. Approximately 85 unstable hemoglobin variants have been described to date. They constitute an important form of congenital nonspherocytic hemolytic anemia. This entity is discussed in Chapter 13.

Table 10–3. **CLINICALLY IMPORTANT HEMOGLOBIN VARIANTS**

I. The Sickle Syndromes
   A. Sickle cell trait
   B. Sickle cell disease
     1. SS
     2. SC
     3. SD$_{Los\ Angeles}$
     4. SO$_{Arab}$
     5. S/β-Thalassemia
II. The Unstable Hemoglobins→Congenital Heinz Body Anemia (~ 90 variants)
III. Hemoglobins with Abnormal Oxygen Affinity
   A. High Affinity→familial erythrocytosis (~ 40 variants)
   B. Low affinity→familial cyanosis (Hbs Kansas, Beth Israel, St. Mandé)
IV. The M Hemoglobins→familial cyanosis (6 variants)
V. Structural Variants that Result in a Thalassemic Phenotype
   A. β-Thalassemia phenotype
     1. Lepore hemoglobins (δβ fusion)
     2. Abnormal mRNA processing: Hbs E, Knossos
     3. Extreme instability: Hb Indianapolis
   B. α-Thalassemia phenotype
     1. Chain termination mutants, i.e., Hb Constant Spring
     2. Extreme instability: Hb Quong Sze

Variants with abnormal oxygen binding are described in Chapter 14. This group has provided a considerable amount of relevant physiological and biochemical information. Individuals with congenital methemoglobinemia may have one of the so-called M hemoglobins. The six M hemoglobins encountered thus far have very interesting properties, which are described in Chapter 15. There are three different Lepore-type hemoglobins, which result in a β-thalassemia phenotype (see Chapters 8 and 9), and four different α-chain termination mutants, which cause α thalassemia. A number of other less common structural variants are also associated with a thalassemic phenotype (see below and Chapters 8 and 9).

GENETIC BASIS OF THE HEMOGLOBIN VARIANTS

Mendelian Inheritance

As explained in Chapter 7, the α and non-α globin polypeptide chains are products of specific genes on separate chromosomes. Thus, a mutant hemoglobin involves a structural abnormality of a particular globin subunit. Hemoglobin variants are inherited as co-dominant traits, according to classic mendelian genetics. An individual inherits one β-chain gene from each parent. As shown in the left panel of Figure 10–3, if both parents are heterozygous for the β-chain variant Hb S (sickle trait or AS), there is a 50 per cent chance that a child will be AS, a 25 per cent chance that it will be AA, and a 25 per cent chance that it will be a sickle homozygote (SS).

If one parent is heterozygous for Hb S and another is heterozygous for Hb C (AC), there

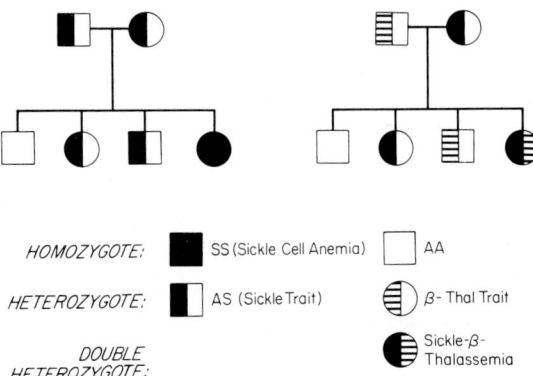

Figure 10–3. Pedigrees showing the inheritance of homozygous sickle cell anemia (left) and the double heterozygous state sickle-β-thalassemia.

is a 25 per cent chance that a child will be a double heterozygote. Its red cells will contain 50 per cent Hb S, 50 per cent Hb C, and no Hb A. The β-thalassemia gene is allelic to the β-chain structural gene. Accordingly, an individual who is a S/β⁰ thalassemia double heterozygote will have red cells containing Hb S (and Hb F) but no Hb A.

The sickle gene results in clinical disease only if inherited as the homozygous state (SS) or as a double heterozygous state (SC, SD$_{Los Angeles}$, SO$_{Arab}$, or S/β thalassemia). In contrast, the unstable variants (see Chapter 13) and those with marked abnormalities of oxygen affinity (see Chapter 14) cause morbidity in heterozygotes. In many cases, the hemoglobin function is so deranged that the homozygous state would be incompatible with life.

As expected, homozygotes have been encountered among variants with high gene frequencies, such as S, C, and E, and among some with moderate gene frequencies, such as D-Los Angeles, O-Arab, and Korle-Bu. The other reported instances of homozygous β-chain variants shown in Table 10–4 are usually the result of consanguineous matings.

Because an individual inherits only two β-chain genes, a functionally abnormal β-chain variant usually constitutes about half of the total hemoglobin in the red cell and is therefore apt to contribute significantly to the function of the red cell. In contrast, most individuals inherit four α-chain genes. Therefore, α-chain variants usually constitute only about 25 per cent of the total hemoglobin and are less likely to cause significant impairment of red cell function. This consideration explains why 50 per cent of the β-chain variants are associated with clinical manifestations, compared with only 20 per cent of the α-chain variants that have been identified to date. As shown in Table 10–1, the α- and β-chain variants that are unassociated with any clinical findings are about equal in number and probably reflect random mutations that result in amino acid substitutions that can be detected by routine electrophoresis.

Occasionally, hemoglobin variants arise as spontaneous mutations.[488a, 488b] Among variants causing clinical manifestations, spontaneous mutants constitute about 15 per cent, a higher frequency than that for variants that are unassociated with clinical abnormalities (see Chapters 13 to 15). Spontaneous mutations are presumed to have arisen at the level of the germ cell. The vast majority of events take place late in germ cell development, so that the mutated egg or sperm is "unique." Accordingly, siblings of individuals with spontaneous mutations would be unaffected. Bradley and colleagues[489] described an interesting exception. They encountered a brother and sister who were each heterozygotes for Hb Köln. Neither parent was affected, however. Exhaustive blood antigen studies effectively established them as true parents. This appears to be a convincing example of gonadal mosaicism in which the mutation took place rela-

Table 10–4. β-CHAIN HEMOGLOBIN VARIANTS FOUND IN THE HOMOZYGOUS STATE THAT HAVE BEEN REPORTED IN THE LITERATURE*

Variant	Substitution	Clinical and Hematological Effects	Location of Homozygote
Hb S	β 6 (A3) Glu→Val	Hemolytic anemia of varying degree, sickle cells	Worldwide
Hb C	β 6 (A3) Glu→Lys	Mild hemolytic anemia, target cells	Worldwide
Hb Siriraj	β 7 (A4) Glu→Lys	None	Thailand
Hb Porto Alegre	β 9 (A6) Ser→Cys	None	South America
Hb G-Coushatta	β 22 (B4) Glu→Ala	None	North American Indians, Koreans, Chinese
Hb E	β 26 (B8) Glu→Lys	Mild microcytic, normocytic anemia	Thailand
Hb G-Galveston	β 43 (CD2) Glu→Ala	None	Ghana
Hb Korle-Bu	β 73 (E17) Asp→Asn	None	Ghana
Hb Tampa	β 79 (EF3) Asp→Tyr	None	United States
Hb G-Szuhu	β 80 (EF4) Asn→Lys	None	Israel
Hb D-Los Angeles	β 121 (GH4) Glu→Gln	Target cells	Punjab
Hb O-Arab	β 121 (GH4) Glu→Lys	Mild anemia with episodes of hemolysis, target cells	Bulgaria, Yugoslavia
Hb K-Woolwich	β 132 (H10) Lys→Gln	None	Ivory Coast

*Compiled by Drs. Ruth Wrightstone and T. H. J. Huisman, International Hemoglobin Information Center (IHIC), Augusta, Georgia.

tively early in the development of the germ line.

As shown in Table 10–1, variants have also been encountered for the other two globin genes, δ and γ, that are found in human red cells in postnatal life. The relatively small number of γ-chain variants is due in part to the fact that hemoglobin F is barely detectable after the first six months of life. Likewise, δ-chain variants may often escape detection, because they are present in small amounts (1 to 2 per cent). No functional significance has been ascribed to any of the γ-chain variants that have been reported, with the exception of Hb F-Poole, an unstable fetal hemoglobin causing hemolytic anemia in the neonatal period,[438] and Hb FM-Osaka, which causes neonatal cyanosis[430] (see Chapter 15).

A heterozygote for both an α-chain variant and a β-chain variant often has four major hemoglobin bands on electrophoresis ($\alpha_2^A \beta_2^A$, $\alpha_2^X \beta_2^A$, $\alpha_2^A \beta_2^X$, and $\alpha_2^X \beta_2^X$). Figure 10–4 shows an electrophoretic pattern of an individual who has an α-chain variant (Hb I) and a β-chain variant (Hb S).

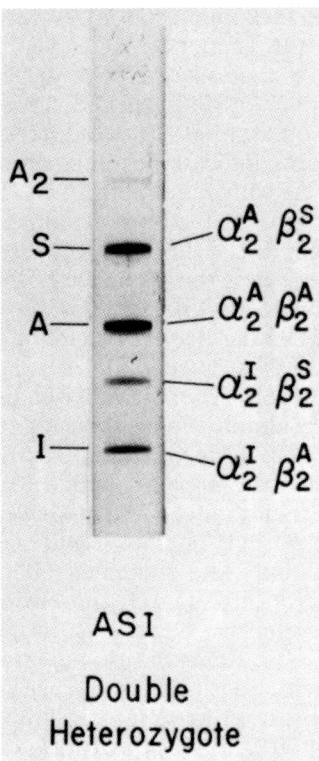

Figure 10–4. Gel electrofocusing pattern of an indivdual doubly heterozygous for an α-chain variant (Hb I) and a β-chain variant (Hb S).

Single Base Substitutions

Of the 400 variants listed in Tables 10–1 and 10–2, the great majority (95%) are single amino acid replacements in a globin polypeptide chain. The structural alteration can be explained by a single base substitution in the corresponding triplet codon of the globin gene DNA (and its corresponding mRNA).* For example, hemoglobins Rainier (β 145 Tyr→Cys), Bethesda (β 145 Tyr→His), and Fort Gordon (β 145 Tyr→Asp) can all be explained by single base substitutions in the triplet UAU, which codes for tyrosine 145 (Table 10–5).

A few variants have amino acid replacements at two different sites on the same subunit (see Table 10–2H). Three of these involve the Hb S substitution (β 6 Glu→Val). These variants arose by one of two mechanisms: new mutation on a variant gene or crossover between two variant genes. For example the C-Harlem gene could have arisen from crossover between genes coding for β^S and $\beta^{Korle-Bu}$.

A total of 2583 single base substitutions are possible for the 141 residues of the α chain and the 146 residues of the β chain (9 × [141 + 146]).[490] Of these, 1690 would result in an amino acid replacement, but only one-third, or 575, would cause a change in charge allowing separation by routine electrophoresis. About 45 per cent of these variants have been discovered thus far.

In a number of cases, the nature of the mutant or variant amino acid substitution indicates a reduction in ambiguity of the nucleotide sequence of the codon for the normal amino acid in the normal globin mRNA. For example, as shown in Figure 10–5, the two mutant hemoglobins Hb Köln and Hb San Diego result from replacement of valine by methionine at positions β 98 and β 109, respectively. There is only one codon for methionine, AUG, but there are four possible codons for the normal valine—GUG, GUA, GUC, or GUU. The codon AUG for methionine could derive from a single base substitution from only one of the four possible valine codons, namely GUG, in which the first nucleotide G is substituted for A. A number of other mutant hemoglobins at different sites of the α and β globin chains suggest similar

---

*For descriptive purposes, in the following discussions, the mutations are described in terms of the nucleotide sequence changes created in the transcription product of the gene: the globin messenger RNA (mRNA). The actual mutation, of course, occurs at the corresponding position in the complementary DNA sequence of the gene.

Table 10–5. **SINGLE BASE SUBSTITUTIONS IN HEMOGLOBIN VARIANTS**

β-Chain Variants		Residue Number 144	145	146	Termination Codon
β^A	Base sequence	AAG	UAU	CAC	UAA
	Amino acid sequence	Lys	Tyr	His	COOH
β Rainier	Base sequence	AAG	UGU	CAC	UAA
	Amino acid sequence	Lys	Cys	His	COOH
β Bethesda	Base sequence	AAG	CAU	CAC	UAA
	Amino acid sequence	Lys	His	His	COOH
β Fort Gordon	Base sequence	AAG	GAU	CAC	UAA
	Amino acid sequence	Lys	Asp	His	COOH

reductions in ambiguity of the sequence of normal globin mRNA codons.[491] At present, there are variants described at 52 amino acid positions of the β globin chain, 29 positions of the α globin chain, four positions of the δ globin chain, and three positions of the γ globin chain that indicate specific reductions in mRNA codon ambiguity.[492, 492a] If the independently derived globin mRNA sequences are compared with the sequences predicted by the variants, it is found that in almost all cases the predictions of mRNA sequence based on the nature of the amino acid replacement are verified by the direct biochemical sequence analysis of the mRNA or gene DNA themselves.[492] In other words, the experimentally derived nucleotide sequences of normal α and β globin mRNAs and gene DNAs confirm the genetic prediction, based on the "single hit" theory of DNA mutation, that amino acid replacements derive from single nucleotide base changes in a unique normal ancestral globin gene DNA (and mRNA) sequence.

A corollary of the observation described above is that most, if not all, individuals share a single unique nucleotide sequence for their

Hb KÖLN β^{98}
Hb SAN DIEGO β^{109}

Val ⟶ Met
GUG
GUA
GUC ⟶ AUG
GUU

Figure 10–5. Example of the origin of an amino acid replacement in the β globin chain of two hemoglobin variants by single nucleotide base substitution in the corresponding mRNA codon. The nature of the amino acid replacement predicts that the third nucleotide of the normal mRNA codon must be G rather than C, A, or U (also allowed by the genetic code), a fact that was verified by direct nucleotide sequence analysis of human β globin mRNA.

globin genes and globin mRNAs, with little or no variability (or polymorphism) from individual to individual in the nucleotide sequence at the third position of various codons. Such third-position changes are theoretically possible without resulting in any abnormality in the amino acid sequence of the gene product. Polymorphism of the coding sequence of normal α and β globin genes must therefore be very rare, although there is evidence that it does, in fact, exist at a low frequency at certain positions of the α and β globin gene. For example, at β-chain position number 50, Hb Edmonton (Thr→Lys) predicts the sequence of the normal threonine codon to be ACA or ACG, but the sequence ACU was found in the sequence analysis of cDNA or gene DNA from a number of different individuals. At β-chain position number 67, two different hemoglobin variants indicate different reductions in ambiguity: As shown in Table 10–6, Hb Bristol (Val→Asp) predicts the normal valine codon to be GUU or GUC, whereas Hb M-Milwaukee (Val→Glu) predicts the sequence of the normal valine codon to be GUA or GUG. Only the sequence GUG has been found in the sequence analysis of cDNA or gene DNA isolated from at least a dozen different individuals. In the case of the α globin chain, a variant at position number 19, Hb J-Kurosh (Ala→Asp), predicts the codon for the normal alanine to be GCU or GCC rather than GCA or GCG, but the analysis of normal α cDNA and gene DNA has yielded only the sequence GCG. These latter observations suggest, therefore, that silent polymorphisms in fact exist in the normal α and β globin genes, with the presence of variable nucleotides in the sequence coding for the third position of codons for amino acids α 19, β 50, and β 67. Base substitutions in the first or second nucleotide positions of these codons could therefore result in the inheritance of different hemoglobin variants in different

Table 10-6. HEMOGLOBIN VARIANTS AFFECTING RESIDUE β 67

Variant	Possible Mutant Codons	Corresponding Normal Valine Codons
Hb Sydney (β 67 Val→Ala)	GCU	GUU
	GCC	GUC
	GCA	GUA
	GCG	GUG
Hb M-Milwaukee (β 67 Val→Glu)	GAA	GUA
	GAG	GUG
Hb Bristol (β 67 Val→Asp)	GAU	GUU
	GAC	GUC

Note that Hb Bristol and Hb M-Milwaukee cannot originate by a single base substitution in a common normal valine codon.

individuals. An alternative explanation for the findings would be that the variants just described resulted from two base substitutions in the involved codon.

Cloning and DNA sequence analysis of globin genes from different individuals have provided direct evidence for occasional silent polymorphisms in the nucleotide sequence of the coding portion of human globin genes. In β globin genes of framework 3 (see pp. 276, 296), the codon for 2 His has the sequence CAU instead of the usual sequence CAC,[493,494] and rare β genes in Asian Indians have the sequence GCA instead of GCC at codon 10.[494a] In the case of the duplicated α globin genes, the nucleotide sequence of the coding portions of the α1 and α2 globin genes in some individuals differ by one nucleotide in two positions (codons 54 and 123) without a resulting change in the amino acid sequence of the encoded α globin polypeptide chain: The sequences are CAG (Gln) and GCC (Ala), respectively, in the α1 (3' or rightward) globin gene,[495-496a] and CAA (Gln) and GCU (Ala) in the α2 (5' or leftward) globin gene of some individuals,[497] but not others.[496a]

Elongated Subunits

One of the more informative developments in the study of human hemoglobins has been the discovery and characterization of variants having elongated subunits. Analysis of these hemoglobins has provided information about the structure of the α and β globin chain genes and about mechanisms underlying the formation of mutant gene products. In addition, the recognition and detection of one of the elongated α-chain variants, Hb Constant Spring, have contributed insights into the pathogenesis and heterogeneity of the α thalassemias.

Ten elongated variants have been described (Tables 10–2F and 10–7). It is likely that they arose by means of one of three different genetic mechanisms: base substitution in the chain termination codon, frameshift mutagenesis, or preservation of initiator methionine.

Mutations of the Chain Termination Codon

In 1971, Milner and associates[498] described a Chinese family containing three members with a phenotype typical of a form of α thalassemia called hemoglobin H disease but with positively charged minor hemoglobin components detected on starch gel electrophoresis (pH 8.6). These abnormal hemoglobins were designated Hb Constant Spring after the village in Jamaica where the family resided. Structural analysis of this variant indicated that the α chain was elongated at the C terminus (141 Arg) by an additional 31 residues[499] (Table 10–8). The fact that the sequence bore no

Table 10-7. VARIANTS HAVING ELONGATED SUBUNITS

	Genetic Mechanism
α Chain Variants	
Constant Spring	Base substitution in termination codon
Icaria	" "
Seal Rock	" "
Koya Dora	" "
Wayne	Frameshift
Grady	Crossover in phase
β Chain Variants	
Marseille	Failure to cleave N-Met
South Florida	" "
Tak	Frameshift
Cranston	" "
Saverne	" "

HUMAN HEMOGLOBIN VARIANTS

Table 10-8. AMINO ACID SEQUENCES AND mRNA NUCLEOTIDE SEQUENCES OF ELONGATED α-CHAIN VARIANTS

		---137	138	139	140	141	142	143	144	145	146	147	148---
α^A		---Thr ---ACC	Ser UCC	Lys AAA	Tyr UAC	Arg CGU	COOH UAA	GCU	GGA	GCC	UCG	GUA	GCA---
α^{CS}		---Thr ---ACC	Ser UCC	Lys AAA	Tyr UAC	Arg CGU	Gln CAA	Ala GCU	Gly GCA	Ala GCC	Ser UCG	Val GUA	Ala--- GCA---
α^{Icaria}		---Thr	Ser	Lys	Tyr	Arg	Lys AAA	Ala	Gly	Ala	Ser	Val	Ala---
$\alpha^{Seal\ Rock}$		---Thr	Ser	Lys	Tyr	Arg	Glu GAA	Ala	Gly	Ala	Ser	Val	Ala---
$\alpha^{Koya\ Dora}$		---Thr	Ser	Lys	Tyr	Arg	Ser UCA	Ala	Gly	Ala	Ser	Val	Ala---
α^{Wayne}		---Thr ---ACC	Ser UC^A_C	Asn AAU	Thr ACC	Val GUU	Lys AAG	Leu CUG	Glu GAG	Pro CCU	Arg CGG	COOH UAG---	

└—Deletion of A or C

resemblance to any portion of normal α chain or any other hemoglobin subunit argued against the occurrence of crossover between two nearby genes. Clegg and Weatherall[499] suggested that the presence of glutamine at position 142, adjacent to α 141 Arg (which is normally the C-terminal residue) was due to a mutation of the termination codon UAA or UAG to CAA or CAG, which code for glutamine. The electrophoretically distinct components of Hb Constant Spring have now been characterized. Hb CS-2 differs from Hb CS-1 by the absence of three residues at the C terminus. Another component, Hb CS-3, which increases on storage, is even more truncated, with α 154 Trp as the C-terminal residue.[499] The electrophoretic heterogeneity of Hb Constant Spring is best explained by proteolytic cleavage of small segments from the C-terminal end of the abnormal subunit.[499]

In retrospect, minor hemoglobins having the electrophoretic behavior of Hb Constant Spring had previously been observed in Asians[500–502] and in Greeks,[503] all in association with Hb H disease.

Three other α-chain variants, like Hb Constant Spring, are present in small amounts and are elongated 31 residues beyond the normal C terminus (see Table 10-8). Hb Icaria, found in Greece, is identical in composition to Hb Constant Spring except that the residue at position 142 is lysine rather than glutamine.[450] This variant is explained by a substitution of A for U in the first base of the termination triplet codon. In like manner, Hb Seal Rock, discovered in a black American,[504] apparently developed because of a substitution of G for U in the termination codon, giving rise to an elongated chain that is identical to that of Hb Constant Spring except that the residue at position 142 is glutamic acid rather than glutamine. In Hb Koya Dora, the elongation of the α chain can be explained by a substitution in the second base of the termination codon (UAA → UCA), resulting in a serine residue at position 142.[451]

Nucleotide sequence analysis of the α globin genes has revealed that the 3′-untranslated sequences of the α1 and α2 genes differ in a number of positions.[497,505] Only the α2 (5′ or leftward) globin gene is consistent with the amino acid sequence of the elongated segments of the α-chain termination variants. Therefore, these mutations occurred only in the α2 and not the α1 globin gene. A chain termination mutation in the α1 globin gene would give rise, after readthrough translation of its mRNA, to an α globin chain having 30 additional C-terminal amino acid residues, in contrast to the 31 additional amino acid residues found in Hb Constant Spring.[505] Although similar in length, the amino acid sequence of the additional polypeptide segment would differ from that of Hb Constant Spring by 14 residues, distributed over the length of the elongated segment. The first six amino acids (residues

143 to 148) would have an identical sequence, whereas the last six amino acids would be totally divergent.[505]

Frameshift Mutants Causing Elongated Subunits

An elongated α-chain variant in small amounts (4 to 6 per cent) was discovered in an American family, unassociated with α thalassemia.[455, 506] The variant was found in two electrophoretic forms (Wayne-I and Wayne-II), with roughly equal amounts of each. Distal to residue 138, α^{Wayne} differed from α^A, having a unique sequence of eight amino acids extending beyond the normal chain length by 5 residues. Knowledge of the Hb Constant Spring sequence provided an explanation of the structure of Hb Wayne. A deletion of one base, either C at codon 138 or A at codon 139, would result in a frameshift.[455, 506] As shown in Table 10–8, the α-chain termination codon (UAA) is now out of phase, and translation continues until a termination codon is encountered in phase. Because of differences in the 3′-untranslated sequences of the α1 and α2 globin genes, Hb Wayne could result from the postulated frame shift only in the α2 globin gene. In the α1 globin gene, a base substitution of A→G changes the new in-phase termination codon at position 147 from UAG to UGG. Therefore, in the event of the same frameshift, the readthrough product of the α1 globin gene would be considerably longer (by 26 additional amino acids) than the α^{Wayne} chain derived from the α2 globin gene. Like Hb Constant Spring, Hb Wayne demonstrated electrophoretic and chromatographic heterogeneity. Hb Wayne-II differs from Hb Wayne-I only at the asparagine residue at position 139, which becomes deamidated at some point following translation.

At the same time that the initial report on Hb Constant Spring appeared,[498] certain members of two Thai families were found to have an elongated β-chain variant composing 40 per cent of the total hemoglobin. No associated hematologic abnormalities were encountered in heterozygotes. Hemoglobin levels and reticulocyte counts were normal. The variant, designated Hb Tak, was reported to be identical to normal β^A through the C-terminal residue (146 His) but was elongated. Subsequent analysis revealed the following structure:[454]

```
              145              150                 155
β^Tak _____ Tyr-His-Thr-Lys-Leu-Ala-Phe-Leu-Leu-Ser-Asn-Phe-Tyr-COOH
```

This sequence ruled out a chain termination mutation such as that responsible for the formation of Hb Constant Spring. Substitution of two bases would be required to convert one of the termination codons (UAA, UAG, or UGA) to a codon for threonine (ACN). Available β globin mRNA sequencing data[508, 509] suggested that Hb Tak arose by a frame shift mutation involving the duplication of two bases, CA at position 146/147 or AC at position 147:[507]

	144	145	146	147	148	149
β^A	Lys	Tyr	His	Term		
	AAG	UAU	CAC	UAA	GCN	
β^{Tak}	Lys	Tyr	His	Thr	Lys	Leu ....
	AAG	UAU	CAC	ACU	AAG	CUN ..
or	AAG	UAU	CAC	ACU	AAG	CUN ..

In an Italian-American family from Cranston, Rhode Island, affected members had well-compensated hemolysis due to the presence of a somewhat unstable hemoglobin variant that composed 30 per cent of the total. A mother, daughter, and grandson all had normal hemoglobin levels and moderate reticulocytosis (5 to 8 per cent). Hb Cranston was shown to have an abnormal β chain, which was identical to β^A through residue 144 but, thereafter, had a sequence extending to a total of 157 residues:[456]

```
            145              150                 155
β^Cr _____ Lys-Ser-Ile-Thr-Lys-Leu-Ala-Phe-Leu-Leu-Ser-Asn-Phe-Tyr-COOH
```

The sequence of the last 11 residues was identical to that of Hb Tak. The structure of Hb Cranston could be explained by a frameshift in which two bases, AG, are inserted at position 145:

	144	145	146	147	148	149
β^A	Lys	Tyr	His	Term		
	AAG	UAU	CAC	UAA	GCN	
β^Cr	Lys	Ser	Ile	Thr	Lys	Leu ....
	AAG	AGU	AUC	ACU	AAG	CUN ...

Thus, it is very likely that both variants arose by means of the postulated frameshifts. Subsequent nucleotide sequence analysis of the β globin gene confirmed the complete agreement between the nucleotide sequence of the 3'-untranslated sequence of the β globin gene and the amino acid sequence of the elongated segments of Hb Tak and Hb Cranston.[510-512] In each case, the postulated insertion of two bases constitutes a tandem repetition of nucleotides in the normal β mRNA sequence. The most likely mechanism for this type of mutation would be the process of frameshift mutagenesis,[513] as detailed below in the section on amino

	142	143	144	145	146
β^A	Ala	His	Lys	Tyr	His .....
	GCC	CAC	AAG	UAU	CAC....
β^Sa	Ala	Pro	Ser	Ile	Thr .....
	GCC	CCA	AGU	AUC	ACU ...

Frameshift in Phase—Internal Reduplication of Sequence

A black American family was found to have an elongated α-chain variant but no other hematologic abnormalities.[457] Hb Grady composed 17 per cent of the total hemoglobin in the propositus and only 7 to 8 per cent in her father. Structural analysis showed that the abnormal α chain had a sequence identical to that of α^A except for the tandem insertion of three residues at position 118:

$$\alpha^{Gr} \ldots \underset{114\ 115\ 116\ 117\ 118}{\text{Pro-Ala-Glu-Phe-Thr}}\text{-}\underset{}{\text{Glu-Phe-Thr}}\text{-}\underset{119\ 120}{\text{Pro-Ala}} \ldots$$

This is the first report of a hemoglobin subunit elongated at a site other than at the C terminus. Huisman and colleagues proposed two possible mechanisms for the origin of α^{Gr}: (1) unequal crossing over between allelic α-chain genes, resulting in a chromosome with two loci, one of which has the elongated α^{Gr} gene; and (2) crossing over between the different α loci, resulting in either three genes ($\alpha 2$-α^{Gr}-$\alpha 1$) or a single gene, $\alpha^{anti-Gr}$. The second mechanism seemed more plausible because the α/β-chain synthesis was greater than unity and Hb Grady composed less than 25 per cent of the total hemoglobin. However, analysis of the α globin genes from an affected individual by means of restriction maps and DNA hybridization did not reveal an extra (fifth) α-chain gene.[514] Therefore, this analysis favors the first mechanism.

An even more likely explanation for the generation of Hb Grady is the process of frameshift mutagenesis,[513] as described below in the section on deletion mutants. The same mechanism of breaking of the DNA strand, mispairing at a short repeated dinucleotide sequence nearby, and subsequent excision or filling-in and repair could lead to the insertion (as well as deletion) of in-phase codons for amino acid residues, depending on the site of the mispairing. In fact, a dinucleotide (CC) is repeated precisely on either side of the sequence for codons 116 to 118 in the α globin gene, as predicted by the frameshift mutagenesis model (Table 10–9 Section B).

A reinvestigation[458] of Hb Dakar,[515] which was encountered among several members of a black family from Senegal, showed that the abnormal α chain was identical to that of Hb Grady. This variant represented about 15 per cent of the total hemoglobin. The fact that the hemoglobin was somewhat unstable when exposed to heat or isopropanol may account for its relatively low amount in red cells.

A third instance of Hb Grady has been encountered in a black male from Mauritania who was hematologically normal. The properties of the hemoglobin were very similar to those reported previously.[458]

NH_2 Terminal Elongation

A 64-year-old woman from Malta was found to have a variant composing 75 per cent of the total hemoglobin. The abnormal subunit, β Marseille, differs from $β^A$ in two respects: β 2 His is replaced by Pro and there is a methionine N-terminal to β 1 Val[106b] (see Table 10–2F). Thus, the sequence is H_2N-Met-Val-Pro-Leu-.

An 8-year-old boy from Florida had a positive chromatographic test for "fast" hemoglobin, suggesting the presence of diabetes (see Chapter 4). However, his blood glucose was normal, and he had no evidence of evidence of glucose intolerance. No hematological abnormalities were noted. A number of relatives had similar findings. They were found to have an electrophoretically and chromatographically silent variant composing 50 per cent of the total hemoglobin. In the abnormal subunit, β South Florida, the N-terminal valine is replaced by methionine, and this residue is preceded by an additional methionine.[160d] Thus, the sequence is H_2N-Met-Met-His-Leu-. About 15 per cent of β South Florida is N-acetylated, like Hb F (see Chapter 4). This modification accounts for the increased "fast" hemoglobin.

These two variants provide insight into the processing of newly synthesized globin chains. Methionine is the first residue to be incorporated. During translation of the nascent polypeptide, the methionine is normally cleaved, making valine the NH_2-terminal residue of α and β chains. It is likely that the amino acid replacements in these two variants inhibit the peptidase that normally leaves the NH_2-terminal methionine.

Biosynthetic Studies

The elongated α-chain variants, except Hb Grady, are all present in very small amounts, composing no more than 5 per cent of the total hemoglobin. This unexpected finding could be due to decreased synthesis of the elongated chain, enhanced degradation, or both. Thus far, biosynthetic studies have been done on three of these variants: Hb Constant Spring,[448, 517-519] Hb Wayne,[520] and Hb Grady.[521] Experiments on the first two variants are difficult to execute and to interpret because of the small amounts of these components and because of post-translational modifications causing chromatographic heterogeneity.

Incubation of reticulocytes with radioisotope-labeled amino acids indicated that the $α^{CS}$ chains are not rapidly destroyed following synthesis.[448] Further experiments ruled out the possibility that low levels of Hb Constant Spring were due to prolonged translation time. It is likely that the synthesis of $α^{CS}$ falls off rapidly as erythroid cells mature, similar to that of the δ chain of Hb A_2[522, 523] and the δβ subunit of Hb Lepore.[523, 524] This conclusion is supported by experiments showing that the specific activity ratio $α^{CS}/α^A$ was 0.68 in reticulocytes and 1.26 in bone marrow cells.[517] The fact that this ratio was greater than unity in erythroblasts indicates that there is some enhancement in the turnover of Hb CS in addition to markedly impaired synthesis. This lability of Hb CS is supported by *in vitro* observations that the variant decreases during storage of the hemolysate.[519] Hbs CS-1 and CS-2 were apparently converted to components having lower isoelectric points, one of which migrated near Hb A_2, while the other co-migrated with Hb A.

Surprisingly, long-term (1 to 3 hours) incubation experiments showed that the α/β synthetic ratio is *increased* in individuals with Hb Constant Spring: 1.2 to 1.4 in heterozygotes and 1.3 to 1.7 in homozygotes.[525, 525a, 543] Subsequent shorter incubations clearly showed that in homozygotes, the α/β ratio is about 0.6, consistent with impaired α globulin synthesis.[525b] During longer incubations, the excess β chains undergo proteolysis, leading to an increase in the ratio. This enhanced turnover of β globin chains probably explains the brisk hemolysis in homozygotes (see below).

Table 10-9. SHORT REPEATED NUCLEOTIDE SEQUENCES FLANKING REGIONS OF THE HUMAN GLOBIN GENES WHERE KNOWN DELETIONS OR INSERTIONS HAVE OCCURRED

A. β-Chain Variants

Hb Leiden	CCT	- - -	- - -	AAG			
Normal	CCT	GAG	GAG	AAG			
	Pro	Glu	Glu	Lys			
		6	7				
Hb Lyon	GGC	- - -	- - -	AAC			
Normal	GGC	AAG	GTG	AAC			
	Gly	Lys	Val	Asn			
		17	18				
Hb Freiburg	GAA	- - -	GGT				
Normal	GAA	GTT	GGT				
	Glu	Val	Gly				
		23					
Hb Niteroi	TT -	- - -	- - -	- - C	TTT	GGG	
Normal	TTC	TTT	GAG	TCC	TTT	GGG	
	Phe	Phe	Glu	Ser	Phe	Gly	
		42	43	44			
Hb Niteroi	TTC	TTT	G - -	- - -	- - -	- GG	
Normal	TTC	TTT	GAG	TCC	TTT	G GG	
	Phe	Phe	Glu	Ser	Phe	Gly	
			43	44	45		
Hb Tochigi	AT-	- - -	- - -	- - -	- - G	GTG	AAG	GCT
Normal	ATG	GGC	AAC	CCT	AAG	GTG	AAG	GCT
	Met	Gly	Asn	Pro	Lys	Val	Lys	Ala
		56	57	58	59			
Hb St. Antoine	GAT	- - -	- - -	GCT			
Normal	GAT	GGT	CTG	GCT			
	Asp	Gly	Leu	Ala			
		74	75				
Hb Vicksburg	GGC	- - -	GCT				
Normal	GGC	CTG	GCT				
	Gly	Leu	Ala				
		75					
Hb Gun Hill	G - -	- - -	- - -	- - -	- - -	- AG	CTG	CAC
Normal	GAG	CTG	CAC	TGT	GAC	AAG	CTG	CAC
	Glu	Leu	His	Cys	Asp	Lys	Leu	His
		91	92	93	94	95		
Hb Tours	GCC	- - -	CTG				
Normal	GCC	A CA	CTG				
	Ala	Thr	Leu				
		87					
Hb Coventry	AAT	GCC	- - -	GCC	CAC		
Normal	AAT	GCC	CTG	GCC	CAC		
	Asn	Ala	Leu	Ala	His		
			141				
Hb McKees Rocks	AAG	- - -	- - -	TAA			
Normal	AAG	TAT	CAC	TAA			
	Lys	Tyr	His	Term			
		145	146				

B. α-Chain Variants

Hb Boyle Heights	GCC	- - -	AAG	ACC			
Normal	GCC	GAC	AAG	ACC			
	Ala	Asp	Lys	Thr			
		6					
Hb Grady	GCC	GAG	TTC	ACC	GAG	TTC	ACC	CCT
Normal	GCC	GAG	TTC	ACC	- - -	- - -	- - -	CCT
	Ala	Glu	Phe	Thr				Pro
		116	117	118				

C. βδ-Chain Variant

Hb Lincoln Park	GCT	GGT	- - -	GCT	
Normal	GCT	GGT	GTG	GCT	
	Ala	Gly	Val	Ala	
			137		

The underlined nucleotide sequences are directly repeated sequences that may serve as foci for intrachoromsomal recombination in the process called frameshift mutagenesis, leading to short deletions or insertions (see text, Figure 10–5B, and reference 513). The numbers under the amino acid sequence refer to the amino acid residues deleted or repeated in the different hemoglobin variants.

Because the 3'-untranslated sequences of the α1 and α2 globin genes are different, it is possible to devise assays to detect and differentiate the transcripts of each gene.[526, 527] Two groups have obtained somewhat different figures for the relative outputs of the normal α1 and α2 globin genes: 40:60[526] and 25:75,[527] respectively. In patients with Hb H disease with Hb Constant Spring and genotype (—/α^{CS}α) (see Chapter 8), it was possible to differentiate the mRNA of the α^{CS} gene. Substantial amounts of α^{CS} mRNA were detectable in bone marrow cells, whereas it was virtually absent in reticulocytes.[527] These results are consistent with instability of the α^{CS} mRNA, but the mechanisms by which a single base substitution could lead to such a dramatic instability are poorly understood. Changes in the secondary structure of the mRNA resulting either from the base substitution or from the readthrough translation may be involved.

The biosynthesis of Hb Wayne has also been examined. Unlike Hb Constant Spring, α$^{Wa-I\ (Asn)}$ was found to have a higher specific activity than α^A, whereas α$^{Wa-II\ (Asp)}$ had a lower specific activity. Thus, the α^{Wa} chains may be slightly unstable. Proteolysis may also play a role in maintaining the higher specific activity. Pulse-chase experiments showed no apparent conversion of α$^{Wa-I\ (Asn)}$ to α$^{Wa-II\ (Asp)}$ over 6 hours, although α$^{Wa-II\ (Asp)}$ labeling was seen in as little as 15 minutes. This suggests that the deamidation step may occur very early in biosynthesis, perhaps at the nascent chain level, and that once assembled into a tetramer, further deamidation occurs very slowly.

The synthesis of Hb Grady has been measured in reticulocytes of two affected individuals. In both cases, the ratio of radioactivity of α^{Gr} to total α chains was slightly higher than the proportion of Hb Grady in the hemolysate. These results are compatible with somewhat enhanced turnover of the variant, in keeping with its modest degree of instability *in vitro*.[458, 516]

Biosynthesis studies have been completed on the fameshift β-chain variants.[454, 528] In reticulocytes, α-chain synthesis was somewhat higher than total β-chain synthesis. The rates of synthesis of β^A and β^{Cr} appeared to be similar if measurements were made following short incubations. During longer incubations, there was a progressive gain in α-chain radioactivity in Hb Cranston, reflecting exchange between unlabeled Hb Cranston and a pool of newly synthesized α chains. Such a phenomenon has been observed in several other unstable hemoglobin variants such as Hb Gun Hill,[529] Hb Sabine[530] and Hb Köln[531] (see Chapter 13).

Functional Studies

Hemoglobins Tak and Cranston have very similar oxygen equilibria. Both hemoglobins, in the purified state, have such high oxygen affinities that they are difficult to deoxygenate. Both variants have absent subunit cooperativity (Hill's $n = 1$) and a nearly absent Bohr effect.[453, 532] The high oxygen affinity of Hb Cranston probably explains the high normal blood hemoglobin levels despite a significant degree of hemolysis. A similar association has been observed in other unstable hemoglobin variants having increased oxygen affinity. (See Chapter 13.)

The striking abnormalities in the oxygen binding of Hb Tak and Cranston are explained by the presence of the hydrophobic tail at the C terminus of the β chain, which probably prevents these molecules from assuming a stable "deoxy" or T structure. In addition, Hb Cranston lacks β 146 His, which normally contributes both to the stabilization of deoxyhemoglobin and to the Bohr effect. X-ray analysis of a deoxygenated mixture of Hbs A and Cranston indicates the presence of hybrid molecules ($α_2β^Aβ^{Cr}$) in which the hydrophobic tail is inserted into the central cavity, relatively protected from a water environment.

Hemoglobins Wayne-I and Wayne-II both have high oxygen affinity and markedly reduced Bohr effect.[532a] The elongation at the C terminus of the α chain also prevents Hb Wayne from forming a stable T quaternary structure.

Hemoglobin Grady has normal oxygen binding[458, 516] although it is slightly unstable *in vitro*.

The fact that functional studies have not been done on the other elongated α-chain variants is understandable, because they are present in such small quantities.

Clinical Significance

Because α-chain variants due to a base substitution in the termination codon are produced in very small amounts, they can contribute to the phenotype designated as α thalassemia. Because the frequencies for both the α-thalassemia genes and the Hb Constant Spring gene are rather high in Southeast Asia, a significant proportion of patients who carry a clinical diagnosis of α thalassemia have Hb Constant Spring. Somewhere between 12 and 50 per cent of Thai and Chinese individuals with Hb H disease have the gene for Hb Constant Spring in association with the gene for α thalassemia 1 in *trans*($--/\alpha^{CS}\alpha$) (see Chapter 8). In addition, homozygotes for Hb Constant Spring have been encountered. Surprisingly, these individuals do not have a thalassemia phenotype. They often have mild jaundice and splenomegaly with mild hemolytic anemia (Hb ~ 10 g/dl).[525–525b] The MCV is slightly elevated (88 to 95 fl), perhaps owing to an increased reticulocyte count. No Hb H or Heinz bodies are demonstrable.

In individuals with elongated β chain variants, the clinical manifestations are less predictable. Those heterozygous for Hb Tak are hematologically normal and show no evidence of hemolysis. The affected members of the Thai family[454] had slightly microcytic red cells, whereas those from a Malay family[533] had normal red cell indices. A child who was doubly heterozygous for Hb Tak and β^0 thalassemia[454] had rather severe anemia and marked disability. The increased oxygen affinity of Hb Tak probably contributed significantly to this child's poor clinical status. As mentioned above, individuals with Hbs Cranston and Saverne have a compensated hemolytic state.

Antibodies against Hb Wayne and Hb Cranston can detect abnormal red cells mixed with normal cells in ratios as low as $1:10^6$.[534] These probes may be useful in detecting somatic cell mutants in which frame shifts have produced elongated subunits with terminal sequences corresponding to these two variants. Such mutants might arise from administration of chemotherapy or some other factor that affects DNA structure or repair.

Shortened Subunits

A few mutant hemoglobins have abnormally short globin chains (see Table 10–2G). In all cases described, one or a few adjacent amino acids are missing from the abnormal chains. The remainder of the subunit is normal. These variants probably involve deletion of one or more intact codons (of the mRNA) that code for the missing amino acids. If an entire codon is deleted, the reading frame will remain in phase, and the remainder of the amino acid sequence will not differ from normal. These variants are generally unstable and are associated with congenital Heinz body hemolytic anemia (see Chapter 13).

Analysis of the nucleotide sequence of β globin mRNA in the regions where deletion mutants have occurred reveals an interesting phenomenon. At virtually all of these sites, there is a reiterated nucleotide sequence, from two to eight base residues in length, with only a few other intervening nucleotides. A model can therefore be constructed by which these deletion mutants may have occurred, as illustrated in Figure 10–6A. Hb Gun Hill has a β chain in which amino acid residues 91 to 95 are deleted (see Table 10–2G). The nucleotide sequence of normal β globin mRNA in this region shows an imperfectly repeated sequence of nine nucleotides (indicated in the boxes in Figure 10–6A) separated by five intervening nucleotides. If these two sets of sequences misaligned during the process of meiosis and nonhomologous crossing over occurred, these phenomena would effectively delete the sequences of the mRNA corresponding to amino acid residues 91 through 95, as shown in Figure 10–6A.

Such an occurrence of nonhomologous crossing over between chromosomes, however, is unlikely to have occurred by misalignment of such short sequences between two homologous chromosomes. A much more likely event that could lead to a deletion in the region of a reiterated nucleotide sequence is the phenomenon of frameshift mutagenesis,[513] which can occur between complementary strands of DNA on a single chromosome and does not require mispairing of the two homologues during meiosis. This process is illustrated in diagrammatic form in Figure 10–6B. A single chromosome is represented with its two complementary strands of DNA: The coding strand is represented as containing the reiterated sequences A and B in black bars, and the complementary sequences A′ and B′ on the noncoding strand are shown in open bars. If a break occurs in the coding strand at the point of the wavy arrow, the strand of DNA that is broken can shift position and rearrange itself until a repair enzyme religates the break; the process of DNA repair following damage occurs continuously in cells. However, if there are two adjacent reiterated sequences, such as A and B, then before religation, sequence B could align with the complementary sequence A′ rather than with sequence B′, leaving sequence A protruding as a redundant strand of DNA on the coding strand and sequence B′ looped out of the complementary strand. Re-

Figure 10–6. Proposed mechanisms for the origin of amino acid deletions in hemoglobin variants. *A,* Nonhomologous crossover between chromosome pairs due to mispairing of chromosomes in the region of reiterated nucleotide sequences, such as those enclosed in the boxes. In the example shown, the indicated crossover would effectively delete codons for amino acids 91 to 95 of the beta globin chain, as has occurred in the variant Hb Gun Hill. *B,* Frame shift mutagenesis due to a break (arrow) in one DNA strand of a gene (on one chromosome) followed by mispairing of a reiterated sequence with the wrong complementary sequence on the second chromosomal DNA strand (i.e., B pairing with A' instead of B'). As a result of excision-repair processes in the cell nucleus, the reiterated sequence block that remains unpaired (i.e., A) is excised by an exonuclease, and the gap in the DNA strand (dashes) is subsequently filled in by a DNA polymerase, thus re-establishing continuity of the gene DNA and repairing the initial chromosomal damage. (From Forget, B. G.: The structure of human globin messenger RNA. Functional, genetic and evolutionary implications. *In* Piomelli, S., and Yachnin, S. [eds.]: Current Topics in Hematology. Vol. 3. New York, Alan R. Liss, Inc., 1980, p. 1.)

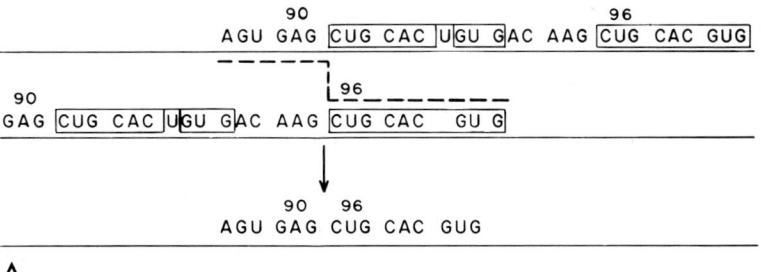

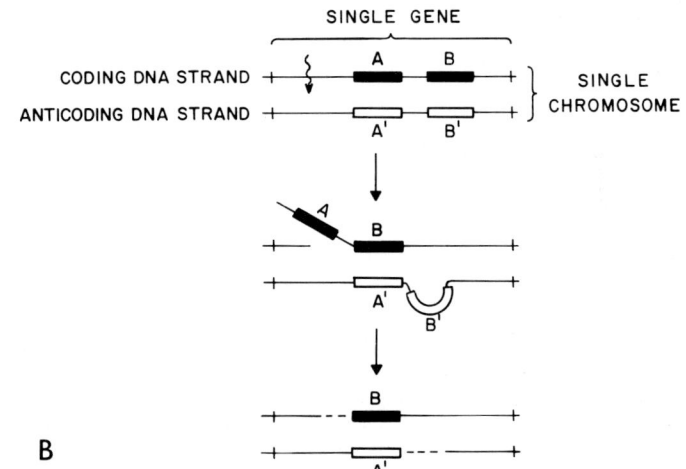

pair enzymes would excise the looped out sequence B' and digest away the redundant sequence A. A repair enzyme such as DNA polymerase would then fill in the gaps according to the complementary sequences of the intact opposing strand. In the process shown in Figure 10–6*B*, sequence A would effectively be deleted in the coding strand of chromosomal DNA. This model can be applied to the example of Hb Gun Hill in the gene for which block A would correspond to the sequence coding for amino acid residues 91 through 95.

Analysis of the nucleotide sequence of normal β globin mRNA in the regions where a number of other deletion mutants have occurred reveals the presence of similar reiterated sequences, as listed in Table 10–9*A*.[535] These deletion mutants probably arose by a mechanism similar to one of those described above: either mispairing and nonhomologous crossing over, or, what is more likely, frameshift mutagenesis during the process of DNA damage and repair. In each case, there is a repeated sequence, two to eight nucleotides long, flanking the nucleotides that are deleted.

A similar short nucleotide sequence repetition occurs in α globin mRNA near the site of the only α globin chain deletion mutant, Hb Boyle Heights[458a] (see Tables 10–2*G* and 10–9*B*).

The process of frameshift mutagenesis could also lead to internal repetition of one or more amino acid residues within the sequence of a globin chain. For instance, in a process similar to that shown in Figure 10–6*B*, if block A misaligned with block B', such an event would lead to the insertion (by repair) of a repeat of sequence A complementary to sequence A' in the resulting gap and repetition in the gene product of the amino acid sequence encoded by block A. As discussed previously, only one human hemoglobin variant has been described that has an internally repeated sequence: Hb Grady, in which amino acid residues 116, 117, and 118 of the α chain are repeated or duplicated.[457] In this case, a dinucleotide sequence flanks the region of the mRNA that is duplicated, supporting the concept of frame-shift mutagenesis (Table 10–9*B*).

One hemoglobin variant, Hb McKees Rocks, has a shortened β subunit that may be due to a nonsense mutation.[407] The β chain of the variant has a structure identical to $β^A$ chains through residue 144 but lacks the two C-terminal residues (Tyr-His). This mutant hemoglobin could be due to a substitution of A or G for U at the third base of the codon UA<u>U</u> for tyrosine at position 145, thus producing a termination codon (UAA or UAG). However, the same structure could have resulted from a frameshift or a deletion. In fact, there is a dinucleotide repeat sequence at the site of the mutation, supporting the possibility of frameshift mutagenesis (Table 10–9A).

Recently, analyses of globin gene structure have shown that both frameshift and nonsense mutations can be responsible for certain types of thalassemia because of premature termination of the affected subunit.[536-538] These studies are discussed in detail in Chapter 8.

Fusion Subunits

The final class of mutant hemoglobins to be considered are those with fused or hybrid globin chains (see Table 10–2E). Hemoglobin Lepore, for example, contains normal α chains and abnormal non-α chains. These non-α chains have a normal length but an abnormal sequence: the first 50 to 80 amino acids have the normal N-terminal amino acid sequence of δ chains, but the last 60 to 90 residues have the normal C-terminal amino acid sequence of β chains. The Lepore chain is thus a fusion or hybrid NH_2-δβ-COOH chain. Three different Lepore chains have been described, in which the transition from δ to β sequences occurs at different points of the sequence. Hemoglobin Kenya is analogous, except that the abnormal hybrid chain contains γ and β sequences (NH_2-γβ-COOH).

Hemoglobin Lepore appears to have arisen through nonhomologous crossing over between part of the δ locus on one chromosome and part of the β locus on the complementary chromosome, as illustrated in Figure 10–7. This phenomenon could occur as a consequence of misalignment of a chromosome pair during meiosis, resulting in the pairing of a δ gene with a β gene instead of with its homologous δ gene. Such an event should give rise to two abnormal chromosomes: the first, the Lepore chromosome, has no normal intact δ or β loci but has instead only the fused δβ Lepore gene.

Such a crossover event should lead to the deletion of normal inter-δβ globin gene DNA on the Lepore chromosome, and the predicted deletion has, in fact, been directly demonstrated by gene mapping techniques in affected individuals.[539-541] The Hb Lepore-Boston globin gene contains the large intervening sequence or intron of the β globin gene.[542, 542a] According to its amino acid sequence, the crossover could

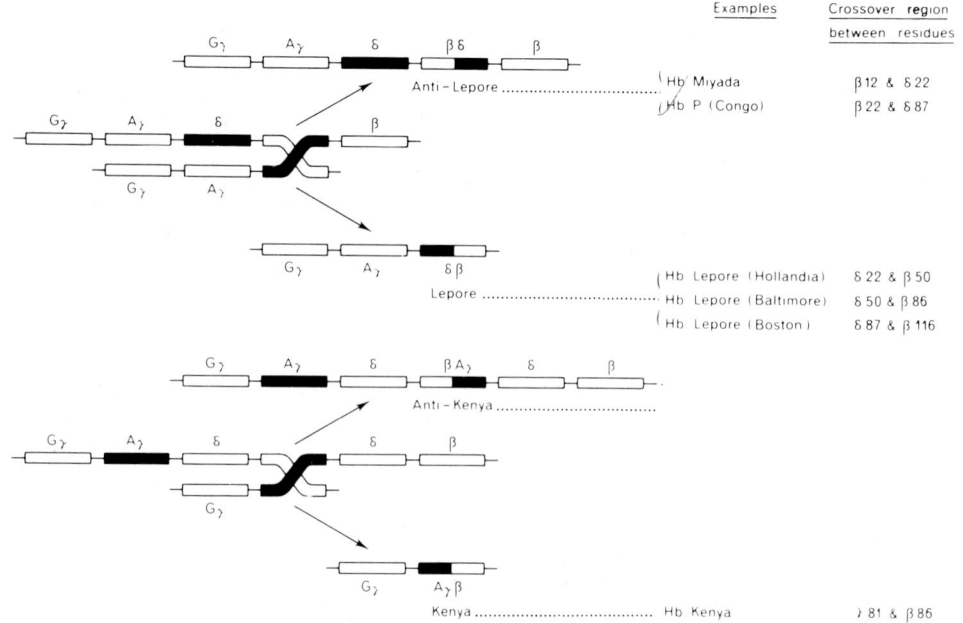

Figure 10–7. Chromosomal crossover responsible for Lepore and anti-Lepore hemoglobins and Hb Kenya. (From Weatherall, D. J., and Clegg, J. B.: The Thalassemia Syndromes. 3rd ed. Oxford, Blackwell Scientific Publications, 1981.)

have occurred anywhere between codon 87 and codon 116. The presence of the β-chain large intron indicates that the crossover in fact occurred at a point at or preceding codon 104. Comparison of the nucleotide sequence of the human β and δ globin genes reveals that both genes have identical sequences from codon 88 to 104 and over the first seven adjoining nucleotides of the large intervening sequence; the crossover could have occurred at any point over that region of the DNA sequence.

The second abnormal chromosome arising from a δβ-gene nonhomologous crossing over event should be an "anti-Lepore" chromosome, which carries normal δ and β loci as well as a gene for an NH$_2$-βδ-COOH anti-Lepore globin chain (see Figure 10–7). Because of the presence of a normal β locus in cis, patients with this chromosome should be clinically normal except for the presence of the anti-Lepore hemoglobin. Such patients have in fact been identified, and four different anti-Lepore hemoglobins have been characterized: Hbs Miyada, P-Nilotic, P-Congo, and Lincoln Park (see Table 10–2E and Figure 10–7). Hb Lincoln Park differs from Hb Nilotic by having a deletion of a valine residue at position 137. The discovery of these anti-Lepore hemoglobins strongly supports the model of nonhomologous crossing over for the origin of Hb Lepore.

Hemoglobin Parchman is a more complex fusion variant.[442] Its non-α subunit has a δ sequence at the N and C termini and a β sequence in the middle. There are no deletions or additions to this subunit. It probably arose by means of a double crossover.

Because of the absence of a normal β locus in cis and the low output of the Lepore gene product, heterozygous Hb Lepore patients have the clinical features of β-thalassemia trait, whereas the clinical characteristics in those with homozygous Hb Lepore syndrome mimic β thalassemia major[543] (see Chapter 9).

The synthesis of the Lepore and anti-Lepore hemoglobins (like that of normal Hb A$_2$) appears to be confined almost entirely to bone marrow and is virtually absent from circulating reticulocytes. The molecular mechanisms responsible for this observation are obscure, but instability of the mRNA has been suggested (see Chapter 8).

Hb Kenya seems to have arisen by nonhomologous crossing over between ^{A}γ and β loci, giving an NH$_2$-γβ-COOH fusion product (see Figure 10–7). Because the γ loci are less homologous to the β loci and are situated farther away from the β loci than are the δ loci, the Kenya crossover must have required a greater degree of mispairing during meiosis. Deletion of normal inter-γβ globin gene sequences has, in fact, been confirmed by gene mapping studies.[542b] Only one type of Hb Kenya has been described so far. The "anti-Kenya" gene has not been identified. The occurrence of both Hb Lepore and Hb Kenya strongly suggested that the γ, δ, and β loci are closely linked on the same chromosome in the order NH$_2$-γδβ-COOH. This gene arrangement has been amply confirmed by isolation and structural analysis of the β globin gene complex (see Chapter 7).

ASSEMBLY OF HEMOGLOBIN VARIANTS

If an individual is heterozygous for a β-chain variant that differs in charge from Hb A, electrophoresis will usually reveal two major components, Hb A ($\alpha_2\beta_2^A$) and Hb X ($\alpha_2\beta_2^X$). However, this analysis gives a misleading impression of the true distribution of hemoglobins in the red cell. Actually, the predominant hemoglobin inside the red cell is the hybrid tetramer $\alpha_2\beta^A\beta^x$ (Fig. 10–8). When analyzed by electrophoresis or chromatography, these hybrid hemoglobins are not detected because they dissociate into dimers of unlike charge that are separated from one another during the analysis. Such hybrid hemoglobins also exist in individuals heterozygous for α-, δ-, and γ-chain variants. Thus, it is best to view the assembly of hemoglobins inside the red cell in terms of formation of αβ dimers (or αδ and αγ dimers), which can then combine with like dimers to form homotetramers or with unlike dimers to form hybrid tetramers.

A number of independent factors influence the relative production of human hemoglobin variants. As shown in Figure 10–9, most α-chain variants compose about 25 per cent of the total hemoglobin, whereas most stable β-chain variants compose about half of the total. As mentioned above, this distribution reflects the presence of four α-chain genes and two β-chain genes. If α thalassemia is also present, the relative amount of the α-chain variant increases in rough proportion to the number of α globin genes that are deleted.[544] Some α-chain variants, such as G-Philadelphia,[545-548] Q,[91, 326, 549, 550] J-Tongariki,[141] J-Cape Town,[551] and J-Mexico,[62] are associated with an α globin gene deletion in cis. In such cases, homozygotes would produce no normal α chains and, therefore, no Hb A.

Many α- and β-chain variants constitute a

418 HUMAN HEMOGLOBIN VARIANTS

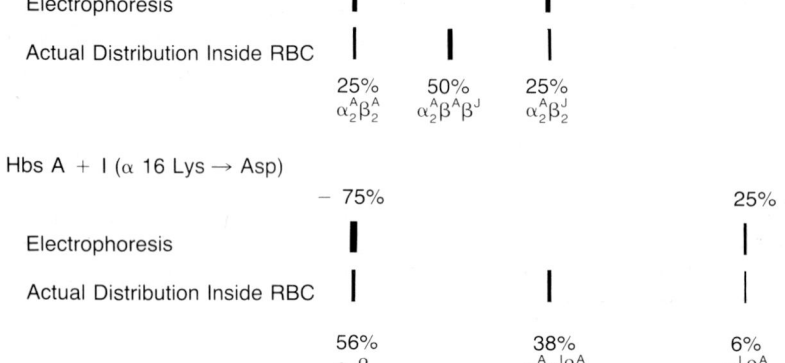

Figure 10–8. Comparison of electrophoretic pattern and actual distribution of hemoglobin inside the red cell. *Top,* Individual heterozygous for a β-chain variant. *Bottom,* Individual heterozygous for an α-chain variant.

smaller proportion of the total hemoglobin than what would be expected from the number of functioning globin chain genes. Conversely, a few variants are present in larger amounts than Hb A. It is apparent that any of the steps in protein synthesis, reviewed in Chapter 7, could affect production of the abnormal globin chain. The mutant mRNA could be transcribed, processed, or transported less efficiently. Alternatively, the abnormal mRNA could be unstable or degraded rapidly. It is unlikely that decreased production of the mutant subunit is due to sluggish translation of the corresponding mRNA, because it contains an abnormal codon that requires a transfer RNA that is in short supply in the cell. Finally, the mutant globin chain could be synthesized normally but could be structurally unstable or unable to associate normally with other chains to form tetramers; as a result, the abnormal chain could be preferentially lost owing to precipitation or catabolism. All of these processes would result in reduced amounts of the abnormal hemoglobin.

Some variant subunits are synthesized at a much lower rate than the corresponding normal subunit. These include Hbs Lepore, Anti-Lepore, and the α-chain termination mutants (see above) as well as Hb E, Hb Knossos,[206a, 206b] Hb K-Woolwich,[551a] and Hb Vicks-

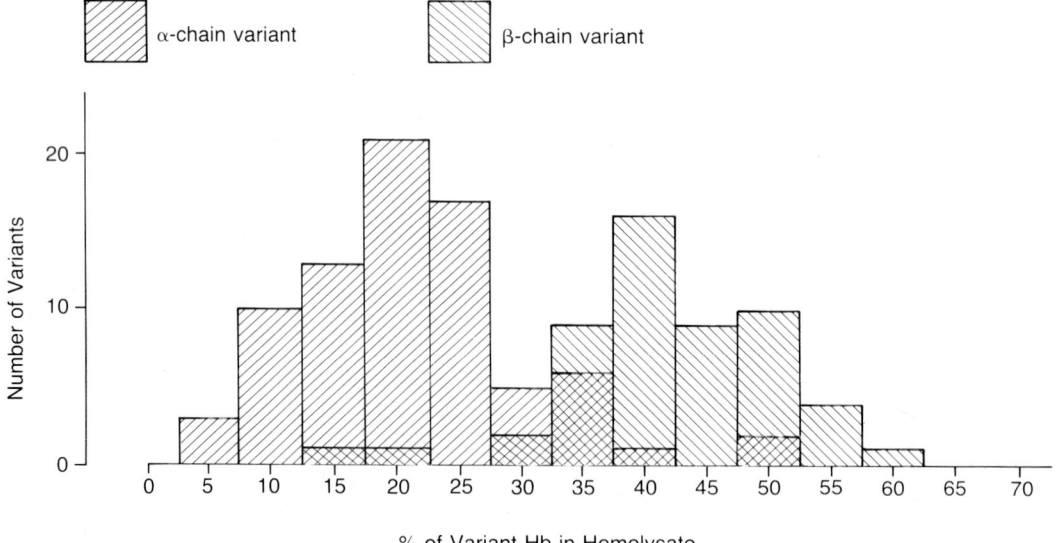

Figure 10–9. Distribution of variant hemoglobins in humans heterozygous for α-chain and β-chain mutant hemoglobins. As an example, variants that compose 17.6 per cent and 22.5 per cent of the total hemoglobin are placed in the section labeled 20. Unstable variants have not been included in this figure.

burg.[465] All of these variants are associated with thalassemia phenotypes. In the case of Hb E[552] and Hb Knossos,[552a] the mutation itself causes a defect in mRNA processing (see below and Chapter 8).

The vast majority of variant subunits are synthesized at a normal rate. The low amounts of the unstable hemoglobin variants can generally be explained by increased catabolism of the newly synthesized hemoglobin owing to one or more of the following: impaired heme binding, abnormal subunit interactions, and decreased solubility. This subject is discussed in detail in Chapter 13. A few variants such as Hb Indianapolis[358] and Hb Quong Sze[149a, 149b] are catabolized so rapidly and so completely that they cannot be detected in circulating red cells. They produce a thalassemia phenotype.

The variability in levels of many, if not most, of the stable hemoglobin variants appears to be due to the differences in the rate of subunit assembly.[553] Following the synthesis of the globin polypeptide on the polyribosome and heme insertion, the subunit must search for an unlike partner in order to form a stable $\alpha\beta$ dimer:

$$\alpha + \beta \rightarrow \alpha\beta$$

This aggregation step confers considerable protection on the newly synthesized subunits because free subunits are less soluble than the $\alpha\beta$ dimer and are much more susceptible to proteolytic digestion (Fig. 10–10). In heterozygotes producing both normal and variant subunits, the rates of $\alpha\beta$ dimer formation could differ significantly, thereby affecting the proportion of the variant hemoglobin in the red cell. For example, in red cells of individuals with sickle trait, Hb S usually composes about 40 per cent of the total hemoglobin. In the presence of α thalassemia, the proportion of Hb S decreases in proportion to the number of α-chain genes deleted (Table 10–10). *In vitro* mixing experiments show that $\alpha\beta^A$ dimers are formed about twice as readily as $\alpha\beta^S$ dimers.[554, 555] Thus, when the concentration of α chains becomes limiting (α thalassemia), relatively less Hb S is produced. Other commonly encountered hemoglobin variants resemble Hb S: The proportion of Hbs C, D-Los Angeles, and E is less than half of the total in normal heterozygotes and decreases further when α thalassemia is also present.[543] In addition, as mentioned above, the production of β^E is decreased, resulting in a β-thalassemia phenotype.

It is not readily apparent why these variant subunits should have slower rates of $\alpha\beta$ dimer assembly compared with $\alpha\beta^A$. The amino acid substitutions are all on the surface of the β chain and far removed from the $\alpha_1\beta_1$ contact surface that is critical for the initial formation of a dimer. Furthermore, none of these variants have impaired stability. Equally puzzling is the fact that certain β-chain variants appear in the red cells of heterozygotes in excess of Hb A. A plausible explanation for these ob-

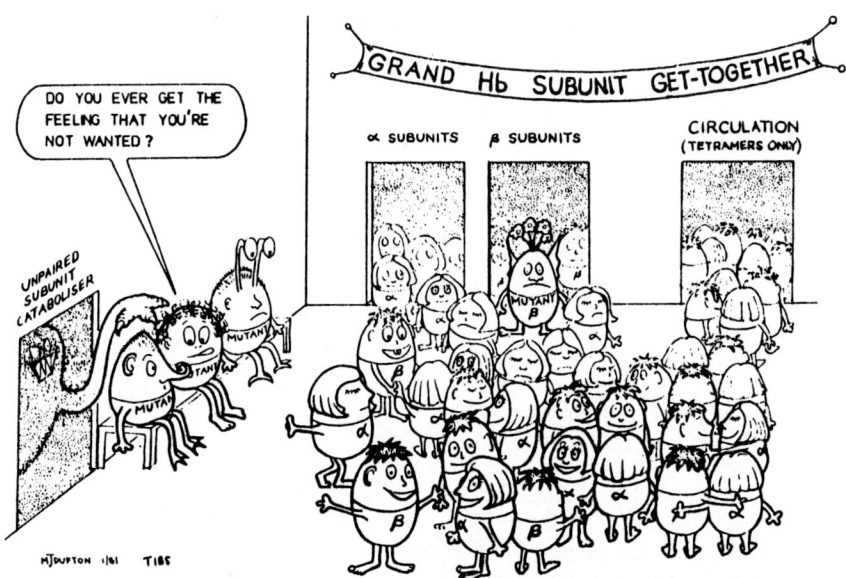

Figure 10–10. The social behavior of hemoglobin subunits. (From Shaeffer, J. R., et al.: Trends in Biochemical Sciences 6:158, 1981.)

Table 10–10. EFFECT OF α THALASSEMIA ON THE PERCENTAGE OF β-CHAIN VARIANT HEMOGLOBIN IN HETEROZYGOTES

	Percentage of Variant in Hemolysate					
	AS	(Ref)	AC	(Ref)	AE	(Ref)
Normal (αα/αα)	41 ± 1.8	(631)	43.8 ± 1.5	(631)	30 ± 1.5	(602)
αα/α-	35.4 ± 1.6	(631)	37.5 ± 1.4	(631)	27 ± 2	(602)
α-/α- or αα/--	28.1 ± 1.4	(631)	32.2 ± 0.8	(631)	22 ± 2	(602)
α-/-- (Hb H)	17	(632)			15	(606)
Iron deficiency*	30→42	(633)			18→27	(608)

*Before and after correction

servations comes from an examination of all the stable β-chain variants for which information is available.[554a] As shown in Figure 10–11, the positively charged variants such as Hbs S, D, C, and E all compose significantly less than half of the total hemoglobin and are reduced further in the presence of α thalassemia. In contrast, many of the negatively charged variants are present in amounts exceeding that of Hb A, and in one case (Hb J-Baltimore), the amount increases when α thalassemia is present. Alpha thalassemia intensifies the competition between normal and variant β chains for binding to α chains. In vitro experiments on purified normal and mutant subunits show that negatively charged $β^{J\text{-Baltimore}}$ and $β^{N\text{-Baltimore}}$ bind more readily to α chains than $β^A$. Conversely, uncharged $β^S$ and positively charged $β^C$ bind progressively less readily to α chains.[554b]

Two conclusions can be drawn from the data shown in Figure 10–11 and the subunit mixing experiments: (1) Chain competition is an important determinant of the distribution of A and non-A hemoglobin in β-variant heterozy-

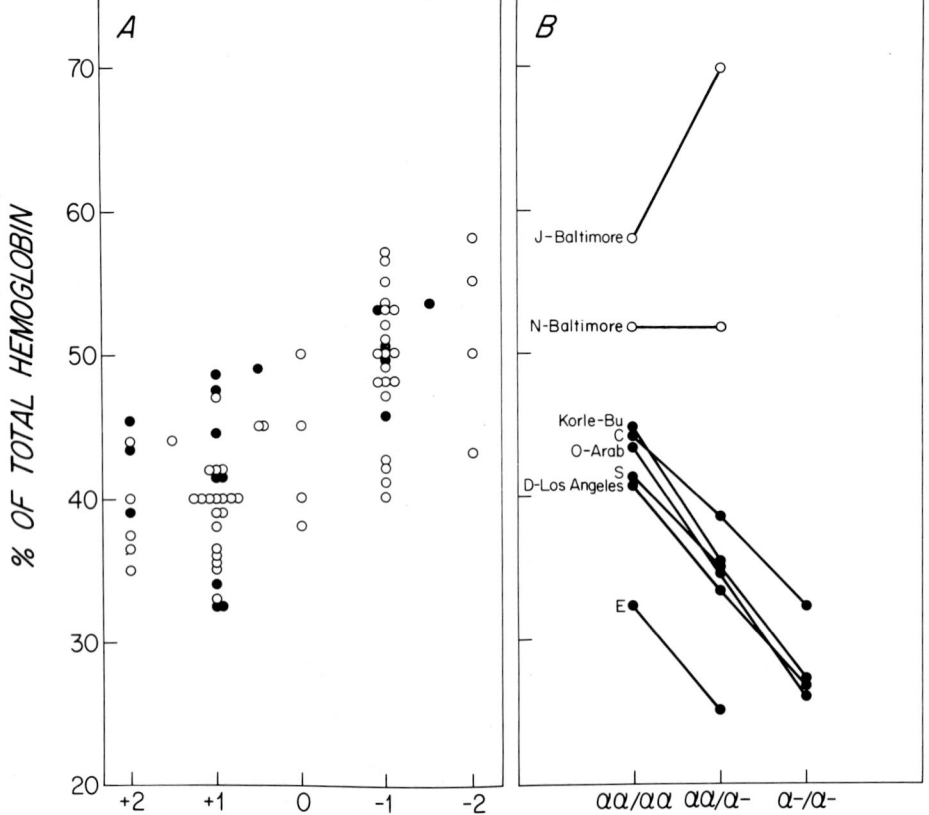

Figure 10–11. A, Effect of charge on the proportion of abnormal hemoglobin in individuals heterozygous for 72 stable β-globin variants. Each data point represents a mean value for a given variant. The solid points (●) denote measurements of Huisman (Am. J. Hematol. 14:393, 1983) utilizing high-resolution chromatography. Substitutions involving a histidine residue were scored as a change of ½ charge. The "−1" group differs significantly from the "+1" group ($p < 0.001$) and from the "0" group ($p \leq 0.05$). B, Effect of α thalassemia on a proportion of six positively charged β-chain variants (●) and of two negatively charged variants (○). (From Bunn, H. F., and McDonald, M. J.: Nature 306:498, 1983.)

gotes. (2) The relative affinity of α chains for β chains is determined in part by the surface charge of the subunits.[554a] In normal Hb A, the β chain is slightly negatively charged (pI = 6.6), whereas the α chain is positively charged (pI = 8.1). The rate of aggregation of α and β monomers to form the αβ dimer depends in part on electrostatic attraction:

$$\alpha^+ + \beta^+ \xrightarrow{slow} \alpha\beta^{2+}$$

$$\alpha^+ + \beta^- \xrightarrow{normal} \alpha\beta$$

$$\alpha^+ + \beta^{3-} \xrightarrow{fast} \alpha\beta^{2-}$$

This scheme explains why the proportion of Hb S is higher in SC red cells than in AS red cells. This difference is an important determinant of the clinical manifestations of SC disease (see Chapter 12). The scheme also provides an explanation for the variable levels of Hb A_2 that accompany certain hematologic disorders. Hb A_2 is decreased in various types of α thalassemia as well as in iron deficiency and sideroblastic anemias, both of which can be considered acquired α thalassemia. It is likely that a deficiency of α-chain production brings out the competition between β^A and the more positively charged δ chains. As the model above predicts, the δ chains would be at a disadvantage, and consequently, less Hb A_2 would be formed. Hb A_2 is increased in β-thalassemia trait. Although these red cells contain reduced mean corpuscular hemoglobin, the absolute levels of Hb A_2 are increased. It is likely that when β-chain production is impaired, δ chains are salvaged by excess α chains, thereby escaping proteolysis.

COMMON HEMOGLOBIN VARIANTS

Hemoglobin C ($\alpha_2\beta_2$ 6 Glu→Lys)

Hb C was the second variant to be identified electrophoretically[555] and structurally.[162] Hb C is found exclusively in blacks. In areas of West Africa, particularly Ghana and Upper Volta, the gene frequency approaches 0.15 (Fig. 10–12). Therefore, about 25 per cent of individuals are heterozygotes (Hb C trait). Among American blacks, the gene frequency ranges between 0.010 and 0.012.[556, 557] Therefore, about 2 to 2.5 per cent of black Americans are AC heterozygotes, and 0.010 to 0.015 per cent are homozygotes (Table 10–11). Hb C is the second most commonly encountered variant in the United States and, next to Hb S and Hb E, the third most prevalent variant worldwide.

Detection. The replacement of lysine for glutamic acid at the sixth position of the β

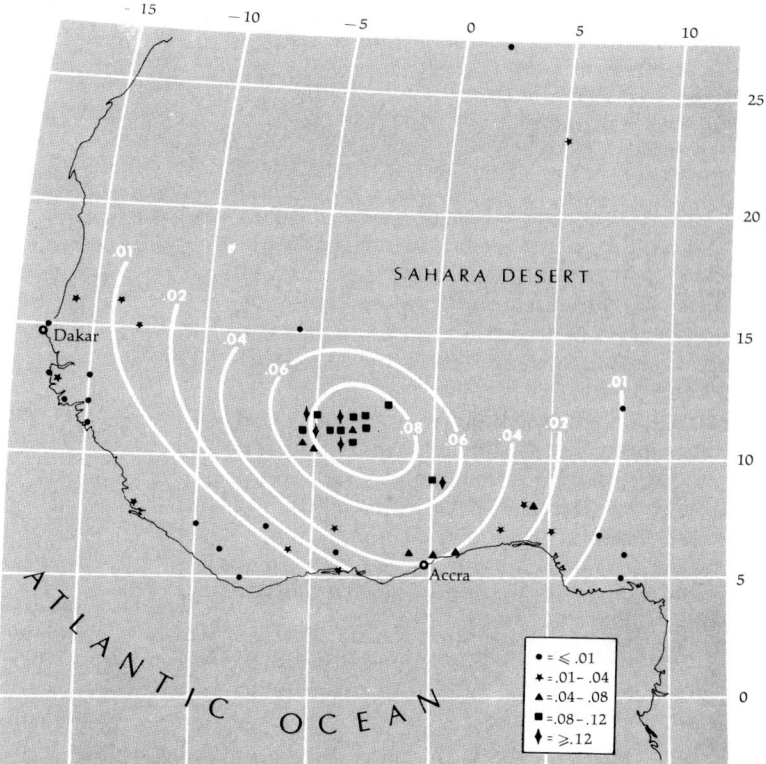

Figure 10–12. Geographical distribution of Hb C gene in West Africa. The numbers .01 to .12 refer to gene frequencies. (From Bodmer, W. F., and Cavalli-Sforza, L. L.: Genetics, Evolution and Man. San Francisco, W. H. Freeman, 1976.)

Table 10–11. FREQUENCY OF HEMOGLOBIN GENOTYPES AMONG BLACK AMERICANS

Genotype	Percentage of Population *	**
AS	8.6	8.0
SS	0.14	0.16
AC	2.4	3.0
CC	0.02	0.02
SC	0.13	0.12

*Survey of 250,000 black Americans[556]
**Review of literature[557]

chain (the same site as the substitution in hemoglobin S) gives Hb C a relatively high positive charge. Accordingly, it has slow mobility upon zone electrophoresis at alkaline pH, identical to that of Hb A_2 and Hb E. These three hemoglobins can be separated by isoelectric focusing on slabs of polyacrylamide gel.[482] When analyzed by electrophoresis on citrate agar at pH 6.0, Hb E has a mobility identical to that of Hb A, whereas Hb C migrates toward the anode (see Figure 10–1). Hbs A_2 and C can be separated by chromatography on CM-Sephadex.[558]

AC Heterozygotes. Individuals who have Hb C trait lack any clinical manifestations. Red cell life span is normal.[559] The red cells contain about 30 to 40 per cent Hb C, 50 to 60 per cent Hb A, and slightly increased amounts of Hb A_2.[558] If alpha thalassemia is also present, the proportion of Hb C is reduced.[543] Stained films of AC blood show increased numbers of target cells, but they are less impressive than those seen in homozygotes (see Color Plate III*I*). AC red cells, like SC red cells, have increased density and increased MCHC intermediate between AA and CC red cells.[560]

SC Compound Heterozygotes. Patients who are doubly heterozygous for Hb C and Hb S have a disease of moderate severity. Hb SC disease is discussed in Chapters 11 and 12.

Hb C–Thalassemia. Individuals who are double heterozygotes for Hb C and β thalassemia have been encountered among Africans, black Americans, Italians, and Turks.[543] There appear to be significant clinical differences among affected individuals in these groups. However, they are generally asymptomatic and have moderate hemolytic anemia. Peripheral blood smear reveals microcytic hypochromic red cells and prominent target cells (see Color Plate III*H*). Those with C/β^+ thalassemia tend to have mild anemia, and the spleen is usually not palpable. In contrast, in individuals with C/β^0 thalassemia, the anemia is more marked, and the spleen is usually enlarged. Some patients will have skeletal abnormalities similar to those of thalassemia intermedia. Anemia may become more severe during pregnancy. The diagnosis of C/β^+ thalassemia is generally straightforward. In addition to the red cell morphologic findings noted above, hemoglobin electrophoresis will reveal 65 to 80 per cent Hb C, 20 to 30 per cent Hb A, and 2 to 5 per cent Hb F. In contrast, the differential between C/β^0 thalassemia and the homozygous CC state may be problematic. In C/β^0 thalassemia, the red cells are more microcytic and show more aniosocytosis than those of CC homozygotes. In C/β^0 thalassemia, the MCV is 55 to 70 fl, and the MCH is 18 to 21 pg; hemoglobin electrophoresis reveals 3 to 10 per cent Hb F, with the remainder being Hb C. In contrast, in CC homozygotes, the MCV averages about 72 fl, and the MCH about 27 pg (Table 10–12); Hb F seldom exceeds 3 per cent.

CC Homozygotes. Patients who are homozygous for Hb C have a mild to moderate congenital hemolytic anemia.[561-568] They are usually asymptomatic. Ill-defined arthralgia and abdominal pain and, rarely, hemorrhagic manifestations have been reported, but their association with Hb CC disease is probably fortuitous. There is no significant fetal or maternal morbidity associated with pregnancy.[569] Splenomegaly is generally present. As in other chronic hemolytic disorders, cholelithiasis and "aplastic crises" may occur. Packed cell vol-

Table 10–12. LABORATORY ABNORMALITIES IN CC HOMOZYGOTES*

	CC	AA
Hematocrit	32.2	45
Hemoglobin (g/dl)	12.4	15
MCHC (g/dl)	38	33
MCV (fl)	72	87
MCH (pg)	27	29
Reticulocytes (%)	3.6	1.0
Mean red cell surface area (μ^3)	131	151
Water—% of cell volume		
Total water	67	71
Solvent water	38	57
Cations (Na+K, meg/l)		
/1 cell volume	101	123
/total cell water	151	173
/1 solvent cell water	266	216
Red cell 2,3-DPG (μmoles/g Hb)	17.3	17.0
mmoles/L solvent H_2O	12.7	9.0
Whole blood P_{50} (mm Hg)	29.5	26.5

*From Murphy, J. R.: J. Clin. Invest. 47:1483, 1968, and Murphy, J. R.: Semin. Hematol. 13:177, 1976.

ume generally ranges between 25 and 37 per cent, accompanied by a moderate reticulocytosis (4 to 8 per cent) (see Table 10–12). Red cell survival is decreased with splenic sequestration.[563, 566] Erythropoiesis is not sufficient to maintain a normal red cell mass[559, 566]; mean corpuscular hemoglobin is normal, but hemoglobin concentration per cell is increased.[570] The majority of erythrocytes on a dried, stained blood film are target cells (see Color Plate IIIG). In addition, a minor population of microspherocytes are seen. The target cells are plumper and of small diameter than those seen in liver disease or biliary obstruction. Hb CC erythrocytes do not appear targeted when examined in a wet preparation.[570] However, their increased resistance to osmotic hemolysis indicates that these red cells have an increased ratio of surface area to volume.[571] A likely mechanism by which red cells containing Hb C (and perhaps Hb D or E) assume a target appearance and have abnormal osmotic fragility is discussed below. On electrophoresis, Hb C constitutes over 90 per cent of the total. Hb F may be slightly increased. No Hb A is present, and no Hb A_2 can be detected because it co-migrates with Hb C.

How does the β 6 Glu→Lys substitution cause the varied and subtle clinical and laboratory abnormalities listed in the previous section as well as in Table 10–12?

Intracellular Crystallization. In 1954, Diggs and colleagues[572] observed the formation of crystals when CC red cells were suspended in a hypertonic medium.[573, 574] These crystals appear in a variety of forms—monoclinic, hexagonal and tetragonal prisms and plates[575]—and exhibit either weak or absent birefringence.[571, 575] Intracellular crystals can be seen in small numbers in routine blood smears on CC individuals, particularly in the dense microspherocytes,[571] or in the cells of individuals who have undergone splenectomy.[572, 576] Furthermore, crystals can be induced more readily and with less dehydration in "older," more viscous microspherocytes compared with the "younger," less viscous target cells.[571] Ultrastructural examination of CC red cells by the freeze fracture technique reveals the presence of aggregates of hemoglobin, 70 Å in diameter, adjacent to the cytoplasmic surface of the membrane.[575] These aggregates were more abundant in the dense microspherocytes than in the younger cells. The formation of intracellular crystals may be preceded by microtubules.[577] More recently, ^{31}P-NMR measurements have suggested the presence of aggregates of C hemoglobin not visualized by light microscopy.[576] This phenomenon was particularly marked in the splenectomized individual.

These observations strongly suggest that Hb C is significantly less soluble than Hb A. Hemolysates from CC individuals form myriads of crystals when the total concentration of hemoglobin exceeds 34 to 36 g/dl, whereas crystals do not appear in normal hemolysates at concentrations of 46 g/dl. A comparison of the solubilities of carboxy and deoxy C and A hemoglobins is shown in Table 10–13.[571] Note that Hb C is less soluble than Hb A except at very high ionic strength and that at physiologic ionic strength, deoxy Hb C is less soluble than carboxy Hb C.

The decreased solubility of Hb C must be due to intermolecular interactions arising from the beta 6 substitution. Precise contacts between molecules can be determined by x-ray diffraction (see Chapter 2). Fitzgerald and Love[578] have prepared five crystal forms of Hb

Table 10–13 **COMPARISON OF SOLUBILITY OF HEMOGLOBINS A AND C IN PHOSPHATE BUFFERS (PH 7.2)**

Temperature	Ionic Strength	Carboxyhemoglobin (g/dl)		Deoxyhemoglobin (g/dl)	
		A	C	A	C
22°C	4.8	4.0	3.6	0.20	0.26
		3.5	4.1	0.28	0.31
	3.6	8.9	5.6	1.3	2.5
		8.6	4.5	1.4	1.9
	2.4	>40	>40	11.0	13.4
				9.3	9.7
	1.2	>40	>40	38.6	30.6
				39.2	28.8
	0.6	>40	>40	40.6	34.2
				42.0	32.4

(From Charache, S., et al.: J. Clin. Invest. 46:1795, 1967.)

25°C	0.4	>35		27	
37°C	0.4	>35		31	

(From Bunn, H. F., and Eaton, W. A.: Unpublished data.)

C: three deoxy and two liganded. They have reported structural details of two of the deoxy forms. The use of difference Fourier analysis permitted a direct comparison with deoxy Hb A. The structure of probable physiologic relevance is a tetragonal crystal that was prepared at neutral pH. This crystal contains two hemoglobin tetramers per asymmetric unit and is isomorphous with crystals of deoxyhemoglobin A grown under similar conditions. The decreased solubility of deoxyhemoglobin C can probably be explained by the finding that three of the four beta 6 lysines in the asymmetric unit are engaged in intermolecular contacts, whereas in deoxyhemoglobin A, only one of the four beta 6 glutamates is involved in a contact.

Crystals of liganded Hb C are generally tetragonal and isomorphous with those of liganded Hbs A and S. Again, the reduced solubility of liganded Hb C must be due to stabilization from intermolecular contacts. Recently, cyanmet Hb C has been analyzed by x-ray diffraction.[579, 580] The resolution of these studies was considerably lower than that obtained in the deoxy crystals described above. The cyanmet crystals assumed an orthorhombic form. The plate-like crystal morphology observed in intact C red cells[575] appears to be due to two dimensional sheets, one molecule thick and stacked over one another so that the spheres of one sheet fill the holes of the other.

In the sickling disorders, Hb S aggregates when the red cell is deoxygenated. In contrast, the crystals found in CC red cells are formed from oxyhemoglobin. These crystals melt when red cells undergo deoxygenation in the capillary circulation.[577a] This oxygen-dependent reversibility of cellular crystallization probably limits the accumulation of crystals as CC red cells circulate *in vivo*.

Cation Leak and Cell Dehydration. Even though intracellular crystallization is a striking and unique feature of Hb CC disease, it is not the prime determinant of the hematological and clinical phenotype. Red cell dehydration is probably the major factor leading to shortened survival of CC red cells and plays an important role in the pathogenesis of SC disease (see Chapter 12). The marked reduction in water in CC red cells results from a parallel decrease in cation content (see Table 10–12). CC red cells have a markedly enhanced potassium efflux that is independent of the Na-K pump, Na-K co-transport, and the Ca-K (Gardos) channel.[580a] It is likely that this potassium leak is activated by the electrostatic interaction of positively charged Hb C with a negatively charged protein on the cytoplasmic surface of the red cell membrane. Indeed, Hb C does bind more readily than Hb A to band 3 on the inner membrane surface.[581] The abnormal K leak in CC red cells probably does not depend on the formation of intracellular aggregates since a similar increase in K efflux can be demonstrated in AC red cells. This phenomenon probably explains why AC and SC cells are targeted and more dense than AA and AS cells. It is likely that the dehydration in Hb C–containing red cells results from the overall surface charge of the hemoglobin rather than a specific interaction at β 6 Lys. Target cells have been noted in other positively charged variants, including homozygotes for Hbs E, D-Los Angeles (see below), and O-Arab. Thus, electrostatic attraction between the positively charged hemoglobin variant and the red cell membrane may open up a potassium efflux channel and lead to dehydration and target cells, a morphologic feature that has traditionally been associated with "hemoglobinopathies."

Because of their increased MCHC and perhaps the presence of inclusions and crystals, CC red cells have a marked reduction in deformability. They traverse Millipore filters more slowly than normal cells,[570, 571] and they have increased bulk viscosity.[570, 571, 575, 582] From the experimental observations discussed at the beginning of this section, it is not surprising that viscosity is further increased in (a) dense microspherocytes; (b) cells suspended in hypertonic medium; (c) cells from a splenectomized patient; and (d) deoxygenated cells.

The decreased deformability of CC red cells is responsible for the moderate reduction in cell life span that has been documented by several investigations.[563, 566, 583-585] Normally, the bone marrow should be able to fully compensate for the mild degree of hemolysis. The fact that CC patients have significant anemia means that the erythropoietic response is suboptimal. Enhanced oxygen delivery to tissues due to a "shift to the right" in the oxyhemoglobin dissociation curve may be responsible for the blunted erythropoietic response.[586]

The mechanism for the decreased oxygen affinity of CC red cells is not obvious. The oxygen saturation curve of dilute solutions of Hb C is normal. Furthermore, Hb C has normal reactivity to 2,3-DPG and CO_2.[587] However, the whole blood oxygen affinity of Hb C is reduced.[586,588] When expressed as a molar ratio to hemoglobin, red cell 2,3-DPG is nor-

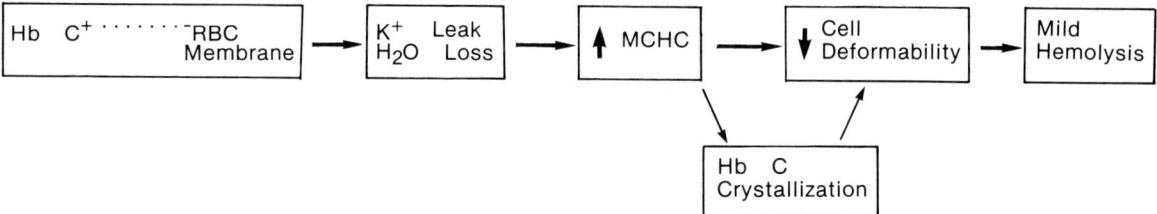

Figure 10–13. Pathogenesis of cell dehydration and hemolysis in Hb CC disease. Lesser degrees of dehydration also occur in AC and SC red cells, but Hb C does not crystallize.

mal in CC homozygotes, unlike most anemic individuals. However, because of the marked reduction in solvent water in CC cells, the activity of 2,3-DPG is considerably higher than normal. This increase in effective concentration of 2,3-DPG in CC red cells probably explains their decreased oxygen affinity.

These pathophysiologic processes are summarized in Figure 10–13. In contrast to the cellular dehydration encountered in SS cells, the loss of cell water in CC red cells is not dependent on deoxygenation. Thus, the CC red cells lack the amplification of intracellular polymerization (the vicious circle) that occurs in the capillary circulation in sickle cell disease. However, as mentioned above, the K and water loss imposed by the presence of Hb C is an important contributor to the pathogenesis of Hb SC disease (see Chapter 12).

The "D" Hemoglobins

In 1951, Itano[590] encountered a new hemoglobin variant that co-migrated with Hb S on moving-boundary electrophoresis but failed to sickle. It was labeled Hb D and was subsequently found to have the structure β 121 Glu→Gln (Hb D-Punjab or D-Los Angeles).[370] Since that time, other variants have been found that also co-migrate with Hb S when electrophoresis is performed at an alkaline pH. A number of these have been named with the prefix D followed by the locale where they were discovered (e.g., D-Ibadan [β 87 Thr →Lys], D-Iran [β 22 Glu→Gln]) or the prefix G (e.g., G-Galveston [β 43 Glu→Ala], G-San Jose [β 7 Glu→Gly]). None of these hemoglobins sickle, yet when they co-exist with Hb S in the double heterozygous state, they can affect sickling to a varying degree. For example, Hb S/D-Los Angeles is a much more severe condition than Hb S/D-Ibadan.[591] The interaction of S and D hemoglobins is covered in detail in Chapter 11. Note that all the D (and G) hemoglobins involve an increase in one unit of positive charge per affected subunit—either a substitution of a neutral amino acid for a negatively charged one or a substitution of a positively charged amino acid for a neutral one. Although they co-migrate with Hb S under standard electrophoretic conditions at alkaline pH, the "D" hemoglobins can be separated from Hb S by electrophoresis on agar gel at pH 6.0; most of them have the same mobility as Hb A. In addition to their failure to sickle, these hemoglobins also differ from Hb S in their solubility properties. Thus, heterozygotes for Hb D (or G) will have negative solubility tests for Hb S.

Hb D-Los Angeles (D-Punjab). This is by far the most commonly encountered "D" hemoglobin.[592] Among Sikhs of the Punjab region of India, 2 to 3 per cent are heterozygous for Hb D-Los Angeles. A number of homozygotes have been reported from various parts of the world.[371, 593-597] These individuals have normal hemoglobin values with no evidence of hemolysis. Red cell indices are generally within normal limits. Some individuals have target cells and decreased osmotic fragility. Hemoglobin electrophoresis shows 95 per cent Hb D and normal amounts of Hb A_2. Tests for sickling are negative. This condition must be distinguished from the double heterozygous state Hb D/$β^0$ thalassemia.[598] Appropriate family studies and careful measurement of red cell indices and Hbs A_2 and F are important in establishing the diagnosis. Individuals doubly heterozygous for Hb D and β thalassemia usually have mild anemia and minimal hemolysis[543] in contrast to those with E/β thalassemia (see below) and S/β thalassemia (see Chapter 12). Hb D-Los Angeles has normal stability and normal or slightly increased oxygen affinity.[599]

Hb E ($α_2β_2$ 26 Glu→Lys)

Hb E is the second most prevalent hemoglobin variant worldwide. It is found primarily in

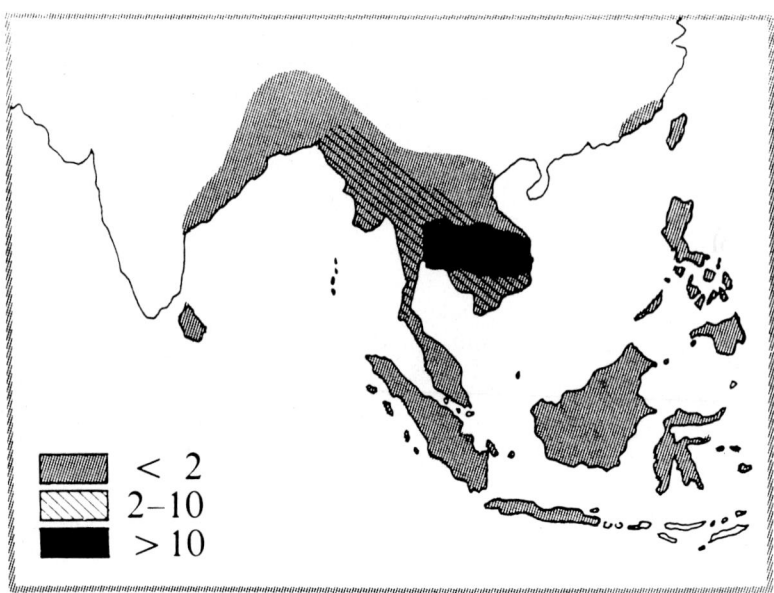

Figure 10–14. Frequency of the β^E gene in Southeast Asia. The key in the lower left corner shows the percentage of the population that bears the gene. (From Cavalli-Sforza, L. L., and Bodmer, W. F.: Genetics of Human Populations. San Francisco, W. H. Freeman, 1971, p. 155.)

Orientals, although it has also been reported in blacks[600, 601] and Caucasians.[190, 602] There is convincing evidence that the β^E gene has arisen independently on a number of occasions.[602a] The gene frequency in Thailand and Burma is 0.05 to 0.10. Accordingly, in Southeast Asia, about 30 million people are heterozygous for Hb E, and about 1 million are homozygous (Fig. 10–14). In China, the gene frequency drops to 0.001.[603, 604] The maintenance of such a high gene frequency in a localized area may be a reflection of some type of balanced polymorphism, in which AE heterozygotes have improved fitness. *In vitro* studies have not revealed any differences in the growth rate of *P. falciparum* in AE versus AA red cells.[604a, 604b] There are conflicting data on whether growth is inhibited in Hb EE red cells.[604a, 604b] Because of the recent emigration of refugees from Southeast Asia, Hb E is encountered quite commonly in the United States.[601a]

Hemoglobin E Trait. Hb E heterozygotes are asymptomatic. Hemoglobin levels are normal, but red cells are microcytic,[605] with an average MCV of 73 fl.[602] There is a corresponding reduction in mean corpuscular hemoglobin. Thus, MCHC is normal. In the presence of concurrent α thalassemia, which is very common in Southeast Asia, the MCV is even lower. Hemoglobin electrophoresis reveals 30 to 35 per cent Hb E; the remainder is Hb A. As in AS and AC heterozygotes, the proportion of Hb E decreases significantly in individuals who also have α thalassemia[606, 607] (see Table 10–10). In addition, the relative amount of Hb E in AE heterozygotes may decrease if they become iron-deficient.[608]

Hemoglobin E Homozygotes. These individuals are also asymptomatic and have normal or slightly decreased hemoglobin levels.[609, 609a] There is no increased morbidity during pregnancy.[610] Red cells are even more microcytic than those from heterozygotes, with a mean MCV of 67 fl. The MCHC is normal. Reticulocyte counts and red cell survival are within normal levels. The hematologic manifestations have been thoroughly reviewed by Fairbanks and associates,[611] who point out that a number of earlier reports of Hb E homozygotes do not clearly rule out E/β thalassemia or concurrent iron deficiency, which is very prevalent in Southeast Asia. Target cells are seen on dried blood smears (see Color Plate III*D*), and in keeping with this observation, there is increased resistance to osmotic lysis.[609, 612] It is curious that homozygotes for hemoglobins S, C, D, and E all have target cells and reduced osmotic fragility, although there are significant differences in red cell indices among these conditions. A plausible mechanism for these morphological abnormalities is discussed in the section above on Hb C.

Hemoglobin E/β Thalassemia. Patients who are doubly heterozygous for Hb E and β thalassemia have an anemia that is variable but is generally more severe than in patients with Hb S/β thalassemia.[612, 613, 613a] E/β thalassemia can be as severe as homozygous β thalassemia. A blood smear is shown in Color Plate III*E*.

Properties of Hemoglobin E. Hb E co-migrates with HbA_2 and Hb C on routine electrophoresis on cellulose acetate or starch gel at pH 8.6. However, these hemoglobins can be separated by gel electrofocusing.[482]* Furthermore, Hbs C and E can be separated by electrophoresis on citrate agar at pH 6.0: Hb E migrates toward the cathode with a mobility similar to Hbs A and D, whereas Hb C moves toward the anode.[478]

An AE hemolysate can also be distinguished from AC by the fact that Hb E is unstable and forms a precipitate when incubated at 50° to 60°C or in the presence of acid,[614] oxidants,[614, 615] or 17 per cent isopropanol.[616] Hb E appears to dissociate into monomers more readily than does Hb A.[617] Nevertheless, there is no evidence that these laboratory phenomena have any significance *in vivo*, because no hemolysis can be detected even in Hb E homozygotes.

Whole blood oxygen dissociation curves of EE homozygotes are shifted slightly to the right.[588, 611, 618] Some have increased red cell 2,3-DPG,[619] whereas others do not.[611] Purified Hb E has normal oxygen affinity, Bohr effect, and reactivity to 2,3-DPG.[601, 619] Thus, the decreased oxygen affinity of EE red cells is unexplained. It would be worthwhile to see whether it is due to a decrease in intracellular pH. The modest enhancement of oxygen delivery due to the right-shifted curve may result in a slightly subnormal rate of red cell production and a corresponding small reduction in red cell mass.[588]

Biosynthesis and Assembly. The synthesis of Hb E in reticulocytes appears to be significantly impaired. Hb E homozygotes who have no accompanying α thalassemia or iron deficiency have an increased α/β synthesis ratio ranging from 1.2 to 2.1.[609a, 611, 620, 621] This ratio is similar to that of individuals with β-thalassemia trait. Reticulocytes from AE heterozygotes synthesize significantly less Hb E than Hb A.[622] These studies do not distinguish between decreased production of $β^E$ versus enhanced catabolism. The findings of decreased levels of $β^E$ mRNA[621, 623] indicates impaired production of $β^E$ chains. Thus, the Hb E structural gene may be viewed as a $β^+$-thalassemia gene. The base substitution at codon 26 creates a new splicing sequence that causes abnormal mRNA processing[552] as well as instability of the mRNA during erythroid maturation.[624] In addition to decreased synthesis of $β^E$, it is likely that enhanced turnover of $β^E$ subunits also contributes to the thalassemic phenotype.[620] Finally, as mentioned earlier in this chapter, variants having positively charged β chains appear to assemble less readily than those having negatively charged β chains. A decreased rate of formation of $αβ^E$ dimers relative to $αβ^A$ explains why the proportion of Hb E in AE heterozygotes is markedly reduced in the presence of α thalassemia[606, 607] or iron deficiency (a form of acquired thalassemia).[608] As explained earlier, identical considerations apply to AS and AC heterozygotes.

Hb Korle-Bu (G-Accra) (β 73 Asp→Asn)

Hemoglobin Korle-Bu is encountered quite frequently in central Africans. There are no clinical or hematological manifestations associated with either the heterozygous or the homozygous state.[625] It is interesting that red cells from an individual homozygous for Hb Korle-Bu had a perfectly normal appearance on blood smear. No target cells were seen.[625] This variant is of additional interest because of its interaction with Hb S. As discussed in detail in Chapter 7, Hb Korle-Bu behaves like Hb F in its failure to participate in the gelation of Hb S.[626] Thus, it is not surprising that individuals who are doubly heterozygous for Hb S and Hb Korle-Bu have no clinical abnormalities.

Hb H ($β_4$)

Hb H is a tetramer composed of four normal β chains. This abnormal hemoglobin is seen in some individuals with α thalassemia (see Chapters 8 and 9).

Hb I ($α_2$ 16 Lys→Glu $β_2$)

Hb I is one of the most commonly encountered α-chain variants. It has been found in individuals of various racial backgrounds. They have no apparent clinical or hematological abnormalities. Heterozygotes usually have about 25 per cent Hb I and 75 per cent Hb A. This proportion is similar to other α-chain variants (see Figure 10–7) and is consistent with the known presence of four copies of the

---

*See beginning of chapter: Detection of Hemoglobin Variants.

α-chain gene. The amount of Hb I in red cells is proportional to its rate of synthesis.[627] In one otherwise normal individual, Hb I constitutes 65 per cent of the total hemoglobin. Genetic analysis revealed three α globin genes.[628] The mutation was present on both the α1 and α2 globin genes. Analysis of the family confirmed that the two affected genes were located *in cis*. This finding probably reflects a recent conversion event within the α globin gene cluster. The amino acid substitution in Hb I is in one of the invariant residues. Nevertheless, Hb I has perfectly normal functional properties.[629] Hemoglobin I may have decreased solubility compared with Hb A. When subjected to the classic metasulfite slide test, red cells containing Hb I assume an elongated shape similar to sickle red cells.[630]

References

1. Zeng, Y.-T., Huang, S.-Z., Qiu, X.-K., Cheng, G.-C., Ren, Z.-R., Jin, Q.-C., Chen, C.-Y., Jiao, C.-T., Tang, Z.-G., Liu, R.-H., Bao, X.-H., Zeng, L.-Z., Duan, Y.-Q., and Zhang, G.-Y.: Hemoglobin Chongqing [α2(NA2)Leu→Arg] and hemoglobin Harbin [α16(A14) Lys→Met] found in China. Hemoglobin, 8:569, 1984.
1a. Crookston, J. H., Beal, D., Irvine, D., and Lehmann, H.: A new haemoglobin J Toronto (α5 Alanine→Aspartic acid). Nature 208:1059, 1965.
2. Vella, F., Hill, J. R., Wiltshire, B., and Lehmann, H.: Hemoglobin J Toronto. Clin. Biochem. 4:137, 1971.
3. Sumida, I., Ohta, Y., Imamura, T., and Yanase, T.: Hemoglobin Sawara: α6(A4) Aspartic acid→Alanine. Biochim. Biophys. Acta 322:23, 1973.
4. Sasaki. J., Imamura, T., Sumida, I., Yanase, T., and Ohya, M.: Increased oxygen affinity for hemoglobin Sawara: αA4(6) Aspartic acid→Alanine. Biochim. Biophys. Acta 495:183, 1977.
5. Jue, D. L., Johnson, M. H., Patchen, L. C., and Moo-Penn, W. F.: Hemoglobin Dunn: α6(A4) Aspartic acid→Asparagine. Hemoglobin 3:137, 1979.
5a. Lee-Potter, J. P., Deacon-Smith, R. A., Lehmann, H., and Robb, L.: Haemoglobin Ferndown (α6 (A4) Aspartic acid→Valine) FEBS Lett. 126:117, 1981.
5b. Como, P. F., Barber, S., Sage, R. E., and Kronenberg, H.: Hemoglobin Woodville—alpha 6 (A4) aspartic acid-tyrosine. Pathology 16:475, 1984.
6. Pootrakul, S., Kematorn, B., Na-Nakorn, S., and Suanpan, S.: A new haemoglobin variant: Haemoglobin Anantharaj alpha 11(A9) Lysine→Glutamic acid. Biochim. Biophys. Acta 405:161, 1975.
6a. Zeng, Y.-T., Huang, S.-Z., Liang, X., Long, G.-F., Lam, H., Wilson, J. B., and Huisman, T. H. J.: Hb Wuming or α₂11 (A9) Lys→Gln β₂. Hemoglobin 5:679, 1981.
6b. Webber, B. B., Lam, H., Wilson, J. B., and Huisman, T. H. J.: Hb Albany-Ga or α₂11(A9) Lys–Asnβ₂. Hemoglobin, 7:257, 1983.
6c. Iuchi, I., Shimasaki, S., and Mizuta, W.: Hb Albany-Suma(alpha-11(A9) Lys→Asn), a hemoglobin variant with slightly elevated oxygen-affinity in Japan. Hemoglobin, 8:343, 1984.
7. Rosa, J., Malekria, N., Vergoz, D., and Dunet, R.: Une nouvelle hémoglobine anormale: l'hémoglobin J α Paris 12 Ala→Asp. Nouv. Rev. Fr. Hématol. 6:423, 1965.
8. Trincao, C., Martins De Melo, J., Lorkin, P. A., and Lehmann, H.: Haemoglobin J Paris in the South of Portugal (Algarve). Acta Haematol. 39:291, 1968.
8a. Honig, G. R., Shamsuddin, M., Vida, L. N., Mompoint, M., Valcourt, E., Bowie, L., Jones, E. C., Powers, P. A., Spritz, R. A., and Guis, M.: Hb Evanston (α14 Trp→Arg): An unstable alpha chain variant expressed as alpha thalassemia. J. Clin. Invest. 73:1740, 1984.
8b. Moo-Penn, W. F., Baine, R. M., Jue, D. L., Johnson, M. H., McGuiffey, J. E., and Benson, J. M.: Hemoglobin Evanston—Alpha 14 (A12) Trp→Arg, a variant hemoglobin associated with α-thalassemia 2. Biochim. Biophys. Acta 747:65, 1983.
9. Marti, H. R., Pik, C., and Mosimann, P.: Eine neue Hämoglobin I Variante: Hb I Interlaken. Acta Haematol. 32:9, 1964.
10. Liddell, J., Brown, D., Beale, D., Lehmann, H., and Huntsman, R. G.: A new haemoglobin-Jα Oxford found during a survey of an English population. Nature 204:269, 1964.
11. Silvestroni, E., Bianco, I., Tentori, L., Vivaldi, G., Carta, S., Sorcini, M., and Brancati, C.: Proc. 10th Congr. Eur. Soc. Hematol., Strasbourg, 1965. Part II. Basel and New York, Karger, 1967, p. 232.
12. Vella, F., Casey, R., Lehmann, H., Labossiere, A., and Jones, T. G.: Haemoglobin Ottawa: α2 15(A13) Gly→Arg β2. Biochim. Biophys. Acta 336:25, 1974.
13. Pootrakul, S., Srichiyanont, S., Wasi, P., and Suanpan, S.: Hemoglobin Siam (α2 15 Arg β2): A new α chain variant. Humangenetik 23:199, 1974.
14. Beale, D., and Lehmann, H.: Abnormal haemoglobins and the genetic code. Nature 207:259, 1965.
15. Schneider, R. G., Alperin, J. B., Beale, D., and Lehmann, H.: Hemoglobin I in an American Negro family: Structural and hematologic studies. J. Lab. Clin. Med. 68:940, 1966.
16. Bowman, B. H., and Barnett, D. R.: Amino-acid substitution in Haemoglobin I (Texas variant). Nature 214:499, 1967.
17. O'Brien, C., Gray, M. J., and Jacobs, A. S.: A survey of cord blood for abnormal hemoglobin with further observations on Hemoglobin I Burlington. Am. J. Obstet. Gynecol. 88:816, 1964.
18. Baur, E. W.: Hb α₂ Glu β₂(Hb I) in a Caucasian family: Independent mutation or common origin? Humangenetik 6:368, 1968.
19. Labossiere, A., and Vella, F.: Hb I in a white family in Saskatoon. Clin. Biochem. 4:104, 1971.
19a. Liang, C. C., Chen, S., Yang, K., Jia, P., Ma, Y., Li, T., Ni, X., Wang, X., Deng, Q., and Yao, S.: Hemoglobin Beijing [α16(A14)Lys–Asn]: A new fast-moving α hemoglobin variant. Hemoglobin 6:629, 1982.
20. Griffiths, K. D., Lang, A., Lehmann, H., Mann, J. R. Plowman, D., and Raine, D. N.: Haemoglobin Handsworth α18 (A16) Glycine→Arginine. FEBS Lett. 75:93, 1977.
21. Rahbar, S., Ala, F., Akhavan, E., Nowzari, G.,

Shoa'i, I., and Zamanianpoor, M. H.: Two new haemoglobins: Haemoglobin Perspolis [α64 (E13) Asp→Tyr] and Haemoglobin J-Kurosh [α19 (AB1) Ala→Asp]. Biochim. Biophys. Acta 427:119, 1976.

21a. Houjun, L., Dexiang, L., Zhiguo, L., Ping, L., Ly, L., Ji, C., and Shaozhi, H.: A new fast-moving hemoglobin variant, Hb J-Tashikuergan [α19 (AB1) Ala→Glu]. Hemoglobin, 8:391, 1984.

22. Wajcman, H., Elion, J., Boissel, J. P., Labie, D., Jos, J., and Girot, R.: A silent hemoglobin variant: Haemoglobin Necker Enfants-Malades α20(B1) His→Tyr. Hemoglobin 4:177, 1980.

22a. Sellaye, M., Blouquit, Y., Galacteros, F., Arous, N., Monplaisir, N., Rhoda, M. D., Braconnier, F., and Rosa, J.: A new silent hemoglobin variant in a black family from French West Indies—Hemoglobin LeLamentin α20 His–Gln. FEBS Lett. 145:128, 1982.

23. Kendall, A. G., Barr, R. D., Lang, A., and Lehmann, H.: Haemoglobin J Nyanza: α21 (B2) Ala→Asp. Biochim. Biophys. Acta 310:357, 1973.

24. Gottlieb, A. J., Restrepo, A., and Itano, H. A.: Hemoglobin J Medellin. Chemical and genetic study. Fed. Proc. 23:172, 1964.

25. Kraus, A. P., Miyaji, T., Iuchi, I., and Kraus, L. M.: Memphis. A new variety of sickle cell anemia with clinically mild symptoms due to an α-chain variant of hemoglobin (α23 Glu NH2). J. Lab. Clin. Med. 66:886, 1965.

26. Boyer, S. H., Crosby, E. F., Fulley, G. F., Ulenurm, L., and Buck, A. A.: A survey of hemoglobins in the Republic of Chad and characterization of hemoglobin Chad. α₂ 23Glu→Lys β₂. Am. J. Hum. Genet. 20:570, 1968.

27. Marengo-Rowe, A. J., Beale, D., and Lehmann, H.: New human haemoglobin variant from southern Arabia: G-Audhali (α23 (B4) Glutamic acid→Valine) and the variability of B4 in human haemoglobin. Nature 219:1164, 1968.

27a. Zeng, Y. T., Huang, S. Z., Zhou, X. D., Qiu, X. K., Dong, Q. Y., Li, M. Y., and Bai, J. H.: Hb Shenyang (α26(B7)Ala→Glu) a new unstable variant found in China. Hemoglobin 6:625, 1982.

28. Schneider, R. G., Brimhall, B., Jones, R. T., Bryant, R., Mitchell, C. B., and Goldberg, A. I.: Hb Fort Worth: α27 Glu→Gly (B8). A variant present in unusually low concentration. Biochim. Biophys. Acta 243:164, 1971.

28a. Liang, C.-C., Tao, H., Lo, H. Y., Huang, S.-Z., Li, R.-Y., and Wang, B.-S.: Hemoglobin Shuangfeng (α27 (B8) Glu→Lys): A new unstable hemoglobin variant. Hemoglobin 5:691, 1981.

29. Ahern, E., Ahern, V., Holder, W., Palomino, E., Serjeant, G. R., Serjeant, B. E., Forbes, M., Brimhall, B., and Jones, R. T.: Haemoglobin Spanish Town, α27 Glu→Val (B8). Biochim. Biophys. Acta 427:530, 1976.

30. Vettore, L, DeSandre, G., Dilorio, E. E., Winterhalter, K. H., Lang, A., and Lehmann, H.: A new abnormal hemoglobin O Padova, α30 (B11) Glu→Lys and a dyserythropoietic anemia with erythroblastic multinuclearity co-existing in the same patient. Blood 44:869, 1974.

31. Schneider, R. G., and Jim, R. T. S.: A new haemoglobin variant (the 'Honolulu Type') in a Chinese. Nature 190:454, 1961.

32. Vella, F., Ager, J. A. M., and Lehmann, H.: An abnormal haemoglobin in a Chinese: Haemoglobin G. Nature 182:460, 1958.

33. Swenson, R. T., Hill, R. L., Lehmann, H., and Jim, R. T. S.: A chemical abnormality in hemoglobin G from Chinese individuals. J. Biol. Chem. 237:1517, 1962.

34. Marinucci, M., Mavilio, F., Massa, A., Gabbianelli, M., Tentori, L., and Ignesti, C.: Haemoglobin Prato: A new amino acid substitution (α31 (B12) Arg→Ser). IRCS Med. Sci. 6:234, 1978.

35. Marinucci, M., Mavilio, F., Massa, A., Gabbianelli, M., Fontanarosa, P. P., Camagna, A., Ignesti, C., and Tentori, L.: A new abnormal human hemoglobin: Hb Prato (α₂31(B12) Arg→Ser β₂). Biochim. Biophys. Acta 578:534, 1979.

36. Tasis, B.: Hemoglobin Queens (α 34 (B15) Leu→Arg): A new variant at the α₁β₁ contact. Blood 54(Suppl. 1):61A, 1979.

36a. Moo-Penn, W. F., Jue, D. L., Johnson, M. H., McGuffey, J. E., Simpkins, H., and Katz, J.: Hemoglobin Queens: α34 (B15) Leu→Arg structural and functional properties and its association with Hb E. Am. J. Hematol. 13:323, 1982.

36b. Harano, T., Harano, H. K., Shibata, S., Ueda, S., Imai, K., Tsuneshi, A., Yamada, H., Seki, M., and Fukui, H.: Hemoglobin Kariya [alpha-40 (C5) Lys-Glu]: A new hemoglobin-variant with an increased oxygen-affinity. FEBS Lett. 153:332, 1983.

37. Beretta, A., Prato, V., Gallo, E., and Lehmann, H.: Haemoglobin Torino—α43 (CD1) phenylalanine replaced by valine. Nature 217:1016, 1968.

38. Ohba, Y., Miyaji, T., Matsuoka, M., Yokoyama, M., Numakura, H., Nagata, K., Takebe, Y., Izumi, Y., and Shibata, S.: Hemoglobin Hirosaki (α43 [CE 1] Phe→Leu), a new unstable variant. Biochim. Biophys. Acta 405:155, 1975.

39. Honig, G. R., Vida, L.N., Shamsuddin, M., Mason, R. G., Schlumpf, H. W. and Luke, R. A.: Hemoglobin Milledgeville (α 44 (CD2) Pro→Leu), a new variant with increased oxygen affinity. Biochim. Biophys. Acta 626:424, 1980.

39a. Harano, T., Harano, K., Ueda, S., Shibata, S., Imai, K., Ohba, Y., Shinohara, T., Horio, S., Nishioka, K., and Shirotani, H.: Hemoglobin Kawachi [α44(CE2)Pro–Arg]: A new hemoglobin variant of high oxygen affinity with amino acid substitution at α₁β₂ contact. Hemoglobin 6:43, 1982.

40. Braconnier, F., Gacon, G., Thillet, J., Wajcman, H., Soria, J., Maigret, P., Labie, D., and Rosa, J.: Hemoglobin Fort de France (α₂⁴⁵(CD3) His→Arg β₂). A new variant with increased oxygen affinity. Biochim. Biophys. Acta 493:228, 1977.

41. Marinucci, M., Mavilio, F., Tentori, L., D'Erasmo, F., Colapietro, A., de Stasio, G., and DiFonzo. S.: A new human hemoglobin variant: Hb Bari (α₂ 45(CD3) His→Gln β₂). Biochim. Biophys. Acta 622:315, 1980.

42. Sumida, I.: Studies of abnormal hemoglobins in western Japan. Frequency of visible hemoglobin variants, and chemical characterization of hemoglobin Sawara (α₂ 6Ala β₂) and hemoglobin Mugino (Hb L Ferrara; α₂ 47Gly β₂). Jpn. J. Hum. Genet. 19:343, 1975.

43. DeVries, A., Joshua, H., Lehmann, H., Hill, R. L., and Fellows, R. E.: The first observation of an abnormal haemoglobin in a Jewish family: Haemoglobin Beilinson. Br. J. Haematol. 9:484, 1963.

43a. Ohba, Y., Hattori, Y., Matsuoka, M., Miyaji, T., and Fuyuno, K.: Hb Kokura [α47 (CE 5) Asp→Gly]: A slightly unstable variant. Hemoglobin 6:69, 1982.

44. Halbrecht, I., Isaacs, W. A., Lehmann, H., and Ben-Porat, F.: Hemoglobin Hasharon (α47 Aspartic acid→Histidine). Israel J. Med. Sci. 3:827, 1967.

45. Ostertag, W., and Smith, E. W.: Hb Sinai: A new α chain mutant α47 His. Humangenetik 6:377, 1968.
46. Schneider, R. G., Ueda, S., Alperin, J. B., Brimhall, B., and Jones, R. T.: Hemoglobin Sealy (α_2 47His β_2): A new variant in a Jewish family. Am. J. Hum. Genet. 20:151, 1968.
47. Bianco, I., Modiano, G., Bottini, E., and Lucci, R.: Alteration in the α-chain of haemoglobin L Ferrara. Nature 198:395, 1963.
48. Tentori, L: Hemoglobin L Ferrara = hemoglobin Hasharon. Hemoglobin 1:602, 1977.
49. Rahbar, S., Mahdavi, N., Nowzari, G., and Mostafavi, I.: Hemoglobin Arya: α_2 47(CD5) Aspartic acid→Asparagine. Biochim. Biophys. Acta 386:525, 1975.
49a. Nakatsuji, T., Wilson, J. B., and Huisman, T. H. J.: Hb Cordele $\alpha_2$47 (CE5) Asp→Ala β_2. A mildly unstable variant observed in black twins. Hemoglobin 8:37, 1984.
50. Brimhall, B., Jones, R. T., Schneider, R. G., Hosty, T. S., Tomlin, G., and Atkins, R.: Two new hemoglobins: Hemoglobin Alabama (β39 (C5) Gln→Lys) and hemoglobin Montgomery (α48 (CD6) Leu→Arg). Biochim. Biophys. Acta 379:28, 1975.
51. Szelényi, J. G., Horányi, M., Földi, J., Hudacsek, J., István, L., and Hollán, S. R.: A new hemoglobin variant in Hungary: Hb Savaria—α49(CE7) Ser→Arg. Hemoglobin 4:27, 1980.
52. Tangheroni, W., Zorcolo, G., Gallo, E., and Lehmann, H.: Haemoglobin J Sardegna: α50 (CD8) Histidine→Aspartic acid. Nature 218:470, 1968.
52a. Harano, T., Harano, K., Shibata, S., Ueda, S., Mori, H., and Seki, M.: Hemoglobin Aichi [α50(CE5)His→Arg]: A new slightly unstable hemoglobin variant discovered in Japan. FEBS Lett. 169:297, 1984.
53. Cabannes, R., Renaud, R., Mauran, A., Pennors, H., Charlesworth, D., Price, B. G., and Lehmann, H.: Deux hémoglobines rapides en Côte-d'Ivoire: l'Hb K Woolwich et une nouvelle hémoglobine, l'Hb J Abidjan (α51 Gly→Asp). Nouv. Rev. Fr. Hematol. 12:289, 1972.
54. Reynolds, C. A., and Huisman, T. H. J.: Hemoglobin Russ or α2 51 Arg β2. Biochim. Biophys. Acta 130:541, 1966.
55. Alberti, R., Mariuzzi, G. M., Artibani, L., Bruni, E., and Tentori, L.: A new haemoglobin variant: J-Rovigo alpha 53 (E-2) Alanine lends to Aspartic acid. Biochim. Biophys. Acta 342:1, 1974.
56. Targino de Araujo, J., Plowman, D., Targino de Aranjo, R. A., de Juza, L. F., and Lehmann, H.: Hemoglobin J Rovigo 53 Alpha (E2) Asp–Ala. Rev. Bras. Pesqui. Med. Biol. 13:37, 1980.
57. Miyaji, T., Iuchi, I., Takeda, I., and Shibata, S.: Hemoglobin Shimonoseki (α2 54 Arg β2A), a slow-moving hemoglobin found in a Japanese family, with special reference to its chemistry. Acta Haematol. Jpn. 26:531, 1963.
58. Imai, K., Morimoto, H., Kotani, M., Shibata, S., Miyaji, T., and Masutomo, K.: Studies on the function of abnormal hemoglobins. II. Oxygen equilibrium of abnormal hemoglobins: Shimonoseki, Ube II, Hikari, Gifu, and Agenogi. Biochim. Biophys. Acta 200:197, 1970.
59. Jones, R. I., Brimhall, B., and Lisker, R.: Chemical characterization of hemoglobin Mexico and hemoglobin Chiapas. Biochim. Biophys. Acta 154:488, 1968.
60. Rosa, J., Labie, D., Maleknia, N., and Blum, N.: Sur quelques hémoglobines anormales nouvelles recemment isolées en France. International Symposium on Comparative Hemoglobin Structure. Thessaloniki, April 11–13, 1966, pp. 140–145.
61. Fessas, P. H., Kaltsoya, A., Loukopoulos, D., and Nilsson, L.-O.: On the chemical structure of haemoglobin Uppsala. Hum. Hered. 19:152, 1969.
62. Trabuchet, G., Benabadji, M., and Labie, D.: Genetic and biosynthetic studies of families carrying hemoglobin Jα Mexico: Association of α-thalassemia with Hb J. Hum. Genet. 42:189, 1978.
63. Pootrakul, S., Boonyarat, D., Kematorn, B., Suanpan, S., and Wasi, P.: Hemoglobin Thailand [α56(E5) Lys→Thr]: A new abnormal human hemoglobin. Hemoglobin 1:781, 1977.
64. Abramov, A., Lehmann, H., and Robb, L.: Hb Shaare Zedek (α56 E5 Lys→Glu). FEBS Lett. 113:235, 1980.
65. Rahbar, S., Kinderlerer, J. L., and Lehmann, H.: Haemoglobin L Persian Gulf: α57(E6) Glycine→Arginine. Acta Haematol. 42:169, 1969.
66. Baglioni, C.: A chemical study of hemoglobin Norfolk. J. Biol. Chem. 237:69, 1962.
67. Imamura, T.: Hemoglobin Kagoshima: An example of hemoglobin Norfolk in a Japanese family. Am. J. Hum. Genet. 18:584, 1966.
68. Yanase, T., Hanada, M., Seita, M., Ohya, I., Ohta, Y., Imamura, T., Fujimura, T., Kawasaki, K., and Yamaoka, K.: Molecular basis of morbidity—from a series of studies of hemoglobinopathies in western Japan. Jpn. J. Hum. Genet. 13:40, 1968.
69. Gerald, P. S., and Efron, M. L.: Chemical studies of several varieties of Hb M. Proc. Natl. Acad. Sci. USA 47:1758, 1961.
70. Shimizu, A., Hayashi, A., Yamamura, Y., Tsugita, A., and Kitayama, K.: The structural study on a new hemoglobin variant, Hb M Osaka. Biochim. Biophys. Acta 97:472, 1965.
71. Hansen, H. A., Jagenburg, O. R., and Johansson, B. G.: Studies on an abnormal hemoglobin causing hereditary congenital cyanosis. Acta Paediatr. 49:503, 1960.
72. Hollán, S. R., Szelényi, J. G., Lehmann, H., and Beale, D.: A Boston-type haemoglobin M in Hungary: Haemoglobin M Kiskunhalas. Haematologia 1:11, 1967.
73. Nakatsuji, T., Miwa, S., Ohba, Y., Miyaji, T., Matsumoto, N., and Matsuoka, I.: Hemoglobin Tottori (α59[E8] Glycine→Valine), a new unstable hemoglobin. Hemoglobin 5:427, 1981.
74. Barclay, G. P. T., Charlesworth, D., and Lehmann, H.: Abnormal haemoglobin in Zambia. A new haemoglobin Zambia α60 (E9) Lysine→Asparagine. Br. Med. J. 4:595, 1969.
75. Spivak, V. A., Molchanova, T. P., Ermakov, N. V., Tokarev, Y. N., Martinez, G., Szelényi, J., Horányi, M., Foldi, J., Hollán, S., Kazieva, H., and Shamov, I. A.: A new hemoglobin variant: Hb Dagestan α60(E9) Lys→Glu. Hemoglobin 5:133, 1981.
76. Brimhall, B., Duerst, M., Hollán, S. R., Stenzel, P., Szelényi, J., and Jones, R. T.: Structural characterizations of hemoglobins J Buda (α61 (E10) Lys→Asn) and G Pest (α74 (EF3) Asp→Asn). Biochim. Biophys. Acta 336:344, 1974.
77. Thillet, J., Blouquit, Y., Perrone, F., and Rosa, J.: Hemoglobin Pontoise α63A1a→Asp (E12). A new fast moving variant. Biochim. Biophys. Acta 491:16, 1977.

78. Blackwell, R. Q., Jim, R. T. S., Tan, T. G. H., Weng, M.-I., Liu, C.-S., and Wang, C.-L.: Hemoglobin G Waimanalo: α64 Asp→Asn. Biochim. Biophys. Acta 322:27, 1973.
79. Ramot, B., Kinderlerer, J. B., and Lehmann, H.: Cited in WHO Technical Report Series No. 509, Annex 1, Geneva, World Health Organization, 1972.
80. Sukumaran, P. K., Merchant, S. M., Desai, M. P., Wiltshire, B. G., and Lehmann, H.: Haemoglobin Q India (α64(E13) Aspartic acid→Histidine) associated with β-thalassemia observed in three Sindhi families. J. Med. Genet. 9:436, 1972.
81. Miyaji, T., Iuchi, I., Yamamoto, K., Ohba, Y., and Shibata, S.: Amino acid substitution of hemoglobin Ube 2 (α2 68 Asp β2): An example of successful application of partial hydrolysis of peptide with 5% acetic acid. Clin. Chim. Acta 16:347, 1967.
82. Baglioni, C., and Ingram, V. M.: Abnormal human haemoglobins. V. Chemical investigation of haemoglobins A, G, C, X from one individual. Biochim. Biophys. Acta 48:253, 1961.
83. Chernoff, A. I., and Pettit, N., Jr.: The amino acid composition of hemoglobin. VI. Separation of the tryptic peptides of hemoglobin Knoxville No. 1 on Dowex-1 X-2 and Sephadex. Biochim. Biophys. Acta 97:47, 1965.
84. Bowman, B., Barnett, D. R., Hodgkinson, K. T., and Schneider, R. G.: Chemical characterization of haemoglobin G St-1. Nature 211:1305, 1966.
85. Minnich, V., Cordonnier, J. K., Williams, W. J., and Moore, C. V.: Alpha, beta and gamma hemoglobin polypeptide chains during the neonatal period with description of a fetal form of hemoglobin D St. Louis. Blood 19:137, 1962.
86. Dance, N., Huehns, E. R., and Shooter, E. M.: The chemical investigation of haemoglobin G Bristol and G Bristol/C. Biochim. Biophys. Acta 86:144, 1964.
87. Colombo, B., Vidal, H., Kamuzora, H., and Lehmann, H.: A new haemoglobin J-Habana α71 (E20) Alanine→Glutamic acid. Biochim. Biophys. Acta 351:1, 1974.
88. Rahbar, S., Nowzari, G., and Daneshmand, P.: Hemoglobin Daneskgah-Tehran α2 72 (EF1) Histidine→Arginine β2A. Nature [New Biol.] 245:268, 1973.
89. Blackwell, R. Q., and Liu, C.-S.: Hemoglobin G Taichung: α74 Asp→His. Biochim. Biophys. Acta 200:70, 1970.
90. Pootrakul, S., and Dixon, G. H.: Hemoglobin Mahidol: A new hemoglobin α-chain mutant. Can. J. Biochem. 48:1066, 1970.
91. Lorkin, P. A., Charlesworth, D., Lehmann, H., Rahbar, S., Tuchinda, S., and Lie-Injo, L. E.: Two haemoglobins Q, α74 (EF3) and α75 (EF4) Aspartic acid→Histidine. Br. J. Haematol. 19:117, 1970.
92. Orringer, E. P., Wilson, J. B., and Huisman, T. H. J.: Hemoglobin Chapel Hill or α2 74 Asp→Gly β2. FEBS Lett. 65:297, 1976.
93. Djoumessi, S., Rousseaux, J., Descamps, J., Goudemand, M., and Dautrevaux, M.: Hemoglobin Lille, α2 [74(EF3) Asp→Ala] β2. Hemoglobin 5:475, 1981.
94. Liang, C.-C., Chen, S.-S., Jia, P.-C., Wang, L.-F., Luo, H.-Y., Liu, G.-Y., Liang, S., Lung, G.-F., Yu, C.-M., Zhuang, L-Z., Liang, B.-L., and Tang, Z.-N.: Hemoglobin Duan, α75(EF4) Asp→Ala, a new variant found in China. Hemoglobin 5:481, 1981.
95. Vella, F., Wiltshire, B., Lehmann, H., and Galbraith, P.: Hemoglobin Winnipeg α2 75 Asp→Tyr β2. Clin. Biochem. 6:66, 1973.
96. Ohba, Y., Miyaji, T., Matsuoka, M., Takeda, I., Fukuba, Y., Shibata, S., and Ohkura, K.: Hemoglobin Matsue-Oki: alpha 75 (EF4) Aspartic acid→Asparagine. Hemoglobin 1:383, 1977.
97. Iuchi, I., Shimasaki, S., Hidaka, K., Harano, T., Ueda, S., Shibata, S., Mizushima, J., and Kubo, N.: Hemoglobin Mizushi (α75[EF4] Asp→Gly): A new hemoglobin variant observed in a Japanese family. Hemoglobin 4:209, 1980.
98. Shibata, S., Ueda, S., Miyaji, T., and Imamura, T.: Hemoglobinopathies in Japan. Hemoglobin 5:509, 1981.
98a. Liang, C.-C., Xiong, F., Yang, K., Chen, S., Jia, P., Zhang, M., and Zhao, Z.: Hemoglobin GuiZhou or α2 77(EF6)Pro→Arg β2, a new slow-moving hemoglobin variant observed in China. Hemoglobin 8:387, 1984.
99. Van Ros, G., Beale, D., and Lehmann, H.: Haemoglobin Stanleyville-II (α78 Asparagine replaced by Lysine). Br. Med. J. 4:92, 1968.
99a. Wong, S. C., Ali, M. A. M., Pond, J. R., Rubin, S. M., Johnson, S. E. N., Wilson, J. B., and Huisman, T. H. J.: Hb J-Singha (α78 Asn→Asp), a newly discovered hemoglobin variant with the same amino acid substitution as one of the two present in Hb J-Singapore (α78 Asn→Asp, α79 Ala→Gly). Biochim. Biophys. Acta 784:187, 1984.
100. Rucknagel, D. L., Brandt, N. J., and Spencer, H. H.: α-Chain mutants of human hemoglobin contributing to the genetics of the α-chain locus. Proceedings of the 1st Inter-American Symposium on Hemoglobins, Caracas, 1969.
101. Adams, J. G., III, Winter, W. P., Rucknagel, D. L., and Spencer, H. H.: Biosynthesis of hemoglobin Ann Arbor: Evidence for catabolic and feedback regulation. Science 176:1427, 1972.
102. Honig, G. R., Shamsuddin, M., Tremaine, L. M., Mason, R. G., Vida, L. N., Sarnwick, R., and Shahidi, N. T.: Hemoglobin Nigeria (α81 Ser→Cys), a new variant having an inhibitory effect on the gelation of sickle hemoglobin. Blood 52(Suppl. 1):113, 1978.
103. Winter, W. P., Rucknagel, D. L., and Fielding, J.: Identification of several rare hemoglobin variants discovered in a population survey, including a new variant Hb Garden State, α82 Ala→Asp. Clin. Res. 26:22A, 1978.
104. Crookston, J. H., Farquharson, H. A., Beale, D., and Lehmann, H.: Hemoglobin Etobicoke: α84 (F5) Serine replaced by Arginine. Can. J. Biochem. 47:143, 1969.
105. Huehns, E. R.: The unstable hemoglobins. Bull. Soc. Chem. Biol. 52:1131, 1970.
106. Lorkin, P. A., Huntsman, R. G., Ager, J. A. M., Lehmann, H., Vella, F., and Darbre, P. D.: Haemoglobin G Norfolk: α85 (F6) Asp→Asn. Biochim. Biophys. Acta 379:22, 1975.
107. Cohen-Solal, M., Manasse, B., Thillet, J., and Rosa, J.: Haemoglobin G Norfolk α85 (F6) Asp→Asn. Structural characterization by sequenator analysis and functional properties of a new variant with high oxygen affinity. FEBS Lett. 50:163, 1975.
108. Fujiwara, N., Maekawa, T., and Matsuda, G.: Hemoglobin Atago (α2 85 Tyr β2), a new abnormal human hemoglobin found in Nagasaki. Int. J. Protein Res. 3:35, 1971.
109. Reed, R. E., Winter, W. P., and Rucknagel, D. L.: Haemoglobin Inkster (α2 85 Aspartic acid→Valine

β2) coexisting with β-thalassemia in a Caucasian family. Br. J. Haemalol. 26:475, 1974.
110. Knuth, A., Pribilla, W., Marti, H. R., and Winterhalter, K. H.: Hemoglobin Moabit: Alpha 86 (F7) Leu→Arg. A new unstable abnormal hemoglobin. Acta Haematol. 61:121, 1979.
111. Miyaji, T., Iuchi, I., Shibata, S., Takeda, I., and Tamura, A.: Possible amino acid substitution in the α-chain (α87 Tyr) of Hb M Iwate. Acta Haematol. Jpn. 26:538, 1963.
112. Heller, P., Weinstein, H. G., Yakulis, V. J., and Rosenthal, I. M.: Hemoglobin M Kankakee, a new variant of hemoglobin M. Blood 20:287, 1962.
113. Pik, C., and Tönz, O.: Nature of haemoglobin M Oldenburg. Nature 210:1182, 1966.
114. Ohba, Y., Miyaji, T., Hattori, Y., Fuyuno, K., and Matsuoka, M.: Unstable hemoglobins in Japan. Hemoglobin 4:307, 1980.
115. De Traverse, P. M., Lehmann, H., Coquelet, M. L., Beale, D., and Isaacs, W. A.: Étude d'une hémoglobine J α non encore décrite, dans une famille française. Compt. R. Scéanc. Soc. Biol. 160:2270, 1966.
116. Vella, F., Charlesworth, D., Lorkin, P. A., and Lehmann, H.: Hemoglobin Broussais, α90 Lys→Asn. Can. J. Biochem. 48:908, 1970.
117. Braconnier, F., Cohen-Solal, M., Schlegel, N., Blouquit, Y., Thillet, J., Cassius De Linval, J., and Rosa, J.: Hemoglobin J Broussais α2 90 Lys→Asn β2A (FG2), découverte dans une famille Martiniquaise. Nouv. Rev. Fr. Hematol. 15:333, 1975.
117a. Harano, T., Harano, K., Shibata, S., Ueda, S., Imai, K., and Seki, M.: Hb Handa (α90 (FG 2) Lys–Met): Structure and biosynthesis of a new slightly higher oxygen affinity variant. Hemoglobin 6:379, 1982.
118. Hyde, R. D., Kinderlerer, J. L., Lehmann, H., and Hall, M. D.: Haemoglobin J Rajappen: α90 (FG2) Lys→Thr. Biochim. Biophys. Acta 243:515, 1971.
119. Brennan, S. O., Tauro, G. P., Melrose, W., and Carrell, R. W.: Haemoglobin Port Phillip α91 (FG3) Leu→Pro. A new unstable haemoglobin. FEBS Lett. 81:115, 1977.
120. Botha, M. C., Beale, D., Isaacs, W. A., and Lehmann, H.: Haemoglobin J Cape Town α2 92 Arginine→Glutamine β2. Nature 212:792, 1966.
121. Lines, J. G., and McIntosh, R.: Oxygen binding by haemoglobin J Cape Town (α2 92 Arg→Gln). Nature 215:297, 1967.
122. Clegg, J. B., Naughton, M. A., and Weatherall, D. J.: Abnormal human haemoglobins. Separation and characterization of the α and β chains by chromatography, and the determination of two new variants, Hb Chesapeake and Hb J (Bangkok). J. Mol. Biol. 19:91, 1966.
123. Charache, S., Weatherall, D. J., and Clegg, J. B.: Polycythemia associated with a hemoglobinopathy. J. Clin. Invest. 45:813, 1966.
124. Wajcman, H., Belkhodja, O., and Labie, D.: Hb Setif: G1 (94) αAsp→Tyr. A new α chain hemoglobin variant with substitution of the residue involved in a hydrogen bond between unlike subunits. FEBS Lett. 27:298, 1972.
125. Schneider, R. G., Atkins, R. J., Hosty, T. S., Tomlin, G., Casey, R., Lehmann, H., Lorkin, P. A., and Nagai, K.: Haemoglobin Titusville: α94 Asp→Asn, a new haemoglobin with a lowered affinity for oxygen. Biochim. Biophys. Acta 400:365, 1975.
126. Schroeder, W. A., Shelton, J. B., Shelton, J. R., and Powars, D.: Hemoglobin Sunshine Seth—α2 (94(G1) Asp→His) β2. Hemoglobin 3:145, 1979.
127. Huisman, T. H. J., Adams, H. R., Wilson, J. B., Efremov, G. D., Reynolds, G. A., and Wrightstone, R. N.: Hemoglobin G Georgia or α2 95 Leu (G2) β2. Biochim. Biophys. Acta 200:578, 1970.
128. Smith, L. L., Plese, C. L., Barton, B. P., Charache, S., Wilson, J. B., and Huisman, T. H. J.: Subunit dissociation of the abnormal hemoglobin G Georgia (α2 95 Leu (G2) β2) and Rampa (α2 95 Ser (G2) β2). J. Biol. Chem. 247:1433, 1972.
129. DeJong, W. W. W., Bernini, L. F., and Meera Khan, P.: Haemoglobin Rampa: α95 Pro→Ser. Biochim. Biophys. Acta 236:197, 1971.
130. Wiltshire, B. G., Clark, K. G. A., Lorkin, P. A., and Lehmann, H.: Haemoglobin Denmark Hill α95 (G2) Pro→Ala, a variant with unusual electrophoretic and oxygen binding properties. Biochim. Biophys. Acta 278:459, 1972.
131. Bannister, W. H., Grech, J. L., Plese, C. F., Smith, L. L., Barton, B. P., Wilson, J. B., Reynolds, C. A., and Huisman, T. H. J.: Hemoglobin St. Luke's or α2 95 Arg (G2) β2. Eur. J. Biochem. 29:301, 1972.
131a. Dysert, P. A., Head, C. G., Shih, T. B., Jones, R. T., and Schneider, R. G.: Hb Dallas α₂97(G4) Asn→Lysβ₂. A new abnormal hemoglobin with high oxygen affinity. Blood 60(Suppl. 1):53A, 1982.
132. Crookston, J. H., Farquharson, H. A., Kinderlerer, J. L., and Lehmann, H.: Hemoglobin Manitoba: α102 (G9) Serine replaced by Arginine. Can. J. Biochem. 48:911, 1970.
132a. Sciarratta, G. V., Ivaldi, G., Parodi, M. I., Sansone, G., Molaro, G. L., Salkie, M. L., Wilson, J. B., Reese, A. L., and Huisman, T. H. J.: The characterization of hemoglobin Manitoba or α₂ 102 (G9) Ser→Arg β₂ and hemoglobin Contaldo or α₂ 103 (G10) His→Arg β₂ by high performance liquid chromatography. Hemoglobin 8:169, 1984.
133. Sanguansermsri, T., Matragoon, S., Changloah, L., and Flatz, G.: Hemoglobin Suan-Dok (α₂ 109 (G16) Leu→Arg β₂): An unstable variant associated with alpha-thalassemia. Hemoglobin 3:161, 1979.
134. Honig, G. R., Shamsuddin, M., Zaizov, R., Steinherz, M., Solar, I., and Kirschmann, C.: Hemoglobin Petah Tikva (α110 Ala→Asp): A new unstable variant with α-thalassemia-like expression. Blood 57:705, 1981.
135. Charache, S., Ostertag, W., and Van Ehrenstein, G.: Clinical studies and physiological properties of Hopkins 2 haemoglobin. Nature [New Biol.] 237:88, 1972.
136. Clegg, J. B., and Charache, S.: The structure of hemoglobin Hopkins-2. Hemoglobin 2:85, 1978.
137. Niazi, G. A., Efremov, G. D., Nikolov, N., Hunter, E., Jr., and Huisman, T. H. J.: Hemoglobin Strumica or α2 112(G19) His→Arg β2. (With an addendum: Hemoglobin J Paris-I α2 12(A10) Ala→Asp β2 in the same population.) Biochim. Biophys. Acta 412:181, 1975.
138. Beksedic, D., Rajevska, T., Lorkin, P. A., and Lehmann, H.: Hb Serbia (α112(G19) His→Arg), a new haemoglobin variant from Yugoslavia. FEBS Lett. 58:226, 1975.
138a. Guis, M., Mentzer, W. C., Jue, D. L., Johnson, M. H., McGuffey, J. E., and Moo-Penn, W. F.: Hemoglobin Twin Peaks α113 (GH1) Leu→His. Hemoglobin 9:175, 1985.
139. Gajdusek, D. C., Guiart, J., Kirk, R. L., Carrell,

R. W., Irvine, D., Kynoch, P. A. M., and Lehmann, H.: Haemoglobin J Tongariki (α115 Alanine→Aspartic acid): The first new haemoglobin variant found in a Pacific (Melanesian) population. J. Med. Genet. *4*:1, 1967.
140. Abramson, R. K., Rucknagel, D. L., Shreffler, D. C., and Seave, J. J.: Homozygous Hb J Tongariki: Evidence for only one alpha chain structural locus in Melanesians. Science *169*:194, 1970.
141. Old, J. M., Clegg, J. B., Weatherall, D. J., and Booth, P. B.: Haemoglobin J Tongariki is associated with α thalassemia. Nature *273*:319, 1978.
142. Baglioni, C., and Lehmann, H.: Chemical heterogeneity of haemoglobin. O. Nature *196*:229, 1962.
143. Lie-Injo, L. E., and Sadono: Haemoglobin O (Buginese X) in Sulawesi. Br. Med. J. *1*:1461, 1958.
144. Sansone, G., Centa, A., Sciarratta, V., Gallo, E., and Lehmann, H.: Haemoglobin O Indonesia (α116 Glu→Lys) in an Italian family. Acta Haematol. *43*:40, 1970.
145. Ohba, Y., Miyaji, T., Matsuoka, M., Morito, M., and Iuchi, I.: Characterization of Hb Ube-4: Alpha 116 (GH4) Glu→Ala. Hemoglobin *2*:181, 1978.
146. Schneider, R. G., Hightower, B., Carpentieri, U., Duerst, M. L., Shih, T. B., and Jones, R. T.: Hb Oleander [α116(GH4) Glu→Gln]: Structural and functional characterization. International Society of Haematology, European and African Division, Sixth Meeting, Athens, Greece, August 30–September 4, 1981.
147. Blackwell, R. Q., Wong Hock Boon, Wang, C.-L., Weng, M.-I., and Liu, C.-S.: Hemoglobin J Meerut: α120 Ala→Glu. Biochim. Biophys. Acta *351*:7, 1974.
148. Kamuzora, H., Lehmann, H., Griffiths, K. D., Mann, J. R., and Raine, D. N.: A new haemoglobin variant—hemoglobin J Birmingham, α120 (H3) Ala→Glu. Ann. Clin. Biochem. *11*:53, 1974.
149. Fleming, P. J., Hughes, W. G., Farmilo, R. K., Wyatt, K., and Cooper, W. N.: Hemoglobin Westmead α2 122(H5) His→Gln β2: A new hemoglobin variant with the substitution in the α1β1 contact area. Hemoglobin *4*:39, 1980.
149a. Goossens, M., Lee, K. Y., Liebhaber, S. A., and Kan, Y. W.: Globin structural mutant α125 Leu—Pro is a novel cause of α-thalassemia. Nature *296*:864, 1982.
149b. Liebhaber, S. A., and Kan, Y. W.: Alpha-thalassemia caused by an unstable alpha-globin mutant. J. Clin. Invest. *71*:461, 1983.
150. Moo-Penn, W. F., Jue, D. L., Johnson, M. H., Wilson, S. M., Therrel, B., Jr., and Schmidt, R. M.: Hemoglobin Tarrant: α126 (H9) Asp→Asn. A new hemoglobin variant in the α1β1 contact region showing high oxygen affinity and reduced cooperativity. Biochim. Biophys. Acta *490*:443, 1977.
151. Vella, F., Galbraith, P., Wilson, J. B., Wong, S. C., Folger, G. C., and Huisman, T. H. J.: Hemoglobin St. Claude or α2 127 (H10) Lys→Thr β2. Biochim. Biophys. Acta *365*:318, 1974.
152. Moo-Penn, W. F., Bechtel, K. C., Johnson, M. H., Jue, D. L., Holland, S., Huff, C., and Schmidt, R. M.: Hemoglobin Jackson, α127 (H10) Lys→Asn. Am. J. Clin. Pathol. *66*:453, 1976.
153. Kleihauer, E. F., Reynolds, C. A., Dozy, A. M., Wilson, J. B., Moores, R. R., Berenson, M. P., Wright, C.-S., and Huisman, T. H. J.: Hemoglobin Bibba or α2 136 Pro β2, an unstable alpha-chain abnormal hemoglobin. Biochim. Biophys. Acta *154*:220, 1968.
153a. Harano, T., Harano, K., Shibata, S., Ueda, S., Imai, K., and Seki, M.: Hemoglobin Tokoname [α139 (HC 1) Lys→Thr]: A new hemoglobin variant with a slightly increased oxygen affinity. Hemoglobin *7*:85, 1983.
154. Clegg, J. B., Weatherall, D. J., Wong Hock Boon, and Mustafa, D.: Two new haemoglobin variants involving proline substitutions. Nature *222*:379, 1969.
155. Poyart, C., Krishnamoorthy, R., Bursaux, E., Gacon, G., and Labie, D.: Structural and functional studies of haemoglobin Suresnes or α2141 (HC3) Arg→His β2, a new high oxygen affinity mutant. FEBS Lett. *69*:103, 1976.
156. Saenz, G. F., Elizondo, J., Alvarado, M. A., Atmetlla, F., Arroys, G., Martinez, G., Lima, F., and Columbo, B.: Chemical characterization of a new haemoglobin variant, haemoglobin J Cubujuqui (α2 141 (HC3) Arg→Ser β2). Biochim. Biophys. Acta *494*:48, 1977.
157. Mavilio, F., Marinucci, M., Tentori, L., Fontanarosa, P. P., Rossi, U., and Biagiotti, S.: Hemoglobin Legnano (α2 141 (HC3) Arg→Leu β2): A new abnormal hemoglobin with high oxygen affinity. Hemoglobin *2*:249, 1978.
158. Martinez, G., Lima, F., Residenti, C., and Columbo, B.: Hb J Camagüey α2 141 (HC3) Arg→Gly β2. A new abnormal human hemoglobin. Hemoglobin *2*:47, 1978.
159. Moo-Penn, W. F., Bechtel, K. C., Schmidt, R. M., Johnson, M. H., Jue, D. L., Schmidt, D. E., Jr., Dunlap, W. M., Opella, S. J., Bonaventura, J., and Bonaventura, C.: Hemoglobin Raleigh (β1 Valine→Acetylalanine). Structural and functional characterization. Biochemistry *16*:4872, 1977.
160. Labossiere, A., Vella, F., Hiebert, J., and Galbraith, P.: Hemoglobin Deer Lodge: α2β2 2 His→Arg. Clin. Biochem. *5*:46, 1972.
160a. Harano, T., Harano, K., Shibata, S., Ueda, S., Mori, H., and Arimasa, N.: Hemoglobin Okayama [β2(NA2) His→Gln]: A new "silent" hemoglobin variant with substituted amino acid residue at the 2,3-diphosphoglycerate binding site. FEBS Lett. *156*:20, 1983.
160b. Blouquit, Y., Lena-Russo, D., Delanoe, J., Arous, N., Bardakjian, J., Lancombe, C., Orsini, A., Rosa, J., and Galacteros, F.: Hb Marseille α2ᴬ β2 1(A1) NH→Met, 2(A2) His→3(A3) Pro: First variant having a N-terminal elongated β chain. (Abstract.) Blood, *64*(Suppl. 1):55a, 1984.
160c. Wilson, C. I. D., Cave, R. J., Lehmann, H., Close, M., and Imai, K.: Haemoglobin Warwickshire (β5[A2]Pro→Arg): A possible "fine tuning" of 2,3-DPG affinity by β5 Pro. FEBS Lett. *176*:331, 1984.
160d. Broissel, J.-P., Kasper, T., Shah, S., Malone, T., and Bunn, H. F.: NH2-terminal processing of protein: Hb South Florida. Proc. Natl. Acad. Sci. USA, in press.
161. Ingram, V. M.: Abnormal human haemoglobins. III. The chemical difference between normal and sickle cell haemoglobins. Biochim. Biophys. Acta *36*:402, 1959.
162. Hunt, J. A., and Ingram, V. M.: Abnormal human haemoglobins. IV. The chemical difference between normal human haemoglobin and haemoglobin C. Biochim. Biophys. Acta *42*:409, 1960.
163. Blackwell, R. Q., Oemijati, S., Pribadi, W., Weng, M.-I., and Liu, C.-S.: Hemoglobin G Makassar: β6 Glu→Ala. Biochim. Biophys. Acta *214*:396, 1970.

163a. Harano, T., Harano, K., Ueda, S., Shibata, S., Imai, K., and Seki, M.: Hemoglobin Machida (β6(A3)Glu→Gln), a new abnormal hemoglobin discovered in a Japanese family: Structure, function and biosynthesis. Hemoglobin 6:531, 1982.
164. Hill, R. L., Swenson, R. T., and Schwartz, H. C.: Characterization of a chemical abnormality in hemoglobin G. J. Biol. Chem. 235:3182, 1960.
165. Tuchinda, S., Beale, D., and Lehmann, H.: A new haemoglobin in a Thai family. A case of haemoglobin Siriraj-β thalassaemia. Br. Med. J. 1:1583, 1965.
166. Blackwell, R. Q., Liu, C.-S., and Wang, C.-L.: Haemoglobin Siriraj β-7 (AA) Glu→Lys in a Chinese subject in Taiwan. Vox Sang 23:433, 1972.
166a. Moo-Penn, W. F., Bechtel, M. H., McGuffey, J. E., Jue, D. L., Therrell, B. L., Jr.: Hemoglobin Rio Grande (β8 (A5)Lys–Thr): A new variant found in a Mexican-American family. Hemoglobin 7:91, 1983.
166b. Cai Yin Lin, Wang, He Be, et al.: A new fast-moving hemoglobin variant, Hb J Luki β8 (A5) Lys→Gln. Chin. Hematol. J. 3:263–265, 1982.
167. Bonaventura, J., and Riggs, A.: Polymerization of hemoglobins of mouse and man. Structural basis. Science 158:800, 1967.
168. Tondo, C. V., Bonaventura, J., Bonaventura, C., Brunori, M., and Antonini, E.: Functional properties of hemoglobin Porto Alegre ($\alpha^A_2\beta^9_2$Ser→Cys) and the reactivity of its extra cysteinyl residue. Biochim. Biophys. Acta 342:15–20, 1974.
169. Arcasoy, A., Casey, R., Lehmann, H., Cavdar, A. O., and Berki, A.: A new haemoglobin J from Turkey—Hb Ankara (β10 (A7) Ala→Asp). FEBS Lett. 42:121, 1974.
169a. Wong, S. C., Ali, M. A. M., Lam, H., Webber, B. B., Wilson, J. B., and Huisman, T. H. J.: Hemoglobin Hamilton or $\alpha_2\beta_2$11(A8)Val→Ile, a silent β-chain variant detected by triton X-100 acid-urea polyacrylamide gel electrophoresis. Am. J. Hematol. 16:47, 1984.
169b. Djoumessi, S., Rousseaux, J., and Dautrevaux, M.: Structural studies of a new hemoglobin: Hb J Lens, β13 (A10) Ala→Asp. FEBS Lett. 136:145, 1981.
170. Monn, E., Gaffney, P. J., and Lehmann, H.: Haemoglobin Sogn (β14 Arginine). A new haemoglobin variant. Scand. J. Haematol. 5:353, 1968.
171. Beuzard, Y., Basset, P., Braconnier, F., El Gammel, H., Martin, L., Oudard, J. L., and Thillet, J.: Haemoglobin Saki $\alpha_2\beta_2$ 14 Leu→Pro (A11) structure and function. Biochim. Biophys. Acta 393:182, 1975.
172. Milner, P. F., Corley C. C., Pomeroy, W. L., Wilson, J. B., Gravely, M., and Huisman, T. H. J.: Thalassemia intermedia caused by heterozygosity for both β-thalassemia and hemoglobin Saki (β14 (A11) Leu→Pro). Am. J. Hematol. 1:283, 1976.
173. Kennedy, C. C., Blundell, G., Lorkin, P. A., Lang, A., and Lehmann, H.: Haemoglobin Belfast 15 (A12) Tryptophan→Arginine: A new unstable haemoglobin variant. Br. Med. J. 4:324, 1974.
174. Gacon, G., Wajcman, H., Labie, D., Varet, B., and Christoforov, B.: A second case of haemoglobin Belfast (β15[A12]Trp→Arg) observed in a French patient. Acta Haematol. 55:313, 1976.
175. Baglioni, C., and Weatherall, D. J.: Abnormal human hemoglobins. IX. Chemistry of hemoglobin J Baltimore. Biochim. Biophys. Acta 78:637, 1963.
176. Weatherall, D. J.: Hemoglobin J (Baltimore) coexisting in a family with hemoglobin S. Johns Hopkins Hosp. Bull. 114:1, 1964.
177. Chernoff, A. I., and Perillie, P. E.: The amino acid composition of Hgb New Haven #2 (Hgb N New Haven). Biochem. Biophys. Res. Commun. 16:368, 1964.
178. Wong, S. C., Bouver, N., Wilson, J. B., and Huisman, T. H. J.: Hb J Georgia = Hb J Baltimore = $\alpha_2\beta_2$16Gly→Asp. Clin. Chim. Acta 35:521, 1971.
179. de Jong, W. W. W., and Wert, L. N.: Haemoglobin J Baltimore and haemoglobin D Punjab in two Dutch families. Acta Genet. (Basel) 18:429, 1968.
180. Wade, P. T., Jenkins, T., and Huehns, E. R.: Haemoglobin variant in a Bushman: Haemoglobin D α Bushman β22 16Gly→Arg. Nature 216:688, 1967.
181. Maekawa, M., Maekawa, T., Fujiwara, N., Tabara, K., and Matsuda, G.: Hemoglobin Nagasaki: $\alpha A2\beta 2$ 17 Glu. A new abnormal human hemoglobin found in one family in Nagasaki. Int. J. Protein Res. 2:147, 1970.
182. Elion, J., Belkhodja, O., Wajcman, H., and Labie, D.: Two variants of hemoglobin D in the Algerian population: Hemoglobin D Ouled Rabah β19 (B1) Asn→Lys and hemoglobin D Iran β22 (B4) Glu→Gln. Biochim. Biophys. Acta 310:360, 1973.
183. Mauran-Sendvail, A., Lefevre-Witier, P., Lehmann, H., and Casey, R.: Haemoglobin D Ouled Rabah (β19 (B1) Asn→Lys) in a Tuareg tribe of the southern Sahara. J. Med. Genet. 14:245, 1977.
184. Lam, H., Wilson, J. B., Harris, H., Gravely, M., and Huisman, T. H. J.: Hemoglobin Alamo [$\alpha_2\beta_2$ 19 (B1) Asn→Asp]. Hemoglobin 1:703, 1977.
185. Stamatoyannopoulos, G., Nute, P. E., Adamson, J. W., Bellingham, A. J., Funk, D., and Hornung, S.: Hemoglobin Olympia (β20 Valine→Methionine): An electrophoretically silent variant associated with high oxygen affinity and erythrocytosis. J. Clin. Invest. 52:342, 1973.
186. Harano, T., Harano, K., Ueda, S., Shibata, S., and Iuchi, I.: Hemoglobin Yusa (β21 (B3) Asp→Tyr), a new abnormal hemoglobin found in Japan. Hemoglobin 5:121, 1981.
186a. Boissel, J.-P., Wajcman, H., Fabritius, H., Cabannes, R., and Labie, D.: Application of high-performance liquid chromatography to abnormal hemoglobin studies. Biochim. Biophys. Acta 670:203, 1981.
187. Moo-Penn, W. F., McPhedran, P., Bobrow, S., Johnson, M. H., Jue, D. L., and Olsen, K. W.: Hemoglobin Connecticut (β21 (B3) Asp→Gly): A hemoglobin variant with low oxygen affinity. Am. J. Hematol. 11:137, 1981.
188. Vella, F., Lorkin, P. A., Carrell, R. W., and Lehmann, H.: A new hemoglobin variant resembling hemoglobin E. Hemoglobin E Saskatoon: β22 Glu→Lys. Can. J. Biochem. 45:1385, 1967.
189. Eng, A. C., Vella, F., and Merry, C. C.: Two possible instances of hemoglobin E Saskatoon in Manitoba. Can. J. Biochem. 48:45, 1970.
190. Vella, F., Labossiere, A., Wiltshire, B., Lehmann, H., Shojania, A. M., and Hill, J. L.: The occurrence of hemoglobins E and E Saskatoon in Central Canada. Am. J. Clin. Pathol. 60:314, 1973.
191. Blackwell, R. Q., Yang, H. J., and Wang, C. C.: Hemoglobin G Taipei: $\alpha_2\beta_2$ 22 Glu→Gly. Biochim. Biophys. Acta 175:237, 1969.
192. Vella, F., Isaacs, W. A., and Lehmann, H.: Hemo-

globin G Saskatoon: β22 Glu→Ala. Can. J. Biochem. 45:351, 1967.
193. Blackwell, R. Q., Liu, C. S., Yang, H. J., Wang, C. C., and Huang, J. T. H.: Hemoglobin variant common to Chinese and North American Indians: α2β2 22 Glu→Ala. Science 161:381, 1968.
194. Bowman, B. H., Barnett, D. R., and Hite, R.: Hemoglobin G Coushatta: A beta variant with a delta-like substitution. Biochem. Biophys. Res. Commun. 26:466, 1967.
195. Blackwell, R. Q., Ro, I. H., Liu, C. S., Yang, H. J., Wang, C. C., and Huang, J. T. H.: Hemoglobin variant found in Koreans, Chinese, and North American Indians. α2β2 22 Glu→Ala. Am. J. Phys. Anthropol. 30:389, 1969.
196. Rahbar, S.: Haemoglobin D Iran: 2 22 Glutamic acid leads to Glutamine (B4). Br. J. Haematol. 24:31, 1973.
197. Garel, M. C., Blouquit, Y., Arous, N., and Rosa, J.: Hb Strasbourg α2β2 20 (B2) Val→Asp: A variant at the same locus as Hb Olympia β20 Val→Met. FEBS Lett. 72:1, 1976.
198. Forget, B. G.: Nucleotide sequence of human globin messenger RNA. Hemoglobin 1:879, 1977.
198a. Nakatsuji, T., Miwa, S., Ohba, Y., Hattori, Y., Miyaji, T., Miyata, H., Shinohara, T., Hori, T., and Takayama, J.: Hemoglobin Miyashiro (β23 (B5) Val→Gly), an electrophoretically silent variant discovered by isopropanol test. Hemoglobin 5:653, 1981.
198b. Brennan, S. O., Williamson, D., Whisson, M. E., and Carrell, R. W.: Hemoglobin Palmerston North β23 (B5) Val–Phe. A new variant identified in a patient with polycythemia. Hemoglobin 6:569, 1982.
199. Ranney, H. M., Jacobs, A. S., Udem, L., and Zalusky, R.: Hemoglobin Riverdale-Bronx, an unstable hemoglobin resulting from the substitution of arginine for glycine at helical residue B6 of the β polypeptide chain. Biochim. Biophys. Acta 33:1004, 1968.
200. Huisman, T. H. J., Brown, A. K., Efremov, G. D., Wilson, J. B., Reynolds, C. A., Uy, R., and Smith, L. L.: Hemoglobin Savannah (B6(24)β-Glycine→Valine): An unstable variant causing anemia with inclusion bodies. J. Clin. Invest. 50:650, 1971.
201. Idelson, L. I., Didkowsky, N. A., Casey, R., Lorkin, P. A., and Lehmann, H.: New unstable haemoglobin (Hb Moscva, β24(B6) Gly→Asp) found in the U.S.S.R. Nature 249:768, 1974.
202. Blackwell, R. Q., and Liu, C.-S.: Hemoglobin G Taiwan-Ami α2β2 25 Gly→Arg. Biochem. Biophys. Res. Commun. 30:690, 1968.
203. Hunt, J. A., and Ingram, V. M.: Abnormal human haemoglobins. VI. The chemical difference between haemoglobins A and E. Biochim. Biophys. Acta 49:520, 1961.
204. Blouquit, Y., Arous, N., Machado, P. E. A., and Garel, M. C.: Hb Henri Mondor: β26 (B8) Glu→Val: A variant with a substitution localized at the same position as that of Hb E β 26 Glu→Lys. FEBS Lett. 72:5, 1976.
205. Idelson, L. I., Didkowsky, N. A., Filippova, A. V., Casey, R., Kynoch, P. A. M., and Lehmann, H.: Haemoglobin Volga, β27 (B9) Ala→Asp, a new highly unstable haemoglobin with a suppressed charge. FEBS Lett. 58:122, 1975.
206. Kuis-Reerink, J. D., Jonxis, J. H. P., Niazi, G. A., Wilson, J. B., Bolch, K. C., Gravely, M., and Huisman, T. H. J.: Hb Volga or α2β2 27(B9) Ala→Asp: An unstable hemoglobin variant in three generations of a Dutch family. Biochim. Biophys. Acta 439:63, 1976.
206a. Arous, N., Galacteros, F., Fessas, P. H., Loukopoulos, D., Blouquit, Y., Komis, G., and Sellaye, M., Boussiou, M., and Rosa, J.: Hemoglobin Knossos. β27 Ala→Ser (B9): A new hemoglobinopathy presenting as a silent β-thalassemia. Blood 60(Suppl. 1):51A, 1982.
206b. Arous, N., Galacteros, F., Fessas, P., Leukopoulos, D., Blouquit, Y., Komis, G., Sellaye, M., Boussiou, M., and Rosa, S.: Structural study of hemoglobin Knossos, β 27 (B9) Ala→Ser. A new abnormal hemoglobin present as a silent β-thalassemia. FEBS Lett. 147:247, 1982.
207. Cohen-Solal, M., Seligmann, M., Thillet, J., and Rosa, J.: Haemoglobin Saint Louis β28 (B10) Leucine→Glutamine. A new unstable haemoglobin only present in a ferri form. Abstract 408, XIV Intl. Cong. Hematol., São Paulo, 1972. FEBS Lett. 33:37, 1973.
208. Thillet, J., Cohen-Solal, M., Seligmann, M., and Rosa, J.: Functional and physicochemical studies of hemoglobin St. Louis β28 (B10) Leucine→Proline. Nature 214:877, 1967.
209. Sansone, G., Carrell, R. W., and Lehmann, H.: Haemoglobin Genova: β28 (B10) Leucine→Proline. Nature 214:877, 1967.
210. Shibata, S., Miyaji, T., and Ohba, Y.: Abnormal hemoglobins in Japan. Hemoglobin 4:395, 1980.
211. Schmidt, B., Bechtel, K. C., Johnson, M. H., Therrell, B. J., Jr., and Moo-Penn, W. F.: Hemoglobin Lufkin: β29(B11) Gly→Asp: An unstable hemoglobin variant involving an internal amino acid residue. Hemoglobin 1:799, 1977.
212. Brimhall, B., Jones, R. T., Baur, E. W., and Motulsky, A. G.: Structural characterization of hemoglobin Tacoma. Biochemistry 8:2125, 1969.
212a. Nakatsuji, T., Miwa, S., Ohba, Y., Hattori, Y., Miyaji, T., Hino, S., and Matsumoto, N.: A new unstable hemoglobin, Hb Yokohama β31 (B13) Leu→Pro, causing hemolytic anemia. Hemoglobin 5:667, 1981.
213. Jackson, J. M., Yates, A., and Huehns, E. R.: Haemoglobin Perth: β32 (B14) Leu→Pro. An unstable haemoglobin causing haemolysis. Br. J. Haematol. 25:607, 1973.
214. Honig, G. R., Green, D., Shamsuddin, M., Vida, L. N., Mason, R. G., Gnarra, D. J., and Maurer, H. S.: Hemoglobin Abraham Lincoln, β32(B14) Leucine→Proline. An unstable variant producing severe hemolytic disease. J. Clin. Invest. 52:1746, 1973.
215. Garel, M. C., Blouquit, Y., and Rosa, J.: Hemoglobin Castilla β32 (B14) Leu→Arg: A new unstable variant producing severe hemolytic disease. FEBS Lett. 58:145, 1975.
216. Blouquit, Y., Braconnier, F., Cohen-Solal, M., Foldi, J., Arous, N., Ankri, A., Binet, J. L., and Rosa, J.: Hemoglobin Pitie-Salpetriere β34(B16) Val→Phe, a new high oxygen affinity variant associated with familial erythrocytosis. Biochim. Biophys. Acta 624:473, 1980.
217. Rieder, R. F., Oski, F. A., and Clegg, J. B.: Hemoglobin Philly (β35 Tyrosine→Phenylalanine): Studies in the molecular pathology of hemoglobin. J. Clin. Invest. 48:1627, 1969.
217a. Jeppsson, J. O., Kallman, I., Lindgren, G., and

Fagerstan, L. G.: Hb Linkoping (Beta-36 Pro→Thr)—a new hemoglobin mutant characterized by reversed-phase high-performance liquid-chromatography. J. Chromatogr. *297*:31, 1984.
218. Yamaoka, K.: Hemoglobin Hirose: α1β2 37(C3) Tryptophan yielding Serine. Blood *38*:730, 1971.
219. Gacon, G., Belkhodja, O., Wajcman, H., and Labie, D.: Structural and functional studies of Hb Rothchild β37 (C3) Trp→Arg. A new variant of the α$_1$β$_2$ contact. FEBS Lett. *82*:243, 1977.
219a. Blouquit, Y., Delanoe-Garin, J., Lacombe, C., Arous, N., Cayre, Y., Peduzzi, J., Braconnier, F., and Galacteros, F.: Structural study of hemoglobin Hazebrouck, β38(C4)Thr→Pro: A new abnormal hemoglobin with instability and low oxygen affinity. FEBS Lett. *172*:155, 1984.
220. Brimhall, B., Jones, R. T., Schneider, R. G., Hosty, T. S., Tomlin, G., and Atkins, R.: Two new hemoglobins: Hemoglobin Alabama (β39 (C5) Gln→Lys) and hemoglobin Montgomery (α48 (CD6) Leu→Arg). Biochim. Biophys. Acta *379*:28, 1975.
221. Kendall, A. G., Pas, A. T., Wilson, J. B., Cope, N., Bolch, K., and Huisman, T. H. J.: Hb Vaasa or α2β2 (39)(C5) Gln→Glu), a mildly unstable variant found in a Finnish family. Hemoglobin *1*:292, 1977.
222. Brown, W. J., Niazi, G. A., Jayalakshmi, M., Abraham, E. C., and Huisman, T. H. J.: Hemoglobin Athens-Georgia, or α$_2$β$_2$ 40(C6) Arg→Lys, a hemoglobin variant with an increased oxygen affinity. Biochim. Biophys. Acta *439*:70, 1976.
223. Moo-Penn, W. F., Johnson, M. H., Bechtel, K. C., Jue, D. L., Therrell, B. L., and Schmidt, R. M.: Hemoglobins Austin and Waco: Two hemoglobins with substitutions in the α1β2 contact region. Arch. Biochem. Biophys. *179*:86, 1977.
224. Burkett, L. B., Sharma, V. S., Pisciotta, A. V., Ranney, H. M., and Bruckheimer, S.: Hemoglobin Mequon β41 (C7) Phenylalanine→Tyrosine. Blood *48*:645, 1976.
225. Dacie, J. V., Shinton, N. K., Gaffney, P. J., Jr., Carrell, R. W., and Lehmann, H.: Haemoglobin Hammersmith (β42(CD1) Phe→Ser). Nature *216*:663, 1967.
226. Ohba, Y., Miyaji, T., Matsuoka, M., Yamaguchi, K., Yonemitsu, H., Ishii, T., and Shibata, S.: Hemoglobin Chiba: Hb Hammersmith in a Japanese girl. Acta Haematol. Jpn. *38*:53, 1975.
227. Keeling, M. M. Ogdon, L. L., Wrightstone, R. N., Wilson, J. B., Reynolds, C. A., Kitchens, J. L., and Huisman, T. H. J.: Hemoglobin Louisville (β42(CD1)Phe→Leu): An unstable variant causing mild hemolytic anemia. J. Clin. Invest. *50*:2395, 1971.
228. Bratu, V., Lorkin, P. A., Lehmann, H., and Predescu, C.: Haemoglobin Bucuresti β42(CD1) Phe→Leu, a cause of unstable haemoglobin haemolytic anaemia. Biochim. Biophys. Acta *251*:1, 1971.
229. Bowman, B. H., Oliver, C. P., Barnett, D. R., Cunningham, J. R., and Schneider, R. G.: Chemical characterization of three hemoglobins G. Blood *23*:193, 1964.
230. Iuchi, I., Ueda, S., Hidaka, K., and Shibata, S.: Hemoglobin Hoshida (β43 (CD-2) Glu→Gln), a new hemoglobin variant discovered in Japan. Hemoglobin *2*:235, 1978.
230a. Adams, J. G., Morrison, W. T., Pullen, D. J., Abney, R. L., and Steinberg, M. H.: Hemoglobin Mississippi (MS): A new hemoglobin variant with three distinct electrophoretic mobilities. Clin. Res. *33*:603A, 1985.
230b. Jue, D. L., Yeager, A. M., Zinkham, W. H., and McGriffey, J. E.: Hemoglobin Cheverly: β45(CD4) Phe→Ser. A silent unstable variant associated with mild anemia. Abstract A4–2, ISH 6th meeting. Athens, Greece, August 1981.
231. Allan, N., Beale, D., Irvine, D., and Lehmann, H.: Three haemoglobins K: Nature *208*:658, 1965
231a. Chen, S. S., Webber, B. B., Wilson, J. B., and Huisman, T. H. J.: HB Gainesville-GA or α$_2$β$_2$46(CD5)Gly→Arg. Hemoglobin *9*:179, 1985.
232. Sick, K., Beale, D., Irvine, D., Lehmann, H., Goodall, P. T., and MacDougall, S.: Haemoglobin G Copenhagen and haemoglobin J Cambridge. Two new β-chain variants of haemoglobin A. Biochim. Biophys. Acta *140*:231, 1967.
233. Marinucci, M., Mavilio, F., Tentori, L., and Alberti, R.: Hemoglobin Gavello α$_2$β$_2$ 47 (CD6) Asp→Gly, a new hemoglobin variant from Polesine (Italy). Hemoglobin *1*:771, 1977.
234. Rahbar, S., Nowzari, G., and Ala, F.: Haemoglobin Avicenna (β47 (CD6) Asp→Ala), a new abnormal haemoglobin. Biochim. Biophys. Acta *576*:466, 1979.
234a. Marinucci, M., Boissel, J. P., Massa, A., Wajcman, H., Tentori, L., and Labie, D.: Hemoglobin Maputo: A new β-chain variant (α$_2$β$_2$47 (CD6) Asp→Tyr) in combination with Hb S identified by high performance liquid chromatography (HPLC). Hemoglobin *7*:423, 1983.
235. Charache, S., Brimhall, B., Milner, P., and Cobb, L.: Hemoglobin Okaloosa (β48(CD7) Leucine→Arginine). An unstable hemoglobin with decreased oxygen affinity. J. Clin. Invest. *52*:2858, 1973.
236. Labossiere, A., Hill, J. R. and Vella, F.: A new TP V hemoglobin variant: Hb Edmonton. Clin. Biochem. *4*:114, 1971.
237. Jones, R. T., Koler, R. D., Duerst, M. L., and Dhindsa, D. S.: Hemoglobin Willamette [α2β2 51 Pro→Arg (D2)]: A new abnormal human hemoglobin. Hemoglobin *1*:45, 1976.
238. Konotey-Ahulu, F. I. D., Kinderlerer, J. L., Lehmann, H., and Ringelhann, B.: Haemoglobin Osu-Christiansborg: A new β-chain variant of haemoglobin A (β52(D3) Aspartic acid→Asparagine) in combination with haemoglobin S. J. Med. Genet. *8*:302, 1971.
239. Beresford, C. H., Clegg, J. B., and Weatherall, D. J.: Haemoglobin Ocho Rios (β52(D3) Aspartic acid→Alanine); a new β-chain variant of haemoglobin A found in combination with haemoglobin S. J. Med. Genet. *9*:151, 1972.
240. Wilkinson, T., Brennan, S. O., Carrell, R. W., Wells, R. M., Como, P., and Kronenberg, H.: Hemoglobin Summer Hill β52 (D3) Asp→His, a new variant from Sydney, Australia. Hemoglobin *4*:185, 1980.
241. Clegg, J. B., Naughton, M. A., and Weatherall, D. J.: Abnormal human haemoglobins. Separation and characterization of the α and β chains by chromatography, and the determination of two new variants. J. Mol. Biol. *19*:91, 1966.
242. Blackwell, R. Q., and Liu, C-S.: The identical structural anomalies of hemoglobins J Meinung and J Korat. Biochem. Biophys. Res. Commun. *24*:732, 1966.
243. Blackwell, R. Q., Liu, C.-S., Lie-Injo, L. E. and

Pribadi, W.: Fast hemoglobin variant in Minahassan people of Sulawesi, Chinese and Thais: α2β2 56 Gly→Asp. Am. J. Phys. Anthropol. 32:147, 1970.
244. Rahbar, S., Nowzari, G., Haydari, H., and Daneshmand, P.: Haemoglobin Hamadan α2Aβ2 56 Glycine→Arginine (D7). Biochim. Biophys. Acta 379:645, 1975.
245. Giardina, B., Brunori, M., Antonini, E., and Tentori, L.; Properties of hemoglobin G Ferrara (β$_{57}$ (E1) Asn→Lys). Biochim. Biophys. Acta 534:1–6, 1978.
245a. Boissel, J. P., Wajcman, H., Labie, D., Fabritius, H., and Cabannes, R.: Hb J Daloa (β57 (E1) Asn–Asp): A new variant found in the Ivory Coast. Hemoglobin 6:433, 1982.
246. Marengo-Rowe, A. J., Lorkin, P. A., Gallo, E., and Lehmann, H.: Haemoglobin Dhofar—a new variant from Southern Arabia. Biochim. Biophys. Acta 168:58, 1968.
247. Boulton, F. E., Huntsman, R. G., Lehmann, H., Lorkin, P., and Romero Herrera, A.: Myoglobin variants. Br. J. Haematol. 20:671, 1971.
248. Blackwell, R. Q., Liu, C.-S., and Shih, T.-B.: Hemoglobin J Kaohsiung: β59 Lys→Thr. Biochim. Biophys. Acta 229:343, 1971.
249. Blackwell, R. Q., Jim, R. T. S., Liu, C.-S., Weng, M.-I., Wang, C.-L., and Shih, T.-B.: Fast hemoglobin variant found in Hawaiian-Chinese-Caucasian family in Hawaii and a Chinese subject in Taiwan. Vox Sang. 22:469, 1972.
250. Wajcman, H., Amegnizin, K. P. E., Belkhodja, O., and Labie, D.: Hemoglobin J Lome β59(E3) Lys→Asn. A new fast moving variant found in a Togolese. FEBS Lett. 84:372, 1977.
251. Kagimoto, T., Morino, Y., and Kishimoto, S.: A new hemoglobin variant Hb Yatsushiro α$^A_2$β$_2^{60}$ Val→Leu. Biochim. Biophys. Acta 532:195, 1978.
251a. Williamson, D., Brennan, S. O., Muir, H., and Carrell, R. W.: Hemoglobin Collingwood β60 (E4) Val→Ala, a new unstable hemoglobin. Hemoglobin 7:511, 1983.
252. Jones, R. T., Brimhall, B., Huehns, E. R., and Motulsky, A. G.: Structural characterization of hemoglobin N Seattle: α2Aβ2 61 Lys→Glu. Biochim. Biophys. Acta 154:278, 1968.
253. Shibata, S., Miyaji, T., Iuchi, I., Ueda, S., and Takeda, I.: Hemoglobin Hikari (α2Aβ2 61 AspNH2): A fast moving hemoglobin found in two unrelated Japanese families. Clin. Chim. Acta 10:101, 1964.
254. Marinucci, M., Giuliani, A., Maffi, D., Massa, A., Giampaolo, A., Mavilio, F., Zannotti, M., and Tentori, L.: Hemoglobin Bologna (α$_2$β$_2$ 61 (E5) Lys→Met), an abnormal human hemoglobin with low oxygen affinity. Biochim. Biophys. Acta 668:209, 1981.
255. Beutler, E., Lang, A., and Lehmann, H.: Hemoglobin Duarte: α2β2 62 (E6) Ala→Pro: A new unstable hemoglobin with increased oxygen affinity. Blood 43:527, 1974.
256. Muller, C. J., and Kingma, S.: Haemoglobin Zürich α2Aβ263 Arg. Biochim. Biophys. Acta 50:595, 1961.
257. Gerald, P. S., and Efron, M. L.: Chemical studies of several varieties of Hb M. Proc. Natl. Acad. Sci. USA 47:1758, 1961.
258. Shibata, S., Miyaji, T., Iuchi, I., and Ueda, S.: A comparative study of hemoglobin M Iwate and hemoglobin M Kurume by means of electrophoresis, chromatography and analysis of peptide chains. Acta Haematol. Jpn. 24:486, 1961.
259. Murawski, K., Szymanowska, Z., and Kozlowska, J.: A new variant of abnormal methaemoglobin: Hb M Radom. Biochim. Biophys. Acta 69:442, 1963.
260. Hobolth, N.: Haemoglobin Marhus: I. Clinical family study. Acta Paediatr. Scand. 54:357, 1965.
261. Josephson, A. M., Weinstein, H. G., Yakulis, V. J., Singer, L., and Heller, P.: A new variant of hemoglobin M disease: Hemoglobin M Chicago. J. Lab. Clin. Med. 59:918, 1962.
262. Betke, K., Gröschner, E., and Bock, K.: Properties of a further variant of haemoglobin M. Nature 188:864, 1960.
263. Hörlein, H., and Weber, G.: Über chronishe familiäre methämoglobinämie und eine neue modifikation des methämoglobins. Dtsch. Med. Wochenschr. 73:476, 1948.
264. Efremov, G. D., Huisman, T. H. J., Stanulovic, M., Zurovec, M., Duma, H., Wilson, J. B., and Jeremic, V.: Haemoglobin M Saskatoon and haemoglobin M Hyde Park in two Yugoslavian families. Scand. J. Haematol. 13:48, 1974.
265. Kohne, E., Grosze, H. P., Versmold, H., Kley, H. P., and Kleihauer, E.: Hb M Erlangen: α2β2 63 (E7) Tyr. Eine neue mutation mit hämolyse und diaphorasemangel. Kinderheilk 120:69, 1975.
266. Wajcman, H., Krishnamoorthy, R., Gacon, G., Elion, J., Allard, C., and Labie, D.: A new hemoglobin variant involving the distal histidine: Hb Bicetre (β63(E7) His→Pro). J. Mol. Med. 1:187, 1976.
267. Tentori, L.: Three examples of double heterozygosis beta-thalassemia and rare hemoglobin variants. Abstract 68. Intl. Symp. Abnormal Hemoglobin and Thalassemia. Istanbul, Turkey, 1974.
268. Ricco, G., Pich, P. G., Mazza, U., Rossi, G., Ajmar, F., Arese, P., and Gallo, E.: Hb J Sicilia: β65(E9) Lys→Asn, a beta homologue of Hb Zambia. FEBS Lett. 39:200, 1974.
269. Garel, M. C., Hassan, W., Coquelet, M. T., Goossens, M., and Rosa, J.: Hemoglobin J Cairo: β65(E9) Lys→Gln, a new hemoglobin variant discovered in an Egyptian family. Biochim. Biophys. Acta 420:97, 1976.
270. Rosa, J., Labie, D., Wajcman, H., Boigne, J. M., Cabannes, R., Bierme, R., and Ruffie, J.: Haemoglobin I Toulose: β66 (E10) Lys→Glu: A new abnormal haemoglobin with a mutation localized on the E10 porphyrin surrounding zones. Nature 223:190, 1969.
271. Steadman, J. H., Yates, A., and Huehns, E. R.: Idiopathic Heinz body anaemia: Hb-Bristol (β67(E11) Val→Asp). Br. J. Haematol. 18:435, 1970.
272. Carrell, R. W., Lehmann, H., Lorkin, P. A., Raik, E., and Hunter, E.: Haemoglobin Sydney: β67(E11) Valine→Alanine: An emerging pattern of unstable haemoglobins. Nature 215:626, 1967.
273. Ohba, Y., Miyaji, T., Matsuoka, M., Sugiyama, K., Suzuki, T., and Sugiura, T.: Hemoglobin Mizuho or beta 68(E12) Leucine→Proline, a new unstable variant associated with severe hemolytic anemia. Hemoglobin 1:467, 1977.
274. Brennan, S. O., Wells, R. M., Smith, H., and Carrell, R. W.: Hemoglobin Brisbane: β68 Leu→His. A new high oxygen affinity variant. Hemoglobin 5:325, 1981.
275. Rahbar, S., Winkler, K., Louis, J., Rea, C., Blume,

K., and Beutler, E.: Hemoglobin Great Lakes (β68[E12] Leucine→Histidine): A new high-affinity hemoglobin. Blood 58:813, 1981.
276. Salomon, H., Tatarski, I., Dance, N., Huehns, E. R., and Shooter, E. M.: A new hemoglobin variant found in a Beduin tribe: Hemoglobin "Rambam." Isr. J. Med. Sci., 1:836, 1965.
276a. Rahbar, S., Asmerom, Y., and Blume, K. G.: A silent hemoglobin variant detected by HPLC. Hemoglobin City of Hope β69 (E13) Gly→Ser. Hemoglobin 8:333,1984.
276b. Delanoe-Garin, J., Arous, N., Blouquit, Y., Hafsia, R., Bardakdjian, J., Lacombe, C., Rosa, J., and Galacteros, F.: Hemoglobin Kenitra $\alpha_2\beta_269$(E13)Gly→Arg. A new β variant of elevated expression associated with α-thalassemia, found in a Moroccan woman. Hemoglobin 9:1, 1985.
277. Kurachi, S., Hermodson, M., Hornung, S., and Stamatoyannopoulos, G.: Structure of haemoglobin Seattle. Nature [New Biol] 243:275, 1973.
278. Carrell, R. W., and Owen, M. C.: A new approach to haemoglobin variant identification. Haemoglobin Christchurch β71(E15) Phenylalanine→Serine. Biochim. Biophys. Acta 236:507, 1971.
279. Jones, R. T., Brimhall, B., Pootrakul, S., and Gray, G.: Hemoglobin Vancouver [$\alpha_2\beta_2$ 73(E17) Asp→Tyr]: Its structure and function. J. Mol. Evol. 9:37, 1976.
280. Konotey-Ahulu, F. I. D., Gallo, E., Lehmann, H., and Ringelhann, B.: Haemoglobin Korle-Bu (β73 Aspartic acid→Asparagine) showing one of the two amino acid substitutions of haemoglobin C Harlem. J. Med. Genet. 5:107, 1968.
281. Bio-Doku, F. S., Kinderlerer, J., and Lehmann, H.: Atlas of Protein Sequence and Structure 5:73, 1972.
282. Schneider, R. G., Hosty, T. S., Tomlin, G., Atkins, R., Brimhall, B., and Jones, R. T.: Hb Mobile [$\alpha_2\beta_2$ 73(E17) Asp→Val]: A new variant. Biochem. Genet. 13:411, 1975.
283. Rieder, R. F., Wolf, D. J., Clegg, J. B., and Lee, S. L.: Rapid post-synthetic destruction of unstable haemoglobin Bushwick. Nature 254:725, 1975.
284. White, J. M., Brain, M. C., Lorkin, P. A., Lehmann, H., and Smith, M.: Mild "unstable haemoglobin haemolytic anaemia" caused by haemoglobin Shepherds Bush (β74 (E18) Gly→Asp). Nature 225:939, 1970.
285. Hubbard, M., Winton, E. F., Lindeman, J. G., Dessauer, P. L., Wilson, J. B., Wrightstone, R. N., and Huisman, T. H. J.: Hemoglobin Atlanta or α2β2 75 Leu→Pro (E19): An unstable variant found in several members of a Caucasian family. Biochim. Biophys. Acta 386:538, 1975.
286. Johnson, C. S., Moyes, D., Schroeder, W. A., Shelton, J. B., Shelton, J. R., and Beutler, E.: Hemoglobin Pasadena, $\alpha_2\beta_2$ 75(E19) Leu→Arg: Identification by high performance liquid chromatography of a new unstable variant with increased oxygen affinity. Biochim. Biophys. Acta 623:360, 1980.
287. Romain, P. L., Schwartz, A. D., Shamsuddin, M., Adams, J. G., III, Mason, R. G., Vida, L. N., and Honig, G. R.: Hemoglobin J-Chicago (β76 (E20) Ala→Asp): A new hemoglobin variant resulting from a substitution of an external residue. Blood 45:387, 1975.
288. Rahbar, S., Beale, D., Isaacs, W. A., and Lehmann, H.: Abnormal haemoglobins in Iran. Observation of a new variant—Haemoglobin J Iran (α2β2 77 His→Arg). Br. Med. J. 1:674, 1967.
288a. Jen, P. C., Chen, L. C., Chen, P. F., Wong, Y., Chen, L. F., Guo, Y. Y., Chang, F. Q., Chow, Y. C., and Chiu, Y.: Hemoglobin Quin-Hai, β78 (EF2) Leu→Arg, a new abnormal hemoglobin found in Guangdong, China. Hemoglobin 7:407, 1983.
289. Blackwell, R. Q., Shih, T.-B., Wang, C.-L., and Liu, C.-S.: Hemoglobin C-Hsi-Tsou: β79 Asp→Gly. Biochim. Biophys. Acta 257:49, 1972.
290. Benesch, R., Edilji, R., and Benesch, R. E.: Oxygenation properties of hemoglobin variants with substitutions near the polyphosphate binding site. Biochim. Biophys. Acta 393:368, 1975.
291. Johnson, M. H., Jue, D. L., Patchen, L. C., Hartwig, E. C., Jr., Schneider, N. J., and Moo-Penn, W. F.: Hemoglobin Tampa: β79 (EF3) Aspartic acid→Tyrosine. Biochim. Biophys. Acta 623:119, 1980.
292. Blackwell, R. Q., Yang, H. T., and Wang, C. C.: Hemoglobin G-Szuhu: β80 Asn→Lys. Biochim. Biophys. Acta 188:59, 1969.
293. Kaufman, S., Leiba, H., Clejan, L., Wallis, K., Lorkin, P. A., and Lehmann, H.: Hemoglobin G-Szuhu, β80 Asn–Lys in the homozygous state in a patient with abetalipoproteinemia. Hum. Hered. 25:60, 1975.
294. Schneider, R. G., Hettig, R. A., Bilunos, M., and Brimhall, B.: Hemoglobin Baylor [α2β2 81 (EF5) Leu→Arg]—an unstable mutant with high oxygen affinity. Hemoglobin 1:85, 1976.
295. Moo-Penn, W. F., Jue, D. L., Bechtel, K. C., Johnson, M. H., Schmidt, R. M., McCurdy, P. R., Fox, J., Bonaventura, J., Sullivan, B., and Bonaventura, C.: Hemoglobin Providence. A human hemoglobin variant occurring in two forms in vivo. J. Biol. Chem. 251:7557, 1976.
296. Bonaventura, J., Bonaventura, C., Sullivan, B., Ferruzzi, G., McCurdy, P. R., Fox, J., and Moo-Penn, W. F.: Hemoglobin Providence. Functional consequences of two alterations of the 2,3-diphosphoglycerate binding site at position β82. J. Biol. Chem. 251:7563, 1976.
297. Lorkin, P. A., Stephens, A. D., Beard, M. E. J., Wrigley, P. F. M., Adams, L., and Lehmann, H.: Haemoglobin Rahere (β82 Lys→Thr): A new affinity haemoglobin associated with decreased 2,3-diphosphoglycerate binding and relative polycythaemia. Br. Med. J. 4:200, 1975.
298. Ikkala, E., Koskela, J., Pikkarainen, P., Rahiala, E.-L., El-Hazmi, M. A. F., Nagai, K., Lang, A., and Lehmann, H.: Hb Helsinki: A variant with high oxygen affinity and a substitution at a 2,3-DPG binding site (β^{82}[EF6] Lys→Met). Acta Haematol. 56:257, 1976.
299. Blackwell, R. Q., Liu, C.-S., and Wang, C.-L.: Hemoglobin Ta-Li: β83 Gly→Cys. Biochim. Biophys. Acta 243:467, 1971.
300. Tatsis, B., Sofroniadou, K., and Stergiopoulos, C. I.: Hemoglobin Pyrgos (α2β2 83(EF7) Gly→Asp). A new hemoglobin (Hb) variant. Abstract 168. Annual Meeting of the American Society of Hematology. Miami, 1972.
301. Tatsis, B., Sofroniadou, K., and Stergiopoulos, C. I.: Hemoglobin Pyrgos α2β2 83)EF7) Gly→Asp: A new hemoglobin variant in double heterozygosity with hemoglobin S. Blood 47:827, 1976.
302. Bradley, T. B., Wohl, R. C., Murphy, S. B., Oski,

F. A., and Bunn, H. F.: Properties of hemoglobin Bryn Mawr, β85 Phe→Ser, a new spontaneous mutation producing an unstable hemoglobin with high oxygen affinity. Abstract 40. Annual Meeting of the American Society of Hematology. Miami, 1972.
303. de Weinstein, B. I., White, J. M., Wiltshire, B. G., and Lehmann, H.: A new unstable haemoglobin: Hb Buenos Aires, β85(F1) Phe→Ser. Acta Haematol. 50:357, 1973.
304. Watson-Williams, E. J., Beale, D., Irvine, D., and Lehmann, H.: A new haemoglobin, D Ibadan (β87 Threonine→Lysine), producing no sickle cell haemoglobin D disease with haemoglobin S. Nature 205:1273, 1965.
305. Hollender, A., Lorkin, P. A., Lehmann, H., and Svensson, B.: New unstable haemoglobin Böras: β88(F4) Leucine→Arginine. Nature 222:953, 1969.
306. Opfell, R. W., Lorkin, P. A., and Lehmann, H.: Hereditary nonspherocytic haemolytic anaemia with post-splenectomy inclusion bodies and pigmenturia caused by an unstable haemoglobin Santa Ana—β88(F4) Leucine→Proline. J. Med. Genet. 5:292, 1968.
307. Thillet, J., Blouquit, Y., Garel, M. C., Dreyfus, B., Reyes, F., Cohen-Solal, M., Beuzard, Y., and Rosa, J.: Hemoglobin Creteil β89(F5) Ser→Asn: High oxygen affinity variant of hemoglobin frozen in a quaternary R-structure. J. Mol. Med. 1:135, 1976.
308. Paniker, N. V., Kuang-Tzu Davis Lin, Krantz, S. B., Flexner, J. M., Wasserman, B. K., and Puett, D.: Haemoglobin Vanderbilt (α2β2 89 Ser→Arg): A new haemoglobin with high oxygen affinity and compensatory erythrocytosis. Br. J. Haematol. 39:249, 1978.
309. Miyaji, R., Suzuki, H., Ohba, Y., and Shibata, S.: Hemoglobin Agenogi (α2β2 90 Lys), a slow moving hemoglobin of a Japanese family resembling Hb-E. Clin. Chim. Acta 14:624, 1966.
310. Schneider, R. G., Satoshi, U., Alperin, J. B., Brimhall, B., and Jones, R. T.: Hemoglobin Sabine, β91(F7) Leu→Pro. An unstable variant causing severe anemia with inclusion bodies. N. Engl. J. Med. 280:739, 1969.
311. Ahern, E., Ahern, C., Hilton, T., Serjeant, G. R., Serjeant, B. E., Seakins, M., Lang, A., Middleton, A., and Lehmann, H.: Haemoglobin Caribbean β91(F7) Leu→Arg: A mildly unstable haemoglobin with low oxygen affinity. FEBS Lett. 69:99, 1976.
312. Heller, P., Coleman, R. D., and Yakulis, V.: Hemoglobin M Hyde Park: A new variant of abnormal methemoglobin. J. Clin. Invest. 45:1021, 1966.
313. Shibata, S., Yamamoto, K., Ohba, Y., Miyaji, R., Karita, K., and Iuchi, I.: Hemoglobin M Akita disease. Acta Haematol. Jpn. 32:311, 1969.
314. Beuzard, Y., Courvalin, J. C., Cohen-Solal, M., Garel, M. C., Rosa, J., Brizard, C. P., and Gibaud, A.: Structural studies of hemoglobin Saint Etienne β92(F8) His→Gln: A new abnormal hemoglobin with loss of β proximal histidine and absence of heme on the chains. FEBS Lett. 27:76, 1972.
315. Aksoy, M., Erdem, S., Efremov, G. D., Wilson, J. B., Huisman, T. H. J., Schroeder, W. A., Shelton, J. R., Shelton, J. B., Ulitin, O. N., and Müftuglü, A.: Hemoglobin Istanbul: Substitution of glutamine for histidine in a proximal histidine (F8(92)β). J. Clin. Invest. 51:2380, 1972.

316. Adams, J. G., III, Przywara, K. P., Shamsuddin, M., and Heller, P.: Hemoglobin J Altgeld Gardens (β92(F8) His→Asp): A new hemoglobin variant involving a substitution of the proximal histidine. Am. Soc. Hematol. 18th Annual Meeting, Dallas, Texas, 1975.
316a. Spivak, V. A., Molchanova, T. P., Yu, V., Postnikov, V., Aseeva, E. A., Lutsenko, I. N., and Tokarev, Y. N.: A new abnormal hemoglobin: Hb Mozhaisk β92(F8)His–Arg. Hemoglobin 6:169, 1982.
317. Finney, R., Casey, R., Lehmann, H., and Walker, W.: Hb Newcastle: β92(F8) His→Pro. FEBS Lett. 60:435, 1975.
317a. Harano, K., Harano, T., Shibata, S., Ueda, S., Mori, H., and Seki, M.: Hb Okazaki [β93 (F8) Cys→Arg], a new hemoglobin variant with increased oxygen affinity and instability. FEBS Lett. 173:45, 1984.
317b. Como, P. F., Kennett, D., Wilkinson, T., and Kronenberg, H.: A new hemoglobin with high oxygen affinity—hemoglobin Bunbury—$\alpha_2\beta_2$ 94(FG1) Asp→Asn. Hemoglobin 7:413, 1983.
318. Clegg, J. B., Naughton, M. A., and Weatherall, D. J.: An improved method for the characterization of human haemoglobin mutants: Identification of α2β2 95 Glu, haemoglobin N (Baltimore). Nature 207:945, 1965.
319. Gottlieb, A. J., Robinson, E. A., and Itano, H. A.: Primary structure of Hopkins-I haemoglobin. Nature 214:189, 1967.
320. Dobbs, N. B., Jr., Simmons, J. W., Wilson, J. B., and Huissman, T. H. J.: Hemoglobin Jenkins or Hemoglobin N-Baltimore or α2β2 95 Glu. Biochim. Biophys. Acta 117:492, 1966.
321. Bayrakci, C., Josephson, A., Singer, L., Heller, P., and Coleman, R. D.: A new fast hemoglobin. Xth Congress of the International Society of Haematology, Stockholm, Sweden, 1964.
322. Hamilton, H. H., Iuchi, I., Miyaji, T., and Shibata, S.: Hemoglobin Hiroshima (β^{143} Histidine→ Aspartic acid): A newly identified fast moving beta chain variant associated with increased oxygen affinity and compensatory erythremia. (Personal communication P. Heller.) J. Clin. Invest. 48:525, 1969.
323. Moo-Penn, W. F., Schneider, R. G., Andrian, S., and Das, D. K.: Hemoglobin Detroit: β95 (FG2) Lysine→Asparagine. Biochim. Biophys. Acta 536:283, 1978.
323a. Devaraj, R., Wilson, J. B., and Huisman, T. H. J.: Hb Regina or $\alpha_2\beta_2$ 96(FG3)Leu→Val, a high oxygen affinity variant disovered by cation-exchange HPLC. Am. J. Hematol., in press.
324. Lorkin, P. A., Lehmann, H., Fairbanks, V. F., Berglund, G., and Leonhardt. T.: Two new pathological haemoglobins: Olmsted β141 (H19) Leu→Arg and Malmö β97 (FG4) His→Gln. Biochem. J. 119:68, 1970.
325. Taketa, F., Huang, Y. P., Libnoch, J. A., and Dessell, B. H.: Hemoglobin Wood β97(FG4) His→Leu: A new high-oxygen-affinity hemoglobin associated with familial erythrocytosis. Biochim. Biophys. Acta 400:348, 1975.
326. Taketa, F., Antholine, W. E., Mauk, A. G., and Libnoch, J. A.: Nitrosylhemoglobin Wood: Effects of inositol hexaphosphate on thiol reactivity and electron paramagnetic resonance spectrum. Biochemistry 14:3229, 1975.

326a. Ohba, Y., Imanaka, M., Matsuoka, M., Hattori, Y., Miyaji, T., Funaki, C., Shibata, K., Shimokata, H., Kuzuya, F., and Miwa, S.: A new unstable, high oxygen affinity hemoglobin: Hb Nagoya or β97(FG4)His→Pro. Hemoglobin 9:11, 1985.

327. Carrell, R. W., Lehmann, H., and Hutchinson, H. E.: Haemoglobin Köln (β98 Valine→Methionine): An unstable protein causing inclusion-body anaemia. Nature 210:915, 1966.

328. Woodson, R. D., Heywood, J. D., and Lenfant, C.: Oxygen transport in hemoglobin San Francisco. Clin. Res. 18:134, 1970.

329. Ohba, Y., Miyaji, T., and Shibata, S.: Identical substitution in Hb Ube-1 and Hb Köln. Nature [New Biol.] 243:205, 1973.

330. Gordon-Smith, E. C., Dacie, J. V., Blecher, T. E., French, E. A., Wiltshire, B. G., and Lehmann, H.: Haemoglobin Nottingham, β98(FG5) Val→Gly: A new unstable haemoglobin producing severe haemolysis. Proc. R. Soc. Med. 66:507, 1973.

331. Gacon, G., Wajcman, H., and Labie, D.: A new unstable hemoglobin mutated in β98(FG5) Val→Ala: Hb Djelfa. FEBS Lett. 58:238, 1975.

332. Reed, C. S., Hampson, R., Gordon, S., Jones, R. T., Novy, M. J., Brimhall, B., Edwards, M. J., and Koler, R. D.: Erythrocytosis secondary to increased oxygen affinity of a mutant hemoglobin, hemoglobin Kempsey. Blood 31:623, 1968.

333. Jones, R. T., Osgood, E. E., Brimhall, B., and Koler, R. D.: Hemoglobin Yakima: I. Clinical and biochemical studies. J. Clin. Invest. 46:1840, 1967.

334. Weatherall, D. J., Clegg, J. B. Callender, S. T., Wells, R. M. G., Gale, R., Huehns, E. R., Perutz, M. F., Viggiano, G., and Ho, C.: Haemoglobin Radcliffe ($\alpha_2\beta_2$ 99(Gl)Ala): A high oxygen-affinity variant causing familial polycythaemia. Br. J. Haematol. 35:177, 1977.

335. Rucknagel, D. L., Glynn, K. P., and Smith, J. R.: Hemoglobin Ypsilanti characterized by increased oxygen affinity, abnormal polymerization and erythremia. Clin. Res. 15:270, 1967.

336. Blouquit, Y., Braconnier, F., Galacteros, F., Arous, N., Soria, J., Zittoun, R., and Rosa, J.: Hemoglobin Hotel-Dieu β99 Asp→Gly (G1). A new abnormal hemoglobin with high oxygen affinity. Hemoglobin 5:19, 1981.

336a. Rochette, J., Poyart, C., Varet, B., and Wajcman, H.: A new hemoglobin variant altering the $\alpha_1\beta_2$ contact: Hb Chemilly $\alpha_2\beta_2$ 99 (G1) Asp→Val. FEBS Lett. 166:8, 1984.

337. Lokich, J. J., Mahoney, C. W., Bunn, H. F., Bruckheimer, S. M., and Ranney, H. M.: Hemoglobin Brigham (α2Aβ2 100 Pro→Leu). Hemoglobin variant associated with familial erythrocytosis. J. Clin. Invest. 52:2060, 1973.

338. Jones, R. T., Brimhall, B., and Gray, G.: Hemoglobin British Columbia [α2β2 101(G3) Glu→Lys]: A new variant with high oxygen affinity. Hemoglobin 1:171, 1976.

339. Adams, J. B., Winter, W. P., Tausk, K., and Heller, P.: Hemoglobin Rush [β-101(G3) Glutamine]: A new unstable hemoglobin causing mild hemolytic anemia. Blood 45:261, 1974.

340. Mant, M. J., Salkie, M. L., Cope, N., Appling, F., Bolch, K., Jayalakshmi, M., Gravely, M., Wilson, J. B., and Huisman, T. H. J.: Hb Alberta or α2β2 (101(G3) Glu→Gly), a new high-oxygen-affinity hemoglobin variant causing erythrocytosis. Hemoglobin 1:183, 1976–77.

341. Charache, S., Jacobson, R., Brimhall, B., Murphy, E. A., Hathaway, P., Winslow, R., Jones, R., Rath, C., and Simkovich, J.: Hb Potomac (β101 Glu→Asp): Speculations on placental oxygen transport in carriers of high-affinity hemoglobins. Blood 51:331, 1978.

342. Efremov, G. D., Huisman, T. H. J., Smith, L. L., Wilson, J. B., Kitchens, J. L., Wrightstone, R. N., and Adams, H. R.: Hemoglobin Richmond, a human hemoglobin which forms asymmetric hybrids with other hemoglobins. J. Biol. Chem. 244:6105, 1969.

343. Bonaventura, J., and Riggs, A.: Hemoglobin Kansas, a human hemoglobin with a neutral amino acid substitution and an abnormal oxygen equilibrium. J. Biol. Chem. 243:980, 1968.

344. Nagel, R. L., Joshua, L., Johnson, J., Landau, L., Bookchin, R. M., and Harris, M. B.: Hemoglobin Beth Israel: A mutant causing clinically apparent cyanosis. N. Engl. J. Med. 295:125, 1976.

345. Arous, N., Braconnier, F., Thillet, J., Bouquit, Y., Galacteros, F., Chevrier, M., Bordahandy, C., and Rosa, J.: Hemoglobin Saint Mande β102(G4) Asn→Tyr: A new low oxygen affinity variant. FEBS Lett. 126:114, 1981.

346. White, J. M., Szur, L., Gillies, I. D. S., Lorkin, P. A., and Lehmann, H.: Familial polycythaemia caused by a new haemoglobin variant. Hb Heathrow β103(G5) Phenylalanine→Leucine. Br. Med. J. 3:665, 1973.

347. Wilkinson, T., Ching Geh Chua, Carrell, R. W., Robin, H., Exner, T., Kit Ming Lee, and Kronenberg, H.: A new haemoglobin variant, haemoglobin Camperdown β104(G6) Arginine→Serine. Biochim. Biophys. Acta 393:195, 1975.

348. Ryrie, D. R., Plowman, D., and Lehmann, H.: Haemoglobin Sherwood Forest β104(G6) Arg→Thr. FEBS Lett. 83:260, 1977.

349. Hyde, R. D., Hall, M. D., Wiltshire, B. G., and Lehmann, H.: Haemoglobin Southampton, β106(G8) Leu→Pro: An unstable variant producing severe hemolysis. Lancet 2:1170, 1972.

350. Koler, R. D., Jones, R. T., Bigley, R. H., Litt, M., Lovrien, E., Brooks, R., Lahey, M. E., and Fowler, R.: Hemoglobin Casper: β106(G8) Leu→Pro, a contemporary mutation. Am. J. Med. 55:549, 1973.

351. Kleihauser, E., Waller, H. D., Benöhr, H. C., Kohne, E., and Gelinsky, P.: Hb Tübingen, eine neue β-kettenvariante (βTp 10–12) mit erhöhter spontanozydation. Klin. Wochenschr. 48:651, 1971.

352. Kohne, E., Kley, H. P., Kleihauer, E., Versmold, H., Benöhr, H. C., and Braunitzer, G.: Structural and functional characteristics of the Hb Tübingen: β^{106} (G8) Lau→Gln. FEBS Lett. 64:443, 1976.

353. Jones, R. T., and Koler, R. D.: Functional studies of seven new abnormal hemoglobins. Abstract No. 1–21. 16th International Congress in Hematology. September 1976.

354. Imamura, T., Fujita, S., Ohta, Y., Hanada, M., and Yanase, T.: Hemoglobin Yoshizuka (G10(108) β Asparagine→Aspartic acid): A new variant with a reduced oxygen affinity from a Japanese family. J. Clin. Invest. 48:2341, 1969.

355. Moo-Penn, W. F., Wolff, J. A., Simon, G., Vacek, M., Jue, D. L., and Johnson, M. H.: Hemoglobin Presbyterian: β108(G10) Asparagine→Lysine. A hemoglobin variant with low oxygen affinity. FEBS Lett. 92:53, 1978.

356. Nute, P. E., Stamatoyannopoulos, G., Hermodson, M. A., Roth, D., and Hornung, S.: Hemoglobinopathic erythrocytosis due to a new electrophoretically silent variant, hemoglobin San Diego (β109(G11) Val→Met). J. Clin. Invest. 53:320, 1974.
357. King, M. A. R., Wiltshire, B. G., Lehmann, H., and Morimoto, H.: An unstable haemoglobin with reduced oxygen affinity: Haemoglobin Peterborough, β111(G13) Valine→Phenylalanine, its interaction with normal haemoglobin and with haemoglobin Lepore. Br. J. Haematol. 22:125, 1972.
358. Adams, J. G., Boxer, L. A., Baehner, R. L., Forget, B. G., Tsistrokis, G. A., and Steinberg, M. H.: Hemoglobin Indianapolis: Post-translational degradation of an unstable β-chain variant producing a phenotype of severe heterozygous β-thalassemia. Clin. Res. 26:501A, 1978.
359. Ranney, H. M., Jacobs, A. S., and Nagel, R. L.: Haemoglobin New York. Nature 213:876, 1967.
360. Sugihara, J., Imamura, T., Imoto, T., and Yanase, T.: Identification of an abnormal hemoglobin with reduced oxygen affinity by high-performance liquid chromatography. Biochim. Biophys. Acta 669:105, 1981.
361. Outeirino, J., Casey, R., White, J. M., and Lehmann, H.: Haemoglobin Madrid, β115(G17) Alanine→Proline: An unstable variant associated with haemolytic anaemia. Acta Haematol. 52:53, 1974.
362. Schneider, R. G., Alperin, J. B., Brimhall, B., and Jones, R. T.: Hemoglobin P ($\alpha_2\beta_2$ 117Arg): Structure and properties. J. Lab. Clin. Med. 73:616, 1969.
362a. Ohba, Y., Hasegawa, Y., Amino, H., Miwa, S., Nakatsuji, T., Hattori, Y., and Miyaji, T.: Hemoglobin Saitama or β117(G19)His→Pro, a new variant causing hemolytic disease. Hemoglobin 7:47, 1983.
362b. Hedlung, B., Paine, S., Smith, C. M., III, Raines, J., Morrison, W. T., and Adams, J., III: Hemoglobin Minneapolis-Laos [β118(GH1) Phe→Tyr]: A new hemoglobin variant with normal functional properties. Hemoglobin 8:47, 1984.
363. Schneider, R. G., Berkman, N. L., Brimhall, B., and Jones, R. T.: Hemoglobin Fannin-Lubbock [$\alpha_2\beta_2^{119}$ (GH$_2$) Gly→Asp]: A slightly unstable mutant. Biochim. Biophys. Acta 453:478, 1976.
364. Moo-Penn, W. F., Bechtel, K. C., Johnson, M. H., Jue, D. L., Therrell, B. L., Jr., Morrison, B. Y., and Schmidt, R. M.: Hemoglobin Fannin-Lubbock [$\alpha_2\beta_2^{119}$ (GH2) Gly→Asp]: A new hemoglobin variant at the $\alpha_2\beta_1$ contact. Biochim. Biophys. Acta 453:472, 1976.
365. Chen-Marotel, J., Braconnier, F., Blouquit, Y., Martin-Caburi, J., Kammerer, J., and Rosa, J.: Hemoglobin Bougardirey-Mali β119 (GH2) Gly→Val. An electrophoretically silent variant migrating in isoelectrofocusing as Hb F. Hemoglobin 3:253, 1979.
366. Miyaji, T., Ohba, Y., Yamamoto, K., Shibata, S., Iuchi, I., and Hamilton, H. B.: Hemoglobin Hijiyama: A new fast-moving hemoglobin in a Japanese family. Science 159:204, 1968.
367. El-Hazmi, M. A. F., and Lehmann, H.: Hemoglobin Riyadh [$\alpha_2\beta_2$ 120(GH3) Lys→Asn]—a new variant found in association with α-thalassemia and iron deficiency. Hemoglobin 1:59, 1976.
368. Miyaji, T., Ohba, Y., Matsuoka, M., Kudoh, H., Asano, M., Yamamoto, K., and Satoh, T.: Hemoglobin Karatsu: Beta 120(GH3) Lysine→Asparagine. An example of Hb Riyadh in Japan. Hemoglobin 1:461, 1977.
369. Iuchi, I., Hidaka, K., Harano, T., Ueda, S., Shibata, S., Shimasaki, S., Mizushima, J., Kubo, N., Miyake, T., and Uchida, T.: Hemoglobin Takamatsu (β120 (GH3) Lys→Gln): A new abnormal hemoglobin detected in three unrelated families in the Takamatsu area of Shikoku. Hemoglobin 4:165, 1980.
369a. Lu, Y. Q., Fan, J. L., Liu, J. F., Hu, H. L., Peng, X. H., Huang, C. H., Huang, P. Y., Chen, S. S., Jia, P. C., and Yang, K. G.: Hemoglobin Jianghua, β120 (GH3) Lys→Ile. A new fast moving variant found in China. Hemoglobin 7:321, 1983.
370. Baglioni, C.: Abnormal human haemoglobins. VIII. Chemical studies on haemoglobin D. Biochim. Biophys. Acta 59:437, 1962.
371. Ozsoylu, S.: Homozygous hemoglobin D Punjab. Acta Haematol. 43:353, 1970.
372. Ramot, B., Rotem, J., Rahbar, S., Jacobs, A. S., Udem, L., and Ranney, H. M.: Hemoglobin D Punjab in a Bulgarian Jewish family. Isr. J. Med. Sci. 5:1066, 1969.
373. Smith, E. W., and Conley, C. L.: Sickle cell–hemoglobin D disease. Ann. Intern. Med. 50:94, 1959.
374. Wasi, P., Pootrakul, S., Na-Nakorn, S., Beale, D., and Lehmann, H.: Haemoglobin D β Los Angeles (D Punjab, $\alpha_2\beta_2$ 121 GluNH$_2$) in a Thai family. Acta Haematol. 39:151, 1968.
375. Imamura, T., and Riggs, A.: Identification of hemoglobin Oak Ridge with hemoglobin D Punjab (Los Angeles). Biochem. Genet. 7:127, 1972.
376. Bowman, B., and Ingram, V. M.: Abnormal human haemoglobins. VII. The comparison of normal human haemoglobin D Chicago. Biochim. Biophys. Acta 53:569, 1961.
377. Baglioni, C., and Lehmann, H.: Chemical heterogeneity of haemoglobin O. Nature 196:229, 1962.
378. Kamel, K., Hoerman, K., and Awny, A.: Ethnological significance of hemoglobin $\alpha_2\beta_2$ 121 Lys. Am. J. Phys. Anthropol. 26:107, 1970.
379. Efremov, G. D., Duma, H., Rudivic, R., Rolovic, Z., Wilson, J. B., and Huisman, T. H. J.: Hemoglobin Beograd or α2β2 121 Glu→Val (GH4). Biochim. Biophys. Acta 328:81, 1973.
380. Clegg, J. B., Weatherall, D. J., Wong Hock Boon, and Mustafa, D.: Two new haemoglobin variants involving proline substitutions. Nature 22:379, 1969.
381. Bursaux, E., Blouquit, Y., Poyart, C., Rosa, J., Arous, N., and Bohn, B.: Hemoglobin Ty Gard ($\alpha_2^A\beta_2$ 124 (H2) Pro→Gln): A stable high O_2 affinity variant at the α1β1 contact. FEBS Lett. 88:155, 1978.
382. Miyaji, T., Ohba, Y., Yamamoto, K., Shibata, S., Iuchi, I., and Takenaka, H. Japanese haemoglobin variant. Nature 217:89, 1968.
383. Strahler, J. R., Rosenbloom, B. B., and Hanash, S. M.: A silent neutral substitution detected by reverse phase high performance liquid chromatography: Hemoglobin Beirut. Science 221:860, 1983.
384. Altay, C., Altinöz, N., Wilson, J. B., Bolch, K. C., and Huisman, T. H. J.: Hemoglobin Hacettepe or α2β2 127 (H5) Gln→Glu. Biochim. Biophys. Acta 434:1, 1976.
385. Martinez, G., Lima, F., and Colombo, B.: Haemoglobin J Guantanamo ($\alpha_2\beta_2$ 128 (H6) Ala→Asp). A new fast unstable haemoglobin found in a Cuban family. Biochim. Biophys. Acta 491:1, 1977.
386. Blackwell, R. Q., Yang, Y.-J., and Wang, C.-C.:

Hemoglobin J Taichung: β129 Ala→Asp. Biochim. Biophys. Acta *194*:1, 1969.

387. Maniatis, A., Bousios, T., Nagel, R. L., Balazs, T., Ueda, Y., Bookchin, R. M., and Maniatis, G. M.: Hemoglobin Crete (β129 Ala→Pro): A new high-affinity variant interacting with β⁰- and δβ⁰-thalassemia. Blood *54*:54, 1979.

388. Lorkin, P. A., Pietschmann, H., Braunsteiner, H., and Lehmann, H.: Structure of haemoglobin Wein β130 (H8) Tyrosine→Aspartic acid: An unstable haemoglobin variant. Acta Haematol. *51*:351, 1974.

389. Wade Cohen, P. T., Yates, A., Bellingham, A. J., and Huehns, E. R.: Amino-acid substitution on the α1β1 intersubunit contact of haemoglobin Camden β131 (H9) Gln→Glu. Nature [New Biol.] *243*:467, 1973.

389a. Moo-Penn, W. F., Johnson, M. H., McGuffey, J. E., and Jue, D. L.: Hemoglobin Shelby [β131(H9) Gln→Lys] a correction to the structure of hemoglobin Deaconess and hemoglobin Leslie.* Hemoglobin *8*:583, 1984. *Annotation: Wilson, J. B., Webber, B. B., and Huisman, T. H. J.: Hb Leslie is the same as Hb Shelby or α₂β₂131(H9)Gln→Lys. Hemoglobin *8*:595, 1984.

390. Ringelhann, B., Konotey-Ahulu, F. I. D., Talapatia, N. C., Nkrumah, F. H., Wilshire, B., and Lehmann, H.: Haemoglobin K Woolwich (α₂β₂¹³² Lysine→Glutamine) in Ghana. Acta Haematol. *45*:250, 1971.

391. Ohba, Y., Miyaji, T., Matsuoka, M., Ueda, S., Iuchi, I., and Shibata, S.: Hemoglobin Toluchi: β131 glutamine leads to glutamic acid, an example of Hb Camden in Japan. Acta Haematol. Jpn. *38*:1, 1975.

392. Arends, T., Lehmann, H., Plowman, D., and Stathopoulou, R.: Haemoglobin North Shore–Caracas β134 (H12) Valine→Glutamic acid. FEBS Lett. *80*:261, 1977.

393. Brennan, S. O., Arnold, B., Fleming, P., and Carrell, R. W.: A new unstable haemoglobin, β134 Val→Glu. Proc. New Zealand Med. J. *85*:398, 1977.

394. Marti, H. R., Winterhalter, K. H., Di Iorio, E. E., Lorkin, P. A., and Lehmann, H.: Hb Altdorf α2β2 135(H13) Ala→Pro: A new electrophoretically silent unstable haemoglobin variant from Switzerland. FEBS Lett. *63*:193, 1976.

395. Minnich, V., Hill, R. J., Khuri, P. D., and Anderson, M. E.: Hemoglobin Hope: A beta chain variant. Blood *25*:830, 1965.

396. Moo-Penn, W. F., Jue, D. L., Johnson, M. H., Bechtel, K. C., and Patchen, L. C.: Hemoglobin variants and methods used for their characterization during 7 years of screening at the Center for Disease Control. Hemoglobin *4*:347, 1980.

396a. Como, P. F., Hockey, D., Trent, R. J., and Kronenberg, H.: Hb Geelong β 139 (H17) Asn→Asp, a new hemoglobin with thalassemia-like characteristics. Abstract. New South Wales Thalassemia Society, 1985.

396b. Rochette, J., Varet, B., Boissel, J. P., Clough, K., Labie, D., Wajcman, H., Bohn, B., Magne, P., and Poyart, C.: Structure and function of Hb Saint-Jacques (α₂β₂ 140 (H18) Ala→Thr): A new high-oxygen-affinity variant with altered bisphosphoglycerate binding. Biochim. Biophys. Acta *785*:14–21, 1984.

397. Moo-Penn, W. F., Schneider, R. G., Shih, T.-B., Jones, R. T., Govindarajan, S., Govindarajan, P. G., and Patchen, L. C.: Hemoglobin Ohio (β142 Ala→Asp): A new abnormal hemoglobin with high oxygen affinity and erythrocytosis. Blood *56*:246, 1980.

398. Hirano, M., Ohba, Y., Imai, K., Ino, T., Morishita, Y., Matsui, T., Shimizu, S., Sumi, H., Yamamoto, K., and Miyaji, T.: Hb Toyoake: β142(H20) Ala→Pro. A new unstable hemoglobin with high oxyten affinity. Blood *57*:697, 1981.

399. Tentori, L., Carta Sorcini, M., and Bucella, C.: Hemoglobin Abruzzo: Beta 143 (H21) His→Arg. Clin. Chim. Acta *38*:258, 1972.

400. Bromberg, P. A., Alben, J. O., Bare, G. H., Balcerzak, S. P., Jones, R. T., Brimhall, B., and Padilla, F.: Hemoglobin Little Rock (β143 His→Gln: (H21)). A high oxygen affinity haemoglobin variant with unique properties. Nature [New Biol.] *243*:177, 1973.

401. Jensen, M., Oski, F. A., Nathan, D. G., and Bunn, H. F.: Hemoglobin Syracuse (α2β2 143 (H21) His→Pro), a new high-affinity variant detected by special electrophoretic methods. J. Clin. Invest. *55*:469, 1975.

402. Zak, S. J., Brimhall, B., Jones, R. T., and Kaplan, M. E.: Hemoglobin Andrew-Minneapolis α2Aβ2 144 Lys→Asn: A new high-oxygen-affinity mutant human hemoglobin. Blood *44*:543, 1974.

403. Hayashim, A., Stamatoyannopoulos, G., Yoshida, A., and Adamson, J.: Haemoglobin Rainier: β145(HC2) Tyrosine→Cysteine and haemoglobin Bethesda: β145(HC2) Tyrosine→Histidine. Nature [New Biol.] *230*:264, 1971.

404. Kleckner, H. B., Wilson, J. B., Lindeman, J. G., Stevens, P. D., Niazi, G., Hunter, E., Chen, C. J., and Huisman, T. H. J.: Hemoglobin Fort Gordon or α2β2 145 Tyr→Asp, a new high-oxygen-affinity hemoglobin variant. Biochim. Biophys. Acta *400*:343, 1975.

405. Charache, S., Brimhall, B., and Jones, R. T.: Polycythemia produced by hemoglobin Osler (β145(HC2) Tyr→Asp). Johns Hopkins Med. J. *136*:132, 1975.

406. Gacon, G., Wajcman, H., and Labie, D.: Structural and functional study of Hb Nancy β145 (HC2) Tyr→Asp: A high oxygen affinity hemoglobin. FEBS Lett. *56*:39, 1975.

407. Winslow, R. M., Swenberg, M.-L., Gross, E., Chervenick, P. A., Buchman, R. R., and Anderson, W. F.: Hemoglobin McKees Rocks (α2β2 145 Tyr→Term): A human "nonsense" mutation leading to a shortened β-chain. J. Clin. Invest. *57*:772, 1976.

408. Perutz, M. F., del Pulsinelli, P., Ten Eyck, L., Kilmartin, J. V., Shibata, S., Iuchi, I., Miyaji, T., and Hamilton, H. B.: Haemoglobin Hiroshima and the mechanisms of the alkaline Bohr effect. Nature [New Biol.] *232*:147, 1971.

409. Barem, G. H., Bromberg, P. A., Alben, J. O., Brimhall, B., Jones, R. T., Mintz, S., and Rother, I.: Altered C-terminal salt bridges in haemoglobin York cause high oxygen affinity. Nature *259*:155, 1976.

410. Wajcman, H., Kilmartin, J. V., Najman, A., and Labie, D.: Hemoglobin Cochin–Port Royal—consequences of the replacement of the β chain C-terminal by an arginine. Biochim. Biophys. Acta *400*:354, 1975.

411. Schneider, R. G., Bremner, J. E., Brimhall, B.,

Jones, R. T., and Shih, T-B.: Hemoglobin Cowtown (β146 HC3 His→Leu). A mutant with high oxygen affinity and erythrocytosis. Am. J. Clin. Pathol. 72:1028, 1979.
412. Jones, R. T., Brimhall, B., Huehns, E. R., and Barnicot, N. A.: Hemoglobin Sphakiá: A delta chain variant of hemoglobin A_2 from Crete. Science 151:1406, 1966.
413. Ranney, H. M., Jacobs, A. S., Ramot, B., and Bradley, T. B., Jr.: Hemoglobin NYU, a delta chain variant, $\alpha_2\delta_2$ 12 Lys. J. Clin. Invest. 48:2057, 1969.
414. Ball, E. W., Meynell, M. J., Beale, D., Kynoch, P., Lehmann, H., and Stretton, A. O. W.: Haemoglobin A_2': $\alpha_2\delta_2$ 16 Glycine→Arginine. Nature 209:1217, 1968.
415. Rieder, R. F., Clegg, J. B., Weiss, H. J., Cristy, N. P., and Rabinowitz, R.: Hemoglobin A_2-Roosevelt: $\alpha_2\delta_2$ 20 Val→Glu. Biochim. Biophys. Acta 439:501, 1976.
416. Jones, R. T., and Brimhall, B.: Structural characterization of two δ chain variants. J. Biol. Chem. 242:5141, 1967.
416a. Brennan, S. O., Williamson, D., Smith, M. B., Cauchi, M. N., MacPhee, A., and Carrell, R. W.: Hb A_2 Victoria δ24(B6) Gly→Asp, a new δ chain occurring with β-thalassemia. Hemoglobin 8:163, 1984.
417. Sharma, R. S., Harding, D. L., Wong, S. C., Wilson, J. B., Gravely, M. E., and Huisman, T. H. J.: A new δ chain variant Haemoglobin A_2Melbourne or $\alpha_2\beta_2$ 43Glu→Lys(CD2). Biochim. Biophys. Acta 359:233, 1974.
418. XIII Meeting Gruppo di Studio Dell'Entrocita, Torino, June 12, 1977.
419. Lie Injo, L. E., Pribada, W., Boerma, F. W., Efremov, G. D., Wilson, J. B., Reynolds, C. A., and Huisman, T. H. J.: Hemoglobin A_2-Indonesia or $\alpha_2\delta_2$ 69 (E13) Gly→Arg. Biochim. Biophys. Acta 229:335, 1971.
419a. Salkie, M. L., Gordon, P. A., Ringal, W. M., Lam, H., Wilson, J. B., Headlee, M. E., and Huisman, T. H. J.: Hb A_2-Canada or $\alpha_2\delta_2$ 99 (G1) Asp→Asn, a newly discovered delta chain variant with increased oxygen affinity occurring in cis to β-thalassemia. Hemoglobin 6:223, 1982.
420. Sharma, R. S., Williams, L., Wilson, J. B., and Huisman, T. H. J.: Hemoglobin A_2-Coburg or $\alpha_2\delta_2$ 116 Arg→His (G18). Biochim. Biophys. Acta 393:379, 1975.
420a. Romero Garcia, C., Navarro, J. L., Lam, H., Webber, B. B., Headlee, M. E., Wilson, J. B., and Huisman, T. H. J.: Hb A_2 Manzanares or $\alpha_2\delta_2$121(GH4) Glu→Val, an unstable δ chain variant observed in a Spanish family. Hemoglobin 7:435, 1983.
420b. Juricic, D., Crepinko, I., Efremov, G. D., Lam, H., Webber, B. B., Headlee, M. G., and Huisman, T. H. J.: Hb A_2 Zagreb or $\alpha_2\delta_2$125-(H3)Gln→Glu in association with δβ-thalassemia in a Yugoslavian female. Hemoglobin 7:443, 1983.
421. DeJong, W. W. W., and Bernini, L. F.: Haemoglobin Babinga (δ136 Glycine→Aspartic acid): A new delta chain variant. Nature 219:1360–1362, 1968.
421a. Williamson, D., Brennan, S. O., Strosberg, H., Whitty, J., and Carrell, R. W. Hemoglobin A_2 Fitzroy δ 142 Ala→Asp: A new delta-chain variant. Hemoglobin 8:325, 1984.
422. Lie-Injo, L. E., Kamuzora, H., and Lehmann, H.

Haemoglobin F Malaysia: $\alpha_2\gamma_2$ 1(NA1) Glycine→Cysteine: 136 Glycine. J. Med. Genet. 11:25, 1974.
423. Jenkins, G. C., Beale, D., Black, A. J., Huntsman, G. R., and Lehmann, H.: Haemoglobin F Texas I ($\alpha_2\gamma_2$ 5 Glu→Lys): A variant of haemoglobin F. Br. J. Haematol. 13:252, 1967.
423a. Ohta, Y., Saito, S., Fujita, S., Wilson, J. B., Lam, H., and Huisman, T. H. J.: Hb F-Meinohama or $\alpha_2\gamma_2$ (5 Glu→Gly; 75 Ile; 136 Gly). Hemoglobin 5:565, 1981.
424. Larkin, I. L. M., Baker, T., Lorkin, P. A., Lehmann, H., Black, A. J., and Huntsman, R. G.: Haemoglobin F Texas II ($\alpha_2\gamma_2$ 6 Glu→Lys): The second of the haemoglobin F Texas variants. Br. J. Haematol. 14:233, 1968.
424a. Yoshinaka, H., Ohba, Y., Hattori, Y., Matsuoka, M., Miyaji, T., and Fuyuno, K.: A new γ chain variant, Hb F Kotobuki or $^A\gamma^I$6 (A3) Glu→Gly. Hemoglobin 6:37, 1982.
424b. Nakatsuji, T., Webber, B., Lam, H., Wilson, J. B., Huisman, T. H. J., Sciarratta, G. V., Sansone, G., and Molaro, G. L.: A new γ chain variant: Hb F-Pordenone [γ6(A3)Glu→Gln: 75 Ile: 136 Ala]. Hemoglobin 6:397, 1982.
425. Carrell, R. W., Owen, M. C., Anderson, R., and Berry, E.: Haemoglobin F Auckland Gγ7 Asp→Asn—further evidence for multiple genes for the gamma chain. Biochim. Biophys. Acta 365:323, 1974.
426. Loukopoulos, D., Kaltsoya, A., and Fessas, P. H.: On the chemical abnormality of Hb "Alexandra," a fetal hemoglobin variant. Blood 33:114, 1969.
426a. Bradley, T.: Personal communication, 1983.
426b. Nakatsuji, T., Lam, H., and Huisman, T. H. J.: Hb F-Calluna or $\alpha_2\gamma_2$ (12 Thr→Arg; 75 Ile; 136 Ala) in a Caucasian baby. Hemoglobin 7:563, 1983.
427. Brennan, S. O., Smith, M. B., and Carrell, R. W.: Haemoglobin F Melbourne Gγ 16 Gly→Arg and Haemoglobin F Carlton Gγ 121 Glu→Lys. Biochim. Biophys. Acta 490:452, 1977.
428. Lie-Injo, L. E., Wiltshire, B. G., and Lehmann, H.: Structural identification of haemoglobin F Kuala Lumpur ($\alpha_2\gamma_2$ 22(B4) Asp→Gly: (136Ala)). Biochim. Biophys. Acta 322:224, 1973.
428a. Chen, S. S., Wilson, J. B., Webber, B. B., and Huisman, T. H. J.: Hb F-Tokyo or $\alpha_2^G\gamma_2$34 (B16)Val→Ile, a silent γ chain variant detected by reverse phase high performance liquid chromatography. Hemoglobin 9:25, 1985.
428b. Chen, S. S., Wilson, J. B., and Huisman, T. H. J.: Hb F-Pendergrass, an $^A\gamma^I$ variant with a Pro→Arg substitution at position γ36(C2). Hemoglobin 9:73, 1985.
428c. Nakatsuji, T., Headlee, M., Lam, H., Wilson, J. B., and Huisman, T. H. J.: Hb F-Bonaire-Ga or $\alpha_2^A\gamma_2$39(C5)Gln–Arg, characterized by high pressure liquid chromatography and microsequencing procedures. Hemoglobin 6:599, 1982.
428d. Honig, G. R., Koshy, M., Schroeder, W. A., Shelton, J. B., and Shelton, J. R.: Hemoglobin F Lòdz ($^G\gamma^I$ 44 Ser→Arg). A newly identified variant from an American infant of Polish descent. Biochim. Biophys. Acta 707:213, 1982.
428e. Serjeant, G. R., Serjeant, B. E., Lehmann, H., Dukes, M., and Robb, L.: Hb F Kingston [$^G\gamma$55(D6)Met→Arg]. FEBS Lett. 150:77, 1982.
429. Ahern, E. J., Jones, R. T., Brimhall, B., and Gray,

R. H.: Haemoglobin F Jamaica ($\alpha_2\gamma_2$ 61 Lys→Glu: 136Ala). Br. J. Haematol. *18*:369, 1970.
430. Hayashi, A., Fujita, T., Fujimura, M., and Titani, K.: A new abnormal fetal hemoglobin, Hb FM-Osaka ($\alpha_2\gamma_2$ 63 His→Tyr). Hemoglobin *4*:447, 1980.
430a. Zeng, Y. T., Huang, S. Z., Nakatsuji, T., and Huisman, T. H. J.: $-^G\gamma^A\gamma-$Thalassemia and γ-chain variants in Chinese newborn babies. Am. J. Hematol. *18*:235, 1985.
431. Fuyuno, K., Torigoe, T., Ohba, Y., Matsuoka, M., and Miyaji, T.: Survey of cord blood hemoglobin in Japan and identification of two new γ chain variants. Hemoglobin *5*:139, 1981.
431a. Nakatsuji, T., Lam, H., and Huisman, T. H. J.: Hb F-Kennestone or $\alpha_2{}^G\gamma_2$ (EFl)77 His→Arg observed in a Caucasian baby. Hemoglobin, *7*:267, 1983.
431b. Al-Awamy, B. H., Niazi, G. A., Al-Mouzan, M. I., Chen, S. S., Wilson, J. B., Webber, B. B., and Huisman, T. H. J.: Hb F-Damman or $\alpha_2{}^A\gamma_2$79(EF3) Asp→Asn. Hemoglobin *9*:171, 1985.
432. Ahern, E., Holder, W., Ahern, V., Serjeant, G. R., Serjeant, B. E., Forbes, M., Brimhall, B., and Jones, R. T.: Haemoglobin F Victoria Jubilee ($\alpha2A\gamma2$ 80 Asp→Tyr). Biochim. Biophys. Acta *393*:188, 1975.
432a. Nakatsuki, T., Lam, H., Carver, J., and Huisman, T. H. J.: Hb F-Marietta, or $^G\gamma^l$80[EF4]Asp→Asn, observed in a Caucasian baby. Hemoglobin *6*:407, 1982.
432b. Nakatsuji, T., Lam, H., Wilson, J. B., Webber, B. B., and Huisman, T. H. J.: Hb F-Columbus-Ga or $\alpha_2{}^G\gamma_2$94(FGl)Asp–Asn. Hemoglobin *6*:593, 1982.
433. Schneider, R. G., Haggard, M. E., Gustavson, L. P., Brimhall, B., and Jones, R. T.: Genetic haemoglobin abnormalities in about 9,000 black and 7,000 white newborns: Haemoglobin F Dickinson (A97 His→Arg), a new variant. Br. J. Haematol. *28*:515, 1974.
433a. Nakatsuji, T., Shimizu, K., and Huisman, T. H. J.: Hb F-La Grange or $\alpha_2\gamma_2$ 101 (G3) Glu→Lys; 75 Ile; 136 Gly; a high oxygen affinity fetal hemoglobin variant observed in a Caucasian newborn. Biochim. Biophys. Acta. *789*:224, 1984.
434. Omura, H., Miyaji, T., and Shibata, S.: Hemoglobin F Ube (108 Asn→Lys), a new abnormal fetal hemoglobin found in a Japanese baby. Chem. Abstr. *83*:266, 1975.
435. Cauchi, M. N., Clegg, J. B., and Weatherall, D. J.: Haemoglobin F (Malta), a new foetal haemoglobin variant with a high incidence in Maltese infants. Nature *223*:311, 1969.
435a. Giardina, B., Condo, S. G., Brunori, M., Bannister, J. V., and Bannister, W. H.: Properties of hemoglobin F-Malta. Bull. Mol. Biol. Med. *5*:33, 1980.
435b. Shelton, J. B., Shelton, J. R., Espinueva, Z., Huynh, V., Schroeder, W. A., and Powars, D.: Hemoglobin F-Caltech:$\alpha_2{}^G\gamma_2$ 120Lys–Gln. Hemoglobin *6*:577, 1982.
436. Sacker, L. S., Beale, D., Black, A. J., Huntsman, R. G., Lehmann, H., and Lorkin, P. A.: Haemoglobin F Hull (γ121 Glutamic acid→Lysine), homologous with haemoglobins O and O Indonesia. Br. Med. J. *3*:531, 1967.
436a. Care, A., Marinucci, M., Massa, A., Maffi, D., Sposi, N. M., Improta, T., and Tentori, L.: Hb F-Siena ($\alpha_2{}^A\gamma^T_2$ 121 (GH4)Glu–Lys). A new fetal hemoglobin variant. Hemoglobin *7*:79, 1983.
437. Brimhall, B., Vedvick, T. S., Jones, R. T., Ahern, E., Palomino, E., and Ahern, V.: Haemoglobin F Port Royal (α2Gγ 125 Glu→Ala). Br. J. Haematol. *27*:313, 1973.
438. Lee-Potter, J. P., Deacon-Smith, R. A., Simpkiss, M. J., Kamuzora, H., and Lehmann, H.: A new cause of haemolytic anemia in the newborn. A description of an unstable fetal haemoglobin: F Poole, α2Gγ2 130 Tryptophan→Glycine. J. Clin. Pathol. *28*:317, 1975.
439. Barnabas, J., and Muller, C. J.: Haemoglobin Lepore Hollandia. Nature *194*:931, 1962.
440. Ostertag, W., and Smith, E. W.: Hemoglobin Lepore-Baltimore, a third type of a $\delta\beta$ crossover (δ50, β86). Eur. J. Biochem. *10*:371, 1969.
441. Baglioni, C.: The fusion of two peptide chains in hemoglobin Lepore and its interpretation as a genetic deletion. Proc. Natl. Acad. Sci. USA *48*:1880, 1962.
442. Adams, J. G., III, Morrison, W. T., and Steinberg, M. H.: Hemoglobin Parchman: Double crossover within a single human gene. Science *218*:291, 1982.
443. Ohta, Y., Yamaoka, K., Sumida, I., and Yanase, T.: Hemoglobin Miyada, a β-δ fusion peptide (anti-Lepore) type discovered in a Japanese family. Nature [New Biol.] *234*:218, 1977.
444. Lehmann, H., and Charlesworth, D.: Observation on haemoglobin P (Congo type). Biochem. J. *119*:43, 1970.
445. Badr, F. M., Lorkin, P. A., and Lehmann, H.: Haemoglobin P-Nilotic: Containing a β-δ chain. Nature [New Biol.] *242*:107, 1973.
446. Honig, G. R., Shamsuddin, M., Mason, R. G., and Vida, L. N.: Hemoglobin Lincoln Park: A $\delta\beta$ fusion (anti-Lepore) variant with an amino acid deletion in the δ chain-derived segment. Proc. Natl. Acad. Sci. USA *75*:1475, 1978.
447. Huisman, T. H. J., Wrightstone, R. N., Wilson, J. B., Schroeder, W. A., and Kendall, A. G.: Hemoglobin Kenya, the product of fusion of γ and β polypeptide chains. Arch. Biochem. Biophys. *153*:850, 1972.
448. Clegg, J. B., Weatherall, D. J., and Milner, P. F.: Haemoglobin Constant Spring—a chain termination mutant. Nature *234*:337, 1971.
449. Weatherall, D. J., and Clegg, J. B.: The α-chain-termination mutants and their relation to the α-thalassemias. Philos. Trans. R. Soc. Lond. [Biol.]:*271*:411, 1975.
450. Clegg, J. B., Weatherall, D. J., Contopolou-Griva, I., Caroutsos, K., Poungouras, P., and Tsevrenis, H.: Haemoglobin Icaria, a new chain-termination mutant which causes α thalassemia. Nature *251*:245, 1974.
451. DeJong, W. W. W., Meera Khan, P., and Bernini, L. F.: Hemoglobin Koya Dora; High frequency of a chain termination mutant Am. J. Hum. Genet. *27*:81, 1975.
452. Flatz, G., Kinderlerer, J. L., Kilmartin, J. V., and Lehmann, H.: Haemoglobin Tak: A variant with additional residues at the end of the β-chains. Lancet *10*:732, 1971.
453. Imai, K., and Lehmann, H.: The oxygen affinity of haemoglobin Tak, a variant with an elongated β chain. Biochim. Biophys. Acta *412*:288, 1975.
454. Lehmann, H., Casey, R., Lang, A., Stathopoulou,

R., Imai, K., Tuchinda, S., Vinae, P., and Flatz, G.: Haemoglobin Tak: A β-chain elongation. Br. J. Haematol. *31*(Suppl): 119, 1975.
455. Seid-Akhavan, M., Winter, W. P., Abramson, R. K., and Rucknagel, D. L.: Hemoglobin Wayne: A frameshift variant occurring in two distinct forms. Abstract No. 9. Ann. Meeting Am. Soc. Hematol., Miami, 1972.
456. Bunn, H. F., Schmidt, G. J., Haney, D. N., and Dluhy, R. G.: Hemoglobin Cranston, an unstable variant having an elongated β chain due to a nonhomologous crossover between two normal beta chain genes. Proc. Natl. Acad. Sci. USA *72*:3609, 1975.
456a. Delanoe, J., North, M. K., Arous, N., Bardakjian, F., Pflumio, F., Brunagel, M. L., Lancombe, C., Poyart, C., Galacteros, F., Rosa, J., and Blouquit, Y.: Hb Saverne: A new variant having an elongated β chain. (Abstract.) Blood, *64*(Suppl. 1):56a, 1984.
457. Huisman, T. H. J., Wilson, J. B., Gravely, M., and Hubbard, M.: Hemoglobin Grady: The first example of a variant with elongated chains due to an insertion of residues. Proc. Natl. Acad. Sci. USA *71*:3270, 1974.
458. Garel, M. C., Goossens, M., Oudart, J. L., Blouquit, Y., Thillet, J., and Rosa, J.: Hemoglobin Dakar = hemoglobin Grady: Demonstration by a new approach to the analysis of the tryptic core region of the α chain and oxygen equilibrium properties. Biochim. Biophys. Acta *453*:459, 1976.
458a. Johnson, C. S., Schoeder, W. A., Shelton J. B., and Shelton, J. R.: The first example of a deletion in the human α chain—Hb Boyle Heights. Hemoglobin *7*:125, 1983.
459. DeJong, W. W. W., Went, L. N., and Bernini, L. F.: Haemoglobin Leiden: Deletion of β6 or 7 glutamic acid. Nature *220*:788, 1968.
460. Cohen-Solal, M., Blouquit, Y., Garel, M. C., Thillet, J., Gaillard, L., Creyssel, R., Gibaud, A., and Rosa, J.: Haemoglobin Lyon (β17–18(A14–15) Lys–Val→0) determination of sequenator analysis. Biochim. Biophys. Acta *351*:306, 1974.
461. Jones, R. T., Brimhall, B., Huisman, T. H. J., Kleihauer, E., and Betke, K.: Hemoglobin Freiburg: Abnormal hemoglobin due to deletion of a single amino acid residue. Science *154*:1024, 1966.
462. Praxedes, H., and Lehmann, H.: Haemoglobin Niteroi—a new unstable variant. Proc. 14th International Congress of Hematology, São Paulo, Brazil, 1972.
463. Shibata, S., Miyaji, T., Ueda, S., Matsuoka, M., Iuchi, I., Yamada, K., and Shinkai, N.: Hemoglobin Tochigi (beta 56–59 deleted). A new unstable hemoglobin discovered in a Japanese family. Proc. Jpn. Acad. *46*:440, 1970.
464. Wajcman, H., Labie, D., and Schapira, G.: Two new hemoglobin variants with deletion. Hemoglobin Tours: Thr β87(F3) deleted and hemoglobin St. Antoine: Gly→Leu β74–75 (E18–19) deleted. Consequences for oxygen affinity and protein stability. Biochim. Biophys. Acta *295*:495, 1973.
465. Adams, J. G., Steinberg, M. H., Newman, M. V., Morrison, W. T., Benz, E. J., and Iyer, R.: β-Thalassemia present in cis to a new β chain structural variant, Hb Vicksburg [β75 (E19) Leu→0]. Proc. Natl. Acad. Sci. USA *78*:469, 1981.
466. Bradley, T. B., Wohl, R. C., and Rieder, R. F.: Hemoglobin Gun Hill: Deletion of five amino acid residues and impaired heme-globin binding. Science *157*:1581, 1967.
467. Lutcher, C. L., and Huisman, T. H. J.: Hb-Leslie, an unstable variant due to deletion of Gln β131, occurring in combination with β⁰-thalassemia, Hb-S, and Hb-C. Clin. Res. *23*:278A, 1975.
468. Lutcher, C. L., Wilson, J. B., Gravely, M. E., Stevens, P. D., Chen, C. J., Linderman, J. G., Wong, S. C., Miller, A., Gottleib, M., and Huisman, T. H. J.: Hb Leslie, an unstable hemoglobin due to deletion of glutaminyl residue β131(H9) occurring in association with β⁰-thalassemia, Hb-C, and Hb-S. Blood *47*:99, 1976.
469. Moo-Penn, W. F., Jue, D. L., Bechtel, K. C., Johnson, M. H., Bemis, E., Brosious, E., and Schmidt, R. M.: Hemoglobin Deaconess, a new deletion mutant: β131(H9) Glutamine deleted. Biochem. Biophys. Res. Commun. *65*:8, 1975.
470. Casey, R., Kynoch, P. A. M., Lang, A., Lehmann, H., Nozari, G., and Shinton, N. K.: Double heterozygosity for two unstable haemoglobins: Hb Sydney (β67[E11] Val→Ala) and Hb Coventry (β141[H19] Leu deleted). Br. J. Haematol. *38*:195, 1978.
471. Bookchin, R. M., Nagel, R. L., and Ranney, H. M. Structure and properties of hemoglobin C Harlem, a human hemoglobin variant with amino acid substitutions in 2 residues of the β-polypeptide chain. J. Biol. Chem. *242*:248, 1967.
472. Lang, A., Lehmann, H., McCurdy, P. R., and Pierce, L.: Identification of haemoglobin C Georgetown. Biochim. Biophys. Acta *278*:57, 1972.
473. Adams, J. G., and Heller, P.: Hemoglobin Arlington Park (β6 Glu→Lys 95 Lys→Glu): Electrophoretically "silent" hemoglobin variant with two amino acid substitutions in the same polypeptide chain. Blood *42*:990, 1973.
474. Blackwell, R. Q., Wong Hock Boon, Liu, C.-S., and Weng, M. I.: Hemoglobin J Singapore: α78Asn→Asp: α79 Ala→Gly. Biochim. Biophys. Acta *278*:482, 1972.
475. Goossens, M., Garel, M. C., Auvinet, J., Basset, P., Gomes, P. F., and Rosa, J.: Hemoglobin C Ziguinchor α2Aβ2 6 (A3) Glu→Val β58 (E2) Pro→Arg: The second sickling variant with amino acid substitutions in 2 residues of the β polypeptide chain. FEBS Lett. *58*:149, 1975.
476. Moo-Penn, W. F., Schmidt, R. M., Jue, D. L., Bechtel, K. C., Wright, J. M., Horne, M. K., III. Haycraft, G. L., Roth, E. F., and Nagel, R. L.: Hemoglobin S Travis. A sickling hemoglobin with two amino acid substitutions [α6 (A3) Glutamic acid→Valine and β142 (H20) Alanine→Valine] Eur. J. Biochem. *77*:561, 1977.
477. Moo-Penn, W. F., Jue, D. L., Johnson, M. H., Bechtel, K. C., and Patchen, L. C.: Hemoglobin variants and methods used for their characterization during 7 years of screening at the Center for Disease Control. Hemoglobin *4*:347, 1980.
478. Schneider, R. G.: Methods for detection of hemoglobin variants and hemoglobinopathies in the routine clinical laboratory. CRC Crit. Rev. Clin. Lab. Sci. *9*:243, 1978.
479. Schneider, R. G., and Barwick, R. C.: Hemoglobin mobility in citrate agar electrophoresis—its relationship to anion binding. Hemoglobin *6*:199, 1982.
479a. Winter, W. P., and Yodh, J.: Interaction of human

hemoglobin and its variants with agar. Science 221:175, 1983.
480. International Committee for Standardization in Hematology: Simple electrophoretic system for presumptive identification of abnormal hemoglobins. Blood 52:1058, 1978.
481. International Committee for Standardization in Hematology: Recommendations of a system for identifying abnormal hemoglobins. Blood 52:1065, 1978.
482. Basset, P., Beuzard, Y., Garel, M. C., and Rosa, J.: Isoelectric focusing of human hemoglobin: Its application to screening, to the characterization of 70 variants, and to the study of modified fractions of normal hemoglobins. Blood 51:971, 1978.
483. Galacteros, F., Kleman, K., Caburi-Martin, J., Beuzard, Y., Rosa, J., and Lubin, B.: Cord blood screening for hemoglobin abnormalities by thin layer isoelectric focusing. Blood 56:1068, 1980.
484. Garver, F. A., Baker, M. M., and Grenett, H. E.: Immunochemical identification and quantitation of variant hemoglobins. Tex. Rep. Biol. Med. 40:167, 1980–81.
485. Reichlin, M.: Amino acid substitution and antigenetic structure in globular proteins. Adv. Immunol. 20:71, 1975.
486. Garver, F. A., Baker, M. B., Jones, C. S., Gravely, M., Altay, G., and Huisman, T. H. J.: Radioimmunoassay for abnormal hemoglobins. Science 196:1334, 1977.
487. Grenett, H. E., and Garver, F. A.: Identification and quantitation of sickle cell hemoglobin with an enzyme-linked immunosorbent assay (ELISA). J. Lab. Clin. Med. 96:597, 1980.
487a. Wada, Y., Hayashi, A., Fujita, T., Matsuo, T., Katakose, I., and Matsuda, H.: Structural analysis of human hemoglobin variants by mass spectrometry. Int. J. Mass Spectrometry and Ion Physics 48:209, 1983.
488. Harris, H.: Genetic heterogeneity in inherited disease. J. Clin. Pathol. 27:32, 1974. (Supplement 8 Royal College of Pathology).
488a. Stamatoyannopoulos, G., Nute, P. E., and Miller, M.: De novo mutations producing unstable hemoglobins or hemoglobin M. Hum. Genet. 58:396, 1981.
488b. Stamatoyannopoulos, G., and Nute, P. E.: Cases of unstable hemoglobin and methemoglobin produced by de novo mutation. (Review.) Hemoglobin 8:85, 1984.
489. Bradley, T. B., Wohl, R. C., Petz, L. D., Perkins, H. A., and Reynolds, R. D.: Possible gonadal mosaicism in a family with hemoglobin Koln. Johns Hopkins Med. J. 146:236, 1980.
490. Sick, K., Beale, D., Irvine, D., Lehmann, H., Goodall, P. T., and MacDougall, S.: Hemoglobin G Copenhagen and haemoglobin J Cambridge. Two new β chain variants of hemoglobin A. Biochim. Biophys. Acta 140:231, 1967.
491. Fitch, W. M.: The restriction of codon ambiguity on the basis of known variants. J. Mol. Evol. 10:97, 1977.
492. Forget, B. G.: The structure of human globin messenger RNA. Functional, genetic and evolutionary implications. In Piomelli, S., and Yachnin, S. (eds.): Current Topics in Hematology. Vol. 3. New York, Alan R. Liss, Inc., 1980, p. 1.
492a. Forget, B. G.: Unpublished observations.
493. Orkin, S. H., Kazazian, H. H., Jr., Antonarakis, S. E., Goff, S. C., Boehm, C. D., Sexton, J. P., Waber, P. G., and Giardina, P. J. V.: Linkage of β-thalassemia mutations and β globin gene polymorphisms with DNA polymorphisms in human β globin gene cluster. Nature 296:627, 1982.
494. Spence, S. E., Pergolizzi, R. G., Donovan-Peluso, M., Kosche, K. A., Dobkin, C. S., and Bank, A.: Five nucleotide changes in the large intervening sequence of a β globin gene in a β^+-thalassemia patient. Nucleic Acids Res. 10:1283, 1982.
494a. Kazazian, H. H., Jr., Orkin, S. H., Antonarakis, S. E., Sexton, J. P., Boehm, C. D., Goff, S. C., and Waber, P. G.: Molecular characterization of seven β-thalassemia mutations in Asian Indians. EMBO J. 3:593, 1984.
495. Wilson, J. T., Wilson, L. B., Reddy, V. B., Cavallesco, C., Ghosh, P. K., deRiel, J. K., Forget, B. G., and Weissman, S. M.: Nucleotide sequence of the coding portion of human α globin messenger RNA. J. Biol. Chem. 255:2807, 1980.
496. Liebhaber, S. A., Goossens, M. J., and Kan, Y. W.: Cloning and complete nucleotide sequence of the human 5'-α globin gene. Proc. Natl. Acad. Sci. USA 77:7054, 1980.
496a. Michelson, A. M., and Orkin, S. H.: Boundaries of gene conversion within the duplicated human α-globin genes: Concerted evolution by segmental recombination. J. Biol. Chem. 258:15245, 1983.
497. Liebhaber, S. A., Goossens, M., and Kan, Y. W.: Homology and concerted evolution at the α1 and α2 loci of human globin. Nature 290:26, 1981.
498. Milner, P. F., Clegg, J. B., and Weatherall, D. G.: Haemoglobin-H disease due to a unique haemoglobin variant with an elogated α-chain. Lancet 1:729, 1971.
499. Clegg, J. B., and Weatherall, D. J.: Hemoglobin Constant Spring, an unusual α-chain variant involved in the etiology of hemoglobin H disease. Ann. N.Y. Acad. Sci. 232:168, 1974.
500. Lie-Injo, L. E., Lopez, C. G., and Lopes, M.: Inheritance of haemoglobin H disease. Acta Haematol. 46:106, 1971.
501. Pootrakul, S., Wasi, P., Pornpatkul, M., and Na-Nakorn, S.: Incidence of alpha thalassemia in Bangkok. J. Med. Assn. Thai. 53:250, 1970.
502. Efremov, G. D., Wrightstone, R. N., Huisman, T. H. J., Schroeder, W. A., Hyman, C., Ortega, J., and Williams, K.: An unusual hemoglobin anomaly and its relation to α-thalassemia and hemoglobin H disease. J. Clin. Invest. 50:1628, 1971.
503. Sofroniadou, K., Kaltsova, A., Loukopoulos, D., and Phessas, P.: Hemoglobin "Athens": An alpha chain variant with unusual properties. Abstract. XII Cong. Inter. Soc. Haemat. New York, 1968, p. 56.
504. Bradley, T. B., Wohl, R. C., and Smith, E. J.: Elongation of the α globin chain in a black family: Interaction with G-Philadelphia. Clin. Res. 23:131A, 1975.
505. Michelson, A. M., and Orkin, S. H.: The 3'-untranslated regions of the duplicated human α globin genes are unexpectedly divergent. Cell 22:371, 1980.
506. Seid-Akhavan, M., Winter, W. P., Abramson, R. K., and Rucknagel, D. L.: Hemoglobin Wayne:

A frame shift mutation detected in human hemoglobin alpha chains. Proc. Natl. Acad. Sci. USA 73:882, 1976.
507. Fitch, W. M.: A comparison between evolutionary substitutions and variants in human hemoglobins. Ann. N.Y. Acad. Sci. 241:439, 1974.
508. Marotta, C. A., Forget, B. G., Weissman, S. M., Verma, I. M., McCaffrey, R. P., and Baltimore, D.: Nucleotide sequences of human globin messenger RNA. Proc. Natl. Acad. Sci. USA 71:2300, 1974.
509. Forget, B. G., Marotta, C. A., Weissman, S. M., and Cohen-Solal, M.: Nucleotide sequences of the 3'-terminal untranslated region of the messenger RNA for the human beta globin chain. Proc. Natl. Acad. Sci. USA 72:3614, 1975.
510. Marotta, C. A., Wilson, J. T., Forget, B. G., and Weissman, S. M.: Human beta-globin messenger RNA. III. Nucleotide sequences derived from complementary DNA. J. Biol. Chem. 252:5040, 1977.
511. Proudfoot, N. J.: Complete 3' noncoding region sequences of rabbit and human β-globin messenger RNAs. Cell 10:559, 1977.
512. Lawn, R. M., Efstratiadis, A., O'Connell, C., and Maniatis, T.: The nucleotide sequence of the human β globin gene. Cell 21:647, 1980.
513. Streisinger, G., Okada, Y., Emrich, J., Newton, J., Tsugita, A., Terzaghi, E., and Inouye, M.: Frame shift mutations and the genetic code. Cold Spring Harbor Symp. Quant. Biol. 31:77, 1966.
514. Scott, A. F., Phillips, J. A., Young, K. E., Kazazian, H. H., Jr., Smith, K. D., Charache, S., and Clegg, J. B.: The molecular basis of hemoglobin Grady. Am. J. Hum. Genet. 33:129, 1981.
515. Rosa, J., Audart, J. C., Pagnier, J., Belkhodja, O., Boigne, J. M., and Labie, D.: A new abnormal hemoglobin: $\alpha^{112\ His\text{-}Gly}$ Hb Dakar. 12th Congress Intern. Soc. Haematol. New York, 1968, p. 73.
516. Labie, D., Bertrand, O., Belkhodja, O., Gacon, G., Wajcman, H., and Varet, B.: A second case of hemoglobin Grady, repetitive in the middle of the α chain. Hemoglobin 1:211, 1976–1977.
517. Kan, Y. W., Todd, D., and Dozy, A. M.: Haemoglobin Constant Spring synthesis in red cell precursors. Br. J. Haematol. 28:103, 1974.
518. Pooktrakul, S., Pongsamart, S., Prawatmuant, P., and Kemathorn, B.: Hb Constant Spring: Degradation and Hb synthesis studies. 16th Inter. Congr. Hematol. Koyoto, 1976, p. 55.
519. Weatherall, D. J., and Clegg, J. B.: The α-chain termination mutants and their relation to the α thalassemias. Philos. Trans. R. Soc. Lond. [Biol.] 271:411m, 1975.
520. Hanash, S., Winter, W. P., and Rucknagel, D. C.: Synthesis of haemoglobin Wayne in erythroid cells. Nature 269:717, 1977.
521. Huisman, T. H. J., and Miller, A.: Hb Grady and α thalassemia: A contribution to the problem of the number of Hb A structural loci in man. Am. J. Hum. Genet. 28:363, 1976.
522. Rieder, R. F., and Weatherall, D. J.: Studies on hemoglobin biosynthesis: Asynchronous synthesis of hemoglobin A and hemoglobin A_2 by erythrocyte precursors. J. Clin. Invest. 44:42, 1965.
523. Roberts, A. V., Weatherall, D. J., and Clegg, J. B.: The synthesis of human hemoglobin A_2 during erythroid maturation. Biochem. Biophys. Res. Commun. 47:81, 1972.
524. Gill, F., Atwater, J., and Schwartz, E.: Hemoglobin Lepore trait: Globin synthesis in bone marrow and peripheral blood. Science 178:623, 1972.
525. Lie-Injo, L. E., Ganesan, J., Clegg, J. B., and Weatherall, D. J.: The homozygous state for Hb Constant Spring. Blood 43:251, 1974.
525a. Wasi, P., Pootrakul, S., Pootrakul, P., Pravatnwang, P., Winichagoon, P., and Fucharoen, S.: Thalassemia in Thailand. Ann. N.Y. Acad. Sci. 344:352, 1980.
525b. Derry, S., Wood, W. G., Pippard, M., Clegg, J. B., Weatherall, D. J., Wickramasinghe, S. N., Darley, J., Fucharoen, S., and Wasi, P.: Hematologic and biosynthetic studies in homozygous hemoglobin Constant Spring. J. Clin. Invest. 73:1673, 1984.
526. Orkin, S. H., and Goff, S. C.: The duplicated human α globin genes: Their relative expression as measured by RNA analysis. Cell 24:345, 1981.
527. Liebhaber, S. A., and Kan, Y. W.: Differentiation of the mRNA transcripts originating from the α1 and α2 globin loci in normals and α-thalassemics. J. Clin. Invest. 68:439, 1981.
528. Shaeffer, J. R., Schmidt, G. J., Kingston, R. E., and Bunn, H. F.: Synthesis of hemoglobin Cranston, an elongated β chain variant. J. Mol. Biol. 140:377, 1980.
529. Rieder, R. F.: Synthesis of hemoglobin Gun Hill: Increased synthesis of the heme-free β^{GH} globin chain and subunit exchange with a free-α-chain pool. J. Clin. Invest. 50:388, 1971.
530. Shaeffer, J. R.: Structure and synthesis of the unstable hemoglobin Sabine ($\alpha_2\beta_2^{91\ Leu\text{-}Pro}$). J. Biol. Chem. 248:7473, 1973.
531. White, J. M., and Dacie, J. V.: The unstable hemoglobins—molecular and clinical features. Prog. Hematol. 7:69, 1971.
532. McDonald, M. J., Lund, D. P., Bleichman, M., Bunn, H. F., DeYoung, A., Noble, R. W., Foster, B., and Arnone, A.: Equilibrium, kinetic and structural properties of hemoglobin Cranston. An elongated β chain variant. J. Mol. Biol. 140:357, 1980.
532a. Moo-Penn, W. F., Jue, D. L., Johnson, M. H., McDonald, M. J., Turci, S. M., Shih, T.-B., Jones, R. T., Therrell, B. L., and Arnone, A.: Structural and functional studies of hemoglobin Wayne: An elongated α-chain variant. J. Mol. Biol. 180:1119, 1984.
533. Lie-Injo, L. E., Raudhawa, Z. I., Ganesan, J., Kane, J., and Peterson, D.: Hemoglobin Tak in a newborn Maylai. Hemoglobin 1:747, 1977.
534. Stamatoyannopoulos, G., Nute, P. E., Papayannopoulou, T., McGuire, T., Lim, G., Bunn, H. F., and Rucknagel, D.: Development of a somatic mutation screening system using Hb mutants. IV. Successful detection of red cells containing the human frame shift mutants Hb Wayne and Hb Cranston using monospecific fluorescent antibodies. Am. J. Hum. Genet. 32:484, 1980.
535. Efstratiadis, A., Posakony, J. W., Maniatis, T., Lawn, R. M., O'Connell, C., Spritz, R. A., deRiel, J. K., Forget, B. G., Weissman, S. M., Slightom, J. L., Blechl, A. E., Smithies, O.,

Baralle, F. E., Shoulders, C. C., and Proudfoot, N. J.: The structure and evolution of the human β globin gene family. Cell 21:653, 1980.
536. Chang, J. C., and Kan, Y. W.: β^0 thalassemia, a nonsense mutation in man. Proc. Natl. Acad. Sci. USA 76:2886, 1979.
537. Orkin, S. H., and Goff, S. C.: Nonsense and frame shift mutations in β^0 thalassemia detected in cloned β globin genes. J. Biol. Chem. 256:9782, 1981.
538. Trecartin, R. F., Liebhaber, S. A., Chang, J. C., Lee, K. Y., Kan, Y. W., Furbetta, M., Angius, A., and Cao, A.: β^0 thalassemia in Sardinia is caused by a nonsense mutation. J. Clin. Invest. 68:1012, 1981.
539. Flavell, R. A., Kooter, J. M., DeBoer, E., Little, P. F. R., and Williamson, R.: Analysis of the βδ-globin gene loci in normal and Hb Lepore DNA: Direct determination of gene linkage and intergene distance. Cell 15:25, 1978.
540. Mears, J. G., Ramirez, F., Leibowitz, D., and Bank, A.: Organization of human δ- and β-globin genes in cellular DNA and the presence of intragenic inserts. Cell 15:15, 1978.
541. Ottolenghi, S., Giglioni, B., Comi, P., Gianni, A. M., Polli, E., Acquaye, C. T., Oldham, J. H., and Masera, G.: Globin gene deletion in HPFH, $\delta^0 \beta^0$ thalassemia and Hb Lepore disease. Nature 278:654, 1979.
542. Baird, M., Schreiner, H., Driscoll, C., and Bank, A.: Localization of the site of recombination in formation of the Lepore Boston globin gene. J. Clin. Invest. 68:560, 1981.
542a. Mavilio, F., Giampaolo, A., Caré, A., Sposi, N. M., and Marinucci, M.: The δβ crossover region in Lepore Boston hemoglobinopathy is restricted to a 59 base pairs region around the 5' splice junction of the large globin gene intervening sequence. Blood 62:230, 1983.
542b. Ojwang, P. J., Nakatsuji, T., Gardiner, M. B., Reese, A. L., Gilman, J. G., and Huisman, T. H. J.: Gene deletion is the molecular basis for the Kenya-^{G}γ-HPFH condition. Hemoglobin 7:115, 1983.
543. Weatherall, D. J., and Clegg, J. B.: The Thalassemia Syndromes. 3rd ed. Oxford, Blackwell Scientific Publications, 1981.
544. Felice, A. E., Webber, B. B., and Huisman, T. H. J.: α-Thalassemia and the production of different α chain variants in heterozygotes. Biochem. Genet. 19:487, 1981.
545. Baine, R. M., Rucknagel, D. L., Dublin, P. A., and Adams, J. G.: Trimodality in the proportion of hemoglobin G Philadelphia in heterozygotes: Evidence for heterogeneity in the number of human alpha chain loci. Proc. Natl. Acad. Sci. USA 73:3633, 1976.
546. Rieder, R. F., Woodbury, D. H., and Rucknagel, D. L.: The interaction of α-thalassaemia and haemoglobin G Philadelphia. Br. J. Haematol. 32:159, 1976.
547. Milner, P. F., and Huisman, T. H. J.: Studies of the proportion and synthesis of haemoglobin G Philadelphia in red cells of heterozygotes, a homozygote and a heterozygote for both haemoglobin G and alpha thalassaemia. Br. J. Haematol. 34:207, 1976.
548. Surrey, S., Ohene-Frempong, K., Rappaport, E., Atwater, J., and Schwartz, E.: α Thalassemia and the expression of hemoglobin G-Philadelphia. Ann. N.Y. Acad. Sci. 344:62, 1980.
549. Lie-Injo, J. E., Dozy, A. M., Kan, Y. W., Lopes, M., and Todd, D.: The α-globin gene adjacent to the gene for Hb Q-α 74 Asp→His is deleted, but not that adjacent to the gene for Hb G-α 30 Glu→Gln; three fourths of the α-globin genes are deleted in Hb Q-α-thalassemia. Blood 54:1407, 1979.
550. Higgs, D. R., Old, J. M., Pressley, L., Clegg, J. B., Pressley, L., and Weatherall, D. J.: The genetic basis of Hb Q-H disease. Br. J. Haematol. 46:387, 1980.
551. Botha, M. C., Stathopoulou, R., Lehmann, H., Rees, J. S., and Plowman, D.: A Hb J Cape Town homozygote—association of Hb Cape Town and alpha thalassaemia. FEBS Lett. 95:331, 1978.
551a. Lang, A., Lehmann, H., and King-Lewis, P. A.: Hb K Woolwich, the cause of a thalassemia. Nature 249:467, 1974.
552. Orkin, S. H., Kazazian, H. H., Jr., Antonarakis, S. E., Ostrer, H., Goff, S. C., and Sexton, J. P.: Abnormal RNA processing due to the exon mutation of β^E globin gene. Nature 300:768, 1982.
552a. Orkin, S. H., Antonarakis, S. E., and Loukopoulos, D.: Abnormal processing of $\beta^{Knossos}$ RNA. Blood 64:311, 1984.
553. Shaeffer, J. R., McDonald, M. J., and Bunn, H. F.: Assembly of normal and abnormal human hemoglobins. Trends in Biochemical Sciences 6:158, 1981.
553a. Mrabet, N. T., McDonald, M. J., Turci, S. M., and Bunn, H. F.: Electrostatic interactions in the subunit assembly of human hemoglobin. Fed. Proc. 43:1577, 1984.
554. Shaeffer, J. R., Kingston, R. E., McDonald, M. J., and Bunn, H. F.: Competition of normal β chains and sickle hemoglobin β chains for α chains as a post-translational control mechanism. Nature 276:631, 1978.
554a. Bunn, H. F., and McDonald, M. J.: Electrostatic interactions in the assembly of human hemoglobin. Nature 306:498, 1983.
554b. Abraham, E. C., and Huisman, T. H. J.: Differences in affinity of variant β chains for α chains—a possible explanation for the variation in the percentages of β-chain variants in heterozygotes. Hemoglobin 1:861, 1977.
555. Itano, H. A., and Neel, J. V.: A new inherited abnormality of human hemoglobin. Proc. Natl. Acad. Sci. USA 36:613, 1950.
556. Schneider, R. G., Hightower, B., Hosty, T. S., Ryder, H., Tomlin, G., Atkins, R., Brimhall, B., and Jones, R. T.: Abnormal hemoglobins in a quarter million people. Blood 48:629, 1976.
557. Motulsky, A. G.: Frequency of sickling disorders in U.S. blacks. N. Engl. J. Med. 288:31, 1973.
558. Huisman, T. H. J.: Chromatographic separation of hemoglobins A_2 and C. The quantities of hemoglobin A_2 in patients with AC trait, CC disease and C-β-thalassemia. Clin. Chim. Acta. 40:159, 1972.
559. Prindle, K. M., and McCurdy, P. R.: Red cell life span in hemoglobin C disorders. Clin. Res. 17:33, 1969.

560. Bunn, H. F., Noguchi, C. T., Hofrichter, J., Schechter, G. P., Schechter, A. N., and Eaton, W. A.: The molecular and cellular pathogenesis of hemoglobin SC disease. Proc. Natl. Acad. Sci. USA, 79:7527, 1982.
561. Ranney, H. M., Larson, D. L., and McCormack, G. II.: Some clinical, biochemical and genetic observations on hemoglobin C. J. Clin. Invest. 32:1277, 1953.
562. Spaet, T. H., Alway, R. H., and Ward, G.: Homozygous type "C" hemoglobin. Pediatrics 12:483, 1953.
563. Singer, K.: Pure (homozygous) hemoglobin C disease. Blood 9:1023, 1954.
564. Terry, D. W., Motulsky, A. G., and Rath, C. E.: Homozygous hemoglobin C: A new hereditary hemolytic disease. N. Engl. J. Med. 251:365, 1954.
565. Hartz, W. H., and Schwartz, S. O.: Hemoglobin C disease, report of four cases. Blood 10:235, 1955.
566. Jensen, W. N., Schofield, R. A., and Agner, R.: Clinical and necropsy findings in hemoglobin C disease. Blood 12:74, 1957.
567. Smith, E. W., and Krevans, J. R.: Clinical manifestations of hemoglobin C disorders. Bull. Johns Hopkins Hosp. 104:17, 1959.
568. Redetzki, J. E., Bickers, J. N., and Samuels, M. S.: Homozygous hemoglobin C disease: Clinical review of 15 patients. South. Med. J. 61:238, 1968.
569. Anderson, M., Bluestone, R., Milner, P. F.: Pregnancy and homozygous haemoglobin C disease. J. Obstet. Gynaecol. Br. Cwlth. 74:694, 1967.
570. Murphy, J. R.: Hemoglobin CC disease: Rheological properties of erythrocytes and abnormalities in cell water. J. Clin. Invest. 47:1483, 1968.
571. Charache, S., Conley, C. L., Waugh, D. F., Ugoretz, R. J., and Spurrell, R. J.: Pathogenesis of hemolytic anemia in homozygous hemoglobin C disease. J. Clin. Invest. 46:1795, 1967.
572. Diggs, C. W., Kraus, A. O., Morrison, D. B., and Rudnicki, R. P. T.: Intra-erythrocytic crystals in a white patient with hemoglobin C in the absence of other types of hemoglobin. Blood 9:1172, 1954.
573. Kraus, A. P., and Diggs, L. W.: In vitro crystallization of hemoglobin occurring in citrated blood from patients with hemoglobin C. J. Lab. Clin. Med. 47:700, 1956.
574. Wheby, M. S., Thorup, O. A., and Leavell, B. S.: Homozygous hemoglobin C disease in siblings: Further comments on intra-erythrocytic crystals. Blood 11:266, 1956.
575. Lessin, L. S., Jensen, W. N., and Ponder, E.: Molecular mechanism of hemolytic anemia in homozygous hemoglobin C disease. J. Exp. Med. 130:443, 1969.
576. Fabry, M. E., Kaul, D. K., Raventos, C., Baez, S., Rieder, R., and Nagel, R. L.: Some aspects of the pathophysiology of homozygous Hb CC erythrocytes. J. Clin. Invest. 67:1284, 1981.
577. White, J. G.: Ultrastructural features of erythrocyte and hemoglobin sickling. Arch. Intern. Med. 133:545, 1974.
577a. Hirsch, R. E., Raventos-Suarez, C., Olson, J. A., and Nagel, R. L.: Ligand state of intraerythrocyte circulating Hb C crystals in homozygote CC patients. Blood, in press.
578. Fitzgerald, P. M. D., and Love, W. E.: Structure of deoxy hemoglobin C (beta six Glu→Lys) in two crystal forms. J. Mol. Biol. 132:603, 1979.
579. Houston, T. E., Girling, R. L., Amma, E. L., and Huisman, T. H. J.: Structure of human hemoglobin C: A disease with intra-erythrocytic crystals. Biochim. Biophys. Acta 576:497, 1979.
580. Girling, R. L., Houston, T. E., Amma, E. L., and Huisman, T. H. J.: An x-ray determination of the molecular interactions in hemoglobin C: A disease characterized by intraerythrocytic crystals. Biochem. Biophys. Res. Commun. 88:768, 1979.
580a. Brugnara, C., Kopin, A., Bunn, H. F., and Tosteson, D. C.: Regulation of cation content and cell volume in erythrocytes from patients with homozygous hemoglobin C disease. J. Clin. Invest. 75:1608, 1985.
581. Reiss, G., Ranney, H. M., and Shaklai, N.: The association of hemoglobin C with red cell ghosts. J. Clin. Invest. 70:946, 1982.
582. Self, F., McIntire, L. V., and Zanger, B.: Rheological evaluation of hemoglobin S and hemoglobin C hemoglobinopathies. J. Lab. Clin. Med. 89:488, 1976.
583. Thomas, E. D., Motulsky, A. G., and Walters, D. H.: Homozygous hemoglobin C disease. Am. J. Med. 18:832, 1955.
584. Dedmon, R. E., Emanuelli, A., and Trobaugh, F. E.: Hemolytic studies in homozygous hemoglobin C disease. Am. J. Clin. Pathol. 31:487, 1959.
585. Movitt, E. R., Pollycove, M., Mangum, J. F., and Porter, W. R.: Hemoglobin C disease: Quantitative determination of iron kinetics and hemoglobin synthesis. Am. J. Med. Sci. 80:558, 1964.
586. Murphy, J. R.: Hemoglobin CC erythrocytes: Decreased intracellular pH and decreased O_2 affinity anemia. Semin. Hematol. 13:177, 1976.
587. Bunn, H. F.: The interaction of sickle hemoglobin with DPG, CO_2 and with other hemoglobins: Formation of asymmetrical hybrids. In Brewer, G. J. (ed.): Hemoglobin and Red Cell Structure and Function. New York, Plenum Press, 1972, p. 41.
588. Bellingham, A. J., and Huehns, E. R.: Compensation in haemolytic anaemias caused by abnormal haemoglobins. Nature 218:924, 1968.
589. Adachi, K., and Asakura, T.: Aggregation and crystallization of hemoglobins A, S and C. J. Biol. Chem. 256:1824, 1981.
590. Itano, H. A.: A third abnormal hemoglobin associated with hereditary hemolytic anemia. Proc. Natl. Acad. Sci. USA 37:775, 1951.
591. Watson-Williams, E. J., Beale, D., Irvine, D., and Lehmann, H.: A new haemoglobin, D-Ibadan (β87 threonine→lysine), producing no sickle cell/haemoglobin D disease with haemoglobin S. Nature 205:1273, 1965.
592. Vella, F., and Lehmann, H.: Haemoglobin D Punjab (D Los Angeles). J. Med. Genet. 11:341, 1974.
593. Bird, G. W. G., and Lehmann, H.: Haemoglobin D in India. Br. Med. J. 1:514, 1956.
594. Chernoff, A. I.: The hemoglobin D syndromes. Blood 13:116, 1958.
595. Stout, C., Holland, C. K., and Bird, R. M.: Hemoglobin D in an Oklahoma family. Arch. Intern. Med. 114:296, 1964.
596. Dutta, R. N., Grover, J., and Lal, M.: Haemoglobin D disease. J. Indian Med. Assoc. 58:42, 1972.
597. Politis-Tsegos, C., Kynoch, P, Lang, A., Lehmann, H., Lorkin, P. A., Stathopoulou, R., and Wakefield, G.: Homozygous haemoglobin D Punjab. J. Med. Genet. 12:269, 1975.

598. Rieder, R. F.: Globin chain synthesis in Hb D (Punjab)-β-thalassemia. Blood 47:113, 1976.
599. Huisman, T. H. J., Still, J., and Nechtman, C. M.: The oxygen equilibria of some "slow moving" human haemoglobin types. Biochim. Biophys. Acta 74:69, 1963.
600. Gatti, F., Vandepitte, J., Lehmann, H., and Gaffney, P. J.: Hemoglobin E in a Congolese family. Ann. Soc. Belg. Med. Trop. 48:527, 1968.
601. Bunn, H. F., Meriwether, W. D., Balcerzak, S. P., and Rucknagel, D. L.: Oxygen equilibrium of hemoglobin E. J. Clin. Invest. 51:2984, 1972.
601a. Monzon, C. M., Fairbanks, V. F., Burgert, E. O., Jr., Sutherland, J. E., and Elliott, S. C.: Hematologic/genetic disorders among the Southeast Asian refugees. Clin. Res. 30:525A, 1982.
602. Fairbanks, V. F., Gilchrist, G. S., Brimhall, B., Jereb, J. A., and Goldston, E. C.: Hemoglobin E trait reexamined: A cause of microcytosis and erythrocytosis. Blood 53:109, 1979.
602a. Kazazian, H. H., Waber, P. G., Boehm, C. D., Lee, J. I., Antonara, S. E., and Fairbank, V. F.: Hemoglobin E in Europeans—further evidence for multiple origins of the beta-E-globin gene. (Technical note.) Am. J. Hum. Genet. 36:212, 1984.
602b. Nagel, R. L., Raventos-Suarez, C., Fabry, M. E., Tanowitz, H., Sicard, D., and Labie, D.: Impairment of the growth of *Plasmodium falciparum* in Hb EE erythrocytes. J. Clin. Invest. 68:303, 1981.
603. Vella, F.: Abnormal haemoglobin variants in 10,441 Chinese subjects. Acta Haematol. 23:393, 1960.
604. Blackwell, R. Q., Huang, J. T.-H., and Chien, L.-C.: Distribution of abnormal hemoglobins among normal Chinese residents of Taiwan. Isr. J. Med. Sci. 1:759, 1965.
604a. Santairanont, R., and Wilairat, P.: Red cells containing hemoglobin E do not inhibit malaria parasite development in man. Am. J. Trop. Med. Hyg. 30:541, 1981.
605. Keller, P., and Kohne, E.: Hypochromie der Erythrozyten bei heterozygotem Hämoglobin E (β26 Glu→Lys). Acta Haematol. 56:276, 1976.
606. Tuchinda, S., Rucknagel, D. L., Minnich, V., et al.: The coexistence of the genes for hemoglobin E and α thalassemia in Thais, with resultant suppression of hemoglobin E synthesis. Am. J. Hum. Genet. 16:311, 1964.
607. Wasi, P., Na-Nakorn, S., Pootrakul, S., et al.: Alpha- and beta-thalassemia in Thailand. Ann. N.Y. Acad. Sci. 165:60, 1969.
608. Wasi, P., Disthasongchan, P., and Na-Nakorn, S.: The effect of iron deficiency on the levels of hemoglobins A_2 and E. J. Lab. Clin. Med. 71:85, 1968.
609. Lehmann, H., Story, P., and Thien, H.: Hemoglobin E in Burmese. Br. Med. J. 1:544, 1956.
609a. Wong, S. C., and Ali, M. A. M.: Hemoglobin E diseases: Hematological, analytical, and biosynthetic studies in homozygotes and double heterozygotes for α-thalassemia. Am. J. Hematol. 13:15, 1982.
610. Ong, H. C.: Maternal and fetal outcome associated with hemoglobin E trait and hemoglobin E disease. Obstet. Gynecol. 45:672, 1975.
611. Fairbanks, V. F., Oliveros, R., Brandabur, J. H., Willis, R. R., and Fiester, R. F.: Homozygous hemoglobin E mimics β-thalassemia minor without anemia or hemolysis: Hematologic, functional and biosynthetic studies of first North American cases. Am. J. Hematol. 8:109, 1980.
612. Chernoff, A. I.: The human hemoglobins in health and disease. N. Engl. J. Med. 253:365, 1955.
613. Sturgeon, P., Itano, H. A., and Bergren, W. R.: Clinical manifestations of inherited abnormal hemoglobins. II. Interaction of hemoglobin E and thalassemia trait. Blood 10:396, 1955.
613a. Mehta, B. C., Agarwal, M. B., Varandan, D. G., Joshi, R. H., and Bhargava, A. B.: Hemoglobin E thalassemia—a study of 16 cases. Acta Haematol. 64:201, 1980.
614. Yuthavong, Y., Ruenwongsa, P., Benyajati, C., and Suttimool, W.: Studies on the structural stability of haemoglobin E. J. Med. Assoc. Thai. 58:351, 1975.
615. Frischer, H., and Bowman, J.: Hemoglobin E, an oxidatively unstable mutation. J. Lab. Clin. Med. 85:531, 1975.
616. Ali, M. A. M., Quinlan, A., and Wong, S. C.: Identification of hemoglobin E by isopropanol solubility test. Clin. Biochem. 13:146, 1980.
617. Ruenwongsa, P., and Yuthavong, Y.: Studies on the subunit dissociation of the abnormal haemoglobins E and New York. J. Med. Assoc. Thai. 58:253, 1975.
618. Kolatat, T.: Oxygen affinity of hemoglobin E Siriraj. Hosp. Gaz. 16:205, 1964.
619. Gacon, G., Wajcman, H., and Labie, D.: Hemoglobin E: Its oxygen affinity in relation with the ionic environment. FEBS Lett. 41:147, 1974.
620. Pagnier, J., Wajcman, H., and Labie, D.: Defect in hemoglobin synthesis possibly due to a disturbed association. FEBS Lett. 45:252, 1974.
621. Traeger, J., Wood, W. G., Clegg, J. B., Weatherall, J. B., and Wasi, P.: Defective synthesis of Hb E is due to reduced levels of β^E mRNA. Nature 288:497, 1980.
622. Feldman, R., and Rieder, R. F.: The interaction of hemoglobin E with β thalassemia: A study of hemoglobin synthesis in a family of mixed Burmese and Iranian origin. Blood 42:783, 1973.
623. Benz, E. J., Berman, B. W., Tonkonow, B. L., Coupal, E., Coates, T., Boxer, L. A., Altman, A., and Adams, J. G.: Molecular analysis of the β-thalassemia phenotype associated with inheritance of hemoglobin E ($\alpha_2\beta_2^{26\ Glu\to Lys}$). J. Clin. Invest. 68:118, 1981.
624. Traeger, J., Winichagoon, P., and Wood, W. G.: Instability of β^E-messenger RNA during erythroid cell maturation in hemoglobin E homozygotes. J. Clin. Invest. 69:1050, 1982.
625. Lehmann, H., and Huntsman, R. G.: Man's Haemoglobins. 2nd ed. Philadelphia, J. B. Lippincott Co., 1974.
626. Bookchin, R. M., Nagel, R. L., and Balazs, T.: Role of hybrid tetramer formation in gelation of haemoglobin S. Nature 256:667, 1975.
627. Esan, G. J. F., Morgan, F. J., and O'Donnell, J. V.: Diminished synthesis of an alpha chain mutant, hemoglobin I (α16 Lys→Glu). J. Clin. Invest. 49:2218, 1970.
628. Liebhaber, S. A., Rappaport, E. F., Cash, F. E., Ballos, S. K., Schwartz, E., and Surrey, S.: Hemoglobin I mutation encoded at both α-globin loci on the same chromosome: Concerted evolution in the human genome. Science 226:1449, 1984.
629. McDonald, M. J., Noble, R. W., Sharma, V. S., and Ranney, H. M.: Equilibrium and kinetic studies of hemoglobin I: Functionally silent amino acid substitution at an invariant residue. J. Mol. Biol. 89:245, 1974.

630. Atwater, J., Schwartz, I. R., Erslev, A. J., Montgomery, T. L., and Tocantins, L. M.: Sickling of erythrocytes in a patient with thalassemia hemoglobin I disease. N. Engl. J. Med. *263*:1215, 1960.
631. Huisman, T. H. J.: Trimodality in the percentages of β chain variants in heterozygotes: The effect of the number of active Hb_α structural loci. Hemoglobin *1*:349, 1977.
632. Matthay, K. K., Mentzer, W. C., Dozy, A. M., Kan, Y. W., and Bainton, D. F.: Modification of hemoglobin H disease by sickle trait. J. Clin. Invest. *64*:1024, 1979.
633. Levere, R. D., Lichtman, H. C., and Levine, J.: Effect of iron deficiency anaemia on the metabolism of the heterogenic haemoglobins in sickle cell trait. Nature *202*:499, 1964.
634. Winter, W. P.: Geographic and ethnic distribution of human hemoglobin variants. Tex. Rep. Biol. Med. *40*:179, 1980–1981.
635. Bodmer, W. F., and Cavalli-Sforza, L. L.: Genetics, Evolution and Man. San Francisco, W. H. Freeman, 1976.
636. Barwick, R. C., Jones, R. T., Head, C. G., et al.: Hb Long Island: A hemoglobin variant with a methionyl extension at the NH_2-terminus and a prolyl substitution for the normal histadyl residue of the beta chain. Proc. Natl. Acad. Sci. USA, in press.

VERNON INGRAM

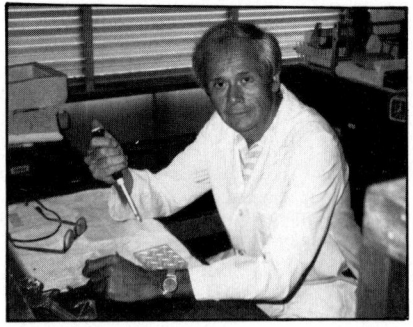

One of the crucial experiments that ushered in the "new biology" was done single-handedly in 1956 by a young biochemist at the Medical Research Council (MRC) Laboratory in Cambridge.

Vernon Ingram, like Perutz, Lehmann, and the Benesches, fled from Central Europe to England, just before the outbreak of World War II. After obtaining his doctorate in organic chemistry at Birkbeck College in London, he spent 2 years in the United States preparing and crystallizing proteins at the Rockefeller Institute and studying peptide chemistry at Yale. Perutz invited him to come to the MRC unit at the Cavendish Laboratory in 1952 in order to place heavy metal atoms in myoglobin and hemoglobin, to facilitate analysis of their crystal structures. The success and significance of their venture are recounted in Chapter 2. Perutz and Francis Crick persuaded Ingram to turn his attention to sickle hemoglobin. Ingram was well prepared for the task. He had already published several papers on amino acid and peptide chemistry. As he recalls, "The Cavendish idea of a biochemical laboratory was a room with a bench and a sink and a Bunsen burner and really very little else." However, he was able to consult with Frederick Sanger, whose laboratory was doing pioneering studies on primary protein structure. Hemoglobins A and S were digested with trypsin to give a mixture of peptides. Separation by either electrophoresis or paper chromatography revealed no apparent differences between the two proteins. However, when Ingram combined the two techniques, with chromatography run perpendicular to the direction of electrophoresis, a two-dimensional "fingerprint" emerged in which Hbs A and S were identical in all but one peptide. A year later, he showed that the abnormal peptide from sickle hemoglobin differed by only a single amino acid: valine instead of the glutamic acid found in Hb A. One can imagine the excitement that this discovery caused, not only in the highly charged environs of the MRC Laboratory but also among biologists worldwide. This experiment provided elegant and convincing proof of the one gene-one protein hypothesis of Beadle and Tatum. Furthermore, the identification of the structural abnormality of Hb S paved the way for understanding the molecular pathogenesis of sickle cell disease. A few years later, Ingram and a graduate student, John Hunt, determined the amino acid replacement in Hb C.

Ingram then became distracted by Crick, who sensed that the key to genetic diversity lay in alterations in protein composition. They searched in vain for amino acid differences among egg-white lysozymes from different strains of hens or indeed among lysozymes from the tears of the laboratory workers!

In 1958, Ingram joined the Biochemistry Department at the Massachusetts Institute of Technology. He is one of distinguished group of scientists at MIT who have built one of the world's leading centers of cell and molecular biology. After arriving there, Ingram continued to investigate hemoglobin variants. He and a graduate student, Anthony Stretton, established that Hb A_2 differed from Hb A at several sites, thus providing structural evidence for tandem globin genes. They developed a valid scheme for the evolution of globin genes and were the first to classify the thalassemias into α and β. Their classic paper on thalassemia shows remarkable clairvoyance. Ingram and Stretton proposed that reduction in globin chain synthesis could be due either to a silent mutation in the structural gene or to a defect in neighboring DNA that regulates gene expression. As discussed in Chapters 7 and 8, these predictions have been fully realized.

During the past two decades, Ingram's laboratory has focused on hemoglobin biosynthesis and erythroid cell differentiation. He and his colleagues have made a series of novel observations in a variety of model systems, including the frog, the chick, and the Friend erythroleukemia cell line. His contributions have ranged broadly from the cellular and organismal levels to chromatin structure and function and the control of gene expression. Thus, Ingram has remained at the forefront of molecular biology since its inception. Despite his accomplishments, Ingram remains unpretentious. He has developed a "proper disregard" for administration, preferring to keep his scientific life simple, just as in the days of the Cavendish Laboratory.

SICKLE CELL DISEASE—MOLECULAR AND CELLULAR PATHOGENESIS

11

HISTORICAL BACKGROUND*

The history of our understanding of sickle cell disease can be likened to the opening of the proverbial Russian egg: at once another egg appears within, and inside that another and yet another and so on. Thus, in the study of sickle cell disease, first we see the ailing and anemic patient, then his deoxygenated, sickled red cell, then its abnormal hemoglobin, and finally, hidden away inside the beta chain of the molecule, a single displaced amino acid.

William B. Castle[2]

The path from man to molecule begins with the recognition of the clinical manifestations of sickle cell disease at the beginning of this century (see Chapter 12). Herrick's initial description in 1910 of elongated crescent-shaped cells led to a variety of *in vitro* experiments that attempted to explain this phenomenon. Emmel[3] showed that virtually all red cells from an affected patient sickled following prolonged anaerobic incubation (see Fig. 12–1). This problem attracted the attention of Vernon Hahn, a young surgeon at the University of Indiana. In 1927, he and an intern, Elizabeth Gillespie, devised a simple but effective apparatus for examining the morphological changes in sickle red cells under carefully controlled conditions.[4] They found that cells suspended in a hanging drop sickled when oxygen tension was reduced below 45 mm Hg. When pH exceeded 7.4, sickling was inhibited. The sickle shape change could be reversed by reoxygenating the red cells or treating them with carbon monoxide. Moreover, cells devoid of hemoglobin (red cell ghosts) could not be induced to sickle. Three years later, Scriver and Waugh demonstrated reversible oxygen-

---

*Dr. C. Lockard Conley[1] has written a detailed account of the history of sickle cell research.

dependent sickling *in vivo*.[4a] In retrospect, these well-designed experiments provide convincing evidence that an abnormality in hemoglobin was responsible for the sickling phenomenon. No further insights into pathogenesis arose until 1940, when Thomas Hale Ham and William Castle[5] established the relationship between sickling and increased viscosity. They proposed that red cells engaged in a vicious circle of deoxygenation and sickling leading to the vaso-occlusive manifestations of the disease. In the same year, Irving Sherman,[6] a student in Wintrobe's laboratory at Johns Hopkins, presented *in vivo* as well as *in vitro* evidence that at reduced oxygen tensions, red cells from anemic patients (those with SS disease) sickled much more readily than those with asymptomatic sickle trait. An observation of even greater importance was the striking birefringence that he noted when deoxygenated sickled red cells were examined with a polarizing microscope. Sherman failed to comment on the significance of this finding, but others readily appreciated that the birefringence meant "that certain molecules of the cell became oriented when the cell undergoes sickling."[7]

Castle introduced sickle cell disease to Linus Pauling during a historic train ride in 1945:

> He and I were both members of a committee that eventuated in the publication of the book by Vannevar Bush, *Science, the Endless Frontier*, which among other places, met in Denver, I think in 1945. On the overnight train between Denver and Chicago, not long after leaving Denver, I had a conversation with Doctor Pauling about the molecular relation of antibody to antigen, etc., which was very informative to me. I then sketched a little bit of the work that Doctor Ham and I had been doing since 1940 on sickle cell disease and mentioned that, as stated by Doctor I. J. Sherman in 1940, when the cells were deoxygenated and sickled they showed birefringence in polarized light. This, I stated, meant to me some type of molecular alignment or orientation, and ventured to suggest that this might be "the kind of thing in which he would be interested." I am equally clear that I did not make the further generalization that it was orientation of the hemoglobin that might be doing this.[8]

The conclusion that hemoglobin was the culprit was inferred by Janet Watson, a hematologist in Brooklyn, New York, who observed that sickling did not become significant until the fetal hemoglobin in the infant was replaced by "adult" hemoglobin.[9]

In 1949, Linus Pauling took up the challenge of the sickle cell. In collaboration with younger colleagues Harvey Itano, S.J. Singer, and I.C. Wells,[10] he analyzed hemolysates by moving

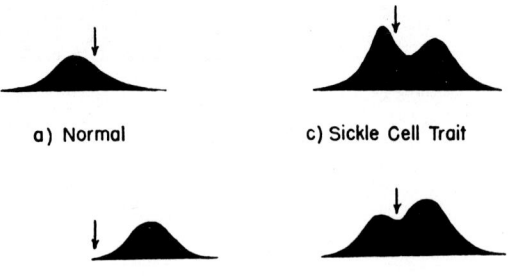

Figure 11–1. First demonstration of a molecular disease: Analysis of hemolysates of sickle cell and sickle trait red cells by moving boundary electrophoresis, 20 hours, pH 6.9. (From Pauling, L., et al.: Science *110*:543, 1949.)

boundary electrophoresis, a technique that had recently been devised by Tiselius. As shown in Figure 11–1, they found that the hemoglobin from a patient with sickle cell anemia had a different mobility from that of a normal individual. Moreover, individuals with sickle trait had both hemoglobins in approximately equal amounts. In one stroke, this experiment provided the first identification of a "molecular disease" as well as a sound explanation for the pattern of inheritance. Moreover, these investigators provided a remarkably coherent assessment of the molecular pathogenesis of the disease:

> Under the appropriate conditions, then, the sickle cell anemia hemoglobin molecules might be capable of interacting with one another at these sites sufficiently to cause at least a partial alignment of the molecules within the cell, resulting in the erythrocyte's becoming birefringent, and the cell membrane's being distorted to accommodate the now relatively rigid structures within its confines.[10]

While a postdoctoral fellow in Castle's laboratory, John Harris "demonstrated that a concentrated solution of sickle hemoglobin upon deoxygenation indeed formed birefringent polymers."[11] He showed that the appearance of liquid crystals or "tactoids"* was accompanied by a marked increase in viscosity. Harris concluded that the sickling of red cells and the accompanying loss of cell deformability was due to polymerization of the abnormal hemoglobin. Simultaneously, Perutz and Mitchison[12] reported that crystals of deoxy-

---

*In this chapter, "gel" and "gelation" refer to the transformation of a liquid to a semisolid that is no longer able to flow. Polymerization and aggregation are used synonymously to denote noncovalently linked arrays of deoxy Hb S. A tactoid is a liquid crystal composed of domains of polymer. "Sickle" refers only to change in red cell shape and not to the state of intracellular hemoglobin.

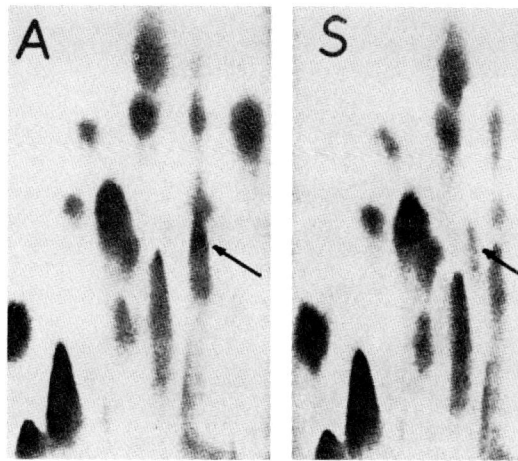

Figure 11–2. Demonstration of structural abnormality in sickle hemoglobin by two-dimensional mapping of tryptic peptides (see Figure 2–1). Arrows show displacement of a single peptide in Hb S. (From Ingram, V. M.: Scientific American *198*:68, 1958).

hemoglobin S were birefringent and had decreased solubility. During this time, Karl and Lily Singer[13] and Anthony Allison[14, 15] examined the gelling properties of Hb S and its interaction with Hbs A, F, and C. The observations of these investigators laid the groundwork for understanding both the structure of the sickle fiber and the mechanisms responsible for polymerization.

In 1957, Vernon Ingram established that sickle hemoglobin differed from Hb A by only a single amino acid substitution: glutamic acid → valine.[16, 17] This was the first important application of two-dimensional peptide mapping (Fig. 11–2). Ingram's remarkable discovery not only provided definitive information on the first "molecular disease" but also lent cogent support to the one gene/one enzyme (polypeptide) theory advanced by Beadle and Tatum. Hemoglobin has remained in the forefront of molecular biology ever since.*

OVERVIEW

The pathophysiologic manifestations of sickle cell disease stem directly from the single base mutation A → T in the triplet codon for the sixth residue of the β globin chain. As shown in Figure 11–3, in concentrated hemoglobin solutions that have undergone partial

---
*The year 1957 seems a logical time to end this historical account. The chapter will discuss in great detail subsequent developments. Interest and progress in research on sickle cell disease grew considerably in the early 1970's, in part coincident with the establishment of the Sickle Cell Disease Branch of the National Institutes of Health.

or full deoxygenation, the substitution of valine for glutamic acid at β 6 leads to polymerization. The formation of intracellular fibers causes a significant reduction in cell deformability and sometimes a distortion of cell shape (sickling). These rigid cells are capable of obstructing flow in the microcirculation. The vaso-occlusive manifestations of sickle cell disease are critically dependent on the intracellular concentration of deoxyhemoglobin S and on the kinetics of polymerization.

Intracellular polymerization of Hb S inflicts damage on the red cell membrane, which may lead to dehydration and the potentiation of hemoglobin polymerization. Because of genetic and cellular modulators, as well as conditioning in the circulation, red cells of patients with sickle cell disease are quite heterogeneous, a feature that greatly complicates our understanding of pathogenesis.

This chapter will begin with a detailed review of current information on the structure of the sickle hemoglobin fiber followed by a description of the mechanism responsible for polymerization. The roles of oxygen binding and nonsickle hemoglobins will be discussed in detail. This information on the properties of sickle hemoglobin in free solution will be useful in understanding the behavior of Hb S–containing red cells, earmarked by various types of cell heterogeneity. The contribution of the membrane lesion will be presented along with a brief account of the fate of sickle cells in the microcirculation. The chapter will end with a consideration of various strategies that can be used to inhibit the polymerization of sickle hemoglobin.

STRUCTURE OF THE SICKLE HEMOGLOBIN FIBER

Knowledge of the structure of hemoglobin has set the stage for understanding how the sickling phenomenon takes place at the molecular level. The following two questions need to be resolved: (1) How are the hemoglobin molecules packed in the polymer? (2) What are the important intermolecular contacts? The sickling phenomenon must ultimately be explained by the substitution of the hydrophobic valine residue for glutamic acid at the sixth position of the β chain. Polymerization of Hb S is due to a localized alteration on the surface of the molecule rather than to any widespread conformational changes. In dilute solution, Hb S has entirely normal functional properties.[18–22] Early studies of Allison[14] and Murayama[23]

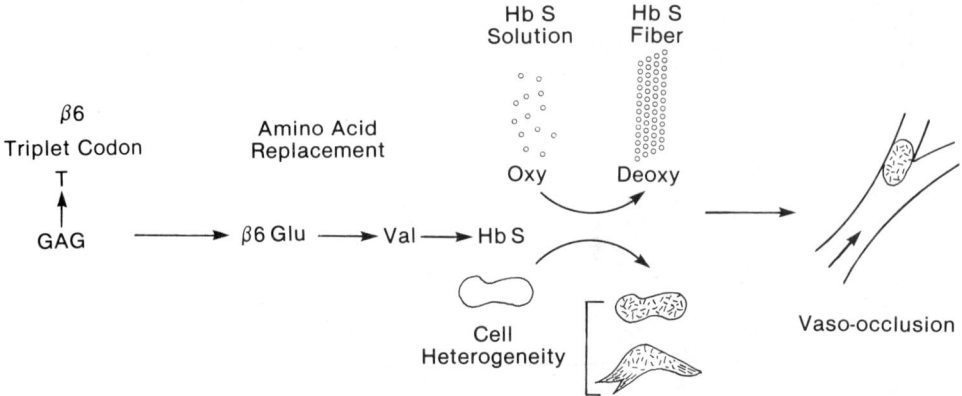

Figure 11–3. Scheme of pathogenesis of sickle cell disease.

indicated that the polymerization of sickle hemoglobin molecules involved hydrophobic bonding. Evidence supporting this conclusion included the demonstration of a negative temperature coefficient of gelation and the ability of nonpolar molecules such as propane and urea to inhibit sickling. Later studies showed that electrostatic bonds are also important in the polymerization of sickle hemoglobin molecules.[24] Thus, the formation of the sickle polymer is complex and must involve multiple types of chemical interactions.

Electron Microscopy and Image Reconstruction

When sickle hemoglobin is deoxygenated, either in intact red cells or in concentrated solution, it forms a gel. Electron micrographs (Fig. 11–4) reveal bundles of long fibers, some of which are aligned in parallel.[23, 25–29] In cells, the fibers correspond to the long axis of the sickled shape. Cross sections of these bundles reveal that the fibers are solid, not hollow, and have a center-to-center distance of about 210 Å.[30] High-resolution electron micrographs, abetted by negative staining, have revealed additional features in the sickle fiber that have been used in constructing a three-dimensional model.[31] The fiber shown in Figure 11–5 has a subtle undulating pattern with variable diameter and a twisted appearance indicative of a right-handed helix of high pitch having a periodicity of 3000 Å. Edelstein and colleagues have made exhaustive analyses of these high-resolution electron micrographs, utilizing optical diffraction and three-dimensional image reconstruction. As shown in Figure 11–5, they propose that the sickle fiber most commonly observed in both cells and in solution consists of 14 strands, a closely packed inner core of four and an outer sheath of ten. By improved methods of fixation and embedding, these investigators obtained cross-sectional images with considerable detail.[32] A number of patterns were observed, including bull's-eyes and concentric crescents. These images were consistent with a 14-stranded fiber in which sections were cut at various angles relative to the fiber axis. Occasional fibers appeared to lack specific strand pairs. As will be discussed later, these anomalous forms have provided insights into the assembly of the sickle fiber and provide additional support for the 14-strand model.

These analyses of electron micrographs do not provide any information per se on the orientation of the sickle hemoglobin molecule in the polymer. Initially, the problem was approached with optical measurements. Perutz and Mitchison[12] studied the absorption of sickled erythrocytes with polarized light. Their results, when interpreted in terms of the later x-ray structural information, indicated that the long molecular X axis of the hemoglobin tetramers was close to the fiber axis. More recent optical data of Hofrichter and Eaton[33, 34] confirm and extend this early conclusion. Their measurements indicate that the X axis of the tetramer (65 Å dimension) is within 22 degrees of the fiber axis. These results impose an important constraint on the orientation of the hemoglobin molecule within the fiber lattice.

X-ray Diffraction

Definitive information on the intermolecular contacts in the sickle polymer have come from x-ray diffraction studies. Love and associates[35] have analyzed crystals of deoxyhemoglobin S

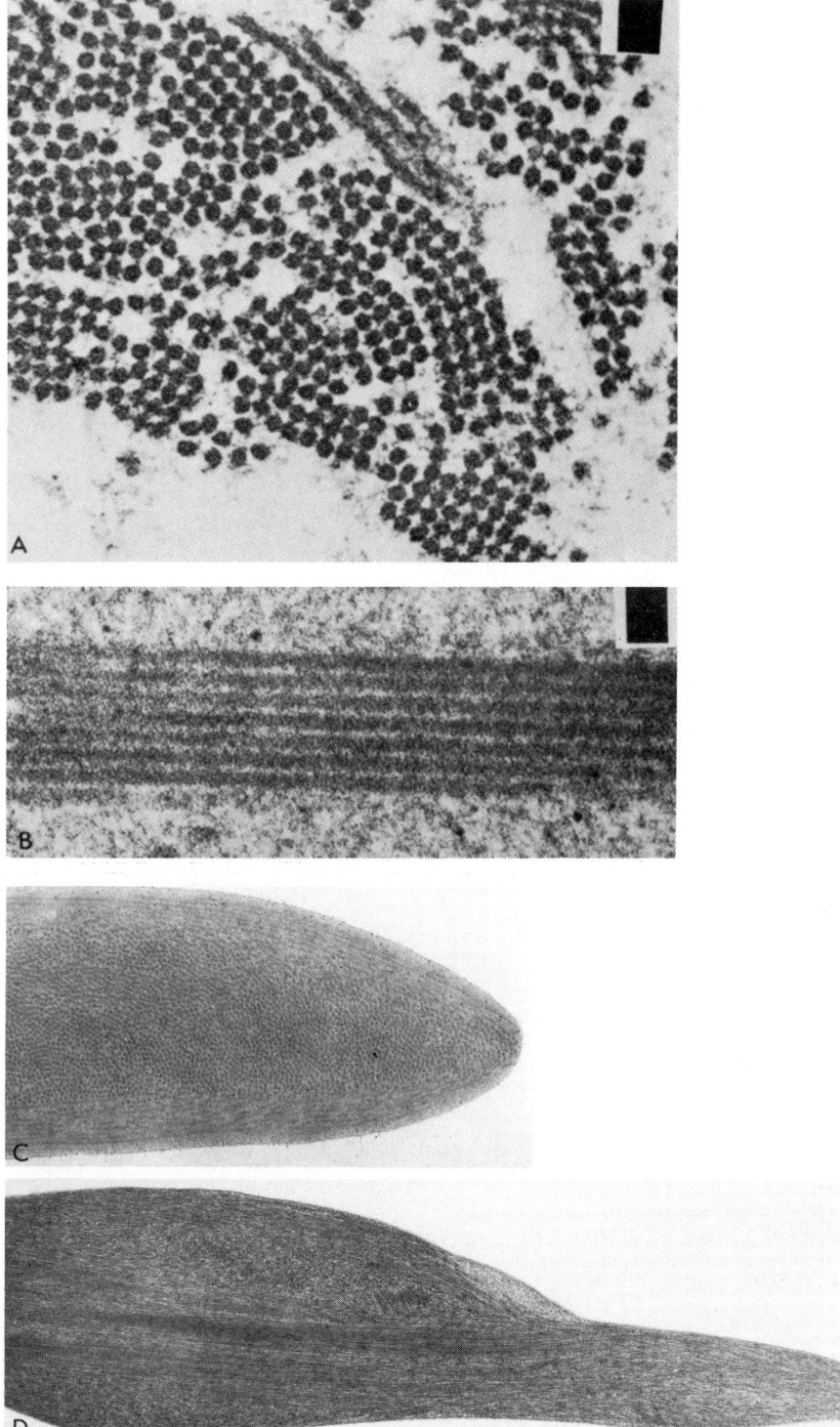

Figure 11-4. A and B, Electron micrographs of a centrifuged pellet of deoxyhemoglobin S ($\times$ 325,000). A, Transverse section showing bundles of Hb S fibers. B, Longitudinal section showing aligned fibers. (From Finch, J. T., et al.: Proc. Natl. Acad. Sci. USA 70:718, 1973.) C and D, Electron micrograph of deoxygenated SS erythrocyte. C, Transverse section. D, Longitudinal section. (Courtesy of Dr. J. F. Bertles and Dr. Joanna Döbler.)

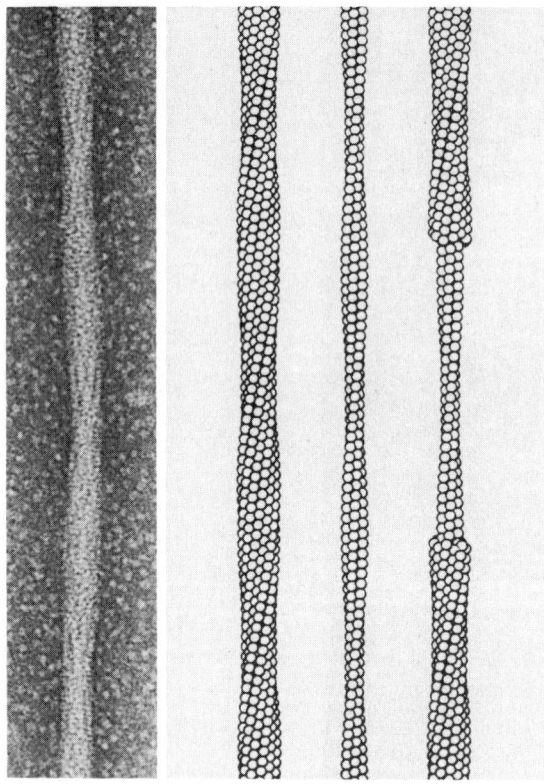

Figure 11–5. *Left,* Electron micrograph of negatively stained sickle fiber. Note twist of the strands within the fiber. *Right,* Three-dimensional image reconstruction of the fiber. Each sphere represents a Hb S tetramer. The inner core of 4 strands and the outer sheath of 10 strands are shown. (From Edelstein, S. J.: Tex. Rep. Biol. Med. *40*:221, 1980–81.)

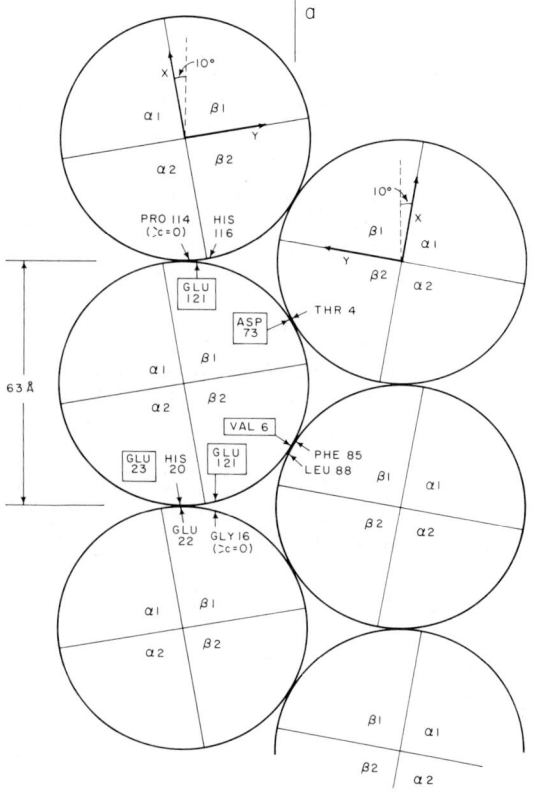

Figure 11–6. Double strand showing intermolecular contacts between neighboring molecules of Hb S. This model was constructed from x-ray crystallographic data of Wishner and associates (J. Mol. Biol. *98*:179, 1975).

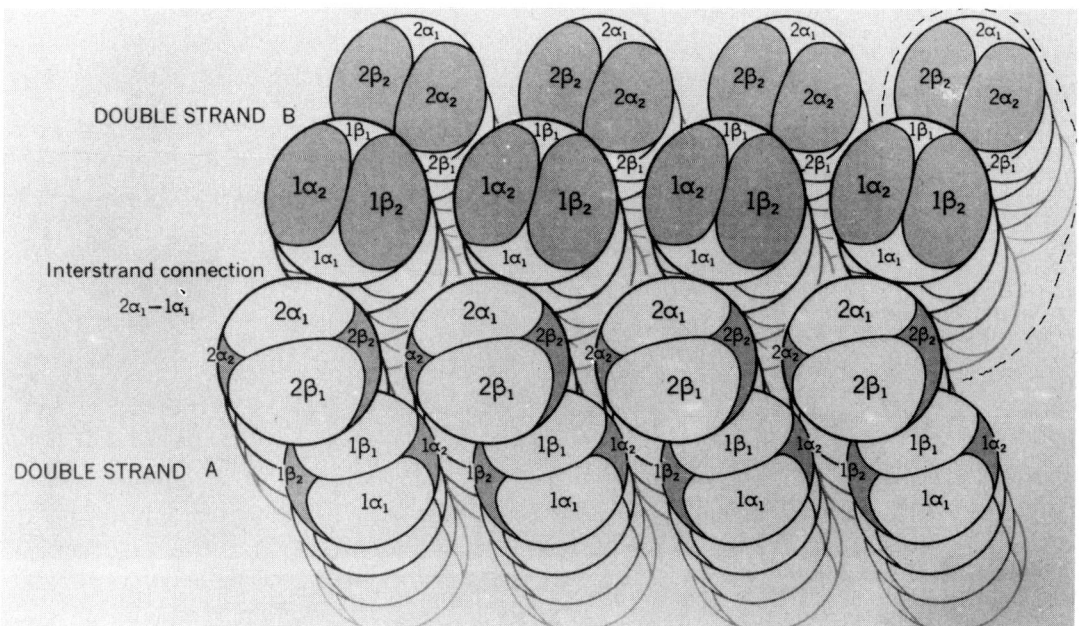

Figure 11–7. Packing of double strands in crystal of deoxyhemoglobin S. The double strands are oriented perpendicular to the plane of the page. One of the double strands has been earmarked with a dotted line. Note that double strand B goes in a direction opposite to double strand A, i.e., antiparallel. The contacts between double strands are primarily α_1–α_1. (From Dickerson, R. E., and Geis, I.: Hemoglobin: Structure, Function, Evolution and Pathology. Menlo Park, California, Benjamin Cummins, 1983.)

grown in 10 to 15 per cent polyethylene glycol. In the crystal, molecules of deoxyhemoglobin S are arrayed in pairs of parallel strands. In each pair, adjacent strands are staggered by half a molecule and rotated by half a turn (Fig. 11–6). Thus, each strand is related to its partner strand by a twofold screw axis running between them. The molecular X axis is 10 degrees from the axis of the double strand (consistent with the optical studies cited previously). As shown in Figure 11–7, each double strand is in contact with another double strand that is oriented in the opposite direction (i.e., antiparallel).

X-ray analysis has enabled the identification of contacts between neighboring molecules. The interactions within each strand are called axial contacts, whereas those between strands in a pair are designated lateral contacts. As depicted in Figures 11–6 and 11–8, β 6 Val makes a lateral contact with β 85 (F1) Phe and β 88 (F4) Leu on the partner strand. Note that only one of the two β 6 sites on the tetramer makes such a contact. Thus, asymmetrical hybrids of the type $\alpha_2\beta^S\beta^A$ should be able to readily enter into the sickle polymer if properly oriented. This hydrophobic interaction requires that hemoglobin be in the deoxy conformation. In oxyhemoglobin S, this stereochemical fit is no longer possible. Another lateral contact includes an interaction between β 73 Asp and β 4 Thr on the partner strand (see Fig. 11–6). Among the axial contacts are those involving β 22 Glu and β 121 Glu with an α chain on the adjacent molecule on the same strand. Experiments involving mixtures of Hb S and various hemoglobin variants have verified the importance of these contacts in stabilizing the sickle fiber (see below). In general, lateral contacts between the paired fibers involve interactions between cis and trans* β chains, whereas axial contacts include both β and α chains. Finally, interactions between antiparallel double strands involve primarily α-chain contacts (see Fig. 11–7).

Padlan and Love[36] have recently completed a 3-Å refinement of the crystal structure of deoxyhemoglobin S. They found that the only significant conformational difference between Hb S and Hb A is in the N-terminal A helix (β 4–β 18), which remains intact in Hb S but undergoes a hinge-like displacement, allowing it to make contact with receptor groups in the β EF region of the adjacent strand.

Intermolecular Contacts in the Fiber

Clearly, the structural analyses of Hb S crystals have provided a wealth of information about intermolecular contacts. The crucial is-

---

*"Cis" refers to the $\alpha\beta$ dimer having the β 6 Val donor site; "trans" refers to the other $\alpha\beta$ dimer.

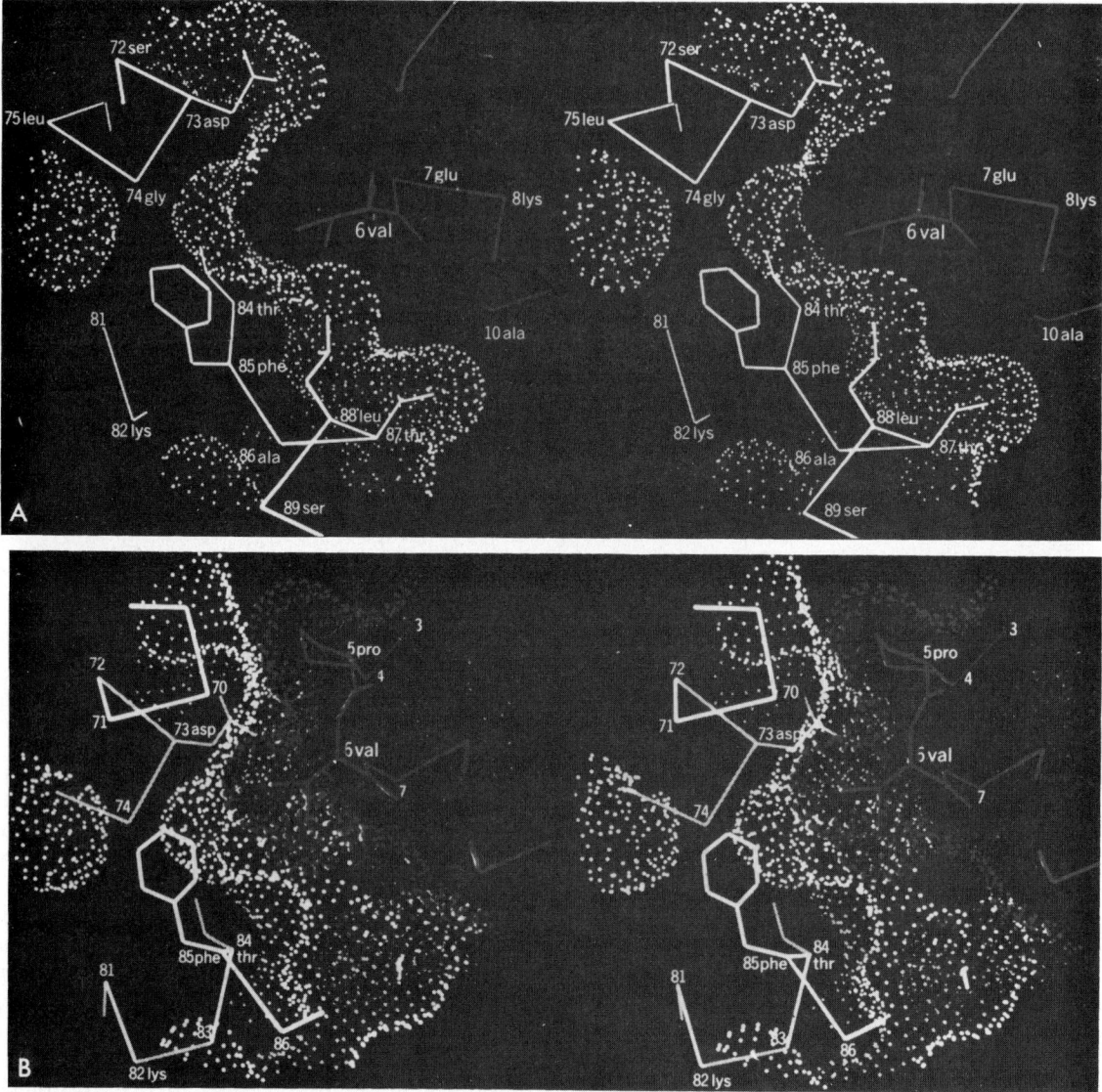

Figure 11–8. *A*, Stereoscopic view showing the interaction between the sickle mutation β 6 Val (donor site) and the acceptor site at the EF region including β 85 Phe and β 88 Leu. *B*, Demonstration of complementarity between donor and acceptor surfaces. (From Dickerson, R. E., and Geis, I.: Hemoglobin: Structure, Function, Evolution and Pathology. Menlo Park, California, Benjamin Cummins, 1983.)

sue is how relevant are these interactions to those present in the sickle fiber formed under physiologic conditions. A number of independent lines of evidence suggest that the fiber, in fact, bears strong structural resemblance to the crystal and that many of the intermolecular contacts present in the crystal also occur in the fiber.

One can view the packing of molecules in the crystal as a continuous lattice of parallel and antiparallel double strands (see Fig. 11–7). It is easy to visualize taking a group of double strands (e.g., 7, to give a 14-stranded fiber) and with a slight twist producing a helical fiber like the one deduced from image reconstruction of electron micrographs.[31] Such a transition might involve only a small change in energy. In fact, Magdoff-Fairchild[37] has shown that sickle fibers can transform spontaneously to a crystal having the same structure as those analyzed by Love and coworkers.[35] With routine storage, this transition requires months or years. However, when stirred, concentrated solutions of deoxyhemoglobin S form crystals quite rapidly.[38] The mechanism by which stirring promotes crystal formation is not understood. Wellems and Josephs[39, 40, 40a] have obtained stunning electron micrographic documentation of the transition from the fiber to the crystal. They observe intermediate forms, including ribbons that appear to be sheets of aligned double strands as well as paracrystals having a clear herringbone pattern (Fig. 11–9) that corresponds precisely to the spacing of antiparallel double strands.

The solubility of the crystal is slightly lower than that of the fiber, indicating that the transition is unidirectional: Fiber can turn to crystal but not vice versa. The fact that the difference in solubility is not large suggests that the energy required for the transition is indeed very small. The notion that the "crystal" double strand is the basic unit of the fiber receives considerable support from the optical measurements (mentioned previously) showing that the orientation of the hemoglobin molecule relative to the fiber axis is very close to its orientation in the crystal double strand (see Fig. 11–6). Moreover, x-ray diffraction patterns obtained by Magdoff-Fairchild and Chiu on sickle fibers have identified the double strand as the basic structural unit in the fi-

ber.[37, 41] The fact that the fiber appears to contain seven double strands must mean that some pairs are oriented in one direction and an unequal number of pairs are antiparallel. In fact, the fiber does have a net polarity.[42] Figure 11–10B shows the polarities of the individual double strands in the model proposed by Edelstein and colleagues. The validity of this arrangement is supported by the observation of occasional fibers appearing like a diamondback snake in longitudinal view, while on cross section two specific peripheral double strands appear to be missing (Fig. 11–10C). These "incomplete" fibers are particularly prominent when prepared from a mixture of Hb S and an α-chain variant (Hb Hasharon [α 47 Asp → His]) known to lower the stability of the sickle polymer (see below.)[43] The best resolution that can be achieved by electron microscopy of sickle fibers is approximately 30 Å. Recent analysis of fibers by x-ray diffraction at 15 Å resolution confirms the 14-stranded model but suggests alternate pairings of the double strands.[43a]

From the cumulative evidence that has been marshalled to date, it is likely that both the axial contacts and the lateral contacts in the crystal double strand are preserved in the fiber with virtually total fidelity. In contrast, the twist required to transform a bundle of seven double strands into a fiber undoubtedly produces a diverse set of contacts between double strands that are not present in the crystal. Edelstein[44] has compared the topology of the helical 14-strand fiber with that of the crystal and has determined what new contacts will be made and what others would be broken upon going from one to the other (see below).

Other structures have been proposed for the sickle fiber. Six-strand[23, 29] and eight-strand[45] models are unlikely candidates because their fiber diameter would be smaller than what is observed on electron micrographs and because they would contain a hollow center, a feature never observed on electron micrographs of cross sections. More recently, Wellems and Josephs[39] have proposed a 16-strand fiber. This structure has considerable appeal because of its symmetry: four antiparallel pairs of double strands. However, a cross-sectional view shown in Figure 11–10D reveals that a large crevice would be present running up the fiber axis. This feature has not been demonstrated on electron micrography. Moreover, the recent demonstration that the fiber has a net polarity[41] would rule out this symmetrical 16-strand model. As discussed earlier, the bulk of the

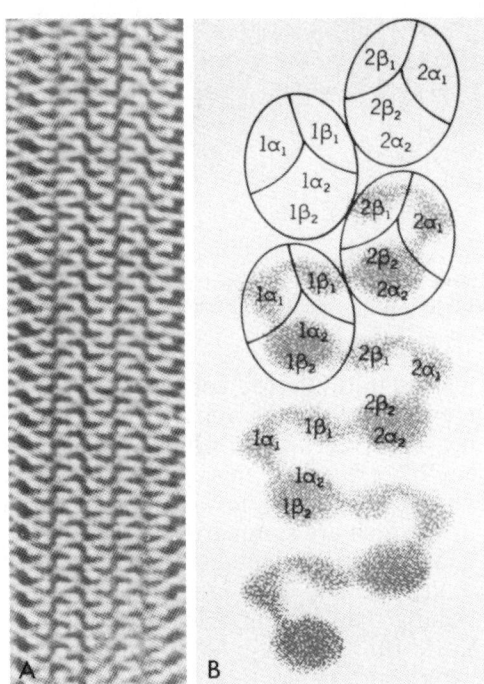

Figure 11–9. A, Electron micrograph of crystal grown in stirred solution of deoxy Hb S. Note the herringbone pattern. Three antiparallel double strands are shown. (Courtesy of Dr. Robert Josephs.) B, Electron-density pattern of a single double strand. The nubbins of increased density represent superimposition of α_2 and β_2 subunits. (From Dickerson, R. E., and Geis, I.: Hemoglobin: Structure, Function, Evolution and Pathology. Menlo Park, California, Benjamin Cummins, 1983.)

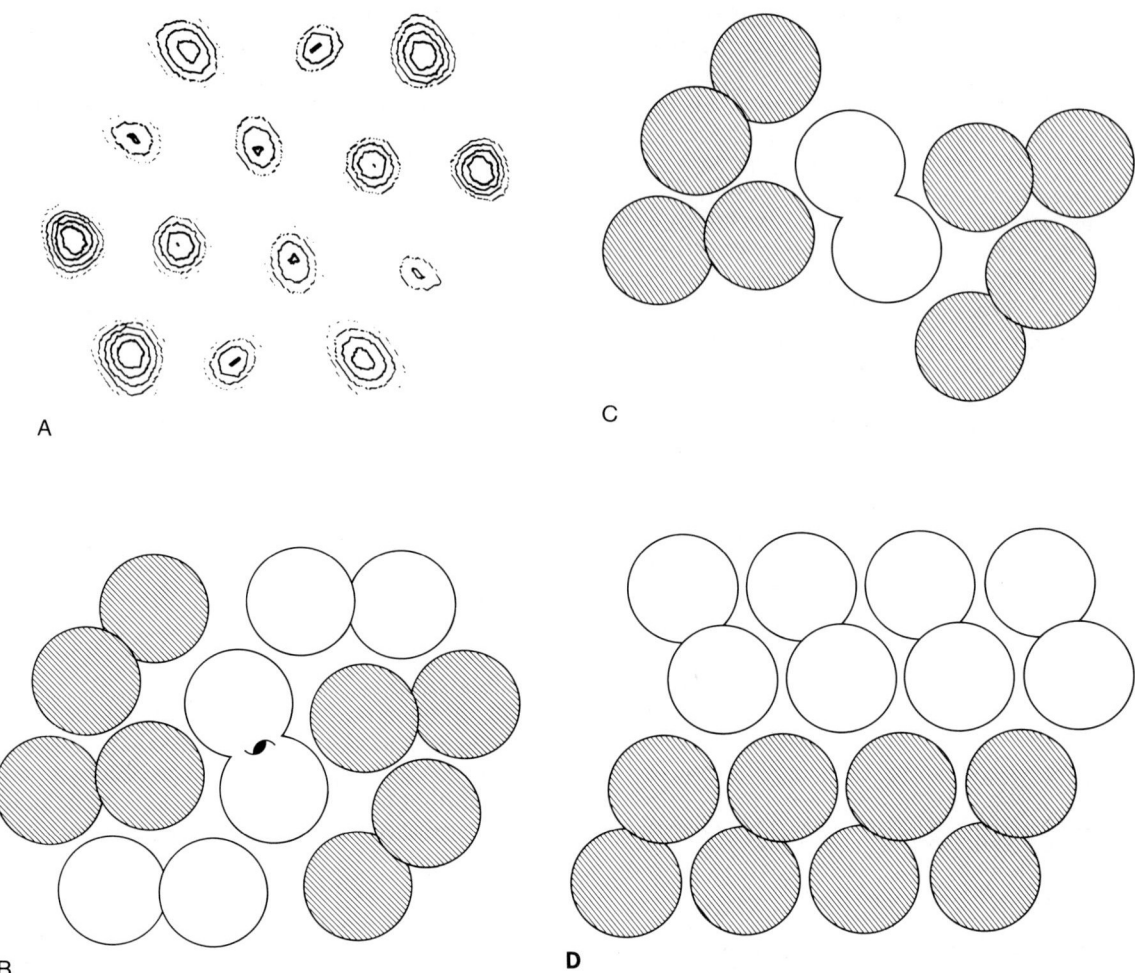

Figure 11–10. Cross sections of sickle fiber. *A*, Electron-density map obtained by Edelstein, showing 14 strands. *B*, Edelstein model showing polarity of double strands, i.e., ○○ and ●● are antiparallel. (From Edelstein, S. J., et al.: Proc. Natl. Acad. Sci. USA 70:1104, 1973.) *C*, Occasional fiber found to lack two peripheral double strands. *D*, Model of a 16-stranded fiber.

ultrastructural and solution data argue strongly that the 14-strand fiber is the predominant form both in red cells and in free solution.

Interaction of S and Non-S Hemoglobins

Studies on the gelation of deoxygenated mixtures of S and non-S hemoglobins have provided crucial information about the contact points between neighboring molecules in the sickle polymer. The early experiments of Singer and Singer[13] established that the presence of hemoglobin F increased the minimum concentration of total hemoglobin required for gelation (MGC). In fact, these MGC results suggested that hemoglobin F failed to participate at all in the sickling phenomenon. Mixtures of Hb S with either Hb A or Hb C gelled at a considerably lower concentration. Thus, these two hemoglobins apparently participate in the polymer. Bookchin, Nagel, and Ranney[46–48] extended this experimental approach to a wide variety of other β-chain variants, which are summarized in Table 11–1. For example, they demonstrated that Hb C-Harlem (β 6 Glu → Val, 73 Asp → Asn) gelled less readily than hemoglobin S. Furthermore, Hb Korle-Bu (β 73 Asp → Asn) participated in gelation with hemoglobin S less readily than did Hb A.[47] These observations indicated that the aspartate residue at position 73 of the β chain is an important site in the polymerization of sickle hemoglobin. In contrast, Hb O-Arab[49] (β 121 Glu→Lys) and Hb D-Los Angeles (β 121 Glu→Gln)[50] both interact particularly strongly with sickle hemoglobin; that is, mixtures gel about as readily as pure Hb S. It can be inferred from these experiments that β 121

Table 11-1. VARIANT HEMOGLOBINS THAT AFFECT POLYMERIZATION OF Hb S*

Variant	Structure	Effect†	Site of Contact‡ Experimental	Site of Contact‡ Edelstein Model
Sawara	α 6 Asp→Ala	↑		$α_1$—inter DS
Anantharaj	α 11 Lys→Glu	↓		0
I	α 16 Lys→Glu	↓	$α_2$	$α_2$—axial
Le Lamentin	α 20 His→Gln	↓	$α_2$	$α_2$—axial
Memphis	α 23 Glu→Gln	↓		0
Hasharon (Sealy)	α 47 Asp→His	↓	$α_1$ and $α_2$	0
J-Mexico	α 54 Gln→Glu	↓		$α_1$ and $α_2$—inter DS
G-Philadelphia	α 68 Asn→Lys	↓		0
Winnipeg	α 75 Asp→Tyr	↑		$α_2$—inter DS
Stanleyville	α 78 Asn→Lys	↓	$α_2$	$α_2$—inter DS
O-Indonesia	α 116 Glu→Lys	↓		$α_2$—axial
J-Baltimore	β 16 Gly→Asp	↓	Prob. $β_1$	$β_1$—axial
J-Amiens	β 17 Lys→Gln	↓	Prob. $β_1$	$β_1$—axial
D-Ouled Rabah	β 19 Asn→Lys	↓	Prob. $β_1$	$β_1$—axial
G-Coushatta	β 22 Glu→Ala	↓	Prob. $β_1$	$β_1$—axial
I-Toulouse	β 66 Lys→Glu	↑	Prob. $β_1$	$β_1$—lateral
Korle-Bu	β 73 Asp→Asn	↓	$β_1$	$β_1$—lateral
G-Szuhu	β 80 Asn→Lys	↓	Prob. $β_1$	0
Pyrgos	β 83 Gly→Asp	↓	Prob. $β_1$	$β_1$—lateral
D-Ibadan	β 87 Thr→Lys	↓	Prob. $β_1$	$β_1$—lateral
Detroit	β 95 Lys→Asn	↓	Prob. $β_1$	Near $β_1$—lateral
N-Baltimore	β 95 Lys→Glu	↓	Prob. $β_1$	Near $β_1$—lateral
O-Arab	β 121 Glu→Lys	↑	Prob. $β_1$	$β_1$—axial; $β_2$—lateral
D-Los Angeles	β 121 Glu→Gln	↑	Prob. $β_1$	$β_1$—axial; $β_2$—lateral

*Compiled from references 44, 48, and 51–53.
† ↑ = potentiates gelation; ↓ = inhibits gelation.
‡The β 6 Val contact is on the $β_2$ subunit. Thus, cis contacts would be on $α_2$ and $β_2$ subunits and trans contacts would be on $α_1$ and $β_1$ subunits. The designation 0 means no contact.
Prob: probably; Inter DS = between double strands.

Glu weakens the axial $α_2β_1$ contact (see Fig. 11-6). Moreover, these observations have striking clinical relevance. Patients who are doubly heterozygous for SO-Arab or SD-Los Angeles have disease comparable in severity to the homozygous state (SS) (see Chapter 12).

Ruth and Reinhold Benesch[51-53] have examined the gelation of mixtures of Hb S with a number of α-chain variants and have identified several sites that are likely to be α-chain contacts in the sickle polymer (see Table 11-1).

Despite their value, gelling experiments on mixtures of S and non-S hemoglobin often fail to provide an unambiguous structural interpretation. In some cases, the structural alteration of the mutant hemoglobin may not be adequate to either establish a contact or rule it out. Furthermore, simple mixing experiments do not reveal whether the contact is cis or trans to the β 6 contact.* More definitive information can be obtained by specific refinements of these gelation experiments. Ordinary mixtures of S and non-S hemoglobins contain the hybrid tetramer $α_2β^Sβ^x$ as well as the two parent hemoglobins (see Chapter 10). The presence of three hemoglobin species sometimes complicates the interpretation of these experiments. If instead the parent hemoglobins are deoxygenated prior to mixing, no hybrid is formed, and therefore, only two species will be present, S and non-S tetramer.[19, 54, 56] Conversely, definitive information can also be obtained from gelation of hybrid hemoglobins $α_2β^Sβ^x$, which have been chemically cross-linked to prevent their dissociation into dimers.[57, 58] Another type of hybrid hemoglobin ($α^x_2β^S_2$) is required to provide precise information about α-chain contacts in the sickle fiber. These hemoglobins seldom occur *in vivo* but can be prepared by isolating α and β hemoglobin subunits and then mixing equal amounts of each to form the tetramer.[52, 53, 58] These approaches have all been useful in determining whether a given site on the alpha chain participates in a contact cis or trans to the β 6 Val contact. For example, the Benesches used a combination of chain recombination and cross-linking to prepare hybrid hemoglobin between Hb S and Hb I in which the α 16 Lys → Glu

*In a simple mixture of Hb S and another β-chain variant, the predominant species is $α_2β^Sβ^x$. Thus, if the gelation of this mixture differs significantly from an S + A mixture, the $β^x$ substitution is likely to be a contact site trans to β 6 Val. However, direct measurements show the incorporation of non-S homotetramers into the polymer.[54, 55] Therefore, a cis effect of the mutant hemoglobin cannot be ruled out.

substitution was either cis or trans to the β 6 Val contact. Their gelling data show unequivocally that this alpha substitution inhibits polymerization only when it is cis to β 6 Val. Similar experiments have been performed with Hb Hasharon (Sealy) (α 47 Asp → His),[58] Hb Stanleyville-II (α 78 Asn → Lys),[59] and Hb LeLamentin (α 20 His → Gln).[59a]

In order to demonstrate β-chain contacts cis to β 6 Val, it is necessary to have mutant β chains containing both β 6 Val and another amino acid substitution. Bookchin and coworkers[46-48] have examined the available double beta mutants. Their experiments comparing Hb C-Harlem and Hb Korle-Bu (mentioned previously) showed unequivocally that the β 73 contact was trans to β 6 Val. Moreover, these experiments provided the first evidence that only one β 6 Val contact was involved in the sickle polymer. This conclusion was subsequently documented by studies on cross-linked hybrids.[57]

Chemical modifications at specific sites provide additional independent evidence on the contacts in the sickle polymer. For example, nitrogen mustard alkylates several histidine residues, including His 116, and markedly inhibits polymerization.[60] X-ray analysis of the crystal indicates that β 116 His is an axial contact site. Glyceraldehyde modifies Hb S primarily at α 16 Lys and also greatly impairs polymerization.[61] This finding supports the aforementioned experiments employing Hb I and indicates that this is also a contact site.

As noted earlier, Edelstein[44] has determined the surfaces on Hb S that would be involved in contacts within the 14-strand fiber. The axial contact areas within a single strand are shown in Figure 11–11A along with the mutant hemoglobins that have been found to either inhibit or potentiate polymerization. The lateral contact areas within the double strand are shown in Figure 11–11B. In addition, Edelstein also determined the areas that are likely involved in contacts between double strands (not shown). The topology of these contacts is less secure because, as mentioned previously, the polarities of each of the seven double strands have not yet been established. In general, there is good agreement between these projected contact areas and the location of mutants that affect gelation.

In summary, the 14-stranded structure of the sickle fiber is consistent with a large body of experimental evidence, including high-resolution electron microscopy and image reconstruction, x-ray diffraction analysis, and studies employing mutant hemoglobins. The determination of this structure is one of the major achievements in the application of modern structural biology to clinical medicine.

POLYMERIZATION OF SICKLE HEMOGLOBIN

A large body of precise and coherent information has been gathered on the mechanisms underlying the polymerization of sickle hemoglobin. These studies involve equilibrium and kinetic measurements in both solution and intact cells as well as rheological studies. They form the cornerstone of our understanding of the pathogenesis of sickle cell disease.

Equilibrium Measurements

When a concentrated solution of deoxyhemoglobin S forms a gel under physiologic conditions, it behaves as a simple two-phase system.* At equilibrium, the rod-like polymers (fibers) coexist with hemoglobin molecules ($\alpha_2\beta_2$) in free solution. The dense polymerized phase can be readily separated from the soluble phase by ultracentrifugation.[62-64] Measurement of the concentration of hemoglobin in the supernatant provides a precise way of determining the solubility of the system (Fig. 11–12). The solubility reflects the stability of the sickle polymer. This equilibrium measurement has been invaluable in examining the effects of solvent conditions, ligand binding, chemical modifications, and other hemoglobins on the polymerization of Hb S. The solubility is a much more precise and meaningful measurement than the minimum gelling concentration (MGC), which, until recently, was used by a number of investigators. The MGC assay involves continuous evaporation of the sample with dry inert gas until the solution ceases to flow because of polymer formation. It is neither an equilibrium nor a kinetic measurement. Furthermore, it cannot be used to study the polymerization of partially oxygenated Hb S.

The gelation of Hb S is dependent on both pH and temperature.[65-67] Solubility is minimal at pH 6.5[54, 68] and increases directly with pH over the range 6.5 to 7.5. This pH dependency is particularly pronounced at higher tempera-

---

*As discussed in the preceding section, the sickle fiber can undergo a transition to the crystal, which has a slightly lower solubility. However, no significant amount of crystal forms under physiologic conditions.

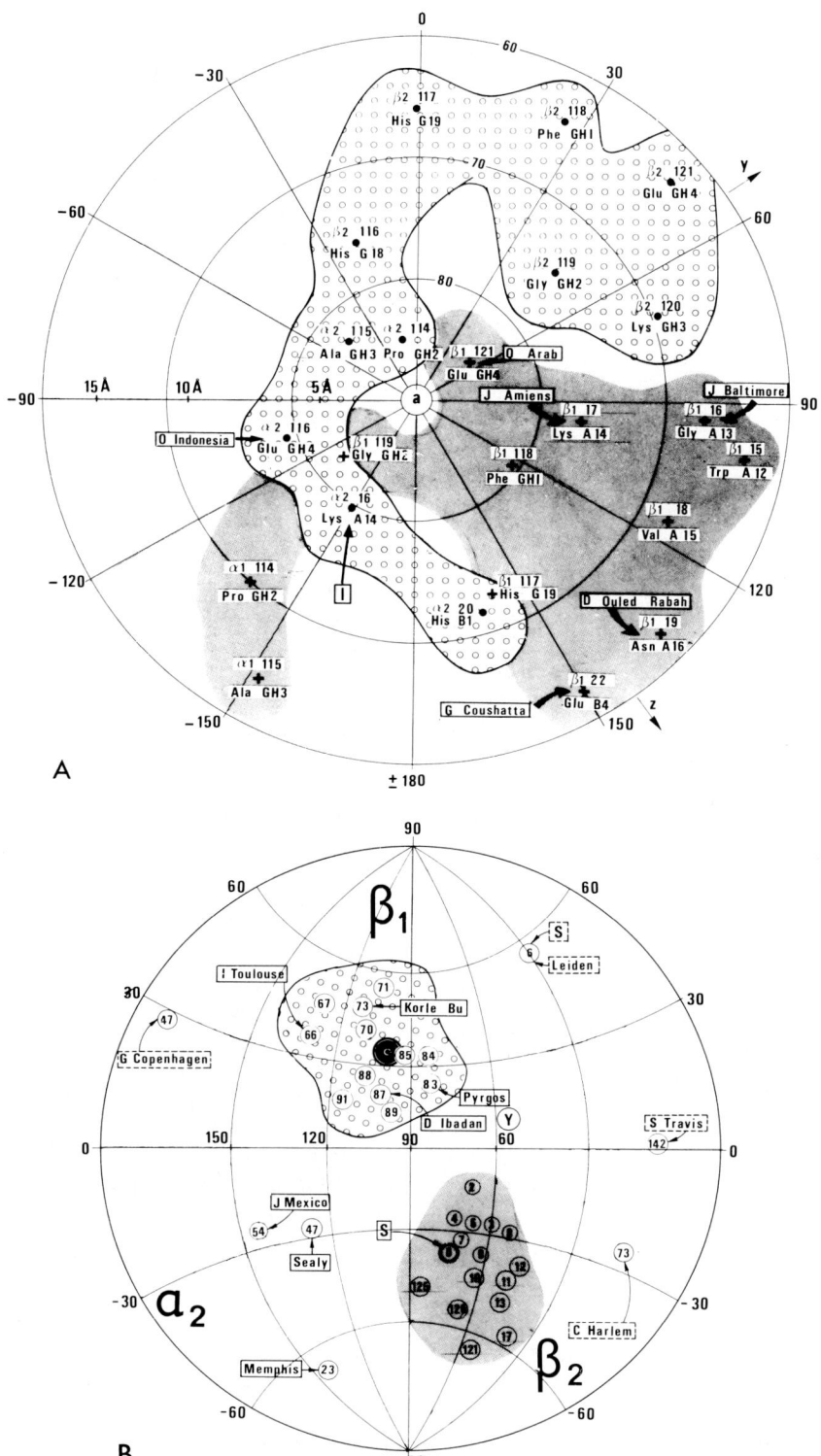

Figure 11–11. Surface maps of deoxy Hb S in 14-strand Edelstein fiber showing axial *(A)* and lateral *(B)* contacts. Variants known to affect polymerization are shown in rectangles. (Modified from Edelstein, S. J.: J. Mol. Biol. *150*:557, 1981.)

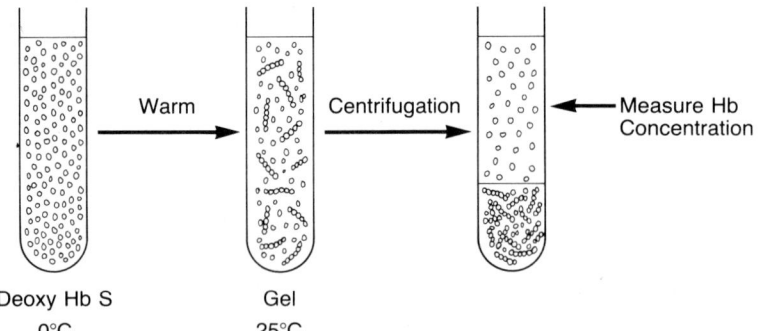

Deoxy Hb S
0°C

Gel
25°C

Figure 11–12. Measurement of solubility of deoxy Hb S.

ture. At intracellular pH (7.2), the solubility decreases considerably from 6° to 25°C (Δ H° = 3.5 kcal/mol) (Fig. 11–13). At higher temperatures, the solubility remains constant (ΔH° = O). In contrast, at lower pH (6.5), the enthalpy remains fairly constant throughout the entire temperature range (ΔH° ≅ 3 kcal/mol). The small heat of polymerization has been confirmed by direct calorimetry and suggests, first, that no large conformational changes are involved when Hb S enters the fiber and, second, that the process is largely entropically driven (ΔS° = 10 cal/deg, mol [37° C]). At first reflection, the process of formation of well-ordered fibers followed by their alignment would suggest a decrease in entropy. However, the aggregation of Hb S molecules to form the fiber may be associated with a significant release of protein-bound water, thereby causing a gain in entropy. Moreover, the alignment of long, synthetic, rod-like polymers is known to be associated with increased entropy. Consider how logs in high density will spontaneously line up as they slowly float downstream to the lumber mill.

Nonideal Behavior of Concentrated Solutions. The assembly of natural rod-like polymers, such as tubulin, is much more favorable than the formation of the sickle fiber. The latter requires a very high concentration of hemoglobin. In general, concentrated solutions of colloid exhibit highly nonideal behavior owing to the large amount of space taken up by the macromolecules, often called the excluded volume. Under these circumstances, the chemical potential or activity of the protein in solution is markedly higher than its concentration.[69] In contrast, the activity of a macromolecule in dilute solution approaches its concentration (activity coefficient becomes unity).

Consideration of nonideality due to excluded volume has led to a deeper understanding of the thermodynamics of sickle hemoglobin polymerization[69] and helps to explain a number of puzzling observations such as the "participation" of non-S hemoglobins in gelation and the solubility of partially liganded Hb S. These will be discussed in detail.

A number of experimental strategies have been used to circumvent the problem of working with high concentrations of hemoglobin. The aggregation of Hb S can be studied in the presence of a noninteracting, space-occupying colloid such as polyethylene glycol.[70, 71] This approach allows measurements with much lower concentrations of Hb S. To a first approximation, the properties of polymerizing sickle hemoglobin are preserved in the polyethylene glycol system.

An alternate and more widely employed approach takes advantage of the marked decrease in solubility of hemoglobin in concentrated (1 to 2 M) phosphate buffers.[72–74] Deoxyhemoglobin S is "salted out" at a lower concentration than other hemoglobins. In general, the relative solubilities of Hb S and mixtures of S and non-S hemoglobins parallels the data on concentrated solutions at more physiologic ionic strength. However, exceptions have been noted.[75] Moreover, the nature of the polymer in concentrated phosphate buffer differs from that of the sickle fiber.[76]

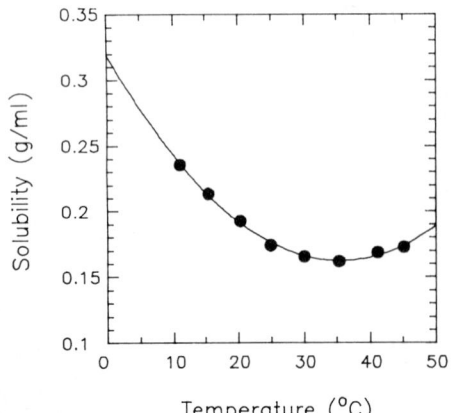

Figure 11–13. Relationship between solubility and temperature. Hb S in 0.15 M potassium phosphate, 0.05 M sodium dithionite, pH 7.15. (Plotted from data of Ross, P. D., et al.: J. Mol. Biol. 115:111, 1977.)

Effect of Hbs F, A, and A$_2$. A considerable amount of information has been collected on the interaction of Hb S with other hemoglobins that coexist in the red cells of common sickling disorders. The solubility or minimum gelling concentration of equimolar mixtures of S and non-S hemoglobins is generally less than twice that of Hb S. This "sparing effect" led many investigators to conclude that these non-S hemoglobins readily copolymerize with Hb S. However, nonideality must be considered in interpreting these mixture experiments. In fact, excluded volume accounts for a considerable portion of the sparing effect of non-S hemoglobins.[67, 77] Therefore, any claim of copolymerization requires direct experimental evidence.

As mentioned already, mixtures of hemoglobins S and F have very high solubility. The primary effect of Hb F is via the asymmetrical hybrid $\alpha_2\beta^S\gamma$.[54, 56] Thus, the inhibition of polymerization is primarily trans to the β 6 Val contact. Nagel and colleagues[78] have concluded that γ 87 and γ 80 are two of the important inhibiting sites. The former residue is located in the trans lateral contact area (see Fig. 11–11B), whereas the latter is not at one of the proposed contact areas. Hb A$_2$ ($\alpha_2 \delta_2$) is an equally potent inhibitor.[78, 79] Because it has much closer structural homology to the β chain (see Table 4–1), the sites of inhibition can be identified with more confidence. By an ingenious comparison of specific mutant hemoglobins, including the Lepore (δβ hybrid) hemoglobins, Nagel and coworkers concluded that δ 22 and δ 87 are the important inhibitory sites. According to Edelstein's topological map[44] (see Fig. 11–11A), residue 22 is in the axial contact area of the trans β chain.

Mixtures of Hb S and Hb A have a much lower solubility than comparable mixtures of Hbs S and F.[77] Thus, Hb A appears to participate in the polymerization. Indeed, measurements of the composition of the polymer formed from S + A mixtures have indicated the presence of Hb A.[54, 55, 80–82]* Even when no $\alpha_2\beta^S\beta^A$ hybrid is present, Hb A probably enters the polymer. It is not surprising that Hb A copolymerizes with Hb S. After all, Hb S and Hb A share all of the multiple contacts in the 14-strand fiber except for the β 6 Val site. Thus, even Hb A tetramers should be able to enter the polymer, althrough less readily than Hb S. Indeed, in 1.5 M phosphate buffer, in which all hemoglobins are less soluble, deoxyhemoglobin A forms a gel with a kinetic pattern and temperature dependence similar to those of Hb S.[84]

The Polymerization of Partially Oxygenated Hb S

Thus far, the discussion of sickle polymerization has been restricted to fully deoxygenated hemoglobins. However, an understanding of *in vivo* sickling requires detailed information on the behavior of partially oxygenated Hb S. This section will describe the equilibrium between sol and gel as influenced by hemoglobin concentration and oxygen saturation.

Effect of Hemoglobin Conformation on Polymerization. Since the early experiments of Hahn and Gillespie,[4] it has been known that deoxygenation favors the sickling of red cells. Harris[11] subsequently demonstrated in cell-free solutions that the deoxy form of hemoglobin S was a prerequisite for the formation of polymer. Because hemoglobin undergoes a marked change in quaternary conformation upon deoxygenation, it has been assumed that this structural transition opens up one or more binding sites on the hemoglobin S molecule necessary for its aggregation. As discussed in a previous section, the structural basis for this assumption is still poorly understood.

Deoxyhemoglobin is not the only form of hemoglobin that is capable of undergoing a transition to the T quaternary structure.* As discussed in Chapter 16, methemoglobin, particularly at low pH and in the presence of organic phosphates, can assume a T-like structure. Concentrated solutions of methemoglobin S can polymerize in the presence of organic phosphates.[85] The binding of nitric oxide (NO) to the heme groups of hemoglobin also results in a species that is capable of assuming the T conformation.[86] Under appropriate conditions, NO-Hb S can polymerize into a gel, documented by both ultracentrifugation data and the demonstration of birefringence.[87] In the presence of the potent organic phosphate inositol hexaphosphate, even oxyhemoglobin can be partially converted to the T quaternary

---

*The analysis of polymers formed under physiologic conditions is technically difficult, owing to the high concentrations of hemoglobin.[54, 55, 80] Under experimental conditions in which solubility is lower,[81, 82] the demonstration of copolymerization is much more convincing. In concentrated phosphate buffer, even Hb F is incorporated into the polymer.[83] However, under these conditions, the polymer probably has a structure different from that formed under physiologic conditions.

*See Chapter 3 for discussion of T and R quaternary structures.

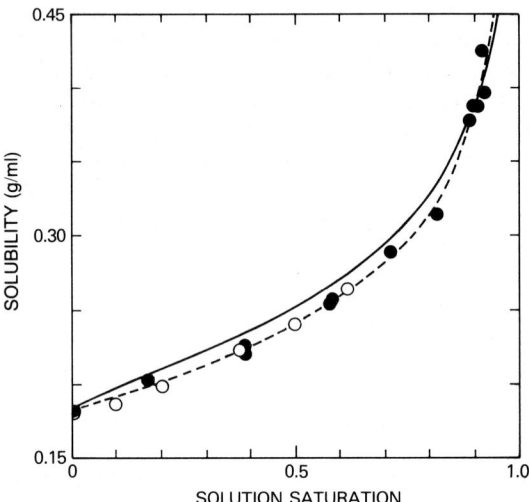

Figure 11–14. Solubility of Hb S at varying degrees of oxygen saturation (●) and carbon monoxide saturation (○) (0.15 M phosphate, pH 7.0). The broken line (– – –) is the best fit using an empirical exponential equation. The unbroken line (—) is based on thermodynamic measurements of solubility at 0 oxygen saturation and oxygen binding to solution and to polymer. (From Sunshine, H. R., et al.: J. Mol. Biol. 158:251, 1982.)

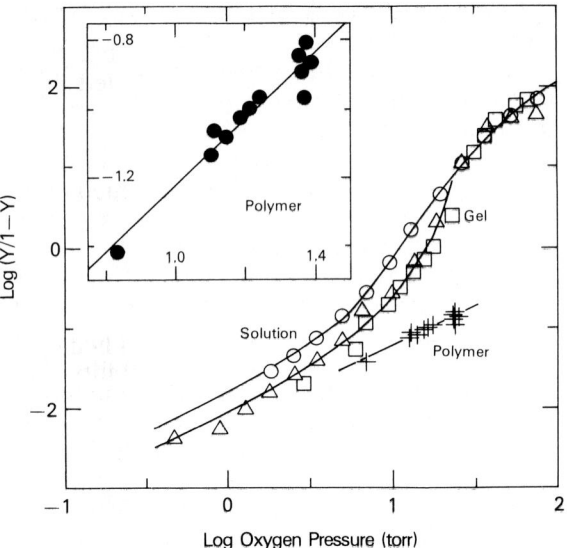

Figure 11–15. Hill plots of oxygen binding of Hb S solution (16 g/dl) (○), gel (37 g/dl) (△, □), and polymer (+) (● in inset). The solution binding curve was determined by Gill and associates.[21] The intersection of the gel and solution curves at about 85 per cent saturation is the crisis point. Note that the polymer binds oxygen noncooperatively ($n=1$) and with very low oxygen affinity. (From Sunshine, H. R., et al.: J. Mol. Biol. 158:251, 1982.)

structure and, as such, can undergo *in vitro* gelation.[88]

Solubility of Partially Oxygenated Hb S. Hofrichter, Eaton, and colleagues at the National Institutes of Health[89, 90] have made rigorous measurements of the solubility of partially liganded Hb S. As shown in Figure 11–14, the solubility of Hb S rises monotonically with increasing oxygen saturation.[90, 91] Spectral analysis of both supernatant and gel indicated that very little oxygen bound to polymerized Hb S. Very similar results have been obtained with carbon monoxide.[89, 92, 93] Although the total hemoglobin concentration of the soluble phase increases directly with oxygen saturation, the solubility of the deoxyhemoglobin actually decreases owing to the excluded volume of the nonpolymerizing hemoglobin. This factor is an important contributor to the presence of polymer in circulating red cells and will be discussed further in the section on the sickling of intact erythrocytes.

Oxygenation of Hb S. In dilute solution, the functional properties of Hb S are indistinguishable from those of Hb A. Relevant studies include both equilibrium and kinetics of ligand binding as well as the Bohr effect and the interaction with CO_2 and organic phosphates.[18–22]*

---

*A direct binding study[94] as well as one report of oxygen equilibria[95] suggests slight differences between Hb S and Hb A in their interaction with 2,3-DPG.

Oxygen equilibrium measurements on concentrated solutions of Hb S reveal an interesting phenomenon.[90, 96] As shown in Figure 11–15, at an oxygen saturation below 80 per cent, the oxygen affinity of a concentrated solution of Hb S is considerably lower than that of a dilute Hb S solution, whereas at high saturations (> 80 per cent), the two solutions have identical oxygen affinities. As a result, the Hill plot of the concentrated Hb S solution has a steeper slope in the middle zone of oxygen binding (30 to 85 per cent). The rightward displacement of the lower portion of the curve can be explained by the preferential aggregation of molecules with the T quaternary structure. This represents a linkage system similar to the effects of protons and organic phosphates on the oxygenation of hemoglobin (see Chapter 3).[18, 21, 91] The following linked equations apply:

$$\begin{array}{ccc} Hb & \rightleftarrows & (Hb)_n \\ + & & + \\ 4O_2 & & O_2 \\ \updownarrow & & \updownarrow \\ Hb(O_2)_4 & \rightleftarrows & (Hb)_n(O_2)_{4n} \end{array}$$

Thus, polymerization of deoxyhemoglobin S and oxygen binding can be viewed as reciprocal processes. The low affinity of the polymer for oxygen leads to a rightward displacement of the O_2 binding curve. The intersection of the two curves in Figure 11–15 at approximately 80 per cent saturation, the crisis point, reflects the completion of polymer melting with increasing oxygenation.

The oxygen binding of concentrated Hb S can be fully defined from measurements of the solubility of partially liganded hemoglobin (see Fig. 11–14) as well as the oxygen binding of Hb S in solution[19-21] and of Hb S polymer. The last measurement poses a formidable technical challenge. Hofrichter and colleagues[89, 90] solved it by the use of linear dichroism, which can yield optical spectra of polymerized hemoglobin. They showed that the polymer present in solutions up to 70 per cent saturated with CO or oxygen was no more than 10 per cent saturated. The oxygen binding curve of the sickle polymer is shown in Figure 11–15. As expected, its oxygen affinity is much lower than that of Hb S in free solution. In fact, it is close to that of T-state hemoglobin (see Chapter 3). Moreover, its oxygen binding is entirely noncooperative. These findings strongly suggest that only the T quaternary structure enters the polymer and are therefore entirely compatible with studies discussed previously on the conformational requirements for Hb S polymerization.

The oxygen binding curve provides an indirect measurement of polymer both in concentrated solutions of Hb S[97*] and in cells (see below). The reduction in oxygen affinity of a gelled solution is directly dependent on hemoglobin concentration. Oxygen binding measurements of gels and Hb S–containing red cells display hysteresis.[21] The oxygenation curve is shifted to the right of the deoxygenation curve. This phenomenon represents a departure from true equilibrium and reflects the time dependency of melting of polymer during oxygenation and formation of polymer during deoxygenation.

In summary, the oxygenation of Hb S can be considered in terms of equilibrium between partially liganded sol and unliganded gel. Figure 11–14 can be viewed as a simple phase diagram. Below a critical oxygen saturation and above a critical hemoglobin concentration, polymeric and soluble phases coexist. Although detailed analyses by analytical ultracentrifugation suggest a more complex situation,[68] this simple two-phase model can accommodate most of the experimental findings on solutions of deoxy and partially liganded Hb S.

Participation of Small Molecules in Hb S Polymerization. In order to understand the sickling of red cells *in vivo*, it is necessary to determine how various intracellular mediators of hemoglobin function affect polymerization. These factors include pH, ionic strength, organic phosphates (particularly 2,3-DPG), and CO_2. The effect of protons on polymerization has been discussed earlier. Because 2,3-DPG stabilizes the quaternary T structure, one might expect that it would potentiate polymerization. However, the most thorough solubility measurements indicate that it has either no effect[98] or a small one[68] on the solubility of deoxyhemoglobin S. CO_2 inhibits gelation of stripped (phosphate-free) deoxyhemoglobin S, probably by forming carbamino adducts at the N terminus of the β chain.[99] However, in the presence of 2,3-DPG, CO_2 binding is displaced, and thus, the antigelling effect is abolished. Accordingly, CO_2 probably has no effect on the polymerization of Hb S under physiologic conditions.

Oxygenation of Sickle Blood. Because the sickling phenomenon depends on the formation of deoxyhemoglobin S, it is important to define the oxygen binding properties of sickle red cells. As mentioned previously, Hb S in dilute solution has normal oxygen equilibria. However, SS blood has markedly decreased oxygen affinity.[100-103] Several independent factors contribute to the low oxygen affinity of sickle red cells. Like patients with other types of anemia, SS homozygotes have elevated red cell 2,3-DPG. As discussed in Chapter 5, 2,3-DPG lowers oxygen affinity not only because of its direct interaction with deoxyhemoglobin but also because it lowers intracellular pH. However, P_{50} values of SS blood are higher than would be predicted from red cell 2,3-DPG values.[104] In fact, there is not a significant correlation between P_{50} and red cell 2,3-DPG.[105] The major cause of decreased oxygen affinity in sickle blood is intracellular polymerization of Hb S. As shown by the aforementioned measurements on concentrated solutions of Hb S (see Fig. 11–15), the right shift in the lower portion of the oxygen binding curve can be explained by aggregation of deoxyhemoglobin S. Accordingly, in red cells, this phenomenon should depend on intracellular hemoglobin concentration. The P_{50} of SS red cells suspended in artificial media rises sharply when the MCHC is increased from 10 g/dl to 30 g/dl, whereas the oxygen affinity of

---

*The change in the P_{50} of solutions of Hb S with increasing hemoglobin concentration provides a practical way of measuring minimum gelling concentration.[97]

AA red cells is unaffected.[106, 107] Therefore, it is not surprising that SS red cells having the highest MCHC (irreversibly sickled cells) have the highest P_{50} values[105] (Fig. 11–16A).

Because of marked red cell heterogeneity, the oxygen binding curves of SS blood samples are much harder to interpret than studies on concentrated solutions of Hb S. As already noted, cells having higher hemoglobin concentration will have more marked decrease in oxygen affinity. Like concentrated solutions, SS blood samples also show a steeper slope in the midportion of the oxygen binding curve. Furthermore, as mentioned earlier, these specimens also often display hysteresis: The oxygenation curve is shifted to the right of the deoxygenation curve,[108–110] owing to the presence of polymer (Fig. 11–16B).* The increased slope as well as the hysteresis indicates that significant amounts of polymer exist in SS red cells having relatively high hemoglobin concentration, even at arterial oxygen tension.[109, 112] As will be discussed later, this observation has been confirmed and extended by nuclear magnetic resonance (NMR) measurements of sickle polymer in partially oxygenated red cells.

The decreased oxygen affinity of SS red cells is a mixed blessing.[20] On the one hand, the right-shifted curve greatly facilitates oxygen unloading (see Chapter 5) and helps to explain why SS homozygotes tolerate severe degrees of anemia surprisingly well when they are free of crisis or infection. On the other hand, decreased oxygen affinity promotes the formation of deoxyhemoglobin and, as a result, favors polymer formation. As the pH drops in the capillary circulation with the uptake of CO_2, the decrease in oxygen affinity is exaggerated, owing to the enhanced polymer formation at low pH.[113] Thus, the increased Bohr effect of SS red cells results in a further increment in polymer formation.

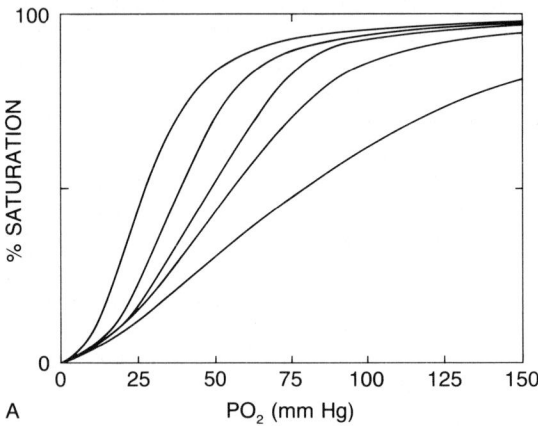

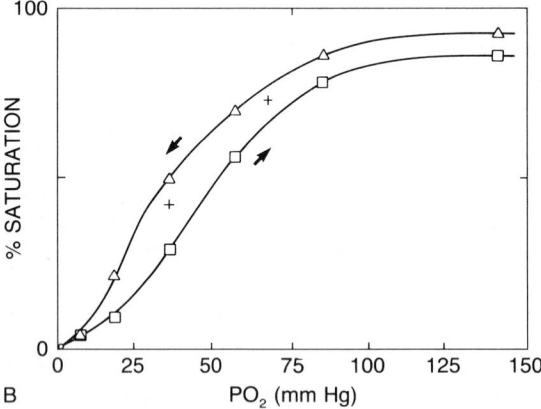

Figure 11–16. *A,* Effect of increasing MCHC on oxygenation of SS red cells at pH 7.40, 37°C. To gradually increase intracellular hemoglobin concentration, 2 M NaCl was added to cell suspension. The O_2 binding curve is progressively shifted to the right with increasing MCHC ranging from 33.0 g/dl to 47.5 g/dl. The left-hand curve is measurement on normal red cells. *B,* Oxygen binding curves of SS blood at pH 7.35, 37°C. Oxygenation is shown by the squares and deoxygenation by the triangles. This loop or hysteresis is not seen in AA blood and reflects a departure from the equilibrium due to the slow melting (□) or formation (△) of polymer. Two *in vivo* points taken from a patient's arterial and venous blood (+) lie between the ascending and descending curves. (From Winslow, R. M.: Hemoglobin interactions and whole blood oxygen equilibrium curves in sickling disorders. *In* Caughey, W. S. (ed.): Clinical and Biochemical Aspects of Hemoglobin Abnormalities. New York, Academic Press, 1978.)

Kinetics of Polymerization of Sickle Hemoglobin

In a concentrated solution of Hb S, polymerization can be induced by rapid deoxygenation or by a sudden increase in the temperature of a deoxygenated sample. The kinetics of this process can be monitored by a number of probes, including turbidity,[114] birefringence,[115] calorimetry,[115] viscosity,[116, 117] and nuclear magnetic resonance.[118–120] After induction, a delay time is followed by sudden formation of polymer (Fig. 11–17A). The rate of polymerization varies exponentially with hemoglobin concentration:

$$1/td = k(C/C_S)^n$$

where td = delay time, C = hemoglobin concentration, and C_S = solubility (see

---

*Hysteresis of oxygen binding curves depends considerably on the technique employed. Hysteresis is minimized by methods that employ long equilibration times and those that put red cells under shear, which tends to break up nascent polymer.[111]

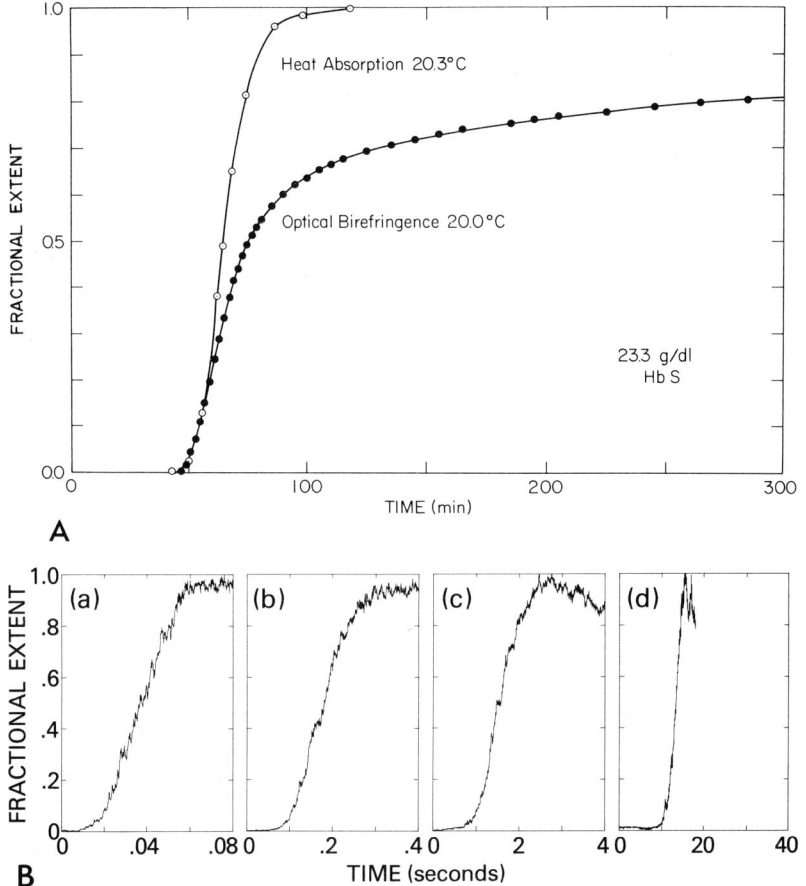

Figure 11–17. *A,* Kinetics of polymerization of deoxy Hb S. The 23 g/dl solution was fully deoxygenated and chilled to melt all polymer. At time 0, the temperature was rapidly increased to 20°C and heat absorption and optical birefringence were continuously monitored. A delay time of 50 minutes was observed. Note that heat absorption was complete within approximately 15 minutes, indicating the rapid formation of polymers. The continuous slow rise in birefringence probably reflects the more gradual alignment of polymers. (From Ross, P. D., et al.: J. Mol. Biol. 96:239, 1975.) *B,* Kinetics of polymerization of concentrated solutions of Hb S. Solutions of HbCO S were exposed to laser light at time 0 in order to rapidly remove carbon monoxide. The onset of scattered light indicates the beginning of polymerization. (a) Hb concentration—35 g/dl; temperature—35°C; delay time—0.018 sec. (b) Hb concentration—35 g/dl; temperature—24°C; delay time—0.09 sec. (c) Hb concentration—27 g/dl; temperature—35°C; delay time—1 sec. (d) Hb concentration—27 g/dl; temperature—24°C; delay time—11 sec. (From Ferrone, F. A., et al.: Biophys. J. 32:361, 1980.)

above). Thus, the delay time is markedly affected by small changes in hemoglobin concentration.

In their initial experiments, Hofrichter, Ross, and Eaton[115] employed Hb S concentrations of 19 to 23 g/dl and obtained highly reproducible delay times ranging from 0.5 to 1000 minutes and an n value of about 30. Subsequent experiments on more concentrated solutions of Hb S, exceeding that of the red cell, have enabled this kinetic scheme to be further refined.[121–121b] A laser light source was used to photodissociate carbon monoxide from carboxyhemoglobin S. The time that elapsed before the deoxyhemoglobin S polymerized was monitored by light scattering with a microspectrophotometer. As shown in Figure 11–17B, unambiguous delay times were noted, similar to those in solutions of lower hemoglobin concentration. Moreover, there was smooth continuity between the kinetic data on concentrated solutions initiated by flash photolysis and earlier measurements initiated by temperature jumps. The n value in these highly concentrated solutions decreases to about 15, a value reflecting the approximate number of molecules in the nucleus. These kinetic measurements on very concentrated solutions can be accommodated by a simple model of homogeneous nucleation followed by fiber growth. In contrast, the kinetics of polymerization of less concentrated solutions of deoxyhemoglobin S probably involve initial homogeneous nucleation followed by heterogeneous nucleation on the surface of existing polymer (Fig. 11–18). This model explains the higher n values obtained for these solutions and also makes predictions about the nature of polymer formation in intact cells under conditions of partial oxygenation (see below). Moreover, the model is testable by application of biophysical and ultrastructural probes.

Any kinetic scheme for the polymerization of Hb S predicts the existence of aggregates intermediate in size between the hemoglobin tetramer and the fiber. However, because the polymerization is such a concerted process, such intermediates are present in low concentration and are therefore very difficult to detect. Nevertheless, their qualitative existence has been demonstrated by a number of probes, including light scattering,[122, 123] viscosity,[124] nuclear magnetic resonance,[125] and electron spin resonance.[126]

Rheology of Sickle Hemoglobin

The transition from a sol to a gel is accompanied by a dramatic increase in viscosity. The viscoelastic properties of the sickle gel depend on both the density and rigidity of the component fibers. Thus, rheological measurements on sickle gels not only provide fresh insights into the structure of the gel but also have clear-cut implications regarding the deformability of sickle cells *in vivo*. The rheological properties of the gel can be regarded as the proximate and most immediate cause of the vaso-occlusive manifestations of sickle cell disease.

Hemoglobin, whether in solution or encased in red cells, is a non-Newtonian fluid. That is, its viscosity (stress/shear rate) is markedly dependent on shear rate. Nevertheless, measurement of viscosity can provide reproducible information on the aggregation of hemoglobin. Figure 11–19A shows the change in viscosity of increasing concentrations of oxy and deoxy Hbs A and S. Above the minimum gelling concentration of deoxyhemoglobin S, the viscosity increases precipitously.[14]

Briehl[127–129] has thoroughly examined the viscoelastic properties of sickle gels. He and others[130] showed that unsheared gels are not viscous but, instead, exhibit solid-like behavior. Slightly sheared gels begin to exhibit intermediate (viscoplastic) behavior, and heavily sheared gels are truly viscous and, as shown in Figure 11–19B and C, exhibit thixotrophy: A gel recently exposed to high shear becomes less viscous than one that has not been so exposed. Ketchup is an annoying example of thixotropy. This hysteresis is reminiscent of that observed in the oxygenation of sickle hemoglobin but has an entirely different mechanism. It reflects the fact that shear breaks up nascent polymer and therefore lowers viscosity. This disruption of polymer significantly shortens the delay time,[37, 116, 124, 128, 129] presumably by creating more nucleation sites for polymer growth.

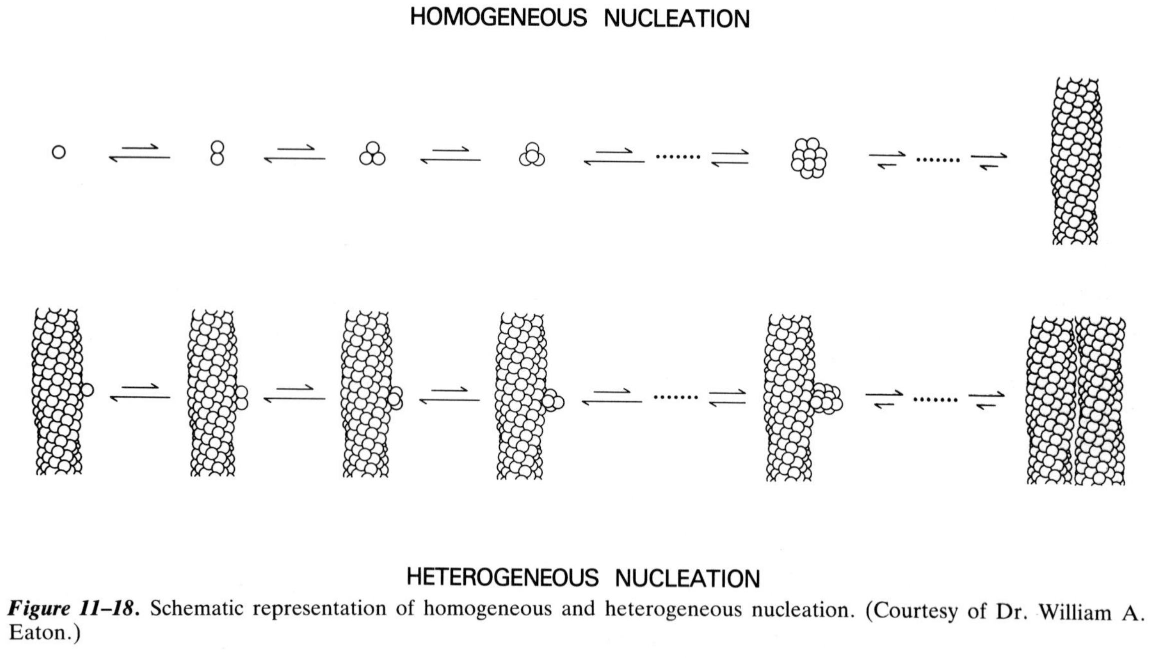

HOMOGENEOUS NUCLEATION

HETEROGENEOUS NUCLEATION

Figure 11–18. Schematic representation of homogeneous and heterogeneous nucleation. (Courtesy of Dr. William A. Eaton.)

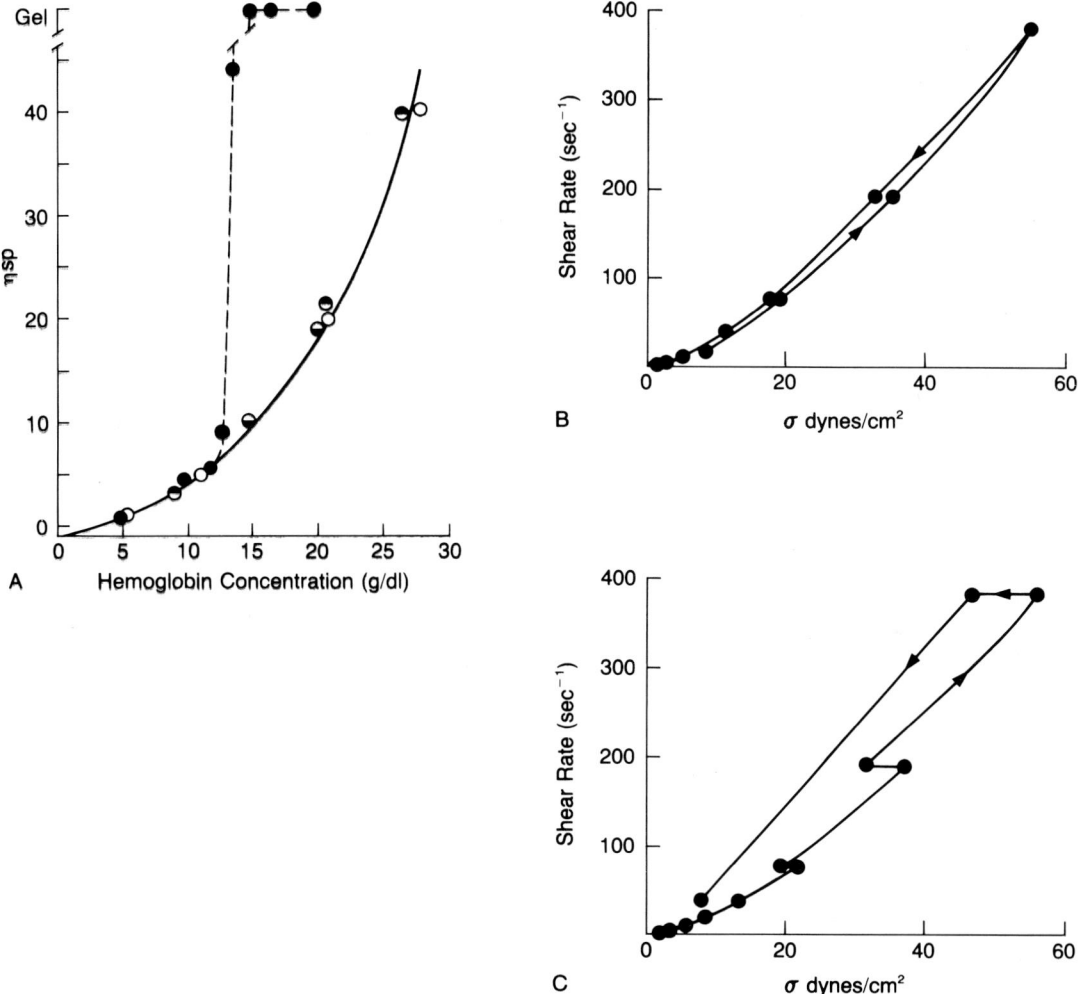

Figure 11-19. A, Comparison of viscosities of oxy Hbs A (◐) and S (◐) and deoxy Hbs A (○) and s (●) at different hemoglobin concentrations. (Redrawn from Allison, A. C.: Biochem. J. 65:212, 1957.) B and C, Relationship between stress (dynes/cm^2) on abscissa and strain (shear rate) on ordinate in Hb S gels. The viscosity is given by stress/shear rate. The fact that the relationship is not linear indicates the non-Newtonian nature of the gels. The loop demonstrates thixotropy or dependence of stress on previous history of shear rate. The wider loop in C reflects the fact that this gel had been less well sheared. (From Briehl, R. W.: Physical chemical properties of sickle cell hemoglobin. *In* Wallach, D. F. H. (ed.): The Function of Red Blood Cells: Erythrocyte Pathobiology. New York, A. R. Liss, Inc., 1981.)

As red cells circulate in large- and narrow-bore vessels under varying pressures and degrees of turbulence, shear may become a critical variable, having contrary effects on intracellular polymerization.[128] On the one hand, shear might be expected to lessen the risk of vaso-occlusion by making the intracellular gel more viscous rather than solid-like. On the other hand, shear may aggravate vaso-occlusion by shortening the delay time.

POLYMERIZATION IN INTACT SICKLE CELLS

The preceding section presented detailed information on polymerization in solutions of Hb S under carefully controlled solvent conditions. To a first approximation, this rigorous and self-consistent body of information makes accurate predictions about equilibrium and kinetic measurements of polymerization in intact red cells. The intrinsic behavior of hemoglobin S per se and its interaction with cofactors and other hemoglobins within the erythrocyte determine its propensity to form sickle polymer. Thus, it is unnecessary to invoke a primary role of the red cell membrane in sickling.[131]

Nevertheless, polymerization in a population of sickle erythrocytes is much more complex than in a homogeneous solution of Hb S. The major reason for this is red cell heterogeneity, particularly in SS disease. In addition, as discussed in the next section of this chapter, the red cell membrane plays an important secondary role, leading to continuous alteration of SS cells as they circulate *in vivo*. This conditioning is an important contributor to cell heterogeneity.

Cell Heterogeneity

A casual inspection of a blood film of a patient with SS disease reveals impressive variation in size, shape, and color among the circulating red cells. Both congenital and acquired factors contribute to this heterogeneity (Fig. 11–20). As explained in Chapter 12, Hb F is distributed unevenly among SS red cells (see Color Plate III*C*). Cells that contain Hb F have proportionally less Hb S. Thus, the total amount of hemoglobin is relatively uniform among SS cells and remains so as they circulate. Because Hb F is such a potent inhibitor of polymerization, it is not surprising that

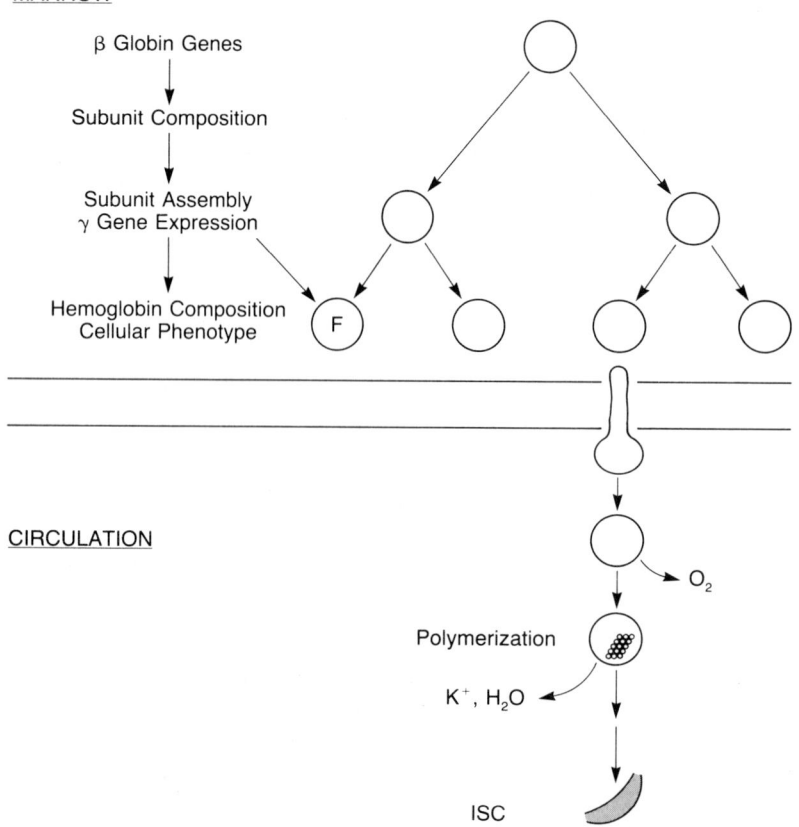

Figure 11–20. Factors that contribute to red cell heterogeneity in SS disease.

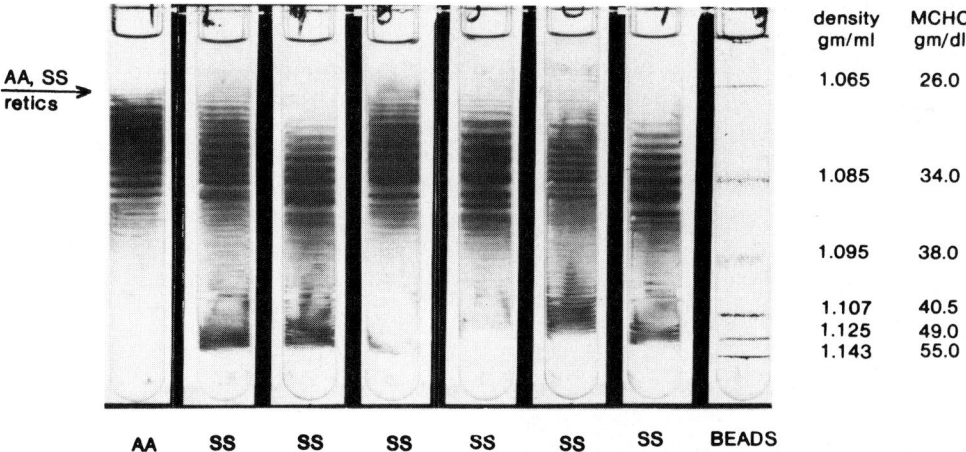

Figure 11–21. Percoll-Renografin continuous density gradients of an AA control and six different SS patients. Note the broad density distribution of SS samples. (Courtesy of Drs. Mary E. Fabry and Ronald L. Nagel.)

F cells have a decreased propensity to sickle and therefore have prolonged *in vivo* survival.[132] In contrast, irreversibly sickled cells tend to have decreased amounts of Hb F and are prone to undergo early destruction.[133] The protective effect of Hb F can be quantitatively assessed by a comparison of F cell production (F reticulocytes) and circulating F cells.[134] In some SS patients, the ratio of F cells to F reticulocytes is as high as 4, indicating marked preferential survival of F cells. Moreover, the amount of Hb F per F cell is often twice that per F reticulocyte. Thus, a rich endowment of Hb F gives a cell protection against early destruction. However, in some SS patients, often those with concomitant α thalassemia, there is no significant enrichment of F cells (F cells/F reticulocytes ≅ 1). Clearly, in these patients, other factors override the influence of Hb F on cell survival.

Another contributor to red cell heterogeneity is 2,3-DPG. Unlike Hb F, 2,3-DPG cannot be measured in individual red cells. However, it is known that the overall level of 2,3-DPG gradually falls as red cells age *in vivo* (see Chapter 5). Furthermore, it is likely that differences in levels of enzymes and metabolic intermediates can affect the concentration of 2,3-DPG in individual red cells. Therefore, 2,3-DPG is likely to be a contributor to heterogeneity of SS red cells and, as such, could have an independent effect on the potential for intracellular polymerization in individual red cells.

The third and most important type of cell heterogeneity involves differences in cell size and hemoglobin concentration. When normal AA blood is fractionated on a density gradient, the young red cells, including reticulocytes, migrate to the top, while cells of increasing age move progressively toward the bottom (Fig. 11–21). Red cells from SS patients show a much broader density distribution.[135, 136, 136a] The increase in cells of low density reflects the high proportion of young red cells. The marked increase in highly dense red cells results from *in vivo* conditioning (see Fig. 11–20). In contrast to normal (AA) red cells, deoxygenation of SS red cells usually causes an increase in density.[137] Moreover, as explained in the following section on the red cell membrane, repetitive cycles of polymerization and depolymerization induce leakage of potassium and water from the red cell, resulting in a further increase in intracellular hemoglobin concentration. The proportion of high-density cells is lower in patients who have concomitant α thalassemia (especially -α/-α)[138–138b] and also in those with increased levels of Hb F.[138a] Thus, the heterogeneity due to genetic and erythropoietic factors and that due to cell conditioning are partially linked. In addition, there are undoubtedly other differences among individual red cells that affect their propensity to sickle.

Equilibrium Measurements of Intracellular Polymerization

When the oxygen tension of the Hb S–containing red cell is lowered to a critical point, intracellular polymerization of hemoglobin occurs, leading to the formation of the classic sickle shape (Fig. 11–22). This phenomenon can be monitored by direct morphological examination. The oxygen saturation at which the sickle shape change occurs is deter-

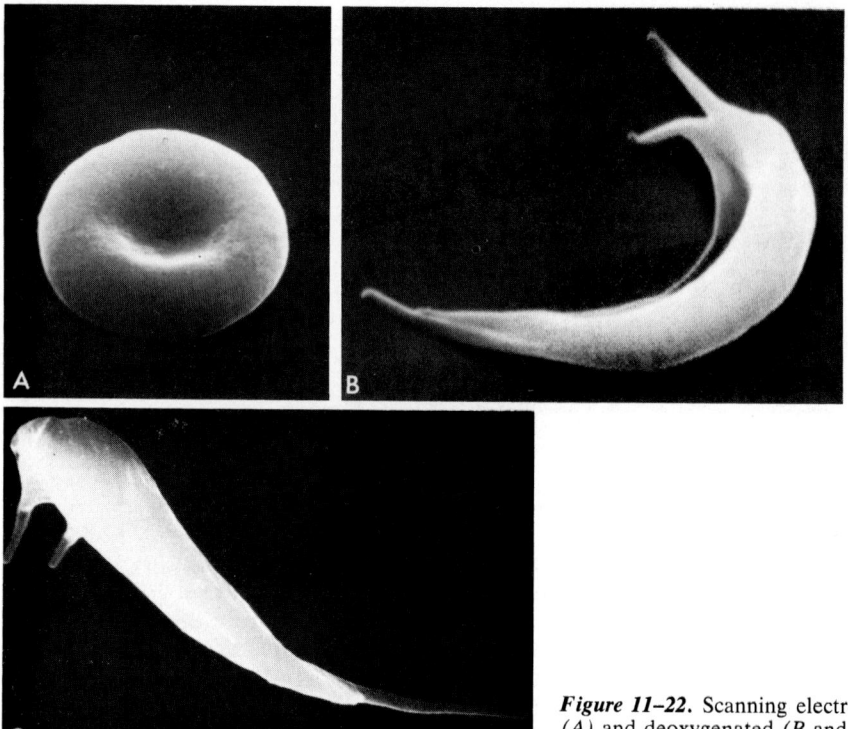

Figure 11–22. Scanning electron micrographs of oxygenated *(A)* and deoxygenated *(B* and *C)* SS erythrocytes. (Courtesy of Dr. James White.)

mined by a number of factors. As Figure 11–23 and Table 11–2 show, the presence of non-S hemoglobin has a profound effect on cellular sickling, comparable to its influence on gelation of the correponding hemolysate. Griggs and Harris[139] demonstrated that, under physiologic conditions, the sickling of red cells from homozygotes was first noted at O_2 saturations below 85 per cent. Sickling was nearly complete at 38 per cent O_2 saturation. A progressive increase in whole blood viscosity paralleled the appearance of sickled cells. In contrast, no sickling of AS red cells was observed until the O_2 saturation fell below 40 per cent. These *in vitro* studies provide a crude assessment of the sickling phenomenon *in vivo*. SS homozygotes would be expected to have a significant amount of sickling at oxygen tensions normally encountered in the capillary and venous circulation. However, kinetic considerations (discussed below) suggest that the amount of sickling *in vivo* is less than that expected from *in vitro* incubations. The fact that AS heterozygotes rarely have clinical manifestations is not surprising in view of the severe and nonphysiologic degree of hypoxemia necessary to induce the sickling deformity.

Experiments involving the quantitation of morphological shape change are of necessity subjective and, therefore, prone to observer bias. It is often difficult to distinguish a sickled cell from a cell deformed by some other mechanism. The shape of fully deoxygenated SS cells is strikingly dependent on the rate at which they undergo deoxygenation[140] as well

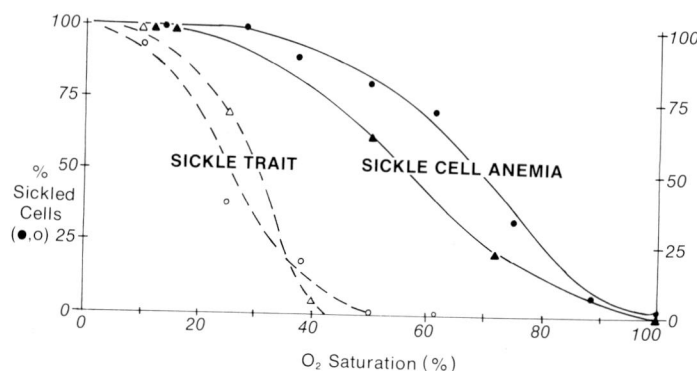

Figure 11–23. Measurement of viscosity and percentage of sickled forms in SS and AS red cell suspensions at different oxygen saturations. (Prepared from data of Griggs, R. C., and Harris, J. W.: Arch. Intern. Med. 97:315, 1956.)

Table 11–2. **FORMATION OF SICKLED CELLS AND INCREASE IN VISCOSITY FOLLOWING PARTIAL DEOXYGENATION OF BLOOD CELL SUSPENSIONS FROM VARIOUS SICKLING DISORDERS***

Genotype	PO_2 (mm Hg)		Solubility of Hemolysate (g/dl)†
	50% Sickled Forms	50% of Maximal Viscosity	
SS	35–50	32–55	19
AS	2–7	3–10	28
SC	10–20	10–22	26
S/β Thal	22–32	20–25	Variable
S/HPFH	~10	12	24

*From Griggs, R. C., and Harris, J. W.: Arch. Intern. Med. 97:315, 1956.
†0.1 M PO_4, pH 7.35, 22°C. Data taken from Sunshine, H. R., et al.: J. Mol. Biol. 133:435, 1979, and Bunn, H. F., et al.: Proc Natl. Acad. Sci. USA 79:7527, 1982.

as on their water content.[141] Slow removal of oxygen results in a high yield of classic banana-shaped cells. Rapid deoxygenation produces cells with a granular or mosaic appearance that lack elongated projections and probably contain multiple domains of randomly oriented polymer. The "holly leaf" cell is intermediate between these extremes. If a cell is sufficiently dehydrated (either by *in vivo* conditioning [Fig. 11–24A] or by *in vitro* manipulation [Fig. 11–24B–E]), it will not readily assume a sickle or spiculated shape, probably because its hemoglobin is so concentrated that it forms multiple domains of polymer.

Although time-honored and useful, the information provided by morphological studies of sickle shape change is indirect and qualitative. A cell may contain a considerable amount of polymer and yet maintain its disc-like shape. In order to obtain more quantitative information, a number of other approaches have been explored, including assays of viscosity[5, 142] and filterability[143–145]* as well as oxygen binding measurements.[112]† However, none of these methods provides direct information on the extent of intracellular polymerization.

Recently, natural abundance ^{13}C nuclear magnetic resonance (NMR) spectroscopy has proved to be useful for quantitation of sickle polymer in intact erythrocytes. Noguchi, Torchia, and Schechter[146–148] have completed a series of NMR measurements on blood specimens from the common sickle syndromes equilibrated at varying oxygen tensions. They have found that the amount of polymer at various levels of oxygen saturation agrees very well with that predicted from the solution studies discussed in the previous section. Figure 11–25 shows data from whole blood specimens of SS homozygotes. Note that there is detectable polymer in cells that appear to be nearly fully oxygenated. On initial reflection, this result seems counterintuitive. Its interpretation depends on two important considerations. The first factor is that partially oxygenated red blood cells depart markedly from ideality owing to the excluded volume of oxyhemoglobin molecules that fail to be incorporated into the polymer.[90, 149] As a result, the activity of the relatively small proportion of deoxyhemoglobin molecules is extremely high, and therefore, polymerization is favored. The contribution of nonideality is illustrated schematically in Figure 11–26. The second major factor that influences the NMR results shown in Figure 11–25 is the marked heterogeneity of SS red cells. The polymer observed at low oxygen saturation is directly proportional to cell density.[148] Only the most dense cells with the highest intracellular hemoglobin concentration formed significant polymer at high oxygen saturation. Even this subset of cells is likely to be quite heterogeneous. The NMR measurements of SC disease[150] and sickle trait[147] again agree very well with solution data on hemoglobin mixtures and are consistent with previous determinations of sickle shape change at partial

---

*There is a large body of research on the rheology of sickle red cells that is not covered in this chapter. For further information see Blood Cells, Volume 8, Issues 1 and 2, 1982.

†From accurate oxygen binding curves (see Fig. 11–15), one can determine the fractional oxygen saturation of hemoglobin S in solution (Y_S) at a given oxygen tension. As shown in Figure 11–14, the solubility (C_S) can be determined at a given value of Y_S. The fraction of polymer (X_P) is obtained from the equation:

$$X_P = \frac{1 - C_S/C_T}{1 - C_S/C_P}$$

where C_T = total hemoglobin concentration and C_P = concentration of hemoglobin in the polymer (69 g/dl). The fractional oxygen saturation of the total solution (Y_T) can be calculated from the polymer fraction and the oxygen binding of the polymer and solution phases (see Fig. 11–15). These calculations give values for X_P and Y_T, the ordinate and abscissa of Figure 11–25.

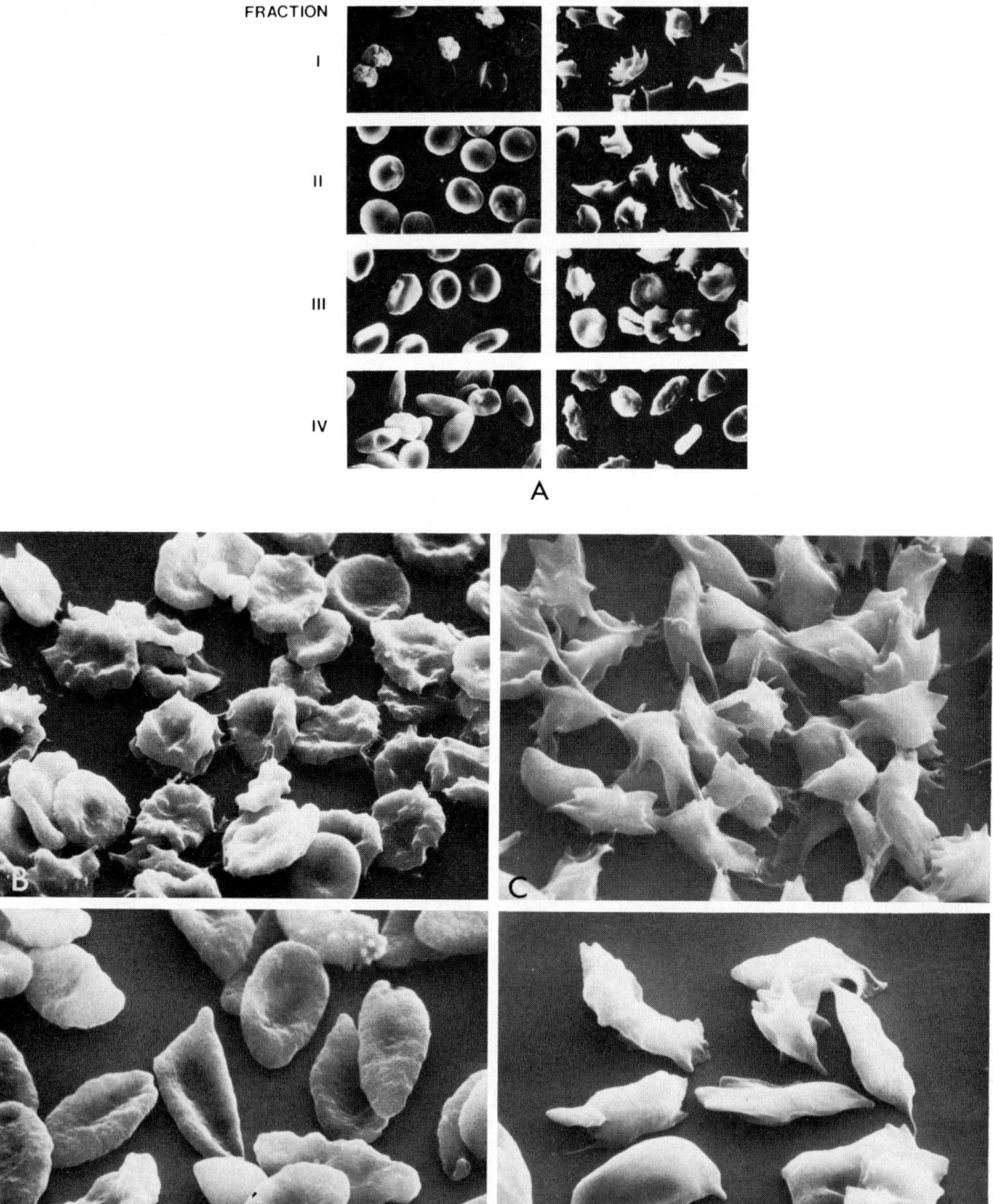

Figure 11–24. *A,* Scanning electron micrographs of SS red cells separated by a density gradient. Note that the least dense fractions (I, II) readily assume a classic sickle shape when deoxygenated. In contrast, the most dense fractions (III, IV), when deoxygenated, fail to undergo this shape change. (From Kaul, D. K., et al.: J. Clin. Invest. 72:22, 1983.) *B–C,* Scanning electron micrographs of deoxygenated SS red cells. *B,* Discoid cells dehydrated with nystatin. Note absence of spicules and sickle shapes. *C,* Rehydrated cells. Note spicules and classic sickle shapes. *D,* Irreversibly sickled cells. Note absence of spicules. *E,* Irreversibly sickled cells hydrated in a hypotonic medium. Note classic spicules and sickle shapes. (Courtesy of Drs. Margaret Clark and Steven B. Shohet.)

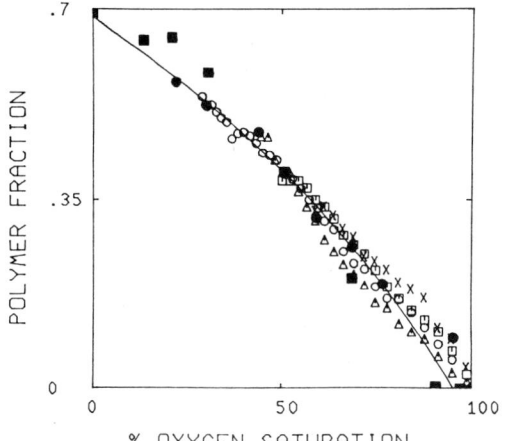

Figure 11–25. Fraction of polymer in samples of SS blood from several patients as a function of oxygen saturation, measured by ^{13}C NMR (pH=7.2). The solid line is calculated from solution data. (See footnote.) (From Noguchi, C. T., et al.: Proc. Natl. Acad. Sci. USA 77:5487, 1980.)

oxygen saturation (see Fig. 11–23 and Table 11–2).

Kinetic Measurements of Intracellular Polymerization

The vaso-occlusive manifestations of sickle cell disease involve a complex and dynamic sequence of events in the microcirculation. Whether a sickle red cell develops sufficient rigidity to cause obstruction of a narrow-bore blood vessel depends on the rate at which deoxygenation and polymer formation occur. The subsequent steps leading to tissue ischemia are not well understood. Obstruction of flow at the distal arteriole or capillary probably promotes local hypoxia, deoxygenation of red cells, and further sickling. In this way, the area of vaso-occlusion is amplified.[5, 151] Local anatomical and physiological factors such as distribution of blood vessels, blood flow, and oxygen consumption help to determine where and when this vicious cycle will occur. Eaton[152] and associates have stressed the importance of the relationship between the rate of sickling of a partially deoxygenated red cell and the duration of its flow through the microcirculation.

Investigation of the kinetics of intracellular polymerization is a vital first step in understanding the pathophysiology of sickle cell disease. In view of the variety of techniques that have been applied to this problem, it is not surprising that markedly conflicting results have appeared in the literature. For example, following rapid deoxygenation of SS red cells, the average time that elapsed before a recognizable change in morphology was 0.03 second in one study[153] and 2 seconds in another.[154] As mentioned earlier, the formation of the classic sickle or holly leaf shape is unlikely to be the physiologically relevant event. A number of investigators have noted morphological changes that preceded the formation of elongated cells.[153, 155] Messer and Harris[144] documented an intermediate phase of cell rigidity by filtration measurements of rapidly deoxygenated SS red cells. Subsequently, Messer, Hahn, and Bradley[156, 157] examined the serial changes in ultrastructure and deformability after SS red cells were suddenly exposed to decreased oxygen tension. As expected,

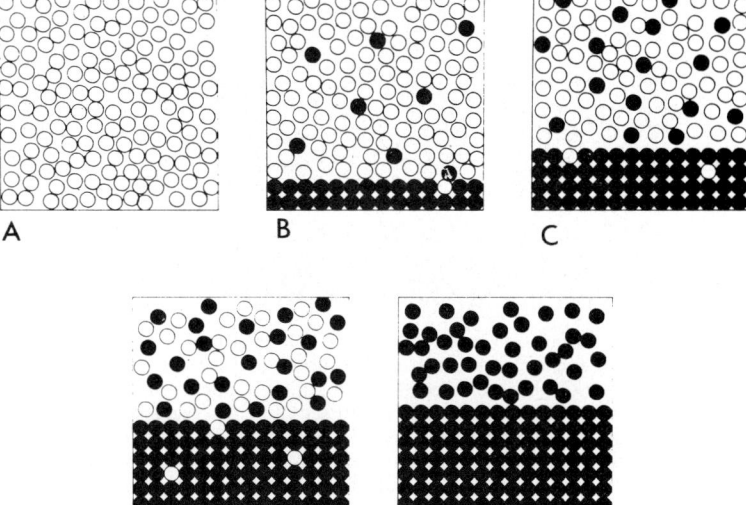

Figure 11–26. Diagram of hemoglobin S solution at various degrees of oxygen saturation. *A*, 100%. *B*, 75%. *C*, 50%. *D*, 25%. *E*, 0%. Open circles represent oxygenated hemoglobin S molecules; filled circles represent deoxygenated hemoglobin S molecules. Polymer is represented by the arrays at the bottoms of panels *B* to *E*. The possibility that a small amount of oxyhemoglobin S enters the deoxyhemoglobin S polymer is indicated in panels *B–D*. (From Noguchi, C. T., and Schechter, A. N.: Blood 58:1057, 1981.)

changes occurred much more rapidly in dense SS red cells compared with lighter cells having a lower mean corpuscular hemoglobin concentration (MCHC). Within 0.5 to 1 second after partial deoxygenation of the dense cells, some developed mottled areas of increased electron density indicating small aggregates of hemoglobin (Fig. 11–27A), while the remainder contained randomly oriented short fibers. Both morphological features coexisted in some cells. At this time, a significant decrease in filterability was noted. At later intervals following deoxygenation, the randomly oriented fibers increased in number and in length. By 15 seconds, a few cells had surface projections, some of which contained aligned polymer (see Fig. 11–27F). Many of the cells retained a normal discoid shape despite the abundance of polymer. In contrast to the dense cells, polymer was not noted in the light cell populations for periods of up to 40 seconds after partial deoxygenation. These elegant studies indicate that under physiologic conditions, fiber formation and decreased deformability occur readily in dense cells prior to any shape change. Comparisons of arterial and central venous blood suggest that a significant proportion of cells do change shape *in vivo*,[158, 159] but probably not until they have escaped from the microcirculation.

Whether a cell obstructs a small-bore blood vessel depends on the rate at which polymerization occurs. The delay times of individual red cells have been measured by laser photolysis and microspectrophotometry[160] similar to that employed for concentrated solutions of Hb S (described above). In keeping with the marked cellular heterogeneity in SS disease, delay times ranged from a few milliseconds to a few seconds (Fig. 11–28). A population of cells with even longer delay times was noted in patients having increased levels of Hb F. By comparison, red cells from a patient with SC disease had delay times ranging between 0.1 and 100 seconds (Fig. 11–28). The delay time of a given cell and the kinetics of polymerization of concentrated solutions of Hb S (discussed in the preceding section) permit an estimation of the hemoglobin concentration of that cell. The estimated distribution of hemoglobin concentrations among red cells in samples of SS blood[160] agrees very well with direct measurements of MCHC and density distribution. Because circulating red cells undergo only partial deoxygenation, the physiologic delay times would be considerably longer. Indeed, their distribution in SS disease would probably span the capillary circulation times for most tissues. Thus, the kinetics of intracellular polymerization are very likely to be rel-

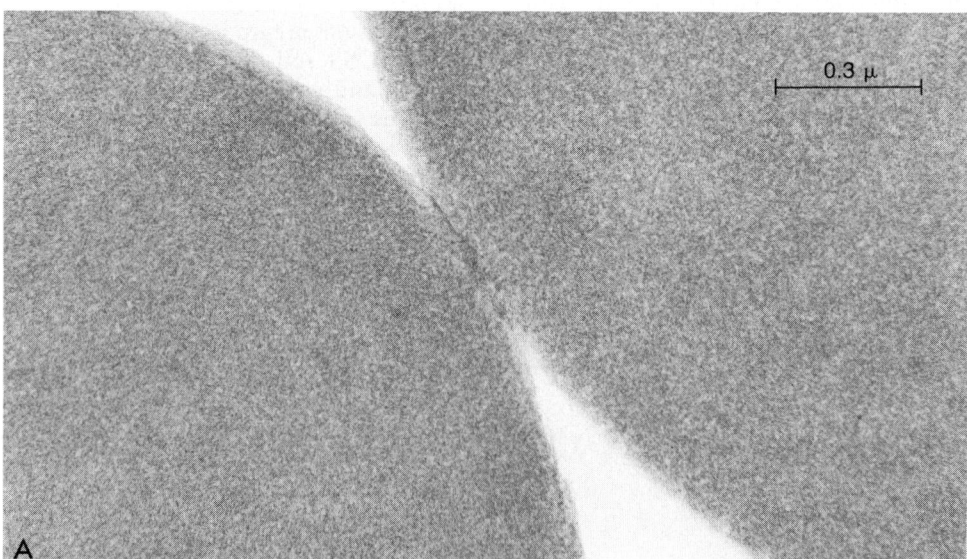

Figure 11–27. Transmission electron micrographs of SS red cells in time-lapse study of Hahn, Messer and Bradley. *A*, Two oxygenated red cells. No hemoglobin fibers are seen. *B*, 0.5 sec after deoxygenation. Note areas of increased electron density. *C*, 0.5 sec after deoxygenation. Upper cell has short, randomly distributed fibers and scattered ribosomes. Lower cell has no fibers. *D*, 10 sec after deoxygenation. Upper cells have increased amount of fibers; no fibers can be seen in the lower cell. *E*, 15 sec after deoxygenation. Fibers are present in high density, yet there is no distortion of sickle shape. *F*, 15 sec after deoxygenation. Fibers are randomly distributed except for alignment and surface projection on upper edge of cell. *G*, 15 sec after *reoxygenation*. ISC on left has persistence of highly organized fiber bundles. In contrast, the reversibly sickled cell on the right shows no fibers. (From Hahn, J. A., et al.: Br. J. Haematol. 34:559, 1976.)

Illustration continued on opposite page

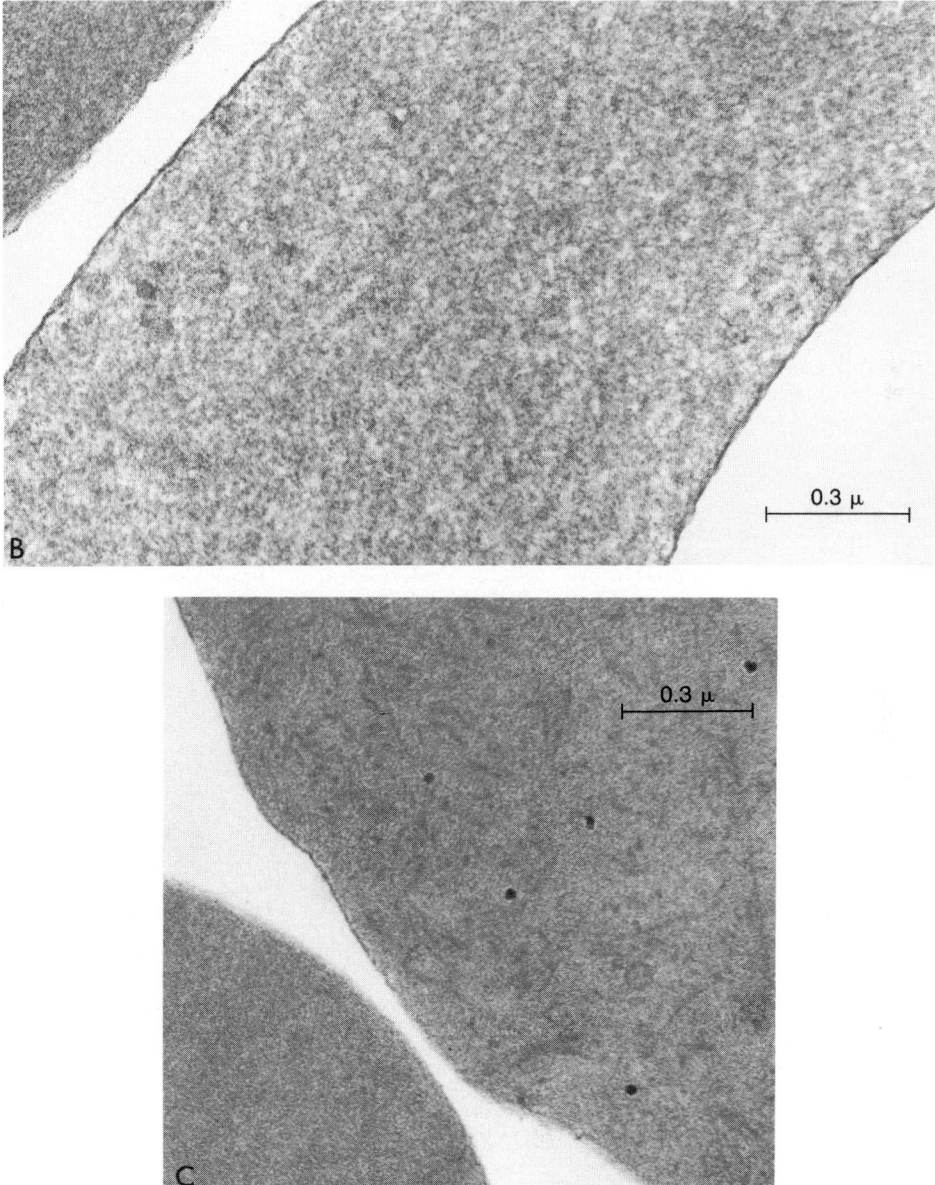

Figure 11–27 Continued. Illustration continued on following page

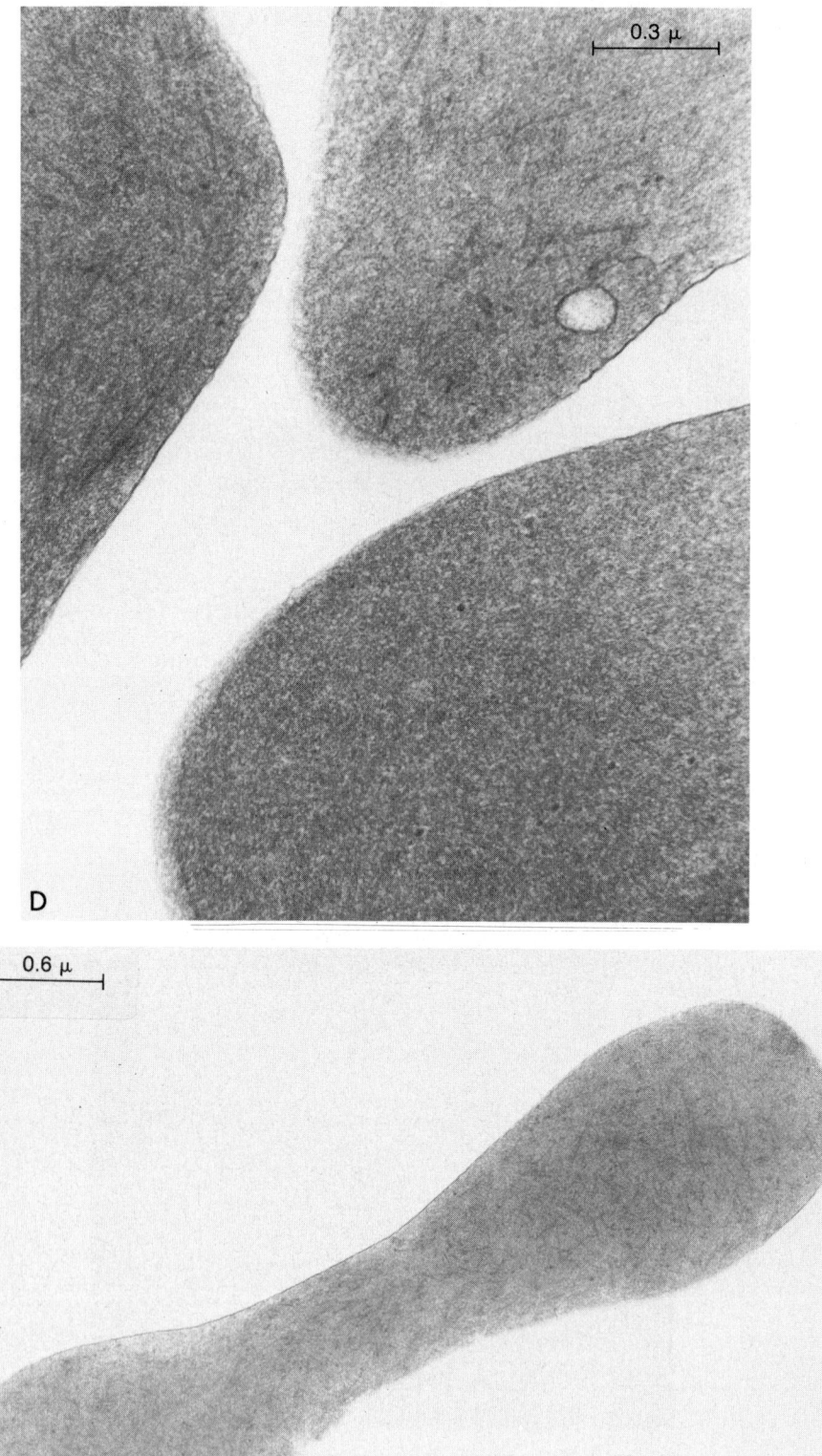

Figure 11-27 Continued. Illustration continued on opposite page.

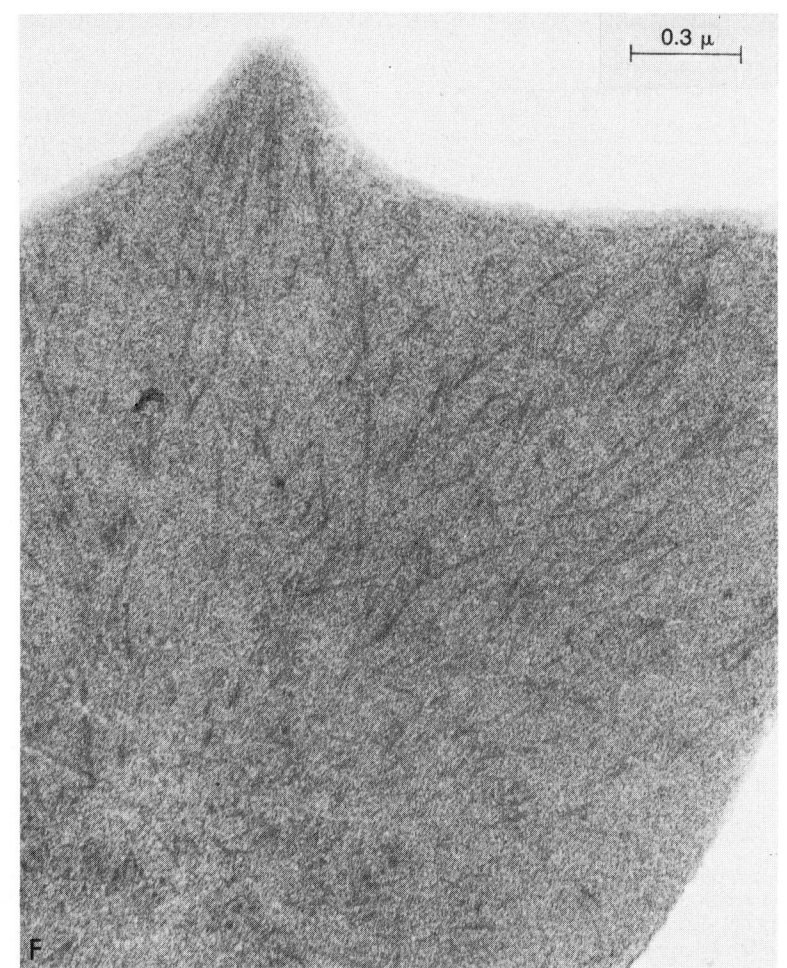

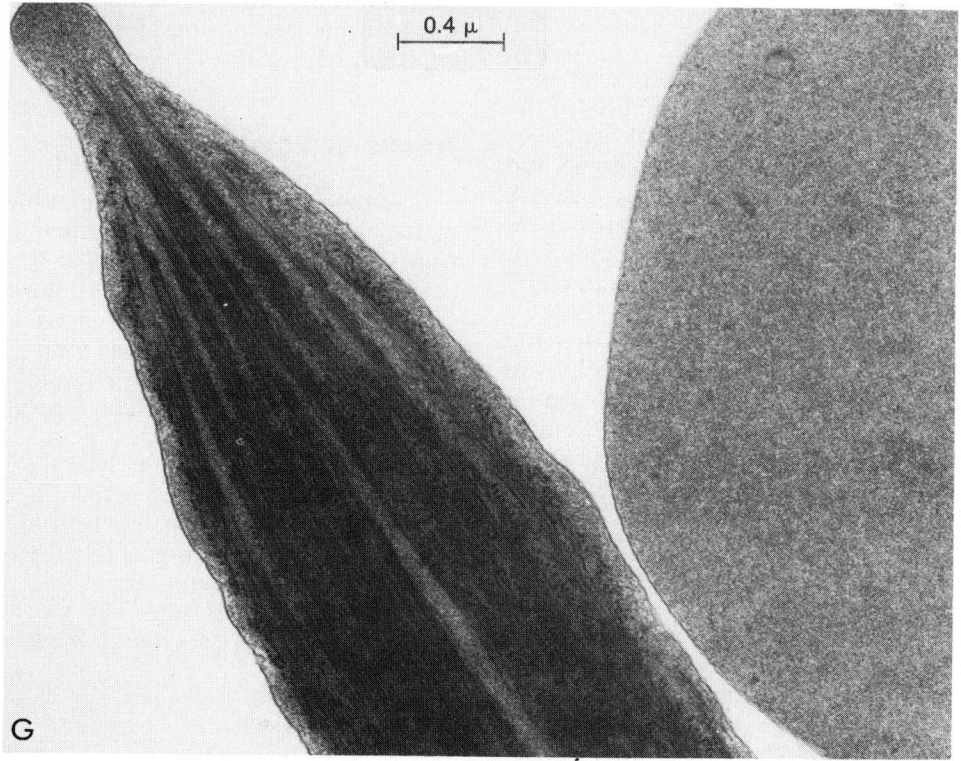

Figure 11-27 Continued.

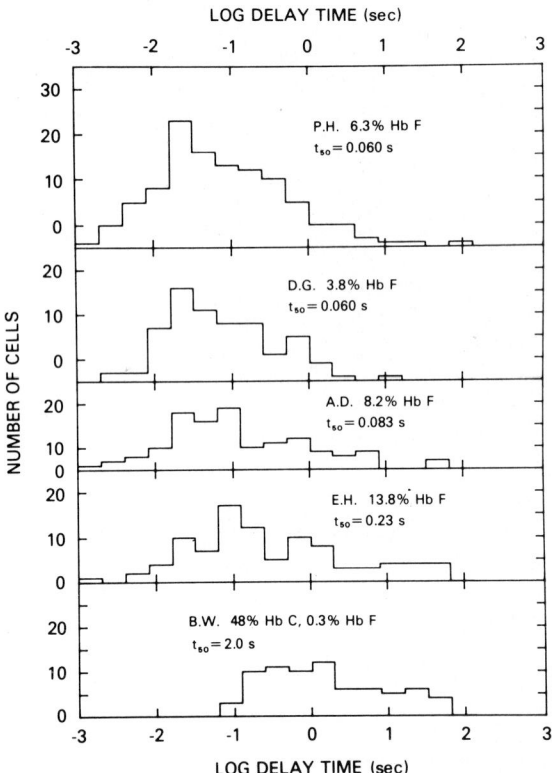

Figure 11–28. Histogram of delay times of individual red cells from four patients with SS disease and one with SC disease plotted on a logarithmic scale. Note that SS patients with elevated Hb F have cells with relatively long delay times. (From Coletta, M., et al.: Nature *300*:194, 1982.)

evant to *in vivo* flow rates. The rate of oxygenation of SS red cells also contributes to the extent of polymer formation at different sites in the circulation. Fully deoxygenated SS red cells bind oxygen much more slowly than AA cells, owing to the slowness of depolymerization.[161, 162] The half-time for oxygenation of dense SS red cells is about 120 milliseconds,[162] whereas the pulmonary circulation time is about 700 milliseconds. Considering that red cells entering the pulmonary circulation are only partially deoxygenated, it is likely that in the great majority of cells that circulate through normal pulmonary alveoli the polymer melts completely. This conclusion is supported by serial electron micrographs that monitor the reoxygenation of fully deoxygenated SS cells.[157]

Equilibrium measurements (discussed in the preceding section) have suggested that some dense SS red cells retain polymer as they pass into the arterial circulation. These probably include cells that were shunted away from pulmonary alveoli. Because these cells already contain nucleation sites, they are unlikely to have a delay time. More ultrastructural studies are needed to establish the proportion of cells containing sickle fibers in arterial blood. It is likely that the great majority of SS cells lack polymer until they undergo deoxygenation in the microcirculation. The delay times of these cells are likely to be a critical determinant of vaso-occlusive manifestations of sickle cell disease.

THE MEMBRANE OF SICKLE RED CELLS*

Considering the gross distortion that is imposed on the cell by polymerization of hemoglobin into aligned fibers, it is not surprising that a number of structural and functional abnormalities have been noted in the membrane of SS red cells. There is compelling evidence that membrane damage plays an important role in pathogenesis. As explained in detail below, under certain circumstances, intracellular polymerization leads to leakage of potassium ion accompanied by water loss. The resulting increase in intracellular hemoglobin concentration greatly accelerates the rate at which further polymerization can occur. Such a vicious circle can eventually lead to the irreversibly sickled cell. Because these cells are the ultimate testament to membrane injury in sickle cells, they will be described first. The mechanisms responsible for their formation will then be discussed.

Irreversibly Sickled Cells

Upon examination of peripheral blood films of patients with sickle cell anemia, anywhere from 2 to 30 per cent of the red cells have the characteristic elongated sickle deformity (see Color Plate III*A*). These cells have a smooth contour with blunt ends, in contrast to the sharp terminal spicules of *reversibly* sickled cells (Fig. 11–29). The striking appearance of these cells probably provided the first clue that sickle cell anemia is a hemolytic disease. The presence of such cells is surprising, because the erythrocytes in a peripheral blood smear are likely to be fully oxygenated and therefore would not be expected to sickle. Electron microscopy of such cells fails to reveal the aligned sickle fibers so characteristic of deox-

---

*This topic has been reviewed recently by Bookchin and Lew.[162a]

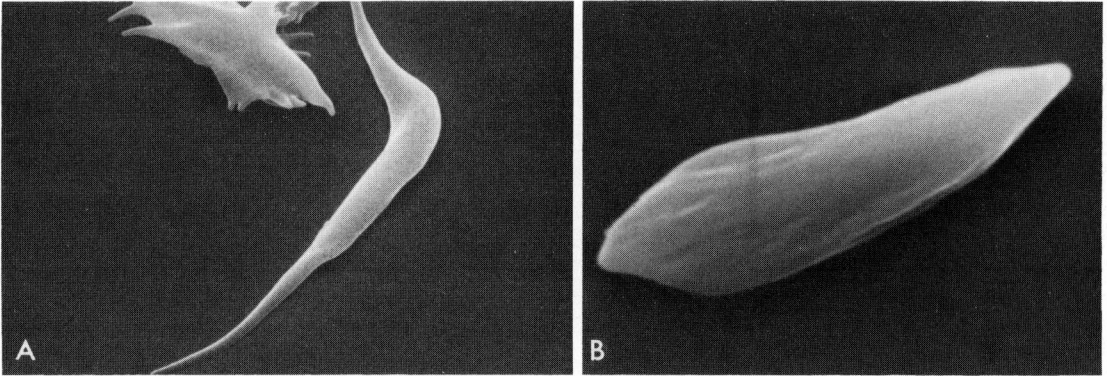

Figure 11–29. Scanning electron micrographs. *A,* Reversibly sickled cells (following deoxygenation) ($\times$ 1400). *B,* A typical irreversibly sickled cell ($\times$ 1400). (Courtesy of Dr. James White.)

ygenated sickle cells.[27] Thus, these cells have a permanently sickled shape even in the absence of any intracellular polymerization of hemoglobin. These observations indicate that irreversibly sickled cells (ISCs) have a damaged membrane that is no longer capable of assuming the normal biconcave disc shape upon reoxygenation.

Enumeration of ISCs has not been a consistent predictor of the clinical severity of sickle cell disease. Estimates may be falsely high because of the presence of dense cells that have very low oxygen affinity and therefore contain sufficient Hb S polymer to produce a sickled shape. Incubation of SS blood with 100 per cent O_2 will reduce the proportion of sickled forms by about 50 per cent.[162b] Incubation with 100 per cent carbon monoxide will lower the count even further, providing an estimate of bona fide ISCs.

ISCs are unduly rigid.[163, 164] Indeed, the presence of these cells explains why oxygenated SS blood has a higher viscosity than normal blood having a comparable packed cell volume.[165] These cells may plug capillaries and thereby initiate or potentiate vaso-occlusive crises. ISCs have a markedly shortened life span[133, 166, 167] and contribute significantly to the hemolytic anemia of patients with SS disease. In an individual patient, the percentage of ISCs in the peripheral blood tends to remain reasonably constant over a prolonged period of time. Among different SS patients, the percentage varies inversely with red cell survival.[166, 167]

Bertles and Milner[133] have identified the important characteristics of ISCs formed *in vivo.* Because of their high MCHC, these cells are dense and can readily be separated from other red cells by centrifugation. They have a relatively low content of Hb F.[133] It is likely that cells that are not well endowed with Hb F are at a distinct disadvantage from the time they emerge from the bone marrow. Without the protection provided by Hb F, these cells have a high probability of repeated sickling and within a few days become ISCs (see Fig. 11–20). They have relatively low levels of 2,3-DPG and ATP when expressed as amount per packed cell volume. However, because these cells are dehydrated, the concentration of these organic phosphates per volume of cell water is probably normal.[178] Because of their high intracellular concentration of Hb S, ISCs have very low oxygen affinity (P_{50} may be twice that of normal red blood cells[105]), for reasons discussed in the preceding section. Accordingly, even in the arterial circulation, ISCs are apt to contain a significant amount of deoxy Hb S in very high concentration* and, therefore, a corresponding amount of polymer.[109, 149] (See Fig. 11–27G.) This process adds to the rigidity of ISCs as they circulate *in vivo.* However, even fully oxygenated ISCs have markedly decreased deformability. Among these cells there is a surprising variability in degree of rigidity.[168] Those that are relatively less deformable do not differ in morphology from the more deformable ISCs. They are somewhat more osmotically fragile, however, perhaps because they have undergone more loss of membrane (see below). The membrane of ISCs is stiffer than that of normal red cells.[168a–169b] However, this abnormality is not an important factor in the rheology of intact ISCs. The deformability of oxygenated ISCs can be virtually normalized if the cells are allowed to swell in a hypotonic medium.[169a, 170, 171] Moreover, ghosts prepared from ISCs and filled

---

*The concentration is high owing to nonideality (see the section entitled "Polymerization of Sickle Hemoglobin").

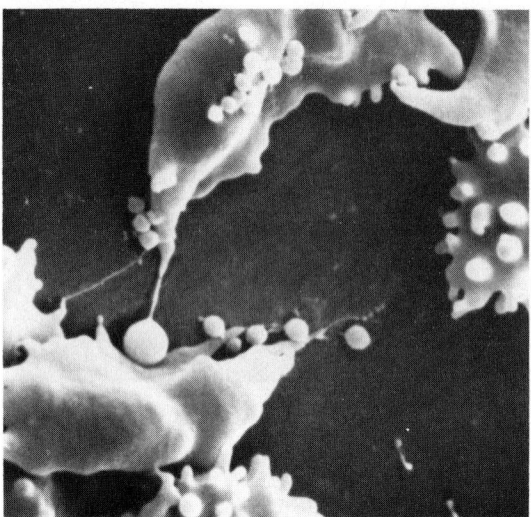

Figure 11–30. Scanning electron micrograph of sickle cells following incomplete reoxygenation. Retraction of long spicules leads to membrane fragmentation. (From Lessin, L. S., et al.: Arch. Intern. Med. *129*:306, 1972.)

with Hb A have near normal deformability.[170] Thus, the abnormal rheology of an ISC is primarily due to its high hemoglobin concentration rather than to a stiff membrane.*

ISCs can be generated *in vitro* by prolonged incubation of deoxygenated SS red cells.[173] Such treatment induces a membrane lesion with potassium and water loss and perhaps loss of membrane as well.

Morphological and Structural Alterations of the Membrane

Following deoxygenation of SS red cells, long filamentous projections commonly appear on the cell surface, producing the sickle or holly leaf shapes. Following repetitive sickling and unsickling, the sickle cell retracts its long filaments and develops terminal spherules, shown in Figure 11–30.[155, 174, 175] Fragmentation of these spherules leads to loss of cell membrane.[169b] These microvesicles contain integral membrane proteins such as Band 3 but no cytoskeletal proteins such as spectrin.[176] Moreover, the hemoglobin composition, specifically the percentage of Hb F, is identical to that of the parent cells.[176] It is unlikely that this loss of membrane spherules observed with *in vitro* sickling plays a significant role in the generation of ISCs *in vivo*. The mean cell hemoglobin in ISCs is not significantly different from the remainder of the cell population.[133, 163, 177] Moreover, ISCs have the same content of membrane lipid as non-ISCs.[178]

Membrane Lipid. In comprison with normal membranes, SS membranes contain 30 per cent more cholesterol per cell.[179] Dense SS erythrocytes exchange cholesterol with plasma less readily than normal red cells[180] and therefore accumulate this lipid. In contrast, SS membranes have normal levels of the four major phospholipids as well as normal distribution of fatty acids.[179] Nevertheless, the orientation of the phospholipids in the lipid bilayer of SS red cells is abnormal (Fig. 11–31). In normal red cells, phosphatidylcholine (lecithin) and sphingomyelin are located primarily on the outer leaflet of the bilayer in contact with plasma. In contrast, phosphatidylserine (PS) and phosphatidylethanolamine (PE) are found in the inner leaflet, in contact with cytoplasm. The functional significance of this phospholipid asymmetry is not known. In contrast to normal cells, when SS red cells are deoxygenated, the movement of phospholipids across the lipid bilayers is enhanced fourfold.[181] Normal movement resumes following reoxygenation. Irreversibly sickled cells and cells that are (reversibly) sickled by deoxygenation exhibit a marked increase of the amino phospholipids PS and PE on their outer surface.[182–184] This phospholipid "flip-flop" may reflect a derangement in the proteins of the cytoskeleton (described below) that normally stabilize the phospholipid asymmetry. The abnormal lipid surface of SS red cells has enhanced procoagulant activity,[185, 185a] which may contribute to the myriad abnormalities in coagulation that have been observed in patients with sickle cell disease (see Chapter 12).

Membrane fatty acids in SS red cells have an enhanced rate of peroxidation. This phenomenon will be discussed in the following section on the interaction of Hb S with the membrane.

Membrane Protein. The striking shape abnormality of oxygenated ISCs cannot be explained either by polymerizing hemoglobin or by abnormalities in membrane lipid. By exclusion, the shape change must reflect a derangement of membrane protein. Indeed, when ISC ghosts are treated with a detergent and rendered free of hemoglobin, lipid, and intrinsic membrane proteins, they still possess the characteristic ISC shape.[186] This observation demonstrates that the cytoskeleton (spectrin-

---

*The viscosity of hemoglobin in solution is very concentration-dependent and rises dramatically when the concentration exceeds 35 g/dl.[172]

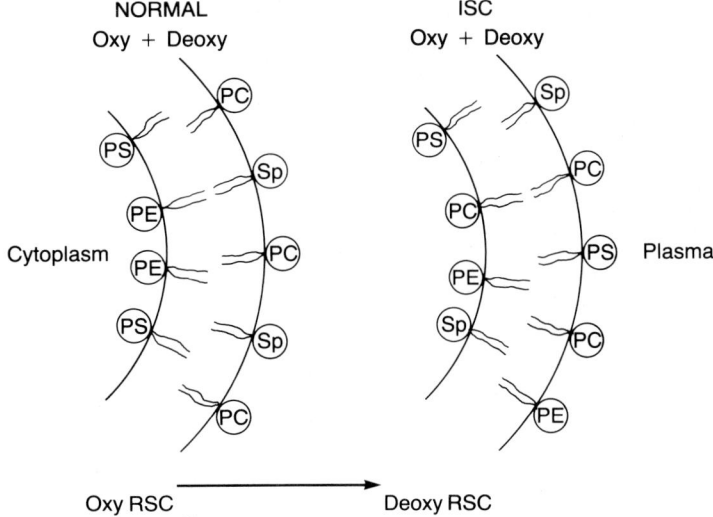

Figure 11–31. Phospholipid "flip-flop" induced by sickling. AA red cells and oxygenated SS red cells (non-ISCs) have normal phospholipid asymmetry with the amino phospholipids phosphatidyl serine (PS) and phosphatidyl ethanolamine (PE) on the inner cytoplasmic surface. The distribution becomes more even in ISCs or after deoxygenation of reversibly sickled cells (RSCs). (PC = phosphatidyl choline [lecithin]; Sp = sphingomyelin.)

actin-Band 4.1 lattice) becomes irreversibly deformed. It is likely that repeated cycles of polymerization and depolymerization result in a cumulative reorganization of the proteins of the cytoskeleton. Recent studies[187, 187a, 188] have not confirmed the report[189] of high–molecular-weight protein aggregates in ISC membranes. However, SS membranes contain increased intraprotein disulfide bonds,[188] probably induced by oxidant stress (see below).

The molecular events leading to the deformity of the cytoskeleton are not well understood. The overall composition of membrane proteins in SS red cells does not appear to differ significantly from that of normal cells.[190] Nevertheless, there are significant differences in the orientation of membrane proteins.[191–194] For example, spectrin binds much less readily to inside-out vesicles prepared from SS red cells compared with vesicles from normal cells.[195] Furthermore, ankyrin, the protein that stabilizes the interaction of spectrin with Band 3, has impaired binding to Band 3 of sickle cell inside-out vesicles.* These perturbations in the interaction of the intrinsic membrane proteins (those that penetrate the lipid bilayer) with the cytoskeleton may lead to the increased *in vitro* mechanical fragility[151] of sickle cells and even to the enhanced hemolysis that has been observed following vigorous exercise.[196] The organization of the cytoskeleton is an important determinant of the surface distribution of intrinsic membrane proteins. There are conflicting reports about whether there is abnormal distribution of glycophorin on the surface of SS red cells.[197–198] These red cells do contain abnormalities in the amounts of surface glycoprotein antigens,[199, 199a] but this finding probably reflects stress erythropoiesis rather than rearrangement of intrinsic membrane proteins.

Interaction of Hb S with the Membrane. The juxtaposition of the cytoplasmic surface of the red cell membrane and intracellular hemoglobin in high concentration raises the question of whether hemoglobin attaches to specific sites on the membrane. Equilibrium experiments using porous red cell ghosts indeed demonstrate that hemoglobin displays saturable binding behavior.[200, 201] However, nonphysiologic conditions of low pH and low ionic strength were required to demonstrate this phenomenon. Nevertheless, it is likely that hemoglobin binds to the inner membrane in intact red cells.[201a] Hemoglobin competes with glyceraldehyde-3-phosphate dehydrogenase for binding to the cytoplasmic surface of Band 3.[202, 203, 203a] Hb S binds more readily to red cell ghosts than Hb A does.[204–207a] Moreover, β^S chains show a higher affinity for membranes than β^A chains do.[208]

The pathophysiologic significance of these experiments has not yet been established. There is growing evidence that Hb S interacts with the erythrocyte membrane *in vivo*. Electron micrographs of membranes from SS red cells reveal small aggregates of hemoglobin studding the cytoplasmic surface.[174, 175, 209] Membrane-bound inclusions, presumed to be precipitated hemoglobin, have also been demonstrated both by darkfield microscopy[210, 211]

---

*Platt, O.: Unpublished observations.

and following acid elution.[211, 212] This hemoglobin appears to be denatured.[213] Electron paramagnetic resonance measurements have shown that some of the Hb S bound to the membrane is in the form of hemichrome.[214] Thus, the accumulation of membrane aggregates of denatured hemoglobin is reminiscent of congenital Heinz body hemolysis due to unstable hemoglobins (see Chapter 13). However, in sickle cell disease, notwithstanding the absence of a functioning spleen, these membrane-bound inclusions do not accumulate to a point where they can be identified as Heinz bodies. It is unclear whether these inclusions contribute to the deformability of SS red cells.

Although the information just presented clearly indicates interaction of Hb S with the red cell membrane, this phenomenon does not appear to influence either the rate or the extent of intracellular polymerization. As mentioned previously, measurements of sickling in intact red cells agree closely with experiments on concentrated solutions of Hb S. Furthermore, the addition of either red cell ghosts or inside-out vesicles (Fig. 11–32) to solutions of Hb S does not affect either solubility or delay time of polymerization.[131] Measurements employing membrane-bound fluorescent probes fail to demonstrate binding of deoxyhemoglobin S polymers to the membrane.[214a] Thus, the cytoplasmic surface of the red cell membrane does not serve as a nucleation site for formation of sickle fibers.

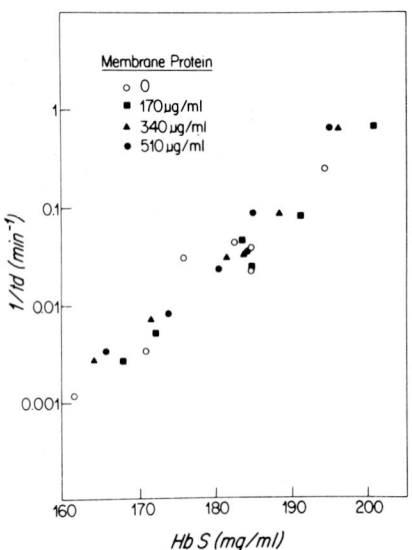

Figure 11–32. Kinetics of polymerization of deoxyhemoglobin S in the absence (○) and presence of increasing amounts (■, ▲, ●) of sealed inside-out vesicles from normal human red cells (td = delay time in minutes). (From Goldberg, M. A., et al.: J. Biol. Chem. 256:193, 1981.)

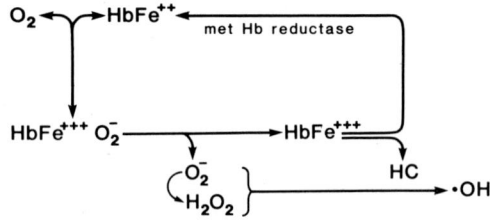

Figure 11–33. Generation of activated oxygen compounds O_2^-, H_2O_2, and ·OH in sickle cells. The formation of ·OH may be catalyzed by hemichrome (HC) bound to the red cell membrane. (From Hebbel, R., et al.: J. Clin. Invest. 70:1253, 1982.)

Oxidant Damage to the Membrane. Compared with normal cells, SS cells spontaneously generate twofold higher levels of activated oxygen compounds—superoxide, peroxide, and hydroxyl radical.[215] As explained in Chapter 16, superoxide is formed as a product of hemoglobin autoxidation:

$$HbFe^{2+}O_2 \rightarrow HbFe^{3+} + O_2^-$$

This reaction proceeds much more readily when hemoglobin is partially (rather than fully) saturated with oxygen. Thus, the low oxygen affinity of SS red cells would enhance the rate of autoxidation and superoxide formation. The fact that no significant amount of methemoglobin accumulates reflects the abundance of the enzymatic reducing system in these young red cells. Peroxide is formed from superoxide in the presence of superoxide dysmutase (SOD), another enzyme abundant in red cells:

$$2O_2^- + 2H^+ \xrightarrow{SOD} H_2O_2 + O_2$$

Hydroxyl radical (·OH) is formed from superoxide by means of the Haber-Weiss reaction:

$$O_2^- + H_2O_2 \rightarrow \cdot OH + OH^- + O_2$$

This reaction is facilitated by ionic iron or iron compounds capable of oxidation and reduction. Hemichrome that is formed in SS red cells[214] may function in this way and thereby facilitate ·OH formation[215] (Fig. 11–33).

These activated oxygen products are highly toxic to biological tissues and therefore may contribute to the membrane injury. Considerable evidence has accumulated that SS red cells of all ages are barraged by undue oxidant stress. The hexose-monophosphate shunt is stimulated,[216] and levels of reduced glutathione are somewhat diminished.[216, 217] Despite such metabolic defense, oxidant damage does occur. Increased levels of malonyldialdehyde[218] and malonyldialdehyde phospholipid adducts[219] indicate that peroxidation of membrane lipids occurs *in vivo*. Lipid peroxidation may be mediated by activated neutrophils.[219a] As mentioned previously, the presence of intraprotein disulfide bonds in SS membranes could also be a footprint of enhanced oxidant stress.[188]

Membrane Function in SS Red Cells

In the 1950s, Tosteson and colleagues[220, 221] demonstrated a fundamental abnormality of membrane function in SS red cells. They showed that deoxygenation increases the passive influx of sodium ion and the efflux of potassium ion. Following prolonged deoxygenation or depletion of ATP,[222, 223] loss of potassium exceeds net gain of sodium and therefore may be responsible for the progressive potassium and water loss that ultimately leads to ISCs (Fig. 11–34). Successive cycles of polymerization and depolymerization in the circulation may be the *in vivo* parallel of the *in vitro* perturbations that are required to dehydrate cells.

When normal cells are depleted of ATP in a calcium-containing medium, they lose potassium and water and gain calcium.[224] How does this well-known Gardos effect relate to the potassium and water loss induced by sickling? There is little convincing evidence that SS red cells are deprived of energy. Even ISCs probably have normal levels of ATP.[178] However, SS red cells contain at least twice as much calcium as normal cells, and the level in ISCs is fourfold that in normal cells.[225–228] Moreover, calcium uptake is markedly enhanced following deoxygenation of SS red cells. Normal red cells are able to maintain a very low level of calcium because they are endowed with a very

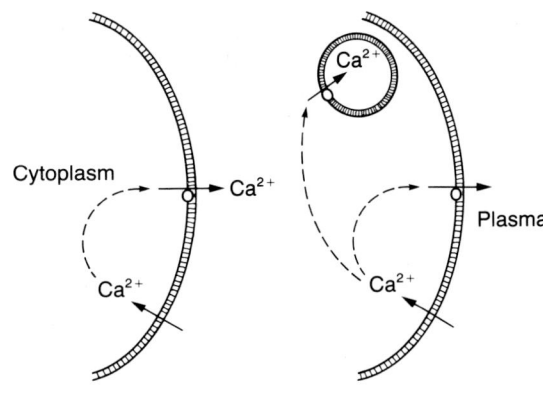

Figure 11–35. Calcium in normal and SS red cells. In normal cells, whatever Ca^{2+} leaks into the cell is pumped out (σ) by the Ca^{2+} ATPase. In addition, SS red cells contain inside-out vesicles, which actively pump Ca^{2+} into the vesicle. This phenomenon probably accounts for the high level of calcium in SS red cells.

efficient Ca^{2+}-ATPase that expels Ca^{2+} out of the cell against a large concentration gradient. Kinetic measurements following a pulse of deoxygenation show a delay in the efflux of calcium, suggesting impairment of the calcium pump.[229, 230] However, recent careful measurements show that in SS red cells, Ca^{2+}-ATPase is entirely normal.[231, 232] Taken together, these observations indicate that SS red cells contain a pool of calcium that is not readily accessible to the calcium pump. In fact, Bookchin and Lew[233] have recently obtained evidence suggesting that the calcium in SS red cells is neither freely distributed in the cytoplasm nor tightly bound but behaves as if it were compartmentalized, possibly within intracellular inside-out vesicles (Fig. 11–35). These probably accumulate during repetitive sickling cycles and represent yet another example of disorganization of the red cell membrane. Sequestered in this way, calcium per se is unlikely to have a significant influence on the function or viability of sickle red cells. In particular, calcium accumulation is unlikely to play a direct role in the development of ISCs. The rate of transformation of SS red cells into ISCs *in vitro* is not influenced by either extracellular Ca^{2+} or intracellular ATP.[234] Moreover, normal red cell ghosts reconstituted with Hb S are able to form irreversibly sickled forms even in the absence of calcium.[235]

Sickle Cells in the Microcirculation

The ultimate understanding of the pathogenesis of the vaso-occlusive manifestations of

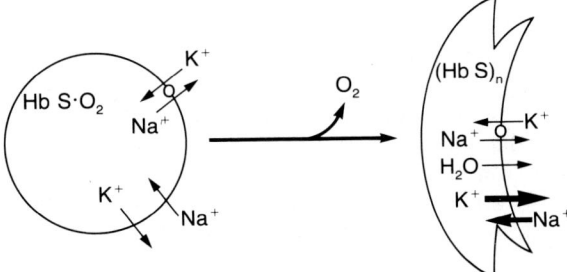

Figure 11–34. Potassium leak and dehydration induced by sickling. The small circle (○) on the membrane represents the sodium-potassium pump.

sickle cell disease will require detailed investigation of the behavior of partially deoxygenated SS cells within the microcirculation. The large and complex body of information on regulation of blood flow and oxygen transport in normal tissues must be applied to the circulation of sickle cells. The anatomical sites of oxygen unloading must be established. In some tissues, a significant amount of oxygen is released in the distal arterioles proximal to precapillary sphincters.[236–238] More information is needed about neural and humoral control of blood flow in various tissues of patients with sickle cell disease as well as the extent to which peripheral arteriolar-venous shunting influences the initiation and progation of vaso-occlusive events.

There is growing evidence that sickle cells have increased adherence to the endothelial surface of blood vessels. Monolayers of either human[197] or bovine[239] endothelial cells bind SS cells more readily than normal cells. ISCs show particularly strong adherence.[239] However, adherence is decreased when SS cells are reversibly sickled by deoxygenation.[197] Experiments on individual red cells utilizing a micropipette indicate that the abnormal adherence is not restricted to a small population of SS red cells and is not dependent on irreversible sickling.[240] The mechanism underlying this phenomenon is not understood. The proposal that SS cells have an alteration in the topography of surface charge[197] has not been confirmed.[198] Perhaps the phospholipid "flip-flop" in SS red cells contributes to their increased adherence. The extent to which red cells adhere to endothelial cells is quite variable among individual patients with SS disease but appears to be less marked in those with relatively mild disease.[241] The interaction is modulated by plasma factors,[240] particularly fibrinogen, which increases adherence.[242] This observation may have bearing on the role of acute infection in precipitating sickle crises. The pathophysiologic significance of this phenomenon is uncertain. The degree of adherence that has been demonstrated by the aforementioned *in vitro* studies may be significantly less than the shear forces generated at capillary endothelial surfaces *in vivo*. The bulk of clinical and experimental evidence collected over the past 40 years strongly indicates that deoxygenation of sickle cells and subsequent polymer formation are the proximal events responsible for vaso-occlusion.

Progress is now being made in studying the flow of sickle red cells in *ex vivo* preparations of circulatory beds such as mesentery[243–245] or cardiac.[245] The rat mesoappendix system is able to discriminate deoxygenated SS red cells of increasing density and hence decreasing deformability.[244] In addition, a variety of noninvasive techniques are now being adapted to examine microcirculation in patients with sickle cell disease.[246] Further experience with these approaches should help to unravel the sequence of events that trigger the development of a vaso-occlusive episode.

INHIBITION OF POLYMERIZATION

Information presented in this chapter on intracellular polymerization of sickle hemoglobin suggests a variety of ways in which the process can be inhibited. A number of laboratories all over the world have focused on this problem. So many different approaches have been taken that a complete account is far beyond the scope of this book.* Instead, only a few well-studied antisickling agents will be discussed, and the molecular mechanisms responsible for inhibition of polymerization will be stressed. The practical aspect of designing effective agents for treating sickle cell disease will be discussed at the end of the next chapter.

Sodium cyanate was the first antisickling agent to undergo systematic investigation. In 1971, Cerami and Manning[249] showed that when SS red cells were incubated with 30 mM cyanate, sickling was inhibited. The CNO^- anion readily traverses the red cell membrane and reacts with amino groups of hemoglobin and other proteins to form covalent adducts:

$$RNH_2 + CNO^- + H^+ \rightarrow RNH\overset{O}{\overset{\|}{C}}NH_2$$

The N-terminal amino groups of the α and β globin chains are preferentially carbamylated because of their low pKa. As shown in Table 11-3, polymerization of Hb S is significantly inhibited when the N terminus of the β chain is selectively carbamylated, whereas modification at the N terminus of the α chain has no effect.[250] It is likely that carbamylation at the β N terminus directly alters the conformation of the nearby β 6 Val donor site. Carbamyl phosphate, a normal metabolic intermediate, also inhibits Hb S polymerization and *in vitro* sickling.[251] It is hydrolyzed to cyanate inside

---

*For more information, see reviews by Dean and Schechter,[247] Klotz et al.,[248] and Acquaye et al.[248a]

Table 11–3. EFFECT OF SPECIFIC CHEMICAL MODIFICATIONS ON THE GELLING OF SICKLE HEMOGLOBIN

Compound	Minimum Gelling Concentration (g/dl)	Reference
None	24	251
Cyanate $\alpha_2\beta_2^{CNO}$	29	
$\alpha_2^{CNO}\beta_2$	24	
$\alpha_2^{CNO}\beta_2^{CNO}$	29	
None	23	254
Pyridoxal phosphate $\alpha_2\beta_2^{PLP}$	26	
Pyridoxal sulfate $\alpha_2^{PLS}\beta_2$	30	
None	23	264
Nitrogen mustard 2 mM	28	
4 mM	35	
None	22	255
bis(3,5-dibromosalicyl) fumarate 1 mM	28	
	Solubility (g/dl)	
None	16	256, 257
bis(3,5-dibromosalicyl) succinate (C4)	24	
bis(3,5-dibromosalicyl) glutarate (C5)	20	
bis(3,5-dibromosalicyl) adipate (C6)	17	

the red cell. Cyanate also increases the oxygen affinity of hemoglobin. This effect contributes more toward cyanate's inhibition of sickling at physiologic oxygen tensions than its direct effect on polymerization of deoxy Hb S.[252] The therapeutic use of cyanate is discussed in Chapter 12.

An alternate approach is modification of Hb S at the 2,3-DPG binding site. The Beneschs and associates[253] have shown that pyridoxal phosphate behaves as an affinity label and reacts selectively at the β-chain N terminus. This site-specific modification has a modest effect on polymerization of sickle hemoglobin (see Table 11–3). In contrast, selective blocking of the α-chain N-terminal amino group with pyridoxal sulfate causes a more marked increase in minimum gelling concentration (see Table 11–3). These results seem to conflict with those of the studies cited previously on carbamylated Hb S. Clearly, the effect[254] of selective modifications at the N termini of α and β chains is strongly dependent on the nature of the blocking groups.

Bifunctional aspirin derivatives also bind selectively at the 2,3-DPG binding site.[255, 256] The compounds bis(3,5-dibromosalicyl) fumarate and bis(3,5-dibromosalicyl) succinate both crosslink Hb S by forming covalent adducts at β 82 lysine of each β chain. As shown in Table 11–3, modification with these agents causes a marked increase in minimum gelling concentration. X-ray analysis shows that β 85 Phe and β 88 Leu, the acceptor sites for β 6 Val, are pulled inward and thus are less available for contact[256, 257] (Fig. 11–36). If the bridging group is longer (e.g., glutarate or adipate), this tension is relaxed and polymerization is no longer inhibited. Walder and colleagues have systematically tested a wide variety of bifunctional aspirin derivatives in order to achieve optimal crosslinking, inhibition of polymerization, and penetration across the red cell membrane.[255] For example, the bromine substitutions enable the compound to enter the red cell. These crosslinked hemoglobins have nearly normal oxygen affinity. However, they are not responsive to organic phosphates because the 2,3-DPG binding site is blocked. Unfortunately, these compounds also react with the red cell membrane and induce spheroechinocytes (see Chapter 12).

The compounds that have been discussed thus far all form covalent adducts with amino groups on hemoglobin. Other covalent inhibitors that react with amino groups include pyridoxal,[258] glyceraldehyde,[259, 260] and acetaldehyde,[261] as well as monofunctional[262] and bifunctional[263] amidoesters. These compounds have less structural specificity than those described above but are nevertheless potent inhibitors. A comparison of their antisickling properties is presented at the end of the next chapter.

A few covalent inhibitors attach to Hb S at sites other than amino groups. The potent alkylating agent nitrogen mustard causes a marked inhibition of polymerization (see Table

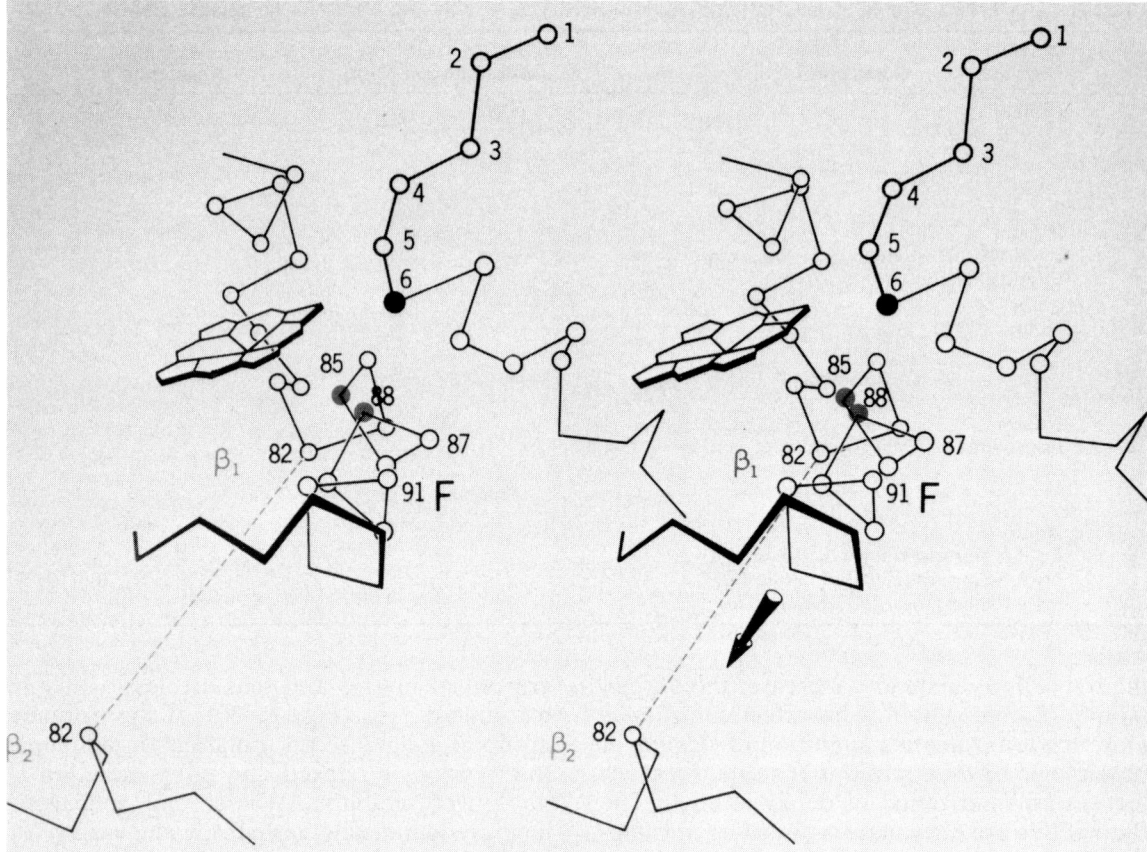

Figure 11–36. Stereodiagram of Hb S crosslinked with bis(3,5-dibromosalicyl) succinate or fumarate. The compound pulls the β 85 Phe and β 88 Leu acceptor site toward the interior of the molecule and therefore inhibits contact with the β 6 Val donor site. (From Dickerson, R. E., and Geis, I.: Hemoglobin: Structure, Function, Evolution and Pathology. Menlo Park, California, Benjamin Cummins, 1983.)

11–3) without a significant alteration in oxygen affinity.[264] Chemical, NMR,[265] and x-ray[60] analyses indicate that the primary sites of stable alkylation are four histidine residues on the β chain: 2, 97, 117, and 143. As discussed previously, β 117 His is one of the contacts in the sickle fiber. Nitrogen mustard is far too toxic to be administered systemically for treatment of sickle cell disease. However, it might be effective if administered by an extracorporeal device.[266] Compounds that bind at the β 93 cysteine sulfhydryl group also inhibit sickling[267, 268] but primarily by increasing oxygen affinity rather than by destabilizing the sickle polymer.

A wide variety of noncovalent inhibitors of polymerization have been reported. They include aromatic amino acids[269, 270, 270a] and peptides,[271–274] benzyl esters,[275] alkyl ureas,[276–278] alcohols,[279] and many other types of compounds. The mechanism underlying the inhibiting effect of the aromatic drug clofibric acid and related compounds has been studied by x-ray analysis.[280] Few, if any, of these agents are realistic candidates for therapy. A noncovalent agent would have to bind to hemoglobin with extremely high specificity and affinity in order for polymerization to be inhibited at an acceptably low concentration of the agent in the plasma. However, investigation of noncovalent inhibitors has provided information on the mechanism of polymerization and may be useful in the design of more specific antisickling agents.

References

1. Conley, C. L.: Sickle cell anemia—the first molecular disease. *In* Wintrobe, M. M. (ed.): Blood Pure and Eloquent. New York, McGraw-Hill, 1980, p. 139.
2. Castle, W. B.: From man to molecule and back to mankind. Semin. Hematol. *13*:159, 1976.
3. Emmel, V. E.: A study of the erythrocytes in a case of severe anemia with elongated and sickle-shaped red blood corpuscles. Arch. Intern. Med. *20*:586, 1917.

4. Hahn, E. V., and Gillespie, E. B.: Sickle cell anemia: Report of a case greatly improved by splenectomy; experimental study of sickle cell formation. Arch. Intern. Med. *39*:223, 1927.
4a. Scriver, J. B., and Waugh, T. R.: Studies on a case of sickle-cell anemia. Can. Med. Assoc. J. *23*:375, 1930.
5. Ham, T. H., and Castle, W. B.: Relation of increased hypotonic fragility and of erythrostasis to mechanism of hemolysis in certain anemias. Trans. Assoc. Am. Physicians *55*:127, 1940.
6. Sherman, I. J.: The sickling phenomenon, with special reference to the differentiation of sickle cell anemia from the sickle cell trait. Bull. Johns Hopkins Hosp. *67*:309, 1940.
7. Murphy, R. C., Jr., and Shapiro, S.: Sickle cell disease. I. Observations on behavior of erythrocytes in sickle cell disease. Arch. Intern. Med. *74*:28, 1944.
8. Castle, W. B., quoted by Strauss, M. B.: Of medicine, men and molecules: Wedlock or divorce? Medicine (Baltimore) *43*:619, 1964.
9. Watson, J., Stahman, A. W., and Bilello, F. P.: The significance of the paucity of sickle cells in newborn Negro infants. Am. J. Med. Sci. *215*:419, 1948.
10. Pauling, L., Itano, H., Singer, S. J., and Wells, I. C.: Sickle cell anemia: A molecular disease. Science *110*:543, 1949.
11. Harris, J. W.: Studies on the destruction of red blood cells. VII. Molecular orientation in sickle cell hemoglobin solutions. Proc. Soc. Exp. Biol. Med. *75*:197, 1950.
12. Perutz, M. F., and Mitchison, J. M.: State of haemoglobin in sickle-cell anaemia. Nature *166*:677, 1950.
13. Singer, K., and Singer, L.: The gelling phenomenon of sickle cell hemoglobin: Its biological and diagnostic significance. Blood *8*:1008, 1953.
14. Allison, A. C.: Properties of sickle-cell haemoglobin. Biochem. J. *65*:212, 1957.
15. Allison, A. C.: Observations on the sickling phenomenon and on the distribution of different haemoglobin types of erythrocyte populations. Clin. Sci. *15*:497, 1956.
16. Ingram, V. M.: A specific chemical difference between the globins of normal human and sickle-cell anaemia haemoglobin. Nature *178*:792, 1956.
17. Ingram, V. M.: Gene mutations in human haemoglobin: The chemical difference between normal and sickle cell haemoglobin. Nature *180*:326, 1957.
18. Allen, D. W., and Wyman, J.: Équilibre de l'hémoglobine de drepanocytose avec l'oxygène. Rev. Hematol. *9*:155, 1954.
19. Bunn, H. F.: The interaction of sickle hemoglobin with DPG, CO_2 and with other hemoglobins: Formation of asymmetrical hybrids. In Brewer, G. J. (ed.): Hemoglobin and Red Cell Structure and Function. New York, Plenum Press, 1972, p. 41.
20. Ross-Bernardi, L., Luzzana, M., Samaja, M., Rossi, F., and Perrella, M.: The functional properties of sickle cell blood. FEBS Lett. *59*:15, 1975.
21. Gill, S. J., Benedict, R. C., Fall, L., Spokane, R., and Wyman, J.: Oxygen binding to sickle cell hemoglobin. J. Mol. Biol. *130*:175, 1979.
22. Pennelly, R. R., and Noble, R. W.: Functional identity of hemoglobins S and A in the absence of polymerization. In Caughey, W. S. (ed.): Biochemical and Clinical Aspects of Hemoglobin Abnormalities. New York, Academic Press, 1978, p. 401.
23. Murayama, M.: Molecular mechanism of red cell "sickling." Science *153*:145, 1966.
24. Bookchin, R. M., and Nagel, R. L.: Molecular interactions of sickling hemoglobins. In Abramson, H., Bertles, J. F., and Wethers, D. L. (eds.): Sickle Cell Disease. St. Louis, C. V. Mosby Co., 1973, p. 140.
25. Stetson, C. A. Jr.: The state of hemoglobin in sickled erythrocytes. J. Exp. Med. *123*:431, 1966.
26. White, J. G.: The fine structure of sickled hemoglobin in situ. Blood *31*:561, 1968.
27. Bertles, J. F., and Döbler, J.: Reversible and irreversible sickling: A distinction by electron microscopy. Blood *33*:884, 1969.
28. Edelstein, S. J., Telford, J. N., and Crepeau, R. H.: Structure of fibers of sickle cell hemoglobin. Proc. Natl. Acad. Sci. USA *70*:1104, 1973.
29. Finch, J. T., Perutz, M. F., Bertles, J. F., and Döbler, J.: Structure of sickled erythrocytes and of sickle-cell hemoglobin fibers. Proc. Natl. Acad. Sci. USA *70*:718, 1973.
30. Crepeau, R. H., Dykes, G., Garrell, R., and Edelstein, S. J.: Diameter of hemoglobin S fibers in sickled cells. Nature *274*:616, 1978.
31. Dykes, G., Crepeau, R. H., and Edelstein, S. J.: Three-dimensional reconstruction of the 14-filament fibers of hemoglobin S. J. Mol. Biol. *130*:451, 1979.
32. Garrell, R. L., Crepeau, R. H., and Edelstein, S. J.: Cross-sectional views of hemoglobin S fibers by electron microscopy and computer modeling. Proc. Natl. Acad. Sci. USA *76*:1140, 1979.
33. Hofrichter, J., Hendricker, D., and Eaton, W. A.: Structure of hemoglobin S fibers: Optical determination of the molecular orientation in sickled erythrocytes. Proc. Natl. Acad. Sci. USA *70*:3604, 1973.
34. Eaton, W. A., and Hofrichter, J.: Polarized absorption and linear dichroism spectroscopy of hemoglobin. Methods Enzymol. *76*:175, 1981.
35. Wishner, B. C., Ward, K. B., Lattman, E. E., and Love, W. E.: Crystal structure of sickle-cell deoxyhemoglobin at 5 Å resolution. J. Mol. Biol. *98*:179, 1975.
36. Padlan, E. A., and Love, W. E.: Refined crystal structure of deoxyhemoglobin S. J. Biol. Chem., in press.
37. Magdoff-Fairchild, B., and Chiu, C. C.: X-ray diffraction studies of fibers and crystals of deoxygenated sickle cell hemoglobin. Proc. Natl. Acad. Sci. USA *76*:223, 1979.
38. Pumphrey, J. G., and Steinhardt, J.: Crystallization of sickle hemoglobin from gently agitated solutions—an alternative to gelation. J. Mol. Biol. *112*:359, 1977.
39. Wellems, T. E., and Josephs, R.: Crystallization of deoxyhemoglobin S by fiber alignment and fusion. J. Mol. Biol. *135*:651, 1979.
40. Wellems, T. E., Vassar, R. J., and Josephs, R.: Polymorphic assemblies of double strands of sickle hemoglobin. J. Mol. Biol. *153*:1011, 1981.
40a. Potel, M. J., Wellems, T. C., Vassar, R. J., Deer, B., and Josephs, R.: Macrofiber structure and the dynamics of sickle cell hemoglobin crystallization. J. Mol. Biol. *177*:819, 1984.
41. Chiu, C. C., and Magdoff-Fairchild, B.: Deoxygenated sickle hemoglobin—phase-transformation from fiber to a new monoclinic crystalline form. J. Mol. Biol. *136*:455, 1980.
42. Crepeau, R. H., and Edelstein, S. J.: Polarity of the

14-strand fibers of sickle cell hemoglobin determined by cross-correlation methods. Ultramicroscopy *13*:11, 1984.
43. Crepeau, R. H., Edelstein, S. J., Szalay, M., Benesch, R. E., Benesch, R., Kwong, S., and Edalji, R.: Sickle cell hemoglobin fiber stucture altered by α-chain mutation. Proc. Natl. Acad. Sci. USA *78*:1406, 1981.
43a. Rosen, L. S., and Magdoff-Fairchild, B.: X-ray diffraction studies of 14-filament models of deoxygenated Hb S fibers. I. Models based on electron micrograph reconstructions. J. Mol. Biol., in press.
44. Edelstein, S. J.: Molecular topology in crystals and fibers of hemoglobin S. J. Mol. Biol. *150*:557, 1981.
45. Josephs, R., Jarosch, H. S., and Edelstein, S. J.: Polymorphism of sickle cell hemoglobin fibers. J. Mol. Biol. *102*:409, 1976.
46. Bookchin, R. M., Nagel, R. L., and Ranney, H. M.: Structure and properties of hemoglobin C-Harlem, a human hemoglobin variant with amino acid substitutions in 2 residues of the β-polypeptide chain. J. Biol. Chem. *242*:248, 1967.
47. Bookchin, R. M., Nagel, R. L., and Ranney, H. M.: The effect of $\beta^{73\,Asn}$ on the interactions of sickling hemoglobins. Biochim. Biophys. Acta *221*:373, 1970.
48. Nagel, R. L., Johnson, J., Bookchin, R. M., Garel, M. C., Rosa, J., Schiliro, G., Wajcman, H., Labie, D., Moo-Penn, W., and Castro, O.: β-Chain contact sites in the haemoglobin S polymer. Nature *283*:832, 1980.
49. Milner, P. F., Miller, C., Grey, R., Seakins, M., DeJong, W. W., and Went, L. N.: Hemoglobin O Arab in four Negro families and its interaction with hemoglobin S and hemoglobin C. N. Engl. J. Med. *283*:1417, 1970.
50. McCurdy, P. R.: Clinical and physiological studies in a Negro with sickle cell hemoglobin D disease. N. Engl. J. Med. *262*:961, 1960.
51. Benesch, R. E., Yung, S., Benesch, R., Mack, J., and Schneider, R. G.: α-Chain contacts in the polymerization of sickle haemoglobin. Nature *260*:219, 1976.
52. Benesch, R. E., Kwong, S., Benesch, R., and Edalji, R.: Location and bond type of intermolecular contacts in the polymerization of haemoglobin. S. Nature *269*:772, 1977.
53. Benesch, R. E., Kwong, S., Edalji, R., and Benesch, R.: α-Chain mutations with opposite effects on the gelation of hemoglobin S. J. Biol. Chem. *254*:8169, 1979.
54. Goldberg, M. A., Husson, M. A., and Bunn, H. F.: The participation of hemoglobins A and F in the polymerization of sickle hemoglobin. J. Biol. Chem. *252*:3414, 1977.
55. Benesch, R. E., Edalji, R., Benesch, R., and Kwong, S.: Solubilization of hemoglobin S by other hemoglobins. Proc. Natl. Acad. Sci. USA *77*:5130, 1980.
56. Bookchin, R. M., Nagel, R. L., and Balazs, T.: Role of hybrid tetramer formation in gelation of hemoglobin S. Nature *256*:667, 1975.
57. Bookchin, R. M., Balazs, T., Nagel, R. L., and Tellez, I.: Polymerization of haemoglobin SA hybrid tetramers. Nature *269*:526, 1977.
58. Benesch, R. E., Kwong, S., and Benesch, R.: The effect of α chain mutations cis and trans to the β6 mutation on the polymerization of sickle cell haemoglobin. Nature *299*:231, 1982.
59. Rhoda, M. D., Martin, J., Bloquit, Y., Garel, M. C., Edelstein, S. J., and Rosa, J.: Sickle cell hemoglobin fiber formation strongly inhibited by the Stanleyville-II mutation (β 78 Asn-Lys). Biochem. Biophys. Res. Commun. *111*:8, 1983.
59a. Rhoda, M. D., Blouquit, Y., Caburi-Martin, J., Monplaisir, N., Galacteros, F., Garel, M. C., and Roas, J.: Effects of the α20 mutation on the polymerization of Hb S. Biochim. Biophys. Acta *786*:62, 1984.
60. Roth, E. F., Arnone, A., Bookchin, R. M., and Nagel, R. L.: Chemical modification of human hemoglobin by antisickling concentrations of nitrogen mustard. Blood *58*:300, 1981.
61. Acharya, A. S., and Manning, J. M.: Reactivity of the amino groups of carbon monoxyhemoglobin S with glyceraldehyde. J. Biol. Chem. *255*:1406, 1980.
62. Bertles, J. F., Rabinowitz, R., and Döbler, J.: Hemoglobin interaction: Modification of solid phase composition in the sickling phenomenon. Science *169*:375, 1970.
63. Briehl, R. W., and Ewert, S.: Effects of pH, 2,3-diphosphoglycerate and salts on gelation of sickle cell deoxyhemoglobin. J. Mol. Biol., *80*:445, 1973.
64. Hofrichter, J., Ross, P. D., and Eaton, W. A.: Supersaturation in sickle cell hemoglobin solutions. Proc. Natl. Acad. Sci. USA *73*:3035, 1976.
65. Ross, P. D., Hofrichter, J., and Eaton, W. A.: Calorimetric and optical characterization of sickle cell hemoglobin gelation. J. Mol. Biol. *96*:239, 1975.
66. Magdoff-Fairchild, B., Poillon, W. N., Li, T.-I., and Bertles, J. F.: Thermodynamic studies of polymerization of deoxygenated sickle cell hemoglobin. Proc. Natl. Acad. Sci. USA *73*:990, 1976.
67. Ross, P. D., Hofrichter, J., and Eaton, W. A.: Thermodynamics of gelation of sickle cell deoxyhemoglobin. J. Mol. Biol. *115*:111, 1977.
68. Briehl, R. W.: Gelation of sickle cell hemoglobin. IV. Phase transitions in hemoglobin S gels: Separate measures of aggregation and solution-gel equilibrium. J. Mol. Biol. *123*:521, 1978.
69. Minton, A. P.: Non-ideality and the thermodynamics of sickle-cell hemoglobin gelation. J. Mol. Biol. *110*:89, 1977.
70. Middaugh, C. R., Tisel, W. A., Haire, R. N., and Rosenberg, A.: Determination of the apparent thermodynamic activities of saturated protein solutions. J. Biol. Chem. *254*:367, 1970.
71. Tisel, W. A., Haire, R. N., White, J. G., Rosenberg, A., and Middaugh, C. R.: Polyphasic linkage between protein solubility and ligand binding in the hemoglobin–polyethylene glycol system. J. Biol. Chem. *255*:8975, 1980.
72. Itano, H. A.: Solubilities of naturally occurring mixtures of human hemoglobins. Arch. Biochem. Biophys. *47*:148, 1953.
73. Cottam, G. L., and Waterman, M. R.: Reversible solubility of deoxyhemoglobin S. Biochem. Biophys. Res. Commun. *54*:1157, 1973.
74. Adachi, K., and Asakura, T.: The solubility of sickle and non-sickle hemoglobins in concentrated phosphate buffer. J. Biol. Chem. *254*:4079, 1979.
75. Roth, E. F., Jr., Bookchin, R. M., and Nagel, R. L.: Deoxyhemoglobin S gelation and insolubility at high ionic strength are distinct phenomena. J. Lab. Clin. Med. *93*:867, 1979.
76. Adachi, K., and Asakura, T.: Multiple nature of polymers of deoxyhemoglobin S prepared by different methods. J. Biol. Chem. *258*:3045, 1983.
77. Sunshine, H. R., Hofrichter, J., and Eaton, W. A.:

Gelation of sickle cell hemoglobin in mixtures with normal adult and fetal hemoglobins. J. Mol. Biol. *133*:435, 1979.

78. Nagel, R. L., Bookchin, R. M., Johnson, J., Labie, D., Wajcman, H., Isaac-Sodeye, W. A., Honig, G. R., Schiliro, G., Crookston, J. H., and Matsutomo, K.: Structural bases of the inhibitory effects of hemoglobin F and hemoglobin A_2 on the polymerization of hemoglobin S. Proc. Natl. Acad. Sci. USA *76*:670, 1979.
79. Cheetham, R. C., Huehns, E. R., and Rosemeyer, M. A.: Participation of haemoglobins A, F, A_2 and C in polymerization of haemoglobin S. J. Mol. Biol. *129*:45, 1979.
80. Bunn, H. F., Noguchi, C. T., Hofrichter, J., Schechter, G. P., Schechter, A. N., and Eaton, W. A.: The molecular and cellular pathogenesis of hemoglobin SC disease. Proc. Natl. Acad. Sci. USA *79*:7527, 1982.
81. Adachi, K., Ozguc, M., and Asakura, T.: Nucleation-controlled aggregation of deoxyhemoglobin S. Participation of hemoglobin A in the aggregation of deoxyhemoglobin S in concentrated buffer. J. Biol. Chem. *255*:3092, 1980.
82. Jones, M. M., and Steinhardt, J.: Evidence of the incorporation of normally nonaggregating hemoglobins into crystalline aggregates of deoxyhemoglobin S. J. Biol. Chem. *257*:1913, 1982.
83. Adachi, K., Segal, R., and Asakura, T.: Nucleation-controlled aggregation of deoxyhemoglobin S. Participation of hemoglobin F in the aggregation of deoxyhemoglobin S in concentrated phosphate buffer. J. Biol. Chem. *255*:7595, 1980.
84. Adachi, K., and Asakura, T.: Gelation of deoxyhemoglobin A in concentrated phosphate buffer. Exhibition of delay time prior to aggregation and crystallization of deoxyhemoglobin A. J. Biol. Chem. *254*:12273, 1979.
85. Briehl, R. W., and Ewert, S.: Gelation of sickle cell hemoglobin. II. Methemoglobin. J. Mol. Biol. *89*:759, 1974.
86. Salhany, J. M., Ogawa, S., and Shulman, R. G.: Spectral-kinetic heterogeneity in reactions of nitrosyl hemoglobin. Proc. Natl. Acad. Sci. USA *71*:3359, 1974.
87. Briehl, R. W., and Salhany, J. M.: Gelation of sickle hemoglobin. III. Nitrosyl hemoglobin. J. Mol. Biol. *96*:733, 1975.
88. Gupta, R. K.: Nuclear relaxation and gelation study of the interaction of organophosphates with human normal and sickle hemoglobins. In vitro gelation of sickle oxyhemoglobin in the presence of inositol hexaphosphate. J. Biol. Chem. *25*:6815, 1976.
89. Hofrichter, J.: Ligand binding and the gelation of sickle cell hemoglobin. J. Mol. Biol. *128*:335, 1979.
90. Sunshine, H. R., Hofrichter, J., Ferrone, F. A., and Eaton, W. A.: Oxygen binding by sickle cell hemoglobin polymers. J. Mol. Biol. *158*:251, 1982.
91. Gill, S. J., Spokane, R., Benedict, R. C., Fall, L., and Wyman, J.: Ligand-linked phase equilibria of sickle cell hemoglobin. J. Mol. Biol. *140*:299, 1980.
92. Chung, L. L., and Magdoff-Fairchild, B.: Extent of polymerization in partially liganded sickle hemoglobin. Arch. Biochem. Biophys. *189*:535, 1978.
93. Christakis, J., Bare, G. H., Balcerzak, S. P., Alben, J. O., and Bromberg, P. A.: Mechanism of inhibition of hemoglobin S polymerization by cyanate. J. Lab. Clin. Med. *89*:992, 1977.
94. Elbaum, D., Hirsch, R., and Nagel, R. L.: Decreased binding of 2,3-diphosphoglycerate to deoxyhemoglobin S: A polymerization-independent functional abnormality. University of Chicago Symposium on SC Disease, Vol. 1. Molecular Basis of Mutant Hemoglobin Dysfunction. New York, Elsevier North Holland, 1981, p. 253.
95. Ueda, Y., Bookchin, R. M., and Nagel, R. L.: A decreased effect of organic phosphates on hemoglobin S at low concentrations. Biochem. Biophys. Res. Commun. *85*:526, 1978.
96. Gill, S. J., Skold, R., Fall, L., Shaeffer, T., Spokane, R., and Wyman, J.: Aggregation effects on oxygen binding of sickle cell hemoglobin. Science *201*:362, 1978.
97. Benesch, R. E., Edalji, R., Kwong, S., and Benesch, R.: Oxygen affinity as an index of hemoglobin S polymerization: A new micromethod. Anal. Biochem. *89*:162, 1978.
98. Swerdlow, P. H., Bryan, R. A., Bertles, J. F., Poillon, W. N., Magdoff-Fairchild, B., and Milner, P. F.: Effect of 2,3-diphosphoglycerate on the solubility of deoxy-sickle hemoglobin. Hemoglobin *1*:527, 1977.
99. Ueda, Y., and Bookchin, R. M.: Effects of carbon dioxide and pH variations in vitro on blood respiratory function, red cell volume, transmembrane pH gradients and sickling in sickle cell anemia. J. Lab. Clin. Med. *104*:146, 1984.
100. Becklake, M. R., Griffiths, S. B., McGregor, M., Goldman, H. I., and Schreve, J. P.: Oxygen dissociation curves in sickle cell anemia and in subjects with sickle cell trait. J. Clin. Invest. *34*:751, 1955.
101. Bromberg, P. A., and Jensen, W. N.: Blood oxygen dissociation curves in sickle cell disease. J. Lab. Clin. Med. *70*:480, 1967.
102. Cawein, M. J., O'Neill, R. P., Dauzer, L. A., Lappat, E. J., and Roach, T.: A study of the sickling phenomenon and oxygen dissociation curve in patients with hemoglobins SS, SD, SF and SC. Blood *34*:682, 1969.
103. Lian, C. V., Roth, S., and Harkness, D. R.: The effect of alteration of intracellular 2,3-DPG concentration upon oxygen binding of intact erythrocytes containing normal and mutant hemoglobins. Biochem. Biophys. Res. Commun. *45*:151, 1971.
104. Charache, S., Grisolia, S., Fiedler, A. J., and Hellegers, A.: Effect of 2,3-diphosphogylcerate on oxygen affinity of blood in sickle cell anemia. J. Clin. Invest. *49*:806, 1970.
105. Seakins, M., Gibbs, W. N., Milner, P. F., and Bertles, J. F.: Erythrocyte Hb S concentration; an important factor in the low oxygen affinity of blood in sickle cell anemia. J. Clin. Invest. *52*:422, 1973.
106. May, A., and Huehns, E. R.: The mechanism of the low oxygen affinity of red cells in sickle cell disease. Haematol. Bluttransfus. *10*:279, 1972.
107. May, A., and Huehns, E. R.: The concentration dependence of the oxygen affinity of haemoglobin S. Br. J. Haematol. *30*:317, 1975.
108. Mizukami, H., Beaudoin, A. G., Bartnicki, D. E., and Adams, B.: Hysteresis-like behavior of oxygen association-dissociation equilibrium curves of sickle cells determined by a new method. Proc. Soc. Exp. Biol. Med. *154*:304, 1977.
109. Winslow, R. M.: Hemoglobin interactions and whole blood oxygen equilibrium curves in sickling disorders. In Caughey, W. S. (ed.): Clinical and Biochemical Aspects of Hemoglobin Abnormalities. New York, Academic Press, 1978, p. 369.
110. Sinet, M., and Pocidalo, J. J.: Blood oxygen affinity and sickling in sickle cell disease: Effect of prior deoxygenation. J. Lab. Clin. Med. *98*:492, 1981.

111. Bookchin, R. M., and Nagel, R. L.: Personal communication, 1983.
112. Winslow, R. M.: Blood oxygen equilibrium studies in sickle cell anemia. In Hercules, J. I., Cottam, G. L., Waterman, M. R., and Schechter, A. N. (eds.): Proceedings of the Symposium on Molecular and Cellular Aspects of Sickle Cell Disease. DHEW Publication (NIH) 76–1007. Bethesda, Maryland, National Institutes of Health, 1976, p. 235.
113. Ueda, Y., Nagel, R. L., and Bookchin, R. M.: An increased Bohr effect in sickle cell anemia. Blood 53:472, 1979.
114. Moffat, K., and Gibson, Q. H.: The rates of polymerization and depolymerization of sickle cell hemoglobin. Biochem. Biophys. Res. Commun. 61:237, 1974.
115. Hofrichter, J., Ross, P. D., and Eaton, W. A.: Kinetics and mechanism of deoxyhemoglobin S gelation: A new approach to understanding sickle cell disease. Proc. Natl. Acad. Sci. USA 71:4864, 1974.
116. Malfa, R., and Steinhardt, J.: A temperature-dependent latent period in the aggregation of sickle cell deoxyhemoglobin. Biochem. Biophys. Res. Commun. 59:887, 1974.
117. Harris, J. W., and Bensusan, H. B.: The kinetics of the sol gel transformation of deoxyhemoglobin S by continuous monitoring of viscosity. J. Lab. Clin. Med. 86:564, 1975.
118. Eaton, W. A., Hofrichter, J., Ross, P. D., Tschudin, R. G., and Becker, E. D.: Comparison of sickle cell hemoglobin gelation kinetics by NMR and optical methods. Biochem. Biophys. Res. Commun. 69:538, 1976.
119. Waterman, M. R., and Cottam, G. L.: Kinetics of the polymerization of hemoglobin S: Studies below normal erythrocyte hemoglobin concentration. Biochem. Biophys. Res. Commun. 73:639, 1976.
120. Shibata, K., Waterman, M. R., and Cottam, G. L.: Alteration of the rate of deoxyhemoglobin S polymerization. Effect of pH and percentage of oxygenation. J. Biol. Chem. 252:7468, 1977.
121. Ferrone, F. A., Hofrichter, J., Sunshine, H. R., and Eaton, W. A.: Kinetic studies on photolysis-induced gelation of sickle cell hemoglobin suggest a new mechanism. Biophys. J. 32:361, 1980.
121a. Ferrone, F. A., Hofrichter, J., and Eaton, W. A.: Kinetics of sickle hemoglobin polymerization. I. Studies using temperature-jump and laser photolysis techniques. J. Mol. Biol., in press.
121b. Ferrone, F. A., Hofrichter, J., and Eaton, W. A.: Kinetics of sickle hemoglobin polymerization. II. A dual nucleation mechanism. J. Mol Biol., in press.
122. Wilson, W. W., Luzzana, M. R., Penniston, J. T., and Johnson, C. S., Jr.: Pregelation aggregation of sickle cell hemoglobin. Proc. Natl. Acad. Sci. USA 71:1260, 1974.
123. Elbaum, D., and Nagel, R. L.: Aggregation of deoxyhemoglobin S at low concentrations. J. Biol. Chem. 251:7657, 1976.
124. Danish, E. H., and Harris, J. W.: Viscosity studies of deoxyhemoglobin S: Evidence for formation of microaggregates during the lap phase. J. Lab. Clin. Med. 101:515, 1983.
125. Russu, I. M., and Ho, C.: Proton longitudinal relaxation investigation of histidyl residues of normal human adult and sickle deoxyhemoglobin: Evidence for the existence of pregelation aggregates in sickle deoxyhemoglobin solutions. Proc. Natl. Acad. Sci. USA 77:6577, 1980.
126. Hu, C. C., and Johnson, M. E.: Spin label detection of aggregation by deoxygenated sickle hemoglobin under non-gelling conditions. FEBS Lett. 125:231, 1981.
127. Briehl, R. W.: Solid-like behaviour of unsheared sickle haemoglobin gels and the effects of shear. Nature 288:622, 1980.
128. Briehl, R. W.: Physical chemical properties of sickle cell hemoglobin. In Wallach, D. F. H. (ed.): The Function of Red Blood Cells: Erythrocyte Pathobiology. New York, A. R. Liss, Inc., 1981, p. 241.
129. Briehl, R. W.: The effects of shear on the delay time for gelation of hemoglobin S. Blood Cells 8:201, 1982.
130. Gabriel, D. A., Smith, L. A., and Johnson, C. S., Jr.: Elastic properties of deoxyhemoglobin S (deoxy-Hb S) gels. Arch. Biochem. Biophys. 211:774, 1981.
131. Goldberg, M. A., Lalos, A., and Bunn, H. F.: The effect of erythrocyte membrane preparations on the polymerization of sickle hemoglobin. J. Biol. Chem. 256:193, 1981.
132. Reed, L. J., Bradley, T. B., and Ranney, H. M.: The effect of amelioration of anemia on the synthesis of fetal hemoglobin in sickle cell anemia. Blood 25:37, 1963.
133. Bertles, J. F., and Milner, P. F.: Irreversibly sickled erythrocytes: A consequence of the heterogeneous distribution of hemoglobin types in sickle cell anemia. J. Clin. Invest. 47:1731, 1968.
134. Dover, G. J., Boyer, S. H., Charache, S., and Heintzelman, K.: Individual variation in the production and survival of F cells in sickle cell disease. N. Engl. J. Med. 299:1428, 1978.
135. Oda, S., Oda, E., and Tanaka, K. R.: Relationship of density distribution and pyruvate kinase electrophoretic pattern of erythrocytes in sickle cell diseases and other disorders. Acta Haematol. 60:201, 1978.
136. Fabry, M. E., and Nagel, R. L.: Heterogeneity of red cells in the sickler: A characteristic with practical clinical and pathophysiological implications. Blood Cells 8:9, 1982.
136a. Weems, H. F., and Lessin, L. S.: Erythrocyte density distribution in sickle cell anemia. Acta Haematol. 71:361, 1984.
137. Fabry, M. E., and Nagel, R. L.: The effect of deoxygenation on red cell density: Significance for pathophysiology of sickle cell anemia. Blood 60:1370, 1982.
138. Embury, S. N., Clark, M. R., Monroy, G., and Mohandas, N.: Concurrent sickle cell anemia and α-thalassemia. Effect on pathological properties of sickle erythrocytes. J. Clin. Invest. 73:116, 1984.
138a. Fabry, M. E., Mears, J. G., Patel, P., Schaefer, K., Carmichael, L. D., Martinez, G., and Nagel, R. L.: Dense cells in sickle cell anemia—the effects of gene interaction. Blood 64:1042, 1984.
138b. Noguchi, C. T., Dover, G. J., Rodgers, G. P., Serjeant, G. R., Antonarakis, S. E., Anagnou, N. P., Higgs, D. R., Weatherall, D. J., and Schechter, A. N.: α-Thalassemia changes erythrocyte heterogeneity in sickle cell disease. J. Clin. Invest. 75:1632, 1985.
139. Griggs, R. C., and Harris, J. W.: Biophysics of the variants of sickle cell disease. Arch. Intern. Med. 97:315, 1956.
140. Asakura, T., and Mayberry, J.: Relationship be-

tween the morphology of sickle cells and the method of deoxygenation. J. Lab. Clin. Med. *104*:987, 1984.
141. Clark, M. R., Guatelli, J. C., Mohandas, N., and Shohet, S. B.: Influence of red cell water content on the morphology of sickling. Blood 55:823, 1980.
142. Charache, S., and Conley, C. L.: Rate of sickling of red cells during deoxygenation of blood from persons with various sickling disorders. Blood *24*:25, 1964.
143. Jandl, J. H., Simmons, R. L., and Castle, W. B.: Red cell filtration and the pathogenesis of certain hemolytic anemias. Blood *18*:133, 1961.
144. Messer, M. J., and Harris, J. W.: Filtration characteristics of sickle cells: Rates of alteration of filtrability after deoxygenation. J. Lab. Clin. Med. *76*:537, 1970.
145. Usami, S., Chien, S., and Bertles, J. F.: Deformability of sickle cells as studied by microsieving. J. Lab. Clin. Med. *86*:274, 1975.
146. Noguchi, C. T., Torchia, D. A., and Schechter, A. N.: Determination of deoxyhemoglobin S polymer in sickle erythrocytes upon deoxygenation. Proc. Natl. Acad. Sci. USA *77*:5487, 1980.
147. Noguchi, C. T., Torchia, D. A., and Schechter, A. N.: Polymerization of hemoglobin in sickle trait erythrocytes and lysates. J. Biol. Chem. *256*:4168, 1981.
148. Noguchi, C. T., Torchia, D. A., and Schechter, A. N.: The intracellular polymerization of sickle hemoglobin: Effects of cell heterogeneity. J. Clin. Invest. *72*:846, 1983.
149. Noguchi, C. T., and Schechter, A. N.: The intracellular polymerization of sickle hemoglobin and its relevance to sickle cell disease. Blood *58*:1057, 1981.
150. Noguchi, C. T.: Polymerization in erythrocytes containing S and non-S hemoglobin. Biophys. J. *45*:1039, 1984.
151. Harris, J. W., Brewster, H. H., Ham, T. H., and Castle, W. B.: Studies on the destruction of red blood cells. The biophysics and biology of sickle cell disease. Arch. Intern. Med. *97*:145, 1956.
152. Eaton, W. A., Hofrichter, J., and Ross, P. D.: Delay time of gelation: A possible determinant of clinical severity in sickle cell disease. Blood *47*:621, 1976.
153. Rampling, M. W., and Sirs, J. A.: The rate of sickling of cells containing sickle cell haemoglobin. Clin. Sci. Mol. Med. *45*:655, 1973.
154. Zarkowsky, H. S., and Hochmuth, R. M.: Sickling times of individual erythrocytes at zero PO_2. J. Clin. Invest. *56*:1023, 1975.
155. Padilla, F., Bromberg, P. A., and Jensen, W. N.: The sickle-unsickle cycle: A cause of fragmentation leading to permanently deformed cells. Blood *41*:653, 1973.
156. Messer, M. J., Hahn, J. A., and Bradley, T. B.: The kinetics of sickling and unsickling of red cells under physiologic conditions: Rheologic and ultrastructural correlations. In Hercules, J. I., Cottam, G. L., Waterman, M. R., and Schechter, A. N. (eds.): Proceedings of the Symposium on Molecular and Cellular Aspects of Sickle Cell Disease. DHEW Publication (NIH) 76–1007. Bethesda, Maryland, National Institutes of Health, 1976, p. 225.
157. Hahn, J. A., Messer, M. J., and Bradley, T. B.: Ultrastructure of sickling and unsickling in time-lapse studies. Br. J. Haematol. *34*:559, 1976.
158. Jensen, W. N., Rucknagel, D. L., and Taylor, W. J.: In vivo study of the sickle cell phenomenon. J. Lab. Clin. Med. *56*:854, 1960.
159. Serjeant, G. R., Petch, M. C., and Serjeant, B. E.: The in vivo sickle phenomenon: A reappraisal. J. Lab. Clin. Med. *81*:850, 1973.
160. Coletta, M., Hofrichter, J., Ferrone, F. A., and Eaton, W. A.: Kinetics of sickle haemoglobin polymerization in single red cells. Nature *300*:194, 1982.
161. Rotman, H. H., Klocke, R. A., Andersson, K. K., D'Alecy, L., and Forster, R. E.: Kinetics of oxygenation and deoxygenation of erythrocytes containing hemoglobin S. Respir. Physiol. *21*:9, 1974.
162. Harrington, J. P., Elbaum, D., Bookchin, R. M., Wittenberg, J. B., and Nagel, R. L.: Ligand kinetics of hemoglobin S containing erythrocytes. Proc. Natl. Acad. Sci. USA *74*:203, 1977.
162a. Bookchin, R. M., and Lew, V. L.: Red cell membrane abnormalities in sickle-cell anemia. Prog. Hematol. *13*:1, 1983.
162b. Rodgers, G. P., Noguchi, C. T., and Schechter, A. N.: Irreversibly sickled erythrocytes in sickle cell anemia. A quantitative reappraisal. Am. J. Hematol., in press.
163. LaCelle, P. L., and Kirkpatrick, F. H.: Determinant of erythrocyte membrane elasticity. In Brewer, G. J. (ed.): Erythrocyte Structure and Function. New York, A. R. Liss Inc., 1975, p. 535.
164. LaCelle, P. L., Weed, R. I., and Santillo, P. A.: Pathophysiologic significance of abnormalities of red cell shape. In Bolis, L., Hoffman, J. F., and Leaf, A. (eds.): Membranes and Disease. New York, Raven Press, 1976, p. 1.
165. Chien, S., Usami, S., and Bertles, J. F.: Abnormal rheology of oxygenated blood in sickle cell anemia. J. Clin. Invest. *49*:623, 1970.
166. Serjeant, G. R., Serjeant, B. E., and Milner, P. F.: The irreversibly sickled cell: A determinant of haemolysis in sickle cell anemia. Br. J. Haematol. *17*:527, 1969.
167. McCurdy, P. R., and Sherman, A. S.: Irreversibly sickled cells and red cell survival in sickle cell anemia. A study with both $DF^{32}P$ and ^{51}Cr. Am. J. Med. *64*:253, 1978.
168. Smith, C. M., Kuettner, J. F., Tukey, D. P., Burris, S. M., and White, J. G.: Variable deformability of irreversibly sickled erythrocytes. Blood *58*:71, 1981.
168a. Rice-Evans, C., Bruckdorfer, K. R., and Dootson, G.: Studies on the altered membrane characteristics of sickle cells. FEBS Lett. *94*:81, 1978.
169. Nash, G. B., and Meiselman, H. J.: Viscoelastic properties of red cells in sickle cell disease. Biophys. J. *41*:118A, 1983.
169a. Evans, E., Mohandas, N., and Leung, A.: Static and dynamic rigidities of normal and sickle erythrocytes. J. Clin. Invest. *73*:477, 1984.
169b. Nash, G. B., Johnson, C. S., and Meiselman, H. J.: Mechanical properties of oxygenated red blood cells in sickle cell (Hb SS) disease. Blood *63*:73, 1984.
170. Clark, M. R., Mohandas, N., and Shohet, S. B.: Deformability of oxygenated irreversibly sickled cells. J. Clin. Invest. *65*:189, 1980.
171. Gully, M. L., Ross, D. W., Feo, C., and Orringer, E. P.: The effect of cell hydration on the deformability of normal and sickle erythrocytes. Am. J. Hematol. *13*:283, 1982.
172. Charache, S., Conley, C. L., Waugh, D. F., Ugoretz, R. J., and Spurrell, R.: Pathogenesis of hemolytic

anemia in homozygous hemoglobin C disease. J. Clin. Invest. 46:1795, 1967.
173. Shen, S. C., Fleming, E. M., and Castle, W. B.: Studies on the destruction of red blood cells. V. Irreversibly sickled erythrocytes: The experimental production *in vitro*. Blood 4:498, 1949.
174. Lessin, L. S., Jensen, W. N., and Klug, P.: Ultrastructure of the normal and hemoglobinopathic red blood cell membrane. Arch. Intern. Med. 129:306, 1972.
175. Lessin, L. S.: Membrane ultrastructure of normal, sickled and Heinz-body erythrocytes by freeze-etching. Nouv. Rev. Fr. Hematol. 12:871, 1972.
176. Allan, D., Limbrick, A. R., Thomas, P., and Westerman, M. P.: Microvesicles from sickle erythrocytes and their relation to irreversible sickling. Br. J. Haematol. 47:383, 1981.
177. Murphy, J. R., Wengard, M., and Brereton, W.: Rheological studies of Hb SS blood: Influence of hematocrit, hypertonicity, separation of cells, deoxygenation, and mixture with normal cells. J. Lab. Clin. Med. 87:475, 1976.
178. Clark, M. R., Unger, R. C., and Shohet, S. B.: Monovalent cation composition and ATP and lipid content of irreversibly sickled cells. Blood 51:1169, 1978.
179. Sasaki, J., Waterman, M. R., Buchanan, G. R., and Cottam, G. L.: Plasma and erythrocyte lipids in sickle cell anaemia. Clin. Lab. Haematol. 5:35, 1983.
180. Jain, S. K., and Shohet, S. B.: Red blood cell (^{14}C) cholesterol exchange and plasma cholesterol esterifying activity of normal and sickle cell blood. Biochim. Biophys. Acta 688:11, 1982.
181. Franck, P. F. H., Chiu, D., Op den Kamp, J. A. F., Lubin, B., van Deenen, L. L. M., and Roelofsen, B.: Accelerated transbilayer movement of phosphatidylcholine in sickled erythrocytes. J. Biol. Chem. 258:8436, 1983.
182. Gordesky, S. E., Marinetti, G. V., and Segel, B. G.: Differences in the reactivity of phospholipids with FDNB in normal RBC, sickle cells and RBC ghosts. Biochem. Biophys. Res. Commun. 47:223, 1972.
183. Chiu, D., Lubin, B., and Shohet, S.: Erythrocyte membrane lipid reorganization during the sickling process. Br. J. Haematol. 41:223, 1979.
184. Lubin, B., Chiu, D., Bastacky, J., Roelofsen, B., and van Deenen, L. L. M.: Abnormalities in membrane phospholipid organization in sickled erythrocytes. J. Clin. Invest. 67:1643, 1981.
185. Chiu, D., Lubin, B., Roelofson, B., and van Deenen, L. L.: Sickled erythrocytes accelerate clotting in vitro: An effect of abnormal membrane lipid asymmetry. Blood 58:398, 1981.
185a. Westerman, M. P., Cole, E. R., and Wu, K.: The effect of spicules obtained from sickle red cells on clotting activity. Br. J. Haematol. 56:557, 1984.
186. Lux, S. E., John, K. M., and Karnovsky, M. J.: Irreversible deformation of the spectrin-actin lattice in irreversibly sickled cells. J. Clin. Invest. 58:955, 1976.
187. Palek, J., and Liu, S. C.: Membrane protein organization in ATP depleted and irreversibly sickled red cells. J. Supramol. Struct. 10:79, 1979.
187a. Palek, J., and Lux, S. E.: Red cell membrane skeletal defects in hereditary and acquired hemolyte anemias. Semin. Hematol. 20:189, 1983.
188. Rank, B., Carlsson, J., and Hebbel, R. P.: Abnormal redox status of membrane protein thiols in sickle erythrocytes. J. Clin. Invest. 75:1531, 1985.
189. Lessin, L. S., Kurantsin-Mills, J., Wallas, C., and Weems, H.: Membrane alterations in irreversibly sickled cells: Hemoglobin-membrane interaction. J. Supramol. Struct. 9:537, 1978.
190. Ballas, S. K., and Burka, E. R.: Failure to demonstrate red cell membrane protein abnormalities in sickle cell anaemia. Br. J. Haematol. 46:627, 1980.
191. Rubin, R. W., Milikowski, C., and Wise, G. E.: Organizational differences in the membrane proteins of normal and irreversibly sickled erythrocytes. Biochim. Biophys. Acta 595:1, 1980.
192. Ro, J., Neilan, B., Magee, P. N., Paik, W. K., and Kim, S.: Reduced erythrocyte membrane protein methylation in sickle cell anemia. J. Biol. Chem. 256:10572, 1981.
193. Green, G. A., and Kalra, V. K.: Carboxymethylation of membrane proteins of irreversibly sickled erythrocytes. J. Biol. Chem. 256:10565, 1981.
194. Dzandu, J. K., and Johnson, R. M.: Membrane protein phosphorylation in intact normal and sickle cell erythrocytes. J. Biol. Chem. 255:6382, 1980.
195. Platt, O. S., Falcone, J. F., and Lux, S. E.: Molecular defect in the sickle erythrocyte cytoskeleton: Abnormal spectrin binding to sickle inside-out vesicles. J. Clin. Invest., 75:266, 1985.
196. Platt, O. S.: Exercise-induced hemolysis in sickle cell anemia: Shear sensitivity and erythrocyte dehydration. Blood 59:1055, 1982.
197. Hebbel, R. P., Yamada, O., Moldow, C. F., Jacob, H. S., White, J. G., and Eaton, J. W.: Abnormal adherence of sickle erythrocytes to cultured vascular endothelium. J. Clin. Invest. 65:154, 1980.
198. Clark, L. J., Chan, L. S., Powars, D. R., and Baker, R. F.: Negative charge distribution and density on the surface of oxygenated normal and sickle red cells. Blood 57:675, 1981.
199. Fukuda, M., Fukuda, M. N., Hakomori, S., and Papayannopoulou, T.: Anomalous cell-surface structure of sickle-cell anemia erythrocytes as demonstrated by cell-surface labeling and endo-beta-galactosidase treatment. J. Supranol. Struct. 17:289, 1981.
199a. Basu, M. K., Lee, M. M., Maniatis, A., and Bertles, J. F.: Characteristics of I and E antigen receptors on the membrane of erythrocytes in sickle cell anemia. J. Lab. Clin. Med., 103:712, 1984.
200. Shaklai, N., Yguerabide, J., and Ranney, H. M.: Interaction of hemoglobin with red blood cell membranes as shown by a fluorescent chromophore. Biochemistry 16:5585, 1977.
201. Shaklai, N., Yguerabide, J., and Ranney, H. M.: Classification and localization of hemoglobin binding sites on the red blood cell membrane. Biochemistry 16:5593, 1977.
201a. Eisenger, J., Flores, J., and Salhany, J. M.: Association of cytosol hemoglobin with the membrane in intact erythrocytes. Proc. Natl. Acad. Sci. USA 79:408, 1982.
202. Salhany, J. M., Cordes, K. A., and Gaines, E. D.: Light-scattering measurements of hemoglobin binding to the erythrocyte membrane. Evidence for a transmembrane effect related to a disulfonic stilbene binding to band 3. Biochemistry 19:1447, 1980.
203. Cassoly, R.: Quantitative analysis of the association

of human hemoglobin with the cytoplasmic fragment of band 3 protein. J. Biol. Chem. 258:3859, 1983.
203a. Walder, J. A., Chatterjee, R., Steck, T. L., Low, P. S., Musso, G. F., Kaiser, E. T., Rogers, P. H., and Arnone, A.: The interaction of hemoglobin with the cytoplasmic domain of band 3 of the human erythrocyte membrane. J. Biol. Chem. 259:238, 1984.
204. Klipstein, F. A., and Ranney, H. M.: Electrophoretic components of the hemoglobin of red cell membranes. J. Clin. Invest. 39:1894, 1960.
205. Fischer, S., Nagel, R., Bookchin, R. M., Roth, E. F., and Tellez-Nagel, I.: The binding of hemoglobin to membranes of normal and sickle erythrocytes. Biochim. Biophys. Acta 375:422, 1975.
206. Shaklai, N., and Ranney, H. M.: Interaction of sickle cell hemoglobin with erythrocyte membranes. Proc. Natl. Acad. Sci. USA 78:65, 1981.
207. Fung, L. W.-M., Litvin, S. D., and Reid, T. M.: Spin-label detection of sickle hemoglobin-membrane interaction at physiological pH. Biochemistry 22:864, 1983.
207a. Sears, D. A., and Luthra, M. G.: Membrane bound hemoglobin in the erythrocytes of sickle cell anemia. J. Lab. Clin. Med. 102:694, 1983.
208. Bank, A., Mears, G., Weiss, R., O'Donnell, J. V., and Natta, C. L.: Preferential binding of β^S globin chains associated with stroma in sickle cell disorder. J. Clin. Invest. 54:805, 1974.
209. Wise, G. E., Miller, E., and Castello, C. M.: High-voltage electron microscopy of normal and irreversibly sickled red blood cells. Cell Tissue Res. 214:129, 1981.
210. Schneider, R. G., Takeda, I., Gustavson, L. P., and Alperin, J. B.: Intraerythrocytic precipitation of haemoglobins S. and C. Nature [New Biol.] 234:88, 1972.
211. Kim, H. C., Friedman, S., Asakura, T., and Schwartz, E.: Inclusions in red blood cells containing Hb S or Hb C. Br. J. Haematol. 44:547, 1980.
212. Kleihauer, E., and Kohne, E.: Application of the acid elution technique for the detection of inclusion bodies. In Schmidt, R. M. (ed.): Abnormal Haemoglobins and Thalassemia. New York, Academic Press, 1975, p. 149.
213. Lau, P., Hung, C., Minakata, K., Schwartz, E., and Asakura, T.: Spin-label studies of membrane-associated denatured hemoglobin in normal and sickle cells. Biochim. Biophys. Acta 552:499, 1979.
214. Asakura, T., Minakata, K., Adachi, K., Russell, M. O., and Schwartz, E.: Denatured hemoglobin in sickle erythrocytes. J. Clin. Invest. 59:633, 1977.
214a. Eisinger, J., Flores, J., and Bookchin, R. M.: The cytosol-membrane interface of normal and sickle erythrocytes: Effect of hemoglobin deoxygenation and sickling. J. Biol. Chem. 259:7169, 1984.
215. Hebbel, R., Eaton, J. W., Balasingam, M., and Steinberg, M. H.: Spontaneous oxygen radical generation by sickle erythrocytes. J. Clin. Invest. 70:1253, 1982.
216. Lachant, N. A., Davidson, W. D., and Tanaka, K. R.: Impaired pentose phosphate shunt function in sickle cell disease: A potential mechanism for increased Heinz body formation and membrane lipid peroxidation. Am. J. Hematol 15:1, 1983.
217. Wetterstroem, N., Brewer, G., Warth, J. A., Mitichin, A., and Near, K.: Relationship of glutathione levels and Heinz body formation to irreversibly sickled cells in sickle cell anemia. J. Lab. Clin. Med. 103:589, 1984.
218. Das, S. K., and Nair, R. C.: Superoxide dismutase, glutathione peroxidase, catalase and lipid peroxidation of normal and sickled erythrocytes. Br. J. Haematol. 44:87, 1980.
219. Jain, S. K., and Shohet, S. B.: A novel phospholipid in irreversibly sickled cells: Evidence for *in vivo* peroxidative damage in sickle cell disease. Blood, 63:362, 1984.
219a. Claster, S., Chiu, D. T.-Y., Quintanilha, A., and Lubin, B.: Neutrophils mediate lipid peroxidation in human red cells. Blood 64:1079, 1984.
220. Tosteson, D. C., Carlsen, E., and Dunham, E. T.: The effects of sickling on ion transport. I. Effect of sickling on potassium transport. J. Gen. Physiol. 39:31, 1955.
221. Tosteson, D. C., Shea, E., and Darling, R. C.: Potassium and sodium of red blood cells in sickle cell anemia. J. Clin. Invest. 31:406, 1952.
222. Segel, G., Mentzer, W. C., Jensen, M. C., Nathan, D. G., and Shohet, S. P.: Abnormal cation fluxes in human erythrocytes: Relation to ATP. In Gerlach, E., Moser, K., Deutsch, E., and Wilmanns, W. (eds.): Erythrocytes, Thrombocytes, Leukocytes. Stuttgart, G. Thieme, 1972, p. 118.
223. Glader, B. E., and Nathan, D. G.: Cation permeability alterations during sickling: Relationship to cation composition and cellular hydration of irreversibly sickled cells. Blood 51:983, 1978.
224. Gardos, G.: The function of calcium in the potassium permeability of human erythrocytes. Biochim. Biophys. Acta 30:653, 1958.
225. Eaton, J. W., Skelton, T. D., Swofford, H. S., Koplin, C. E., and Jacob, H. S.: Elevated erythrocyte calcium concentrations in sickle cell disease. Nature 246:105, 1973.
226. Palek, J.: Calcium accumulation during sickling of hemoglobin S (Hb SS) red cells. (Abstract.) Blood 42:988, 1973.
227. Eaton, J. W., Berger, E., White, J. G., and Jacob, H. S.: Calcium-induced damage of haemoglobin SS and normal erythrocytes. Br. J. Haematol. 38:57, 1978.
228. Palek, J.: Red cell calcium content and transmembrane calcium movements in sickle cell anemia. J. Lab. Clin. Med. 89:1365, 1977.
229. Bookchin, R. M., and Lew, V. L.: Progressive inhibition of the Ca^{++} pump and Ca^{++}-Ca^{++} exchange in sickle red cells. Nature 284:561, 1980.
230. Bookchin, R. M., and Lew, V. L.: Effect of a "sickling pulse" on calcium and potassium transport in sickle cell trait red cells. J. Physiol. 312:265, 1981.
231. Litosch, I., and Lee, K. S.: Sickle red cell calcium metabolism: Studies on Ca^{2}-Mg^{2+} ATPase and Ca-binding properties of sickle red cell membranes. Am. J. Hematol. 8:377, 1980.
232. Luthra, M. G., and Sears, D. A.: Increased Ca^{++}, Mg^{++}, and $Na^{+} + K^{+}$ ATPase activities in erythrocytes of sickle cell anemia. Blood 60:1332, 1982.
233. Bookchin, R. M., Ortiz, O. E., and Lew, V. L.: Silent intracellular calcium in sickle cell anemia red cells. In Brewer, G. J. (ed.): The Red Cell. Proceedings of the Sixth International Conference of Red Cell Metabolism and Function. New York, Alan R. Liss, Inc., 1984.
234. Palek, J., Church, A., and Fairbanks, G.: Transmembrane movements and distribution of calcium

in normal and hemoglobin S erythrocytes. *In* Leaf, A., Hoffman, J. F., and Bolis, L. (eds.): Membranes and Diseases. Craus-sur-Sierre, Switzerland, 1975.
235. Clark, M. R., and Shohet, S. B.: Hybrid erythrocytes for membrane studies in sickle cell disease. Blood 47:121, 1976.
236. Duling, B. R., and Berne, R. M.: Longitudinal gradients in periarteriolar oxygen tension: A possible mechanism for the participation of oxygen in local regulation of blood flow. Circ. Res. 27:669, 1970.
237. Pittman, R. N., and Duling, B. R.: Effects of altered carbon dioxide tension on hemoglobin oxygenation in hamster cheek pouch microvessels. Microvasc. Res. 13:211, 1977.
238. Duling, B. R., Kuschinsky, W., and Wahl, M.: Measurements of the perivascular PO_2 in the vicinity of the pial vessels of the cat. Pflugers Arch. 383:29, 1979.
239. Hoover, R., Rubin, R., Wise, G., and Warren, R.: Adhesion of normal and sickle erythrocytes to endothelial monolayer cultures. Blood 54:4, 1979.
240. Mohandas, N., and Evans, E.: Adherence of sickle erythrocytes to vascular endothelial cells: Requirement for both cell membrane changes and plasma factors. Blood 64:282, 1984.
241. Hebbel, R. P., Boogaerts, M. A. B., Eaton, J. W., and Steinberg, M. H.: Erythrocyte adherence to endothelium in sickle-cell anemia. N. Engl. J. Med. 302:992, 1980.
242. Hebbel, R. P., Moldow, C. F., and Steinberg, M. H.: Modulation of erythrocyte-endothelial interactions and the vasocclusive severity of sickling disorders. Blood 58:947, 1981.
243. Kaul, D. K., Nagel, R. L., and Baez, S.: Pressure effects on the flow behavior of sickle (Hb SS) red cells in isolated *(ex vivo)* microvascular system. Microvasc. Res. 26:170, 1983.
244. Kaul, D. K., Fabry, M. E., Windisch, P., Baez, S., and Nagel, R. L.: Erythrocytes in sickle cell anemia are heterogeneous in their rheological and hemodynamic characteristics. J. Clin. Invest. 72:22, 1983.
245. Vargas, F. F., and Blackshear, G. L.: Vascular resistance and transit time of sickle red blood cells. Blood Cells 8:139, 1982.
246. Rodgers, G. P., Schechter, A. N., Noguchi, C. T., Klein, H. G., Nienhuis, A. W., and Bonner, R. F.: Periodic microcirculatory flow in patients with sickle cell disease. N. Engl. J. Med. 311:1534, 1984.
247. Dean, J., and Schechter, A. N.: Sickle cell anemia: Molecular and cellular bases of therapeutic approaches. N. Engl. J. Med. 299:752, 804, 863, 1978.
248. Klotz, I. M., Haney, D. N., and King, L. C.: Rational approaches to chemotherapy: Antisickling agents. Science 213:724, 1981.
248a. Acquaye, C., Wilchek, M., and Gorecki, M.: Strategies for tackling sickle cell disease. Trends Biochem. Sci., 6:146, 1981.
249. Cerami, A., and Manning, J. M.: Potassium cyanate as an inhibitor of the sickling of erythrocytes *in vitro*. Proc. Natl. Acad. Sci. USA 68:1180, 1971.
250. Nigen, A. M., Njikam, N., Lee, C. K., and Manning, J. M.: Studies on the mechanism of action of cyanate in sickle cell disease: Oxygen affinity and gelling properties of hemoglobin S carbamylated on specific chains. J. Biol. Chem. 249:6611, 1974.
251. Kraus, L. M., and Kraus, A. P.: Carbamyl phosphate mediated inhibition of the sickling of erythrocytes in vitro. Biochem. Biophys. Res. Commun. 44:1381, 1971.
252. Diederich, D.: Relationship between the oxygen affinity and *in vitro* sickling propensity of carbamylated erythrocytes. Biochem. Biophys. Res. Commun. 46:1255, 1972.
253. Benesch, R. E., Yung, S., Suzuki, T., Bauer, C., and Benesch, R.: Pyridoxal compounds as specific reagents for the α and β N termini of hemoglobin. Proc. Natl. Acad. Sci USA 70:2595, 1973.
254. Benesch, R., Benesch, R. E., and Yung, S.: Chemical modifications that inhibit gelation of sickle haemoglobin. Proc. Natl. Acad. Sci. USA 71:1504, 1974.
255. Walder, J. A., Zaugg, R. H., Walder, R. Y., Steele, J. M., and Klotz, I. M.: Diaspirins that cross-link β chains of hemoglobin: bis(3,5-dibromosalicyl) succinate and bis(3,5-dibromosalicyl) fumarate. Biochemistry 18:4265, 1979.
256. Walder, J. A., Walder, R. Y., And Arnone, A.: Development of antisickling compounds that chemically modify hemoglobin S specifically with 2,3-diphosphoglycerate binding site. J. Mol. Biol. 141:195, 1980.
257. Chatterjee, R., Walder, R. Y., Arnone, A., and Walder, J. A.: Mechanism for the increase in solubility of deoxyhemoglobin S due to cross-linking the β chains between lysine-82 $β_1$ and lysine-82 $β_2$. Biochemistry 21:5901, 1982.
258. Kark, J. A., Kale, M. P., Tarassoff, P. G., Woods, M., and Lessin, L. S.: Inhibition of erythrocyte sickling *in vitro* by pyridoxal. J. Clin. Invest. 62:888, 1978.
259. Nigen, A. M., and Manning, J. M.: Inhibition of erythrocyte sickling *in vitro* by DL-glyceraldehyde. Proc. Natl. Acad. Sci. USA 74:367, 1977.
260. Nigen, A. M., and Manning, J. M.: Effects of glyceraldehyde on the structural and functional properties of sickle erythrocytes. J. Clin. Invest. 61:11, 1978.
261. Abraham, E. C., Stallings, M., Abraham, A., and Garbutt, G. J.: Modification of sickle hemoglobin by acetaldehyde and its effect on oxygenation, gelation and sickling. Biochim. Biophys. Acta 705:76, 1982.
262. Chao, T. L., Berenfeld, M. R., and Gabuzda, T. G.: Inhibition of sickling by methyl acetimidate. FEBS Lett. 62:57, 1976.
263. Lubin, B. H., Pena, V., Mentzer, W. C., Bymun, E., Bradley, T. B., and Packer, L.: Dimethyl adipimidate: A new antisickling agent. Proc. Natl. Acad. Sci. USA 72:43, 1975.
264. Roth, E. F., Nagel, R. L., Bookchin, R. M., and Grayzel, A. I.: Nitrogen mustard: An *in vitro* inhibitor of erythrocyte sickling. Biochem. Biophys. Res. Commun. 48:612, 1972.
265. Fung, L. W.-M., Ho, C., Roth, E. F., and Nagel, R. L.: The alkylation of hemoglobin S by nitrogen mustard. J. Biol. Chem. 250:4786, 1975.
266. Charache, S., Dreyer, R., Zimmerman, I., and Hsu, C.-K.: Evaluation of extracorporeal alkylation of red cells as a potential treatment for sickle cell anemia. Blood 47:481, 1976.
267. Zak, S. J., Geller, G. R., Finkel, B., Tukey, D. P., McCormack, M. K., and Krivit, W.: Bis-(N-maleimidomethyl) ether: An antisickling reagent. Proc. Natl. Acad. Sci. USA 72:4153, 1975.
268. Hassan, W., Beuzard, Y., and Rosa, J.: Inhibition

of erythrocyte sickling by cystamine, a thiol reagent. Proc. Natl. Acad. Sci. USA 73:3288, 1976.
269. Noguchi, C. T., and Schechter, A. N.: Inhibition of sickle hemoglobin gelation by amino acids and related compounds. Biochemistry 17:5455, 1978.
270. Poillon, W. N.: Noncovalent inhibitors of sickle hemoglobin gelation: Effects of aryl-substituted alanines. Biochemistry 21:1400, 1982.
270a. Votano, J. R., Altman, J., Wilchek, M., Gorecki, M., and Rich, A.: Potential use of biaromatic l-phenylalanyl derivates as therapeutic agents in the treatment of sickle-cell disease. Proc. Natl. Acad. Sci. USA 81:3190, 1984.
271. Votano, J. R., Gorecki, M., and Rich, A.: Sickle hemoglobin aggregation: A new class of inhibitors. Science 196:1216, 1977.
272. Kubota, S., and Yang, J. T.: Oligopeptides as potential antiaggregation agents for deoxyhemoglobin S. Proc. Natl. Acad. Sci. USA 74:5431, 1977.
273. Gorecki, M., Votano, J. R., and Rich, A.: Peptide inhibitors of sickle hemoglobin aggregation: Effect of hydrophobicity. Biochemistry 19:1564, 1980.
274. Franklin, I. M., Cotter, R. I., Cheetham, R. C., Pardon, J. F., Hale, A. J., and Huehns, E. K.: A potent new dipeptide inhibitor of cell sickling and hemoglobin S. gelation. Eur. J. Biochem. 136:209, 1983.
275. Gorecki, M., Acquaye, C. T., Wilchek, M., Votano, J., and Rich, A.: Antisickling activity of amino acid benzyl esters. Proc. Natl. Acad. Sci. USA 77:181, 1980.
276. Elbaum, D., Nagel, R. L., Bookchin, R. M., and Herskovits, T. T.: Effect of alkylureas on the polymerization of hemoglobin S. Proc. Natl. Acad. Sci. USA 71:4718, 1974.
277. Elbaum, D., Roth, E. F., Neumann, G., Jaffe, E. R., Bookchin, R. M., and Nagel, R. L.: Molecular and cellular effects of antisickling concentrations of alkylureas. Blood 48:273, 1976.
278. Herskovits, T. T., and Elbaum, D.: The inhibitory effect of alkylureas and alkylamides on the gelation of hemoglobin S. Biochim. Biophys. Acta 622:36, 1980.
279. Poillon, W. N.: Noncovalent inhibitors of sickle hemoglobin gelation: Effects of aliphatic alcohols, amides and ureas. Biochemistry 19:3194, 1980.
280. Abraham, D. J., Perutz, M. F., and Phillips, S. E. V.: Physiological and x-ray studies of potential antisickling agents. Proc. Natl. Acad. Sci. USA 80:324, 1983.

SICKLE CELL DISEASE—CLINICAL AND EPIDEMIOLOGICAL ASPECTS

12

HISTORICAL BACKGROUND*

The clinical spectrum of sickle cell disease has been recognized in West Africa for several centuries. The disease was given specific vernacular names by different tribes, such as *chwechweechwe* (Ga tribe), *nwiiwii* (Faute tribe), *nuidudui* (Ewe tribe), and *ahotutuo* (Twi tribe).[2] Many generations of West Africans were familiar with the varying degrees of clinical severity and knew that the disease "ran in families." In one family from the Krobo tribe in Ghana, sickle cell disease had been traced back through nine successive generations. Because of the coexistence of malnutrition, endemic infections, and lack of medical care in West and Central Africa, SS homozygotes seldom survived beyond infancy. This led to the mistaken conclusion that the homozygous state was rare in Africa and that some type of additional genetic or environmental factor was responsible for higher prevalence of SS individuals in America.[3]

The first account of sickle cell anemia to appear in the medical literature was provided by James B. Herrick,[4] a prominent Chicago physician, who subsequently published one of the first accounts of coronary artery occlusion. In 1910, he described a 20-year-old black male from Grenada, West Indies, who was attending one of the professional schools in Chicago. The patient complained of breathlessness, palpitations, and occasional bouts of icterus. His past history included no mention of pain crises. Physical examination revealed pulmonary rales and an enlarged, forceful heart. The presence of anemia was documented, and a photomicrograph that accompanied the case report showed for the first time "thin sickle-shaped and crescent-shaped" red cells.[4] One year after this clinical evaluation, the patient was hospi-

---

*Dr. C. Lockard Conley's chapter in *Blood, Pure and Eloquent*[1] contains a detailed and enthralling narrative of the major events and personalities in the history of sickle cell disease.

talized because of malaise and back pain extending to the muscles of the extremities. In comparison to most initial descriptions of specific diseases, this one is unusually clear, complete, and prescient. Herrick ended his report with the suggestion that the cause of the disease may be "some unrecognized change in the corpuscle itself."

Following this report, additional descriptions of similar patients began to appear in the literature. The designation "sickle cell anemia" was first applied in 1922 by Verne Mason,[5] who subsequently became the personal physician of Howard Hughes and a founder of the Howard Hughes Institute for Medical Research.

The first experimental studies on sickle cells were performed by Victor Emmel,[6] an anatomist at Washington University in St. Louis. In 1915, he studied the first patient with sickle cell disease recognized at that institution. He sealed a suspension of the patient's red cells between a microscope slide and a coverslip and noted that, with time, all the red cells assumed the peculiar sickle shape. Moreover, he observed that the red cells of the patient's nonanemic father also became sickled while in this sealed chamber, even though no abnormal forms were seen when fresh blood samples were examined (Fig. 12–1). This observation was the first documentation of the inheritance of "sickling." Emmel's *in vitro* "sickle cell preparation" was used by Guthrie and Huck[7] in the first genetic study documenting the transmission of sickling through three generations. However, they and subsequent observers failed to distinguish between sickle trait and sickle cell anemia. A compilation of the literature prior to 1947 indicated that about 7.5 per cent of black Americans had "sickling" as defined by an *in vitro* preparation. The ratio of asymptomatic cases to those with anemia was estimated to be somewhere between 9:1 and 50:1. Clinicians wondered whether asymptomatic cases with "sicklemia" developed into sickle cell anemia and vice versa.

The mode of inheritance of sickle cell disease was not established until 1947 to 1949, when investigators from three widely distant parts of the world independently arrived at the same conclusion. By far the most complete and convincing proof came from James Neel,[8–10] who established simple but definitive clinical and hematological criteria for distinguishing sickle trait from sickle cell anemia. He first completed a thorough review of the literature, which provided suggestive but not conclusive evidence of the mode of inheritance.[8] He then examined 42 parents of 29 patients with sickle cell anemia and showed that they all had a positive sickle preparation.[9, 10] Moreover, he showed the presence of a positive sickle preparation in about half of the asymptomatic siblings of patients with sickle cell anemia. From these observations, Neel concluded that those with anemia were homozygous for a sickle gene, whereas their asymptomatic nonanemic parents were heterozygous. In 1947, Accioly published a family study in a Portuguese journal that clearly shows the correct inheritance pattern for sickle cell disease[11] (Fig. 12–2). Two years later, a medical officer in northeastern Rhodesia, E.A. Beet,[12] independently arrived at the same conclusion from observations on a family that included a child with sickle cell anemia and asymptomatic par-

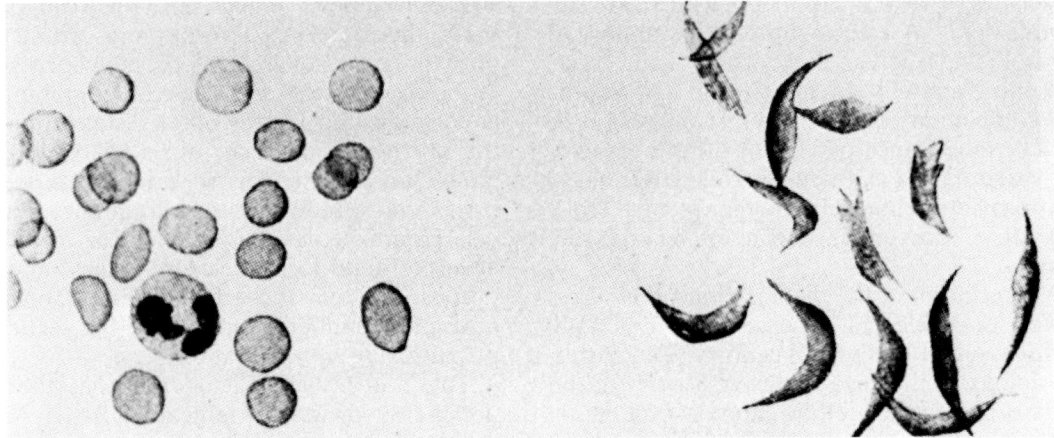

Figure 12–1. Smears prepared by V. E. Emmel on fresh blood from an individual with sickle cell trait. *Left,* Immediately after making airtight seal. *Right,* After the sealed preparation had been stored for 8 days. These experiments represent the first *in vitro* demonstration of erythrocyte sickling. (From Emmel, V. E.: Arch. Intern. Med. *20*:586, 1917.)

JESSÉ ACCIOLY

ficamos a imaginar o que aconteceria a um indivíduo filho de dois outros "sickle cell trait", e que herdasse de ambos os progenitores o gen responsável pelo estigma falciforme, isto é, que fôsse homozigoto. Daí nasceu uma hipótese que apresentámos em nota prévia em uma das sessões realizadas por ocasião da inauguração do Instituto Brasileiro para Investigação da Tuberculose, e que assim se resume:

a) — o fenômeno da falcemia decorre da existência de um gen S+, aparecido por mutação;
b) — o fenotipo falcêmico seria portanto um heterozigoto e genotipo S+S—;
c) — o indivíduo homozigoto, genotipo S+S-|- seria um fenotipo "anemia falciforme".

Daí se infere que do cruzamento de dois falcêmicos, genotipo S+S—, poder-se-ia prever que de cada quatro filhos, um teria anemia falciforme, (S+S-|-), dois seriam falcêmicos, (S+S—), e um seria normal, (S—S—), conforme o esquema:

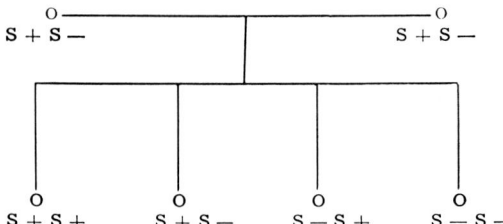

Entretanto, para que a nossa hipótese fôsse verdadeira, seria preciso que todos os portadores de anemia falciforme fôssem filhos de dois falcêmicos. Uma simples revisão bibliográfica, porém, nega de logo o seu fundamento genético, pois são inúmeros os casos em que um dos pais é falcêmico, mas o outro é normal. De outro lado, porém, êstes trabalhos não referem a técnica usada, nem quantos "tests" foram feitos para a pesquisa da falcemia.

Figure 12–2. First published account of the mode of inheritance of sickle cell disease by Jesse Accioly. Facsimile of page 172 of Arquivos da Faculdade de Medicina da Universidade Federal da Bahia, Vol. 2, 1947. (Cited by Azevedo, E.: Am. J. Hum. Genet. *25*:457, 1973.)

ents who had positive sickle preparations. The conclusions drawn from these studies of families received dramatic and compelling confirmation by the discovery of Pauling, Itano, and colleagues in 1949 that patients with sickle cell anemia had an electrophoretically abnormal hemoglobin, whereas those with "sickle trait" had equal amounts of the normal and abnormal components (see Chapter 11 and Fig. 11–1). The inheritance pattern of other hemoglobin variants was clarified by Helen Ranney,[13] who provided convincing evidence that Hb S and Hb C are either allelic or very closely linked.

Appreciation of the diverse clinical manifestations of sickle cell disease grew gradually during the first half of this century. The pathophysiology of the vaso-occlusive aspects of the disease became a lifelong interest of Lemuel Diggs, a pathologist who was a student of John Huck at Johns Hopkins and of George Whipple at Rochester. During his long tenure as Director of Clinical Pathology at the University of Tennessee, he compiled careful clinical and hematological profiles on large numbers of patients. Diggs was able to distinguish sickle cell anemia from sickle trait. He was the first pathologist to collate postmortem findings on patients with sickle cell anemia.[14] This information provided new insights into the vaso-occlusive manifestations of the disease and the ubiquity of tissue involvement. As suggested by the passage that follows, Diggs developed an intuitive grasp of the dynamics of this process.

A possible explanation of the capillary engorgement is that the elongated and spiked cells interlock and pass with more difficulty through narrow spaces than do normal cells. . . . Experimental confirmation of this tendency to mat together is found in the test tube, where difficulty of resuspension of centrifugalized blood is encountered. . . . Since the distortion is increased under conditions of anoxemia, it is reasonable to assume that it will be greatest in tissue where there is stasis. . . . The sudden pains experienced by patients with sickle cell anemia, which often disappear as mysteriously as they come, may in part be explained by this capillary blockade.[14]

This pathogenetic sequence was established by subsequent incubation experiments of Castle and colleagues, discussed in Chapter 11.

EPIDEMIOLOGY OF THE SICKLE GENE

The geographical distribution of the β^S gene is shown in Figure 12–3. The gene is most concentrated in two areas of West Central Africa; one encompasses what is now Nigeria and Ghana, and the other Gabon and Zaire. In these locales, the gene frequency can exceed 0.14. Therefore, AS heterozygotes would compose over one quarter of the newborn population. In addition, the sickle hemoglobin gene is concentrated in two other distant areas. In the northeastern corner of Saudi Arabia (the Shia Oasis) as well as in a localized area of East Central India, the gene frequency is about 0.1. Homozygotes from Africa (or of African ancestry) tend to have severe clinical manifestations, whereas those from Arabia and India have much milder disease. (See the section on prognosis at end of chapter.)

There is historical evidence that the high prevalence of the sickle gene in Saudi Arabia and India may have arisen from migrations out of East Africa.[15] Transport of slaves from East Africa to the Persian Gulf flourished from 200

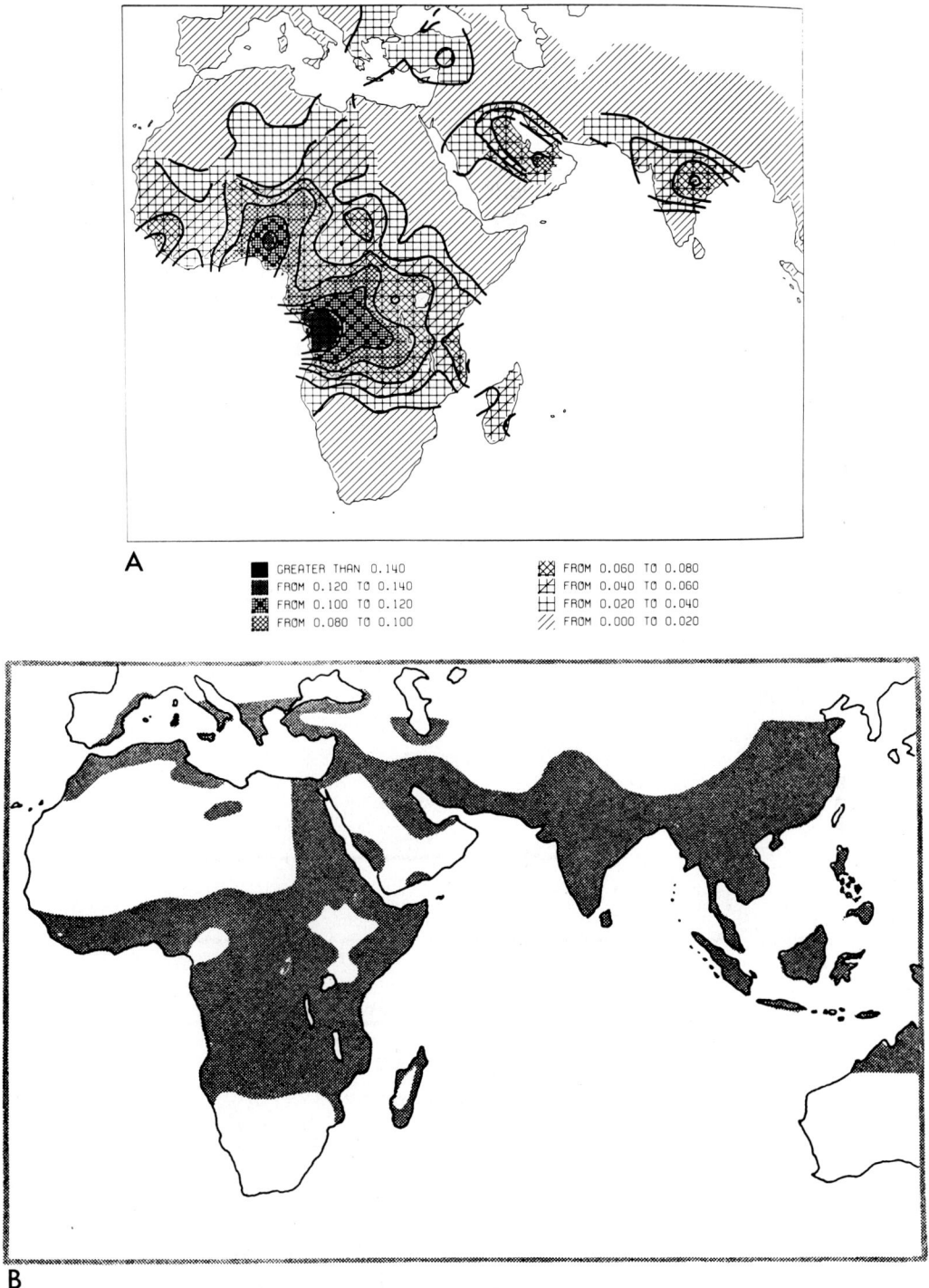

Figure 12–3. *A,* Distribution of hemoglobin S gene in the Old World. This computer-generated map shows the frequency of the β^s gene as indicated by the key. (Data from compilation of F. B. Livingstone, courtesy of D. E. Schreiber, IBM Research Labooratory, San Jose. From Bodmer, W. F., and Cavalli-Sforza, L. L.: Genetics, Evolution and Man. San Francisco, W. H. Freeman, 1976.) *B,* Distribution of falciparum malaria in the Old World approximately 150 years ago. (From Boyd, M. F. (ed.): Malariology. Philadelphia, W. B. Saunders Company, 1949.)

to 1500 A.D. In the year 1051, the Persian writer Naser-i-Khusraw commented, "When I was in Lahsa, these princes possessed 30,000 Negro Abyssinian slaves, purchased with money, which were employed in agriculture and gardening."[15] Likewise, there was active transport of East African slaves to India until the nineteenth century.

The distribution of the β^S gene in the New World is based entirely on emigration from West Africa. The gene frequency among American blacks is about 0.04 (see Table 10–11). A similar frequency has been encountered among blacks in areas of Central and South America, where there was active slave trade.[16]

Recent investigations of globin gene structure have provided further insight into the origins and migration of the β^S gene. Restriction endonuclease maps that employ Hpa I revealed a polymorphism that is closely linked with the β^S mutation.[17] Nearly all Caucasians and 97 per cent of blacks with a Hb AA phenotype have a 7.6 kilobase (kb) or, less commonly, a 7.0 kb Hpa I fragment that encompasses the entire β globin gene. Only 3 per cent have a 13 kb fragment. In contrast, among American blacks who have Hb S, nearly 70 per cent have the 13 kb fragment. As mentioned at the end of this chapter, this linkage disequilibrium has been exploited for the antenatal diagnosis of sickle cell anemia (SS disease). Among blacks with Hb C (β 6 Glu→Lys), virtually all have the 13 kb fragment. It is likely that β^S and β^C mutations both arose on a β gene carrying the 13 kb mutation (Fig. 12–4) and that the 13 kb mutation arose in a small geographical area corresponding to what is now Upper Volta and Ghana.[18, 19] Although the β^S gene has widespread geographical distribution, it is highly concentrated in this area (Fig. 12–3), and the β^C gene is localized to this area (see Fig. 10–12). Because the β^S and β^C genes protected against malaria (see below), the frequency of these genes increased and, along with it, the linked 13 kb mutation. This is an example of "genetic hitch-hiking."[18] In contrast, the incidence of the ancestor 13 kb β^A gene remained low because it lacks any selective advantage. The association of β^S with the 13 kb fragment has also been noted in North Africans[20] and Sicilians,[18] providing strong evidence that the β^S gene in these individuals originated in the Ghana-Nigeria region and spread northward.

In Central and East Africa as well as in Saudi Arabia and India, the β^S gene is associated with the wild-type 7.6 kb fragment.[18] As shown in Figure 12–4, the best explanation for

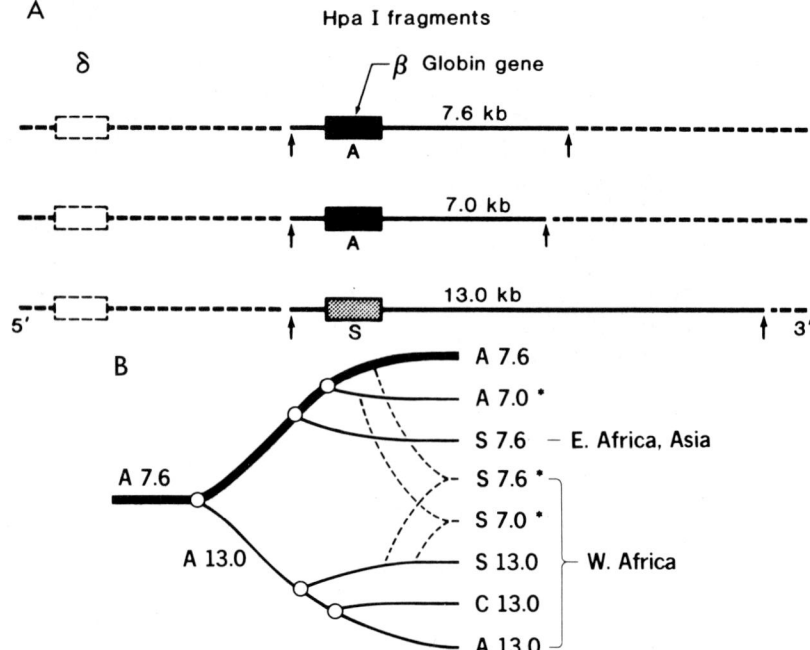

Figure 12–4. *A*, Polymorphism of the human β globin gene as recognized by the restriction endonuclease Hpa I. In West Africans, the sickle gene is strongly associated with the 13 kb DNA fragment. *B*, Evolution of the Hpa I polymorphism and the β globin genes. The letters A, S, and C represent the β globin genotypes, and the numbers indicate the lengths of the Hpa I fragments in kilobases. No time scale is implied in this diagram. The divergence of the S gene before the C gene indicated in this diagram is arbitrary. (Asterisks denote where the precise mode of evolution is not certain. ——— = normal; ——— = variants; ------ = recombinants.) (From Kan, Y. W., and Dozy, A. M.: Science 209:388, 1980.)

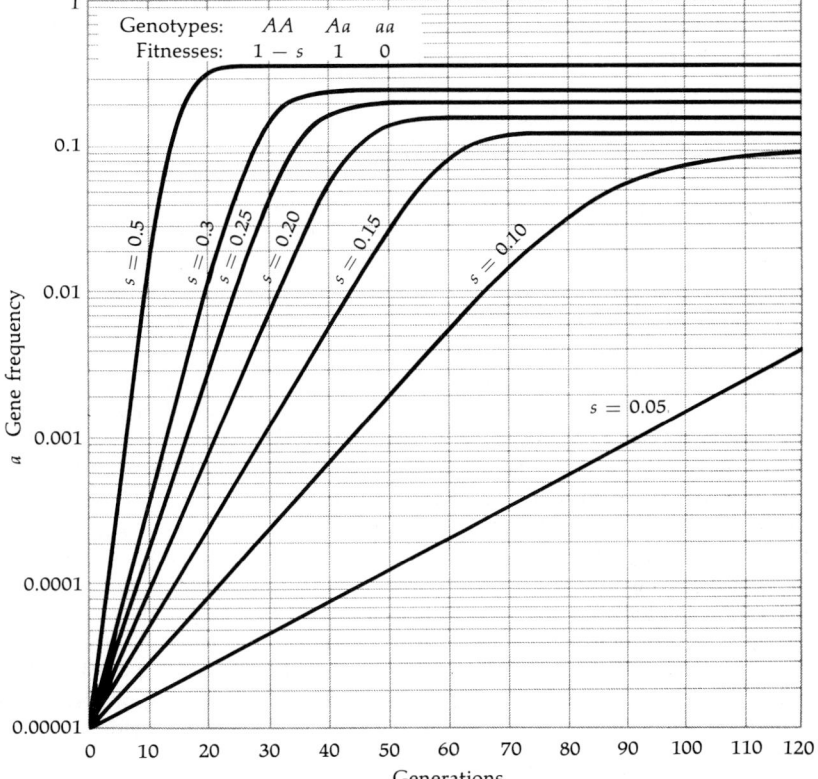

Figure 12–5. Theoretical plot of the change in gene frequency in a population over a prolonged time period for a gene that confers improved fitness (s) in the heterozygote (Aa) but is lethal in the homozygote (aa). Note that the gene frequency is on a log scale. (From Bodmer, W. F., and Cavalli-Sforza, L. L.: Genetics, Evolution and Man. San Francisco, W. H. Freeman, 1976.)

these findings is that the β^S gene in these areas arose independently from that in West Africa. In view of the slave trade, which was mentioned earlier, the β^S gene in the latter areas could have arisen from a single mutation occurring in East Africa. However, the marked differences in blood groups and other genetic markers among these people suggest that separate and independent β^S mutations may have occurred in each of these areas. In fact, a recent survey of restriction-site polymorphisms in various populations of Africa suggests multiple independent β^S mutations.[20a, 20b]

Hb S and Malaria. As shown in Figure 12–3, the distribution of the Hb S gene in the Old World corresponds closely to that of falciparum malaria. In 1949, J.B.S. Haldane[21] (see Fig. 1–7) first suggested that individuals with various red cell disorders might be protected against fatal malaria infections. Subsequent epidemiological evidence indicated that sickle hemoglobin heterozygotes (AS) were protected against *Plasmodium falciparum,* the organism causing the most severe form of human malaria.[22] A recent field survey in Nigeria demonstrated a prevalence of AS of 24 per cent in newborns compared with 29 per cent in those over the age of 5 years.[23] From these data, it appears that the presence of sickle trait confers a relative improved fitness of 0.20 compared with normal AA individuals. In a stable population, a gene providing improved fitness of the heterozygous state and lethality in the homozygous state should reach an equilibrium.[24] Figure 12–5 shows theoretical plots for the time required for the mutation to reach equilibrium as well as the gene frequency at equilibrium. In the aforementioned Nigerian population, the improved fitness of 0.20 is calculated to give a gene frequency of about 0.15, a value very close to the measured gene frequency. Moreover, if a β^S mutation should occur in this environment, about 50 generations (or 1000 years) would be required to reach equilibrium.

The protection of sickle trait against falciparum malaria applies almost entirely to infants.[24, 25] Infants with sickle trait become infected with *P. falciparum,* but their infections occur less frequently and are milder than those in AA infants.[22, 25] In an endemic area, AS individuals 30 to 60 weeks of age were noted to have a lower frequency of trophozoites in their circulating red cells as well as a considerable reduction in parasite density compared with AA infants.[23] This difference was not observed in older children. It is likely that the acquisition of immunity to the parasite blunts differences in susceptibility between older AS and AA individuals.

Even though there is conclusive evidence that AS individuals are partially protected against falciparum malaria, the cellular mechanisms underlying this phenomenon are not at all clear. Luzzato and associates[26] showed that during anaerobic incubations AS cells containing *P. falciparum* parasites sickled more readily than nonparasitized red cells. This observation suggested that *in vivo* sickling might provide a means for rapid clearance of parasitized red cells and subsequent destruction in the reticuloendothelial system.

The recent development of continuous culture systems for *P. falciparum*[27] has permitted more detailed studies on how sickle hemoglobin affects resistance to malaria. When the parasites are grown at ambient oxygen tension, their growth in AS and SS red cells is the same as that in AA red cells.[28, 29] However, when the oxygen tension is reduced (1 to 5 per cent), the invasion by parasites[29] and their growth[28, 29] are markedly inhibited in AS and SS red cells (Fig. 12–6). When subjected to low oxygen tension, AS cells containing small parasites (ring forms) sickled more rapidly than nonparasitized red cells.[30] Those containing large parasites (trophozoites and schizonts) did not show increased sickling but were found to contain intracellular polymers of hemoglobin. The enhanced sickling of parasitized red cells appears to be due in part to decreased intracellular pH (about 0.4 units below that of unaffected cells).[31] As explained in Chapter 11, decreased pH favors polymerization of Hb S by reduction of oxygen affinity (the Bohr effect). The death of the parasites in deoxygenated AS red cells appears to be due to reduction of intracellular potassium that accompanies Hb S polymerization[31] (see Chapter 11). In addition, aggregates of deoxyhemoglobin S may disrupt the parasite membrane.[32]

In summary, there is convincing epidemiological and experimental evidence that infants with sickle cell trait are endowed with partial protection against falciparum malaria.

SICKLE CELL TRAIT

Clinical Features

There is a large cumulative body of information on the natural history of sickle cell trait. AS individuals have entirely normal growth and development.[33] There is no increased morbidity or mortality of pregnant women with sickle cell trait, and their offspring have normal weight and viability.[34] Moreover, AS individuals have normal exercise tolerance,[35, 36] even though a small percentage of sickled cells (< 0.5 per cent) can be detected in the peripheral blood after vigorous exercise.[37] The fact that the prevalence of Hb AS in black professional football players is the same as that in the black population in the United States[38] attests to the benign nature of sickle cell trait.

When the Veterans Administration com-

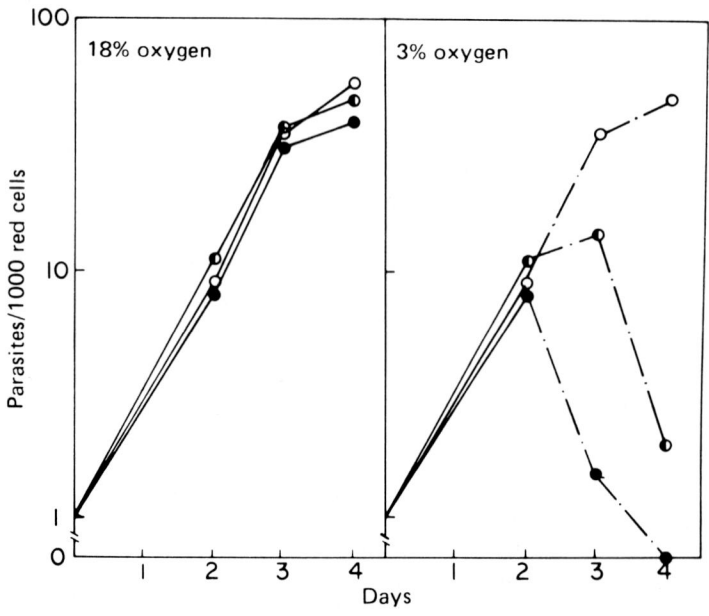

Figure 12–6. Growth of *Plasmodium falciparum* in Hb S–containing erythrocytes. Cultures were grown under an atmosphere of 18% O_2/3% CO_2 for 2 days and then either maintained in this gas mixture *(left)* or shifted to 3% O_2/3% CO_2 *(right)*. (○ = AA red cells; ◐ = SA red cells; ● = SS red cells.) (From Friedman, M. J.: Proc. Natl. Acad. Sci. USA 75:1994, 1978.)

pleted a cooperative study of 65,154 hospitalized black male patients,[39] there was no age-dependent difference in the frequency of sickle cell trait and sickle cell trait had no effect on the average age at hospitalization or age at death. Thus, the overall mortality of AS individuals was indistinguishable from that of normal individuals. This conclusion was confirmed in a cohort study of 574 AS individuals.[40] In the cooperative study of veterans,[37] there were no differences in the frequencies of specific illnesses, except pulmonary embolism and hematuria (see below). The absence of significant morbidity was confirmed in a comprehensive health survey of 600 Navy enlistees with sickle cell trait.[41]

Despite the benign nature of sickle cell trait, a number of associated clinical abnormalities have been reported (Table 12–1).[42, 43] Most of these reports are anecdotal, and therefore, the association with sickle cell trait may be coincidental. Very few studies include a fair comparison between AS and AA individuals at risk.

In the Veterans Administration cooperative study cited earlier, unexplained hematuria was noted among 2.5 per cent of AS individuals compared with 1.3 per cent of AA individuals. Because the difference is so small, hematuria should not be attributed to sickle cell trait unless other causes have been ruled out. The presence of sickle cell trait may lower the threshold for hematuria in individuals with bleeding disorders such as von Willebrand's disease.[44] In the few patients with totally unexplained painless hematuria (including rare white individuals[45]), sickle cell trait may be responsible. The hematuria probably reflects small medullary infarcts. The renal medulla in AS individuals has diminished vasa recta.[46] The ability to make concentrated urine is impaired,[47] but acidification of urine is normal.[48]

The Veterans Administration study also found a higher frequency of pulmonary embolism among AS patients (2.2 per cent) compared with AA patients (1.5 per cent). Again, this difference is small, so that the pathogenetic role of sickling is uncertain. As with hematuria, the coexistence of two risk factors may lead to increased morbidity. For example, women with sickle cell trait who are taking oral contraceptives may be at slightly increased risk of developing pulmonary emboli.[49]

If general anesthesia is properly administered, AS individuals are not subject to any added risk.[50] Surgeons may be concerned about the application of a tourniquet to an injured extremity because of sickling induced by prolonged stasis.[51, 51a] However, AS individuals usually tolerate this procedure very well.[52, 52b]

The incidence of bone and joint disease in those with sickle cell trait is not higher than that in normal individuals.[53] However, the coexistence of sickle cell trait and erythrocytosis may increase the risk of developing avascular necrosis of bone.[54]

Individuals with sickle cell trait occasionally develop vaso-occlusive complications during periods of hypoxia. A few patients have sustained splenic infarction when flying at high altitude in unpressurized aircraft. According to *in vitro* measurements, AS red cells begin to sickle when the oxygen pressure falls below 10 to 15 mm Hg, corresponding to an altitude of 21,500 to 23,500 feet. Some U.S. Air Force cargo transport missions demand flight in unpressurized cabins at altitudes of up to 10,000 feet.[55] At higher altitudes, pressurized cabins are mandatory.* Cabin or cockpit decompression occurs about 60 times a year during peace time. Among such mishaps that have occurred recently in USAF aircraft, nearly half were at less than 15,000 feet[55] and therefore should pose no threat to the individual with sickle cell trait. When decompression occurs at very high altitude, both AA and AS individuals are at immediate risk of severe hypoxia. Thus, there will be very few instances when someone with sickle cell trait will be at a significantly greater risk than one with normal hemoglobin.

Table 12–1. ABNORMALITIES REPORTED WITH SICKLE CELL TRAIT*

I. Association with Sickle Cell Trait Very Likely
   Splenic infarction at high altitude
   Hyposthenuria
   Hematuria
   Bacteriuria and pyelonephritis in pregnancy

II. Association with Sickle Cell Trait Possible
   Pulmonary embolism
   Complications induced by prolonged use of tourniquet
   Renal papillary necrosis
   Proliferative retinopathy
   Avascular necrosis of bone
   Intravascular sickling with strenuous exertion (especially in untrained subjects)

*Modified from Sears, D. A.: Am. J. Med. *64*:1021, 1978 and Johnson, L. N.: J. Natl. Med. Assoc. *74*:751, 1982.

---

*Even pressurized cabins in commercial airplanes flying at high altitudes (40,000 feet) have a relatively low cabin PO_2 (120 mm Hg), corresponding to an alveolar PO_2 of 66 mm Hg (normal = 107 mm Hg).[58]

The armed services as well as commercial airlines have an abiding interest in this problem. No consistent position has emerged thus far. In 1979, five cadets with sickle cell trait were expelled from the Air Force Academy on the grounds that rigorous training might endanger their health. Two years later, the Department of Defense lifted occupational bans, including flight service, for all those having less than 41 per cent Hb S. However, the individual military services have not fully complied with this ruling. Commercial airlines have adopted a middle ground. Many will hire AS individuals for all types of flight duty except pilot and co-pilot. In summary, AS individuals are exposed to very little added risk by flying in commercial or military aircraft.[56–57a] In general, they should not be given a special liability status. Certainly, there is no justification for denial of employment[57] or life insurance to individuals with sickle cell trait on the grounds of increased morbidity or mortality.

Diagnosis

Individuals with sickle cell trait have normal blood counts. Red cell morphology is usually normal, although some AS individuals have occasional target cells. The diagnosis of sickle cell trait is established by the combination of a positive test for sickling (such as the metabisulfite slide test or solubility test [Sickledex]) and a characteristic pattern on hemoglobin electrophoresis. If performed properly, the metabisulfite test is highly reliable, but because it requires a microscope and a skilled observer it is not suitable for large-scale screening or field studies. When deoxygenated, red cells from AS individuals who have severe iron deficiency may fail to sickle, owing to decreased intracellular hemoglobin concentration.[58a] Several solubility tests are commercially available in kit form. They are easy to perform and quite reliable, but occasional false-positive results have been noted in individuals with unstable hemoglobins.[59] A false-negative test may be encountered in AS individuals who also have homozygous α thalassemia-2 ($-\alpha/-\alpha$).[59a] Hemoglobin electrophoresis usually reveals about 60 per cent Hb A, 40 per cent Hb S, and slightly elevated Hb A_2. As discussed in detail in Chapter 10, the proportion of Hb S in AS individuals is decreased in the presence of α thalassemia. Heterozygotes who have one α gene deleted ($-\alpha/\alpha\alpha$) have about 35 per cent Hb S, whereas homozygotes who have two gene deletions ($-\alpha/-\alpha$) have about 30 per cent Hb S. The proportion of Hb S in AS individuals may also be diminished in the presence of folic acid deficiency and iron deficiency (see Chapter 10). In contrast, AS individuals with the $\alpha\alpha\alpha/\alpha\alpha$ genotype have a slightly higher level of Hb S than those with the normal $\alpha\alpha/\alpha\alpha$ genotype.[59b]

Screening Programs

The advisability of screening programs is a controversial issue. Certainly, the appropriate tests should be available to all individuals who want to know if they or their children have a sickling disorder. Occasionally, screening clinics detect individuals with clinically significant disorders such as SS, SC, or S/β thalassemia.

A person derives no obvious benefit from the knowledge that he has sickle cell trait unless he is engaged in one of the few occupations that may confer increased risk. Establishing the diagnosis of sickle cell trait may be useful to some individuals who are planning families. If screening programs are employed, it is very important that confidentiality be preserved and that affected individuals have the benefit of adequate education and counseling.[60] Such services are now being provided in a number of Sickle Centers as well as in large hospitals throughout the United States.

SICKLE CELL DISEASE*

The term sickle cell disease usually refers to the homozygous state (SS or sickle cell anemia) but may also include other doubly heterozygous states in which the presence of Hb S causes significant morbidity. Sickle/β thalassemia and sickle C (SC) disease are discussed in detail at the end of this chapter. In addition, patients may be doubly heterozygous for Hb S and another β-chain variant that readily copolymerizes with Hb S, such as Hb D-Los Angeles or Hb O-Arab. In all these doubly heterozygous conditions, patients have hemolytic anemia and vaso-occlusive episodes similar to those encountered in homozygous SS disease.

---

*For additional information on the clinical manifestations of sickle cell disease, the reader should consult the monograph by G.R. Serjeant entitled *The Clinical Features of Sickle Cell Disease*[61] and the collaborative study of the natural history of sickle cell disease sponsored by the National Institutes of Health.[62]

The manifestations of sickle cell disease can be grouped in four major categories:
1. Chronic hemolytic anemia.
2. Systemic manifestations, including impairment of growth and development, and increased susceptibility to infections.
3. Vaso-occlusive or painful "crises" of varying severity and frequency, affecting different parts of the body. The pain is attributed to the occlusion of small vessels by cells containing polymerized Hb S.
4. Organ damage that is the consequence of multiple vaso-occlusive events and of chronic anemia. Organ damage is cumulative to some extent, and adults with severe sickle cell anemia may have impairment of a number of different organ systems: cardiac, pulmonary, renal, skeletal, cerebral, and hepatic damage may be present.

Anemia of Sickle Cell Disease

The anemia of sickle cell disease is due to accelerated red cell destruction. Average red cell survival in SS disease is about 15 per cent that of normal.[63] Because of marked heterogeneity, the survival of individual SS red cells varies considerably. Destruction appears to be random rather than secondary to red cell senescence. The extent of hemolysis and therefore the severity of anemia in various sickling disorders correlate very well with a calculation of intracellular polymerization of sickle hemoglobin, based on the concentration of hemoglobin inside red cells and the relative amounts of Hb S and other hemoglobins.[64] Because the presence of irreversibly sickled cells also reflects increased intracellular polymerization of Hb S (see Chapter 11), it is not surprising that the severity of hemolysis correlates with the number of irreversibly sickled cells.[61,65] Hemolysis is also more marked in the occasional SS patient with persistent splenomegaly.

Because the bone marrow is capable of increasing red cell production about eightfold, one might expect that it could fully compensate for the sevenfold reduction in red cell survival in SS disease. However, red cell production, as measured by iron kinetics, is generally only three to six times normal.[66,67] Therefore, these patients have severe anemia. Among 438 SS patients studied by Serjeant,[61] the mean hematocrit was 24.6 ± 3.8 (S.D.). Failure of the marrow to compensate could be due to either faulty erythropoiesis or a submaximal stimulus. There is no evidence of ineffective erythropoiesis in sickle cell disease. However, the stimulus to red cell production appears to be blunted. As explained in Chapter 5, erythropoietin-mediated control of red cell production is markedly affected by the position of the oxyhemoglobin dissociation curve. As shown in Figure 11–16, the oxygen affinity of SS red cells is markedly decreased owing to intracellular polymerization of Hb S (see Chapter 11). The relatively enhanced oxygen unloading from SS red cells provides a higher tissue PO_2 and therefore reduces the rate of erythropoietin production. Thus, it is likely that the decrease in oxygen affinity in sickle cell disease is the primary reason for the marrow's failure to fully compensate for the enhanced red cell destruction. In addition, the plasma volume appears to be expanded in SS disease more than in other hemolytic anemias with comparable hematocrits.[61] Thus, the measured hematocrit or hemoglobin level in SS patients is often lower than that expected from their actual red cell mass.

The anemia of sickle cell disease is probably a blessing in disguise. Because of the right-shifted oxygen binding curve, patients tolerate anemia surprisingly well (see Chapter 5). Moreover, the viscosity of the blood is inversely proportional to the degree of anemia. Thus, the vaso-occlusive manifestations of the disease would probably be more pronounced if the anemia were less marked.

Factors That Aggravate the Anemia. Infections, both viral and bacterial, cause suppression of erythropoiesis. When individuals with normal red cell survival become infected, their hematocrit generally remains stable. In contrast, the development of infection in patients with sickle cell disease often leads to a rapid and pronounced fall in hematocrit due to the coexistence of suppressed red cell production and continued hemolysis. This is known as an "aplastic crisis."[68] How infection causes a reduction in erythropoiesis is not well understood. There is no measurable decrement in erythroid stem cells.[69] Moreover, erythropoietin levels rise during the aplastic crisis.[70] Prospective serological studies suggest that infection with parvovirus may be responsible for a sizable portion of aplastic crises in both Jamaica[71] and the United States.[72] This agent also causes acute suppression of erythropoiesis in a variety of other kinds of hemolytic anemia.[72a] Human sera containing parvo-like virus selectively inhibit erythroid progenitor cells *in vitro*.[73]

Aplastic crises are not always caused by

infection. One SS patient developed prolonged pancytopenia as a result of widespread bone marrow infarction and necrosis.[73a]

Infants and young children with SS disease and sickle/β thalassemia sometimes develop acute splenic enlargement accompanied by pain, fever, and a rapid fall in hematocrit. The worsening of anemia can be explained by marked pooling of red cells in the rapidly enlarging spleen. This complication is known as "acute splenic sequestration." Fulminant episodes may be accompanied by cardiovascular collapse, and sometimes death. Children and adolescents with persistent splenomegaly often develop a worsening of anemia and mild thrombocytopenia owing to hypersplenism.

Glucose-6-phosphate dehydrogenase (G-6-PD) deficiency has the same incidence in SS patients as in otherwise normal blacks. SS homozygotes with coexisting G-6-PD deficiency may have an increased rate of hemolysis following infection or exposure to an oxidant drug. This constitutes the best documented mechanism for "hemolytic crisis" in sickle cell disease. Many references to "hemolytic crisis" in the older literature probably represent recovery from aplastic crises.

SS patients occasionally have superimposed immune hemolysis.[74] This association is probably greater than that dictated by chance. Although only a small minority (<5 per cent) of SS patients have a positive direct Coombs test, a surprising number (63 per cent) have increased immunoglobulin G on the surface of the red cell membrane, as detected by the sensitive complement-fixing antibody consumption test.[74a] This phenomenon is probably a sequela of the marked alteration in structure and topography of SS erythrocyte membranes (see Chapter 11) and may explain enhanced ingestion of SS red cells by macrophages, which is inhibited by the addition of IgG.[74b]

Anemia may be aggravated by nutritional deficiencies. As in other chronic hemolytic anemias, patients with sickle cell disease have an increased requirement for folic acid. Those with decreased dietary intake of folate coupled with the added demand imposed by infancy or pregnancy are very likely to become folate-deficient and may develop more severe anemia, the so-called "megaloblastic crisis." Mild folate deficiency is not uncommon among patients with SS disease,[61, 75, 75a] but deficiency sufficient to produce megaloblastic morphology is unusual.[75a]

Similarly, a sizable proportion of patients with sickle cell disease have mild iron deficiency,[61, 76–78b] whereas only a rare patient has sufficient lack of iron to cause worsening of anemia. Serum ferritin is of greater diagnostic value than bone marrow iron stores.[78c] Iron deficiency may be more severe among SS patients in India.[76] If iron deficiency is sufficient to cause microcytosis and hypochromia, the patient may be misdiagnosed as having sickle/β thalassemia.[78, 78a] The cause of iron deficiency is unclear. These patients have increased urinary iron excretion (> 1 mg/day) owing to chronic hemoglobinemia and hemosiderinuria.[79] In addition, episodes of hematuria or epistaxis may lead to further loss of iron. When SS patients become anemic from iron deficiency, they may have less hemolysis[79a] and may experience fewer pain crises,[80, 81] perhaps because the reduction of intracellular hemoglobin concentration inhibits intracellular polymerization of sickle hemoglobin.

If patients with sickle cell disease develop renal failure, their anemia worsens, owing to impaired red cell production. Erythropoietin levels fall, proportional to the decrease in creatinine clearance.[82] Many of these patients become transfusion-dependent. Some respond to androgen therapy.

Systemic Manifestations

Two features of sickle cell disease that can be considered systemic are (1) increased susceptibility to infections, particularly bacterial infections, and (2) impaired growth and development. They are much more important in homozygotes than in the doubly heterozygous states. In this section, a third systemic manifestation, abnormalities of coagulation, will also be discussed.

Susceptibility to Infection. Infection plays a dominant role in the clinical spectrum of sickle cell disease. In the United States, bacterial sepsis is the leading cause of death among children with SS disease.[83–86] In Africa, infection assumes even more importance and encompasses a much wider range of pathogens, including malarial and various other parasites.

In both America[87, 88] and Africa,[89] pneumococcal sepsis is the leading cause of life-threatening infection. *Streptococcus pneumoniae* is isolated much more frequently in young SS children with respiratory symptoms and fever[83, 90] than in adult homozygotes with the same symptoms. Children may present with coryza or cough or with unexplained fever and irritability.[88] These symptoms can progress at an alarming rate to meningitis and overwhelming septicemia and shock. Hemorrhagic necrosis of the adrenal glands (Waterhouse-Friderichsen syndrome) is commonly noted on postmortem examination.[88] Among SS children who develop meningitis, pneumococci can be isolated in about 80 per cent of cases.[91] The incidence of meningitis in SS children is 200- to 300-fold higher than in normal children.

Other prevalent bacterial pathogens include *Escherichia coli*,[89, 92] *Hemophilus influenzae*,[89, 90, 93, 94] and *Salmonella*[89, 90] and *Shigella*[89] species. In addition, SS patients may have an increased susceptibility to infection with *Mycoplasma pneumoniae*. *E. coli* is the leading cause of urinary tract infections among patients with sickle cell disease, just as it is among normal individuals. Surprisingly, in Africa, the incidence of both clinically overt infections and of asymptomatic bacteriuria is no greater in SS patients than in normal individuals.[95]

Perhaps the primary cause for the increased susceptibility to infection is generalized reticuloendothelial blockade, and impaired splenic function in particular. Beginning at the age of 9 to 12 months, a time when the spleen is regularly palpable in infants with sickle cell anemia, the phagocytic function of the spleen, as measured by uptake of isotopes, is impaired.[96] The demonstration of Howell-Jolly bodies and "pits" in circulating red cells also attests to the absence of spleen function.[97, 98] SS infants who show an early rise in pitted red cells are more likely to develop life-threatening infections.[98a] As a result of successive infarctions, the spleen slowly decreases in size and is usually not palpable in children with sickle cell anemia after the age of 7 years. Children with sickle cell anemia are prone to the same kinds of life-threatening bacterial infections as other asplenic children. SS children who undergo splenectomy do not appear to be at further risk of developing sepsis.[99] In young children, the spleen plays a major role in host defense, a role that diminishes with advancing age. In addition, decreasing incidence of infections with age may reflect immunity induced by previous infection. The incidence of repeated infection varies widely among reported series.[83, 90, 93] It is unclear whether the spleen is responsible for synthesis of proteins important in host defenses in young children. A functioning spleen may be necessary for the formation of antibodies to particulate antigens. SS children fail to develop a normal rise in antibody titer following the intravenous injection of antigen.[100]

Patients with sickle cell anemia have a moderate leukocytosis (white blood cell count = 12,300 ± 3000/µl) with 40 to 50 per cent granulocytes.[101] During crisis, the white blood cell count rises somewhat (16,400 ± 5000/µl). Following bacterial infection, a marked leukocytosis generally occurs (22,000 ± 10,000/µl), with a significant increase in band cells.[101] It is unclear whether granulocytes of SS patients function normally. Reports of impaired oxidative metabolism[102, 103] have not been confirmed in another laboratory.[104] The function of SS neutrophils appears to depend on the plasma environment. Defective microbicidal activity of SS granulocytes may be corrected when the cells are resuspended in normal plasma.[103] Moreover, serum of patients in sickle cell crises appears to retard migration of granulocytes.[105] The serum of SS patients is deficient in tuftsin,[106] a polypeptide that stimulates phagocytic activity.

There is also some controversy as to whether immune function is impaired in sickle cell disease. Levels of IgM are normal, and levels of IgG and IgA are normal or elevated.[107] However, the synthesis of antibodies is probably inhibited by functional asplenia. Circulating immune complexes are generally not elevated except in the presence of hepatic crisis.[108] Some patients with sickle cell anemia have a deficiency in opsonization of pneumococci[109-111] and salmonellae,[112] which may be due to an abnormality of the alternative (properdin) pathway of complement activation.[110] However, defective function of this pathway is documented in only 16 per cent of SS patients and in 10 per cent of splenectomized individuals.[113] Defective opsonization is not affected by pain crises.[111] Both the molecular basis and the clinical significance of these abnormalities await future investigation.

Growth and Development. Patients with sickle cell disease have significant impairment of growth and development.[114-119] No abnormalities are encountered until late infancy. In a multi-institutional study of 2064 American children with SS, SC, S/β^+ thalassemia, and S/β^0 thalassemia, all had significantly delayed growth and maturation compared with black controls.[114] SS and S/β^0 thalassemia patients showed more delay than SC and S/β^+ thalassemia patients (Fig. 12–7). The groups differed in weight more than height. By the end of adolescence, the patients with sickle cell disease nearly caught up with the controls in height but not in weight. Both boys and girls showed significant delays in sexual maturation

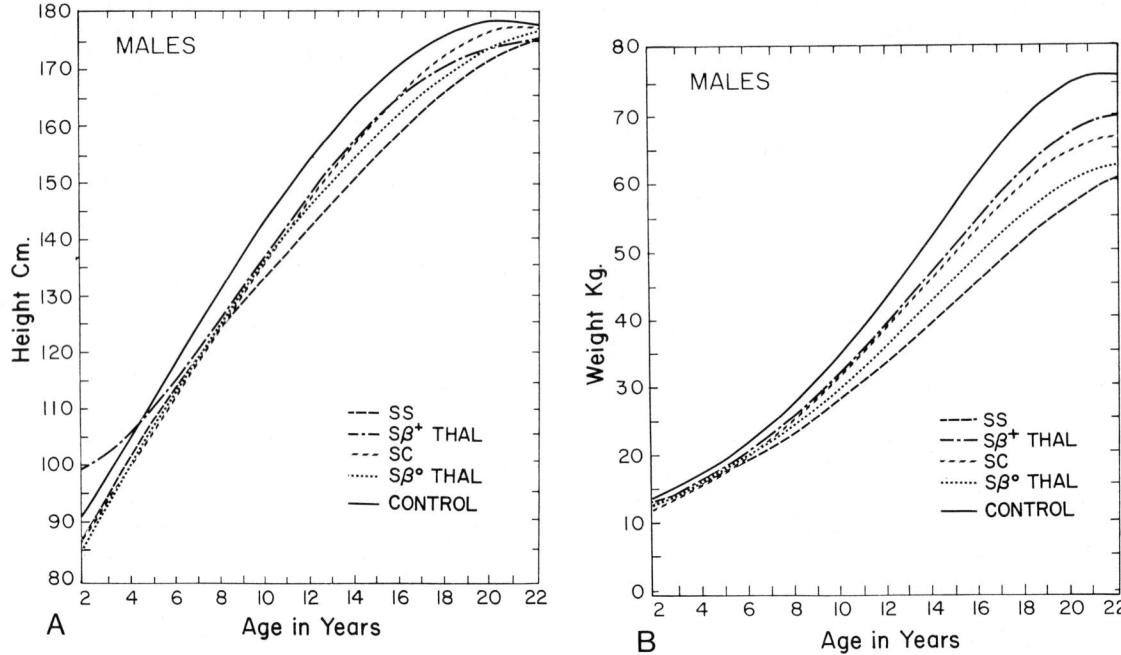

Figure 12–7. Growth of boys with various sickle cell disorders. *A*, Height in centimeters. *B*, Weight in kilograms. Control data were obtained from a study of normal black children conducted at Howard University. (From Platt, O. S., et al.: N. Engl. J. Med. *311*:7, 1984.)

(Fig. 12–8). The fact that the relationship between onset of menarche and height and weight matched that of controls suggests a constitutional rather than a primary endocrine basis for the delay in sexual maturation. Although most patients achieve full sexual maturation, some SS homozygotes have mild primary hypogonadism.[120]

Even though they have normal primary and secondary sexual development, a sizable mi-

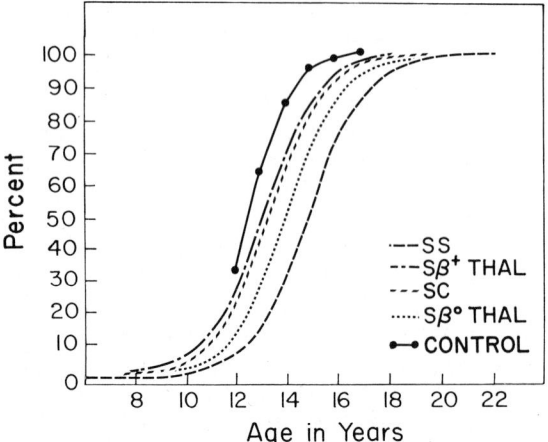

Figure 12–8. Onset of puberty of boys with various sickle cell disorders as determined by development of pubic hair. Control data were obtained from a study of normal black children conducted at Howard University. (From Platt, O. S., et al.: N. Engl. J. Med. *311*:7, 1984.)

nority of SS males are subfertile, with decreased sperm count, subnormal sperm motility, and abnormal sperm morphology.[121, 122] Fertility in females is more difficult to assess but is probably normal.[123] SS women appear to have significantly fewer pregnancies when compared with a normal population.[61] However, multiple social factors contribute to this phenomenon.

Some SS patients may be deficient in zinc,[123a, 123b] probably because of hemolysis and urinary loss of red cell carbonic anhydrase, an abundant zinc-containing enzyme. Replacement of this important trace metal has been associated with improvement in growth and development, sexual maturation, red cell morphology, and dark adaptation.[123b] A large controlled therapeutic trial is needed to assess the overall significance of zinc deficiency in sickle cell disease.

Coagulation Abnormalities. Considerable attention has been focused on the coagulation system in sickle cell disease because of its possible role in vaso-occlusive phenomena. As discussed in Chapter 11, alteration in the organization of the membrane in SS red cells may provide a source of procoagulant. Despite a large number of clinical studies, no clear pattern emerges. It is difficult to discern whether the reported abnormalities contribute to vascular obstruction or are merely epiphenomena. The platelet count is generally elevated in SS patients but may decline significantly during vaso-occlusive crises.[124, 125] Measurements with radiolabeled platelets indicate a moderate shortening of survival during crises.[126] However, platelet production does not change significantly.[127] Reports of abnormalities of platelet function during crises[128–130] have not been confirmed.[127, 130a] There are similar inconsistencies in studies of the soluble coagulation system between and during crises. Plasma fibrinogen increases during crises but no more so than in AA individuals who develop infections.[131] During crises, fibrinogen turnover appears to be enhanced,[132] accompanied by elevated levels of fibrin degradation products,[133] fibrin monomer,[134] fibrinopeptide A,[135] and β-thromboglobulin,[136] as well as complexes of fibrinogen[137] and Factor VIII.[138] Although these findings suggest intravascular coagulation, a full coagulation profile rarely documents that the process is generalized or extensive. There is no consensus as to whether fibrinolytic activity is decreased,[139, 140] normal,[124] or increased[141] during pain crises. It is likely that the complex and often inconsistent coagulation abnormalities in sickle cell disease are secondary to vaso-occlusive events, initiated by rigid red cells containing polymers of Hb S.

Sickle Cell Crises

Acute pain crises constitute the most prominent manifestation of sickle cell disease in the United States. Various forms of pain crises account for the vast majority of hospital admissions among the adult population of homozygotes and are also an important problem in children. In contrast, pain crises are a less important cause of morbidity among the Jamaican population with sickle cell disease[61] and are not considered a major problem in Africa. The reason for the differences among these populations is not obvious.

Although sickle cell crisis in young children is often associated with evident bacterial or presumed viral infections, clear evidence for infection is frequently absent in older children or adults. Overall, about one third of acute painful crises in adults are probably associated with a concurrent or preceding infection. Shortened survival of SS red cells has been noted for a few days after the appearance of fever.[142] An associated enhancement of sickling may be responsible for precipitating a vaso-occlusive crisis. Changes in plasma proteins that accompany infections, such as increased fibrinogen, may enhance the adherence of sickle cells to capillary endothelium[143, 144] (see Chapter 11), thereby presenting potential sites for obstruction in blood flow. Crises can also be precipitated by acidosis, hypoxia, and dehydration, factors that are known to potentiate intracellular polymerization (see Chapter 11).

The occurrence of pain crises appears to be sporadic. In Jamaica, the incidence of crises increases with seasonal decline in temperature,[145] but this relationship has not been observed in the central United States (e.g., Chicago).[146]

The frequency and severity of painful crises vary considerably among patients and even in a given patient. Crises may occur rather infrequently in some patients, whereas in others recurrent episodes of painful crises interfere with schooling or steady employment. In any group of sickle cell patients, a few account for most of the hospital admissions.[83] Although cerebral thrombosis carries grave implications for recurrence, particularly in children, and recurrent bone infarctions may lead to bone changes on radiographs (but minimal clinical sequelae, except in the hips and shoulders), organ damage in adult patients does not correlate very well with the observed frequency or severity of sickle crises.

The diagnosis of sickle cell crisis is often one of exclusion. As explained in detail later, acute pain crises may mimic a variety of clinical disorders. The primary dilemma often involves distinguishing a sickle cell crisis from some type of local infection. In general, there is no significant change in hematological parameters during crises. Hemoglobin, hematocrit, and reticulocyte counts remain constant. The plasma hemoglobin and serum bilirubin are unchanged during crisis.[147] Red cell survival is probably unchanged unless there is an associated infection.[143] No consistent change in irreversibly sickled cells has been noted during pain crises.[147a, 147b] There are conflicting reports on the effect of crisis on red cell density distribution.[147c, 147d] The filterability of partially[147e] and fully[147b, 147f] oxygenated red cell suspensions is significantly decreased for several days following the onset of crisis. The pathophysiologic mechanism for this phenomenon is unclear. As mentioned previously, a modest increase in white blood cell count and a fall in platelet count often accompany the pain crisis. Two serum tests may be useful in distinguishing crisis from infections: myoglobin and α-hydroxybutyrate dehydrogenase. Patients with sickle cell anemia have increased levels of the latter, but during pain crises a further increase (60 to 100 per cent) is noted.[148, 149] In contrast, the enzyme level remains unchanged during infection.

The effects of recurrent episodes of severe painful crises on the mental state of the affected patient and on the structure of the family are variable in the extreme. The sporadic and unpredictable nature of sickle crises makes it impossible for many patients to hold jobs or to make long-range plans.[150] There is a close, although ill-defined, relationship between stressful life events and sickle cell crises. Some patients are psychologically incapacitated. Many become dependent on narcotic drugs. Others with similar histories of painful crises have succeeded in attending school and have had permanent employment thereafter. That such contrasts can be observed in affected siblings reflects unknown variations in the disease and in the response of affected individuals.

Table 12–2. DIFFERENTIATION BETWEEN PNEUMONIA AND PULMONARY INFARCTION*

Common features
  Chest pain
  Cough
  Fever
  Infiltrate
  Leukocytosis
  Hypoxemia
  Pleural effusion

Features Favoring Pneumonia
  Age ≤ 5 years
  Shaking chills
  Upper lobe disease
  Bands > 1000 cells/mm^3
  ESR > 20 mm
  Sputum Gram stain ⎫
  Cultures   ⎬ Positive
  Cold agglutinins   ⎭

Features Favoring Infarction
  Associated painful bone crisis
  Clear radiograph at onset
  Lower lobe disease

*Modified from Platt, O. S.: *In* Nathan, D. G., and Oski, F. A. (eds.): Hematology of Infancy and Childhood. 2nd ed. Philadelphia, W. B. Saunders Company, 1981.

Chest Crises

The "acute chest syndrome" is one of the common manifestations of sickling vaso-occlusive crises and accounts for a large number of hospital admissions. Affected patients have sudden onset of pleural pain with fever. Although cough is common, hemoptysis is surprisingly uncommon. Radiographic findings may be absent initially, but pulmonary infiltrates usually appear. Leukocytosis is common. The obvious problem is the difficulty in distinguishing between pulmonary infection and infarction (Table 12–2).

Children less than 5 years old are more likely to have pneumonia. The susceptibility of young children with sickle cell anemia to bacterial infections, particularly pneumococcal sepsis, has been mentioned earlier. In addition, severe bouts of mycoplasmal pneumonia are frequently encountered in these patients.[151] In contrast, microbial pathogens are less frequently identified in adults with pulmonary symptoms.[152] When pneumonia is present in adults, it is usually caused by *Staphylococcus aureus* or *Hemophilus* species rather than *Pneumococcus*. Most episodes diagnosed as "pneumonia" in adults with sickle cell disease are actually pulmonary infarction.[152, 152a] Pulmonary vascular occlusion has been demonstrated in sickle cell anemia as well as in the doubly heterozygous states. Although vascular occlusion may occasionally be caused by marrow or fat emboli from infarcted bone,[152b] it is much more likely to be caused by thrombosis of sickled cells in situ.[153–155] Infection and infarction of the lung in these patients share so many clinical features (e.g., fever, leukocytosis, pleurisy with or without pleural effusion) that it may be difficult to distinguish the two pathological processes definitively. Because infection may be accompanied by microinfarctions and thrombosis may be accompanied by superimposed infection, the distinction in clinically severe examples of the chest syndrome may be somewhat academic. Upper lobe infiltrates are more likely to be infection rather than infarction. Pulmonary angiography is unlikely to be helpful in establishing the diagnosis and carries added risk because of possible induction of sickling by the hypertonic contrast media. Unusual erythrocytes called "blister cells" may be seen in peripheral blood films of patients during acute chest crises.[156, 157] The specificity and pathogenetic significance of this finding are not clear. The increased frequency of episodes of chest pain in the last trimester of pregnancy in patients with SC disease has been noted by many observers. Anticoagulation has been of no demonstrated value in the acute chest syndrome.

Musculoskeletal Crises

Musculoskeletal crises occur in all age groups. An erroneous diagnosis of acute rheumatic fever or "arthritis" is occasionally made at the time of the initial crisis. The frequency of objective findings such as swelling and tenderness appears to be higher in children.

Dactylitis (hand-foot syndrome) may be the initial manifestation of SS disease in infants. It is characterized by the rather sudden onset of painful swelling of the dorsum of the hands and feet (Fig. 12–9). Usually, at least two and frequently all four extremities are involved. Dactylitis most often occurs between 3 and 20 months of age and rarely after 48 months.[158]

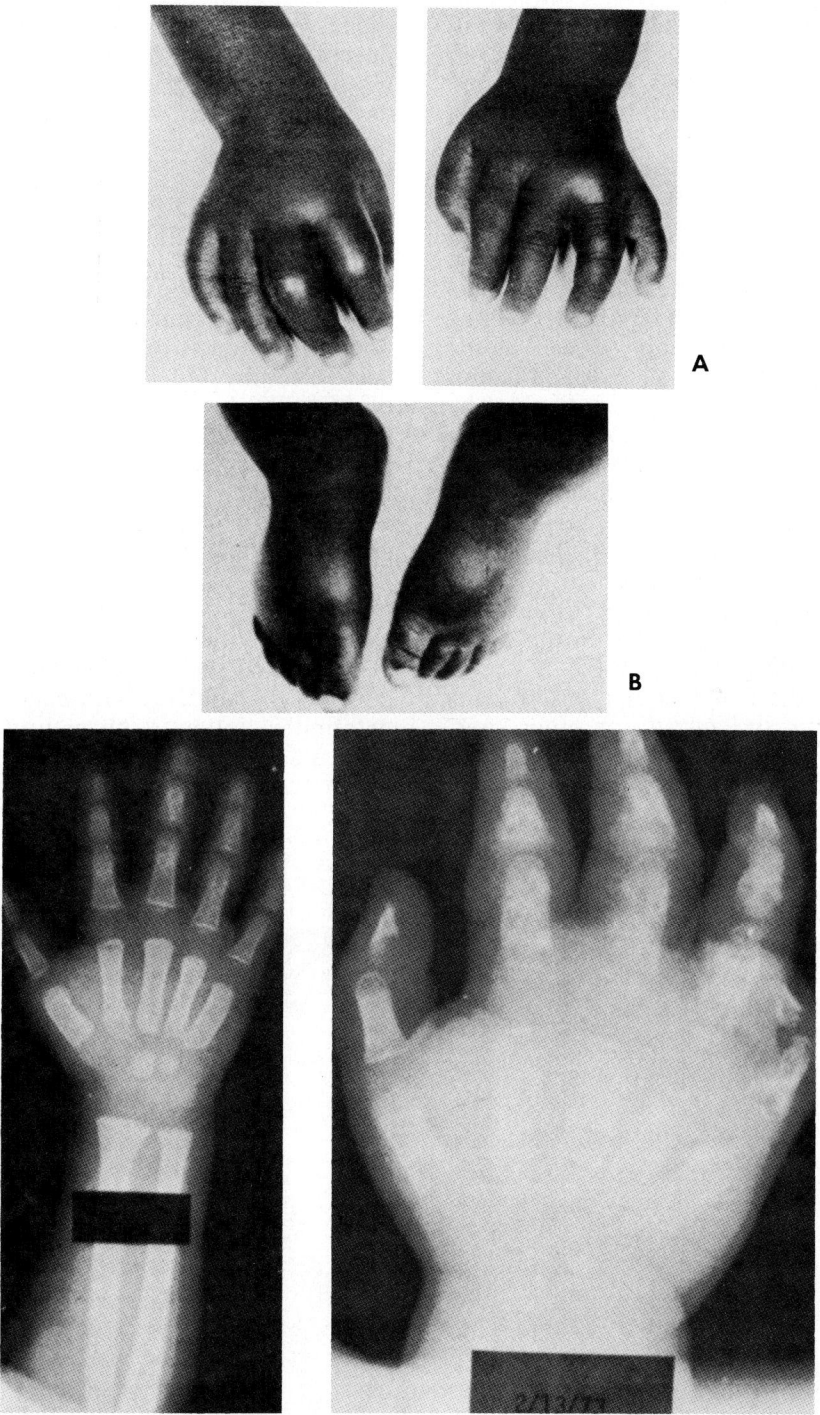

Figure 12–9. Acute dactylitis. *A* and *B,* Hands and feet of a 2-year-old child with SS disease and the "hand-foot syndrome." (From Konotey-Akulu, F. I.: Arch. Intern. Med. *133*:611, 1974.) *C,* Radiographs of a child's hand during *(left)* and 2 weeks following *(right)* an attack of dactylitis. Note the development of destructive bony lesions. (From Nathan, D. G., and Oski, F. A.: Hematology of Infancy and Childhood. Philadelphia, W. B. Saunders Company, 1981.)

Episodes are more common in the colder months of the year. A single episode usually lasts 1 or 2 weeks and may recur one or two times during the next several months or years. Patients with relatively low levels of Hb F are more likely to develop this complication. Children with dactylitis usually have fever and, as might be expected, irritability. Radiographs may show no abnormalities, but evidence of cortical thinning and marked bone destruction with healing may be seen (Fig. 12–9). Most episodes subside without sequelae, but deformity of the hand due to infarction and destruction of the carpal or metacarpal bones may rarely occur. A shortened digit secondary to infarcted bone has been reported.[159] Two factors probably account for the age predilection of dactylitis: the rapid growth of bone that has a limited blood supply as well as the rich supply of marrow in the hands and feet of young children. The occlusion of a vessel by sickled cells may not be easily compensated by a collateral blood supply in bone. The regular features of symmetrical local swelling and involvement of more than one extremity are, admittedly, not so readily explained. The growing bones appear to be a site at which sickling is particularly likely to occur once the proportion of sickle hemoglobin in the infant has greatly exceeded that of Hb F.

In older children and adults, acute bone infarctions occur sporadically at other sites. About 10 per cent of SS children will sustain one or more clinically identifiable acute bone infarctions.[160] The most commonly involved sites include the humerus (38 per cent), tibia (23 per cent), and femur (19 per cent), often the distal segment. Patients usually develop tenderness and prominent swelling over the site of infarction and sometimes limitation of joint motion as well as local warmth and erythema. Most patients have minimal fever and do not appear ill. At the onset of pain, plain radiographs are usually normal. After several days have elapsed, bone infarctions can sometimes be demonstrated by aspiration[160, 161] or by radiographs.[162, 163] Sometimes, ^{99m}Tc–sulfur colloid scans can localize bone infarction[164, 165] (Fig. 12–10) that cannot be detected by plain radiograph or ^{99m}Tc-methyldiphosphonate scans.[165, 166] In patients with fever, leukocytosis, and pain localized to a single site, acute bone infarction is difficult to distinguish from acute osteomyelitis, a much less common complication. (Table 12–3). There are conflicting reports[167–167b] about whether radionuclide imaging is of value in this diagnostic dilemma. Negative bacterial cultures and improvement within several days of supportive therapy favor acute bone infarction. Therefore, it is usually advisable to wait for a day or two rather than to undertake a long course of probably unnecessary antibiotic therapy for osteomyelitis.

Occasional musculoskeletal vaso-occlusive crises begin suddenly with pain in the back or extremities followed by pleuritic chest pain. Such a sequence of symptoms may reflect an initial bone infarct, followed by fat emboliza-

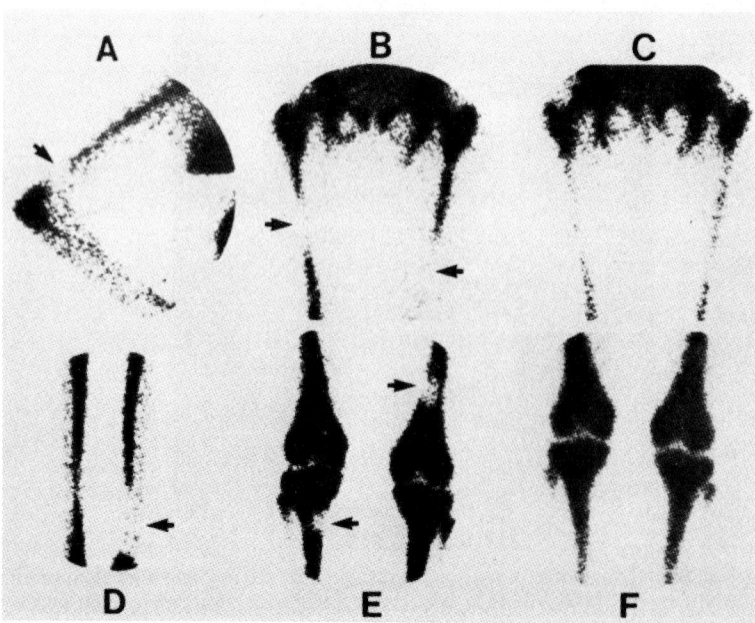

Figure 12–10. High-resolution ^{99m}Tc-sulfur colloid images of long bones to demonstrate bone marrow infarcts. *A,* Small defect in the distal right humerus, which was matched by roentgenographic evidence of bone infarction. *B,* Defects in both femora. *C,* Image in the same patient 3 months later shows resolution of marrow defects. *D,* Defect in the distal left tibia. *E,* Defects in the proximal right tibia and distal left femur. *F,* Image in the same patient 7 months later shows resolution of the marrow defects. (From Milner, P. F., and Brown, M.: Blood *60*:1411, 1982.)

Table 12-3. DIFFERENTIATION BETWEEN BONE INFARCTION AND OSTEOMYELITIS*

Common Features
   Local pain, tenderness, swelling, and erythema
   Fever
   Leukocytosis

Features Favoring Infarction
   Multiple sites
   Patient description of "crisis"
   History of predisposing factor
   Negative cultures
   Response without antibiotics

Features Favoring Osteomyelitis
   Single site
   Bands > 1000 cells/mm^3
   ESR > 20 mm
   Positive cultures
   No response without antibiotics

*Modified from Platt, O. S.: *In* Nathan, D. G., and Oski, F. A. (eds.): Hematology of Infancy and Childhood. 2nd ed. Philadelphia, W. B. Saunders Company, 1981.

tion to the lung. Fat emboli have been documented in a few patients, but it is not known how often they occur in nonfatal crises.

Sometimes, a sickle cell crisis may present as an acute monarticular or polyarticular arthritis. The elbows and knees are most often involved. The presence of signs of inflammation and joint effusion may mimic rheumatoid arthritis, gout, or acute septic arthritis.[168–169b] Examination of the joint fluid is helpful in this differential diagnosis. If the effusion is due to sickling, the synovial fluid usually reflects a noninflammatory or mildly inflammatory process. The fluid will be clear and yellow with normal viscosity. Microscopic examination reveals a low white cell count (~100 to 1000/mm^3) with a predominance of mononuclear cells and an absence of bacteria or uric acid crystals. Synovial biopsy may show sickled erythrocytes in the lumen of small vessels. Some SS patients present with an acute inflammatory arthritis. The joint fluid is an exudate and often has low levels of complement. Noninflammatory arthritis may lead to erosive bone lesions.[170] SS patients have a higher incidence of gout than normal individuals,[171, 171a] but the gouty arthritis is usually neither inflammatory nor tophaceous.[171a, 172] This complication is much less common than sickle arthropathy.

Splenic Sequestration Crises

The frequent "autosplenectomy" that results in the absence of splenic function in older children and adults with sickle cell anemia was mentioned earlier. Only about 10 per cent of adult patients with sickle cell anemia have splenomegaly. In contrast, more than half the patients with SC disease and S/β thalassemia have enlarged spleens. Splenic calcifications are sometimes visualized roentgenographically in SS patients with splenomegaly.

As discussed in the preceding section on anemia, the presence of continuing splenomegaly in young children seems to predispose to life-threatening episodes of so-called "sequestration crises."[173, 174] In such crises, the already enlarged spleen rapidly enlarges over several hours as the child becomes progressively more anemic. A child with splenic sequestration is usually admitted to the hospital with impending or actual shock, grossly enlarged spleen, and severe anemia. The sequence of events indicates that blood has collected in the spleen. Prompt transfusion and supportive measures are necessary. There is some uncertainty as to whether a single episode of acute splenic sequestration is an indication for splenectomy when the patient's condition has stabilized. A history of one episode implies an increased risk for a second. (See discussion of splenectomy in the section on treatment at the end of this chapter.) Minor episodes may also occur, in which an enlarging spleen is accompanied by increasing anemia.[174]

Abdominal Crises

When the sole manifestations of sickle cell crises are abdominal symptoms and signs, the differential diagnosis includes other causes of acute abdomen. Patients with sickle cell crises may have classic rebound tenderness. The presence of bowel sounds favors the diagnosis of sickle cell crisis rather than an acute process requiring surgical intervention. Although the white blood cell count tends to be higher in patients with surgical abdomens,[175] it cannot be relied on in making this differential diagnosis. Because of these uncertainties, SS patients have often undergone unnecessary abdominal surgery. After the age of 10 years, many patients have similar pain patterns with recurrent crises, and the perceptive patient's assessment of his or her pain is frequently helpful. The hepatobiliary manifestations of sickle cell disease are discussed later.

Neurological Crises

Occlusion of vessels in the brain by sickle cells may cause seizures or the sudden onset of neurological deficits, such as hemiplegia. Such occlusive events, although not common, occur in young individuals; dramatic improvement in the initial symptoms may be seen over the course of days or weeks, although affected children often have continuing or recurring neurological deficits. Neurological complications are discussed in more detail in a section that follows.

Sudden Death

Death of patients with sickle cell anemia is frequently sudden, occurring within minutes or hours following symptoms of crisis. The information that the patient died suddenly at home or on the way to the hospital is occasionally obtained when efforts are made to secure information about patients who have failed to keep appointments with physicians. Sometimes, the historical sequence of events suggests that the patient had an infection followed by a major vaso-occlusive event. Autopsy findings of massive occlusion of vessels by sickle cells are difficult to interpret because postmortem sickling will lead to similar findings. In many of these patients, particularly young children, pneumococcal sepsis or other infection is the most common precipitating cause of the fatal outcome.

Chronic Organ Damage in Sickle Cell Disease

Manifestations of specific organ damage appear in SS patients after mid-childhood and contribute significantly to the illness of adult patients. Many different organs may be affected; the heart, lungs, kidneys, liver, skin, bones, eyes, and central nervous system all bear the scars of the disease.

Heart*

Patients with sickle cell disease often have cardiovascular symptoms, including palpitations, dyspnea, and fatigue, along with cardiovascular signs such as cardiomegaly and cardiac murmurs. These findings are shared by most patients with chronic severe anemia. Two additional features of sickle cell disease contribute to its cardiovascular manifestations: vaso-occlusive phenomena and a marked reduction in red cell oxygen affinity.

---

*Falk and Hood[176] have recently published a detailed review of this topic.

Patients with SS disease usually have normal sinus rhythm and a normal heart rate at rest unless they are compromised by pain crises, infection, or congestive heart failure. Their blood pressure is lower than that of age- and sex-matched blacks and does not rise with advancing age.[177] The reduced blood pressure in these patients may be explained by increased sodium and water excretion (see the section on the genitourinary system that follows), which blunts the plasma volume expansion necessary for sustained hypertension.[177] A forceful apical impulse can be palpated owing to increased stroke volume and sometimes to an asthenic body build. Less commonly, the examiner will note a left parasternal heave and an impulse at the second left intercostal space, over the pulmonary artery. Moderate cardiomegaly is usually apparent on physical examination and can be verified by an increased cardiothoracic ratio on an upright chest radiograph or on an echocardiogram.[178] The heart size varies directly with the severity of anemia[61] (Fig. 12–11). Cardiac output is augmented as a result of an increase in stroke volume rather than heart rate.[179, 180] This hyperdynamic state also increases with the severity of the anemia[61] (Fig. 12–11) and represents an important compensation for the reduction in the oxygen-carrying capacity of the blood. Nearly all patients have a midsystolic ejection murmur, probably as a result of increased flow out of the left ventricle. Diastolic murmurs have been reported in a number of clinical reviews of sickle cell disease, but their hemodynamic origin or significance has not been documented. The pulmonic contribution to the second heart sound is usually prominent and will be further accentuated if pulmonary hypertension is present (see below). A third heart sound is often noted. The various murmurs encountered in these patients have sometimes led to the mistaken diagnosis of acute rheumatic fever,[181] especially in children with musculoskeletal complaints.

Noninvasive evaluation of left ventricular function in SS patients has revealed a puzzling difference between children and adults. In a thorough study of 44 children, those with significant dyspnea and fatigue tended to have reduction of the ejection fraction of the left ventricle as well as diminished contraction velocity.[178] In contrast, the asymptomatic children, who were no less anemic than those with symptoms, had normal left ventricular function. Comparable evaluations of adults have revealed normal volume and velocity of left ventricular contraction in both asymptomatic

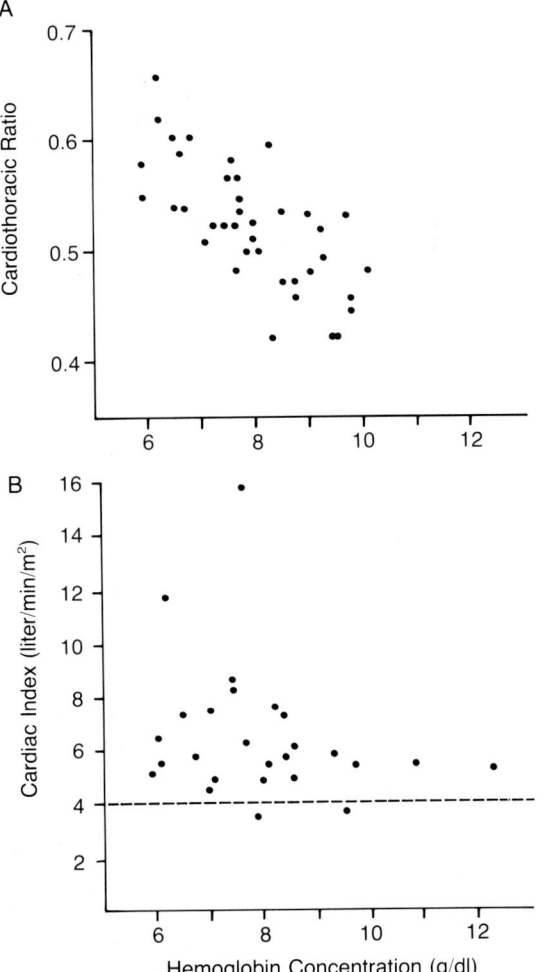

Figure 12–11. Relationship between severity of anemia in SS disease and heart size *(A)* and cardiac output *(B)*. The cardiothoracic ratios were obtained on plain chest radiographs by Serjeant.[61] The upper limit of normal is 0.5. The data on cardiac index were collected by Lindsay and associates.[180] The upper limit of normal is 4 liters/min/m².

and symptomatic patients.[182–184a] Moreover, there is no worsening of left ventricular function during crises.[185] It is unlikely that the differences between these studies can be explained by the failure of symptomatic children to survive into adulthood, because myocardial failure is an uncommon cause of death among SS children.

Even though the myocardium extracts more oxygen than any other tissue, clinically detectable vaso-occlusion (i.e., myocardial infarction) is an uncommon event in sickle cell disease. When it occurs, there is usually no evidence of coronary artery occlusion.[185a, 185b] Indeed, SS patients have considerably less coronary atherosclerosis than age-matched controls. Very few patients complain of angina pectoris. Blood from the coronary sinus contains no more sickled forms than mixed venous blood.[186] The best explanation for this apparent paradox is that blood flow through the myocardium is very rapid, especially in a hyperdynamic heart. Thus, there may be insufficient time for morphologic sickling to occur, despite the high levels of deoxyhemoglobin S in these cells. Nevertheless, the oxygenation of the myocardium may be compromised in some SS patients. When a group of SS children were evaluated during graded exercise, about half showed ischemic electrocardiographic responses.[187]

Postmortem examination fails to identify specific cardiac pathology in sickle cell disease. Moderate increases in heart weight and wall thickness have been noted.[180] Histologic sections often reveal interstitial edema, fiber hypertrophy, variable fibrosis, and occasional vacuolar degeneration, nuclear hypertrophy, and foci of nonspecific lymphocytic infiltration.[188] In a clinicopathologic study of 52 patients, no evidence was found for a specific "sickle" myocardiopathy.[189] Moreover, in another postmortem series of 53 patients, no significant increase in ischemic myocardial injury was revealed.[190] Cardiac hemosiderosis, which is so common in β thalassemia major (see Chapter 9), is seldom observed in sickle cell disease, in keeping with the fact that most patients have normal or diminished iron stores unless they have received a large number of blood transfusions.

Patients with sickle cell anemia often have significant reduction in arterial oxygen saturation.[180, 191] Two factors contribute to this abnormality: (1) arteriovenous shunting in the lungs, presumably resulting from multiple pulmonary infarctions, and (2) decreased affinity of SS red cells for oxygen. Resting arterial PO_2 generally ranges between 70 and 90 mm Hg, and oxygen saturation is usually 80 to 90 per cent. Arterial hypoxemia may contribute to the enhanced cardiac output in these patients. In some patients, sleep induces a further decrease in arterial oxygen saturation and thus could trigger a vaso-occlusive event.[192]

Despite the increased cardiac output encountered in patients with chronic anemia, pulmonary artery pressure remains normal, owing to a large reserve of cross-sectional area in the pulmonary circulation. Cardiac catheterization of patients with sickle cell anemia usually reveals normal resting pulmonary artery pressures and low pulmonary vascular resistance.[180] However, noninvasive evaluation of right ventricular function has revealed decreased ejection fraction.[184a] If SS patients sustain repeated pulmonary infarctions, pulmonary vascular resistance may increase to such an extent that the occasional patient can develop pulmonary hypertension and, eventually, cor pulmonale.[193] This complication rarely occurs before the fourth decade. It has also been reported in a number of patients with SC disease.

Lungs

As mentioned previously, the acute chest syndrome is one of the chief forms of pain crisis in sickle cell disease. In adolescents and adults, these episodes generally represent occlusion of pulmonary vessels, accompanied by local thrombosis rather than infection or pulmonary emboli.[152] Some patients are particularly prone to repeated chest crises. Over a prolonged period of time, multiple lung infarctions can lead to significant ventilation-perfusion mismatch and thus to arterial hypoxemia.[194] The calculated alveolar-arterial (A-a) PO_2 difference in these patients may exceed 20 mm Hg, a higher value than that seen in patients with comparable degrees of anemia of other cause.[191] The widened alveolar-arterial PO_2 difference apparently reflects a large contribution of intrapulmonary shunting because such gradients are observed in SS patients breathing 100 per cent oxygen.[195] Decreased oxygen diffusion does not appear to be a major factor in the etiology of the oxygen unsaturation,[196] although some impairment in gas diffusion is sometimes noted.*

Pulmonary function tests in SS patients are sometimes normal[197] but often reveal a modest reduction in vital capacity and total lung capacity.[194, 196, 198, 198a] These abnormalities do not correlate with history of past chest crises. A minority of patients also display some degree of obstructive lung disease.

Postmortem series confirm that pulmonary emboli from venous thrombi are no more common in SS patients than in an age- and sex-matched control group.[155] However, the sickle cell group is distinguished by occasional cases of bone marrow and fat emboli following marrow infarction.[152b] This complication is observed in about 15 per cent of SS patients examined post mortem and is the direct cause of death in about half of these patients.[155, 161]

---

*Reduction of diffusing capacity as measured by CO methods is generally demonstrable in anemia of any cause; the observed reduction is attributed to decreased numbers of red cells in capillaries.

In "sickle-type" pulmonary vascular occlusion, clinically apparent infarction is the exception rather than the rule. However, microatelectasis or other functional changes may occur in the absence of abnormalities apparent on chest radiograph.[194] Postmortem examination commonly demonstrates occlusion of alveolar air spaces with edema fluid and inflammatory exudate, often accompanied by alveolar wall necrosis.[155] These pathological changes probably contribute to arterial hypoxemia and help to explain the protracted clinical course associated with the acute chest syndrome.

Because intracellular polymerization of Hb S is favored by reduced oxygen tension, the development of hypoxemia is of particular concern in patients with sickle cell disease. In adults with sickle cell disease, gas exchange is frequently abnormal, even during stable periods between crises.[194] As mentioned earlier, resting arterial PO_2 is usually decreased in adult patients with sickle cell disease, although it is seldom at dangerously low levels. Because the oxygen affinity of the blood in sickle cell anemia is shifted to the right, the reduction in arterial PO_2 produces a more marked decrease in arterial blood oxygen saturation.[194, 195] To compensate for the anemia, larger volumes of oxygen per red cell must be delivered to the tissues than is the case in normal individuals. Despite these considerations, the values for pulmonary arterial oxygen saturation have been found to be higher than would be expected from systemic arterial PO_2 in SS patients, suggesting peripheral arteriovenous shunting.[195]

It is likely that the decreased arterial oxygen saturation is a significant factor in the morbidity of sickle cell disease. Hypoxemia promotes the polymerization of deoxyhemoglobin S, leading to the rigid red cells that are responsible for the vaso-occlusive manifestations of the disease.

Hepatobiliary System

Mild jaundice is commonly encountered among patients with sickle cell disease. The mean serum bilirubin is 3.1 mg/dl.[61] The chronic jaundice reflects accelerated red cell destruction. The enzyme bilirubin UDP-glucuronyl transferase, which is responsible for conjugation of bilirubin, is increased twofold in SS disease.[199] Otherwise, these patients would be even more icteric. Hepatic injury in sickle cell disease sometimes occurs as a result of transfusion-induced hepatitis. In addition, these patients may develop hepatic infarcts, which occasionally become infected, resulting in hepatic abscess.[200] If a significant portion of hepatic parenchyma becomes infarcted, fibrosis and deterioration of liver function may result.[201] Most patients with sickle cell disease have slight to moderate hepatomegaly and modest abnormalities in liver function tests.[202] Two types of hepatic crises are recognized. About 10 per cent of SS patients develop a transient form of intrahepatic obstruction, the usual "hepatic crisis." Generally, these episodes are self-limited, lasting 3 to 7 days. Acute right upper quadrant pain is accompanied by increased jaundice. However, serum bilirubin seldom exceeds 15 mg/dl, and serum glutamic-oxaloacetic transaminase remains below 300 IU/l.[203, 204] It is likely that these episodes are caused by obstruction to blood flow as red cells become deoxygenated and sickled during passage from the sinusoids to hepatic venules. Sinusoids may be further obstructed by the engorgement of Kupffer cells with sickled red cells.[204] Postmortem examination often reveals patches of necrosis and regenerating nodules. It is likely that these lesions represent prior hepatic infarcts followed by repair with fibrosis and regeneration.[204]

A considerably more serious but much rarer complication has been termed sickle cell intrahepatic cholestasis.[188, 205, 206] Patients develop sudden onset of right upper quadrant pain accompanied by progressive hepatomegaly and extreme jaundice. The highest levels of serum bilirubin recorded in any disease (100 to 300 mg/dl) are noted in these patients, resulting from a combination of complete biliary obstruction and continued hemolysis. Patients generally develop hepatic encephalopathy and shock. Of the 13 patients that have been reported to date, 11 died as a result of liver failure and/or bleeding. Postmortem examination reveals extensive obstruction of hepatosinusoids due to sickle cells accompanied by plugging of canaliculi with bile. Antemortem diagnosis by liver biopsy is generally precluded because of coagulation abnormalities. One patient recovered following exchange transfusion.[205] Intrahepatic cholestasis may be confused with choledocholithiasis and cholangitis. However, the latter are seldom encountered among patients with sickle cell disease.

Like patients with other types of congenital hemolytic anemia, patients with sickle cell disease have a high incidence of cholelithiasis.[207, 208] Surveys employing ultrasonography[209-212] or oral cholecystography[209, 210, 213] indicate that about one third of SS patients more than 10 years old have gallstones, and another 20 per cent have sludge in the gallbladder.[210-212] Considering the fact that these stones originate from calcium bilirubinate crystals, it is not surprising that in the majority of cases, the gallstones are radiopaque. The incidence of gallstones increases with age (11 to 12 per cent in young children to 40 to 50 per cent in adults).[210, 211] The presence of gallstones correlates with the level of bilirubin[211] but not with hematological values.[211, 212] African SS patients have a much lower incidence of gallstones[214] compared with American[209-212] or Jamaican[213] patients, perhaps because of differences in diet.

The clinical significance of gallstones is difficult to assess in otherwise normal individuals and even more so in patients with sickle cell disease. In patients with documented gallstones, only a small minority develop clear-cut cholecystitis. It is often very difficult to discern whether right upper quadrant pain is caused by cholecystitis rather than a sickle cell crisis. If a HIDA* radionuclide scan fails to reveal the gallbladder, the diagnosis of acute cholecystitis is favored. Because of this uncertainty, SS patients with recurrent episodes of abdominal pain and gallstones should undergo elective cholecystectomy.[215-217] This operation is quite safe if performed electively. In contrast, the operation carries significant risk if undertaken when SS patients have acute cholecystitis.[217]

Genitourinary System

The kidney is involved in virtually all individuals who inherit sickle hemoglobin. In the hypertonic, hypoxic, and acidotic environment of the renal medulla, the increased concentration of deoxyhemoglobin S in red cells leads to enhanced polymerization.[218, 219] As a result, there is obstruction to blood flow in vasa recta of the medulla and progressive infarction of medullary papillae (Fig. 12–12), leading to abnormalities in tubular function and bouts of hematuria.

Tubular Function. Several defects of renal tubular function have been identified in sickle cell disease: loss of ability to make concentrated urine (hyposthenuria) and decreased reabsorption of sodium in the distal nephron coupled with decreased secretion of hydrogen ion and potassium.

The impairment in concentrating ability occurs in all the sickle disorders, including sickle cell trait. This defect is more pronounced in

---
*6-dimethylacetanilide imino diacetic acid.

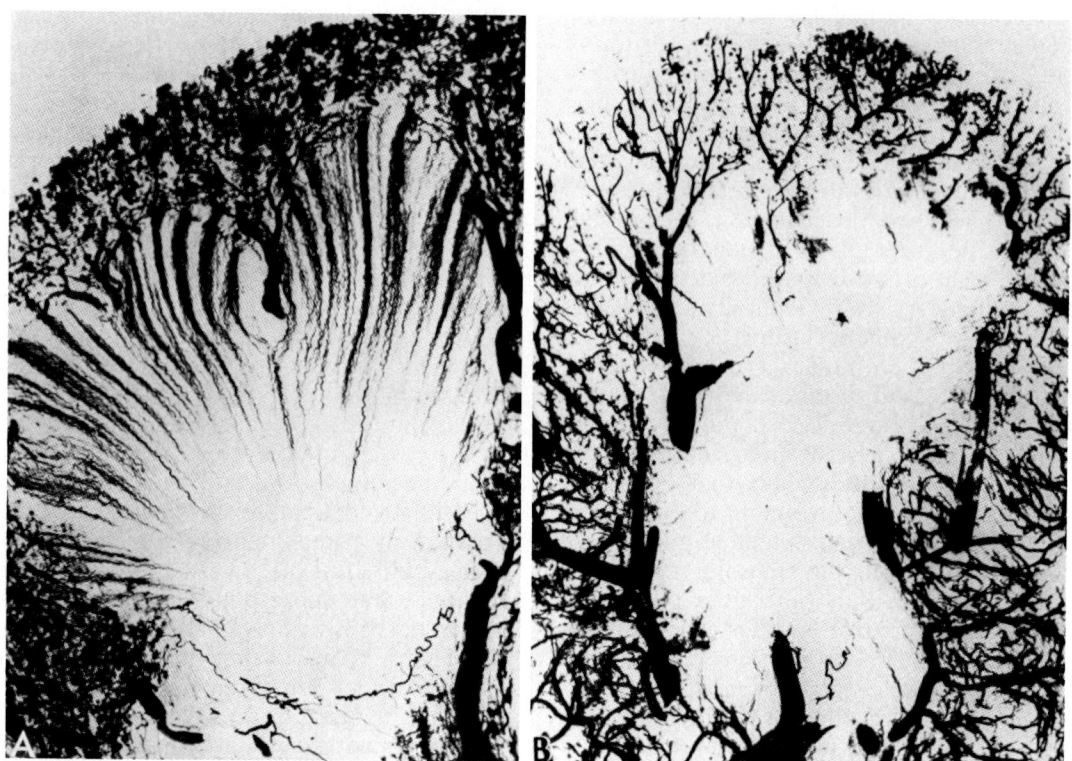

Figure 12–12. Microangiographic studies of the vasa recta in a normal individual *(A)* and a patient with sickle cell anemia *(B)*. (From Statius van Eps, L. W., et al.: Lancet *1*:450, 1970.)

sickle cell disease (SS, SC, S/β thalassemia). In children, renal concentrating ability can be restored following blood transfusions.[220, 221] However, in adult patients, the defect is irreversible. Derangement of the countercurrent distributor in the medullary circulation is responsible for the concentrating defect. Cells of the thick ascending limb of Henle in the inner and outer medulla are metabolically active and are therefore particularly sensitive to hypoxic damage.[218] Here, active sodium reabsorption is thought to be responsible for establishing an osmotic corticomedullary gradient and a hypertonic urine. In sickle cell disease, blood flow to the glomeruli is maintained (or enhanced), whereas flow to vasa recta in the medulla is reduced. Injection of kidneys at autopsy has demonstrated decreased filling of medullary vasa recta, dilated capillaries, and extravasation of contrast material from ruptured capillaries. The renal concentrating defect is unusual because tubular reabsorption of free water during osmotic diuresis appears to be normal or decreased only slightly.[222] Following papillectomy in rats, maximum tubular reabsorption of free water (as measured during osmotic diuresis) is also normal despite a marked defect in maximum urine osmolality.[223] In contrast to the universal reduction in concentrating ability, the abilty to excrete dilute urine is unimpaired. It is likely that the concentration defect is due to decreased perfusion of nephrons with long loops of Henle extending into the papillae. The normal maximum tubular reabsorption of free water reflects normal function of the shorter ascending loops of Henle in the outer medulla, which are not affected by the damage to papillae.[224]

Because patients are unable to make concentrated urine, they tend to drink large volumes of water and, therefore, may complain of polyuria and nocturia. Enuresis is a common problem among children with sickle cell disease.[61]

Patients with sickle cell disease have a mild form of distal renal tubular acidosis. They have impaired ability to acidify their urine following an acid load.[225] This phenomenon poses a potential problem because systemic acidosis may trigger a sickle cell crisis. In addition, these patients have impaired excretion of potassium following a potassium load.[226] Accordingly, some patients with sickle cell disease develop bouts of hyperkalemic hyperchloremic metabolic acidosis.[227] These defects in excretion of hydrogen ion and potassium are linked to impaired reabsorption of sodium in the distal nephron. Patients with sickle cell disease usually have normal serum electrolytes. However, during crisis or infection, they frequently develop mild hyponatremia. About one third will have serum sodium less than 135 mEq/l.[228] The hyponatremia is accompanied by a negative sodium balance. These patients compensate for renal sodium loss by maintaining increased production of renin and aldosterone.[229] As mentioned in the section on the heart, the relatively low blood pressures encountered in these patients are probably explained by increased urinary loss of sodium. Mild sodium depletion may be responsible for modest elevations in serum phosphate.[230] The distal tubular defect in SS disease also appears to be responsible for decreased secretion of uric acid that is encountered in the minority of SS patients who become hyperuricemic[231] (see below).

Hematuria. Patients with the various sickle cell disorders, including some with sickle cell trait, may have bouts of gross hematuria. Intravenous pyelography generally reveals papillary erosion (Fig. 12–13). However, this finding is of little diagnostic value because it is seen in about one quarter of SS patients in the absence of hematuria.[232] The anatomical lesion is papillary necrosis and ulceration.[14] In addition, peritubular extravasation of blood has been observed in kidneys surgically removed for hematuria. The papillary lesion, like the concentrating defect, is secondary to impaired blood supply. Although hematuria has been rather common in patients with SS and SC disease, it is distinctly uncommon in sickle cell trait when one considers the number of individuals at risk in each of the two groups. As mentioned in the section on sickle cell trait, causes of painless hematuria other than sickling should be carefully evaluated in such patients. In some patients with hematuria, blood loss continuing over many weeks may lead to iron deficiency anemia. Oral iron administration should not be overlooked in the frustration of both the physician and the patient during the prolonged hematuria. The use of diuretic agents and of water diuresis to decrease medullary hypertonicity has been recommended in the attempt to stop prolonged hematuria. Occasionally, renal bleeding has been so extensive and prolonged that nephrectomy was performed.[223, 234] However, nephrectomy has largely been abandoned because in many patients, bleeding has occurred on separate occasions from each kidney. Epsilon-aminocaproic acid (EACA) has been effective in selected patients with prolonged refractory hematuria[235–237]; however, it should be used with caution, because it may prevent the dissolution of clots in the renal pelvis or ureters. Glycopressin, a synthetic analogue of vaso-

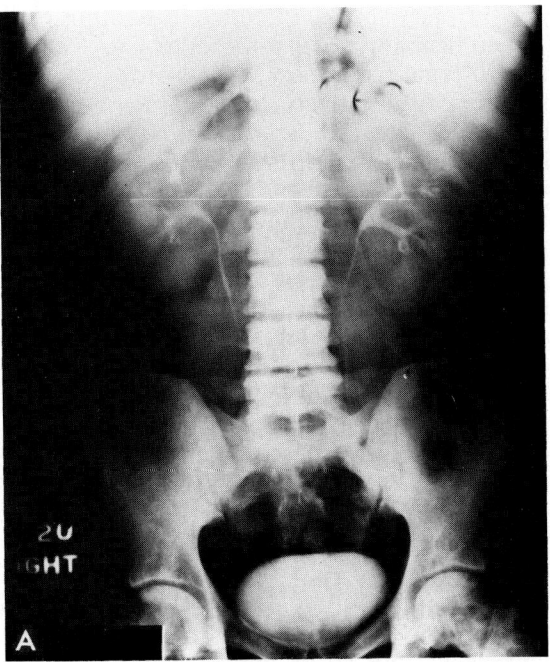

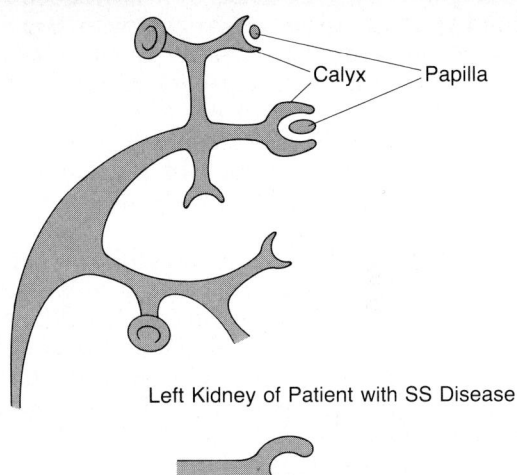

Figure 12–13. A, Intravenous pyelogram of a patient with SS disease. Note the cavity in the papilla that has filled with radiopaque dye. This cavity has been caused by sloughing of necrotic tissue from the papilla. Note also the dense vertebral bodies and the mottled density of the left femoral head. (Courtesy of the Department of Radiology, Brigham and Women's Hospital, Boston, Massachusetts.) B, Diagram of the left kidney of the patient in A and a normal calyx and papilla.

pressin, may also be effective in treating prolonged hematuria.[238] It appears to cause reduction in renal blood flow while sparing cortical function. Alternatively, local therapy has been employed. One AS patient with severe bleeding responded to irrigation of the renal pelvis with oxychlorosene.[238a]

Renal Failure and the Nephrotic Syndrome. Morphological abnormalities in the kidneys of patients with sickle cell disease extend beyond the renal medulla. The glomerular capillaries, afferent arterioles, and interlobular arteries are distended with erythrocytes, some of which appear sickled.[222] The juxtamedullary glomeruli appear particularly enlarged.[239] These glomeruli may have electron-dense material in the mesangial cytoplasm.[240] These changes are especially evident in renal sections of patients with sickle cell anemia and the nephrotic syndrome.[241, 242] The electron-dense deposits may represent some form of iron that remains from phagocytosis of red cells or hemoglobin by mesangial cells.[241] Because iron is frequently found in renal tissues in patients with hemolytic anemia (primarily in proximal tubular cells), it is difficult to attribute renal insufficiency to the presence of the metal. The glomerular lesion in SS disease may be due to an immune complex composed of renal tubular epithelial antigen and antibody directed toward that antigen.[243, 244]

Frank renal failure, sometimes following the nephrotic syndrome, occurs in a relatively small number of patients with sickle cell anemia. Among 25 Jamaican SS patients over age 40, 6 had creatinine clearances below the fifth percentile for age and sex.[245] Patients who become uremic usually develop a transfusion requirement, which is reduced if the patient undergoes chronic hemodialysis.[246] Increasing numbers of uremic patients are receiving renal transplants. A survey of renal transplant centers in the United States revealed nine SS patients who had received a kidney graft, all of whom survived.[247] The graft failed in only one patient. In another patient, the increase in erythropoiesis that followed renal transplant led to re-emergence of pain crises.[248] Patients with sickle cell anemia who have survived to the fourth and fifth decades commonly develop mild nitrogen retention. Some of the patients have elevated levels of uric acid due to impaired renal clearance as well as increased purine turnover,[231, 249] but uric acid stones are rare. It is likely that renal insufficiency of variable degree will be encountered more frequently as longer average life span leads to an older population of sickle cell patients.

Oliguria in patients with sickle cell disease need not imply renal failure. Occasionally, a painful crisis is accompanied by urinary retention in an acutely distended bladder.[250] These episodes cannot be explained on any anatomical or neurological basis. It is possible that in some cases, analgesic medication is responsible.

Priapism. Male patients with sickle cell disease occasionally develop spontaneous and painful engorgement of the penis caused by obstruction of normal venous drainage of the corpora cavernosa. This distressing symptom occurs in about 40 per cent of SS male patients[251] and accounts for about 4 per cent of hospital admissions.[252, 253] The median age of onset is 21 years.[251] Two patterns have been noted: short "stuttering" episodes lasting less than 3 hours and severe prolonged attacks lasting more than 24 hours. Rarely, attacks appear to be provoked by ethanol ingestion.[254] Repeated attacks may lead to a massively enlarged penis owing to hypertrophy of the corpora cavernosa.[253, 255] Priapism occurs with about equal frequency in prepubertal and postpubertal patients, although the latter are more difficult to treat. About 25 per cent develop impotence, particularly following a severe prolonged episode. Initial management should be conservative.[256] As with other types of sickle cell crises, the patient should be given sedation, analgesia, and adequate intravenous fluids. Packed red cell transfusion may provide additional benefit.[257, 258] Surgical intervention is indicated only when conservative measures fail.[259] If surgery is to be performed, the creation of a fistula between the glans penis and the corpora cavernosa is probably more effective than simple incision and drainage or irrigation.[259] It is uncertain whether surgery decreases[260] or increases[256] the likelihood of impotence. Patients who develop long-standing impotence may benefit from a penile prosthesis.

Central Nervous System

Stroke is the most dreaded complication of sickle cell disease. Two thirds of these strokes occur in children, with a mean age at onset of 8 years.[261] About 5 per cent of children with SS disease will sustain a cerebral infarction.[261-264] Among those affected, the great majority (85 per cent) survive, but about two thirds of these will develop a second stroke, usually within 3 years.[261, 262] Most of these strokes occur spontaneously. However, a few predisposing factors can be identified. Children who have had bacterial meningitis in the past are at higher risk of developing a stroke. Acute precipitating events include shock, worsening of anemia, infection,[263] pain crises,[263] hyperventilation,[265] and various kinds of hypoxic stress such as severe pneumonia or inadequate ventilation during surgery. The great majority of cerebral infarcts involve the large blood vessels, particularly the internal carotid artery, the circle of Willis, and the middle cerebral artery.[266–269] Pathological examination generally reveals intimal hyperplasia, leading to stenosis of the lumen and secondary obstruction with thrombus. Often, multiple vessels are involved. The role of "sickled" cells in this process is not clear. It is possible that rigid erythrocytes obstruct flow in the vasa vasorum of these large vessels, leading to a degenerative response that includes intimal hyperplasia. In regions of stenosis, adherence of sickle erythrocytes to the vascular endothelium may further reduce blood flow and potentiate stasis and thrombosis.[143] The higher incidence of cerebral infarcts among children is difficult to explain. Children have relatively higher cerebral blood flow than adults, in keeping with higher cerebral oxygen requirement. It is likely that the combination of severe anemia and vaso-occlusion leads to cerebral infarction.[262] The development of collateral vessels[267, 268] is probably responsible for the high recovery rate. Sometimes, the angiographic pattern consists of a telangiectatic network of collateral circulation, usually in the basal ganglion (called moyamoya).[267, 270] Children who develop strokes do not appear to share any distinguishing hematological or clinical features.[261, 262] They may form a subset of SS patients based on anatomical differences that put them at higher risk for developing cerebral infarction.

In adults, strokes are as likely to be caused by intracerebral hemorrhage. These patients have an immediate 50 per cent mortality rate.[262] In some cases, subarachnoid hemorrhage may be due to rupture of a thin-walled collateral vessel. In a surprising number of patients with sickle cell disease, subarachnoid hemorrhage is caused by rupture of a berry aneurysm. It is possible that some of these lesions are acquired, perhaps as a result of damage to a portion of the wall of a large cerebral artery.

Neurological findings vary considerably among SS patients who develop a stroke.[271] Hemiplegia is the most common manifestation, followed by coma, convulsion, and visual disturbances.[61, 271] Computerized tomography (CT scan) is useful in the initial diagnosis of cerebral infarct and hemorrhage. Angiography is required for identification of stenotic blood vessels and aneurysms.[268, 269] Because hypertonic radiopaque contrast agents can potentiate sickling, patients should undergo exchange transfusion and be well hydrated prior to cerebral angiography. Spontaneous recovery of brain function generally occurs within 3 to 6 months following a cerebral infarct or hemorrhage. However, many children are left with significant defects in cognitive and sensorimotor function.[261, 272] They often fail to return to school, and become invalids.

The major thrust of treatment of strokes in sickle cell disease is preventive. Because the recurrence rate is so high among children,[261, 262] in many clinics, patients have been maintained on a hypertransfusion regimen following their initial stroke. There is mounting evidence that this therapy is effective in preventing recurrences.[272–274] Unfortunately, many patients sustain another stroke shortly after the transfusions have been discontinued.[272] It is likely that the efficacy of transfusion therapy is based primarily on maintaining enhanced oxygen delivery to the brain.[262] It is possible[273–274a] but unlikely[272, 275] that chronic transfusion therapy reverses the vascular abnormalities seen in angiography. The clinician faces a difficult dilemma in the continued care of these patients. The efficacy of transfusion therapy in preventing strokes must be weighed against the cumulative risks of hepatitis, iron overload, and antigenic sensitization.

Other kinds of neurological complications are encountered in sickle cell disease. The high incidence and mortality of meningitis are discussed in a preceding section on infection. Patients may have other treatable neurological disorders, such as subdural hematoma, which must be distinguished from vaso-occlusive episodes. One well-documented case of spinal cord infarction has been reported.[276]

Bone

Skeletal abnormalities result both from infarction and from the marrow hyperplasia secondary to accelerated red cell destruction.[162] A skull radiograph reveals thickening of the calvarium and widening of the diploetic space in about 20 per cent of SS patients; the "hair on end" appearance so often encountered in thalassemia is seen in only 5 per cent.[277] The "tower skull" of chronic hemolytic anemia is occasionally seen. Gnathopathy, an overgrowth of the maxillary portion of the skull

(Fig. 12–14), occurs frequently in African patients with SS disease, but it is less commonly encountered in Americans.[278] All of these findings are caused by expansion of hyperplastic marrow.

Certain skeletal sites such as vertebral bodies and the femoral head are particularly prone to infarction. Radiographs of the spine may reveal sclerosis consequent to old infarcts as well as the characteristic biconcave deformity of the vertebrae known as H-shaped or "fishmouth" vertebrae (Fig. 12–15). This abnormality is generally encountered in older patients with sickle cell disease and is distinguished from a similar nonspecific deformity of a number of skeletal disorders by the flat "floor" or "roof" on the depressed area, sparing the peripheral bone, and by the coarse bony trabeculae of sickle cell disease. As shown in Figure 12–15, the deformity arises because the central position of the vertebral body is less well perfused with blood than the outer portion. This radiographical appearance is not entirely pathognomonic of sickle cell disease. A similar abnormality may be seen in Gaucher's disease.[279]

Bone abnormalities occur most often in patients who have frequent skeletal crises during childhood.[83] Bony changes may be seen in any of the long bones,[280] but the most symptomatic changes occur in the hip, where avascular necrosis of the femoral head may lead to disability. Some patients require a total hip prosthesis.[280a] As Figure 12–16 shows, nuclear magnetic imaging may prove to be useful in the early diagnosis of aseptic necrosis of the hip. This complication occurs almost as frequently in SC disease as in SS disease.[280a] The enhanced blood viscosity in SC disease, owing to higher hematocrit levels, may be responsible for this association. This argument is supported by the observation that avascular necrosis of the femoral head is more commonly encountered among those SS patients who have relatively high hematocrits.[281] The management of osteonecrosis in sickle cell disease has been reviewed.[282] Acute attacks of anterior chest pain in SS children may represent infarction of one or more of the ossification centers of the infused sternum.[283] Previous sternal infarctions can be detected by a cup-shaped radiolucency apparent on plain radiograph.[284]

Osteomyelitis has been found in sickle cell disease of all types. Acute osteomyelitis is discussed in the section on acute skeletal crises. Chronic osteomyelitis appears to be less common than formerly, probably because of the administration of effective antibiotics earlier in the course of the disease. The infection probably begins in a nidus of infarcted bone. In both Africa[285] and America,[286, 287] *Salmonella* species are by far the most common organisms responsible for osteomyelitis in SS patients, accounting for about 75 per cent of positive cultures. Only about 10 per cent are due to *Staphylococcus*. In contrast, *Staphylococcus* accounts for about 80 per cent of osteomyelitis in the general population.[288] The peculiar susceptibility of SS patients to *Salmonella* infections is not well understood.

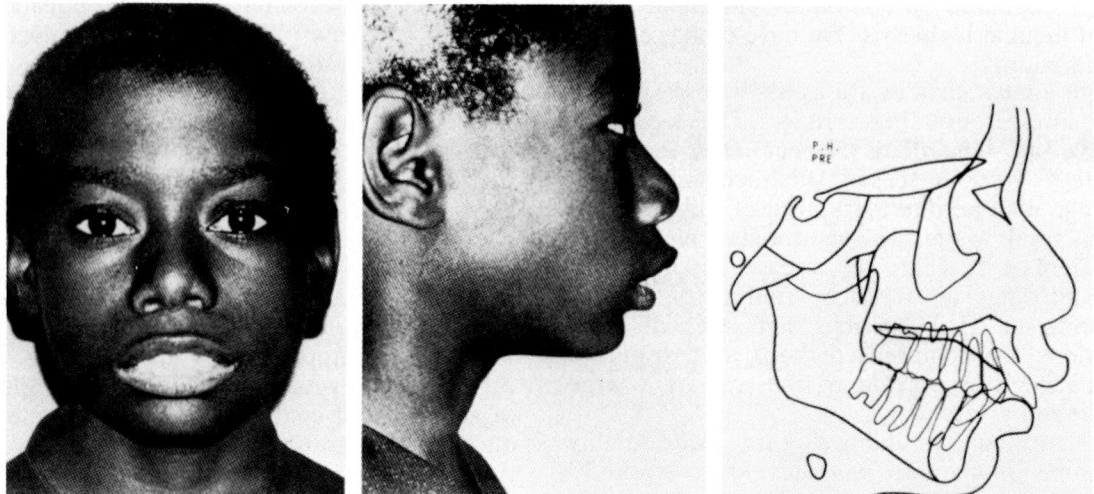

Figure 12–14. Maxillary hypertrophy and dental malocclusion in a boy with sickle cell anemia. (From Wessberg, G. A., et al.: J. Maxillofac. Surg. 8:187, 1980.)

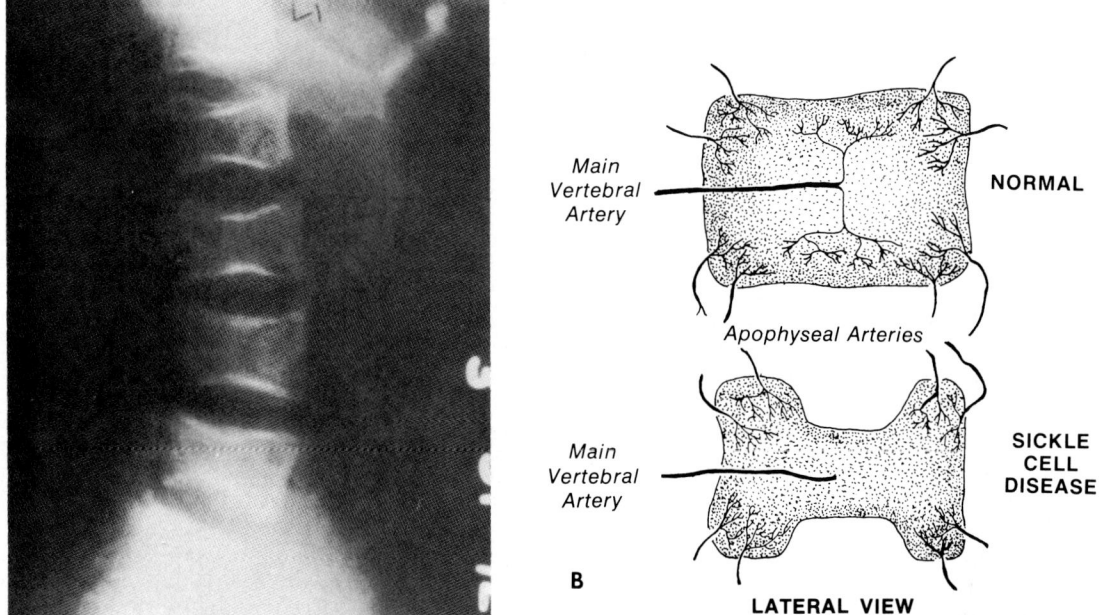

Figure 12–15. *A*, Lateral radiograph of the lumbosacral spine of a patient with SS anemia. Note the classic "H" deformity. (Courtesy of Dr. Charles Peterson.) *B*, Pathogenesis of "H" deformity. The central depression of the vertebral end-plates is caused by local inhibition of bone growth from ischemia. The central portion of the growth plate suffers ischemic damage owing to impaired circulation through the main vertebral artery. In contrast, the ring epiphyses and outer portion of the vertebral plates are spared because of numerous perforating apophyseal arteries.

It may be that the high frequency of gallstones favors the harboring of *Salmonella* in the gallbladder. Chronic hemolysis in both man and experimental animals appears to be associated with enhanced susceptibility to infection by this organism.[61]

Skin Ulcers

Many patients with sickle cell disease are handicapped by recurrent chronic skin ulcers of the lower extremities.[289] The lesions usually begin around the ankle and may become very large (Color Plate IV*E*). Ulcers are more common in those patients with the most severe anemia. Similar lesions have been encountered, although rarely, in patients with thalassemia major and in other types of congenital hemolytic anemia. Most of the leg ulcers are found in patients with SS disease or S/β thalassemia. The finding of scars of healed ulcers on the lower extremities of young black patients strongly suggests one of the sickling diseases. Leg ulcers may be more common in

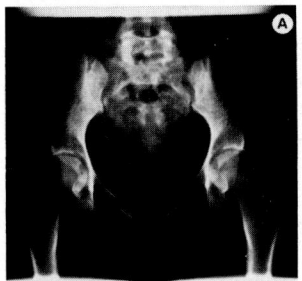 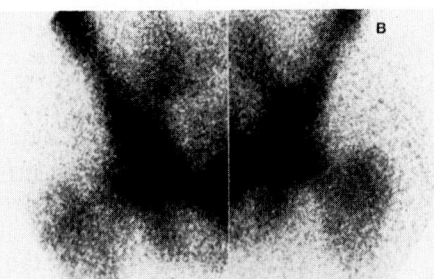 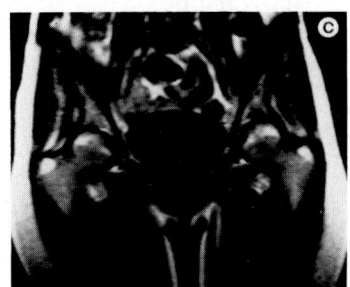

Figure 12–16. Imaging studies on a patient with SS disease who has bilateral hip pain. *A*, A standard radiograph that a bone and joint radiologist interpreted as being normal. *B*, A pinhole collimated bone scan (^{99m}Tc-methyldiphosphonate) was also considered normal. *C*, A proton nuclear magnetic resonance image in the sagittal plane of the pelvis showing inhomogeneity of marrow fat in the femoral heads and prominent low-intensity signals (dark, mottled areas) bilaterally. A normal femoral head has homogeneous intensity. The abnormalities in *C* represent early aseptic necrosis. (Courtesy of Griffin P. Rodgers, National Institutes of Health.)

tropical areas. Among the large group of SS patients in Jamaica, 63 per cent have had leg ulcers at some time in their history.[290] The incidence is considerably less among patients living in the United States and, surprisingly, among Africans (in Nigeria).[291] Leg ulcers occur most commonly between 10 and 25 years of age.[290, 291] Unfortunately, the ulcers heal very slowly, and healing is not infrequently followed by the appearance of another ulcer months or years later. Both the frequency and the chronicity may reflect difficulty in keeping the ulcer clean. The development or deterioration of an ankle ulcer is sometimes associated with an effusion in the ankle joint.[169a]

Some ulcers heal fairly well with frequent simple clean dressing changes and the use of a mild debriding agent such as Dakin's solution. The application of beads made of cross-linked dextran has been effective in removing debris and thus promoting wound healing.[292] The surface of the ulcer can be protected by the weekly application of supportive paste (Unna) boots or a newly developed membrane wrapping, Opsite, which is permeable to water but not to bacteria. If these measures are ineffective, transfusions may be added to the regimen to reduce the circulating Hb S to less than 50 per cent. Rarely, skin grafting is necessary. Skin grafting should be undertaken only after conservative measures (including transfusion) have failed, because both prolonged elevation and transfusions are usually used as adjuncts to grafting, and the simpler measures make the graft unnecessary. The oral administration of zinc sulfate may hasten the healing of leg ulcers.[293]

Eyes

Sickle cell disease can affect a number of sites in the complex anatomy of the eye. Because its multiple vascular beds are so readily accessible to direct inspection, the eye provides special insights into the abnormal rheology of sickle cell disease.

The most important ocular problems involve the retina. Sickle cell retinopathy can be divided into two broad categories—proliferative and nonproliferative.[294] Proliferative sickle retinopathy (PSR) is most characteristic of SC disease and sickle/β thalassemia. As shown in Figure 12–17, the prevalence of this complication among individuals with SC disease greatly exceeds that among SS patients.[295] It is likely that the increased viscosity of SC blood, caused by higher hematocrit, is responsible for this higher prevalence. However, among SC

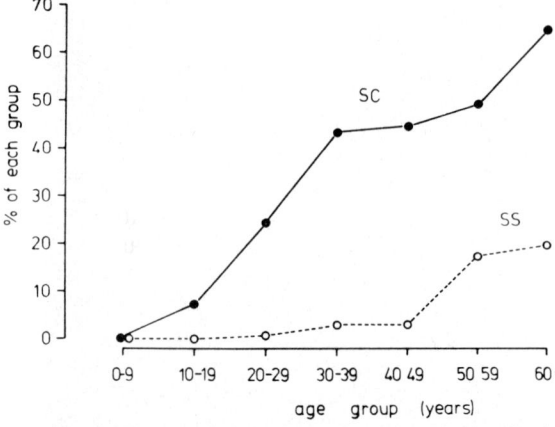

Figure 12–17. Prevalence of proliferative retinopathy in patients with SS (○——○) and SC (●——●) disease in different age groups. (From Condon, P. I., et al.: Trans. Ophthalmol. Soc. UK *100*:434, 1980.)

individuals in a given age group, the presence of PSR does not correlate with hemoglobin level.[296] In the Jamaican population, about one third of SC individuals have PSR.[296] It develops most frequently between the ages of 20 and 30 years. Among those older than 40 years, half are affected. SC males develop this complication more often than females.

Ophthalmoscopic and fluorescence angiographical examinations have established five successive stages of PSR:

Stage I. *Peripheral arteriolar occlusions.* A narrow-bore peripheral arteriole, usually at the equator of the fundus, becomes obstructed by sludging of sickle red cells. At this stage, the vessel may assume a white or "silver-wire" appearance, while the adjacent retina thins and appears greyish-brown.

Stage II. *Peripheral arteriolar-venular anastomoses.* Following arteriolar occlusion, normal capillaries that branch from the arteriole proximal to the occlusion become dilated, perhaps owing to increased hydrostatic pressure.

Stage III. *Neovascularization.* This stage is most characteristic of SC disease. As a result of local tissue ischemia, new capillary buds begin to sprout, often from the A-V anastomoses. These new vessels often assume a "sea-fan" appearance (see Color Plate IV*F*). Early lesions can be detected more readily by fluorescein angiography than by direct inspection. Although spontaneous regression may occur, these lesions can progress over an extended period of time, sometimes leading to Stages IV and V.

Stage IV. *Vitreous hemorrhage.* Hemorrhage may occur with mild ocular trauma or even spontaneously. Because most proliferative lesions are in the periphery of the retina, the hemorrhage may not cause symptoms. However, the hemorrhage occasionally affects central vision. Clotted blood from recurrent hemorrhages may organize.

Stage V. *Retinal detachment.* Progressive vitreous degeneration or recurrent hemorrhage into the vitreous may lead to membrane formation and traction bands that pull on the retina and sometimes leave retinal holes, which can progress to detachment. By this mechanism, sickle cell disease is a significant cause of monocular blindness among blacks.

Nonproliferative retinopathy of sickle cell disease includes a variety of lesions, most of which can be diagnosed by direct inspection. Salmon patch hemorrhages (see Color Plate IV*H*) occur adjacent to peripheral arteriolar occlusion. These small oval-shaped lesions are initially red but with time become pink, orange, and white and eventually disappear. Black sunbursts are commonly seen in SS patients (see Color Plate IV*G*). They represent proliferation of retinal pigment epithelium. Venous distention, venous tortuosity, isolated silver-wire arterioles, and retinal holes are also observed in sickle cell disease. Less commonly, patients may develop an occlusion of the central retinal artery or macular arterioles. Other abnormalities include angioid streaks[297] and infarction of the choroid due to posterior ciliary artery occlusion.[298]

When proliferative sickle retinopathy reaches Stage III, it may be treated with photocoagulation, diathermy, or cryopexy measures, which destroy the feeder vessels and thereby prevent complications of the neovascularization. Unfortunately, photocoagulation can cause neovascularization from the choroid[299, 300] and, on occasion, retinal breaks,[301] which pose the threat of retinal detachment. If retinal detachment does occur, either as Stage V PSR or iatrogenically, a scleral buckling procedure may be effective in restoring or salvaging vision.[302]

Following blunt head trauma, there may be significant hemorrhage into the anterior chamber of the eye (hyphema). If the red cells contain Hb S (i.e., SS, SC, S/thal, AS), they become sickled and obstruct the outflow of fluid from the anterior chamber.[303–305] This obstruction can cause severe secondary glaucoma, and if untreated, blindness may follow. Thus, if a black individual develops hyphema, the possibility of this complication should be strongly considered. In contrast, the incidence of chronic open-angle glaucoma is no greater in AS individuals than in age- and sex-matched black AA individuals.[305a]

If a patient with sickle cell disease develops frontal headaches, proptosis, and lid edema, it is likely that he has developed an infarction of the orbital bone accompanied by compression of vessels and nerves at the orbital apex.[306, 307] The primary differential diagnosis is bone infarct versus infection. If the orbital apex syndrome is caused by the former, it is usually self-limited and regresses with supportive therapy.

Two other ocular abnormalities are encountered in patients with sickle cell disease, but unlike the problems discussed thus far, they do not cause morbidity. Careful examination of the inferior region of the bulbar conjunctiva with a 40-diopter magnifying lens or, preferably, a slit lamp reveals the presence of irregular comma-shaped or corkscrew blood vessels.[308, 309] (See Color Plate IV*I*.) This sign is most prominent in patients with increased numbers of irreversibly sickled cells. Patients with SS disease also have delayed dark adaptation, a finding that may reflect relative zinc deficiency.[310]

Ears

Audiometry has revealed sensorineural hearing loss in about 12 per cent of patients with sickle cell anemia.[311, 312] However, the patients are rarely aware of impaired hearing. This subclinical abnormality probably arises from sludging of sickle red cells in the venous system of the cochlea.[311] On rare occasions, a patient may develop sudden deafness during a pain crisis.[313]

Differential Diagnosis

The diagnosis of moderate or severe forms of homozygous sickle cell anemia is usually quite straightforward. Such patients will have recurrent painful crises, marked anemia, fixed sickle forms on peripheral smear, and > 80 per cent Hb S. However, as discussed later and as noted in Table 12–4, these findings may also be present in patients doubly heterozygous for Hb S and Hb D-Los Angeles, a variant that comigrates with Hb S on routine hemoglobin electrophoresis at pH 8 to 9. Agar-gel electrophoresis at low pH is required to separate these two variants. In severe cases of S/β⁰ thalassemia, the same clinical findings may be present, but the mean corpuscular volume is decreased and microcytosis is evident on blood smears.

Table 12–4. DIFFERENTIAL DIAGNOSIS OF SS DISEASE

Diagnosis	Clinical Severity	Hematocrit	RBC Morphology	Electrophoresis	Distribution of Hb F
SS	Marked	18 to 30	Targets; 2 to 30% ISC's	80 to 95% S 2 to 20% F 2 to 4% A_2	Uneven
SD Los Angeles	Moderate to marked	20 to 30	Targets; frequent ISC's	~50% S ~50% D*	
S/β^0 thal	Moderate to marked	20 to 35	Hypochromic; microcytic; targets; rare ISC's	80 to 95% S 0% A 1 to 15% F 3 to 6% A_2	Uneven
S/β^+ thal	Mild to moderate	25 to 40	Slightly microcytic; targets; rare ISC's	55 to 75% S 10 to 30% A 1 to 13% F 3 to 6% A_2	Uneven
S/HPFH	Mild	38 to 48	Targets	70 to 80% S 20 to 30% F 1 to 3% A_2	Even

*Agar-gel electrophoresis.

In patients who have milder clinical manifestations, other forms of the "sickle syndrome" must be considered. Some of these entities are listed in Table 12–4 and are discussed in the next section. Studies of family members can provide important additional information that may prove vital in establishing the diagnosis. If the diagnosis remains in doubt after the routine hematological evaluation is completed, it may be necessary to perform structural analysis of the patient's hemoglobin.

SICKLING DISORDERS OTHER THAN SS DISEASE

As might be expected of a gene with a high frequency of Hb S, sickle cell hemoglobin is frequently encountered in association with other genetically determined abnormalities of the α or β polypeptide chains (Table 12–5).

Hemoglobin SC Disease

Hb C (β 6 Glu → Lys) is the second most common hemoglobin variant among individuals of African ancestry. As discussed in Chapter 10, the $β^C$ gene is localized to a relatively small area encompassing northern Ghana and the Upper Volta and has a frequency of 0.1. The $β^S$ gene is equally prevalent in this area. Accordingly, the incidence of the doubly heterozygous state, SC, is about 1 per cent in this part of Africa. About 0.04 per cent of black Americans have SC disease. Because it is a relatively benign disorder, the prevalence of SC disease is quite close to its incidence at birth. Among black adults in western Africa, SC disease is much more prevalent than SS disease, owing to the high mortality of the latter condition. Among American blacks, the $β^S$ gene occurs about 3 times as frequently as the $β^C$ gene. However, because of the higher mortality of the homozygous state, the prevalence of SC among black adults in the United States is almost as great as that of SS.

SC individuals generally have a mild hemolytic anemia. In the Jamaican group, the average hemoglobin level is 11.7 ± 1.7 g/dl, with 3.1 ± 1.5 per cent reticulocytes.[314] Red cell survival is about 25 per cent of normal (the mean life span is 29 ± 4 days).[315, 316] The peripheral blood film reveals plump target cells replete with hemoglobin (see Color Plate III*B*). Some cells are pointed at opposite ends and look like broad-beamed canoes. Classic irreversibly sickled cells are not seen. Occasionally, intracellular crystals can be detected.[317]

Patients with SC disease have normal growth and development, normal body habitus, and only a modest reduction in longevity.[318, 319] As discussed in the later section on pregnancy, SC women have increased morbidity during child bearing. Physical examination of individuals with SC disease is generally normal except for moderate splenomegaly, which is noted in about 65 per cent of patients.[61] Although mild sequestration crises occasionally occur,[319a] splenic enlargement does not usually contribute to the degree of anemia. Infarction of the spleen is encountered quite frequently, particularly in patients who have been subjected to hypoxia, such as travel in an unpressurized airplane cabin.

The diagnosis of SC disease is established by hemoglobin electrophoresis that reveals approximately 50 per cent Hb S, with the remainder having slower mobility characteristic of Hb C.[316] More precise analyses by high-resolution chromatography confirm this distribution.[320] Because Hb A_2 comigrates with Hb C, SC red cells actually contain somewhat more Hb S than Hb C. Hb F rarely exceeds 2 per cent of the total hemoglobin.[318] The proportion of Hb S is unchanged in SC individuals who have α thalassemia.[321, 322] Because of the presence of Hb S, sickle cell preparations and solubility tests are positive. If the patient under evaluation is of West African ancestry, these simple laboratory measures strongly suggest the diagnosis of SC disease. However, the doubly heterozygous conditions Hb SE and Hb S/O-Arab may be misdiagnosed as SC disease because Hbs C, E, and O-Arab have similar mobilities on routine electrophoresis. Hb S/O-Arab results in significant anemia and vaso-occlusive complications (see below), whereas Hb SE is benign. Hb C can be distinguished from Hbs E and O-Arab by isoelectric focusing or agar-gel electrophoresis pH 6.5 (see Chapter 10).

Patients with SC disease may develop all of the vaso-occlusive complications seen in SS homozygotes. Most of these events are less common and less severe in SC patients. However, a few exceptions are worth noting. As discussed in the section on the eye, proliferative retinopathy is more common in SC individuals. Aseptic necrosis of the femoral head, bone marrow embolism, and hematuria from renal medullary infarction are additional complications that seem to occur as frequently in SC disease as in the homozygous state.

Why is Hb SC a disease while the more

Table 12–5. SICKLING DISORDERS*

	Genotype Adult Hb	Hemoglobins Present	Clinical Expression
Group I. Homozygous for Hb S			
A. Without other Hb abnormality (sickle cell anemia)	$\alpha\alpha\beta^S\beta^S$	S, F (2–20%), A_2	Severe anemia, vaso-occlusive crises and complications
B. With α thalassemia	$-\alpha/\alpha\alpha,\beta^S\beta^S$ $-\alpha/-\alpha,\beta^S\beta^S$	S, F, A_2	Less severe hemolysis
C. With α-chain structural variant			
1. With Hb Memphis	$\alpha\alpha^{23\,Gln}\beta^S\beta^S$	S, Memphis/S, F, A_2	Hemolytic anemia but milder course and few crises
2. With Hb G-Philadelphia	$\alpha\alpha^{68\,Lys}\beta^S\beta^S$	S, G/S, F, A_2, G_2	Like severe sickle cell anemia
3. With Hb Stanleyville-II	$\alpha\alpha^{78\,Lys}\beta^S\beta^S$	S, Stanleyville/S F, A_2, Stanleyville-II	Like severe sickle cell anemia
Group II. Heterozygous for Hb S			
A. Without other Hb abnormality	$\alpha\alpha\beta^A\beta^S$	A, S, A_2	Asymptomatic; rare complications
B. With α thalassemia	$-\alpha/\alpha\alpha,\beta^A\beta^S$ $-\alpha/-\alpha,\beta^A\beta^S$	A, S (< 40%), A_2	Asymptomatic; RBC microcytic, hypochromic
C. With β thalassemia (1)	$\alpha\alpha\beta^S\beta^{Thal\,0}$	S, F, A_2 (increased)	Moderate to severe anemia and crises; RBC microcytic; may be mistaken for SS
(2)	$\alpha\alpha\beta^S\beta^{Thal\,+}$	A (10–30%), S, F, A_2 (increased)	Mild to severe
(3)	$\alpha\alpha\beta^S\delta\beta^{Thal}$	S, F (10–25%) A_2 (decreased)	Mild anemia without crises
D. With hereditary persistence of Hb F	$\alpha\alpha\beta^S-$	S, F (20–30%), A_2 (decreased)	Hb F homogeneously distributed in RBC; asymptomatic

E. With β-chain structural variants

Hb C**	$\alpha\alpha\beta^S\beta^{6\ Lys}$	C, S, A_2**
Hb G-San José†	$\alpha\alpha\beta^S\beta^{7\ Gly}$	G,† S, A_2
Hb J-Baltimore	$\alpha\alpha\beta^S\beta^{16\ Asp}$	J, S, A_2
Hb D-Iran†	$\alpha\alpha\beta^S\beta^{22\ Gln}$	D-Iran,† S, A_2
Hb E**	$\alpha\alpha\beta^S\beta^{26\ Lys}$	S, E, A_2**
Hb Tacoma	$\alpha\alpha\beta^S\beta^{40\ Ser}$	Tacoma, S, A_2
Hb K-Ibadan	$\alpha\alpha\beta^S\beta^{46\ Glu}$	K, S, A_2
Hb Maputo†	$\alpha\alpha\beta^S\beta^{47\ Tyr}$	Maputo,† S, A_2
Hb Osu-Christiansborg†	$\alpha\alpha\beta^S\beta^{52\ Asn}$	Osu-Christiansborg†, S, A_2
Hb Ocho-Ríos†	$\alpha\alpha\beta^S\beta^{52\ Ala}$	Ocho-Ríos,† S, A_2
Hb Korle-Bu†	$\alpha\alpha\beta^S\beta^{73\ Asn}$	Korle-Bu,† S, A_2
Hb Mobile†	$\alpha\alpha\beta^S\beta^{73\ Val}$	Mobile,† S, A_2
Hb D-Ibadan†	$\alpha\alpha\beta^S\beta^{87\ Lys}$	D,† S, A_2
Hb Caribbean	$\alpha\alpha\beta^S\beta^{91\ Arg}$	Caribbean, S, A_2
Hb Richmond	$\alpha\alpha\beta^S\beta^{102\ Lys}$	Richmond, S, A_2
Hb D-Los Angeles†	$\alpha\alpha\beta^S\beta^{121\ Gln}$	D,† S, A_2
Hb O-Arab**	$\alpha\alpha\beta^S\beta^{121\ Lys}$	O, S, A_2**
Hb Camden	$\alpha\alpha\beta^S\beta^{131\ Glu}$	Camden, S, A_2
Hb K-Woolwich	$\alpha\alpha\beta^S\beta^{132\ Gln}$	K, S, A_2
Hb Hope	$\alpha\alpha\beta^S\beta^{136Asp}$	S, Hope, A_2
Hb Lepore†	$\alpha\alpha\beta^S\beta^{\delta\times\beta}$	S, F, Lepore,† A_2
Hb Kenya	$\alpha\alpha\beta^S\beta^{\gamma\times\beta}$	S, Kenya, F
Hb C-Harlem	$\alpha\alpha\beta^S\beta^{6\ Val,\ 73\ Asn}$	S, C-Harlem

	Moderate anemia, occasional crises, retinopathy
	Asymptomatic
	Asymptomatic
	Moderate anemia
	Asymptomatic
	Asymptomatic
	Asymptomatic
	Asymptomatic
	Asymptomatic
	Asymptomatic
	Asymptomatic
	Asymptomatic
	Asymptomatic
	Asymptomatic
	Moderate to severe anemia, crises
	Moderate to severe anemia, crises
	Asymptomatic
	Mild anemia
	Moderate anemia
	Asymptomatic
	Moderate to severe anemia, crises

*Modified from Milner, P. F.: Clin. Haematol. 3:289, 1974.
**Hb C, Hb O-Arab, and Hb E are not separated from Hb A_2 on routine alkaline electrophoresis.
†Not separated from Hb S on routine alkaline electrophoresis.

common sickle cell trait (Hb AS) is almost entirely benign? The fact that SC individuals have vaso-occlusive complications suggests that their red cells "sickle" more readily than AS red cells. Indeed, during *in vitro* incubations, SC red cells assume a sickled shape at oxygen tensions that do not affect AS red cells.[323] Viscosity,[324] kinetics[325–327] and NMR[328] measurements also indicate that SC cells form more polymer than AS cells when subjected to a comparable degree of deoxygenation. It has been generally assumed that the enhanced tendency of SC red cells to sickle was due to increased copolymerization of Hb S with C.[329] However, both equilibrium and kinetic measurements of mixtures of Hbs S and C indicate that they behave identically to comparable mixtures of Hbs S and A.[330] Moreover, in these mixtures, polymerization takes place by the same mechanism as in solutions of pure Hb S. There is no evidence for independent crystallization of Hb C in SC red cells. Thus, SC red cells do not display abnormal aggregation of intracellular hemoglobins.

The increased tendency of SC red cells to sickle can be explained by two independent phenomena.[330] First, these red cells contain significantly more hemoglobin S than that found in sickle trait red cells. This difference results in approximately a sevenfold increase in the rate of polymerization. Second, the intracellular concentration of hemoglobin is higher in SC cells than in AS cells when measured on whole blood specimens[314] or when determined more precisely by separation of red cells on density gradients (Fig. 12–18).[330–332] Because polymerization of Hb S is so markedly dependent on hemoglobin concentration, the higher hemoglobin concentration in SC red cells contributes significantly toward their enhanced tendency to sickle. When SC cells are suspended in a hypotonic medium, so that their mean intracellular hemoglobin concentration falls to that of AS red cells, much less sickling is noted.[332] The increased intracellular hemoglobin concentration of SC red cells can be explained by the presence of Hb C, because red cells of individuals with Hb C trait (AC) are denser than normal[330] and presumably have increased mean corpuscular hemoglobin concentration (MCHC).

Sickle/β Thalassemia

Sickle/β thalassemia is next in frequency to Hb SC disease among the doubly heterozygous sickle disorders. Because β thalassemia is com-

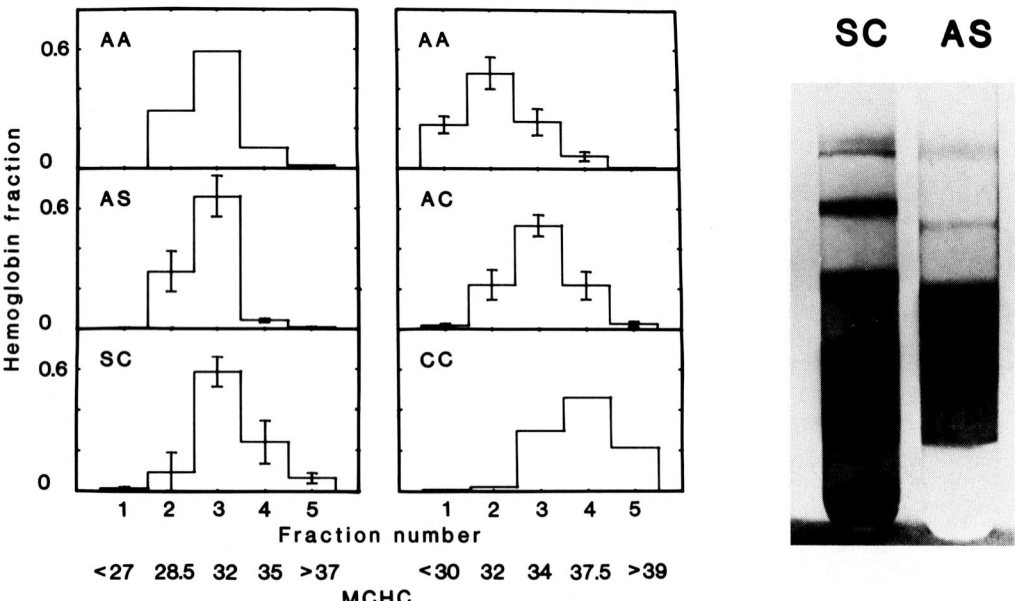

Figure 12–18. Left, Separation of erythrocytes of differing densities by discontinuous Stractan gradients. The ordinate is the fraction of the applied sample in successive layers as measured by the fraction of the total Hb. The mean intracellular Hb concentration of each layer is shown. The error bars represent 1 standard deviation from the mean. Four specimens were used in constructing the histograms with error bars, and one was used for the histograms without error bars. *Right,* Stractan gradient separation of SC and AS cells. (From Bunn, H. F., et al.: Proc. Natl. Acad. Sci. USA 79:7527, 1982.)

mon in the Mediterranean area while the incidence of sickle cell trait is lower, S/β thalassemia is the most common type of sickling disorder in individuals from this region. Beta thalassemia is also found in Africans, with a gene frequency ranging between 0.001 and 0.01. The expression of S/β thalassemia in Africans is generally milder than in the Mediterranean populations. This difference is also seen in thalassemia: Thalassemia major is generally an incapacitating disease in Greeks and Italians, whereas among Africans, it it is considerably milder (see Chapter 9).

It is sometimes difficult to distinguish between sickle cell anemia and S/β thalassemia (see Table 12–4). The finding of an enlarged spleen in an older patient may be useful in the differential diagnosis. Splenomegaly is much more likely to be encountered in patients (> 6 years old) with sickle/β thalassemia than in SS homozygotes. Among 56 patients with S/β thalassemia from Jamaica, half had a palpable spleen.[333] The hypochromia and microcytosis of erythrocytes of patients with sickle/β thalassemia (see Color Plate II*F*) are usually established by the age of 1 year. Furthermore, there are fewer irreversibly sickled cells.[334] Hemoglobin electrophoresis provides important independent evidence. If the proportion of Hb A_2 is significantly increased (e.g., 6 per cent), the diagnosis of sickle/β thalassemia is suggested. Of course, the presence of 10 to 30 per cent hemoglobin A in a patient who has not been transfused, together with Hb S, strongly suggests the presence of S/β$^+$ thalassemia (Fig. 12–19). The differential diagnosis between SS and S/β^0 thalassemia is more difficult, because the elevation in hemoglobin A_2 may not be accurately measured, and in either disorder, the sum of Hb S and Hb F accounts for nearly all the hemoglobin. SS patients with α thalassemia, especially $-\alpha/-\alpha$, have somewhat microcytic red cells and elevated Hb A_2, characteristics that resemble those in patients with S/β thalassemia.[335] Sometimes, family studies are needed to distinguish between the two disorders. The diagnosis of S/β thalassemia can also be made by measuring the biosynthesis of α and β subunits in blood reticulocytes. In S/β thalassemia, the β^S/α ratio is about 0.5, whereas it is close to unity in SS disease.

Sickle/β thalassemia varies in its severity and outlook; the degree of anemia may be as marked as in sickle cell anemia, or the hemoglobin concentration may be nearly normal. As shown in Table 12–4, S/β° thalassemia tends to be more severe than S/β$^+$ thalassemia:

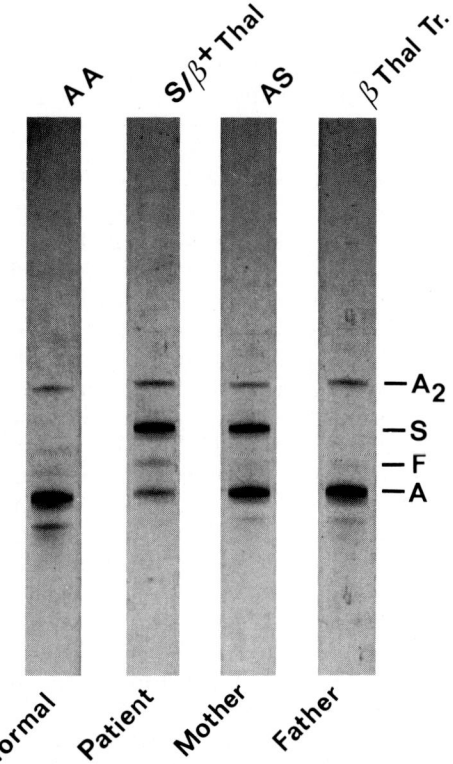

Figure 12–19. Hemoglobin electrophoresis of patient with sickle/β$^+$ thalassemia and his parents. The mother has sickle trait (AS) and the father has β-thalassemia trait. Note that both the patient and his father have elevated Hb A_2. In addition, the patient has elevated Hb F. The presence of Hb A in the patient's hemolysate indicates that he has S/β$^+$ thalassemia rather than S/β^0 thalassemia. Hemolysates were analyzed by electrofocusing on polyacrylamide gels.

the anemia is worse; there are more irreversibly sickled cells; and patients have more frequent vaso-occlusive problems.[333] Ocular and bony manifestations may be present in S/β^0 thalassemia, and splenic sequestration crises have been described.

Other Doubly Heterozygous Disorders

Hb S/D-Los Angeles. Sickle cell/Hb D disease is usually due to the presence of Hb S and Hb D-Los Angeles (or Hb D-Punjab) (in which the glutamic acid residue at β 121 is replaced by glutamine). The combination of Hbs S and D-Los Angeles has been encountered in a number of patients of African origin who have occasional crises and moderate hemolytic anemia. The clinical manifestations of Hb SD disease can be explained by enhanced copolymerization of Hb D-Los Angeles with Hb S due to the β 121 substitution at an important contact in the sickle fiber (see Chapter 11). The electrophoretic pattern of SD disease at alkaline pH is identical to that of SS disease. Hemoglobins S and D-Los Angeles can be separated by electrophoresis at pH 6.2 in citrate agar. In this acid medium, Hb D migrates like hemoglobin A and is distinct from Hb S.

Hb S/Lepore. Seven individuals from different geographical areas have been identified as double heterozygotes for Hb S and Hb Lepore-Boston.[337] These individuals have occasional vaso-occlusive episodes and a moderate hemolytic anemia with microcytic red cells. Because Hb Lepore has an electrophoretic mobility similar to that of Hb S, these individuals may be misdiagnosed as having SS disease or S/β thalassemia. The presence of a normal or low proportion of Hb A_2 provides a clue to the diagnosis, which can be confirmed by appropriate family studies.

At least nine hemoglobin variants with electrophoretic properties similar to Hb D (or S) have been found in association with Hb S[336] (see Table 12–5). Of these, only two, Hb D-Los Angeles and Hb Lepore, have given rise to symptomatic sickle cell disease. The definitive diagnosis of those hemoglobins with the electrophoretic properties of Hb D requires detailed structural analysis.

Hb S/O-Arab. Some patients have a disorder resembling homozygous sickle cell anemia (SS) with vaso-occlusive manifestations, severe hemolytic anemia and irreversibly sickled forms on blood film and yet have an electrophoretic pattern suggesting SC disease. These individuals are likely to be doubly heterozygous for Hb S and Hb O-Arab (β 121 Glu → Lys).[338, 339] Children with Hb S/O-Arab may develop hand-foot syndrome and acute splenic sequestration crisis,[340] complications characteristic of SS disease. Like Hb D-Los Angeles, Hb O-Arab copolymerizes with Hb S more readily than does Hb A because β 121 is an important contact in the sickle fiber (see Chapter 11). As mentioned previously, Hb O-Arab can be distinguished from Hb C by gel electrofocusing or by agar-gel electrophoresis at pH 6.5.

Other doubly heterozygous states can also give an electrophoretic pattern resembling that of SC disease. One patient has been found to be doubly heterozygous for hemoglobin S and hemoglobin C-Harlem.[341] In this disorder, all the β chains have the β 6 Glu → Val substitution and half of the β chains have an additional substitution: β 73 Asp → Asn. The patient suffered numerous crises as a child and became less symptomatic as she approached adulthood. The clinical manifestations of Hb S/C-Harlem disease resemble those of SS disease.

There are a number of reports of Hb SE double heterozygotes.[342, 343] Although their electrophoretic pattern resembles SC and S/O-Arab, the proportion of Hb S is higher owing to impaired synthesis of Hb E (see Chapter 10). Unlike the other "SC-like" disorders mentioned previously, SE individuals appear to be asymptomatic.

Coexistence of an Alpha-Chain Variant. The combination of α-chain variants with heterozygosity for Hb S has not resulted in sickle cell disease. These combinations can generally be recognized by the appearance of multiple major components ($\alpha_2^A\beta_2^A$, $\alpha_2^A\beta_2^S$, $\alpha_2^X\beta_2^A$, $\alpha_2^X\beta_2^S$) as well as two minor components ($\alpha_2^A\delta_2$, $\alpha_2^X\delta_2$) on electrophoresis. Depending on the charge of the α-chain variant, three or four major bands may be visualized on electrophoresis in alkaline media (see Figure 10–4).

Hb Memphis (α_2 23 Gln β_2^S) has been observed in SS homozygotes. These patients have severe anemia but mild symptoms of sickling.[344, 345] These red cells exhibit less morphological sickling and have lower viscosity than ordinary SS red cells.[345]

HbS/HPFH. As explained in Chapter 9, hereditary persistence of fetal hemoglobin (HPFH) is a heterogeneous disorder. One type, commonly called *pancellular HPFH*, involves deletion of a portion of the β globin gene complex. Heterozygotes have about 25 per cent Hb F distributed relatively evenly among red cells. About 0.1 per cent of American blacks are heterozygous for pancellular HPFH.[346] Thus, it is not surprising that occasional individuals have been encountered who are doubly heterozygous for Hb S and pancellular HPFH.[323, 347, 348] Affected individuals have about 70 per cent Hb S, 20 to 30 per cent Hb F, low Hb A_2, and no Hb A. Peripheral blood counts are usually normal, with no evidence of anemia or hemolysis. Red cells are normochromic and normocytic. The peripheral blood film reveals target cells but no fixed sickle forms. Although the sickle preparation and sickling solubility tests are positive, there is rarely clinical evidence of sickling. The mild expression of Hb S/HPFH is due to the fact that the fetal hemoglobin is evenly distributed, thereby protecting all red cells from sickling. The nearly uniform distribution can be demonstrated by differential staining of red cells by acid elution (Kleihauer-Betke stain) or by the use of fluorescently labeled anti-Hb F antibody.

Individuals heterozygous for *heterocellular HPFH* have about 5 to 15 per cent Hb F that is unevenly distributed among red cells. The genetic and cellular basis of this disorder is unknown. The β globin gene complex is intact. Thus, individuals can inherit heterocellular HPFH in cis to HB S[349-352] or any other β-chain variant. Some cases of heterocellular HPFH appear to be closely linked to the β globin gene complex,[353-355a] whereas others are not.[353, 355b, 355c] Some SS homozygotes have elevated levels of Hb F because they are heterozygous for heterocellular HPFH.[351, 355a] They often have a relatively benign clinical course. Indeed, the mild nature of SS disease among the Shi Arabs and Veddoid Indians may be due to the presence of this genetic modulator (see the following section on prognosis).

PROGNOSIS

In many of the early reviews of sickle cell anemia, the assessment of prognosis was unduly pessimistic. This was due in part to case selection. Only patients with relatively severe disease tend to require frequent emergency room visits and hospital admissions. A surprisingly large group of SS homozygotes remain relatively symptom-free and do not solicit medical attention. Furthermore, during the past 30 years, there has been a marked improvement in the care of patients with sickle cell anemia. Infections are treated more promptly with increasingly effective antibiotics. More careful attention is devoted to the maintenance of fluid balance and the prevention of dehydration. In addition, maternal mortality among pregnant SS patients has decreased in recent years. In underdeveloped nations, particularly in Africa, the mortality rate for sickle cell anemia remains high. Children from rural areas have an alarmingly high death rate.[356] However, in certain parts of Africa, better living conditions, nutrition, and medical care have resulted in a significant reduction in mortality.[357]

In the United States, the prognosis for children with sickle cell disease continues to improve. Surveys from Chicago[358] and Los Angeles[83] conducted in the early 1970's indicated a mortality rate of about 10 per cent during the first decade of life. The causes of death are listed in Table 12-6. The modal age of death was 2 years. Nearly half of the children died from infection, primarily sepsis, pneumonia, meningitis, and gastroenteritis. As mentioned in the section on infection, *Pneumococcus* accounted for the majority of the fatal infections. Deaths due to splenic sequestration occurred between 1 and 4 years of age. Many occurred in children not yet known to have sickle cell disease. In Jamaica, gastroenteritis was the major cause of death in infants less than 6 months of age.[359] With the advent of cord blood screening of black newborns, those with sickle cell disease can be identified prior to the development of any clinical manifestations and can be given special medical attention.[360] (See the section on therapy that follows). It is likely that these measures will result in a further reduction in childhood mortality.

Table 12-6. CAUSES OF DEATH AMONG CHILDREN WITH SICKLE CELL DISEASE*

Cause	Percentage of Total Deaths
Infection	44
Splenic sequestration	16
Sudden, unexpected death	14
Cerebrovascular accident	12
Congestive heart failure	7
Miscellaneous	7
	100

*From Mentzer, W. C., and Wang, W. C.: Pediatr. Ann. 9:297, 1980. Compiled from data on 43 children followed by Powars[83] and Seeler.[358]

The causes of death among Jamaican patients of all ages are depicted in Figure 12-20.[361] Serjeant and colleagues have identified a large fraction of all Jamaicans with sickle cell disease and provide regular follow-up care. Therefore, these autopsy findings provide a reliable assessment of the natural history of sickle cell disease on the island. The causes of death among infants and young children are similar to those shown in Table 12-6. Among the adult patients, renal failure becomes a common terminal event.

The prognosis for sickle cell homozygotes may be influenced by a number of coexisting genetic factors that can modulate the severity of the disease. Thus far, two have been identified: α thalassemia and heterocellular hereditary persistence of Hb F.

As discussed in Chapter 9, α thalassemia is prevalent among populations that carry the sickle gene. About 30 per cent of American blacks are heterozygous for α thalassemia 2 ($-\alpha/\alpha\alpha$), and about 2 per cent are homozygous ($-\alpha/-\alpha$). The development of restriction endonuclease mapping has allowed the unequivocal identification of these types of α thalassemia in patients with sickle cell disease.[335, 362]

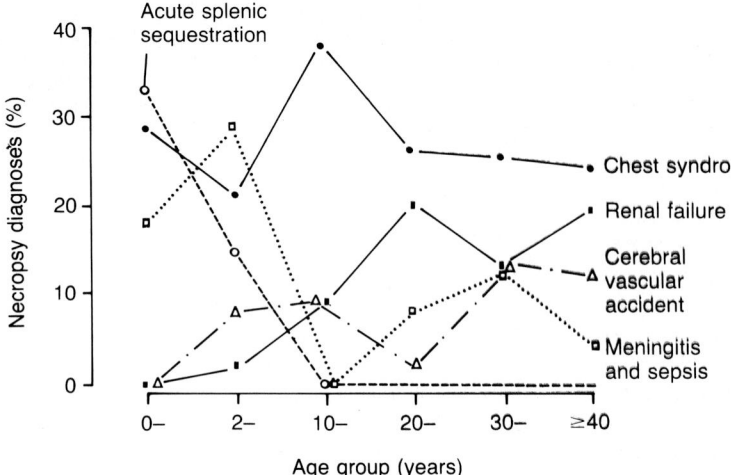

Figure 12–20. Relative frequencies of causes of death among 240 Jamaican patients with SS disease. (From Thomas, A. N., et al.: Br. Med. J. 285:633, 1982.)

The coinheritance of α thalassemia has much more effect on the hematological findings in SS disease than on vaso-occlusive manifestations.[335, 362a] As shown in Figure 12–21, the number of α-chain genes correlates directly with mean corpuscular volume and mean corpuscular hemoglobin concentration and inversely with hemoglobin level. Thus, SS homozygotes with coexisting α thalassemia tend to have less anemia and smaller and paler red cells than those who have all four α-chain genes.[335, 362, 363] The degree of hemolysis is sig-

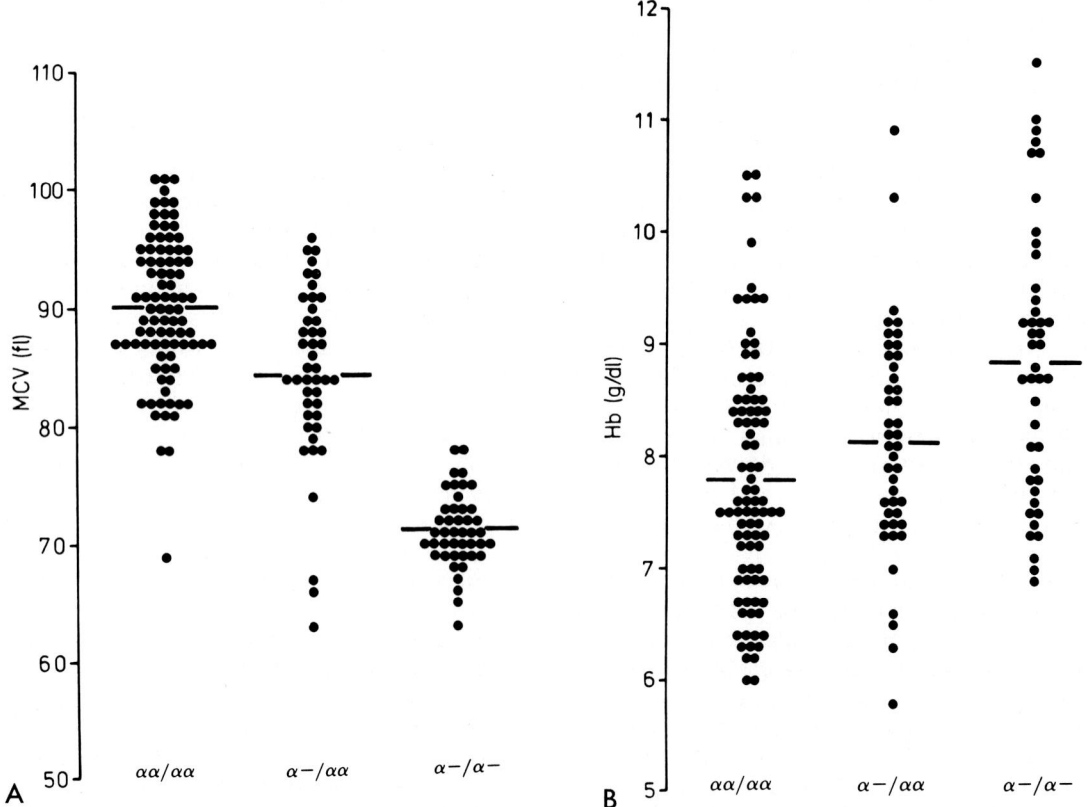

Figure 12–21. Effect of α thalassemia on hematological values in SS homozygotes. *A*, Mean corpuscular volume (MCV) in femtoliters (fl). *B*, Hemoglobin levels (g/dl). (From Higgs, D. R., et al.: N. Engl. J. Med. 306:1441, 1982.)

nificantly reduced in those with α thalassemia, as indicated by lower reticulocyte counts and fewer dense and irreversibly sickled cells.[364-364b] The deformability of SS red cells is enhanced if α thalassemia is also present.[364c, 364d] Despite the lesser degree of anemia and the reduced hemolysis in SS patients with α thalassemia, there is no significant reduction in overall vaso-occlusive manifestations.[335, 362a] This group is more likely to have splenomegaly and may have fewer episodes of acute chest syndrome and chronic leg ulcers,[335] but more information is needed to establish these differences. There is some epidemiological evidence that the coinheritance of α thalassemia confers improved survival upon patients with SS disease.[364a, 365]

Heterocellular hereditary persistence of fetal hemoglobin is a second genetic factor that appears to be a modulator of sickle cell disease. This kind of HPFH is inherited in cis to the β-chain gene[349-352] (see the preceding section on Hb S/HPFH). Patients with SS disease and heterocellular HPFH have significantly higher levels of Hb F than unaffected SS patients. The fact that the Hb F is unevenly distributed among red cells precludes it from having a maximal antisickling effect. Nevertheless, the two populations who are known to have mild SS disease, Shi Arabs[366, 367] and Veddoid Indians,[368, 369] have markedly increased levels of Hb F (mean values of 28 per cent and 20 per cent, respectively), probably as a consequence of this genetic modulator. There is also a high incidence of α thalassemia in these populations.

Among SS patients of African ancestry, the great majority lack any evidence of heterocellular HPFH. The level of Hb F is quite variable, with a mean somewhere between 6 per cent[61] and 10 per cent.[369a] It is unclear whether patients with a relatively low level of Hb F have more severe disease. Among young children, those with a relatively low level of Hb F at 6 months of age had increased mortality, more episodes of dactylitis, and a larger spleen with more frequent splenic sequestration crises.[370] However, the level of Hb F was not a good predictor of hematological or clinical severity among a group of 214 older individuals with SS disease.[371] There may be a threshold of about 20 per cent Hb F, above which the morbidity of SS disease is ameliorated.[369a]

Studies of the clinical and laboratory manifestations of sickle cell disease in the United States and Jamaica involve individuals of diverse African ancestry. Therefore, it is difficult to identify genetic modulators of disease severity. Labie and Nagel[371a, 371b] have circumvented this problem by a detailed comparison of two distinct African populations. They found that SS patients from Benin in Central West Africa have relatively severe disease with a high proportion of dense erythrocytes and a low proportion of Hb F. In contrast, SS patients from Senegal (Atlantic West Africa) have a lower proportion of dense cells and higher levels of Hb F, which has a high $^G\gamma/^A\gamma$ ratio. Sickle cell disease appears to be less severe in this population. The high $^G\gamma$ Hb F expression is associated with a common haplotype for the β globin gene cluster. This genetic modulator apparently ameliorates sickle cell disease through increased levels of Hb F.

Other genetic modulators could contribute to the prognosis of sickle cell disease but have not yet been identified. It is well established that glucose-6-phosphate dehydrogenase deficiency, a very common abnormality among blacks, has no effect on survival of SS patients. Genetic or acquired heterogeneity in the red cell membrane or in the microcirculation may influence clinical severity. Adherence of oxygenated SS erythrocytes to cultured endothelial cells correlates with the frequency and severity of vaso-occlusive complications.[143] These in vitro studies raise the possibility that genetic heterogeneity in the red cell membrane among SS patients may be a significant prognostic determinant. Alternatively, the enhanced endothelial cell adherence in the patients with more severe disease may reflect membrane damage resulting from more frequent cycles of intracellular polymerization and depolymerization. The central thrust of Chapter 11 is that the pathological manifestations of sickle cell disease are a direct consequence of intracellular polymerization of Hb S. Indeed, the extent of hemolysis and anemia among diverse populations with various types of sickling disorders is closely proportional to a theoretical prediction of intracellular polymerization based on the hemoglobin composition as well as intracellular hemoglobin concentration.[64]

TREATMENT OF SICKLE CELL DISEASE

The growing body of information on the molecular pathogenesis of sickle cell disease has raised expectations that specific and effective therapy could be devised to inhibit intracellular polymerization of Hb S. Despite an intense international research effort over the past decade, this goal has not yet been realized. The management of sickle cell disease consists primarily of supportive care. In addition to a review of conventional treatment, this section will discuss newer approaches to therapy that are currently being investigated.

Supportive Therapy

Health Maintenance. The identification of newborns with sickle cell disease by means of cord blood screening will enable them and their parents to be incorporated into a comprehensive program consisting of education, counseling, prevention, and acute health care.

Because of the varied and unpredictable manifestations of sickle cell disease, patients require regular and meticulous medical attention. It is important to see the patient when he is free of crisis and to establish baseline physical findings, such as cardiac murmurs and organomegaly, and laboratory data, including a complete blood count, sedimentation rate, chest x-ray, and electrocardiogram. This information is invaluable in assessing the patient when he becomes ill. Both patients and their parents, when appropriate, should be thoroughly educated about various practical aspects of sickle cell disease. They should understand the importance of early detection and treatment of infection. Proper hygiene should be discussed, with special attention to bruises and abrasions in the lower extremities that could lead to ankle ulcers. Patients should be warned that crises may be induced by hypoxia accompanying high-altitude exposure,[372] air travel, or anesthesia. They should be aware of the importance of adequate fluid intake, especially during hot summer months and periods of fever. They should also be cautioned that acute exposure to cold can bring on pain crises. Yearly or biannual ophthalmological examination is recommended to detect early retinopathy. Women may need to be advised about appropriate methods of birth control. Oral contraceptives probably increase the risk of cerebral and pulmonary thrombosis. An intrauterine device is preferable[372a] even though it may provide a site for infection. Both men and women may seek counseling about fertility problems.

Infections. Because patients with sickle cell disease have increased susceptibility to infection, antibiotics should be administered at the earliest sign of infection, particularly to children, in whom bacterial sepsis is a major hazard.

In the vaso-occlusive crises, the most common reason for hospital admission of adults, evidence of bacterial infection is frequently absent. The clinician is often uncertain whether or when to institute antibiotics and how long to continue treatment. These decisions arise most often in patients with acute chest syndrome and in those with bone infarctions. The clinical characteristics of these complications are reviewed in previous sections of this chapter.

Polyvalent pneumococcal vaccine plays an important role in the treatment of sickle cell disease. Effective immunization against *Streptococcus pneumoniae* would abolish the major cause of mortality in children. Vaccination is safe and associated with only mild local reactions.[373] Unfortunately, the vaccines are not entirely effective.[374] Children under the age of 2 years, the group most susceptible to pneumococcal sepsis, are often unable to mount an effective antibody response[375, 376] Moreover, some strains of pneumococcus are such poor antigens that SS patients of all ages fail to achieve a rise in antibody titers.[376, 377] Finally, even the most comprehensive vaccine contains only 14 polysaccharide antigens and therefore fails to protect against other subtypes, which account for 20 per cent of pneumococcal infections. For these reasons, it is estimated that pneumococcal vaccination provides about 50 per cent protection.[374] Recent mortality figures indicate that this estimate is roughly correct. Currently, it is recommended that SS infants be given polyvalent pneumococcal vaccine at the age of 6 to 12 months, with a booster dose 6 to 12 months later.[375] It is possible that newly developed vaccines for hemophilus and meningococcus will also provide effective protection to patients with sickle cell disease, although these organisms pose much less of a problem than pneumococcus.

Because vaccination fails to confer full protection, it is wise to maintain SS children on oral prophylactic penicillin from 6 months to 6 years of age. It is difficult to assess the efficacy of this prophylaxis because compliance is a major problem.

Antimalarial prophylaxis is indicated in endemic areas.

Anemia. Patients with sickle cell anemia usually tolerate anemia quite well. Worsening of anemia because of folic acid deficiency is readily prevented by administering a daily supplement of this vitamin. Androgen treatment results in a significant increase in red cell mass[378-380] and has been used in selected patients who appear to be symptomatic because of severe anemia. The rise in red cell 2,3-DPG and the decrease in oxygen affinity during androgen therapy (see Chapter 5) would theoretically enhance sickling. However, treatment has no significant effect on red cell survival. The possible benefits of long-term oral androgen therapy must be weighed against adverse effects, chief among which is hepatotoxicity. Furthermore, male patients have a tendency to develop priapism during treatment.[378]

Transfusion Therapy. Blood transfusions play a controversial role in the treatment of anemia of sickle cell disease. Some experienced clinicians believe that vaso-occlusive complications can be prevented by transfusions. Moreover, hypertransfused patients often gain considerable subjective improvement with significantly enhanced exercise tolerance, perhaps owing to superior flow properties of transfused cells.[381, 382] In order to be effective, at least 50 per cent of the patient's red cells should be of donor origin. This clinical impression is supported by whole blood viscosity measurements.[383] An effective protocol for partial blood exchange is shown in Table 12–7.[384] More rapid and efficient exchange can be accomplished by an automated pheresis technique.[385, 386]

Patients who are chronically transfused to hemoglobin levels of 12 g/dl or greater will develop reticulocytopenia and yet maintain increased marrow erythropoiesis. This ineffective erythropoiesis is probably caused by the inability of the SS reticulocytes to cross the sinusoidal barrier from marrow to blood.[382]

Hypertransfusion therapy should not be undertaken lightly, because it entails a considerable commitment of time and resources as well as the familiar risks of hepatitis, iron overload, and red cell sensitization. Delayed transfusion reactions are commonly observed and may mimic a sickle cell crisis.[387] Despite these problems, exchange transfusion may be indicated in selected patients, particularly if they are going through a period of increased risk, such as major surgery[388] or pregnancy.[389] (See below.) When possible, patients should receive blood lacking red cell antigens that have a relatively low frequency in blacks. The most commonly encountered alloantibodies in black patients who have had multiple transfusions include anti-E, C, Lewis, and Kell.[390] Patients receiving more than 100 units of blood are at risk of developing clinically significant iron overload.[391] Measurement of serum ferritin is useful in monitoring the iron status of transfused patients.[392, 393] Those with iron overload will enter negative iron balance when treated with intravenous[393] or continuous subcutaneous deferoxamine.

Painful Crises. The management of the painful vaso-occlusive crisis is best achieved by vigorous hydration, analgesics, and appropriate antibiotics if there is any evidence of infection. Because of their inability to produce concentrated urine, SS patients have an increased fluid requirement and are prone to dehydration. Therefore, if a patient cannot drink an adequate amount of fluid, he should be given an intravenous infusion. Careful attention should also be paid to the patient's acid-base status. Acidosis should be promptly corrected, because it can trigger a painful crisis.[394] However, alkali therapy does not appear to be effective either in the treatment of acute painful crises[395] or in their prevention.[396] Oxygen is usually administered during acute

---

Table 12–7. **PROCEDURE FOR PARTIAL EXCHANGE TRANSFUSION***ᵃ

1. Use at least a No. 16 needle connected to a blood bag via an extension tube and a tube with a bayonet adapter.ᵇ Do not remove any blood until 1 unit of donor cells is on hand. Have 1000 ml of normal saline solution ready for infusion.
2. Remove 500 ml of blood. Inexperienced phlebotomists should ask the Blood Bank what a filled blood bag looks like, and a scale can be used (1 ml of blood weighs about 1.06 g). In *emergency* situations, blood can be "pulled" out and "pushed" in through a jugular or femoral venous catheter.
3. Infuse 500 ml of saline solution.
4. Remove a second 500 ml of blood. Save both units—they are valuable reagents for those studying sickle cells.
5. Infuse 5 units of packed red cells as fast as they will flow without prior dilution.
6. In extremely urgent situations, use a No. 14 needle, pull the blood out with a 50-ml syringe, and push in the normal cells (or use a pressure apparatus). Because rapid infusion of 1000 ml of red cells at 4°C produces severe shaking chills, pre-warm the blood.
7. If a cell separator is available and the extra expense can be justified, elegant exchange transfusions can be performed with little risk.

*From Charache, S.: Ann. Rev. Med. *32*:195, 1981.
ᵃFor a 50-kg adult with a hematocrit of 20 to 27 per cent.
ᵇAE-2—Fenwal Corporation.

painful crises, but its efficacy is doubtful unless the patient has significant ventilatory hypoxia. In contrast, hyperbaric oxygen may be an effective, albeit cumbersome, form of treatment.[397] Oxygen therapy induces a reduction in irreversibly sickled cells, which re-emerge following cessation of therapy, sometimes accompanied by the onset of acute pain crisis.[397a]

Prompt and adequate relief of pain is of prime importance. This is probably the most difficult aspect of the management of patients with sickle cell disease. Those who require admission to the hospital generally require narcotic-type analgesia such as Demerol, Dilaudid, or morphine. Many physicians fail to prescribe adequate amounts of narcotic drugs.[398] A regular schedule of pain medicine is preferable to administration on an as-needed basis, because the anxiety associated with anticipation of recurrence of pain augments pain perception, a classic example of operant conditioning.[399] As the painful episode abates, the dose of analgesic should be gradually lowered and then replaced by a less potent drug such as codeine, aspirin, or acetaminophen (Tylenol). Alternative approaches to pain control, including acupuncture,[400] transcutaneous stimulation,[401] and hypnosis,[402] are being evaluated but have not gained wide acceptance as adequate substitutes for analgesics. Unfortunately, many patients who have frequent painful crises become dependent on, if not addicted to, a variety of narcotics and analgesics. A surprising number of patients become habituated to propoxyphene. Despite the high incidence of addiction, these patients deserve the benefit of the doubt and should not be denied analgesic therapy when they appear to have pain.

Blood transfusion has been recommended in the management of acute painful crises,[403] but the efficacy of this treatment is doubtful. In contrast, in selected patients, exchange transfusion may be effective in the prevention of painful crises.

Surgery. Because patients with sickle cell disease usually do not tolerate major surgery very well, hematologists are conservative in recommending surgical procedures. Close attention should be paid to maintenance of adequate hydration and acid-base balance as well as to optimal oxygenation before, during, and after surgery.[404–406] If extensive surgery is planned on an elective basis, such as a total hip replacement, it is reasonable to prepare the patient with exchange transfusion. In some centers, patients with sickle cell disease are routinely transfused prior to major surgery, but the initial withdrawal of blood is omitted. The value of preoperative transfusion is unproved.

Splenectomy. Most patients with homozygous sickle cell anemia sustain recurrent splenic infarcts, with gradual transformation of the organ into a nubbin of fibrotic tissue. However, under certain circumstances, the spleen can pose sufficient problems to a patient with sickle cell disease that its removal is indicated. As mentioned previously, splenectomy may be necessary in the management of children with recurrent acute splenic sequestration syndrome. Certain patients, especially those with S/β thalassemia or SC disease, have sustained splenomegaly. If an enlarged spleen becomes a site for infarction and subsequent abscess, it should be removed. If splenomegaly is accompanied by hypersplenism, splenectomy may be indicated.[407] Rarely, splenectomy may be required for relief of splenic pain.[408]

During the past 30 years, 60 SS children in Jamaica have undergone splenectomy.[408a] Fourteen patients (all less than 2 years old) had acute splenic sequestration. The remainder (children and adolescents) had chronic hypersplenism. In these patients, hemoglobin levels increased 70 per cent following surgery. Since 1978, all patients have received prophylaxis against infection. None have developed sepsis following surgery.

Pregnancy. The management of pregnancy in patients with sickle cell disease has been somewhat controversial. During the past 15 to 20 years, there has been a marked reduction in both fetal and maternal morbidity and mortality. Older surveys report both fetal and maternal mortality as high as 50 per cent.[409] Because of the larger proportion of pregnant women undergoing prenatal check-ups and because of improved standards of nutrition and medical care, the statistics have improved considerably.[409–412] In most contemporary series, maternal deaths are less than 2 per cent, and the incidence of stillborns and neonatal deaths is usually less than 15 per cent. An additional 25 per cent of pregnant women with sickle cell disease have spontaneous abortions.[411, 412] Women with SC disease have a much lower incidence of stillbirths and neonatal deaths than those with SS disease but have an equal incidence of spontaneous abortions.[411] No special therapeutic measures are indicated during pregnancy. Both iron therapy and folate therapy are indicated. Babies should be delivered through the vagina unless there are strong indications for cesarean section. Adequate analgesia should be given, but as mentioned earlier, special attention must be directed toward maintaining adequate ventilation and oxygenation of tissues.

Some studies suggest that maternal and fetal mortality is further reduced if the mother undergoes exchange transfusions during the last trimester.[410] In other centers, prophylactic transfusions (without exchange) are administered throughout pregnancy.[413, 414] However, in view of the general improvement in care of these patients, the efficacy of transfusions is unproved.[415] Indeed, a large prospective controlled study[416] still under way in Chicago indicates that exchange transfusion has no significant effect on fetal and maternal outcome.[417]

Antisickling Agents

During the past 30 years, a variety of remedies have been proposed for the treatment of sickle cell anemia.[417a] Many of these are listed in Table 12–8. Usually, an initial wave of enthusiasm has been followed by the sober realization that the drug was either ineffective or, in some cases, unsafe. Currently, none of these treatments appear to be of clinical value.

Present-day knowledge of the molecular basis of sickling should enable the design of specific antisickling agents. Inhibition of sickle hemoglobin polymerization could result from three independent mechanisms: (1) increase in oxygen affinity, thereby favoring the oxy conformation; (2) interference with the intermolecular contacts involved in polymerization of deoxyhemoglobin S; and (3) reduction in the intracellular concentration of hemoglobin.

Agents that are direct inhibitors of polymerization or that lower intracellular hemoglobin concentration are preferable to those that act by means of increasing oxygen affinity. It is likely that any compound that significantly raises oxygen affinity will induce an increase in red cell production similar to that observed in individuals with high O_2 affinity variants (see Chapter 14). The enhanced viscosity that would accompany the increase in hematocrit could potentiate vaso-occlusive complications. Moreover, if the red cells are not uniformly modified, the treated cells, having high oxygen affinity, would carry a disproportionate share of oxygen, thereby inducing sickling in the untreated cells that are less well oxygenated.

Various compounds that have been proposed as antisickling agents are listed in Table 12–9. They fall into two broad categories: covalent and noncovalent inhibitors of polymerization. Compounds that bind covalently to hemoglobin are more likely to have thera-

Table 12–8. AGENTS THAT HAVE BEEN PROPOSED FOR THE TREATMENT OF SICKLE CELL ANEMIA

Agents	Proposed	Efficacy Contested
Priscoline	Smith et al. (1953)[454]	
Cobalt	Gross et al. (1955)[455]	
Methemoglobin	Beutler (1961)[456]	
Anticoagulants		Salvaggio et al. (1963)[457]
CO	Sirs (1975)[458] Beutler (1975)[460]	Purugganan and McElfresh (1964)[459]
Alkali		Schwartz and McElfresh (1964)[461]
Dextran	Watson-Williams (1963)[462] Barnes et al. (1965)[464]	Oski et al. (1965)[463]
Carbonic anhydrase inhibitors	Hilkovitz (1957)[465]	dos Santos and Lehman (1959)[466] Finney and Hatch (1965)[467]
Phenothiazines	Hathorn and Lewis (1966)[468]	Pearson and Noyes (1967)[469] Oski et al. (1970)[470]
Androgens	Isaacs and Hayhoe (1967)[471]	Raper et al. (1970)[472]
Urea	Nalbandian et al. (1971)[473]	Cooperative Urea Trials Group (1974)[395]
Cyanate	Gillette et al. (1974)[474]	Harkness and Roth (1975)[423]
Aspirin	Chaplin et al. (1980)[475]	Greenberg et al. (1983)[476], Zago et al. (1984)[477]
Hyponatremia-dDAVP	Rosa et al. (1980)[432]	Charache and Walker (1981)[433]
Medroxyprogesterone acetate	deCeulaer et al. (1982)[478]	

Table 12-9. ANTISICKLING AGENTS*

Compound	Concentration (mM)	Increases Solubility of Deoxy Hb S	O_2 Affinity of Dilute Hb	O_2 Affinity of AA RBC	O_2 Affinity of SS RBC	% Sickled Forms at 50% O_2 Sat. (Agent/ No Agent)	Effect on MCHC
Noncovalent							
Urea	100–200	+	SI ↑	SI ↑	SI ↑	0.95	0
Butylurea	20–50	+	SI →	SI →	↑	0.55	→
L-Phenylalanine	25–50	+	SI ↑	0	SI ↑	1.0	0
Cetiedil	0.15–5	0	0	0	0	1.0	SI ↓†
Covalent							
Cyanate	25–100	+	↑	↑	↑	0.60	0
Carbamyl PO_4	25–50	SI +	↑	SI ↑	↑	1.0	0
Cystamine	5–10	0	↑	↑	↑	1.0	SI SE‡
Pyridoxal	10–20	SI +	↑	↑	↑	0.95	SI SE
Methylacetimidate	5–10	+	↑	↑	SI ↑	0.80	SI SE
Dimethyladipimidate	5–10	+	↑	↑	SI ↑	0.55	SI SE
Glyceraldehyde	10–20	+	↑	↑	↑	0.7	SI SE
Dibromoacetylsalicylic acid	5–10	+	SI ↑	↑	↑	NE§	SE
Bis(3,5-dibromosalicyl) fumarate	2–5	+	↑		↑	NE	SE
Bis(3,5-dibromosalicyl) succinate	2–5	+	↑	↑↑	↑	NE	SE
Nitrogen mustard	5–10	+	↑	SI ↑	SI ↑	0.45	0

*This table was prepared from the report of Chang and associates,[431] in which 15 antisickling agents are compared. Solubility was determined from the concentration of the sol phase after centrifugation of the fully deoxygenated gel (see Chapter 11). An increase in solubility implies that the agent is a direct inhibitor of sickle hemoglobin polymerization. Data on intact red cells provide information on whether the agent penetrates the red cell membrane. If the agent significantly reduces the percentage of sickled forms at 50 per cent O_2 saturation, it is likely to penetrate the red cell and directly inhibit polymerization. Conversely, if the agent has no effect (Agent/No Agent > 0.8), it is likely that it inhibits sickling by another mechanism, such as increasing O_2 affinity.

†See reference 434.
‡SE = spheroechinocytosis.
§NE = not possible to measure owing to SE.

peutic potential. None of the noncovalent inhibitors described to date and listed in Table 12–9 would be effective drugs because they bind relatively weakly to sickle hemoglobin and therefore require a high concentration in the plasma in order to be effective. It is possible, although unlikely, that a stereospecific noncovalent inhibitor could be designed that binds to Hb S with such high affinity that a low and presumably nontoxic concentration of drug in the plasma would suffice.

Among the covalent inhbitors, sodium cyanate has received the most attention. This small anion binds irreversibly to amino groups of proteins:

$$RNH_2 + CNO^- + H^+ \rightarrow RNH\overset{O}{\overset{\|}{C}}NH_2$$

Cerami and Manning[418] showed that cyanate was an effective inhibitor of sickling *in vitro*. Moreover, patients treated with cyanate in low doses generally exhibited prolongation of the red cell life span and a higher hematocrit with increased oxygen affinity.[419, 420] Unfortunately, the appearance of reversible peripheral neuropathy made it impossible to evaluate the effects of higher doses of this agent on the incidence of crises or on the long-term course of sickle cell disease.[421, 422] It is likely that orally administered sodium cyanate has a low therapeutic index. In a double-blind crossover study, patients on oral cyanate for 6 months had the same incidence of painful crises as when they received a placebo.[423]

Extracorporeal carbamylation of the patient's blood has been proposed as a means of increasing an agent's therapeutic index. This approach permits more extensive chemical modification of the hemoglobin without risk of toxic side effects. A small number of patients seem to have derived benefit from batch-type extracorporeal treatment with cyanate.[424] Recently, continuous flow devices have been developed for the incubation of blood with a covalent antisickling agent, followed by dialysis of excess drug and return of the blood to the patient.[425, 426] Such an approach may be potentially useful for the administration of antisickling agents, such as cyanate and nitrogen mustard,[427] that cannot be administered systemically. However, covalent inhibitors, such as imidoesters, may react with the external surface of the red cell membrane, forming neoantigens. Once the patient is sensitized, the modified red cells become coated with immunoglobulin and are rapidly cleared from the circulation. The problem poses a potential obstacle to extracorporeal therapy.

A number of other antisickling drugs are now being investigated, and a safe pharmacological approach to sickle cell disease may emerge in the next decade. A variety of chemical strategies have been considered.[428–430] Despite increasing sophistication in the design and testing[431] of antisickling agents, many investigators are discouraged about the prospect of developing a drug that will be a safe and effective inhibitor of sickling. The ideal agent should be easily absorbed by the gastrointestinal tract, enter the plasma, and readily penetrate the red cell membrane so that it can covalently bind to Hb S in such a way that polymerization is inhibited but the hemoglobin continues to bind and unload oxygen normally. Equally important, this ideal compound should have minimal interaction with molecules in other tissues and therefore would have minimal toxicity.

Because the task of developing a "magic bullet" is so formidable, investigators are exploring alternate approaches to therapy. One strategy that has attracted particular interest is to exploit the marked dependence of the rate of polymerization on hemoglobin concentration (see Chapter 11). The simplest way to lower the intracellular concentration of hemoglobin is by reducing the osmolarity of plasma. Sustained hyponatremia can be induced by a regimen consisting of a low-salt diet, a high fluid intake, diuretics, and the synthetic vasopressin analogue desmopressin.[432] In a limited clinical trial, this therapy resulted in a significant inhibition of *in vitro* sickling. However, there was an insufficient period of observation to determine whether patients were benefited during periods of hyponatremia. Unfortunately, the therapy is difficult to administer[433] and requires both careful laboratory monitoring and supervision by physicians experienced in managing fluid and electrolyte balance. Moreover, the therapy is not well tolerated by outpatients,[433] and as a result, compliance is poor. Nevertheless, this approach to therapy seems sufficiently promising that other pharmacological means should be sought for reduction of intracellular hemoglobin concentration. Certain membrane-active agents such as cetiedil[434] and ticlopidine[435, 435a] are capable of lowering MCHC when incubated with red cells *in vitro*. Cetiedil may retard the exit of potassium and water from sickle erythrocytes by inhibition of the Gardos phenomenon.[436, 437] However, it remains to be demonstrated whether these agents, when administered *in vivo*, can effectively lower MCHC. Current clinical trials with both of these agents should provide this information.

Because irreversibly sickled cells contribute to the anemia and perhaps to the vaso-occlusive manifestations of sickle cell disease, another therapeutic strategy involves attempts to prevent the membrane lesion that causes progressive cellular dehydration and eventually leads to the irreversibly sickled cell. Inhibitors of calmodulin may fulfill this role.[438] *In vitro* experiments suggest a rough correlation between the interaction of various agents with calmodulin and their ability to prevent the *in vitro* production of irreversibly sickled cells.[438, 439] Pentoxifylline (Trental) may be a particularly promising agent because it enhances the deformability of deoxygenated SS red cells.[440] However, the mechanism by which this and other membrane-active agents inhibit sickling is still poorly understood.

Manipulation of Hemoglobin Composition

The most definitive approach to the treatment of sickle cell disease involves a permanent alteration in the hemoglobin phenotype. Three strategies have been considered: marrow transplantation, induction of Hb F synthesis, and gene replacement.

Bone marrow transplantation is one of the major advances in recent biomedical research. It has saved the lives of hundreds of patients with severe aplastic anemia as well as a smaller number of children with congenital immune deficiency states. It has also proved to be effective in the treatment of acute leukemias. As mentioned in Chapter 9, several patients with β thalassemia major have received bone marrow transplants. One patient with SS disease and acute leukemia was successfully engrafted with bone marrow from a sibling with sickle trait.[440a] After recovery, the patient's red cells had the expected AS phenotype. Successful engraftment generally requires that the donor and recipient be identical at the major histocompatibility locus. There is a 25 per cent chance that each of a patient's siblings will be a potential donor. The major complications of marrow transplantation are graft-versus-host disease and the development of opportunistic infections. Until these problems can be minimized, marrow transplantation cannot be recommended for diseases such as sickle cell anemia that have reasonably long life expectancy and unpredictable prognosis.

Because Hb F is such a potent inhibitor of sickle hemoglobin polymerization (see Chapter 11), SS patients with unusually high levels of Hb F tend to have a benign clinical course (see the earlier section on prognosis). Therefore, the induction of Hb F synthesis might be expected to ameliorate sickle cell disease, provided it was not accompanied by an increase in intracellular hemoglobin concentration. Extensive studies in primates showed that the antineoplastic agents 5-azacytidine,[441] cytosine arabinoside,[441a] and hydroxyurea[441b] cause a prompt increase in synthesis of γ chains. In anemic baboons given 5-azacytidine, Hb F levels have risen as high as 85 per cent.[441] A small number of patients with SS disease have been treated with 5-azacytidine,[442, 443] and hydroxyurea.[444] All have developed an increase in the proportion of Hb F, one as high as 30 per cent. Moreover, measurements of F cells and F reticulocytes indicate that following therapy, Hb F was distributed more evenly among red cells. It is not yet clear whether 5-azacytidine acts by causing demethylation of the γ-chain gene, enabling it to be more readily expressed. The increase in Hb F following treatment could represent proliferation of less well differentiated erythroid cells that produce a relatively high proportion of Hb F. As shown in Figure 12–22, there appears to be a reduction in the degree of hemolysis and, in some cases, an increase in hemoglobin level. It is not yet clear whether there is any reduction in pain crises or other vaso-occlusive manifestations as a result of this therapy. The long-term potential for oncogenesis is a serious concern with regard to this and other agents that act directly on cell division.

The ultimate goal in genetic engineering is to replace the defective β^S gene with a normal β^A gene. Clearly, this is a Herculean task, posing a series of independent hurdles. First, an adequate amount of normal β globin gene must be transfected into the patient's hematopoietic cells. These cells and their progeny must then be capable of expressing this gene in a well-regulated fashion so that α- and β^A-chain production is balanced and normal Hb A is produced in adequate amounts. Moreover, these transfected cells should have a selective growth advantage, so that they will gradually replace the patient's own erythroid cells and continue to proliferate under the constraints of physiologic erythroid regulation. As discussed in more detail in Chapter 8, these

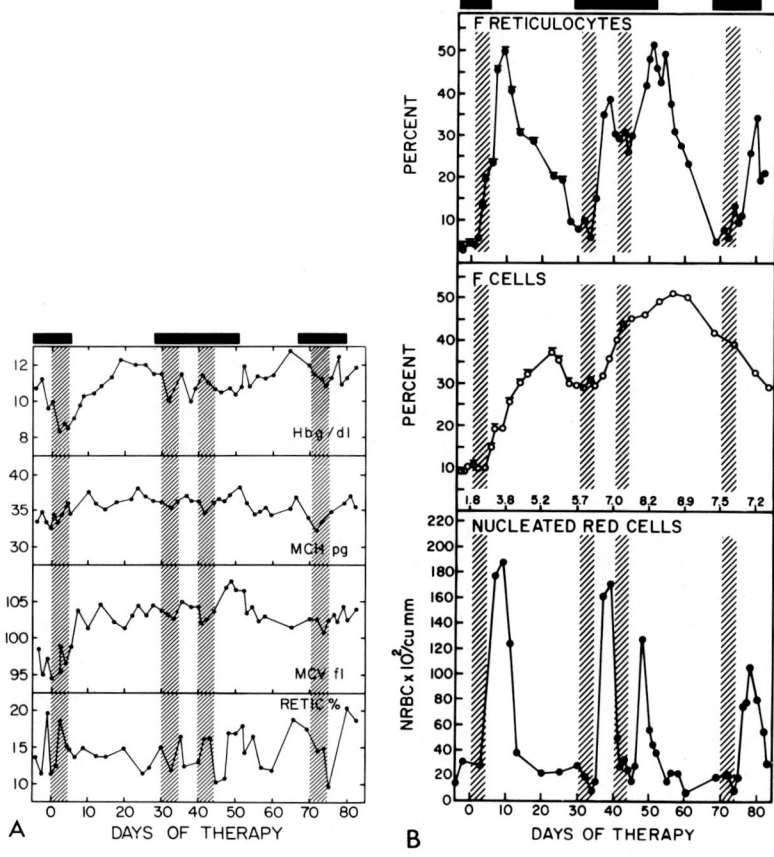

Figure 12–22. *A*, and *B*, Clinical and laboratory findings in a patient with sickle cell anemia treated with 5-azacytidine. Cross-hatched bars indicate treatment periods. Solid black bars indicate pain crises. (From Charache, S., et al.: Proc. Natl. Acad. Sci. USA 80:4842, 1983.)

Figure 12–23. Antenatal diagnosis of sickle cell disease by use of restriction endonuclease Mst II. *A*, Diagram of the flanking region and the 5' portion of the β globin structural gene. Arrows indicate the Mst II sites, including the one corresponding to amino acid position 5, 6, and 7. The 1.15 kb fragment is seen in normal DNA, and the 1.35 kb fragment is seen in sickle DNA. IVS denotes intervening sequences. *B*, Autoradiograph of Mst II–digested DNA, showing samples from parents (AS, AS), a previous child (AA), and cultured amniotic-fluid cells, which demonstrate that the fetus is a SS homozygote.

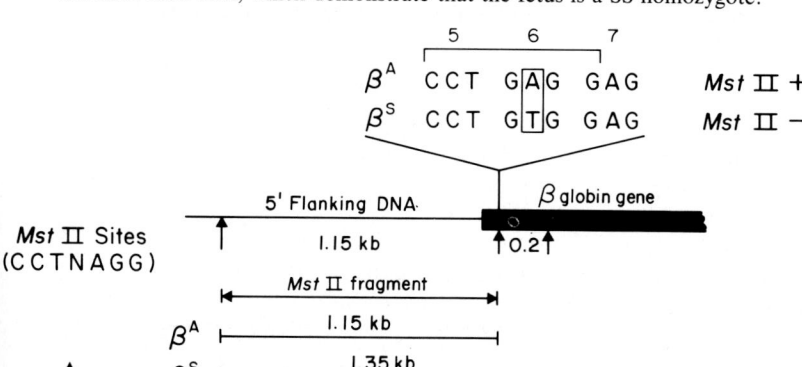

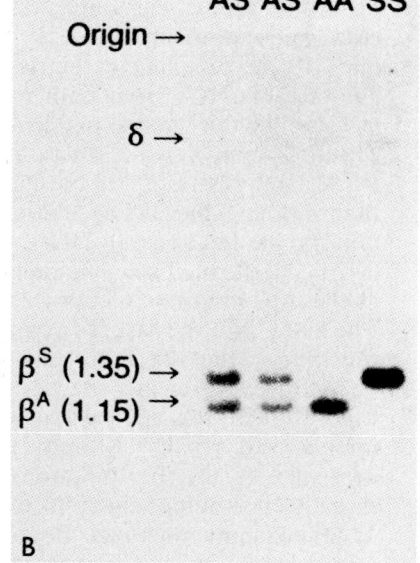

PREVENTION

Genetic counseling can play an important role in the prevention of sickle cell anemia. If both marital partners are known to be AS heterozygotes, they may elect not to have children, knowing that there is a 25 per cent chance that their offspring will be homozygous for Hb S. Obviously, this is a complex and sensitive issue. The counselor must be able to present the pertinent information clearly and thoughtfully, so that the prospective parents can make a rational and guilt-free decision.

Considerable progress has been made on antenatal diagnosis of sickle cell anemia. Initially (1976–1978), it was necessary to obtain a sample of fetal blood from the umbilical vein or from the placenta (if situated anteriorly) in order to measure the synthesis of radioactively labeled β globin chains.[445, 446] Unfortunately, this procedure could not be performed until the twentieth week of gestation and in many cases required the use of fetoscopy, an invasive procedure that entails a 5 per cent risk of fetal mortality. Moreover, the time constraints of this procedure posed an additional problem because elective abortions are seldom performed after the twenty-second week of gestation.

The discovery of linkages between the β^S gene and restriction endonuclease polymorphisms[17, 18] enabled the antenatal diagnosis to be made by analysis of genomic DNA of fetal cells obtained by amniocentesis,[447, 448] a procedure that carries only a 0.5 per cent fetal risk. This approach could be applied to the majority of pregnancies at risk but required analyses of DNA from both parents in order to establish the linkage patterns.

Subsequently, two restriction enzymes (Dde I[449, 450] and Mst II[451–453]) have been identified that will cut normal DNA directly at the β 6 Glu site but fail to cut β^S DNA. This procedure can be performed on amniotic fluid obtained at the fifteenth or sixteenth week of gestation. The assay with the Mst II enzyme is sufficiently sensitive so that the fetal cells do not need to be cultured prior to analysis. As shown in Figure 12–23, this approach provides clear and unequivocal results. Moreover, because the presence of the β^S mutation is determined directly, it is unnecessary to examine parents or other family members. Because of its safety and accuracy, this method should supplant preexisting ones for the antenatal diagnosis of sickle cell anemia. As with genetic counseling in general, the decision to seek prenatal diagnosis as well as the information obtained must be handled with the utmost care and sensitivity.

References

1. Conley, C. L.: Sickle cell anemia—the first molecular disease. In Wintrobe, M. M. (ed.): Blood, Pure and Eloquent. New York, McGraw Hill, 1980, p. 139.
2. Konotey-Ahulu, F. I.: The sickle cell diseases: clinical manifestations including the "sickle crises." Arch. Intern. Med. 133:611, 1974.
3. Raper, A. B.: Sickle cell disease in Africa and America—a comparison. J. Trop. Med. Hyg. 53:49, 1950.
4. Herrick, J. B.: Peculiar elongated and sickle-shaped red blood corpuscles in a case of severe anemia. Arch. Intern. Med. 6:517, 1910.
5. Mason, V. R.: Sickle cell anemia. J.A.M.A. 79:1318, 1922.
6. Emmel, V. E.: A study of the erythrocytes in a case of severe anemia with elongated and sickle-shaped red blood corpuscles. Arch. Intern. Med. 20:586, 1917.
7. Guthrie, C. G., and Huck, J. G.: On the existence of more than four isoagglutinin groups in human blood. Bull. Johns Hopkins Hosp. 34:37, 1923.
8. Neel, J. V.: The clinical detection of the genetic carriers of inherited disease. Medicine (Baltimore) 26:115, 1947.
9. Neel, J. V.: The inheritance of sickle cell anemia. Science 110:64, 1949.
10. Neel, J. V.: The inheritance of the sickling phenomenon with particular reference to sickle cell disease. Blood 6:389, 1951.
11. Accioly, J.: Cited by Azevedo, E.: Historical note on inheritance of sickle cell anemia. Am. J. Hum. Genet. 25:457, 1973.
12. Beet, E. A.: The genetics of the sickle-cell trait in a Bantu tribe. Ann. Eugenics 14:279, 1949.
13. Ranney, H. M.: Observations on the inheritance of sickle cell hemoglobin and hemoglobin C. J. Clin. Invest. 33:1634, 1954.
14. Diggs, L. W., and Ching, R. E.: Pathology of sickle cell anemia. South. Med. J. 27:839, 1934.
15. Gelpi, A. P.: Migrant populations and the diffusion of the sickle cell gene. Ann. Intern. Med. 79:258, 1973.
16. Serjeant, G. R.: Observations on the epidemiology of sickle cell disease. Trans. R. Soc. Trop. Med. Hyg. 75:228, 1981.
17. Kan, Y. W., and Dozy, A. M.: Polymorphism of DNA sequence adjacent to human β-globin structural gene: Relationship to sickle mutation. Proc. Natl. Acad. Sci. USA 75:5631, 1978.
18. Kan, Y. W., and Dozy, A. M.: Evolution of the hemoglobin S and C genes in world populations. Science 209:388, 1980.
19. Mears, J. G., Lachman, H. M., Cabannes, R., Amegnizi, K. P., Labie, D., and Nagel, R. L.: Sickle gene—its origin and diffusion from West Africa. J. Clin. Invest. 68:606, 1981.
20. Mears, J. G., Beldjord, C., Benabadji, M., Belghiti,

Y. A., Baddou, M. A., Labie, D., and Nagel, R. L.: The sickle gene polymorphism in North Africa. Blood 58:599, 1981.
20a. Antonarakis, S. E., Boehm, C. D., Serjeant, G. R., Theisen, C. E., Dover, G. J., and Kazazian, H. H.: Origin of the β^S-globin gene in blacks: The contribution of recurrent mutation or gene conversion or both. Proc. Natl. Acad. Sci. USA 81:853, 1984.
20b. Pagnier, J., Mears, J. G., Dundabel, O., Schaefer, K. E., Beldjord, C., Nagel, R. L., and Labie, D.: Evidence for the multicentric origin of the sickle hemoglobin gene in Africa. Proc. Natl. Acad. Sci. USA 81:1771, 1984.
21. Haldane, J. B. S.: The rate of mutation of human genes. Proceedings of the VIII International Congress on Genetics and Heredity Suppl. 35:367, 1949.
22. Allison, A. C.: Protection afforded by sickle cell trait against subtertian malarial infection. Br. Med. J. 1:290, 1954.
23. Fleming, A. F., Storey, J., Molineaux, L., Iroko, E. A., and Attai, E. D. E.: Abnormal haemoglobins in the Sudan savanna of Nigeria. I. Prevalence of haemoglobins and relationships between sickle cell trait, malaria and survival. Ann. Trop. Med. Parasitol. 73:161, 1979.
24. Bodmer, W. F., and Cavalli-Sforza, L. L.: Genetics, Evolution and Man. San Francisco, W. H. Freeman, 1976, p. 307.
25. Power, H. W.: A model of how the sickle cell gene produces malaria resistance. J. Theor. Biol. 50:121, 1975.
26. Luzzato, L., Nwachuku-Jarrett, E. S., and Reddy, S.: Increased sickling of parasitized erythrocytes is mechanism of resistance against malaria in the sickle trait. Lancet 1:319, 1970.
27. Trager, W., and Jensen, J. B.: Human malaria parasites in continuous culture. Science 193:673, 1976.
28. Friedman, M. J.: Erythrocytic mechanism of sickle cell resistance to malaria. Proc. Natl. Acad. Sci. USA 75:1994, 1978.
29. Pasvol, G., Weatherall, D. J., and Wilson, R. J. M.: Cellular mechanism for the protective effect of haemoglobin S against *P. falciparum* malaria. Nature 274:701, 1978.
30. Roth, E. F., Jr., Friedman, M., Ueda, Y., Tellez, I., Trager, W., and Nagel, R. L.: Sickling rates of human AS red cells infected *in vitro* with *Plasmodium falciparum* malaria. Science 202:650, 1978.
31. Friedman, M. J., Roth, E. F., Nagel, R. L., and Trager, W.: *Plasmodium falciparum*: Physiological interactions with the human sickle cell. Exp. Parasitol. 47:73, 1979.
32. Friedman, M. J.: Ultrastructural damage to the malaria parasite in the sickled cell. J. Protozool. 26:195, 1979.
33. Kramer, M. S., Rooks, Y., and Pearson, H. A.: Growth and development in children with sickle cell trait. A prospective study of matched pairs. N. Engl. J. Med. 299:686, 1978.
34. Blattner, P., Dar, H., and Nitowsky, H. M.: Pregnancy outcome in women with sickle cell trait. J.A.M.A. 238:1392, 1977.
35. Toni, F. B., Dosso, Y., Freminet, A., Leclerc, L., and Poyart, C.: Réactions cardio-respiratoires et métaboliques à un exercice sous-maximal de sujets africains porteurs du trait drepanocytaire. Nouv. Rev. Fr. Hematol. 22:37, 1980.
36. Robinson, J. R., Stone, W. J., and Asendorf, A. C.: Exercise capacity of black sickle cell trait males. Med. Sci. Sports 8:244, 1976.
37. Ramirez, A., Hartley, L. H., Rhodes, D., and Abelmann, W. H.: Morphological features of red blood cells in subjects with sickle cell trait. Arch. Intern. Med. 136:1064, 1976.
38. Murphy, J. R.: Sickle cell hemoglobin (Hb AS) in black football players. J.A.M.A. 225:981, 1973.
39. Heller, P., Best, W. R., Nelson, R. B., and Becktel, J.: Clinical implications of sickle cell trait and glucose-6-phosphate dehydrogenase deficiency in hospitalized black male patients. N. Engl. J. Med. 300:1001, 1979.
40. Stark, A. D., Janerich, D. T., and Jereb, S. K.: The incidence and causes of death in a follow-up study of individuals with haemoglobin AS and AA. Int. J. Epidemiol. 9:325, 1980.
41. Hoiberg, A., Ernst, J., and Uddin, D. E.: Sickle cell trait and glucose-6-phosphate dehydrogenase deficiency. Effects on health and military performance in black navy enlistees. Arch. Intern. Med. 141:1485, 1981.
42. Sears, D. A.: The morbidity of sickle cell trait. A review of the literature. Am. J. Med. 64:1021, 1978.
43. Johnson, L. N.: Sickle cell trait: An update. J. Natl. Med. Assoc. 74:751, 1982.
44. Brody, J. I., Levison, S. P., and Jung, C. J.: Sickle cell trait and hematuria associated with von Willebrand syndromes. Ann. Intern. Med. 86:529, 1977.
45. Richie, J. P., and Kerr, W. S., Jr.: Sickle cell trait: Forgotten cause of hematuria in white patients. J. Urol. 122:134, 1979.
46. Statius van Eps, L. W., Pinedo-Veels, C., DeVries, G. H., and de Koning, J.: Nature of concentrating defect in sickle cell nephropathy. Lancet 1:450, 1970.
47. Schlitt, L. E., and Keitel, H. G.: Renal manifestations of sickle cell disease. A review. Am. J. Med. Sci. 239:773, 1960.
48. Oster, J. R., Lee, S. M., Lespier, L. E., Pellegrini, E. L., and Vaamonde, C. A.: Renal acidification in sickle cell trait. Arch. Intern. Med. 136:30, 1976.
49. Hargus, E. P., Shearin, R., and Colon, A. R.: Pulmonary embolism in a female adolescent with sickle cell trait and oral contraceptive use. Am. J. Obstet. Gynecol. 129:697, 1977.
50. Searle, J. F.: Anaesthesia and sickle cell haemoglobin. Br. J. Anaesth. 44:1335, 1972.
51. Stein, R. E., and Urbaniak, J. R.: Sickle cell disease and the tourniquet. Is there a risk? J. Bone Joint Surg. 57:1027, 1975.
51a. Willinsky, J. S., and Lepow, R.: Sickle cell trait and the use of the pneumatic tourniquet—a case report. J. Am. Podiatry Assoc. 74:38, 1984.
52. Stein, R. E., and Urbaniak, J.: Use of the tourniquet during surgery in patients with sickle cell hemoglobinopathies. Clin. Orthop. 151:231, 1980.
52a. Martin, W. J., Green, D. R., Dougherty, N., Morgan, D., Oheir, D., and Zarro, M.: Tourniquet use in sickle cell disease patients. J. Am. Podiatry Assoc. 74:291, 1984.
53. Dorwart, B. B., Goldberg, M. A., Schumacher, H. R., and Alavi, A.: Absence of increased frequency

of bone and joint disease with hemoglobin AS and AC. Ann. Intern. Med. 86:66, 1977.
54. Keeling, M. M., Lockwood, W. B., and Harris, E. A.: Avascular necrosis and erythrocytosis in sickle-cell trait. N. Engl. J. Med. 290:442, 1974.
55. Rayman, R. B.: Sickle cell trait and the aviator. Aviat. Space Environ. Med. 50:1170, 1979.
56. McKenzie, J. M.: Evaluation of the hazards of sickle trait in aviation. Aviat. Space Environ. Med. 48:753, 1977.
57. Gunby, P.: Military enlists otherwise-qualified sickle trait carriers; research continues. Arch. Intern. Med. 144:901, 1984.
57a. McKenzie, J. M.: Vocational options for those with sickle cell trait. Am. J. Pediatr. Hematol. Oncol. 4:172, 1982.
58. Liebman, J., Lucas, R., Moss, A., Cotton, E., Rosenthal, A., and Ruttenberg, H.: Airline travel for children with chronic pulmonary disease. Pediatrics 57:408, 1976.
58a. Greenberg, M. S., Kass, E. H., and Castle, W. B.: Studies on the destruction of red blood cells. XII. Factors that play a role in the hemolysis and pathologic physiology of sickle cell anemia and related disorders. J. Clin. Invest. 36:833, 1957.
59. Fairbanks, V. F., and Pettit, R. M.: Sickledex test in unstable hemoglobin disorders. J.A.M.A. 220:128, 1972.
59a. Knauss, J. S., and Hahn, D. A.: Homozygous α thalassemia 2 causing a false negative solubility test in sickle cell trait. Clin. Chem. 27:1146, 1981.
59b. Higgs, D. R., Clegg, J. B., Weatherall, D. J., Serjeant, B. E., and Serjeant, G. R.: Interaction of the ααα globin gene haplotype and sickle hemoglobin. Br. J. Haematol. 58:671, 1984.
60. Whitten, C. F., Thomas, J. F., and Nishiura, E. N.: Sickle cell trait counseling—evaluation of counselors and counselees. Am. J. Hum. Genet. 33:802, 1981.
61. Serjeant, G. R.: The Clinical Features of Sickle Cell Disease. New York, Elsevier North-Holland, 1974.
62. Gaston, M., Rosse, W., and the Cooperative Group: The cooperative study of sickle cell disease: Review of study design and objectives. Am. J. Pediatr. Hematol. Oncol. 4:197, 1982.
63. McCurdy, P. R., and Sherman, A. S.: Irreversibly sickled cells and red cell survival in sickle cell anemia. A study with both DF^{32}P and ^{51}Cr. Am. J. Med. 64:253, 1978.
64. Brittenham, G. M., Schechter, A. N., and Noguchi, C. T.: Hemoglobin S polymerization—primary determinant of the hemolytic and clinical severity of the sickling syndromes. Blood, 65:183, 1985.
65. Serjeant, G. R., Serjeant, B. E., and Milner, P. F.: The irreversibly sickled cell: A determinant of hemolysis in sickle cell anemia. Br. J. Haematol. 17:527, 1969.
66. Bothwell, T. H., Hurtado, A. B., Donahue, D. M., and Finch, C. A.: Erythrokinetics. IV. The plasma iron turnover as a measure of erythropoiesis. Blood 12:409, 1957.
67. McCurdy, P. R.: Erythrokinetics in abnormal hemoglobin syndromes. Blood 20:686, 1962.
68. MacIver, J. E., and Parker-Williams, E. J.: The aplastic crisis in sickle cell anemia. Lancet 1:1086, 1961.
69. Lutton, S. D., Schmalzer, E. A., Rao, A. N., Rao, S. P., and Levere, R. D.: Erythroid colony studies in sickle cell anemia in hypoproliferative crisis. Am. J. Hematol. 8:15, 1980.
70. Haddy, T. B., Lusher, J. M., Hendricks, S., and Trosko, B. K.: Erythropoiesis in sickle cell anaemia during acute infection and crisis. Scand. J. Haematol. 22:289, 1979.
71. Serjeant, G. R., Topley, J. M., Mason, K., Serjeant, B. E., Pattison, J. R., Jones, S. E., and Mohamed, R.: Outbreak of aplastic crises in sickle cell anaemia associated with parvovirus-like agent. Lancet 2:595, 1981.
72. Rao, K. R. P., Patel, A. R., Anderson, M. J., Hodgson, J., Jones, S. E., and Pattison, J. R.: Infection with parvovirus-like virus and aplastic crisis in chronic hemolytic anemia. Ann. Intern. Med. 98:930, 1983.
72a. Davis, L. R.: Aplastic crisis in haemolytic anaemia: The role of a parvovirus-like agent. Br. J. Haematol. 55:391, 1983.
73. Mortimer, P. P., Humphries, R. K., Moore, J. G., Purcell, R. H., and Young, N. S.: A human parvovirus-like virus inhibits haematopoietic colony formation in vitro. Nature 302:426, 1983.
73a. Pardoll, D. M., Rodeheffer, R. J., Smith, R. R. L., and Charache, S.: Aplastic crisis due to extensive bone marrow necrosis in sickle cell disease. Arch. Intern. Med. 142:2223, 1982.
74. Chaplin, H., Jr., and Zarkowsky, H.: Combined sickle cell disease and autoimmune hemolytic anemia. Arch. Intern. Med. 141:1091, 1981.
74a. Petz, L. D., Yam, P., Wilkinson, L., Garratty, G., Lubin, B., and Mentzer, W.: Increased IgG molecules bound to the surface of red blood cells of patients with sickle cell anemia. Blood 64:301, 1984.
74b. Hebbel, R. P., and Miller, W. J.: Phagocytosis of sickle erythrocytes: Immunologic and oxidative determinants of hemolytic anemia. Blood 64:733, 1984.
75. Watson-Williams, E. J.: Folic acid deficiency in sickle cell anaemia. E. Afr. Med. J. 39:213, 1962.
75a. Rabb, L. M., Grandison, Y., Mason, K., Hayes, R. J., Sergeant, B., and Sergeant, G. R.: A trial of folate supplementation in children with homozygous sickle cell disease. Br. J. Haematol. 54:589, 1983.
76. Rao, J. N.: Iron deficiency in sickle cell disease. Acta Paediatr. Scand. 69:337, 1980.
77. Peterson, C. M., Graziano, J. H., de Ciutiis, A., Grady, R. W., Cerami, A., Worwood, M., and Jacobs, A.: Iron metabolism, sickle cell disease and response to cyanate. Blood 46:583, 1975.
78. Natta, C., Weiner, M. A., Chang, H., Wolff, J. A., and Fawaz, R.: Sickle cell anemia and iron deficiency. J.A.M.A. 247:1442, 1982.
78a. Davies, S., Henthorn, J., and Brozovic, M.: Iron deficiency in sickle cell anaemia. J. Clin. Pathol. 36:1012, 1983.
78b. Rao, K. R., Patel, A. R., McGinnis, P., and Patel, M. K.: Iron stores in adults with sickle cell anemia. J. Lab. Clin. Med. 103:792, 1984.
78c. Natta, C., Creque, L., and Navarvo, C.: Compartmentalization of iron in sickle cell anemia—an autopsy study. Am. J. Clin. Pathol. 83:76, 1985.
79. Washington, R., and Boggs, D. A.: Urinary iron in patients with sickle cell anemia. J. Lab. Clin. Med. 86:17, 1975.
79a. Castro, O., and Haddy, T. B.: Improved (red cell) survival of iron deficient patients with sickle erythrocytes. N. Engl. J. Med. 308:527, 1983.
80. Vichinsky, E., Klemon, K., and Embury, S.: The diagnosis of iron deficiency anemia in sickle cell disease. Blood 58:963, 1981.
81. Haddy, T. B., and Castro, O.: Overt iron deficiency

in sickle cell disease. Arch. Intern. Med. *142*:1621, 1982.
82. Morgan, A. G., Gruber, C. A., and Serjeant, G. R.: Erythropoietin and renal function in sickle cell disease. Br. Med. J. *285*:1686, 1982.
83. Powars, D. R.: The natural history of sickle cell disease—the first ten years. Semin. Hematol. *12*:267, 1975.
84. Jenkins, M. E., Scott, R. B., and Baird, R. L.: Studies in sickle cell anemia. XVI. Sudden death during sickle cell anemia crises in young children. J. Pediatr. *56*:30, 1960.
85. Pearson, H. A.: Routine screening of umbilical cord blood for sickle cell diseases. J.A.M.A. *227*:420, 1974.
86. Seeler, R. A., Metzger, W., and Mufson, M. A.: *Diplococcus pneumoniae* infections in children with sickle cell anemia. Am. J. Dis. Child. *123*:8, 1972.
87. Robinson, M. G., and Watson, R. J.: Pneumococcal meningitis in sickle cell anemia. N. Engl. J. Med. *74*:1006, 1966.
88. Lobel, J. S., and Bove, K. E.: Clinicopathologic characteristics of septicemia in sickle cell disease. Am. J. Dis. Child. *136*:543, 1982.
89. Eeckels, E., Gatti, F., and Renoirte, A. M.: Abnormal distribution of haemoglobin genotypes in Negro children with severe bacterial infections. Nature *216*:382, 1967.
90. Barrett-Conner, E.: Bacterial infection and sickle cell anemia. Medicine (Baltimore) *50*:97, 1971.
91. Johnston, R. B., Jr.: Increased susceptibility to infection in sickle cell disease: Review of its occurrence and possible causes. South. Med. J. *67*:1342, 1974.
92. Robinson, M. G., and Halpern, C.: Infections, *Escherichia coli*, and sickle cell anemia. J.A.M.A. *230*:1145, 1974.
93. Ward, J., and Smith, A. L.: *Hemophilus influenzae* bacteremia in children with sickle cell disease. J. Pediatr. *88*:261, 1976.
94. Powars, D., Overturf, G., and Turner, E.: Is there an increased risk of *Hemophilus-influenzae* septicemia in children with sickle cell anemia? Pediatrics *71*:927, 1983.
95. Akinyanju, O.: Urinary tract infection and asymptomatic bacteriuria in sickle cell disease. Niger. Med. J. *9*:593, 1979.
96. Pearson, H. A., Spencer, R. P., and Cornelius E. A.: Functional asplenia in sickle cell anemia. N. Engl. J. Med. *281*:923, 1969.
97. Casper, J. T., Koethe, S., Roney, G. E., and Thatcher, L. G.: A new method for studying splenic reticuloendothelial dysfunction in sickle cell disease patients and its clinical application: A brief report. Blood *47*:183, 1976.
98. Pearson, H. A., McIntosh, S., Ritchey, A. K., Lobel, J. S., Rooks, Y., and Johnston, D.: Developmental aspects of splenic function in sickle cell diseases. Blood *53*:358, 1979.
98a. Rogers, D. W., Serjeant, B. E., and Serjeant, G. R.: Early rise in pitted red cell count as a guide to susceptibility to infection in childhood sickle-cell anemia. Arch. Dis. Child. *57*:338, 1982.
99. Pegelow, C. H., Wilson, B., Overturf, G. D., Tigner-Weeks, L., and Powars, D.: Infection in splenectomized sickle cell disease patients. Clin. Pediatr. *19*:102, 1980.
100. Schwartz, A. D., and Pearson, H. A.: Impaired antibody response to intravenous immunization in sickle cell anemia. Pediatr. Res. *6*:145, 1972.
101. Buchanan, G. R., and Glader, B. E.: Leukocyte counts in children with sickle cell disease. Am. J. Dis. Child. *132*:396, 1978.
102. Dimitrov, N. V., Douwes, F. R., Bartolotta, B., Nochumson, S., and Toth, M. A.: Metabolic activity of polymorphonuclear leukocytes in sickle cell anemia. Acta Haematol. *47*:283, 1972.
103. Kaplan, S. S., and Nardi, M.: Impairment of leukocyte function during sickle cell crisis. J. Reticuloendothel. Soc. *22*:499, 1977.
104. Strauss, R. G., Johnson, R. B., Jr., Asbrock, T., Moreno, H., and Lehmeyer, J.: Neutrophil oxidative metabolism in sickle cell disease. J. Pediatr. *89*:391, 1976.
105. Akenzua, G. I., and Amiengheme, O. R.: Inhibitor of *in vitro* neutrophil migration in sera of children with homozygous sickle cell gene during pain crisis. Br. J. Haematol. *47*:345, 1981.
106. Spirer, Z., Weisman, Y., Zakuth, V., Fridkin, M., and Bogair, N.: Decreased serum tuftsin concentrations in sickle cell disease. Arch. Dis. Child. *55*:566, 1980.
107. Ballas, S. K., Burka, E. R., Lewis, C. N., and Krasnow, S. H.: Serum immunoglobulin levels in patients having sickle cell syndromes. Am. J. Clin. Pathol. *73*:394, 1980.
108. Henandez, P., Carnot, J., Cruz, C., Dorticos, E., Espinosa, E., Gonzales, A., Santos, M. N., and Villaescusa, R.: Circulating immune complexes in sickle cell hepatic crises. Acta Haematol. *65*:15, 1981.
109. Winkelstein, J. A., and Drachman, R. H.: Deficiency of pneumococcal serum opsonizing activity in sickle cell disease. N. Engl. J. Med. *279*:459, 1968.
110. Johnston, R. B., Jr., Newman, S. L., and Struth, A. G.: An abnormality of the alternate pathway of complement activation in sickle cell disease. N. Engl. J. Med. *288*:803, 1073.
111. Bjornson, A. B., Lobel, J. S., and Lampkin, B. C.: Humoral components of host defense in sickle cell disease during painful crisis and asymptomatic periods. J. Pediatr. *96*:259, 1980.
112. Hand, W. L., and King, N. L.: Deficiency of serum bactericidal activity against *Salmonella typhimurium* in sickle cell anaemia. Clin. Exp. Immunol. *30*:262, 1977.
113. Corry, J. M., Polhill, R. B., Jr., Edmonds, S. R., and Johnston, R. B., Jr.: Activity of the alternative complement pathway after splenectomy: Comparison to activity in sickle cell disease and hypogammaglobulinemia. J. Pediatr. *95*:964, 1979.
114. Platt, O. S., Rosenstock, W., and Espeland, M. A.: Impact of sickle hemoglobinopathies on growth and development. N. Engl. J. Med. *311*:7, 1984.
115. Jimenez, C. T., Scott, R. B., Henry, W. L., Sampson, C. C., and Ferguson, A. D.: Studies in sickle cell anemia. Am. J. Dis. Child. *111*:497, 1966.
116. Ashcroft, M. T., Serjeant, G. R., and Desai, P.: Heights, weights and skeletal age of Jamaican adolescents with sickle cell anemia. Arch. Dis. Child. *47*:519, 1972.
117. Luban, N. L. C., Leikin, S. L., and August, G. A.: Growth and development in sickle cell anemia. Am. J. Pediatr. Hematol. Oncol. *4*:61, 1982.
118. Whitten, C. F.: Growth status of children with sickle cell anemia. Am. J. Dis. Child. *102*:101, 1961.
119. Olambiwonnu, N. O., Penny, R., and Frasier, S.

D.: Sexual maturation in subjects with sickle cell anemia: Studies of serum gonadotropin concentration, height, weight, and skeletal age. J. Pediatr. 87:459, 1975.
120. Abbasi, A. A., Prasad, A. S., Ortega, J., Congco, E., and Oberleas, D.: Gonadal function abnormalities in sickle cell anemia. Ann. Intern. Med. 85:601, 1976.
121. Nahoum, C. R. D., Fontes, E. A., and Freire, F. R.: Semen analysis in sickle cell disease. Andrologia 12:542, 1980.
122. Osegbe, D. N., Akinyanju, O., and Amaku, E. O.: Fertility in males with sickle cell disease. Lancet 3:275, 1981.
123. Alleyne, S. I., Raseo, R. D., and Serjeant, G. R.: Sexual development and fertility of Jamaican female patients with homozygous sickle cell disease. Arch. Intern. Med. 141:1295, 1981.
123a. Subramanian, L., and Prasad, A. S.: Zinc-deficiency in a patient with sickle-cell disease. (Review.) Nutr. Rev. 41:217, 1983.
123b. Prasad, A. S., and Cossack, Z. T.: Zinc in sickle-cell disease. Trans. Assoc. Am. Physicians 96:246, 1983.
124. Gordon, P. A., Breeze, G. R., Mann, J. R., and Stuart, J.: Coagulation fibrinolysis in sickle cell disease. J. Clin. Pathol. 27:485, 1974.
125. Freedman, M. L., and Karpatkin, S.: Short communication: Elevated platelet count and megathrombocyte number in sickle cell anemia. Blood 46:579, 1975.
126. Haut, M. J., Cowan, D. H., and Harris, J. W.: Platelet function and survival in sickle cell disease. J. Lab. Clin. Med. 82:44, 1973.
127. Buchanan, G. R., and Holtkamp, C. A.: Platelet aggregation, malondialdehyde generation and production time in children with sickle cell anaemia. Thromb. Haemost. 46:690, 1981.
128. Stuart, M. J., Stockman, J. A., and Oski, F. A.: Abnormalities of platelet aggregation in the vaso-occlusive crisis of sickle cell anemia. J. Pediatr. 85:629, 1974.
129. Leichtman, D. A., and Brewer, G. J.: A plasma inhibitor of ristocetin-induced platelet aggregation in platelets with sickle hemoglobinopathies. Am. J. Hematol. 2:251, 1977.
130. Mehta, P., and Mehta, J.: Abnormalities of platelet aggregation in sickle cell disease. J. Pediatr. 96:209, 1980.
130a. Buchanan, G. R., and Holtkamp, C. A.: Evidence against enhanced platelet activity in sickle cell anaemia. Br. J. Haematol. 54:595, 1983.
131. Richardson, S. G. N., Matthews, K. B., Stuart, J., Geddes, A. M., and Wilcox, R. M.: Serial changes in coagulation and viscosity during sickle-cell crisis. Br. J. Haematol. 41:95, 1979.
132. Mattii, R., Weinger, R., and Sisc, H. S.: Coagulation, fibrinogen survival and fibrin split products in sickle cell disease. Blood 42:1004, 1973.
133. Leslie, J., Langler, D., Serjeant, G. R., Serjeant, B. E., Desai, P., and Gordon, Y. B.: Coagulation changes during the steady state in homozygous sickle cell disease in Jamaica. Br. J. Haematol. 30:159, 1975.
134. Ittyerah, R., Alkjaersig, N., Fletcher, A., and Chaplin, H.: Coagulation factor XIII concentration in sickle cell disease. J. Lab. Clin. Med. 88:546, 1976.
135. Leichtman, D. A., and Brewer, G. J.: Elevated plasma levels of fibrinopeptide A during sickle cell anemia pain crisis—evidence for intravascular coagulation. Am. J. Hematol. 5:183, 1978.
136. Mehta, P.: Significance of plasma β-thromboglobulin values in patients with sickle cell disease. J. Pediatr. 97:941, 1980.
137. Alkjaersig, N., Fletcher, A., Joist, H., and Chaplin, H., Jr.: Hemostatic alterations accompanying sickle cell pain crises. J. Lab. Clin. Med. 88:440, 1976.
138. Mackie, I., Bull, H., and Brozovic, M.: Altered factor VIII complexes in sickle cell disease. Br. J. Haematol. 46:499, 1980.
139. Green, D., Dwaan, H. C., and Ruiz, G.: Impaired fibrinolysis in sickle cell disease. Thromb. Haemost. 24:10, 1970.
140. Walsh, R. T., Lusher, J. M., and Barnhart, M. I.: Coagulation and fibrinolysis studies in sickle cell anemia. In Mammen, E. F., Anderson, G. F., and Barnhart, M. I. (eds.): Sickle Cell Disease. Stuttgart, Schattauer Verlag, 1973, p. 271.
141. Hilgartner, M. W., Horowitz, H., Erlandson, M., Ferguson, A., and Smith, C. H.: Studies of the coagulation mechanism in patients with sickle cell anemia. Am. J. Dis. Child. 102:591, 1961.
142. Basu, A. K., and Woodruff, A. W.: Effect of pyrexia on sicklaemic states. Lancet 2:1088, 1963.
143. Hebbel, R. P., Boogaert, M. A., Eaton, J. W., and Steinberg, M. H.: Erythrocyte adherence to endothelium in sickle cell anemia. A possible determinant of disease severity. N. Engl. J. Med. 302:992, 1980.
144. Hebbel, R. P., Moldow, C. F., and Steinberg, M. H.: Modulation of erythrocyte endothelial interactions and the vaso-occlusive severity of sickling disorders. Blood 58:947, 1981.
145. Redwood, A. M., Williams, E. M., Desai, P., and Serjeant, G. R.: Climate and painful crisis of sickle cell disease in Jamaica. Br. Med. J. 1:66, 1976.
146. Seeler, R. A.: Non-seasonality of sickle cell crisis. Lancet 2:743, 1973.
147. Iuchi, I., Diggs, L. W., and Upshaw, J. D., Jr.: Benzidine-positive pigments in serum of patients with sickle cell anemia during painful crises. Ann. Intern. Med. 60:1022, 1964.
147a. Westerman, M. P., and Bacus, J. W.: Red blood cell morphology in sickle cell anemia as determined by image processing analysis: The relationship to painful crisis. Am. J. Clin. Pathol. 79:667, 1983.
147b. Kenny, M. W., Meaken, M., Worthington, D. J., and Stuart, J.: Erythrocyte deformability in sickle crisis. Br. J. Haematol. 49:103, 1981.
147c. Fabry, M. E., Benjamin, L., Lawrence, C., and Nagel, R. L.: An objective sign of painful crisis in sickle cell anemia: Concomitant reduction of high density red cells. Blood 62:56a, 1983.
147d. Warth, J. A., and Rucknagel, D. L.: Echinocytic change in sickle cell pain crisis. Blood 62:62a, 1983.
147e. Rieber, E. E., Veliz, G., and Pollack, S.: Red cells in sickle cell crisis: Observations on the pathophysiology of crisis. Blood 49:967, 1977.
147f. Lucas, G. S., Caldwell, N. M., and Stuart, J.: Fluctuating deformability of oxygenated sickle erythrocytes in the asymptomatic state and in painful crisis. Br. J. Haematol. 59:363, 1985.
148. Roth, E. F., Jr., Bardfeld, P. A., Goldsmith, S. J., Radel, E., and Williams, J. C.: Sickle cell crisis as evaluated from measurements of hydroxybutyrate dehydrogenase and myoglobin in plasma. Clin. Chem. 27:314, 1981.
149. Karayalcin, G., Lanzkowsky, P., and Kazi, A. B.: Serum α-hydroxybutyrate dehydrogenase levels in

children with sickle cell disease. Am. J. Pediatr. Hematol. Oncol. *3*:169, 1981.
150. Leavell, S. R., and Ford, C. V.: Psycho-pathology in patients with sickle cell disease. Psychosomatics *24*:23, 1983.
151. Shulman, S., Bartlett, J., Clyde, W. A., and Ayoub, E. M.: The unusual severity of mycoplasmal pneumonia in children with sickle cell disease. N. Engl. J. Med. *287*:164, 1972.
152. Charache, S., Scott, J. C., and Charache, P.: "Acute chest syndrome" in adults with sickle cell anemia. Arch. Intern. Med. *139*:67, 1979.
152a. Davies, S. C., Luce, P. J., Win, A. A., Riordan, J. F., and Brozovic, M.: Acute chest syndrome in sickle cell disease. Lancet *1*:36, 1984.
152b. Shapiro, M. P., and Hayes, J. A.: Fat embolism in sickle cell disease—report of a case with a brief review of the literature. Arch. Intern. Med. *144*:181, 1984.
153. Moser, K. M., and Shea, J. C. L.: The relationship between pulmonary infarction, cor pulmonale and sickle states. Am. J. Med. *22*:561, 1957.
154. Diggs, L. W.: Pulmonary lesions in sickle cell anemia. Blood *34*:734, 1969.
155. Haupt, H. M., Moore, G. W., Bauer, T. W., and Hutchins, G. M.: The lung in sickle cell disease. Chest *81*:332, 1982.
156. Barreras, L., Diggs, L. W., and Bell, A.: Erythrocyte morphology in patients with sickle cell anemia and pulmonary emboli. J.A.M.A. *203*:569, 1968.
157. Karayalcin, G., Imram, M., and Rosner, F.: "Blister cells": Association with pregnancy, sickle cell disease, and pulmonary infarction. J.A.M.A. *219*:1727, 1972.
158. Stevens, M. C. G., Padwick, M., and Serjeant, G. R.: Observations on the natural history of dactylitis in homozygous sickle cell disease. Clin. Pediatr. *20*:311, 1981.
159. Serjeant, G. R., and Ashcroft, M. T.: Shortening of the digits in sickle cell anaemia—a sequela of the hand-foot syndrome. Trop. Geogr. Med. *23*:341, 1971.
160. Keeley, K., and Buchanan, G. R.: Acute infarction of long bones in children with sickle cell anemia. J. Pediatr. *101*:170, 1982.
161. Charache, S., and Page, D. L.: Infarction of bone marrow in the sickle cell disorders. Ann. Intern. Med. *67*:1195, 1967.
162. Reynolds, J.: Roentgenological Features of Sickle Cell Disease and Related Hemoglobinopathies. Springfield, Illinois, Charles C Thomas, 1965.
163. Bohrer, S. P.: Acute long bone diaphyseal infarcts in sickle cell disease. Br. J. Radiol. *43*:685, 1970.
164. Alavi, A., Bond, J. P., Kuhl, D. E., and Creech, R. H.: Scan detection of bone marrow infarcts in sickle cell disorders. J. Nucl. Med. *15*:1003, 1974.
165. Milner, P. F., and Brown, M.: Bone marrow infarction in sickle cell anemia: Correlation with hematologic profiles. Blood *60*:1411, 1982.
166. Sain, A., Sham, R., and Silver, L.: Bone scan in sickle cell crisis. Clin. Nucl. Med. *3*:85, 1978.
167. Fleisher, G. R., Paradise, J. E., Plotkin, S. A., and Borden, S.: Falsely normal radionuclide scans for osteomyelitis. Am. J. Dis. Child. *134*:499, 1980.
167a. Koren, A., Garty, I., and Katzuni, E.: Bone infarction in children with sickle cell disease. Early diagnosis and differentiation from osteomyelitis. Eur. J. Pediatr. *142*:93, 1984.
167b. Amundsen, T. R., Siegel, M. J., and Siegel, B. A.: Osteomyelitis and infarction in sickle cell hemoglobinopathies—differentiation by combined technetium and gallium scintigraphy. Radiology *153*:807, 1984.
168. Schumacher, H. R., Andrews, R., and McLaughlin, G.: Arthropathy in sickle cell disease. Ann. Intern. Med. *78*:203, 1973.
169. Espinoza, L. R., Spilbert, I., and Osterland, C. K.: Joint manifestations of sickle cell disease. Medicine *53*:295, 1974.
169a. deCeulaer, K., Forbes, M., Roper, D., and Serjeant, G. R.: Non-gouty arthritis in sickle cell disease—report of 37 consecutive cases. Ann. Rheum. Dis. *43*:599, 1984.
169b. Kaklamanis, P.: Osteoarticular manifestations in sickle cell disorders. Clin. Rheumatol. *3*:419, 1984.
170. Rothschild, B. M., and Sebes, J. I.: Calcaneal abnormalities and erosive bone disease associated with sickle cell anemia. Am. J. Med. *71*:427, 1981.
171. Ball, G. V., and Sorenson, L. B.: The pathogenesis of hyperuricemia and gout in sickle cell anemia. Arthritis Rheum. *13*:846, 1970.
171a. Reynolds, M. D.: Gout and hyperuricemia associated with sickle cell disease. Semin. Arthritis Rheum. *12*:404, 1983.
172. Rothschild, B. M., Sienknecht, C. W., Kaplan, S. B., and Spindler, J. S.: Sickle cell disease associated with uric acid deposition disease. Ann. Rheum. Dis. *39*:392, 1980.
173. Seeler, R. A., and Shwiaki, M. Z.: Acute splenic sequestration crisis (ASSC) in young children with sickle cell anemia. Clinical observations in 20 episodes in 14 children. Clin. Pediatr. *11*:701, 1972.
174. Topley, J. M., Rogers, D. W., Stevens, M. C. G., and Serjeant, G. R.: Acute splenic sequestration and hypersplenism in the first five years in homozygous sickle cell disease. Arch. Dis. Child. *56*:765, 1981.
175. Kudsk, K. A., Tranbaugh, R. F., and Sheldon, G. F.: Acute surgical illness in patients with sickle cell anemia. Am. J. Surg. *142*:113, 1981.
176. Falk, R. H., and Hood, W. B.: The heart in sickle cell anemia. Arch. Intern. Med. *142*:1680, 1982.
177. Johnson, C. S., and Giorgio, A. J.: Arterial blood pressure in adults with sickle cell disease. Arch. Intern. Med. *141*:891, 1981.
178. Rees, A. H., Stefadouros, M. A., Strong, W. B., Miller, M. D., Gilman, P., Rigby, J. A., and McFarlane, J.: Left ventricular performance in children with homozygous sickle cell anaemia. Br. Heart J. *40*:690, 1978.
179. Varat, M. A., Adolph, R. J., and Fowler, N. O.: Cardiovascular effects of anemia. Am. Heart J. *83*:415, 1972.
180. Lindsay, J., Meshel, J. C., and Patterson, R. H.: The cardiovascular manifestations of sickle cell disease. Arch. Intern. Med. *133*:643, 1974.
181. Klinefelter, H. F.: The heart in sickle cell anemia. Am. J. Med. Sci. *203*:34, 1942.
182. Gerry, J. L., Baird, M. G., and Fortuin, N. J.: Evaluation of left ventricular function in patients with sickle cell anemia. Am. J. Med. *60*:968, 1976.
183. Covarrubias, E. A., Sheikh, M. U., Solanki, D. L., Morjaria, M., and Fox, L. M.: Left ventricular function in sickle cell anemia: A noninvasive evaluation. South. Med. J. *73*:342, 1980.
184. Denenberg, B. S., Criner, G., Jones, R., and Spann, J. F.: Cardiac function in sickle cell anemia. Am. J. Cardiol. *51*:1674, 1983.
184a. Manno, B. V., Burka, E. R., Hakki, A. H., Manno, C. S., Iskandrian, A. S., and Noone, A. M.:

Biventricular function in sickle cell anemia—radionuclide angiographic and Tl-201 scintigraphic evaluation. Am. J. Cardiol. *52*:584, 1983.
185. Val-Mejias, J., Lee, W. K., Weisse, A. B., and Regan, T. J.: Left ventricular performance during and after sickle cell crisis. Am. Heart J. *97*:585, 1979.
185a. Barrett, O., Saunders, D. E., McFarland, D. E., and Humphries, J. O.: Myocardial infarction in sickle cell anemia. Am. J. Hematol. *16*:139, 1984.
185b. Martin, C., Cobb, C., Johnson, C., Tatter, D., and Haywood, L. J.: Myocardial infarction in sickle cell disease without atherosclerosis. Circulation *68*:III–324a, 1983.
186. Jensen, W. N., Rucknagel, D. L., and Taylor, W. J.: In vivo study of the sickle cell phenomenon. J. Lab. Clin. Med. *56*:854, 1960.
187. Alpert, B. S., Gilman, P. A., Strong, W. B., Ellison, M. F., Miller, M. D., McFarlane, J., and Hayashidera, T.: Hemodynamic and ECG responses to exercise in children with sickle cell anemia. Am. J. Dis. Child. *135*:362, 1981.
188. Song, J.: Pathology of Sickle Cell Disease. Springfield, Illinois, Charles C Thomas, 1971.
189. Gerry, J. L., Burkley, B. H., and Hutchings, G. M.: Clinicopathologic analysis of cardiac dysfunction in 52 patients with sickle cell anemia. Am. J. Cardiol. *42*:211, 1978.
190. Baroldi, G.: High resistance of the human myocardium to shock and red blood cell aggregation (sludge). Cardiology *54*:271, 1969.
191. Bromberg, P. A., and Jensen, W. N.: Arterial oxygen unsaturation in sickle cell disease. Am. Rev. Respir. Dis. *96*:400, 1967.
192. Scharf, M. B., Lobel, J. S., Caldwell, E., Cameron, B. F., Kramer, M., Demarchis, J., and Paine, C.: Nocturnal oxygen desaturation in patients with sickle cell anemia. J.A.M.A. *249*:1753, 1983.
193. Collins, F. S., and Orringer, E. P.: Pulmonary hypertension and cor pulmonale in the sickle hemoglobinopathies. Am. J. Med. *73*:814, 1982.
194. Bromberg, P. A.: Pulmonary aspects of sickle cell disease. Arch. Intern. Med. *133*:652, 1974.
195. Sproule, B. J., Halden, E. R., and Miller, W. F.: A study of cardiopulmonary alterations in patients with sickle cell disease and its variants. J. Clin. Invest. *37*:486, 1958.
196. Elegbele, O. O.: Pulmonary function studies in sickle cell anemia. Trop. Geogr. Med. *30*:473, 1978.
197. Wall, M. A., Platt, O. S., and Strieder, D. J.: Lung function in children with sickle cell anemia. Am. Rev. Respir. Dis. *120*:210, 1979.
198. Miller, G. J., and Serjeant, G. R.: An assessment of lung volumes and gas transfer in sickle cell anemia. Thorax *26*:309, 1971.
198a. Walker, B. K., Ballas, S. K., and Burka, E. R.: The diagnosis of pulmonary thromboembolism in sickle cell disease. Am. J. Hematol. *7*:219, 1979.
199. Maddrey, W. C., Cukier, J. O., Maglalang, A. C., Boitnott, J. K., and Odell, G. B.: Hepatic bilirubin UDP-glucuronyltransferase in patients with sickle cell anemia. Gastroenterology *74*:193, 1978.
200. Brittain, H. P., de la Torre, A., and Willey, E. N.: A case of sickle cell disease with an abscess arising in an infarct of the liver. Ann. Intern. Med. *65*:560, 1966.
201. Green, T. W., Conley, C. L., and Berthrong, M.: The liver in sickle cell anemia. Bull. Johns Hopkins Hosp. *92*:99, 1953.
202. Isichi, U. P.: Liver function and the diagnostic significance of biochemical changes in the blood of African children with sickle cell disease. J. Clin. Pathol. *33*:626, 1980.
203. Sheehy, T. W.: Sickle cell hepatopathy. South. Med. J. *70*:533, 1977.
204. Bauer, T. W., Moore, G. W., and Hutchins, G. M.: The liver in sickle cell disease. A clinicopathologic study of 70 patients. Am. J. Med. *69*:833, 1980.
205. Sheehy, T. W., Law, D. E., and Wade, B. H.: Exchange transfusion for sickle cell intrahepatic cholestasis. Arch. Intern. Med. *140*:1364, 1980.
206. Klion, F. M., Weiner, M. J., and Schaffner, F.: Cholestasis in sickle cell anemia. Am. J. Med. *37*:829, 1964.
207. Weens, H. S.: Cholelithiasis in sickle cell anemia. Ann. Intern. Med. *22*:182, 1945.
208. Barrett-Conner, E.: Cholelithiasis in sickle anemia. Am. J. Med. *45*:889, 1968.
209. Karayalcin, G., Hassani, N., Abrams, M., and Lanzkowsky, P.: Cholelithiasis in children with sickle cell disease. Am. J. Dis. Child. *133*:306, 1979.
210. Lachman, B. S., Lazerson, J., Starshak, R. J., Vaughters, F. M., and Werlin, S. L.: The prevalence of cholelithiasis in sickle cell disease as diagnosed by ultrasound and cholecystography. Pediatrics *64*:601, 1979.
211. Sarnaik, S., Slovis, T. L., Corbett, D. P., Emami, A., and Whitten, C. F.: Incidence of cholelithiasis in sickle cell anemia using the ultrasonic gray-scale technique. J. Pediatr. *96*:1005, 1980.
212. Cunningham, J. J., Houlihan, S. M., and Altay, C.: Cholecystosonography in children with sickle cell disease: Technical approach and clinical results. J. Clin. Ultrasound *9*:231, 1981.
213. McCall, I. W., Desai, P., Serjeant, B. E., and Serjeant, G. R.: Cholelithiasis in Jamaican patients with homozygous sickle cell disease. Am. J. Hematol. *3*:15, 1977.
214. Akinyanju, O., and Ladapo, F.: Cholelithiasis and biliary tract disease in sickle cell disease in Nigerians. Postgrad. Med. J. *55*:400, 1979.
215. Ariyan, S., Shessel, F. S., and Pickett, L. K.: Cholecystitis and cholelithiasis masking as abdominal crises in sickle cell disease. Pediatrics *58*:252, 1976.
216. Solanki, D. L., and McCurdy, P. R.: Cholelithiasis in sickle cell anemia: A case for elective cholecystectomy. Am. J. Med. Sci. *277*:319, 1979.
217. Stephens, C. G., and Scott, R. B.: Cholelithiasis in sickle cell anemia. Surgical or medical management. Arch. Intern. Med. *140*:648, 1980.
218. Perillie, P. E., and Epstein, F. H.: Sickling phenomenon produced by hypertonic solutions: A possible explanation for the hyposthenuria of sicklemia. J. Clin. Invest. *42*:570, 1963.
219. Chaplin, H.: Hematuria in hemoglobin S disorders. Arch. Intern. Med. *140*:1573, 1980.
220. Keitel, A. G., Thompson, D., and Itano, H. A.: Hyposthenuria in sickle cell anemia: A reversible renal defect. J. Clin. Invest. *35*:998, 1958.
221. Statius van Eps, L. W., Schouten, H., La Porte-Wijsman, L. W., and Struyker Boudier, A. M.: The influence of red blood cell transfusions on the hyposthenuria and renal hemodynamics of sickle cell anemia. Clin. Chim. Acta *17*:449, 1967.
222. Heinemann, H. O., and Cheung, M. W.: Renal concentrating mechanism in sickle cell anemia. J. Lab. Clin. Med. *49*:923, 1957.
223. Lief, P. D., Sullivan, A., and Goldberg, M.: Phys-

223. iological contributions of thin and thick loops of Henle to the renal concentrating mechanism. (Abstract.) J. Clin. Invest. 48:52, 1969.
224. Buckalew, V. M., and Someren, A.: Renal manifestations of sickle cell disease. Arch. Intern. Med. 133:660, 1974.
225. Oster, J. R., Lespier, L. E., Lee, S. M., Pellegrini, E. L., and Vaamonde, C. A.: Renal acidification in sickle cell disease. J. Lab. Clin. Med. 88:389, 1976.
226. DeFronzo, R. A., Taufield, P. A., Black, H., McPhedran, P., and Cooke, C. R.: Impaired renal tubular potassium secretion in sickle cell disease. Ann. Intern. Med. 90:310, 1979.
227. Batille, D., Itsarayoungyuen, K., Arruda, J. A. L., and Kurtzman, N. A.: Hyperkalemic hyperchloremic metabolic acidosis in sickle cell hemoglobinopathies. Am. J. Med. 72:188, 1982.
228. Radel, E. G., Kochen, J. A., and Finberg, L.: Hyponatremia in sickle cell disease. J. Pediatr. 88:800, 1976.
229. Matustik, M. C., Carpentieri, U., Corn, C., and Meyer, W. J., III: Hyperreninemia and hyperaldosteronism in sickle cell anemia. Pediatrics 95:206, 1979.
230. Smith, E. C., Valika, K. S., Woo, J. E., O'Donnell, J. G., Gordon, D. L., and Westerman, M. P.: Serum phosphate abnormalities in sickle cell anemia. Proc. Soc. Exp. Biol. Med. 168:254, 1981.
231. Diamond, H. S., Meisel, A. D., and Holden, D.: The natural history of urate overproduction in sickle cell anemia. Ann. Intern. Med. 90:752, 1979.
232. McCall, I. W., Moule, N., Desai, P., and Serjeant, G. R.: Urographic findings in homozygous sickle cell disease. Radiology 129:99, 1978.
233. Mostofi, F. K., and Bruegge, C. F. V.: Lesions in kidneys removed for unilateral hematuria in sickle cell disease. Arch. Pathol. 63:336, 1957.
234. Lucas, W. M., and Bullock, W.: Hematuria in sickle cell disease. J. Urol. 83:733, 1960.
235. Bilinski, R. T., Kandel, G. L., and Rabiner, S. F.: Epsilon aminocaproic acid therapy of hematuria due to heterozygous sickle cell diseases. J. Urol. 102:93, 1969.
236. Black, W. D., Hatch, F. E., and Acchiardo, S.: Aminocaproic acid in prolonged hematuria of patients with sicklemia. Arch. Intern. Med. 136:678, 1976.
237. McInnes, B. K.: The management of hematuria associated with sickle hemoglobinopathies. J. Urol. 124:171, 1980.
238. John, E. G., Schaile, S. G., Spigos, D. G., Cort, J. H., and Rosenthal, I. M.: Effectiveness of triglycyl vasopressin in persistent hematuria associated with sickle cell hemoglobin. Arch. Intern. Med. 140:1539, 1980.
238a. Goodman, M. S., and Jacobs, J. A.: Sickle cell hematuria controlled by intrarenal oxychlorosene irrigation. J. Urol. 130:326, 1983.
239. Bernstein, J., and Whitten, C. F.: A histologic appraisal of the kidney in sickle cell anemia. Arch. Pathol. 70:407, 1960.
240. Pitcock, J. A., Muirhead, E. E., Hatch, F. E., Johnson, J. G., and Kelly, B. J.: Early renal changes in sickle cell anemia. Arch. Pathol. 90:403, 1970.
241. McCoy, R. C.: Ultrastructural alterations in the kidney of patients with sickle cell disease and the nephrotic syndrome. Lab. Invest. 21:85, 1969.
242. Antonovych, T. T.: Ultrastructural changes in glomeruli of patients with sickle cell disease and nephrotic syndrome. In Abstracts, Fifth Annual Meeting of the American Society of Nephrology, Washington, D.C., 1971, p. 3.
243. Strauss, J., Pardo, V., Koss, M. N., Griswold, W., and McIntosh, R. M.: Nephropathy associated with sickle cell anemia: An autologous immune complex nephritis. Am. J. Med. 58:382, 1975.
244. Pardo, V., Straus, J., Kramer, H., Ozawa, T., and McIntosh, R. M.: Nephropathy associated with sickle cell anemia: An autologous immune complex nephritis. Am. J. Med. 59:650, 1975.
245. Morgan, A. G., and Serjeant, G. R.: Renal function in patients over 40 with homozygous sickle cell disease. Br. Med. J. 282:1181, 1981.
246. Friedman, E. A., Rao, T. K., Sprung, C. L., Smith, A., Manis, T., Bellevue, R., Butt, K. M. H., Levere, R. D., and Holden, D. M.: Uremia in sickle cell anemia treated by maintenance hemodialysis. N. Engl. J. Med. 291:431, 1974.
247. Chatterjee, S. N.: National study on natural history of renal allografts in sickle cell disease or trait. Nephron 25:199, 1980.
248. Spector, D., Zachary, J. B., and Sterioff, S.: Painful crises following renal transplantation in sickle cell anemia. Am. J. Med. 64:835, 1978.
249. Walker, B. R., and Alexander, F.: Uric acid excretion in sickle cell anemia. J.A.M.A. 215:255, 1971.
250. Walker, B. K., Brownstein, P. K., Burka, E. R., and Ballas, S. K.: Urinary retention in sickle cell syndromes. Urology 16:33, 1980.
251. Emond, A. M., Holman, R., Hayes, R. J., and Serjeant, G. R.: Priapism and impotence in homozygous sickle cell disease. Arch. Intern. Med. 140:1434, 1980.
252. Campbell, J. H., and Cummins, S. D.: Priapism in sickle cell anemia. J. Urol. 66:697, 1951.
253. Hasen, H. B., and Raines, S. L.: Priapism associated with sickle cell disease. J. Urol. 88:71, 1962.
254. Conrad, M. E., Perrine, G. M., Barton, J. C., and Durant, J. R.: Provoked priapism in sickle cell anemia. Am. J. Hematol. 9:121, 1980.
255. Datta, N. S.: Megalophallus in sickle cell disease. J. Urol. 117:672, 1977.
256. Karayalcin, G., Imran, M., and Rosner, F.: Priapism in sickle cell disease: Report of five cases. Am. J. Med. Sci. 264:289, 1972.
257. Seeler, R. A.: Intensive transfusion therapy for priapism in boys with sickle cell anemia. J. Urol. 110:360, 1973.
258. Rifkind, S., Waisman, J., Thompson, R., and Goldfinger, D.: RBC exchange pheresis for priapism in sickle cell disease. J.A.M.A. 242:2317, 1979.
259. Noe, H. N., Wilimas, J., and Jerkins, G. R.: Surgical management of priapism in children with sickle cell anemia. J. Urol. 126:770, 1981.
260. Grace, D. A., and Winter, C. C.: Priapism: An appraisal of management of twenty-three patients. J. Urol. 99:301, 1968.
261. Powars, D., Wilson, B., Imbus, C., Pegelow, C., and Allen, J.: The natural history of stroke in sickle cell disease. Am. J. Med. 65:461, 1978.
262. Powars, D., and Imbus, C.: Cerebral vascular accidents in sickle cell anemia. Tex. Rep. Biol. Med. 40:293, 1980.
263. Seeler, R. A., and Royal, J. E.: Acute and chronic management of children with sickle cell anemia

and cerebrovascular occlusive crisis. Ill. Med. J. *151*:267, 1977.
264. Wood, D. H.: Cerebrovascular complications of sickle cell anemia. Stroke *9*:73, 1978.
265. Arnow, P. M., Panwalker, A., Garvin, J. S., and Rodriguez-Erdmann, F.: Aspirin, hyperventilation, and cerebellar infarction in sickle cell disease. Arch. Intern. Med. *138*:148, 1978.
266. Stockman, J. A., Nigro, M. A., Mishkin, M. M., and Oski, F. A.: Occlusion of large cerebral vessels in sickle cell anemia. N. Engl. J. Med. *287*:846, 1972.
267. Merkel, K. H. H., Ginsberg, P. L., Parker, J. C., Jr., and Post, M. J. D.: Cerebrovascular disease in sickle cell anemia: A clinical, pathological and radiological correlation. Stroke *9*:45, 1978.
268. Gerald, B., Sebes, J. I., and Langston, J. W.: Cerebral infarction secondary to sickle cell disease: Arteriographic findings. Am. J. Roentgenol. *134*:1209, 1980.
269. Jeffries, B. F., Lipper, M. H., and Kishore, P. R. S.: Major intracerebral arterial involvement in sickle cell disease. Surg. Neurol. *14*:291, 1980.
270. Seeler, R. A., Royal, J. E., Powe, L., and Goldberg, H. R.: Moyamoya in children with sickle cell anemia and cerebrovascular occlusion. J. Pediatr. *93*:808, 1978.
271. Portnoy, B. A., and Herion, J. C.: Neurological manifestations in sickle-cell disease; with a review of the literature and emphasis on the prevalence of hemiplegia. Ann. Intern. Med. *76*:643, 1972.
272. Wilimas, J., Goff, J. R., Anderson, H. R., Jr., Langston, J. W., and Thompson, E.: Efficacy of transfusion therapy for one to two years in patients with sickle cell disease and cerebrovascular accidents. Pediatrics *96*:205, 1980.
273. Russell, M. O., Goldberg, H. I., Reis, L., Friedman, S., Slater, R., Reivich, M., and Schwartz, E.: Transfusion therapy for cerebrovascular abnormalities in sickle cell disease. J. Pediatr. *88*:382, 1976.
274. Russell, M. O., Goldberg, H. I., Hodson, A., Kim, H. C., Halus, J., Reivich, M., and Schwartz, E.: Effect of transfusion therapy on arteriographic abnormalities and on recurrence of stroke in sickle cell disease. Blood *63*:162, 1984.
274a. Huttenlocher, P. R., Moohr, J. W., Johns, L., and Brown, F. D.: Cerebral blood flow in sickle-cell cerebrovascular disease. Pediatrics *73*:615, 1984.
275. Seeler, R. A., and Royal, J. E.: Commentary: Sickle cell anemia, stroke, and transfusion. J. Pediatr. *96*:243, 1980.
276. Rothman, S. M., and Nelson, J. S.: Spinal cord infarction in a patient with sickle cell anemia. Neurology *30*:1072, 1980.
277. Sebes, J. I., and Diggs, L. W.: Radiographic changes of the skull in sickle cell anemia. Am. J. Radiol. *132*:373, 1979.
278. Wessberg, G. A., Epker, B. N., Bordelon, J. H., and Hyer, R. L.: Correction of sickle cell gnathopathy by total maxillary osteotomy. J. Maxillofac. Surg. *8*:187, 1980.
279. Schwartz, A. M., Homer, M. J., and McCauley, R. G. K.: "Step-off" vertebral body: Gaucher's disease versus sickle cell hemoglobinopathy. Am. J. Radiol. *132*:81, 1979.
280. Weinberg, S.: Severe sclerosis of the long bones in sickle cell anemia. Radiology *145*:41, 1982.
280a. Sebes, J. I., and Kraus, A. P.: Avascular necrosis of the hip in the sickle cell hemoglobinopathies. J. Can. Assoc. Radiol. *34*:136, 1983.
281. Hawker, H., Neilson, H., Hayes, R. J., and Serjeant, G. R.: Haematological factors associated with avascular necrosis of the femoral head in homozygous sickle cell disease. Br. J. Haematol. *50*:29, 1982.
282. Chung, S. M. K., Alavi, A., and Russell, M. O.: Management of osteonecrosis in sickle cell anemia and its genetic variants. Clin. Orthop. *130*:158, 1978.
283. Harcke, H. T., Capitanio, M. A., and Naiman, J. L.: Sternal infarction in sickle cell anemia: Concise communication. J. Nucl. Med. *22*:322, 1981.
284. Levine, M. S., Borden, S., IV, and Gill, F. M.: Sternal cupping: A new finding in childhood sickle cell anemia. Radiology *142*:367, 1982.
285. Adeyokunnu, A. A., and Hendrickse, R. G.: Salmonella osteomyelitis in childhood. Arch. Dis. Child. *55*:175, 1980.
286. Diggs, L. W.: Bone and joint lesions in sickle cell disease. Clin. Orthop. *52*:119, 1967.
287. Givner, L. B., Luddy, R. E., and Schwartz, A. D.: Etiology of osteomyelitis in patients with major sickle hemoglobinopathies. J. Pediatr. *99*:411, 1981.
288. Waldvogel, F. A., and Vasey, H.: Osteomyelitis: The past decade. N. Engl. J. Med. *303*:360, 1980.
289. Serjeant, G. R.: Leg ulceration in sickle cell anemia. Arch. Intern. Med. *133*:690, 1974.
290. Gueri, M., and Serjeant, G. R. Leg ulcers in sickle cell anaemia. Trop. Geogr. Med. *22*:155, 1970.
291. Akinyanju, O., and Akinsete, I.: Leg ulceration in sickle cell disease in Nigeria. Trop. Geogr. Med. *31*:87, 1979.
292. Sawyer, P. N., Haque, S., Reddy, K., Sophie, Z., and Feller, J.: Wound healing effects of Debrisan on varicose, postoperative, decubitus, and sickle cell ulcers in man. Surgery *13*:251, 1979.
293. Serjeant, G. R., Galloway, R. E., and Gueri, M. C.: Oral zinc sulfate in sickle cell ulcers. Lancet *2*:891, 1970.
294. Graham, S. J., and Gartner, S. A.: Sickle cell retinopathy. J. Am. Optom. Assoc. *51*:575, 1980.
295. Condon, P. I., Hayes, R. J., and Serjeant, G. R.: Retinal and choroidal neovascularization in sickle cell disease. Trans. Ophthal. Soc. UK *100*:434, 1980.
296. Hayes, R. J., Condon, P. I., and Serjeant, G. R.: Haematological factors associated with proliferative retinopathy in sickle cell haemoglobin C disease. Br. J. Ophthalmol. *65*:712, 1981.
297. Hamilton, A. M., Pope, F. M., Condon, P. I., Slavin, G., Sowter, C., Ford, S., Hayes, R. J., and Serjeant, G. R.: Angioid streaks in Jamaican patients with homozygous sickle cell disease. Br. J. Ophthalmol. *65*:341, 1981.
298. Dizon, R. V., Jampol, L. M., Goldberg, M. F., and Juarez, C.: Choroidal occlusive disease in sickle cell hemoglobinopathies. Surv. Ophthalmol. *23*:297, 1979.
299. Condon, P. I., and Serjeant, G. R.: Photocoagulation in proliferative sickle retinopathy: Results of a 5-year study. Br. J. Ophthalmol. *64*:832, 1980.
300. Dizon-Moore, R. V., Jampol, L. M., and Goldberg, M. F.: Chorioretinal and choriovitreal neovascularization. Their presence after photocoagulation of proliferative sickle cell retinopathy. Arch. Ophthalmol. *99*:842, 1981.

301. Jampol, L. M., and Goldberg, M. F.: Retinal breaks after photocoagulation of proliferative sickle cell retinopathy. Arch. Ophthalmol. 98:676, 1980.
302. Jampol, L. M., Green, J. L., Jr., Goldberg, M. F., and Peyman, G. A.: An update on vitrectomy surgery and retinal detachment repair in sickle cell disease. Arch. Ophthalmol. 100:591, 1982.
303. Goldberg, M. F.: Sickled erythrocytes, hyphema, and secondary glaucoma: I. The diagnosis and treatment of sickled erythrocytes in human hyphemas. Ophthalmic Surg. 10:17, 1979.
304. Goldberg, M. F., Dizon, R., and Raichand, M.: Sickled erythrocytes, hyphema, and secondary glaucoma: II. Injected sickle cell erythrocytes into human, monkey, and guinea pig anterior chambers: The induction of sickling and secondary glaucoma. Ophthalmic Surg. 10:32, 1979.
305. Goldberg, M. F., Dizon, R., Raichand, M., Goldbaum, M., and Jampol, L. M.: Sickled erythrocytes, hyphema, and secondary glaucoma: III. Effects of sickle cell and normal human blood samples in rabbit anterior chambers. Ophthalmic Surg. 10:52, 1979.
305a. Steinmann, W., Stone, R., Nichols, C., Werner, E., Schweitzer, J., Keates, E., and Knorr, R.: A case control study of the association of sickle-cell trait and chronic open angle glaucoma. Am. J. Epidemiol. 118:288, 1983.
306. Al-Rashid, R. A.: Orbital apex syndrome secondary to sickle cell anemia. J. Pediatr. 95:426, 1979.
307. Blank, J. P., and Gill, F. M.: Orbital infarction in sickle cell disease. Pediatrics 67:879, 1981.
308. Armaly, M. F.: Ocular manifestations in sickle cell disease. Arch. Intern. Med. 133:670, 1974.
309. Nagpal, K. C., Asdourian, G. K., Goldbaum, M. H., Raichand, M., and Goldberg, M. F.: The conjunctival sickling sign, hemoglobin S, and irreversibly sickled erythrocytes. Arch. Ophthalmol. 95:808, 1977.
310. Warth, J. A., Prasad, A. S., Zwas, F., and Frank, R. N.: Abnormal dark adaptation in sickle cell anemia. J. Lab. Clin. Med. 98:189, 1981.
311. Serjeant, G. R., Norman, W., and Todd, G. B.: The internal auditory canal and sensorineural hearing loss in homozygous sickle cell disease. J. Laryngol. Otol. 89:453, 1975.
312. Friedman, E. M., Luban, N. L. C., Herer, G. R., and Williams, I.: Sickle cell anemia and hearing. Ann. Otol. Rhinol. Laryngol. 89:342, 1980.
313. Orchik, D. J., and Dunn, J. W.: Sickle cell anemia and sudden deafness. Arch. Otolaryngol. 103:369, 1977.
314. Serjeant, G. R., and Serjeant, B. E.: A comparison of erythrocyte characteristics in sickle cell syndromes in Jamaica. Br. J. Haematol. 23:205, 1972.
315. McCurdy, P. R., Mahmood, L., and Sherman, A. S.: Red cell life span in sickle cell hemoglobin C disease with a note about sickle cell hemoglobin O_{Arab}. Blood 45:273, 1975.
316. Bannerman, R. M., Serjeant, B., Seakins, M., England, J. M., and Serjeant, G. R.: Determinants of haemoglobin level in sickle cell haemoglobin C disease. Br. J. Haematol. 43:49, 1979.
317. Diggs, L. W., and Bell, A.: Intraerythrocytic hemoglobin crystals in sickle cell hemoglobin C disease. Blood 25:218, 1965.
318. Sergeant, G. R., Ashcroft, M. T., and Serjeant, B. E.: The clinical features of haemoglobin SC disease in Jamaica. Br. J. Haematol. 24:491, 1973.
319. Ballas, S. K., Lewis, C. N., Noone, A. M., Krasnow, S. H., Kararulzaman, E., and Burka, E. R.: Clinical, hematological and biochemical features of Hb SC disease. Am. J. Hematol. 13:37, 1982.
319a. Andrews, J., and Buchanan, G. R.: Mild splenic sequestration crises in sickle–hemoglobin-C disease. Clin. Pediatr. 23:354, 1984.
320. Huisman, T. H. J.: The percentages of abnormal hemoglobins in adults with a heterozygosity for an α chain and/or a β chain variant. Am. J. Hematol. 14:393, 1983.
321. Steinberg, M. H., Coleman, M. B., Adams, J. G., Platica, O., Gillette, P., and Rieder, R. F.: The effects of alpha thalassemia in Hb SC disease. Br. J. Haematol. 55:487, 1983.
322. Honig, G. R., Gunay, U., Mason, R. G., Vida, L. N., and Ferenc, C.: Sickle cell syndromes. I. Hemoglobin SC-α-thalassemia. Pediatr. Res. 10:613, 1976.
323. Griggs, R. C., and Harris, J. W.: The biophysics of the variants of sickle cell disease. Arch. Intern. Med. 97:315, 1956.
324. Charache, S., and Conley, C. L.: Rate of sickling of red cells during deoxygenation of blood from persons with various sickling disorders. Blood 24:25, 1964.
325. Zarkowsky, H. S., and Hochmuth, R. M.: Sickling times of individual erythrocytes at zero PO_2. J. Clin. Invest. 56:1023, 1975.
326. Harrington, J. P., Elbaum, D., Bookchin, R. M., Wittenberg, J. B., and Nagel, R. L.: Ligand kinetics of hemoglobin S containing erythrocytes. Proc. Natl. Acad. Sci. USA 74:203, 1977.
327. Coletta, M., Hofrichter, J., Ferrone, F. A., and Eaton, W. A. Kinetics of sickle hemoglobin polymerization in single red cells. Nature 300:194, 1982.
328. Noguchi, C. T.: Polymerization in erythrocytes containing S and non-S hemoglobin. Biophys. J., 415:1153, 1984.
329. Singer, K., and Singer, L.: The gelling phenomenon of sickle cell hemoglobin: Its biological and diagnostic significance. Blood 8:1008, 1953.
330. Bunn, H. F., Noguchi, C. T., Hofrichter, J., Schechter, G. P., Schechter, A. N., and Eaton, W. A.: Molecular and cellular pathogenesis of hemoglobin SC disease. Proc. Natl. Acad. Sci. USA 79:7527, 1982.
331. Oda, S., Oda, E., and Tanaka, K.: Relationship of density distribution and pyruvate kinase electrophoretic pattern of erythrocytes in sickle diseases and other disorders. Acta Haematol. 60:201, 1978.
332. Fabry, M. E., Kaul, D. K., Raventos-Suarez, C., Chang, H., and Nagel, R. L.: SC erythrocytes have an abnormally high intracellular hemoglobin concentration: Pathophysiological consequences. J. Clin. Invest. 70:1315, 1982.
333. Serjeant, G. R., Ashcroft, M. T., Serjeant, B. E., and Milner, P. F.: The clinical features of sickle cell β-thalassemia in Jamaica. Br. J. Haematol. 24:19, 1973.
334. Serjeant, G. R., Sommereux, A. M., Stevenson, M., Mason, K., and Serjeant, B. E.: Comparison of sickle cell β° thalassemia with homozygous sickle cell disease. Br. J. Haematol. 41:83, 1979.
335. Higgs, D. R., Aldridge, B. E., Lamb, J., Clegg, J. B., Weatherall, D. J., Hayes, R. J., Grandison, Y., Lowrie, Y., Mason, K. P., Serjeant, B. E., and Serjeant, G. R.: The interaction of alpha

336. McCurdy, P. R., Lorkin, P. A., Casey, R., Lehmann, H., Uddin, D. E., and Dickson, L. G.: Hemoglobin S-G (S-D) syndrome. Am. J. Med. 57:665, 1974.
337. Stevens, M. C. G., Lehmann, H., Mason, K. P., Serjeant, B. E., and Serjeant, G. R.: Sickle cell-Hb Lepore$_{Boston}$ syndrome. Am. J. Dis. Child. 136:19, 1982.
338. Milner, P. F., Miller, C., Grey, R., Seakins, M., DeJong, W. W., and Went, L. N.: Hemoglobin O$_{Arab}$ in four Negro families and its interaction with hemoglobin S and hemoglobin C. N. Engl. J. Med. 283:1417, 1970.
339. Charache, S., Zinkham, W. H., Dickerman, J. D., Brimhall, B., and Dover, G. J.: Hemoglobin SC, SS/G$_{Philadelphia}$ and SO$_{Arab}$ diseases. Diagnostic importance of an integrative analysis of clinical, hematologic and electrophoretic findings. Am. J. Med. 62:439, 1977.
340. Gilman, P. A., and Abel, A. S.: Acute splenic sequestration in hemoglobin O-Arab disease. Johns Hopkins Med. J. 146:285, 1980.
341. Moo-Penn, W., Bechtel, K., Jue, D., Chan, M. S., Hopkins, G., Schneider, N. J., Wright, J., and Schmidt, R. M.: The presence of hemoglobin S and C Harlem in an individual in the United States. Blood 46:363, 1975.
342. Aksoy, M.: The hemoglobin E syndromes. II. Sickle cell hemoglobin E disease. Blood 15:610, 1960.
343. Altay, C., Niazi, G. A., and Huisman, T. H. J.: The combination of Hb S and Hb E in a black female. Hemoglobin 1:100, 1976.
344. Kraus, L. M., Miyaji, T., Iuchi, I., and Kraus, A. P.: Characterization of α23GluNH$_2$ in hemoglobin Memphis. Hemoglobin Memphis/S, a new variant of molecular disease. Biochemistry 5:3701, 1966.
345. Cooper, M. R., Kraus, A. P., Felts, J. H., Ramseur, W. L., Myers, R., and Kraus, L. M.: A third case of hemoglobin Memphis/sickle cell disease. Am. J. Med. 55:535, 1973.
346. Motulsky, A. G.: Frequency of sickling disorders in U.S. Blacks. N. Engl. J. Med. 288:31, 1973.
347. Edington, G. M., and Lehmann, H.: Expression of the sickle gene in Africa. Br. Med. J. 1:1308, 1955.
348. Bradley, T. B., Brawner, J. N., and Conley, C. L.: Further observations on an inherited anomaly characterized by persistence of fetal hemoglobin. Bull. Johns Hopkins Hosp. 108:242, 1961.
349. Martinez, G., and Colombo, B.: A new type of hereditary persistence of foetal haemoglobin: Is a diffusible factor regulating γ-chain synthesis? Nature 252:735, 1974.
350. Huisman, T. H. J., Miller, A., and Schroeder, W. A.: A ^{G}γ type of hereditary persistence of fetal hemoglobin with β chain production in cis. Am. J. Hum. Genet. 27:765, 1975.
351. Stamatoyannopoulos, G., Wood, W. G., Papayannopoulou, T., and Nute, P. E.: A new form of hereditary persistence of fetal hemoglobin in Blacks and its association with sickle cell trait. Blood 46:683, 1975.
352. Friedman, S., and Schwartz, E.: Hereditary persistence of foetal haemoglobin with γ-chain synthesis in cis position (^{G}γβ$^+$-HPFH) in a Negro family. Nature 259:138, 1976.
353. Wood, W. G., Weatherall, D. J., and Clegg, J. B.: Interaction of heterocellular hereditary persistence of foetal haemoglobin with β-thalassemia and sickle cell anemia. Nature 264:247, 1976.
354. Dover, G. J., Boyer, S. H., and Pembrey, M. E.: F cell production in sickle cell anemia; regulation by genes linked to β-hemoglobin locus. Science 211:1441, 1981.
355. Old, J. M., Ayyub, H., Wood, W. G., Clegg, J. B., and Weatherall, D. J.: Linkage analysis of nondeletion hereditary persistence of fetal hemoglobin. Science 215:981, 1982.
355a. Milner, P. F., Leibfarth, J. D., Ford, J., Barton, B. P., Grenett, H. E., and Garver, F. A.: Increased Hb F in sickle cell anemia is determined by a factor linked to the β^S gene from one parent. Blood 63:64, 1984.
355b. Gianni, A. M., Bregni, M., Capelli, M. D., Fiorelli, G., Taramelli, R., Giglioni, B., Comi, P., and Ottolengi, S.: A gene controlling fetal hemoglobin expression in adults is not linked to the non alpha-globin cluster. Embo. J. 2:921, 1983.
355c. Boyer, S. H., Dover, G. J., Serjeant, G. R., Smith, K. D., Antonarakis, S. E., Embury, S. H., Margolet, J., Noyes, A. N., Boyer, M. L., and Bias, W. B.: Production of F cells in sickle cell anemia: Regulation by a genetic locus separate from the β-globin gene cluster. Blood 64:1053, 1984.
356. Attah, E. B., and Ekere, M. C.: Death patterns in sickle cell anemia. J.A.M.A. 233:889, 1975.
357. Konotey-Ahulu, F. I. D.: Effect of environment on sickle cell disease in West Africa: Epidemiologic and clinical considerations. In Abramson, H., Bertles, J. F., and Wethers, D. L. (eds.): Sickle Cell Disease: Diagnosis, Management, Education and Research. St. Louis, C. V. Mosby Co., 1973, p. 20.
358. Seeler, R. A.: Deaths in children with sickle cell anemia. A clinical analysis of 19 fatal instances in Chicago. Clin. Pediatr. 11:634, 1972.
359. Rogers, D. W., Clarke, J. M., Cupidore, L., Ramlal, A. M., Sparke, B. R., and Serjeant, G. R.: Early deaths in Jamaican children with sickle cell disease. Br. Med. J. 1:1515, 1978.
360. O'Brien, R. T., and McIntosh, S.: Prospective study of sickle cell anemia in infancy. J. Pediatr. 89:205, 1976.
361. Thomas, A. N., Pattison, C., and Serjeant, G. R.: Causes of death in sickle cell disease in Jamaica. Br. Med. J. 285:633, 1982.
362. Embury, S. H., Dozy, A. M., Miller, J., Davis, J. R., Jr., Kleman, K. M., Preisler, H., Vichinsky, E., Lande, W. N., Lubin, B. H., Kan, Y. W., and Mentzer, W. C.: Concurrent sickle cell anemia and α-thalassemia. Effect on severity of anemia. N. Engl. J. Med. 306:270, 1982.
362a. Steinberg, M. H., Rosensto, W., Coleman, M. B., Adams, J. G., Platica, O., Cedeno, M., Rieder, R. F., Wilson, J. T., Milner, P., and West, S.: Effects of thalassemia and microcytosis on the hematologic and vaso-occlusive severity of sickle-cell anemia. Blood 63:1353, 1984.
363. Altay, C., Gravely, M. E., Joseph, B. R., and Williams, D. F.: Alpha-thalassemia-2 and the variability of hematological values in children with sickle cell anemia. Pediatr. Res. 15:1093, 1981.
364. deCeulaer, K., Higgs, D. R., Weatherall, D. J., Hayes, R. J., Serjeant, B. E., and Serjeant, G. R.: α-Thalassemia reduces the hemolytic rate in homozygous sickle cell disease. N. Engl. J. Med. 309:189, 1983.

364a. Fabry, M. E., Mears, J. G., Patel, P., Schaefer, K., Carmichael, L.D., Martinez, G., and Nagel, R. L.: Dense cells in sickle cell anemia—the effects of gene interaction. Blood 64:1042, 1984.

364b. Noguchi, C. T., Dover, G. J., Rodgers, G. P., Serjeant, G. R., Antonarakis, S. E., Anagnou, N. P., Higgs, D. R., Weatherall, D. J., and Schechter, A. N.: α-Thalassemia changes erythrocyte heterogeneity in sickle cell disease. J. Clin. Invest., 75:1632, 1985.

364c. Serjeant, B. E., Mason, K. P., Kenny, M. W., Stuart, J., Higgs, D. R., Weatherall, D. J., Hayes, R. J., and Serjeant, G. R.: Effect of alpha thalassemia on the rheology of homozygous sickle cell disease. Br. J. Haematol. 55:479, 1983.

364d. Embury, S. H., Clark, M. R., Monroy, G., and Mohandas, N.: Concurrent sickle cell anemia and thalassemia. Effect on pathological properties of sickle erythrocytes. J. Clin. Invest. 73:116, 1984.

365. Mears, J. G., Lachman, H., Labie, D., and Nagel, R. L.: Alpha-thalassemia is related to prolonged survival in sickle cell anemia. Blood 62:286, 1983.

366. Perrine, R. P., Pembrey, M. E., John, P., Perrine, S., and Shoup, F.: Natural history of sickle cell anemia in Saudi Arabs. Ann. Intern. Med. 88:1, 1978.

367. Wood, W. G., Pembrey, M. E., Serjeant, G. R., Perrine, R. P., and Weatherall, D. J.: Hb F synthesis in sickle cell anemia: A comparison of Saudi Arab cases with those of African origin. Br. J. Haematol. 45:431, 1980.

368. Brittenham, G., Lozoff, B., Harris, J. W., Sharma, V. S., and Narasimhan, S.: Sickle cell anemia and trait in a population of Southern India. Am. J. Hematol. 2:25, 1977.

369. Brittenham, G., Lozoff, B., Harris, J. W., Mayson, S. M., Miller, A., and Huisman, T. H. J.: Sickle cell anemia and trait in Southern India: Further studies. Am. J. Hematol. 6:107, 1979.

369a. Powars, D. R., Weiss, J. N., Chan, L. S., and Schroeder, W. A.: Is there a threshold level of fetal hemoglobin that ameliorates morbidity in sickle cell anemia? Blood 63:921, 1984.

370. Stevens, M. C. G., Hayes, R. J., Vaidya, S., and Serjeant, G. R.: Fetal hemoglobin and clinical severity of homozygous sickle cell disease in early childhood. J. Pediatr. 98:37, 1981.

371. Powars, D. R., Schroeder, W. A., Weiss, J. N., Chan, L. S., and Azen, S. P.: Lack of influence of fetal hemoglobin levels of erythrocytes indices on the severity of sickle cell disease. J. Clin. Invest. 65:732, 1980.

371a. Labie, D., Pagnier, J., Lapoumeroulie, C., Rouabhi, F., Dunda-Belkhodja, O., Chardin, P., Beldjord, C., Wajcman, H., Fabry, M. E., and Nagel, R. L.: Common haplotype dependencyof high $^G\gamma$ gene expression and high Hb F levels in beta thalassemia and sickle cell anemia. I. North and West African patients. Proc. Natl. Acad. Sci. USA, 82:2111, 1985.

371b. Nagel, R. L., Fabry, M. E., Pagnier, J. Zohoun, I., Wajcman H., Baudin, V., and Labie, D.: Hematologically and genetically distinct forms of sickle cell anemia in Africa: The Senegal type and the Benin type. N. Engl. J. Med., 312:880, 1985.

372. Claster, S., Godwin, M. J., and Embury, S. H.: Risk of altitude exposure in sickle cell disease. West. J. Med. 135:364, 1981.

372a. Sergeant, G. R.: Sickle haemoglobin and pregnancy. Br. Med. J. 287:628, 1983.

373. Overturf, G. D., Rigau-Perez, J. G., Selzer, J., Field, R. J., Powars, D., Pang, E. J., Uy, C., Honig, G., Weiss, J., Chan, L., and Portnoy, B.: Pneumococcal polysaccharide immunization of children with sickle cell disease. I. Clinical reactions to immunization and relationship to preimmunization antibody. Am. J. Pediatr. Hematol. Oncol. 4:19, 1982.

374. Ahonkhai, V. I., Landesman, S. H., Fikrig, S. M., Schmalzer, E. A., Brown, A. K., Cherubin, C. E., and Schiffman, G.: Failure of pneumococcal vaccine in children with sickle-cell disease. N. Engl. J. Med. 301:26, 1979.

375. Buchanan, G. R., and Schiffman, G.: Antibody responses to polyvalent pneumococcal vaccine in infants with sickle cell anemia. J. Pediatr. 96:264, 1980.

376. Overturf, G. D., Selzer, J. W., Chan, L., Weiss, J., Field, R., Rigau-Perez, J. G., Powars, D., Uy, C., Pang, E. J., Honig, G., Steele, R., Edmonds, R., and Portnoy, B.: Pneumococcal polysaccharide immunization of children with sickle cell disease. II. Serologic response and pneumococcal disease following immunization. Am. J. Pediatr. Hematol. Oncol. 4:25, 1982.

377. Kaplan, J., Frost, H., Sarnaik, S., and Schiffman, G.: Type-specific antibodies in children with sickle cell anemia given polyvalent pneumococcal vaccine. J. Pediatr. 100:404, 1982.

378. Lundh, B., and Gardner, F. H.: The hematological response to androgens in sickle cell anemia. Scand. J. Haematol. 7:389, 1970.

379. Alexanian, R., and Nadell, J.: Oxymetholone treatment for sickle cell anemia. Blood 45:769, 1975.

380. Zanger, B., Alfrey, C. P., McIntire, L. V., and Leverett, L. B.: The effects of dromostanolone in sickle cell anemia. J. Lab. Clin. Med. 84:889, 1974.

381. Miller, D. M., Winslow, R. M., Klein, H. G., Wilson, K. C., Brown, F. L., and Statham, N. J.: Improved exercise performance after exchange transfusion in subjects with sickle cell anemia. Blood 56:1127, 1980.

382. Finch, C. A., Lee, M. Y., and Leonard, J. M.: Continuous RBC transfusions in a patient with sickle cell disease. Arch. Intern. Med. 142:279, 1982.

383. Charache, S., and Conley, C. L.: Factors leading to vascular occlusion in sickle cell anemia. In Brewer, G. J. (ed.): Erythrocyte Structure and Function. (Third International Conference on Red Cell Metabolism and Function, University of Michigan, 1974–75.) New York, A. R. Liss, 1975, p. 243.

384. Charache, S.: Treatment of sickle cell anemia. Ann. Rev. Med. 32:195, 1981.

385. Kernoff, L. M., Bothia, M. C., and Jacobs, P.: Exchange transfusion in sickle cell disease using a continuous-flow blood cell separator. Transfusion 17:269, 1977.

386. Kleinman, S., Thompson-Breton, R., Breen, D., Hurvitz, C., and Goldfinger, D.: Exchange red blood cell pheresis in a pediatric patient with severe complications of sickle cell anemia. Transfusion 21:443, 1981.

387. Diamond, W. J., Brown, F. L., Jr., Bitterman, P., Klein, H. G., Davey, R. J., and Winslow, R. M.: Delayed hemolytic transfusion reaction presenting as sickle-cell crisis. Ann. Intern. Med. 93:231, 1980.

388. Lanzkowsky, P., Shende, A., Karayalcin, G., Kim, Y-J., and Aballi, A. J.: Partial exchange transfu-

sion in sickle cell anemia. Am. J. Dis. Child. *132*:1206, 1978.
389. Davey, R. J., Esposito, D. J., Jacobson, R. J., and Corn, M.: Partial exchange transfusion as treatment for hemoglobin SC disease in pregnancy. Arch. Intern. Med. *138*:937, 1978.
390. Orlina, A. R., Unger, P. J., and Koshy, M.: Post-transfusion alloimmunization in patients with sickle cell disease. Am. J. Hematol. *5*:101, 1978.
391. Schafer, A. I., Cheron, R. G., Dluhy, R., Cooper, B., Gleason, R., Soeldner, J. S., and Bunn, H. F.: Clinical consequences of acquired transfusional iron overload in adults. N. Engl. J. Med. *304*:319, 1981.
392. Buffone, G. J., Luban, N. L. C., and Leiken, S. L.: Transfusion therapy and serum ferritin in sickle cell disease. Am. J. Pediatr. Hematol./Oncol. *2*:307, 1980.
393. Cohen, A., and Schwartz, E.: Iron chelation therapy in sickle cell anemia. Am. J. Hematol. *7*:69, 1979.
394. Greenberg, M. S., and Kass, E. H.: Studies on the destruction of red blood cells. XIII. Observation on the role of pH in the pathogenesis and treatment of painful crisis in sickle cell disease. Arch. Intern. Med. *101*:355, 1958.
395. Cooperative Urea Trials Group: Clinical trials of therapy for sickle cell vaso-occlusive crises. J.A.M.A. *228*:1120, 1974.
396. Mann, J. R., and Stuart, J.: Sodium bicarbonate prophylaxis of sickle cell crisis. Pediatrics *53*:414, 1974.
397. Reynolds, J. D. H.: Painful sickle cell crisis—successful treatment with hyperbaric oxygen therapy. J.A.M.A. *216*:1977, 1971.
397a. Embury, S. H., Garcia, J. F., Mohandas, N., Pennathu, R., and Clark, M. R.: Effects of oxygen inhalation on endogenous erythropoietin kinetics, erythropoiesis, and properties of blood cells in sickle-cell anemia. N. Engl. J. Med. *311*:291, 1984.
398. Marks, R. M., and Sacher, E. J.: Undertreatment of medical inpatients with narcotic analgesics. Ann. Intern. Med. *78*:173, 1973.
399. Reuler, J. B., Girard, D. E., and Nardone, D. A.: The chronic pain syndrome: Misconceptions and management. Ann. Intern. Med. *93*:588, 1980.
400. Co, L. L., Schmitz, T. H., Havdala, H., Reyes, A., and Westerman, M. P.: Acupuncture: An evaluation in the painful crises of sickle cell anaemia. Pain *7*:181, 1979.
401. Loeser, J. D., Black, R. G., and Christman, A.: Relief of pain by transcutaneous stimulation. J. Neurosurg. *42*:308, 1975.
402. Zeltzer, L., Dash, J., and Holland, J. P.: Hypnotically induced pain control in sickle cell anemia. Pediatrics *64*:533, 1979.
403. Brody, J. I., Goldsmith, M. H., Park, S. K., and Soltys, H. D.: Symptomatic crises of sickle cell anemia treated by limited exchange transfusion. Ann. Intern. Med. *72*:327, 1970.
404. Flye, M. W., and Silver, D.: The role of surgery in sickle cell disease. Surg. Gynecol. Obstet. *137*:115, 1973.
405. Searle, J. F.: Anaesthesia and sickle-cell haemoglobin. Br. J. Anaesth. *44*:1335, 1972.
406. Janik, J., and Seeler, R. A: Perioperative management of children with sickle hemoglobinopathy. J. Pediatr. Surg. *15*:117, 1980.
407. Szwed, J. J., Yum, M.-N., and Hogan, R.: Case report: A beneficial effect of splenectomy in sickle cell anemia and chronic renal failure. Am. J. Med. Sci. *279*:169, 1980.
408. Ballester, O. F., and Warth, J.: Sickle cell anemia: Recurrent splenic pain relieved by splenectomy. Ann. Intern. Med. *90*:349, 1979.
408a. Emond, A. M., Venugopal, S., Morais, P., Carpenter, R. G., and Serjeant, G. R.: Role of splenectomy in homozygous sickle cell disease in childhood. Lancet *1*:88, 1984.
409. Morrison, J. C., Propst, M. G., and Blake, P. G.: Sickle hemoglobin and the gravid patient: A management controversy. Clin. Perinatol. *7*:273, 1980.
410. Morrison, J. C., Schneider, J. M., Whybrew, W. D., Bucovaz, E. T., and Menzel, D. M.: Prophylactic transfusions in pregnant patients with sickle hemoglobinopathies: Benefit versus risk. Obstet. Gynecol. *56*:274, 1980.
411. Milner, P. F., Jones, B. R., and Dobler, J.: Outcome of pregnancy in sickle cell anemia and sickle cell–hemoglobin C disease. Am. J. Obstet. Gynecol. *138*:239, 1980.
412. Charache, S., Scott, J., Niebyl, J., and Bonds, D.: Management of sickle cell disease in pregnant patients. Obstet. Gynecol. *55*:407, 1980.
413. Cunningham, F. G., and Pritchard, J. A.: Prophylactic transfusions of normal red blood cells during pregnancies complicated by sickle cell hemoglobinopathies. Am. J. Obstet. Gynecol. *135*:994, 1979.
414. Cunningham, F. G., Pritchard, J. A., and Mason, R.: Pregnancy and sickle cell hemoglobinopathies: Results with and without prophylactic transfusions. Obstet. Gynecol. *62*:419, 1983.
415. Miller, J. M., Jr., Horger, E. O., III, Key, T. C., and Walker, E. M., Jr.: Management of sickle hemoglobinopathies in pregnant patients. Am. J. Obstet. Gynecol. *141*:237, 1981.
416. Koshy, M., and Ashenhurst, J.: Management of pregnancy in sickle cell anemia. Tex. Rep. Biol. Med. *40*:273, 1981.
417. Koshy, M.: Personal communication.
417a. Aluoch, J. R.: The treatment of sickle cell disease—a historical and chronological literature review of the therapies applied since 1910. Trop. Geogr. Med. *36*(Suppl.):1, 1984.
418. Cerami, A., and Manning, J. M.: Potassium cyanate as an inhibitor of the sickling of erythrocytes *in vitro*. Proc. Natl. Acad. Sci. USA *68*:1180, 1971.
419. Gillette, P. N., Lu, Y. S., and Peterson, C. M.: The pharmacology of cyanate with a summary of its initial usage in sickle cell disease. Prog. Hematol. *8*:181, 1973.
420. Peterson, C. M., de Ciutiis, A. C., and Cerami, A.: Sodium cyanate and sickle cell disease: Efficacy vs. toxicity. *In* Hercules, J. I., Schechter, A. N., Eaton, W. A., et al. (eds.): Proceedings of the 1st National Symposium on SC Disease. Washington, D.C., DHEW Pub. No. 75–723 (NIH), Bethesda, Maryland, 1974, pp. 37–38.
421. Peterson, C. M., Tsairis, P., Ohnishi, A., Lu, Y. S., Grady, R., Cerami, A., and Dyek, P. J.: Sodium cyanate induced polyneuropathy in patients with sickle cell disease. Ann. Intern. Med. *81*:152, 1974.
422. Charache, S., Duffy, T. R., Jander, N., Scott, J. C., Bedine, M., and Morrell, R.: Toxic-therapeutic ratio of sodium cyanate. Arch. Intern. Med. *135*:1043, 1975.
423. Harkness, D. R., and Roth, S.: Clinical evaluation of cyanate in sickle cell anemia. Prog. Hematol. *9*:157, 1975.

424. Diederich, D. A., Trueworthy, R. C., Gill, P., Cader, A. M., and Larsen, W. E.: Hematologic and clinical responses in patients with sickle cell anemia after chronic extracorporeal carbamylation. J. Clin. Invest. 58:642, 1976.
425. Balcerzak, S. P., Grever, M. R., Sing, D. E., Bishop, J. N., and Segal, M. L.: Preliminary studies of continuous extracorporeal carbamylation in the treatment of sickle cell anemia. J. Lab. Clin. Med. 100:345, 1982.
426. Lee, M. Y., Uvelli, D. A., Agodoa, L. C. Y., Scribner, B. H., Finch, C. A., and Babb, A. L.: Clinical studies of a continuous extracorporeal cyanate treatment system for patients with sickle cell disease. J. Lab. Clin. Med. 100:334, 1982.
427. Roth, E. F., Nagel, R. L., Bookchin, R. M., and Grayzel, A. L.: Nitrogen mustard: An "in vitro" inhibitor of erythrocyte sickling. Biochem. Biophys. Res. Commun. 48:612, 1972.
428. Dean, J., and Schechter, A. N.: Sickle-cell anemia: Molecular and cellular bases of therapeutic approaches. N. Engl. J. Med. 299:752, 804, 863, 1978.
429. Klotz, I. M., Haney, D. N., and King, L. C.: Rational approaches to chemotherapy: Anti-sickling agents. Science 213:724, 1981.
430. Acquaye, C., Wilchek, M., and Gorecki, M.: Strategies for tackling sickle cell disease. Trends Biochem. Sci. 6:146, 1981.
431. Chang, H., Ewert, S. M., Bookchin, R. M., and Nagel, R. L.: Comparative evaluation of fifteen anti-sickling agents. Blood 61:693, 1983.
432. Rosa, R. M., Bierer, B. E., Thomas, R., Stoff, J. S., Kruskall, M., Robinson, S., Bunn, H. F., and Epstein, F. H. A study of induced hyponatremia in the prevention and treatment of sickle cell crises. N. Engl. J. Med. 303:1138, 1980.
433. Charache, S., and Walker, W. G.: Failure of desmopressin to lower serum sodium or prevent crisis in patients with sickle cell anemia. Blood 58:892, 1981.
434. Asakura, T., Ohnishi, S. T., Adachi, K., Ozguc, M., Hashimoto, K., Singer, M., Russell, M. O., and Schwartz, E.: Effect of cetiedil on erythrocyte sickling: New type of anti-sickling agent that may affect erythrocyte membranes. Proc. Natl. Acad. Sci. USA 77:2955, 1980.
435. Labie, D., Sablayrolles, M., Castaigne, J. P., and Wajcman, H.: Ticlopidine: A membrane active in vitro anti-sickling agent modifying intra-erythrocytic hemoglobin concentration. Blood 60:46a, 1982.
435a. Semple, M. J., Alhasani, S. F., Kioy, P., and Savidge, G. F.: A double-blind trial of ticlopidine in sickle-cell disease. Thrombos. Haemostas. 51:303, 1984.
436. Berkowitz, L. R., and Orringer, E. P.: Effects of cetiedil on mono-valent cation permeability in the erythrocyte—and explanation for the efficacy of cetiedil in the treatment of sickle cell anemia. Blood Cells 8:283, 1982.
437. Schmidt, W. F., III, Asakura, T., and Schwartz, E.: Effect of cetiedil on cation and water movements in erythrocytes. J. Clin. Invest. 69:589, 1982.
438. Brewer, G. J., Bereza, U., Mizukami, U., Aster, J. C., and Brewer, L. F.: Drug action hypothesis: How membrane expansion, calmodulin inhibition and sickle cell therapy relate. In Brewer, G. J. (ed.): The Red Cell 5th Ann Arbor Conference. New York, A. R. Liss, Inc., 1982, p. 187.
439. Ohnishi, S. T.: Inhibition of the in vitro formation of irreversibly sickled cells. Presented at Workshop on the Development of Therapeutic Agents for Sickle Cell Disease. Bethesda, Maryland, National Institutes of Health, May 1983.
440. Kaul, D. K., Fabry, M. E., and Nagel, R. L.: Pentoxifylline modifies the rheology of SS cells but does not inhibit polymerization of Hb S. Presented at Workshop on the Development of Therapeutic Agents for Sickle Cell Disease. Bethesda, Maryland, National Institutes of Health, May 1983.
440a. Johnson, F. L., Look, A. T., Gockerman, J., Ruggiero, M. R., Dallapozi, L., and Billings, F. T.: Bone marrow transplantation in a patient with sickle cell anemia. N. Engl. J. Med. 311:780, 1984.
441. DeSimone, J., Heller, P., Hall, L., and Zwiers, D.: 5-Azacytidine stimulates fetal hemoglobin synthesis in anemic baboons. Proc. Natl. Acad. Sci. USA 79:4428, 1982.
441a. Papayannopoulou, T., Deron, A. T., Veith, R., Knitter, G., and Stamatoyannopoulos, G.: Arabinosylcytosine induces fetal hemoglobin in baboons by perturbing erythroid cell-differentiation kinetics. Science 224:617, 1984.
441b. Letvin, N. L., Linch, D. C., Beardsley, P., McIntyre, K. W., and Nathan, D. G.: Augmentation of fetal-hemoglobin production in anemic monkeys by hydroxyurea. N. Engl. J. Med. 310:869, 1984.
442. Ley, T. J., DeSimone, J., Noguchi, C., Turner, P., Schechter, A., Heller, P., and Nienhuis, A. W.: 5-Azacytidine increases γ-globin synthesis and reduces the proportion of dense cells in patients with sickle cell anemia. Blood 62:370, 1983.
443. Charache, S., Dover, G. J., Smith, K. D., Talbot, C. C., Mayer, M., and Boyer, S.: Treatment of sickle cell anemia with 5-azacytidine results in increased fetal hemoglobin production and is associated with nonrandom hypomethylation of DNA around the gamma-delta-beta globin gene complex. Proc. Natl. Acad. Sci. USA 80:4842, 1983.
444. Platt, O. S., Orkin, S. H., Dover, G., Beardsley, G. P., Miller, B., and Nathan, D. G.: Hydroxyurea enhances fetal hemoglobin production in sickle-cell anemia. J. Clin. Invest. 74:652, 1984.
445. Kan, Y. W., Golbus, M. S., and Trecartin, R.: Prenatal diagnosis of sickle cell anemia. N. Engl. J. Med. 294:1039, 1976.
446. Alter, B. P.: Prenatal diagnosis of hemoglobinopathies: A status report. Lancet 2:1152, 1981.
447. Kan, Y. W., and Dozy, A. M.: Antenatal diagnosis of sickle cell anaemia by DNA analysis of amniotic fluid cells. Lancet 2:910, 1978.
448. Phillips, J. A., III, Panny, S. R., Kazazian, H. H., Jr., Boehm, C. D., Scott, A. F., and Smith, K. D.: Prenatal diagnosis of sickle cell anemia by restriction endonuclease analysis: Hind III polymorphisms in β-globin genes extend test applicability. Proc. Natl. Acad. Sci. USA 77:2853, 1980.
449. Geever, R. F., Wilson, L. B., Nallaseth, F. S., Milner, P. F., Bittner, M., and Wilson, J. T.: Direct identification of sickle cell anemia by blot hybridization. Proc. Natl. Acad. Sci. USA 78:5081, 1981.
450. Chang, J. C., and Kan, Y. W.: Antenatal diagnosis of sickle cell anaemia by direct analysis of the sickle mutation. Lancet 2:1127, 1981.
451. Wilson, J. T., Milner, P. F., and Summer, M. E.: Use of restriction endonucleases for mapping the allele for $β^s$ globin. Proc. Natl. Acad. Sci. USA 79:3628, 1982.
452. Chang, J. C., and Kan, Y. W.: A sensitive new

prenatal test for sickle cell anemia. N. Engl. J. Med. *307*:30, 1982.
453. Orkin, S. H., Little, P. F. R., and Kazazian, H. H.: Improved detection of the sickle mutation by DNA analysis. N. Engl. J. Med. *307*:32, 1982.
454. Smith, E., Rosenblatt, P., and Bedo, A. V.: Sickle cell anemia crisis: Report on seven patients treated with priscoline. J. Pediatr. *43*:655, 1953.
455. Gross, R. T., Kriss, J. P., and Spaet, T. H.: The hematopoietic and goitrogenic effects of cobaltous chloride in patients with sickle cell anemia. Pediatrics *15*:284, 1955.
456. Beutler, E.: The effect of methemoglobin formation in sickle cell disease. J. Clin. Invest. *40*:1856, 1961.
457. Salvaggio, J. E., Arnold, C. A., and Banov, C. H.: Long-term anticoagulation in sickle-cell disease: A clinical study. N. Engl. J. Med. *269*:182, 1963.
458. Sirs, J. A.: The use of carbon monoxide on red cell life span in sickle cell disease. Blood *46*:253, 1975.
459. Purugganan, H. B., and McElfresh, A. E.: Failure of carbonmonoxy sickle-cell haemoglobin to alter the sickle state. Lancet *1*:79, 1964.
460. Beutler, E.: The effect of carbon monoxide on red cell life span in sickle cell disease. Blood *46*:253, 1975.
461. Schwartz, E., and McElfresh, A. E.: Treatment of painful crises of sickle cell disease: A double-blind study. J. Pediatr. *64*:132, 1964.
462. Watson-Williams, E. J.: Sickle-cell crisis treated with Rheomacrodex. Lancet *1*:1053, 1963.
463. Oski, F. A., Viner, E. D., Purugganan, H. B., and McElfresh, A. E.: Low molecular weight dextran in sickle cell crisis. J.A.M.A. *191*:43, 1965.
464. Barnes, P. M., Hendrickse, R. G., and Watson-Williams, E. J.: Low-molecular-weight dextran in treatment of bone-pain crises in sickle cell disease: A double-blind trial. Lancet 2:1271, 1965.
465. Hilkovitz, G.: Sickle cell disease: New method of treatment. Preliminary report. Br. Med. J. *2*:266, 1957.
466. dos Santos, W. D., and Lehmann, H.: Acetazolamide in sickle-cell anemia. Br. Med. J. *2*:139, 1959.
467. Finney, R. A., Jr., and Hatch, F. E., Jr.: Effect of a carbonic anhydrase inhibitor (dichlorphenamide) on sickle cell anemia. Am. J. Med. Sci. *250*:154, 1965.
468. Hathorn, M., and Lewis, R. A.: Inhibition of sickling by phenothiazines. Effect on red cell survival. Br. J. Haematol. *12*:195, 1966.
469. Pearson, H. A., and Noyes, W. D.: Failure of phenothiazines in sickle cell anemia. J.A.M.A. *199*:33, 1967.
470. Oski, F. A., Call, F. L., and Lessin, L.: Failure of promazine HCl to prevent the painful episodes in sickle cell anemia. J. Pediatr. *73*:265, 1968.
471. Isaacs, W. A., and Hayhoe, F. G. J.: Steroid hormones in sickle-cell disease. Nature *215*:1139, 1967.
472. Raper, A. B., Black, A. J., Huntsman, R. G., and Pollack, M.: Sickling and steroid hormones. Trans. R. Soc. Trop. Med. Hyg. *64*:293, 1970.
473. Nalbandian, R. M., Schultz, G., Lusher, J. M., Anderson, J. W., and Henry, R. L.: Sickle cell crisis terminated by intravenous urea in sugar solutions—a preliminary report. Am. J. Med. Sci. *261*:309, 1971.
474. Gillette, P. N., Peterson, C. M., Lu, Y. S., and Cerami, A.: Sodium cyanate as a potential treatment for sickle-cell disease. N. Engl. J. Med. *290*:654, 1974.
475. Chaplin, H., Alkjaersig, N., Fletcher, A. P., Michael, J. M., and Joist, J. H.: Aspirin-dipyridamole prophylaxis of sickle-cell disease pain crises. Thrombos. Haemost. *43*:218, 1980.
476. Greenberg, J., Ohenefre, K., Halus, J., Way, C., and Schwartz, E.: Trial of low doses of aspirin as prophylaxis in sickle-cell disease. J. Pediatr. *102*:781, 1983.
477. Zago, M. A., Costa, F. F., Ismael, S. J., Tone, L. G., and Bottura, C.: Treatment of sickle cell diseases with aspirin. Acta Haematol. *72*:61, 1984.
478. deCeulaer, K., Hayes, R., Gruber, C., and Serjeant, G. R.: Medroxyprogesterone acetate and homozygous sickle-cell disease. Lancet *2*:229, 1982.

UNSTABLE HEMOGLOBIN VARIANTS—CONGENITAL HEINZ BODY HEMOLYTIC ANEMIA

13

INTRODUCTION

As mentioned in Chapter 10, most human hemoglobin variants are not associated with detectable clinical manifestations. Many are discovered by chance or during the screening of large populations. However, a substantial number of variants are known to have an enhanced propensity to denature. As a result, the abnormal hemoglobin tends to aggregate within the red cell, forming an amorphous mass or Heinz body that can be detected by a supravital stain. These patients have a disorder of varying clinical severity that is generally called congenital Heinz body hemolytic anemia (CHBA).

In 1952, Cathie[113] described a child with congenital nonspherocytic hemolytic anemia. At 10 months of age, the patient had anemia, jaundice, splenomegaly, and pigmenturia. Splenectomy, performed six months later, resulted in no significant clinical improvement. Subsequently, large Heinz bodies were demonstrated in the patient's red cells. Following this report, a number of similar cases have been encountered throughout the world. In most of these cases, a hemoglobin abnormality was suggested by the demonstration of a copious precipitate upon heating the patient's hemolysate (for details, see below). Nearly all these patients have been shown to have a hemoglobin variant. Cathie's patient was found to have Hb Bristol (β 67 Val $\rightarrow$ Asp).[59]

At present, over 90 different unstable variants have been reported (see Table 13–1). Some, such as Hb Köln, have been encountered repeatedly in unrelated families from widely scattered parts of the world. The term "unstable hemoglobin" is reserved for those variants whose instability is sufficient to cause clinically recognizable hemolysis. The resulting CHBA represents an important type of congenital hemolytic disease. Other variants may display *in vitro* instability but are unassociated with any evidence of hemolysis. Hb E and Hb H both give positive precipitation tests, but neither is regarded as an "unstable hemoglobin." In this chapter, we will review the pathogenesis of CHBA at the molecular and cellular levels, its clinical manifestations, and its laboratory diagnosis and treatment.

PATHOGENESIS

The understanding of the mechanism underlying the hemolysis in CHBA was considerably enhanced when Grimes and associates[114, 115] showed that hemolysates from these patients formed a flocculent precipitate when incubated at 50°C. Such precipitation in stroma-free hemoglobin solutions indicated that an abnormality in soluble cell constituents, probably hemoglobin, was responsible for Heinz body formation. Subsequently, it was shown that heat-labile hemoglobin could be synthesized by reticulocytes.[115] Hence, its presence was not due to some type of aberrant catabolism or denaturation of aged normal hemoglobin. Hb Zürich was the first unstable variant to be analyzed structurally: β 63 (E7) histidine was replaced by arginine.[54] The intimate steric relationship between this residue and the heme group was not known at this time (see Chapter 2). Subsequently, many other patients with CHBA and heat-labile hemoglobin were shown to have electrophoretically abnormal hemoglobins. It became apparent that the great majority of patients whose clinical and laboratory findings suggest the diagnosis of CHBA have structurally abnormal hemoglobin variants. In a few patients with the clinical findings of CHBA, current methods may not permit the delineation of a structural abnormality.

A list of the unstable hemoglobin variants appears in Table 13–1. There are about four times as many β-chain as α-chain variants. The relatively large number of unstable β-chain variants can be best explained by the fact that there are four α-chain genes but only two β-chain genes (see Chapter 7). Accordingly, a structural mutation of an α-chain gene would result in the synthesis of only 25 per cent of abnormal α chains. There may be a relatively high incidence of unstable α-chain variants that escape clinical recognition because they make up only a small proportion of the total hemoglobin in the red cell and therefore result in less significant hemolysis. Indeed, most of the α-chain variants listed in Table 13–1 are associated with mild clinical manifestations. It is noteworthy that of the 40-odd *stable* hemoglobin variants associated with increased O_2 affinity and familial polycythemia, all but six are β-chain variants (see Chapter 14).

Structural Basis of Instability

As discussed in Chapters 2 and 3, considerable knowledge has been amassed on the three-dimensional structure of normal human hemoglobin, allowing rather precise structure-function interpretations. Thus, the properties of a number of human hemoglobin variants have been explained in terms of the stereochemical consequences arising from an amino acid substitution (or deletion) at a specific site in a globin subunit.[116, 117] The instability of most of the variants listed in Table 13–1 can be attributed to one of the following five mechanisms:

1. *Amino Acid Substitution in the Vicinity of the Heme Pocket.* The binding of heme to globin involves a very specific stereochemical fit that helps to stabilize the tertiary conformation of the subunit (see Chapter 2). The heme is inserted into a hydrophobic cleft on the surface of the subunit. The porphyrin interacts with certain nonpolar amino acids in the CD, E, F, and FG regions of the subunits. Most of these nonpolar amino acids are invariant residues. Thus, it is not surprising that substitutions of these residues may result in a decrease in the stability of the heme-globin linkage and, secondarily, of the entire subunit. Figure 13–1A is a three-dimensional diagram of a β chain. Unstable hemoglobin variants in the vicinity of the heme pocket are shown. A number of the unstable hemoglobins have substitutions or deletions in the heme pocket. In some, such as hemoglobins Hammersmith, Zürich, Köln,[118, 119] and Sabine,[75] experimental evidence supports the prediction that heme binding is impaired. Four of these variants (Bristol, Borås, Olmsted, and Shepherds Bush) involve the substitution of a polar for a nonpolar residue. Such substitutions may allow the entrance of water into the normally hydrophobic heme pocket and thereby weaken heme-globin linkage. The consequences of displacement of heme from its normal binding site will be discussed below in further detail.

Three unstable variants have amino acid substitutions at the proximal (heme-linked) histidine (Hbs Istanbul or Saint Etienne [β 92

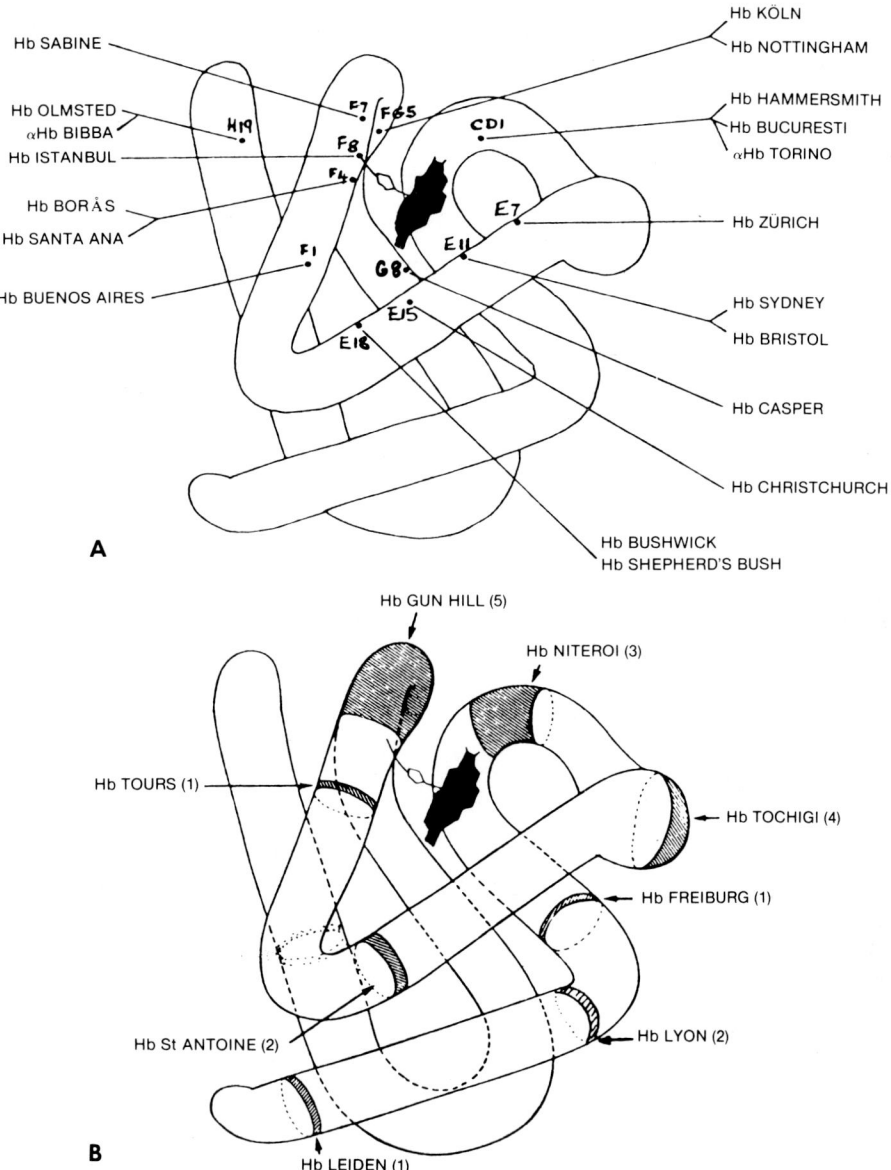

Figure 13–1. *A*, Three-dimensional representation of β chain showing sites of amino acid substitutions at the heme pocket that cause unstable variants. *B*, Three-dimensional representation of β chain showing sites of amino acid deletions causing unstable hemoglobins. (From Milner P. F. and Wrightstone R. N.: *In* Wallach, D. (ed.): The Function of Red Blood Cells. New York, Alan R. Liss, Inc. 1981.)

His → Gln], Mozhaisk [β 92 His→Arg], and Newcastle [β 92 His → Pro]). These abnormal subunits cannot bind heme. Two others (Hbs Zürich and Bicetre) have substitutions at the distal histidine.

The structural alteration in Hb Zürich leads to particularly interesting functional and clinical consequences. The substitution of arginine for the distal histidine at β E7 causes a marked change in the space where ligand binding occurs.[120] As shown in Figure 13–2A, the positively charged arginine attaches to the propionate of the heme, leaving the heme pocket wide open and allowing sulfanilamide ready access to the heme iron. This explains the propensity for individuals with this variant to have hemolytic episodes following ingestion of sulfa drugs (see Clinical Presentation below). Phenazopyridine also causes denaturation of Hb Zürich *in vitro* and hemolysis *in vivo*.[120a] Both of these effects can be reversed by increased levels of carboxyhemoglobin. Carbon monoxide binds to the β-heme iron of Hb Zürich even more strongly than to the β hemes

Text continued on page 572

Table 13–1. UNSTABLE HEMOGLOBIN VARIANTS*

Name	Structure		Molecular Basis for Instability†	Per Cent Abnormal Hb	Hb g/dl‡	Reticulocytes (%)	Inclusion Bodies§	Heat-Labile	Dark Urine	Oxygen Affinity	Comments	Reference
I. α-Chain Variants												
Boyle Heights	α 6	(A4)	Asp→0									1a
Shuangfen	α 27	(B8)	Glu→Lys									1b
Torino	α 43	(CE1)	Phe→Val	13	4.5	5		+		→	Moderately severe; aggravated by drugs	1b
				8	8→12‡	6–16		+	?			
Hirosaki	α 43	(CE1)	Phe→Leu		8	15	+			Nl		2
Umi, Mugino	α 47	(CE5)	Asp→Gly	14–20		9		+		Nl	Mild	3, 4
Hasharon	α 47	(CE5)	Asp→His	14–19	Normal	1–5	0	±	0	Nl	Mild	5–7
J-Rovigo	α 53	(E2)	Ala→Asp	35–49	13.2	1–3		+		Nl	Mild	8
Tottori	α 59	(E8)	Gly→Val		12–13	6–15	+	+				9
Pontoise	α 63	(E12)	Ala→Asp	12	12	10		+		Nl		10
Ann Arbor	α 80	(F1)	Leu→Arg	2–12	11–14	1–3		+		←	Mild	11, 12
Etobicoke	α 84	(F5)	Ser→Arg	15	12–14	6–10	+	+		Nl	Mild	13
Moabit	α 86	(F7)	Leu→Arg	15	Normal	3.6	+	0				14
Iwata	α 87	(F8)	His→Arg	5	11	4		+			Hemichrome, heme loss	15
Port Phillip	α 91	(FG3)	Leu→Pro	7				+				16
Setif	α 94	(G1)	Asp→Tyr	15			+	+	0	Sl ↓	Associated with Hb H	17, 18
Suan-Dok	α 109	(G16)	Leu→Arg								Associated with Hb H	19
Petah Tikva	α 110	(G17)	Ala→Asp		12.3	1.2						20
Hopkins-2	α 112	(G19)	His→Asp	22	Normal					Nl		21, 22
Bibba	α 136	(H19)	Leu→Pro	5–11	6–7.5	6–16	+	+			Severe	23
II. γ-Chain Variant												
F-Poole	γ 130	(H8)	Trp→Gly				+	+			Hemolysis in newborn	24
III. β-Chain Variants												
Leiden	β 6 or 7	(A3 or A4)	Glu→0	30	11–13	3–6	?			→	Mild; one residue deletion	25
Saki	β 14	(A11)	Leu→Pro	41	11–15	2–8		+		Nl	Double heterozygote with Hb S; with β thal	26, 27
Belfast	β 15	(A12)	Trp→Arg	28	11–13	4	+	+		Sl ↑		28, 29
Lyon	β 17, 18	(A14, 15)	Lys, Val→0	37	14.5	4	+	+		←		30
Freiburg	β 23	(B5)	Val→0	30	13	9		+		←	Cyanosis; ↑ methemoglobin	31
Riverdale-Bronx	β 24	(B6)	Gly→Arg	30	11–12	10	+	+	0			32
Savannah	β 24	(B6)	Gly→Val	15–30	4→6‡	50	+	+			Severe	33
Moscva	β 24	(B6)	Gly→Asp	17			+	+			Patient also had leukemia	34
Volga	β 27	(B9)	Ala→Asp	17	9→12	30	+	+		←		35, 36
St. Louis	β 28	(B10)	Leu→Gln	30	10→12	20	+	+		←	15% methemoglobin	37
Genova	β 28	(B10)	Leu→Pro	10–25	8–14	10–50	+	+	±			38, 39

Hb	Position	Helix	Substitution										Ref
Lufkin	β 29	(B11)	Gly→Asp										40
Tacoma	β 30	(B12)	Arg→Ser	B	40	12	7	+	+	0	SI↑	No clinical abnormality	41
Yokohama	β 31	(B13)	Leu→Pro	G		13	4	0	+		←		41a
Perth, Abraham Lincoln	β 32	(B14)	Leu→Pro	G	38	8, 9	40–50	+	+	+	NI		42, 43
Castilla	β 32	(B14)	Leu→Arg	A	~20	8→11	27	+	+	+	NI		44
Philly	β 35	(C1)	Tyr→Phe	B	31	9.6	High	+	+		←		45
Hazebrouck	β 38	C4	Thr→Pro		33	12–14	2–8	+	+	?	←		45a
Vassa	β 39	C5	Gln→Glu	G		11	8				→		45b
Mequon	β 41	(C7)	Phe→Tyr			12	2–5				NI	Severe hemolysis during infection	46
Hammersmith	β 42	(CD1)	Phe→Ser	A	30	15	20–50	+	+	+	→	Severe	47, 48
Louisville	β 42	(CD1)	Phe→Leu	A	30–35	6→7	7–9	+	+	+	→		49, 50
Cheverly	β 45	(CD4)	Phe→Ser		40–50	11–13	3–4	+	+	+	→	Mild	50a
Okaloosa	β 48	(CD7)	Leu→Arg	A	36	9–10	3.6	+	+	+	→	Heterozygous with β⁰ thalassemia	51
G-Ferrara	β 57	(E1)	Asn→Lys	B	92	13		0	+	+		Heterozygous with β⁰ thalassemia	52
Duarte	β 62	(E6)	Ala→Pro	G	~100	15	10	+	+		←		53
Zürich	β 63	(E7)	His→Arg		25	11–12	5–6	+	+	+	+	Mild; drug-sensitive	54
Bicetre	β 63	(E7)	His→Pro	G	20	8–10	15	+	+	+	←		55
J-Calabria	β 64	(E8)	Gly→Asp		33–42	12–14	0.7	+	+	+		Heterozygous with β⁺ thalassemia	56
I-Toulouse	β 66	(E10)	Lys→Glu	A	40	16	1.4	+	+	+	→	Mild	57
Sydney	β 67	(E11)	Val→Ala	D	30	12	8	+	+				58
Bristol	β 67	(E11)	Val→Asp	C	36	7→7	37	+	+	+	→	Severe hemolysis	59
Mizuho	β 68	(E12)	Leu→Pro	G	?	7–9.5		+	+				60
Seattle	β 70	(E14)	Ala→Asp	A	40	9–10	3	+	+	+	→		61
Christchurch	β 71	(E15)	Phe→Ser	D	22	7–13	8–15	+	+	+	→	Moderate hemolysis	62
Shepherds Bush	β 74	(E18)	Gly→Asp	E		12–13	5–8	+	+	+	←	Impaired reactivity of Hb with 2,3-DPG	63, 64
Bushwick	β 74	(E18)	Gly→Val	K			1–2	+	+	0			65
St. Antoine	β 74, 75	(E18, 19)	Gly, Leu→0	G	25	11	8	+	+	+	NI	Mild; drug-sensitive	66
Atlanta	β 75	(E19)	Leu→Pro			9.6	31	+	+	+			67
Pasadena	β 75	(E19)	Leu→Arg	A	31	16	10	0	+	+	←		68
Baylor	β 81	(EF5)	Leu→Arg	D		16	4	+	+	+	←		69
Buenos Aires	β 85	(F1)	Phe→Ser	K		12–14	8–15	+	+	+	←	Compensated hemolysis	70, 71
Tours	β 87	(F3)	Thr→0	A	20	13–14	9	+	0	0	←		66
Borås	β 88	(F4)	Leu→Arg	G	10	8–12		+	+	+	←		72
Santa Ana	β 88	(F4)	Leu→Pro		10	8–13	16–28	+	+	+		Two hemes per molecule	73

Table continued on following page

Table 13–1. UNSTABLE HEMOGLOBIN VARIANTS* Continued

Name	Structure		Molecular Basis for Instability†	Per Cent Abnormal Hb	Hb g/dl‡	Reticulo- cytes (%)	Inclusion Bodies§	Heat- Labile	Dark Urine	Oxygen Affinity	Comments	Reference
Gun Hill	β 91–95	(F7–FG2)	→0	30	13.5	4–10	0	+	←		Two hemes per molecule	74
Sabine	β 91	(F7)	Leu→Pro	8	8–10	35–65	+	+	→		Two hemes per molecule	75
Caribbean	β 91	(F7)	Leu→Arg		10	1		+	←		No clinical manifestations	76
Mozhaisk	β 92	(F8)	His→Arg	32	7	14	+	+	←		Heme loss	76a
Instanbul, St. Etienne	β 92	(F8)	His→Gln	12–15	9→13‡	4	+	+			Two hemes per molecule	77, 78
Newcastle	β 92	(F8)	His→Pro	26	7→9	18	+				Heme loss	79
Köln	β 98	(FG5)	Val→Met	15–25	11→14	5–16	+	+	←		Commonest of unstable hemoglobin variants	80, 81
Nottingham	β 98	(FG5)	Val→Gly		6.7; 9→12	50	+	+	←		Severe hemolysis	82, 83
Djelfa	β 98	(FG5)	Val→Ala					0				84, 85
Rush	β 101	(G3)	Glu→Gln	34	11–12	3–7	+	+	NI			86
Southampton, Casper	β 106	(G8)	Leu→Pro		4–7→13	20–90	+	+	←		Severe hemolysis	87, 88
Tübingen	β 106	(G8)	Leu→Gln	23	15	16–40	0	+	←		Cyanosis due to methemoglobin	89, 90
Burke	β 107	(G9)	Gly→Arg	30	10–12	8–15	+	+	→		?Drug-induced heme crisis	91
Peterborough	β 111	(G13)	Val→Phe		12	3.5	0	+	→		Mild	92
Indianapolis	β 112	(G14)	Cys→Arg	0	5–6	14–45	0	0			Thalassemic phenotype	93, 94
Madrid	β 115	(G17)	Ala→Pro	23	9.7	33	+	+			Severe hemolysis	95
Saitama	β 117	(G19)	His→Pro		10	34		+				95a
Khartoum	β 124	(H2)	Pro→Arg				0	+	NI		Very mild	96
J-Guantanamo	β 128	(H6)	Ala→Asp		10–11	3–4	+	+				97
Wein	β 130	(H8)	Tyr→Asp		10	43	+	+				98
Shelby (Leslie)	β 131	(H9)	Gln→Lys					+	→			99–101
North Shore	β 134	(H12)	Val→Glu	30	13.5	NI	+	+	NI		Mild	102, 103
Altdorf	β 135	(H13)	Ala→Pro	35	9–12	2–17	+	+	←			104

Name	Position	Helix	Substitution	Cat						Comment	Refs
Hope	β 136	(H14)	Gly→Asp		30	10.5			→		105
Brockton	β 138	(H16)	Ala→Pro		5–10	5→6‡			NI		106, 106a
Olmsted	β 141	(H19)	Leu→Arg	A	<10	10	+	+		Severe hemolysis	107, 108
Coventry	β 141	(H19)	Leu→0	K	7	NI	3–8	+	+	May be βδ fusion	109, 110
Toyoake	β 142	(H20)	Ala→Pro	G	35	14	6–8	+	0	↑ Heme loss	111
Cranston	β 144		C terminus					0	0	↑ Elongated β chain	112

*This table was prepared from the list of hemoglobin variants compiled by Dr. Ruth Wrightstone at the International Hemoglobin Information Center, Augusta, Georgia. The laboratory and clinical data were obtained from primary sources (see references in right-hand column). Hb H (β 4) is also an unstable hemoglobin, although not a variant. It is discussed in Chapters 2 and 9.

†Information obtained from G. Fermi and M. F. Perutz: Hemoglobin and myoglobin. In Phillips, D. C., and Richards, F. M. (eds.): Atlas of Molecular Structures in Biology. Oxford, Clarendon Press, 1981.

A: Loss of nonpolar "plug" that normally reaches the protein surface
B: Loss of hydrogen bonds or salt bridges
C: Introduction of interior charge or dipole
D: Introduction of interior gap
E: Introduction of wedge between helices
F: Misfit at subunit contact
G: Introduction of Pro into α helix
H: Unclear
J: Introduction of side chain at position of invariant Gly in β bend
K: Deletion

‡Values separated by an arrow indicate hemoglobin levels before and after splenectomy.

§Inclusion bodies are seen most often and most prominently in splenectomized patients. In nonsplenectomized individuals, incubation was usually required to demonstrate inclusion bodies.

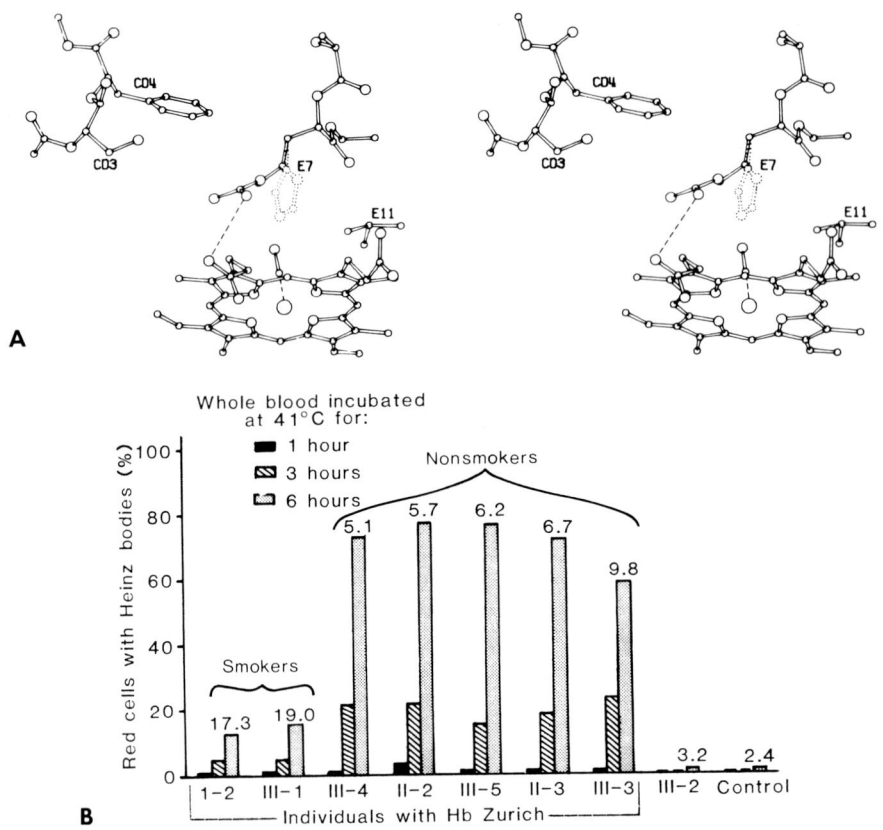

Figure 13–2. *A,* Stereochemical view of the heme pocket in Hb Zürich. Note that the absence of the distal histidine (E7) allows perpendicular bonding of CO to the heme iron. (From Tucker, P. W., et al.: Proc. Natl. Acad. Sci. USA 75:1076, 1978.) *B,* Demonstration of reduced Heinz body formation Hb Zürich heterozygotes who have elevated levels of carboxyhemoglobin due to smoking. The number above each vertical bar is the percentage of carboxyhemoglobin in the blood. (From Zinkham, W. H., et al.: Science *209*:406, 1980.)

of Hb A.[120] The distal histidine in Hb A prevents CO from binding perpendicular to the plane of the porphyrin, and thus, the CO-iron bond in Hb A is weaker than that in β Zürich. The abnormally high affinity of Hb Zürich for carbon monoxide enables this ligand to protect the variant from oxidant denaturation (Fig. 13–2B). Individuals with Hb Zürich who smoke tend to accumulate high levels of carboxyhemoglobin, and they have less hemolysis than affected family members who do not smoke.[121, 121a] In this striking paradox, the pathology of a mutant protein is ameliorated by a normally toxic pollutant.

2. *Disruption of Secondary Structure.* The primary amino acid sequence of a protein determines how much of it will be ordered into some form of secondary structure such as alpha helix or beta pleated sheet. As mentioned in Chapter 2, about 75 per cent of native hemoglobin is in the form of an alpha helix. The remaining segments of the chains are in random coil. Certain residues have a higher probability of forming an alpha helix than others. Thus, an analysis of primary structure can give a prediction of secondary structure.[122] Certain amino acid substitutions could shift the equilibrium between alpha helix and random coil in a given segment of the subunit. This would have a marked effect on tertiary structure and the overall stability of the subunit. Proline cannot participate in an alpha helix except as one of the initial three residues. Eleven of the unstable variants are substitutions of proline for leucine. In addition, five unstable variants involve a substitution of proline for alanine, and three have a substitution of proline for histidine. In 17 out of 19 of these variants, the substitution involves a residue beyond the third place in the helix. Among the 160 stable hemoglobin variants with no associated clinical manifestations, only one involves a proline substitution, and this is at the C-terminal residue of the alpha chain, where it should have no effect on secondary structure: Hb Singapore (α 141 Arg → Pro). Thus, the

disruption of the alpha helix probably accounts for the instability of the 17 variants mentioned above.

3. *Substitution in the Interior of the Subunit.* As mentioned in Chapter 2, the globin subunits are folded in such a way that all the charged amino acids such as lysine, arginine, glutamic acid, and aspartic acid are situated on the surface of the molecule, allowing their ionized groups to be in contact with solvent water. In contrast, the residues oriented toward the interior of the molecule have nonpolar side groups. The interior of the molecule is thus stabilized by hydrophobic interactions. About one third of the unstable variants involve the substitution of a charged for an uncharged residue. As mentioned above, in several of these variants (Bristol, Borås, Shepherds Bush, and Olmsted), these substitutions are near the heme pocket. The introduction of a charged group into the interior of the molecule could result in significant alterations in tertiary structure if water is allowed access to the hydrophobic interior of the subunit. In addition, a variant having a neutral amino acid substitution may owe its instability to an alteration of the stereochemical fit of the residue's side group. This is difficult to predict without very precise atomic coordinates. Nevertheless, it is interesting that 36 of 85 unstable variants (42 per cent) involve the substitution of one noncharged residue for another (including the 11 Leu → Pro substitutions), whereas only 3 per cent of functionally normal and clinically silent variants involve such a substitution. Of course, clinically silent variants are detected primarily because of an alteration of charge.

As mentioned in Chapter 2, hemoglobin readily dissociates symmetrically into αβ dimers: $\alpha_2\beta_2 \rightleftharpoons 2\alpha\beta$. The subunits cleave at the interface between the α_1 and β_2 subunits. In contrast, the bonding between the α_1 and β_1 subunits is considerably stronger. In normal Hb A, the dissociation of the subunits at this interface takes place very slowly.[122a] Measurable amounts of α and β monomer are observed only under extremes of pH or ionic strength or in solutions that favor disruption of secondary and tertiary structure, such as concentrated urea. Seven unstable variants* have substitutions at the $\alpha_1\beta_1$ interface. In some of these, the dissociation of the αβ dimer into monomers allows hidden sulfhydryl groups to become reactive. Hb Philly is the best studied of this type of unstable variant.[45, 123] X-ray analyses have been performed on both Hb Philly[123] and Hb Tacoma.[124]

4. *Amino Acid Deletion(s).* To date, 11 hemoglobin variants have been reported to have deletions from one to five residues in sequence: Boyle Heights, Leiden, Lyon, Freiburg, St. Antoine, Vicksburg, Tours, Gun Hill, Niteroi, Tochigi, and Coventry.† All of these are unstable variants (see Figure 13–1B and Table 13–1). Deletions of more than one residue have been encountered only at or near interhelical corners. Such an alteration in structure can have a marked effect on the overall conformation of the molecule involving intrasubunit and intersubunit interactions.

5. *Elongation of Subunit.* A few hemoglobin variants have elongated subunits, owing either to an error in chain termination or to a frame shift (see Chapter 10). Most of these are present only in small amounts. Hb Cranston and Hb Saverne are associated with a compensated hemolytic state.[112] The instability of these variants is probably due to a hydrophobic segment attached to the C-terminal end of the beta chain.[126] The stability of the other elongated beta-chain variant, Hb Tak, has not yet been determined.

Mechanism of Hemoglobin Denaturation

The mechanisms underlying the formation of intracellular inclusions in CHBA have been studied extensively, particularly by Winterbourn and Carrell,[127-131] Rachmilewitz,[132-134] and Jacob and associates.[118, 119, 135, 136] Their experiments were done on selected variants, but the results are relevant to many of the other unstable hemoglobins.

As explained in detail in Chapter 16, oxyhemoglobin can autoxidize into methemoglobin by dissocation of superoxide anion (O_2^-):

$$Hb\ Fe^{2+}O_2 \rightarrow Hb\ Fe^{3+} + O_2^-$$

Both superoxide anion and its reduction product, hydrogen peroxide, are capable of generating more methemoglobin. Winterbourn

---

*Hbs Petah Tikva, Philly, Tacoma, Indianapolis, Madrid, Khartoum, Shelby, and J-Guantanamo.

†Hb McKees Rocks is a *stable* variant with a deletion of the two C-terminal residues of the beta chain (beta 145–146 Tyr-His→0). A deletion at this site would not impair the folding or solubility of the subunit. Distortion of structure is particularly marked in Hb Gun Hill, in which no heme binding to the beta chain is possible because of the deletion of five residues in the F-FG region. Despite this, individuals with Hb Gun Hill have relatively mild hemolysis.[74, 125]

and colleagues[130] have shown that unstable hemoglobins autoxidize faster than Hb A, with rates roughly proportional to their degree of instability. Furthermore, they found that the unstable hemoglobins were converted from methemoglobin to hemichromes much more rapidly than was Hb A.

Hemichrome Formation. Hemichromes are a common intermediate in various types of hemoglobin denaturation.[132–134] They are characterized by a specific absorption in the visible spectrum (Fig. 13–3) and are formed when the globin undergoes sufficient internal distortion to allow direct bonding of an amino acid side chain to the distal aspect of the heme iron (Fig. 13–4). The incubation of methemoglobin can lead to the formation of hemichromes, particularly under circumstances in which hemoglobin lacks its normal stabilizing interactions. For example, isolated hemoglobin subunits (alpha or beta chains), certain chemically modified hemoglobins, and a number of unstable hemoglobin variants form hemichromes readily.[137] Electron paramagnetic (spin) resonance (EPR) has proved a very useful physical measurement in the further characterization of these intermediates.[137] The bonding of the distal (E7) histidine imidazole to the oxidized heme results in the transition from high spin to low spin state having a characteristic EPR signal (Fig. 13–4). This type of hemichrome has been shown to be reversible (see Figure 13–6). Further distortion of the subunit's conformation allows other groups to form an internal ligand with the heme, resulting in the formation of irreversible hemichromes that have distinguishing EPR spectra (see Figure 13–6). The formation of irreversi-

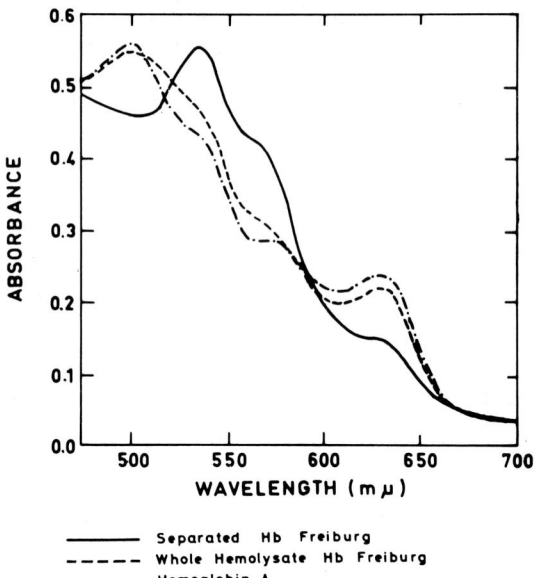

Figure 13–3. Absorption spectra of whole hemolysate and purified hemoglobins from a patient with Hb Freiburg (β 23 Val → 0) 48 hours after oxidation with ferricyanide (0.05 M phosphate, pH 7.0, 4°C). Purified Hb A (—·—·—·) has an absorption spectrum indicating methemoglobin. Purified Hb Freiburg (———) has an absorption spectrum of a hemichrome. (With permission of Dr. E. A. Rachmilewitz.)

ble hemichromes is accompanied by precipitation of the hemoglobin.

A number of unstable hemoglobin variants have been shown to form hemichromes, particularly following incubation of the oxidized (methemoglobin) form. These include hemoglobins Köln, β 98 Val→Met[132]; Hammersmith, β 42 Phe→Ser[138]; Louisville (Bucuresti), β 42 Phe→Leu[134]; Freiburg, β 23 Val→0[132];

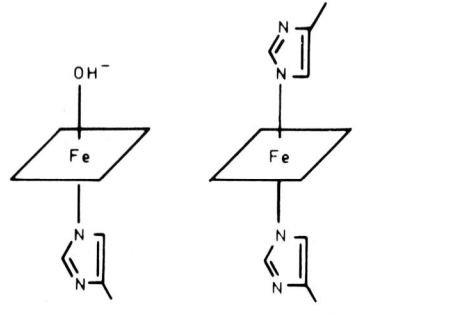
Reversible Hemichromes

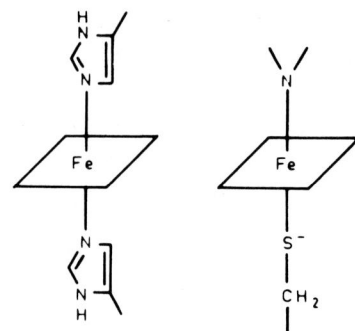
Irreversible Hemichromes

Figure 13–4. Diagrammatic structure of hemichromes showing proximal histidine below the plane of the porphyrin ring and distal histidine above the plane. (From Peisach, J., Blumberg, W. E., and Rachmilewitz, E. A.: Biochim. Biophys. Acta *393*:404, 1975.)

Riverdale-Bronx, β 24 Gly→Arg[132]; Seattle, β 70 Ala→Asp[134]; Sydney, β 67 Val→Ala[129]; Christchurch, β 71 Phe→Ser[129]; and St. Louis, β 28 Leu→Gln.[37] It is likely that such hemichromes are formed during the denaturation of other unstable variants. The amino acid substitution apparently causes sufficient disruption in the tertiary structure of the subunit to permit the apposition of the iron atom of the ferriheme group to certain nearby groups of the globin chain. The formation of hemichromes involves a marked reduction in absorption at 540 nm, in comparison to oxyhemoglobin, and probably contributes to the decreased optical density observed for several unstable variants (↓ OD-540/OD-280).[135, 136]

Displacement of the Heme Group. The stability of the heme-globin linkage is dependent on the precise stereochemical fit conferred by the surrounding residues in the heme pocket (see Chapter 2). As mentioned above, this fit is perturbed in a number of the unstable variants because of amino acid substitutions or deletions in this region. Furthermore, the oxidation state of the heme iron has an important influence on the stability of the heme-globin linkage. In normal oxyhemoglobin and deoxyhemoglobin, the ferrous heme group remains tightly bound to globin. In contrast, the ferriheme group in methemoglobin has a much lower affinity for globin.[139] Ferriheme dissociates more readily from methemoglobin Köln than from methemoglobin A.[119, 139a] During incubation of hemolysates at 50°C, those containing certain unstable hemoglobin variants (Köln, Zürich, Hammersmith) show a rapid decrease in the ratio of absorptions at 540 nm and 280 nm.[135, 136] These results do not necessarily mean "heme loss." Free hematin is very insoluble at neutral pH and binds avidly and nonspecifically to a number of proteins. It is likely that in many cases the heme group is displaced from its normal position in the subunit during the incubation, and, as mentioned above, may form hemichromes. As a result its absorption in the visible spectrum is significantly altered.

Some unstable variants have increased rates of reaction with glutathione to form the mixed disulfide.[118, 119] Red cell glutathione has been found to be decreased in a few patients with CHBA,[43, 140, 141] although normal or elevated in others.[140, 141] The enhanced sulfhydryl reactivity of some of the unstable variants may explain their tendency to become highly labeled with radioactive chromium. When intact CHBA red cells were incubated with ^{51}Cr-labeled sodium chromate, the variant β chains (Köln, Hammersmith, and Shepherds Bush) had two- to sixfold higher specific activity than the β^A chains.[141] Some experiments suggested that in patients with Hb Köln, Heinz bodies may be attached to the inner surface of the red cell membrane by a disulfide bond between hemoglobin and a membrane protein.[118, 119] The inclusions could be released from erythrocyte ghosts by the addition of mercaptoethanol, a reagent capable of reducing disulfide bonds.[118]

Subsequent studies have raised doubt about the importance of sulfhydryl oxidation in the pathogenesis of CHBA.[127–129] Experiments on three unstable variants (Köln, Sydney, Christchurch) revealed no blocked cysteines and no protection by reduced glutathione. Although precipitation of the oxy and carboxy forms of these hemoglobins was accompanied by the formation of intermolecular disulfide bonds, there was no evidence that this phenomenon affected the rate of precipitation. Furthermore, these investigators examined red cells containing inclusions of Hb Christchurch and failed to demonstrate the presence of any covalent linkage (such as disulfide bonds) between globin and membrane protein. They concluded that the adherence of the Heinz body to the inner surface of the red cell membrane is due to hydrophobic bonding.[128]

The two phenomena—dissociation of heme and enhanced sulfhydryl reactivity—may be linked according to the following scheme:

$$\begin{array}{ccc}
\text{Globin—Fe}^{3+}\text{heme} & \rightleftharpoons & \text{Globin} + \text{Fe}^{3+}\text{heme} \\
\mid & K_1 & \mid \\
\text{SH} & & \text{SH} \\
K_2 \updownarrow + \text{RSH} & & K_4 \updownarrow + \text{RSH} \\
\text{Globin—Fe}^{3+}\text{heme} & \rightleftharpoons & \text{Globin} + \text{Fe}^{3+}\text{heme} \\
\mid & K_3 & \mid \\
\text{SSR} & & \text{SSR}
\end{array}$$

The following observations support such a relationship: (1) the dissociation of ferriheme from normal methemoglobin A is enhanced when the β 93 sulfhydryl group is blocked by N-ethylmaleimide ($K_3 > K_1$)[139]; (2) hemoglobin lacking heme groups on the β chains ($\alpha_2\beta_2^0$) has markedly enhanced sulfhydryl reactivity ($K_4 > K_2$)[135]; and (3) in several of the unstable variants both of these reactions are favored. From these considerations, it is not surprising that the rate of denaturation of the unstable hemoglobins can be enhanced by sulfhydryl blockade[118, 119] and that it can be reduced by the addition of a heme ligand such as cyanide[135, 142] that stabilizes the heme-globin

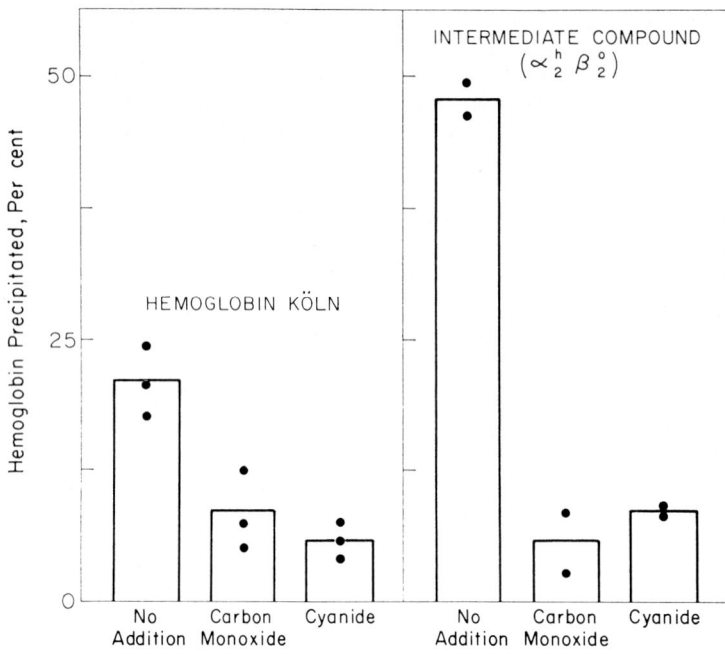

Figure 13–5. Inhibition of heat precipitation of hemoglobin Köln (left) and $\alpha_2^{heme} \beta_2^0$ (right) by cyanide or carbon monoxide. Both heme proteins precipitate copiously when heated at 50°C for 2 hours unless the heme ligands cyanide or carbon monoxide are present. (From Jacob, H. S., and Winterhalter, K. H.: J. Clin. Invest. 49:2008, 1970.)

linkage[139] (Fig. 13–5). Cyanide also inhibits the denaturation of normal hemoglobin.[142]

The unstable hemoglobins have properties very similar to the artificial semihemoglobin Hb $\alpha_2\beta_2^0$.[135] As mentioned above, both have enhanced sulfhydryl reactivity. Both form a flocculent precipitate when incubated at 50°C. This denaturation is inhibited by the addition of heme ligands (carbon monoxide or cyanide [Fig. 13–5]). Both $\alpha_2\beta_2^0$ and many of the unstable variants have an increased degree of dissociation from tetramer to dimer: $\alpha_2\beta_2 \rightarrow 2\alpha\beta$.[143, 144]

During the circulation of the CHBA red cell *in vivo* or the incubation of the hemolysate *in vitro*, the three-dimensional structure of the hemoglobin variant is altered sufficiently so that its solubility decreases and it forms a precipitate. It seems unnecessary to postulate that the hemoglobin tetramer dissociates into individual subunits prior to the precipitation of the abnormal chain.[132, 134] Amino acid analyses and peptide mapping of precipitates of several variants, including Christchurch, Sydney, Köln, and Hammersmith, have demonstrated the presence of equal amounts of α and β chains.[127] Furthermore, some α chain polymerized with β chain by means of disulfide bond formation. The precipitates of hemoglobins Christchurch and Sydney contained a full complement of heme, whereas Hb Köln appeared to be depleted of half the heme. Thus, the precipitation of most unstable variants probably involves the entire molecule rather than the abnormal globin subunit.

The scheme proposed by Winterbourn and Carrell[129] for the denaturation of unstable hemoglobins is depicted in Figure 13–6. Oxyhemoglobin is converted to methemoglobin. The release of superoxide anion (O_2^-) or its product, H_2O_2, may result in oxidant damage to globin thiols and to the membrane (see the following section on Mechanism of Hemolysis). Because of its structural abnormality, the unstable methemoglobin is converted first to a reversible hemichrome intermediate and then to an irreversible hemichrome.

Mechanism of Hemolysis in CHBA

There is both morphological[145, 146] and experimental[118] evidence that in CHBA, Heinz bodies become adherent to the inner surface of the red cell membrane. As mentioned above, this attachment is probably due to hydrophobic rather than covalent interactions.[127, 147] The membrane-bound inclusions cause crater-like indentations on the surface of the cell.[146] Red cells containing Heinz bodies have been shown to have decreased pliability and filterability.[148, 149] It is not surprising that they have difficulty negotiating the microcirculation. Red cells containing Heinz bodies

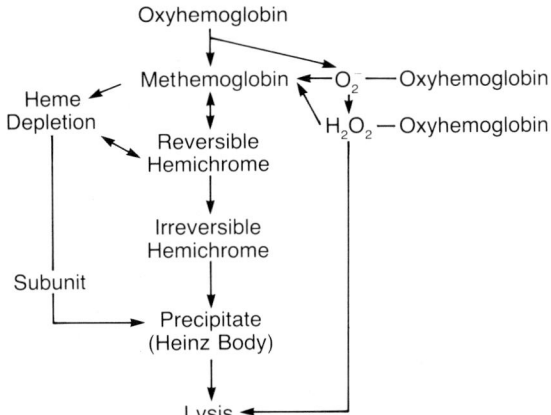

Figure 13-6. Scheme proposed by Winterbourn and Carrell[129] for intracellular denaturation of unstable hemoglobins.

become trapped during their transit between the cords and sinuses of the spleen.[145] The membrane-bound Heinz body may be removed or "pitted" during this passage. The remainder of the red cell then reseals its membrane after it has been relieved of this "excess baggage." These considerations help to explain why the number of Heinz bodies increases markedly after patients with CHBA have undergone splenectomy.

The metabolism of CHBA red cells has been studied by a number of investigators. In general, specific enyzme activities have either been normal or increased in keeping with a young population of red cells. In some cases, glucose consumption is increased in conjunction with decreased levels of ATP.[141, 149] Indeed, one case of CHBA[75] was initially reported as a defect in red cell metabolism.[150] Red cell 2,3-DPG is usually found to be normal. The enhanced potassium efflux[118, 149] found in erythrocytes from certain patients with CHBA has been attributed to the adherence of Heinz bodies to the inner surface of the red cell membrane. However, this increased potassium efflux is rather nonspecific and has been reported in a diverse group of hemolytic states, including sickle cell anemia, Hb CC disease, β thalassemia, pyruvate kinase deficiency, and hereditary stomatocytosis. In order to maintain osmotic equilibrium, the energy-dependent Na-K pump is stimulated to the extent that CHBA red cells leak potassium, thereby increasing ATP utilization. Osmotic fragility is generally normal in CHBA.

The activity of the hexose monophosphate shunt has been increased in some cases of CHBA. Nevertheless, as mentioned above, red cell glutathione is more often normal or increased than decreased[141] and does not have an enhanced turnover rate.[141]

The intracellular release of heme from unstable hemoglobin variants may contribute to the rate of hemolysis. Free ferriheme will induce potassium loss in normal red cells, followed by colloid osmotic lysis.[150a] The molecular basis for membrane damage by ferriheme is uncertain but appears to involve oxidation of sulfhydryl groups. In these *in vitro* experiments, at least 2 μM of ferriheme was required to show a hemolytic effect. It is unlikely that comparable levels of ferriheme are reached in red cells of patients with CHBA.

Unstable hemoglobins release reactive oxidants such as hydrogen peroxide, superoxide, and hydroxyl radical. These toxic compounds damage the red cell membrane by two mechanisms: lipid peroxidation and crosslinking of membrane proteins.[150b] Malondialdehyde, a product of lipid peroxidation, can crosslink proteins, mainly at lysine residues. Proteins from the membrane of Hb Köln red cells are crosslinked in a manner similar to those in malondialdehyde-treated red cells.[150c]

Biosynthesis of Unstable Variants

As shown in Table 13–1, the unstable hemoglobin variant usually makes up only a minority of the total hemoglobin. The remainder is Hb A, Hb A_2, and perhaps some Hb F. The level of Hb F will be significantly increased if an enhanced potential for producing fetal hemoglobin has also been inherited (such as the Swiss type of heterocellular HPFH[151]). Furthermore, in hemolysates of some individuals with unstable beta-chain variants, a very small amount of free alpha chains is observed on electrophoresis.[115, 134, 152-156] The presence of free alpha chains can be explained by either decreased synthesis or enhanced destruction of the unstable beta subunit. As the previous discussion on the pathogenesis of CHBA implies, the latter mechanism predominates.

A significant reduction in δ-aminolevulinic acid synthetase has been noted in four patients with Hb Köln, whereas the enzyme activity was enhanced in red cells of individuals with other types of hemolysis.[157] The increased level of free heme dissociated from the unstable hemoglobin may suppress the synthesis of this rate-limiting enzyme in heme synthesis. Nevertheless, there is no evidence of true heme deficiency in CHBA.

The biosynthesis of a number of unstable variants has been studied. As shown in Table 13–2, the rate of synthesis of normal and variant chains is equal in most cases. In all cases, the specific activity of the abnormal beta chain greatly exceeded that of β^A. The low proportion of unstable hemoglobin in circulating red cells and its high specific radioactivity are due primarily to proteolysis of the affected subunit during erythroid maturation in the bone marrow.[159] This breakdown in the bone marrow cells occurs rapidly and appears to reflect the instability of the isolated, freshly synthesized globin chain before it has folded and joined with other subunits to give the hemoglobin tetramer. In addition to this initial rapid breakdown of the globin subunit by proteolysis, there is also a slower breakdown of the formed tetramer due to denaturation, which continues in the circulation to give Heinz body formation and hemolysis. Thus, there are two different processes involved: the breakdown of the nascent globin, which is a measure of the stability of the tertiary structure; and the breakdown of the hemoglobin, which reflects quaternary stability. The two may not necessarily be affected to the same degree. These different modes of catabolism help to explain the diversity of findings among the unstable hemoglobins.[159a] An abnormality that primarily affects the folding of the globin subunit will cause considerable disturbance of bone marrow erythropoiesis and result in a very low proportion of the variant in the circulation, but it may not cause a severe hemolytic anemia. An abnormality whose major

Table 13–2. **SYNTHESIS OF GLOBIN CHAINS OF UNSTABLE HEMOGLOBIN VARIANTS**

Variant	Per Cent Abnormal Hb	Subunit Specific Activity Var/A	Rate of Synthesis of Variant Chain*	Total $\alpha:\beta$ Synthesis	Reference
Ann Arbor α 80 Leu→Arg	2–15	2.5	20	4.0	Adams, 1974[210]
Suan-Dok α 109 Leu→Arg	9		20	0.59	Sanguansermsri et al., 1979[19]
Petah Tikva α 110 Ala→Asp	31		13–35	0.6–1.4	Honig et al., 1981[20]
Leiden β 6, 7→0	24	1.5	100	1.8	Rieder and James, 1974[165]
Riverdale-Bronx β 24 Gly→Arg	28	1.4–1.5	56–59	~1.2	Zalusky et al., 1970[162]
Abraham Lincoln β 32 Leu→Pro	18	2.5	50	1.18	Honig et al., 1973[43]
Hammersmith β 42 Phe→Ser	40	1.5	100	1.1	White and Dacie, 1970[160]
Zürich β 63 His→Arg	32		110		Rieder et al., 1965[173]
Bristol β 67 Val→Asp	36	1.4	98		Steadman et al., 1979[59]
Shepherds Bush β 74 Gly→Asp	25		100		White and Dacie, 1971[140]
Bushwick β 74 Gly→Val	1–2	20–60	~100	1.0	Rieder et al., 1975[156]
Borås β 88 Leu→Arg	10		33		White 1974[187]
Sabine β 91 Leu→Pro	12	~1.5–3	~100		Shaeffer, 1973[163]
Gun Hill β 91–95 deleted	32	2.4	120	1.0	Rieder, 1971[158]
Köln β 98 Val→Met	12	7.4	100	1.2–1.4	White and Brain, 1970[161]
Nottingham β 98 Val→Gly	16	2.5–2.7	>40	1.0–1.3	Orringer et al., 1978[83]
Indianapolis β 112 Cys→Arg	0		>80	0.4	Adams et al., 1979[93]
Cranston Elongated β chain	30	1.4	100	1.0	Shaeffer et al., 1980[164]

*Expressed as percentage of the rate of synthesis of normal subunit.

effect is on the stability of the tetramer may be present in the circulation in higher proportions but will also produce more marked hemolysis. Usually, of course, there is a mixed pattern with loss occurring in the bone marrow along with subsequent selective loss of the unstable hemoglobin with accompanying hemolysis, as the Heinz body–containing red cells pass through the RE system.

In red cells containing very unstable variants, a small pool of free alpha chains may readily exchange with the alpha chains of the variant. Observations on Hb Gun Hill provide a striking illustration of this point.[158] Following incubation of the reticulocyte-rich blood with ^{14}C leucine, hemoglobins A and Gun Hill were separated by electrophoresis. The alpha chains of the purified hemoglobin A had virtually no radioactivity, whereas the alpha chains of Gun Hill were highly labeled. Thus, the newly synthesized alpha chains appeared to be diluted by a pre-existing pool of unlabeled alpha chains, thereby lowering alpha^A radioactivity. The high activity of the alpha^{GH} chains must have been due to exchange of the partially labeled free alpha-chain pool with the alpha chains of the unlabeled (but labile) Hb Gun Hill. A similar phenomenon has been noted for hemoglobins Hammersmith,[160] Köln,[161] Shepherds Bush,[141] Riverdale-Bronx,[162] Sabine,[163] Abraham Lincoln,[43] Nottingham,[83] and Cranston.[164] Because of this exchange of alpha chains, the ratio of the total radioactivity of the normal and variant hemoglobins is not a reliable indication of the relative synthetic rates. It is curious that despite the marked distortion of primary structure of Hb Gun Hill, which has a deletion of the 5 residue segment at the proximal heme binding site, the rate of translation of beta$^{Gun Hill}$ was equal to that of beta^A.[158] Thus, if heme normally binds to the nascent polypeptide chain, it has no apparent effect on the rate of translation.

As shown in Table 13–2, in most of the synthesis studies done on reticulocytes containing unstable hemoglobins, total alpha- and beta-chain production is balanced. However, some interesting exceptions have been noted. In reticulocytes containing Hb Leiden, the overall alpha/beta synthetic ratio was about 1.8, whereas the ratio was 1.2 in marrow.[165] These values are similar to what has been encountered in individuals with beta thalassemia. This imbalance in subunit synthesis cannot be explained by differences in translation times of alpha and beta chains[166] and is probably due to quantitative differences in specific mRNAs or (less likely) in differential rates of initiation. Thus, the individual with Hb Leiden may also have beta thalassemia in cis. Recently, a mildly unstable variant, Hb Vicksburg (β 75 Leu→0), has been described in cis to a β^+ thalassemia gene.[167] In contrast, a variant may be so unstable that it cannot be detected in circulating red cells and can be documented only by biosynthetic studies using radiolabeled precursors. Adams and colleagues[93, 94] employed elegant radiolabeling experiments to show that an individual presenting as a thalassemic phenotype with a decreased beta/alpha synthetic ratio was producing an extremely labile variant (Hb Indianapolis, β 112 Cys→Arg). This important study raises the question as to whether other families who appear to have thalassemia may actually be harboring an extremely unstable hemoglobin variant.

One variant, Hb Quong Sze (α 125 Leu → Pro), is so unstable that it cannot be detected by any means.[167a] The substitution at the $\alpha_1\beta_1$ interface prevents the formation of $\alpha\beta$ dimers and apparently leads to total destruction of the variant subunit. Accordingly, base sequencing of DNA was required to demonstrate this mutation. The affected individual had an α-thalassemia phenotype.

CLINICAL MANIFESTATIONS

Inheritance

Congenital Heinz body hemolytic anemia exhibits an autosomal dominant pattern of inheritance. Thus, affected individuals are heterozygotes. Because of proteolysis of the abnormal subunit in the bone marrow, the unstable hemoglobin makes up only a minority (10 to 30 per cent) of the total. As expected in the heterozygous state, the remainder is predominantly normal hemoglobin A.

Exceptions include cases in which a beta-chain unstable variant is inherited along with beta thalassemia. Such double heterozygotes have been described for Hbs G-Ferrara,[168] J-Calabria,[168] and Duarte.[53] In these individuals, the production of beta^A chains is completely or partially suppressed, so that the great majority of the hemoglobin is the beta-chain variant. Fortunately, in all of these cases, the variant is only slightly unstable, so that the affected individuals have mild or moderate hemolysis. Indeed, the co-inheritance of beta thalassemia is a means of unmasking variants that might otherwise escape detection. The proportion of alpha-chain unstable variants in the total hemoglobin is generally much lower than that for the beta-chain variants, consistent with the fact that individuals normally inherit four alpha-chain genes (see Chapter 7). As expected, the relative amount of the alpha-chain variant is increased when the affected individual also has alpha thalassemia. Examples include Hb Petah Tikva[20] and Hb Suan-Dok.[19]

Because of the low gene frequency for unstable variants, homozygosity would be very rare (except in offspring of consanguineous marriages) and often incompatible with life. Such genetic considerations also apply to hemoglobin variants with abnormally high oxygen affinity (see Chapter 14).

A sizable minority of cases of CHBA appear to have arisen because of a spontaneous mutation, both parents being unaffected. Viewed another way, of the 22 instances of apparent spontaneous mutations among hemoglobin variants reported until 1973, 17 involved patients with CHBA.[168a] Subsequently, an additional 22 spontaneous mutations with CHBA have been encountered.[168b] This is not surprising, because most cases have clinical manifestations requiring medical attention and evaluation. In contrast, the chances are very remote of finding an asymptomatic individual with a hemoglobin variant due to a spontaneous mutation. Furthermore, the reproductive potential of patients with severe CHBA may be decreased.

Presentation

Congenital Heinz body hemolytic anemia varies widely in clinical severity (see Table 13–1). The variability depends primarily on the structural differences among the unstable variants. A given variant tends to produce similar clinical sequelae in affected individuals whether they are within the same family or are unrelated. Thus far, Hb Köln has been the most frequently encountered unstable variant. At least 10 unrelated kindred or sporadic cases from various parts of the world have been reported to have Hb Köln. These patients all have a moderate hemolytic state that is well compensated, particularly following splenectomy.

On rare occasions, hemolytic anemia in the newborn may be caused by an unstable hemoglobin variant. An unstable γ-chain variant (Hb F-Poole, $^G\gamma$ 130 Trp→Gly) has been reported to cause hemolysis that disappeared when Hb F switched to Hb A in the first few months of life.[24] Significant hemolysis has been noted in newborns with Hb Hasharon (α 47 Asp→His).[169, 170] This variant has been commonly encountered around the world and does not cause significant hemolysis in adults. Perhaps $\alpha_2^{Hash}\gamma_2$ is less stable than $\alpha_2^{Hash}\beta_2$. Alternatively, the formation of methemoglobin Hasharon in the newborn may lead to its enhanced denaturation.[170a]

Patients with severe CHBA usually present with anemia in early childhood. Occasionally, clinical manifestations emerge at approximately six months of age when the transition from γ to β chain production is complete. More commonly, patients present at different ages with unexplained hemolytic anemia. In some cases, patients come to a physician's attention during an "aplastic" crisis, in which erythropoiesis has been temporarily suppressed by either infection or folic acid deficiency. Like other patients with chronic hemolysis, individuals with CHBA have an increased tendency to develop pigmented gallstones.

More often, anemia may be aggravated by hemolytic crises associated with viral or bacterial infections or following exposure to an oxidant agent such as sulfonamides.

Pyrexia may cause a significant increase in the rate of hemolysis. *In vitro* incubations of CHBA red cells[131, 171] or hemoglobin solutions[131] have revealed an increase in autoxidation and a more marked increase in Heinz body formation when the temperature is raised from 37° to 40°C. In addition, the denaturation of the unstable hemoglobin may be enhanced by the release of oxidants (O_2^- and H_2O_2) from activated leukocytes.[131]

Hemolytic crises have been reported in a number of carriers of unstable hemoglobins following the administration of oxidant drugs. In some cases, the hemolytic episode first brings the patient to the attention of the physician. The association of Hb Zürich (β 63 His→Arg) and drug-induced hemolysis is well established. This variant has been encountered in a number of unrelated families.[172-174] Affected individuals have normal hematocrits and absent or minimal hemolysis unless they are exposed to an oxidant stress. A few days of treatment with a sulfa drug can result in a hemolytic crisis with a 50 per cent drop in hematocrit, the emergence of Heinz bodies, and marked hyperbilirubinemia. The anemia remits promptly upon withdrawal of the drug. Those affected family members who have not been exposed to oxidant drugs have no history of hemolysis. The molecular mechanism responsible for sulfonamide-induced hemolysis in Hb Zürich is explained above (see Structural Basis of Instability). Sulfonamides have also been found to exacerbate hemolysis in individuals with hemoglobins Torino,[1, 175, 176] Shepherds Bush,[63] Peterborough,[92] and Hasharon.[177] Other agents besides sulfonamides may also aggravate hemolysis. Increased nitrate content of drinking water has been implicated in a child with Hb Abraham Lincoln (Perth) with severe hemolysis.[178] Oxidant drugs do not affect hemolysis in patients with Hb Köln.[149]

A significant proportion of patients with CHBA give a history of passing dark urine. In the absence of liver disease, patients with hemolytic anemia do not have bilirubinuria. Indeed, an outmoded term for hemolytic anemia is "acholuric jaundice." Furthermore, patients with CHBA do not have enough intravascular hemolysis to produce hemoglobinuria. It turns out that the pigmenturia in such patients with CHBA is probably due to dipyrrolmethenes of the mesobilifuscin group.[179] Fluorescent dipyrroles can also be detected in the Heinz bodies.[179a] The structure of this pigment is not yet definitely established. Pigmenturia is an inconsistent finding in CHBA. As shown in Table 13–1, pigmenturia is not well correlated with the severity of hemolysis. Dipyrroluria has also been encountered in β thalassemia (major),[180, 181] another disorder associated with Heinz body production (see Chapter 9). It is likely that the urinary pigment is a reflection of aberrant heme catabolism, perhaps via a pathway that bypasses heme oxygenase, an enzyme responsible for the physiological catabolism of heme.[182] Experimentally induced Heinz bodies are also broken down aberrantly with decreased conversion of heme to bilirubin and the formation of a urinary pigment having properties indicative of dipyrroles.[183] It may be that during the autoxidation of the unstable hemoglobin *in vivo,* sufficient superoxide anion or peroxide is generated that heme (or its porphyrin) is oxidized in a nonspecific, nonenzymatic fashion, leading to these abnormal products.

A number of the unstable hemoglobin variants are unassociated with any clinical manifestations and have been discovered fortuitously or during surveys of large populations. The frequency of finding these mild unstable variants is uncreasing because of the development of more sensitive and specific methods for detection (see below)

Physical Findings

The physical findings of patients with CHBA are variable and depend primarily on the severity of the disease. Those with moderate or severe hemolysis have jaundice and splenomegaly. Some patients may have hypersplenism with significant thrombocytopenia.[184, 185] Severe hypersplenic hemolysis has been observed in newborns with Hb Hasharon.[186] A few patients with CHBA may be mildly cyanotic, owing either to the presence of methemoglobinemia (as encountered in Hb Freiburg)[31] or to decreased oxygen affinity leading to deoxygenation of the peripheral blood (Hb Hammersmith). Some patients with CHBA have leg ulcers.[42, 187]

LABORATORY DIAGNOSIS OF CHBA

General Parameters of Hemolysis

Patients with CHBA, like those with other types of chronic hemolysis, will have reticulocytosis accompanied by increased serum bilirubin and decreased haptoglobin. However, the extent of hemolysis is often difficult to evaluate in patients having an unstable hemoglobin. Because the precipitated variant takes up supravital stains, Heinz body–containing cells may be mistaken for reticulocytes. Thus, the estimate of reticulocytes by ordinary methods may be falsely high. As shown in Figure 13–7, measurement of red cell RNA will give a truer indication of reticulocyte number.[88] In like manner, measurements of red cell life span by tagging red cells with ^{51}Cr are very difficult to interpret. There is no correlation between ^{51}Cr-labeled red cell survival and degree of hemolysis in CHBA.[188] First, as mentioned above, ^{51}Cr will bind preferentially to the variant hemoglobin, compared with Hb A.[141] Second, the isotope appears to elute more readily from the abnormal hemoglobin.[185] Finally, as we have discussed, precipitates containing the unstable variant are selectively pitted from red cells during *in vivo* circulation. These factors make the rate of disappearance of ^{51}Cr radioactivity greatly exceed the rate of red cell destruction. The use of radioactive amino acid precursor[43] (Fig. 13–8) or DF^{32}P labeling[188] will give a more reliable indication of red cell survival.

Red Cell Morphology

Congenital Heinz body anemia red cells may appear entirely normal on a Wright-stained

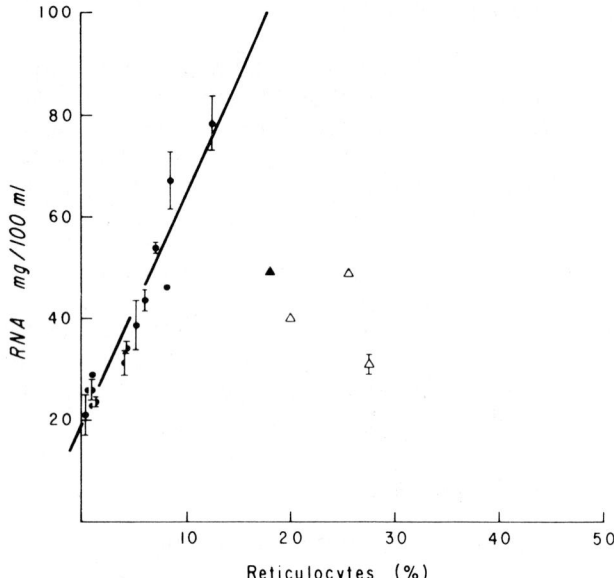

Figure 13–7. The relationship between reticulocytes estimated by supravital stain (abscissa) and by measurement of RNA (ordinate). Normal reticulocytes (●) have a linear relationship between these two measurements. Patients with an unstable hemoglobin variant (Hb Casper) have a falsely high reticulocyte count both prior to (△) and following (▲) splenectomy. (From Koler, R. T., et al.: Am. J. Med. 55:549, 1973.)

blood film. Often, however, the cells are hypochromic (low MCHC), despite having a normal mean corpuscular volume. This may be a reflection of the pitting function of the spleen. The red cells often show more variation in size and shape than normal, and prominent basophilic stippling may be seen (Fig. 13–9). In some patients, the red cells appear as if a bite had been taken from the margin (see Color Plate III*J*). Again, this may be a morphological sequela of splenic pitting.

The demonstration of Heinz bodies requires the use of a supravital stain such as crystal violet or new methylene blue (see Color Plate III*K*). Their presence is highly variable.

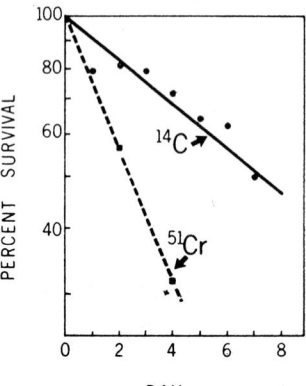

Figure 13–8. Red cell survival of a patient with an unstable hemoglobin variant (Hb Abraham Lincoln) measured by ^{14}C–amino acid labeling of reticulocytes and ^{51}Cr labeling of whole blood. (From Honig, G., et al.: J. Clin. Invest. 52:1746, 1973.)

In the most mild forms of CHBA, it may be necessary to incubate red cells for long periods, either in the presence of an oxidant such as acetylphenylhydrazine or in the absence of substrate (glucose), before Heinz bodies can be demonstrated. It is important to have normal controls for comparison, because Heinz bodies may be elicited in normal red cells by these maneuvers. Heinz bodies are more readily demonstrable in patients with severe CHBA. In all cases, they are much more abundant following splenectomy. They usually appear as irregular blue-purple inclusions, 0.5 to 2.0 μ, often solitary and adjacent to the inner surface of the red cell membrane (Fig. 13–9). Inclusions generated by the oxidant dye tend to be smaller and multiple and may closely resemble Hb H inclusions. Heinz bodies are not specific for CHBA. They can also be seen in the red cells of patients with some forms of α or β thalassemia and in the red cells of patients exposed to an oxidant stress, particularly those deficient in an enzyme involved in the pentose-phosphate pathway (HMP shunt) or in the synthesis of glutathione.

In some patients, the platelet count may be falsely elevated when measured by an automated cell counter.[83] It is likely that free red cell inclusions are "counted" as platelets.

Hemoglobin Denaturation

The diagnosis of CHBA can often be established by the demonstration of denatured

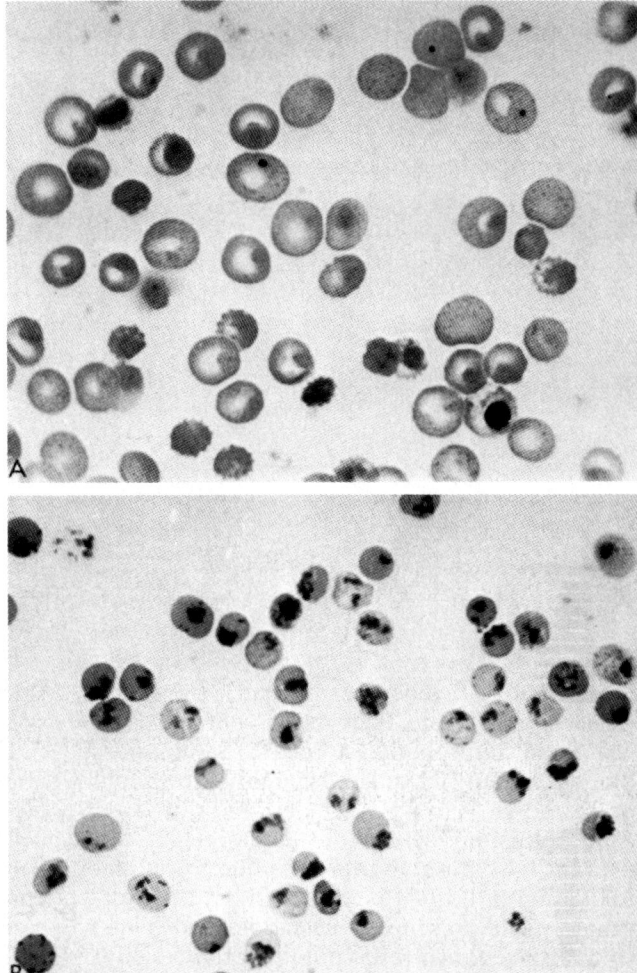

Figure 13–9. *A*, Photomicrograph of peripheral blood from a patient with an unstable hemoglobin variant (Hb Abraham Lincoln). Note basophilic stippling, Howel-Jolly bodies, and normoblast. *B*, Following incubation of blood for 30 minutes with new methylene blue. Most red cells contain large Heinz bodies. (From Honig, G., et al.: J. Clin. Invest. 52:1746, 1973.

hemoglobin in the hemolysate. Table 13–3 lists various laboratory procedures that are useful in revealing an unstable hemoglobin variant. In most cases, the hemoglobin variant will form a flocculent precipitate when a 1 per cent solution of the hemolysate is incubated in a neutral phosphate buffer at 50°C for 1 to 2 hours.[114, 115] In the preparation of the hemolysate, the stroma should not be removed with organic solvents. The sensitivity of the test may be enhanced by the use of TRIS buffer,[189] although we have been unable to notice any advantage in this method for the unstable variants that we have tested. As shown in Figure 13–10, the temperature required for thermal denaturation varies markedly among hemoglobin variants. Note that Hb Christchurch, when oxidized to methemoglobin, denatures at body temperature. In contrast, much higher temperatures are required for the denaturation of Hbs, F, E, and A.

Incubation of hemolysates in 17 per cent isopropanol at 37°C provides enhanced sensitivity[190] (see Color Plate IIIL). This test is easy to perform and should be available in clinical laboratories for routine screening.

Table 13–3. LABORATORY TESTS FOR DEMONSTRATION OF UNSTABLE HEMOGLOBIN VARIANTS

Test	Reference
Heat	Grimes and Meisler, 1962[114]; Grimes et al., 1964[115]
Isopropanol	Carrell and Kay, 1972[190]
Sulfhydryl reagent	Rieder et al., 1969[45]; Huisman et al., 1971[33]
Mechanical agitation	Asakura et al., 1975[192]; Vella, 1975[193]
Zinc acetate	Carrell and Lehmann, 1981[195]

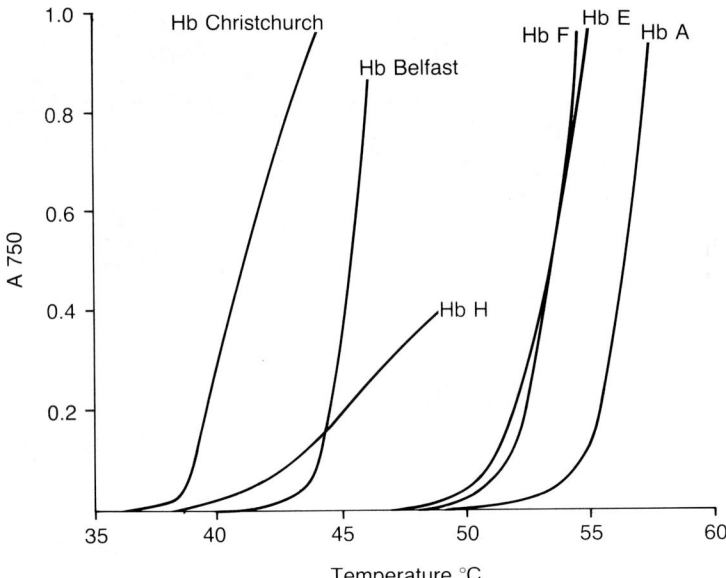

Figure 13–10. Thermal denaturation of hemolysates that have been oxidized to methemoglobin. (From Carrell, R. W., and Winterbourn, C. C.: The unstable hemoglobins. *In* Schneider, R., et al. (eds.): Texas Reports on Biology and Medicine: Human Hemoglobins and Hemoglobinopathies. 1981, pp. 431–446.)

False-positive reactions can occur if the specimen contains more than 4 per cent Hb F or has been improperly stored.[191] Samples of blood, washed red cells, or hemolysate should be stored at 0° to 4° C. The addition of 2 per cent potassium cyanide to hemolysates will prevent false-positive reactions due to the autoxidation of normal hemoglobin.[142, 191] Unfortunately, the presence of cyanide can also lead to a false-negative test; consequently, a significantly unstable variant could be overlooked.

Mechanical agitation, a test originally developed for the detection of Hb S (see Chapter 12), also gives positive results for specimens containing unstable hemoglobin variants.[192-194] However, a few stable variants besides Hb S can also form precipitates after mechanical shaking.[194] The test may be used for quantifying the amount of the variant in a hemolysate. The addition of the sulfhydryl reagent *p*-mercuribenzoate to the hemolysate can also result in the precipitation of the abnormal hemoglobin.[33, 43, 45, 95a] Those unstable variants that have an increased tendency to dissociate into subunits can be readily attacked by sulfhydryl reagents. This approach has been used to prepare unstable hemoglobin subunits that cannot be separated by conventional means.[33,43, 95a] Zinc acetate can also be used to precipitate unstable hemoglobins.[195] In view of the tendency of unstable hemoglobins to denature under a variety of experimental conditions, it is not surprising that the Sickledex test may give a false-positive result in CHBA.[196]

Hemoglobin Electrophoresis

The diagnosis of CHBA is confirmed if an abnormal band is demonstrated on hemoglobin electrophoresis. However, only about 45 per cent of the unstable variants have substitutions (or deletions) that involve an alteration in charge. Even those with a substitution conferring an alteration in charge may have anomalous electrophoretic behavior owing to charge compensation. This phenomenon has been well documented in the x-ray analysis of Hb Tacoma (β 30 Arg→Ser), which has electrophoretic mobility identical to that of Hb A despite its loss of a positive charge.[124] Thus, many of these abnormal hemoglobins are very difficult to separate by ordinary electrophoretic techniques. It may be necessary to try electrophoresis in different media and at several pH values before an optimal separation can be achieved. If hemes are lost or displaced from the abnormal subunit, one or more bands (or a smear) migrating less rapidly toward the anode than the intact hemoglobin (i.e., a more positive net charge) may appear. The anomalous electrophoretic behavior of a number of the unstable variants may be related to heme depletion of the abnormal subunits. Another type of electrophoretic heterogeneity was demonstrated in studies on Hb Rush.[86] Analysis of the hemolysate on cellulose acetate at pH 8.6 revealed two bands migrating cathodally to Hb A. Re-electrophoresis of the middle band produced a pattern similar to that of the whole hemolysate, suggesting that this component was the hybrid tetramer $\alpha_2\beta^A\beta^{Rush}$, and on re-electrophoresis it dissociated and recombined to form the two parent tetramers. (See discussion of asymmetrical hybrid hemoglobins in Chapter 10.)

Hb A_2 may be increased somewhat in patients with CHBA.[34, 43, 63, 79, 83, 97, 98, 141] This is probably a reflection of the fact that the variant hemoglobin is selectively removed from the red cell, as discussed previously, leaving a higher ratio of Hb A_2 to total hemoglobin.[173] As in other types of chronic hemolysis, Hb F levels may be modestly elevated in CHBA.[151] In some unstable variants, free α chains can be demonstrated on electrophoresis, because the unstable β chains may be selectively precipitated (see previous section on biosynthesis).

If an unstable variant is difficult to separate electrophoretically, it will also be difficult to purify by standard preparative procedures such as column chromatography. For this reason, it may be necessary to take advantage of the relative insolubility or enhanced denaturation of the variant in order to purify it and study its properties. This has been done by precipitation with isopropanol,[71] p-mercuribenzoate, or zinc acetate (see above).

Oxygen Equilibria

The unstable hemoglobins tend to have abnormal oxygen affinity. Whole blood oxygen saturation curves have been determined for about half the various unstable variants (see Table 13–1). Of these, the oxygen affinity is normal in 20 per cent, decreased in 30 per cent, and increased in 50 per cent. The last finding is not surprising, because the tertiary structure of the variant subunit may be so altered that it cannot form a stable t structure. If the oxygen affinity of the variant hemoglobin differs significantly from that of Hb A, the whole blood oxygen saturation curve will be biphasic (Fig. 13–11).

Oxygen affinity may be an important determinant of red cell mass in patients with CHBA.[197] The hemoglobin of individuals with Hb Köln exhibits significantly increased oxygen affinity and, as a consequence, impaired release of oxygen during capillary circulation. The resultant tissue hypoxia stimulates erythropoiesis, presumably via regulation by erythropoietin. As a result, individuals with Hb Köln have minimal anemia, despite a significant amount of hemolysis. One patient actually

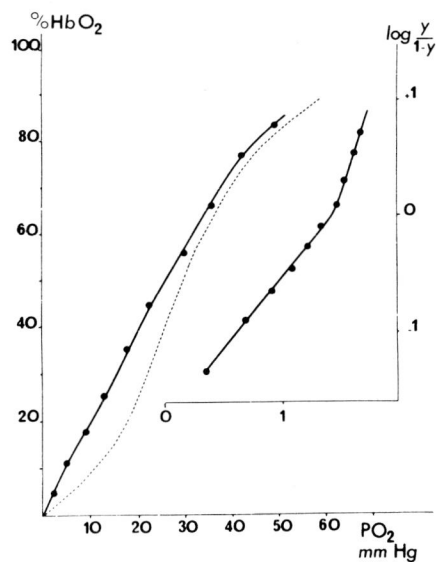

Figure 13–11. Oxygen dissociation curve of blood of a patient with Hb Tours. (Dotted line indicates normal curve.) The Hill plot in the inset on the right shows a biphasic curve. The left-hand portion of the curve shows increased oxygen affinity due to the presence of the hemoglobin variant. The right-hand portion of the curve reflects oxygenation of Hb A in the patient's red cells. (From Wajcman, H., et al.: Biochim. Biophys. Acta 295:495, 1973.)

developed an increase in oxygen affinity and erythrocytosis following splenectomy.[198] Thus, oxygen delivery may not have been improved by the operation.[199] Woodson and associates[200] have studied oxygen transport in two individuals with Hb Köln. These patients had normal oxygen consumption, hemoglobin concentration, and cardiac output. From the Fick equation discussed in Chapter 5, it follows that A-V oxygen extraction must also be normal. However, because of the increase in red cell oxygen affinity, oxygen delivery could be achieved only at the expense of a significant reduction in mixed venous PO_2. This was documented by direct measurement. The marked increase in urinary erythropoietin in one patient and evidence for redistribution of blood flow to vital organs indicated that these individuals had some degree of tissue hypoxia.

In contrast, patients with Hb Hammersmith have decreased O_2 affinity[138] and severe anemia. Those with Hb Seattle also have a "shift to the right,"[201] although much less hemolysis than the patients with Hammersmith. Because oxygen unloading is enhanced, there is less stimulation to erythropoiesis. The red cell mass of these individuals is thus set at a subnormal level appropriate for their hemoglobin function.[201] This relationship appears to be a gen-

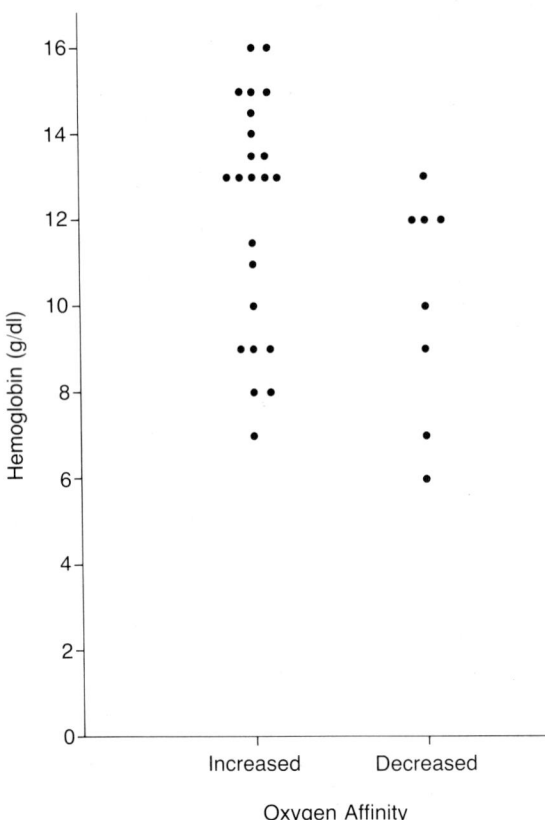

Figure 13–12. Comparison of hemoglobin levels in individuals with CHBA and abnormal oxygen affinity.

eral phenomenon among patients with CHBA. As shown in Figure 13–12, those individuals who have unstable variants with increased oxygen affinity tend to have normal or near-normal hemoglobin values, whereas those with decreased oxygen affinity may have significant anemia.

It is often difficult to study the functional properties of unstable hemoglobins in detail. During the process of separation from normal Hb A, the variant may become irreversibly denatured. Some unstable variants such as Hb Köln,[185, 202, 203] Hb Savannah,[33] Hb Bibba,[204] and Hb Istanbul[78] have an increased tendency to dissociate into dimers. This process appears to be related to the displacement or loss of heme from the β chains. Initial measurements of the oxygen equilibria of purified Hb Köln showed it to have high oxygen affinity, low heme-heme interaction, and decreased reactivity with 2,3-DPG.[202] In contrast, in the presence of added hemin, hemoglobin Köln had a higher degree of heme-heme interaction and normal 2,3-DPG reactivity.[205] Kinetic measurements of binding of carbon monoxide to Hb Köln revealed that in the absence of added hemin, the reaction was fast and monophasic, indicating the deoxy Köln was largely in the R structure.[203] Following the addition of hemin, a biphasic curve was obtained, with the slow component resembling Hb A. These results indicate that the addition of hemin permits Hb Köln to assume the T ("deoxy") conformation and help to explain the conflicting observations on oxygen equilibria noted above. Hb Djelfa (β 98 Val→Ala) has a substitution at the same site as Hb Köln and has very similar functional properties.[206]

Besides Hb Köln and Hb Djelfa, two other unstable hemoglobins have been shown to have impaired interaction with 2,3-DPG. Hb Leiden ($\alpha_2\beta_2$ 6 or 7 Glu→0)[207] probably has weak binding to 2,3-DPG because the deletion increases the distance between the two N termini of the β chains (see Chapters 2 and 6). The mechanism for the diminished response of Hb Shepherds Bush ($\alpha_2\beta$ 74 Gly→Asp) to 2,3-DPG is not clear.[208]

TREATMENT

Most individuals with CHBA do not require treatment. Those with severe hemolysis derive benefit from general supportive measures such as the administration of folic acid and prompt attention to infections. High fever should be prevented by the use of a nonoxidant antipyretic such as aspirin and, if necessary, by physical cooling.[131] Oxidant drugs should be avoided. Transfusions are indicated only rarely, such as during an aplastic crisis in which erythropoiesis has been suppressed.

As discussed in the section on pathogenesis, the spleen has been shown to sequester CHBA red cells. During the circulation through the spleen, Heinz bodies may be "pitted" from the cell, leaving the remainder of the red cell intact. Other cells do not escape from the splenic cords and are destroyed in situ. From these considerations, splenectomy seems to be a reasonable approach in selected cases. After reviewing the literature, Koler and associates[88] concluded that splenectomy may be beneficial in severely affected patients. This conclusion is corroborated by the extensive personal experience of Carrell.* As shown in Figure 13–13, some patients have achieved a significant increase in hemoglobin following splenectomy. It is difficult to predict preoperatively how well

---

*R. Carrell, Personal communication, 1982.

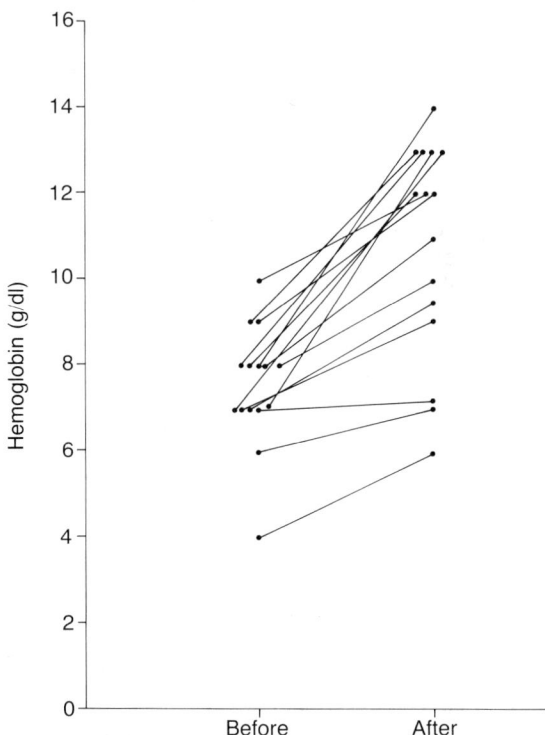

Figure 13–13. Effect of splenectomy on hemoglobin levels of individuals with CHBA.

patients will respond. Measurements of ^{51}Cr-labeled red cell survival and splenic uptake are very difficult to interpret (see above). The decision about whether a patient with CHBA should undergo splenectomy may sometimes be resolved by ascertaining whether other patients with the same variant were benefited (see Table 13–1).[88] As mentioned earlier, one patient with Hb Köln actually developed polycythemia following splenectomy,[198] probably as a result of the increased oxygen affinity of this variant (see above). Sustained thrombocytosis has been observed in patients with CHBA following splenectomy.[209] It is difficult to appraise the reported deaths following splenectomy of two patients presumed to have Hb Duarte, because many relevant details of the hematological status of the individuals either preoperatively or postoperatively are not known.[53] Young children (< six years of age) are at increased risk of developing septicemia following surgery. One six-year-old child with Hb Hammersmith died of pneumococcal septicemia four years after undergoing a splenectomy.[187] The incidence of this complication is reduced by the administration of pneumococcal vaccine.

References

1. Johnson, C. S., Schroeder, W. A., Shelton, J. B., and Shelton, J. R.: The first example of a detection in the human α chain: Hb Boyle Heights. Hemoglobin 7:125, 1983.
1a. Liang, C., Tao, H., Lo, H., Huang, S., Li, R., and Wang, B.: Hemoglobin Shuangfeng (α27 (B8) Glu→Lys): A new unstable hemoglobin variant. Hemoglobin 5:691, 1982.
1b. Beretta, A., Prato, V., Gallo, E., and Lehmann, H.: Haemoglobin Torino—α43 (CD1) Phenylalanine → Valine. Nature 217:1016, 1968.
2. Ohba, Y., Miyaji, T., Matsuoka, M., Yokoyama, M., Numakura, H., Nagata, K., Takebe, Y., Izumi, Y., and Shibata, S.: Hemoglobin Hirosaki (α43 [CE 1] Phe→Leu), a new unstable variant. Biochim. Biophys. Acta 405:155, 1975.
3. Sumida, I.: Studies of abnormal hemoglobins in western Japan. Frequency of visible hemoglobin variants, and chemical characterization of hemoglobin Sawara ($α_2$ 6 Ala $β_2$) and hemoglobin Mugino (Hb L Ferrara; $α_2$ 47 Gly $β_2$). Jpn. J. Hum. Genet. 19:343, 1975.
4. DeVries, A., Joshua, H., Lehmann, H., Hill, R. L., and Fellows, R. E.: The first observation of an abnormal haemoglobin in a Jewish family: Haemoglobin Beilinson. Br. J. Haematol. 9:484, 1963.
5. Halbrecht, I., Isaacs, W. A., Lehmann, H., and Ben-Porat, F.: Hemoglobin Hasharon (α47 Aspartic acid–Histidine). Israel J. Med. Sci. 3:827, 1967.
6. Tentori, L.: Hemoglobin L Ferrara = hemoglobin Hasharon. Hemoglobin 1:602, 1977.
7. Charache, S., Mondzac, A. M., Gessner, U., and Gayle, E. E.: Hemoglobin Hasharon ($α_2^{47His}$ (CD5) $β_2$): A hemoglobin found in low concentration. J. Clin. Invest. 48:834, 1969.
8. Alberti, R., Mariuzzi, G. M., Artibani, L., Bruni, E., and Tentori, L.: A new haemoglobin variant: J-Rovigo alpha 53 (E-2) Alanine–Aspartic acid. Biochim. Biophys. Acta 342:1, 1974.
9. Nakatsuji, T., Miwa, S., Ohba, Y., Miyaji, T., Matsumoto, N., and Matsuoka, I.: Hemoglobin Tottori (α59 [E8] Glycine–Valine)—a new unstable hemoglobin. Hemoglobin 5:427, 1981.
10. Thillet, J., Blouquit, Y., Perrone, F., and Rosa, J.: Hemoglobin Pontoise α63 Ala→Asp (E12). A new fast moving variant. Biochim. Biophys. Acta 491:16, 1977.
11. Rucknagel, D. L., Brandt, N. J., and Spencer, H. H.: α-Chain mutants of human hemoglobin contributing to the genetics of the α-chain locus. Proceedings of the 1st Inter-American Symposium on Hemoglobins, Caracas, 1969.
12. Adams, J. G., III, Winter, W. P., Rucknagel, D. L., and Spencer, H. H.: Biosynthesis of hemoglobin Ann Arbor: Evidence for catabolic and feedback regulation. Science 176:1427, 1972.
13. Crookston, J. H., Farquharson, H. A., Beale, D., and Lehmann, H.: Hemoglobin Etobicoke: α84 (F5) serine replaced by arginine. Can. J. Biochem. 47:143, 1969.
14. Knuth, A., Pribilla, W., Marti, H. R., and Winterhalter, K. H.: Hemoglobin Moabit: Alpha 86 (F7) Leu→Arg. A new unstable abnormal hemoglobin. Acta Haematol. 61:121, 1979.
15. Ohba, Y., Miyaji, T., Hattori, Y., Fuyuno, K., and Matsuoka, M.: Unstable hemoglobins in Japan. Hemoglobin 4:307, 1980.

16. Brennan, S. O., Tauro, G. P., Melrose, W., and Carrell, R. W.: Haemoglobin Port Phillip α91 (FG3) Leu→Pro. A new unstable haemoglobin. FEBS Lett. *81*:115, 1977.
17. Wajcman, H., Belkhodja, O., and Labie, D.: Hb Setif: α G1 (94) Asp–Tyr. A new α chain hemoglobin variant with substitution of the residue involved in a hydrogen bond between unlike subunits. FEBS Lett. *27*:298, 1972.
18. Nozari, G., Rahbar, S., Darbre, P., and Lehmann, H.: Hemoglobin Setif (α94 (G1) Asp→Tyr) in Iran, a report of 9 cases. Hemoglobin *1*:289, 1977.
19. Sanguansermsri, T., Matragoon, S., Changloah, L., and Flatz, G.: Hemoglobin Suan-Dok ($α_2$109 (G16) Leu→Arg $β_2$): An unstable variant associated with α-thalassemia. Hemoglobin *3*:161, 1979.
20. Honig, G. R., Shamsuddin, M., Zaizov, R., Steinherz, M., Solar, I., and Kirschmann, C.: Hemoglobin Petah Tikva (α110 Ala–Asp): A new unstable variant with α-thalassemia-like expression. Blood *57*:705, 1981.
21. Charache, S., and Ostertag, W.: Hemoglobin Hopkins-2 (α112 Asp) 2 β2): "Low output" protects from potentially harmful effects. Blood *36*:852, 1970.
22. Clegg, J. B., and Charache, S.: The structure of hemoglobin Hopkins-2. Hemoglobin *2*:85, 1978.
23. Kleihauer, E. F., Reynolds, C. A., Dozy, A. M., Wilson, J. B., Moores, R. R., Berenson, M. P., Wright, C.-S., and Huisman, T. H. J.: Hemoglobin Bibba or alpha-2–136Pro-beta-2, an unstable-chain abnormal hemoglobin. Biochim. Biophys. Acta *154*:220, 1968.
24. Lee-Potter, J. P., Deacon-Smith, R. A., Simpkiss, M. J., Kamuzora, H., and Lehmann, H.: A new cause of haemolytic anemia in the newborn. A description of an unstable fetal haemoglobin: F Poole, alpha2-G-gamma2 130 tryptophan yields glycine. J. Clin. Pathol. *28*:317, 1975.
25. DeJong, W. W. W., Went, L. N., and Bernini, L. F.: Haemoglobin Leiden: Deletion of β6 or 7 glutamic acid. Nature *220*:788, 1968.
26. Beuzard, Y., Basset, P., Braconnier, F., El Gammel, H., Martin, L., Oudard, J. L., and Thillet, J.: Haemoglobin Saki $α_2 β_2^{14Leu→Pro}$ (A11) structure and function. Biochim. Biophys. Acta *393*:182, 1975.
27. Milner, P. F., Corley, C. C., Pomeroy, W. L., Wilson, J. B., Gravely, M., and Huisman, T. H. J.: Thalassemia intermedia caused by heterozygosity for both β-thalassemia and hemoglobin Saki (β14 (A11) Leu→Pro). Am. J. Hematol. *1*:283, 1976.
28. Kennedy, C. C., Blundell, G., Lorkin, P. A., Lang, A., and Lehmann, H.: Haemoglobin Belfast 15 (A12) Tryptophan→Arginine: A new unstable haemoglobin variant. Br. Med. J. *4*:324, 1974.
29. Gacon, G., Wajcman, H., Labie, D., Varet, B., and Christoforov, B.: A second case of haemoglobin Belfast (β15 [A12] Trp→Arg) observed in a French patient. Acta Haematol. *55*:313, 1976.
30. Cohen-Solal, M., Blouquit, Y., Garel, M. C., Thillet, J., Gaillard, L., Creyssel, R., Gibaud, A., and Rosa, J.: Haemoglobin Lyon (β17–18 (A14–15) Lys-Val→0). Determination by sequenator analysis. Biochim. Biophys. Acta *351*:306, 1974.
31. Jones, R. T., Brimhall, B., Huisman, T. H. J., Kleihauer, E., and Betke, K.: Hemoglobin Freiburg: Abnormal hemoglobin due to deletion of a single amino acid residue. Science *154*:1024, 1966.
32. Ranney, H. M., Jacobs, A. S., Udem, L., and Zalusky, R.: Hemoglobin Riverdale-Bronx, an unstable hemoglobin resulting from the substitution of arginine for glycine at helical residue B6 of the β polypeptide chain. Biochim. Biophys. Acta *33*:1004, 1968.
33. Huisman, T. H. J., Brown, A. K., Efremov, G. D., Wilson, J. B., Reynolds, C. A., Uy, R., and Smith, L. L.: Hemoglobin Savannah (B6 (24) β-Glycine→Valine): An unstable variant causing anemia with inclusion bodies. J. Clin. Invest. *50*:650, 1971.
34. Idelson, L. I., Didkowsky, N. A., Casey, R., Lorkin, P. A., and Lehmann, H.: New unstable haemoglobin (Hb Moscva, β24 (B6) Gly→Asp) found in the U.S.S.R. Nature *249*:768, 1974.
35. Idelson, L. I., Didkowsky, N. A., Filippova, A. V., Casey, R., Kynoch, P. A. M., and Lehmann, H.: Haemoglobin Volga, β27 (B9) Ala–Asp, a new highly unstable haemoglobin with a suppressed charge. FEBS Lett. *58*:122, 1975.
36. Kuis-Reerink, J. D., Jonxis, J. H. P., Niazi, G. A., Wilson, J. B., Bolch, K. C., Gravely, M., and Huisman, T. H. J.: Hb Volga or alpha 2 beta 2 27(B9) Ala→Asp: An unstable hemoglobin variant in three generations of a Dutch family. Biochim. Biophys. Acta *439*:63, 1976.
37. Thillet, J., Cohen-Solal, M., Seligmann, M., and Rosa, J.: Functional and physicochemical studies of hemoglobin St. Louis β28 (B10) Leu→Gln. J. Clin. Invest. *58*:1098, 1976.
38. Sansone, G., Carrell, R. W., and Lehmann, H.: Haemoglobin Genova: β28 (B10) Leucine→Proline. Nature *214*:877, 1967.
39. Kendall, A., Young, S., Oune, N., Wiltshire, B., and Lehmann, H.: The unstable Hb Genova (β28 Leu–Pro) in an East African family. Acta Haematol. *61*:278, 1979.
40. Schmidt, B., Bechtel, K. C., Johnson, M. H., Therrell, B. J., Jr., and Moo-Penn, W. F.: Hemoglobin Lufkin: β29 (B11) Gly–Asp: An unstable hemoglobin variant involving an internal amino acid residue. Hemoglobin *1*:700, 1977.
41. Brimhall, B., Jones, R. T., Baur, E. W., and Motulsky, A. G.: Structural characterization of hemoglobin Tacoma. Biochemistry *8*:2125, 1969.
41a. Nakatsuji, T., Miwa, S., Ohba, Y., Hattori, Y., Miyaji, T., Hino, S., and Matsumoto, N.: A new unstable hemoglobin, Hb Yokohama β31 (B13) Leu→Pro, causing hemolytic anemia. Hemoglobin *5*:667, 1981.
42. Jackson, J. M., Yates, A., and Huehns, E. R.: Haemoglobin Perth: β32 (B14) Leu–Pro. An unstable haemoglobin causing haemolysis. Br. J. Haematol. *25*:607, 1973.
43. Honig, G. R., Green, D., Shamsuddin, M., Vida, L. N., Mason, R. G., Gnarra, D. J., and Mauer, H. S.: Hemoglobin Abraham Lincoln, β32 (B14) Leucine–Proline. An unstable variant producing severe hemolytic disease. J. Clin. Invest. *52*:1746, 1973.
44. Garel, M. C., Blouqit, Y., and Rosa, J.: Hemoglobin Castilla β32 (B14) Leu–Arg: A new unstable variant producing severe hemolytic disease. FEBS Lett. *58*:145, 1975.
45. Rieder, R. F., Oski, F. A., and Clegg, J. B.: Hemoglobin Philly (β35 Tyrosine→Phenylalanine): Studies in the molecular pathology of hemoglobin. J. Clin. Invest. *48*:1627, 1969.
45a. Blouquut, Y., Delanoe-Garin, J., Lacombe, C.,

Arous, N., Cayre, Y., Peduzzi, J., Braconnier, F., and Galacteros, F.: Structural study of hemoglobin Hazebrouck, β38 (C4) Thr→Pro: A new abnormal hemoglobin with instability and low oxygen affinity. FEBS Lett. *172*:155, 1984.

45b. Kendall, A. G., ten Pas, A., Wilson, J. B., Cope, N., Bolch, K., and Huisman, T. H. J.: Hb Vassa or $\alpha_2\beta_2$ (39 (C5) Gln→Glu), a mildly unstable variant found in a Finnish family. Hemoglobin *1*:292, 1977.

46. Burkett, L. B., Sharma, V. S., Pisciotta, A. V., Ranney, H. M., and Bruckheimer, S.: Hemoglobin Mequon β41 (C7) Phenyl-alanine→Tyrosine. Blood *48*:645, 1976.

47. Dacie, J. V., Shinton, N. K., Gaffney, P. J., Jr., Carrell, R. W., and Lehmann, H.: Haemoglobin Hammersmith (β42 (CD1) Phe–Ser). Nature *216*:663, 1967.

48. Ohba, Y., Miyaji, T., Matsuoka, M., Yamaguchi, K., Yonemitsu, H., Ishii, T., and Shibata, S.: Hemoglobin Chiba: Hb Hammersmith in a Japanese girl. Acta Haematol. Jpn. *38*:53, 1975.

49. Keeling, M. M., Ogdon, L. L., Wrightstone, R. N., Wilson, J. B., Reynolds, C. A., Kitchens, J. L., and Huisman, T. H. J.: Hemoglobin Louisville (β42 (CD1) Phe→Leu): An unstable variant causing mild hemolytic anemia. J. Clin. Invest. *50*:2395, 1971.

50. Bratu, V., Lorkin, P. A., Lehmann, H., and Predescu, C.: Haemoglobin Bucuresti β42 (CD1) Phe–Leu, a cause of unstable haemoglobin haemolytic anemia. Biochim. Biophys. Acta *251*:1, 1971.

50a. Yeager, A. M., Zinkham, W. H., Jue, D. L., Winslow, R. M., Johnson, M. H., McGuffey, J. E., and Moo-Penn, W. F.: Hemoglobin Cheverly: An unstable hemoglobin associated with mild anemia. Pediatr. Res. *17*:503, 1983.

51. Charache, S., Brimhall, B., Milner, P., and Cobb, L.: Hemoglobin Okaloosa (β48 (CD7) Leucine–Arginine). An unstable hemoglobin with decreased oxygen affinity. J. Clin. Invest. *52*:2858, 1973.

52. Giardina, B., Brunori, M., Antonini, E., and Tentori, L.: Properties of hemoglobin G Ferrara (β57 (E1) Asn→Lys). Biochim. Biophys. Acta *534*:1, 1978.

53. Beutler, E., Lang, A., and Lehmann, H.: Hemoglobin Duarte: $\alpha_2 \beta_2^{62\,(E6)Ala\rightarrow Pro}$: A new unstable hemoglobin with increased oxygen affinity. Blood *43*:527, 1974.

54. Muller, C. J., and Kingma, S.: Haemoglobin Zurich $\alpha_2^A \beta_2^{63\,Arg}$. Biochim. Biophys. Acta *50*:595, 1961.

55. Wajcman, H., Krishnamoorthy, R., Gacon, G., Elion, J., Allard, C., and Labie, D.: A new hemoglobin variant involving the distal histidine: Hb Bicetre (β63 (E7) His→Pro). J. Mol. Med. *1*:187, 1976.

56. Marinucci, M., Mavilio, F., Fontanarosa, P. P., Tentori, L., and Brancati, C.: Studies on a family with Hb J Calabria ($\alpha_2 \beta_2$ 64(E8) Gly→Asp. Hemoglobin *3*:327, 1979.

57. Rosa, J., Labie, D., Wajcman, H., Boigne, J. M., Cabannes, R., Bierme, R., and Ruffie, J.: Haemoglobin I Toulouse: β66 (E10) Lys–Glu: A new abnormal haemoglobin with a mutation localized on the E10 porphyrin surrounding zones. Nature *223*:190, 1969.

58. Carrell, R. W., Lehmann, H., Lorkin, P. A., Raik, E., and Hunter, E.: Haemoglobin Sydney: β67 (E11) Valine–Alanine: An emerging pattern of unstable haemoglobins. Nature *215*:626, 1967.

59. Steadman, J. H., Yates, A., and Huehns, E. R.: Idiopathic Heinz body anaemia: Hb-Bristol (β67 (E11) Val–Asp). Br. J. Haematol. *18*:435, 1970.

60. Ohba, Y., Miyaji, T., Matsuoka, M., Sugiyama, K., Suzuki, T., and Sugiura, T.: Hemoglobin Mizuho or beta 68 (E12) leucine–proline, a new unstable variant associated with severe hemolytic anemia. Hemoglobin *1*:467, 1977.

61. Kurachi, S., Hermodson, M., Hornung, S., and Stamatoyannopoulos, G.: Structure of haemoglobin Seattle. Nature [New Biol.] *243*:275, 1973.

62. Carrell, R. W., and Owen, M. C.: A new approach to haemoglobin variant identification. Haemoglobin Christchurch β71 (E15) phenylalanine-serine. Biochim. Biophys. Acta *236*:507, 1971.

63. White, J. M., Brain, M. C., Lorkin, P. A., Lehmann, H., and Smith, M.: Mild "unstable hemoglobin haemolytic anaemia" caused by haemoglobin Shepherds Bush (β74 (E18) Gly–Asp). Nature *225*:939, 1970.

64. Sansone, G., Sciarratta, G. V., Genova, R., Darbre, P., and Lehmann, H.: Haemoglobin Shepherds Bush (β74 E18 Gly–Asp) in an Italian family. Acta Haematol. *57*:102, 1977.

65. Rieder, R. F., Wolf, D. J., Clegg, J. B., and Lee, S. L.: Rapid post-synthetic destruction of unstable haemoglobin Bushwick. Nature *254*:725, 1975.

66. Wajcman, H., Labie, D., and Schapira, G.: Two new hemoglobin variants with deletion. Hemoglobin Tours: Thr β87 (F3) deleted and hemoglobin St. Antoine: Gly–Leu β74–75 (E18–19) deleted. Consequences for oxygen affinity and protein stability. Biochim. Biophys. Acta *295*:495, 1973.

67. Hubbard, M., Winton, E. F., Lindeman, J. G., Dessauer, P. L., Wilson, J. B., Wrightstone, R. N., and Huisman, T. H. J.: Hemoglobin Atlanta or $\alpha_2 \beta_2^{75\,Leu\rightarrow Pro}$ (E19): An unstable variant found in several members of a Caucasian family. Biochim. Biophys. Acta *386*:538, 1975.

68. Johnson, C. S., Moyes, D., Schroeder, W. A., Shelton, J. B., Shelton, J. R., and Beutler, E.: Hemoglobin Pasadena, $\alpha_2\beta_2 75(E19)$ Leu-Arg: Identification by high performance liquid chromatography of a new unstable variant with increased oxygen affinity. Biochim. Biophys. Acta *623*:360, 1980.

69. Schneider, R. G., Hettig, R. A., Bilunos, M., and Brimhall, B.: Hemoglobin Baylor [$\alpha_2\beta_2 81(EF5)$ Leu-Arg]—an unstable mutant with high oxygen affinity. Hemoglobin *1*:85, 1976.

70. Bradley, T. B., Wohl, R. C., Murphy, S. B., Oski, F. A., and Bunn, H. F.: Properties of hemoglobin Bryn Mawr, β85 Phe→Ser, a new spontaneous mutation producing an unstable hemoglobin with high oxygen affinity. Abstract 40. Annual Meeting of the American Society of Hematology, Miami, 1972.

71. de Weinstein, B. I., White, J. M., Wiltshire, B. G., and Lehmann, H.: A new unstable haemoglobin: Hb Buenos Aires, β85 (F1) Phe→Ser. Acta Haematol. *50*:357, 1973.

72. Hollender, A., Lorkin, P. A., Lehmann, H., and Svensson, B.: New unstable haemoglobin Boras: β88 (F4) Leucine→Arginine. Nature *222*:953, 1969.

73. Opfell, R. W., Lorkin, P. A., and Lehmann, H.: Hereditary non-spherocytic haemolytic anaemia with post-splenectomy inclusion bodies and pigmenturia caused by an unstable haemoglobin Santa

Ana—β88 (F4) leucine→proline. J. Med. Genet. 5:292, 1968.
74. Bradley, T. B., Wohl, R. C., and Rieder, R. F.: Hemoglobin Gun Hill: Deletion of five amino acid residues and impaired heme-globin binding. Science 157:1581, 1967.
75. Schneider, R. G., Satoshi, U., Alperin, J. B., Brimhall, B., and Jones, R. T.: Hemoglobin Sabine, β91(F7) Leu→Pro. An unstable variant causing severe anemia with inclusion bodies. N. Engl. J. Med. 280:739, 1969.
76. Ahern, E., Ahern, C., Hilton, T., Serjeant, G. R., Serjeant, B. E., Seakins, M., Lang, A., Middleton, A., and Lehmann, H.: Haemoglobin Caribbean β91 (F7) Leu–Arg: A mildly unstable haemoglobin with low oxygen affinity. FEBS Lett. 69:99, 1976.
76a. Spivak, V. A., Molchanova, T. P., Postniker, Y. V., Aseeva, E. A., Lutsenko, I. N., and Tokaren, Y. N.: A new abnormal hemoglobin: Hb Mozhaisk β92 (F8) His→Arg. Hemoglobin 6:169, 1982.
77. Beuzard, Y., Courvalin, J. C., Cohen-Solal, M., Garel, M. C., Rosa, J., Brizard, C. P., and Gibaud, A.: Structural studies of hemoglobin Saint Etienne β92 (F8) His–Gln: A new abnormal hemoglobin with loss of β proximal histidine and absence of heme on the β chains. FEBS Lett. 27:76, 1972.
78. Aksoy, M., Erdem, S., Efremov, G. D., Wilson, J. B., Huisman, T. H. J., Schroeder, W. A., Shelton, J. R., Shelton, J. B., Ulitin, O. N., and Muftuglu, A.: Hemoglobin Istanbul: Substitution of glutamine for histidine in a proximal histidine (F8(92) β). J. Clin. Invest. 51:2380, 1972.
79. Finney, R., Casey, R., Lehmann, H., and Walker, W.: Hb Newcastle: β92 (F8) His–Pro. FEBS Lett. 60:435, 1975.
80. Carrell, R. W., Lehmann, H., and Hutchison, H. E.: Haemoglobin Koln (β98 Valine–Methionine): An unstable protein causing inclusion-body anaemia. Nature 210:915, 1966.
81. Ohba, Y., Miyaji, T., and Shibata, S.: Identical substitution in Hb Ube-1 and Hb Köln. Nature [New Biol.] 243:205, 1973.
82. Gordon-Smith, E. C., Dacie, J. V., Blecher, T. E., French, E. A., Wiltshire, B. G., and Lehmann, H.: Haemoglobin Nottingham, β98 (FG5) Val–Gly: A new unstable haemoglobin producing severe haemolysis. Proc. R. Soc. Med. 66:507, 1973.
83. Orringer, E. P., Felice, A., Reese, A., Wilson, J. B., Lam, H., Gravely, M. E., and Huisman, T. H. J.: Hb Nottingham (α₂β₂ (FG5) 98 Val–Gly) in a Caucasian male: Clinical and biosynthetic studies. Hemoglobin 2:315, 1978.
84. Gacon, G., Wajcman, H., and Labie, D.: A new unstable hemoglobin mutated in β98 (FG5) Val–Ala: Hb Djelfa. FEBS Lett. 58:238, 1975.
85. Gacon, G., Krishnamoorthy, R., Wajcman, H., Labie, D., Tapon, J., and Cosson, A.: Hemoglobin Djelfa β98 (FG5) Val–Ala: Isolation and functional properties of the heme saturated form. Biochim. Biophys. Acta 490:156, 1977.
86. Adams, J. B., Winter, W. P., Tausk, K., and Heller, P.: Hemoglobin Rush [β-101 (G3) Glutamine]: A new unstable hemoglobin causing mild hemolytic anemia. Blood 45:261, 1974.
87. Hyde, R. D., Hall, M. D., Wiltshire, B. G., and Lehmann, H.: Haemoglobin Southampton, β106 (G8) Leu–Pro: An unstable variant producing severe haemolysis. Lancet 2:1170, 1972.

88. Koler, R. D., Jones, R. T., Bigley, R. H., Litt, M., Lovrien, E., Brooks, R., Lahey, M. E., and Fowler, R.: Hemoglobin Casper: β106 (G8) Leu–Pro, a contemporary mutation. Am. J. Med. 55:549, 1973.
89. Kleihauer, E., Waller, H. D., Benöhr, H. C., Kohne, E., and Gelinsky, P.: Hb Tubingen, eine neue β-kettenvariante (βTp 10–12) mit erhöhter spontanozydation. Klin. Wochenschr. 48:651, 1971.
90. Kohne, E., Kley, H. P., Kleihauer, E., Versmodl, H., Beñohr, H. C., and Braunitzer, G.: Structural and functional characteristics of the Hb Tübingen: β106 (G8) Leu–Gln. FEBS Lett. 64:443, 1976.
91. Turner, J. W., Jr., Jones, R. T., Brimhall, B., DuVal, M. C., and Koler, R. D.: Characterization of hemoglobin Burke [β107 (G9) Gly–Arg]. Biochem. Genet. 14:577, 1976.
92. King, M. A. R., Wiltshire, B. G., Lehmann, H., and Morimoto, H.: An unstable haemoglobin with reduced oxygen affinity: Haemoglobin Peterborough, β111 (G13) Valine–Phenylalanine, its interaction with normal haemoglobin and with haemoglobin Lepore. Br. J. Haematol. 22:125, 1972.
93. Adams, J. G., III, Boxer, L. A., Baehner, R. L., Forget, G. B., Tsistrakis, G. A., and Steinberg, M. H.: Hemoglobin Indianapolis (β112 [G14] Arginine). An unstable β-chain variant producing the phenotype of severe β-thalassemia. J. Clin. Invest. 63:931, 1979.
94. Adams, J. G., Steinberg, M. H., Boxer, L. A., Baehner, R. L., Forget, B. G., and Tsistrakis, G. A.: The structure of hemoglobin Indianapolis [β112 (G14) Arginine]. An unstable variant detectable only by isotopic labeling. J. Biol. Chem. 254:3479, 1979.
95. Outeirino, J., Casey, R., White, J. M., and Lehmann, H.: Haemoglobin Madrid, β115 (G17) Alanine–Proline: An unstable variant associated with haemolytic anaemia. Acta Haematol. 52:53, 1974.
95a. Ohba, Y., Hasegawa, Y., Amino, H., Miura, S., Nakatsuji, T., Hattori, Y., and Miyagi, T.: Hemoglobin Saitama or β117 (G19) His→Pro: A new variant causing hemolytic disease. Hemoglobin 7:47, 1983.
96. Clegg, J. B., Weatherall, D. J., Wong Hock Boon, and Mustafa, D.: Two new haemoglobin variants involving proline substitutions. Nature 22:379, 1969.
97. Martinez, G., Lima, F., and Colombo, B.: Haemoglobin J Guantanamo (α₂β₂ 128 (H6) Ala–Asp). A new fast unstable haemoglobin found in a Cuban family. Biochim. Biophys. Acta 491:1, 1977.
98. Lorkin, P. A., Pietschmann, H., Braunsteiner, H., and Lehmann, H.: Structure of Haemoglobin Wien β130 (H8) Tyrosine–Aspartic acid: An unstable haemoglobin variant. Acta Haematol. 51:351, 1974.
99. Lutcher, C. L., and Huisman, T. H. J.: Hb-Leslie, an unstable variant due to deletion of Gln β131, occurring in combination with β⁰-thalassemia, Hb-S, and Hb-C. Clin. Res. 23:278A, 1975.
100. Lutcher, C. L., Wilson, J. B., Gravely, M. E., Stevens, P. D., Chen, C. J., Linderman, J. G., Wong, S. C., Miller, A., Gottleib, M., and Huisman, T. H. J.: Hb Leslie, an unstable hemoglobin due to deletion of glutaminylresidue β131 (H9) occurring in association with β⁰-thalassemia, Hb-C, and Hb-S. Blood 47:99, 1976.

101. Moo-Penn, W. F., Jue, D. L., Bechtel, K. C., Johnson, M. H., Bemis, E., Brosious, E., and Schmidt, R. M.: Hemoglobin Deaconess, a new deletion mutant: β131 (H9) glutamine deleted. Biochem. Biophys. Res. Commun. 65:8, 1975.
102. Arends, T., Lehmann, H., Plowman, D., and Stathopoulou, R.: Haemoglobin North Shore–Caracas β134 (H12) Valine→Glutamic acid. FEBS Lett. 80:261, 1977.
103. Brennan, S. P. Jones, K. O. A., Crethar, L., Arnold, B. J., Fleming, P. J., and Winterbourn, C. C.: Haemoglobin North Shore, β134 Val→Glu. A new unstable hemoglobin. Biochim. Biophys. Acta 494:403, 1977.
104. Marti, H. R., Winterhalter, K. H., Di Iorio, E. E., Lorkin, P. A., and Lehmann, H.: Hb Altdorf $\alpha_2\beta_2$ 135(H13) Ala→Pro: A new electrophoretically silent unstable haemoglobin variant from Switzerland. FEBS Lett. 63:193, 1976.
105. Minnich, V., Hill, R. J., Khuri, P. D., and Anderson, M. E.: Hemoglobin Hope: A beta chain variant. Blood 25:830, 1965.
106. Moo-Penn, W. F., Lux, S. E., Alter, B. P., Jones, R. T., Shih, T. B., and Olsen, K. W.: Hemoglobin Brockton: β138 Ala–Pro. An unstable hemoglobin with normal functional properties. Abstract. International Society of Haematology Meeting, Athens, Greece, 1981.
106a. Moo-Penn, W. F., Jue, D. L., Johnson, M. H., Bechtel, K. C., and Patchen, L. C.: Hemoglobin variants and methods used for their characterization during 7 years screening at the Center for Disease Control. Hemoglobin 4:347, 1980.
107. Lorkin, P. A., Lehmann, H., Fairbanks, V. F., Berglund, G., and Leonhardt, T.: Two new pathological haemoglobins: Olmsted β141 (H19) Leu–Arg and Malmö β97 (FG4) His–Gln. Biochem. J. 119:68, 1970.
108. Lorkin, P. A., Lehmann, H., and Fairbanks, V. F.: The amino acid substitution in Hb Olmsted: β141 (H19) Leucine–Arginine. Biochim. Biophys. Acta 386:256, 1975.
109. Casey, R., Kynoch, P. A. M., Lang, A., Lehmann, H., Nozari, G., and Shinton, N. K.: Double heterozygosity for two unstable haemoglobins: Hb Sydney (β67 [E11] Val-Ala) and Hb Coventry (β141 [H19] Leu deleted). Br. J. Haematol. 38:195, 1978.
110. Nozari, G., Rahbar, S., and Lehmann, H.: Haemoglobin Coventry (β141 deleted) in Iran. FEBS Lett. 95:88, 1978.
111. Hirano, M., Ohba, Y., Imai, K., Ino, T., Morishita, Y., Matsui, T., Shmizu, S., Sumi, H., Yamamoto, K., and Miyaji, T.: Hb Toyoake: β142 (H20) Ala–Pro. A new unstable hemoglobin with high oxygen affinity. Blood 57:697, 1981.
112. Bunn, H. F., Schmidt, G. J., Haney, D. N., and Dluhy, R. G.: Hemoglobin Cranston, an unstable variant having an elongated β chain due to a nonhomologous crossover between two normal β chain genes. Proc. Natl. Acad. Sci. USA 72:3609, 1975.
113. Cathie, I. A. B.: Apparent idiopathic Heinz body anemia. Great Ormond St. J. 3:43, 1952.
114. Grimes, A. J., and Meisler, A.: Possible cause of Heinz bodies in congenital Heinz body anaemia. Nature 194:190, 1962.
115. Grimes, A. J., Meisler, A., and Dacie, J. V.: Congenital Heinz-body anaemia: Further evidence on the cause of Heinz-body production in red cells. Br. J. Haematol. 10:281, 1964.
116. Perutz, M. F., and Lehmann, H.: Molecular pathology of human haemoglobin. Nature 219:902, 1968.
117. Morimoto, H., Lehmann, H., and Perutz, M. F.: Molecular pathology of human haemoglobin: Stereochemical interpretation of abnormal oxygen affinities. Nature 232:408, 1971.
118. Jacob, H. S., Brain, M. K., and Dacie, J. V.: Altered sulfhydryl reactivity of hemoglobins and red blood cell membranes in congenital Heinz body hemolytic anemia. J. Clin. Invest. 47:2664, 1968.
119. Jacob, H. S., Brain, M. C., Dacie, J. V., Carrell, R. W., and Lehmann, H.: Abnormal haem binding and globin SH group blockade in unstable haemoglobins. Nature 218:1214, 1968.
120. Tucker, P. W., Phillips, S. E. V., Perutz, M. F., Houtchens, R., and Caughey, W. S.: Structure of hemoglobins Zürich [His E7(63) β-Arg] and Sydney [Val E11(67) β-Ala] and role of the distal residues in ligand binding. Proc. Natl. Acad. Sci USA 75:1076, 1978.
120a. Virshup, D. M., Zinkham, W. H., Sirota, R. L., and Caughey, W. S.: Unique sensitivity of Hb Zürich to oxidative injury by phenazopyridine: Reversal of the effects by elevating carboxyhemoglobin in vivo and in vitro. Am. J. Hematol. 14:315, 1983.
121. Zinkham, W. H., Houtchens, R. A., and Caughey, W. S.: Carboxyhemoglobin levels in an unstable hemoglobin disorder (Hb Zurich): Effect on phenotypic expression. Science 209:406, 1980.
121a. Zinkham, W. H., Houtchens, R. A., and Caughey, W. S.: Relation between variations in the phenotypic expression of an unstable hemoglobin disorder (hemoglobin Zürich) and carboxyhemoglobin levels. Am. J. Med. 74:23, 1983.
122. Chou, P. Y., and Fasman, G. D.: Prediction of protein conformation. Biochemistry 13:222, 1974.
122a. Shaeffer, J. R., McDonald, M. J., Turci, S. M., Dhinda, D. M., and Bunn, H. F.: Dissociation of αβ dimer of human hemoglobin A. J. Biol. Chem. 259:14544, 1985.
123. Asakura, T., Adachi, K., Wiley, J. S., Fung, L. W.-M., Ho, C., Kilmartin, J. V., and Perutz, M. F.: Structure and function of haemoglobin Philly (Tyr C1 (35) β-Phe). J. Mol. Biol. 104:185, 1976.
124. Tucker, P. W., and Perutz, M. F.: Mechanism of charge compensation and impairment of co-operative functions in haemoglobin Tacoma (Arg B12(30) β-Ser). J. Mol. Biol. 114:415, 1977.
125. Bradley, T. B., and Rieder, R. F.: Hemoglobin Gun Hill: A β chain abnormality associated with a hemolytic state. Blood 28:975, 1966.
126. McDonald, M. J., Lund, D. P., Bleichman, M., Bunn, H. F., DeYoung, A., Noble, R. W., Foster, B., and Arnone, A.: Equilibrium, kinetic and structural properties of hemoglobin Cranston, an elongated beta chain variant. J. Mol. Biol. 140:357, 1980.
127. Winterbourn, C. C., and Carrell, R. W.: Characterization of Heinz bodies in unstable haemoglobin haemolytic anaemia. Nature 240:150, 1972.
128. Winterbourn, C. C., and Carrell, R. W.: The attachment of Heinz bodies to the red cell membrane. Br. J. Haematol. 25:585, 1973.
129. Winterbourn, C. C., and Carrell, R. W.: Studies of hemoglobin denaturation and Heinz body formation in the unstable hemoglobins. J. Clin. Invest. 54:678, 1974.
130. Winterbourn, C. C., McGrath, B. M., and Carrell, R. W.: Reactions involving superoxide and normal

and unstable haemoglobins. Biochem. J. *155*:503, 1976.
131. Winterbourn, C. C., Williamson, D., Vissers, M. C. M., and Carrell, R. W.: Unstable haemoglobin haemolytic crises: Contributions of pyrexia and neutrophil oxidants. Br. J. Haematol. *49*:111, 1981.
132. Rachmilewitz, E. A., and Harari, E.: Intermediate hemichrome formation after oxidation of three unstable hemoglobins (Freiburg, Riverdale-Bronx and Köln). Haematol. Bluttransfus. *10*:241, 1972.
133. Rachmilewitz, E. A., and White, J. M.: Haemichrome formation during the in vitro oxidation of haemoglobin Koln. Nature [New Biol.] *241*:115, 1973.
134. Rachmilewitz, E. A.: Denaturation of the normal and abnormal hemoglobin molecule. Semin. Hematol. *11*:441, 1974.
135. Jacob, H. S., and Winterhalter, K. H.: The role of hemoglobin heme loss in Heinz body formation: Studies with a partially heme-deficient hemoglobin and with genetically unstable hemoglobin. J. Clin. Invest. *49*:2008, 1970.
136. Jacob, H. S., and Winterhalter, K. H.: Unstable hemoglobins: The role of heme loss in Heinz body formation. Proc. Natl. Acad. Sci. USA *65*:697, 1970.
137. Rachmilewitz, E. A., Peisach, J., and Blumberg, W. E.: Studies on the stability of oxyhemoglobin A and its constituent chains and their derivatives. J. Biol. Chem. *246*:3356, 1971.
138. Wajcman, H., Leroux, A., and Labie, D.: Functional properties of hemoglobin Hammersmith. Biochimie *55*:119, 1973.
139. Bunn, H. F., and Jandl, J. H.: Exchange of heme among hemoglobins and between hemoglobin and albumin. J. Biol. Chem. *243*:465, 1968.
139a. Smith, M. L., Hjortsberg, K., Romeo, P.-H., Rosa, J., and Paul, K.-G.: Mutant hemoglobin stability depends upon location and nature of single point mutation. FEBS Lett. *169*:147, 1984.
140. Fairbanks, V. F., Opfell, R. W., and Burgert, E. O.: Three families with unstable hemoglobinopathies (Köln, Olmsted and Santa Ana) causing hemolytic anemia with inclusion bodies and pigmenturia. Am. J. Med. *46*:344, 1969.
141. White, J. M., and Dacie, J. V.: The unstable hemoglobins—molecular and clinical features. Prog. Hematol. *7*:69, 1971.
142. Rieder, R. F.: Hemoglobin stability: Observations on the denaturation of normal and abnormal hemoglobins by oxidant dyes, heat and alkali. J. Clin. Invest. *49*:2369, 1970.
143. Winterhalter, K. H., Amiconi, G., and Antonini, E.: Functional properties of a hemoglobin carrying heme only on alpha chains. Biochemistry *7*:2228, 1968.
144. Waks, M., Yip, Y. K., and Beychok, S.: Influence of prosthetic groups on protein folding and subunit assembly. Recombination of separated human alpha- and beta-globin chains with heme and alloplex interactions of globin chains with heme-containing subunits. J. Biol. Chem. *248*:6462, 1973.
145. Rifkind, R. A.: Heinz body anemia: An ultrastructural study. II. Red cell sequestration and destruction. Blood *26*:433, 1965.
146. Schnitzer, B., Rucknagel, D. L., Spencer, H. H., and Aikawa, M.: Erythrocytes: Pits and vacuoles as seen with transmission and scanning electron microscopy. Science *173*:251, 1971.
147. Chan, E., and Desforges, J.: Role of disulfide bonds in Heinz body attachment to membranes. Blood *44*:921, 1974.
148. Jandl, J. H., Simmons, R. L., and Castle, W. B.: Red cell filtration and the pathogenesis of certain hemolytic anemias. Blood *18*:133, 1961.
149. Miller, D. R., Weed, R. I., Stamatoyannopoulos, G., and Yoshida, A.: Hemoglobin Koln disease occurring as a fresh mutation: Erythrocyte metabolism and survival. Blood *38*:715, 1971.
150. Mills, G. C., Levin, W. C., and Alperin, J. B.: Hemolytic anemia associated with low erythrocyte ATP. Blood *32*:15, 1968.
150a. Chou, A. C., and Fitch, C. D.: Mechanism of hemolysis induced by ferriprotoporphyrin IX. J. Clin. Invest. *68*:1981.
150b. Flynn, T. P., Allen, D. W., Johnson, G. J., and White, J. G.: Oxidant damage of the lipids and proteins of the erythrocyte membranes in unstable hemoglobin disease. Evidence for the role of lipid peroxidation. J. Clin. Invest. *71*:1215, 1983.
150c. Allen, D. W., Burgoyne, C. F., Groat, J. D., Smith, C. M., and White, J. G.: Comparison of hemoglobin Köln erythrocyte membranes with malondialdehyde-reacted normal erythrocyte membranes. Blood *64*:1263, 1984.
151. Testa, U., Beuzard, Y., Vainchenker, W., Goossens, M., Dubart, A., Monplaisir, N., Brizard, C. P., Papayannopoulou, T., and Rosa, J.: Elevated HbF associated with an unstable hemoglobin, hemoglobin Saint Etienne: Hb synthesis in blood BFUe in culture. Blood *54*:334, 1979.
152. Sansone, G., and Pik, C.: Familial haemolytic anemia with erythrocyte inclusion bodies, bilifuscinuria and abnormal haemoglobin (haemoglobin Galliera Genova). Br. J. Haematol. *11*:511, 1965.
153. Raik, E., Hunter, E. G., and Lindsay, D. A.: Compensated hereditary haemolytic disease resulting from an unstable haemoglobin fraction. Med. J. Aust. *1*:955, 1967.
154. Monn, E., Gaffney, P. J., Jr., and Lehmann, H.: Haemoglobin Sögn (beta 14 arginine). A new haemoglobin variant. Scand. J. Haematol. *5*:353, 1968.
155. Rieder, R. F., and Bradley, T. B.: Hemoglobin Gun Hill: An unstable protein associated with chronic hemolysis. Blood *32*:355, 1968.
156. Rieder, R. F., Wolf, D. J., Clegg, J. B., and Lee, S. L.: Rapid postsynthetic destruction of unstable haemoglobin Bushwick. Nature *254*:725, 1975.
157. Kolski, G. B., and Miller, D. R.: Heme synthesis in hereditary hemolytic anemias: Decreased δ-aminolevulinic acid synthetase in hemoglobin Köln disease. Pediatr. Res. *10*:702, 1976.
158. Rieder, R. F.: Synthesis of hemoglobin Gun Hill: Increased synthesis of the heme-free beta[GH] globin chain and subunit exchange with a free alpha chain pool. J. Clin. Invest. *50*:388, 1971.
159. Carrell, R. W., Vissers, M., and Winterbourn, C. C.: Unstable haemoglobin catabolism primarily occurs in the bone marrow. Abstract. International Meeting on Genetic Disorders of Hemoglobin, Jerusalem, Israel, 1981.
159a. Carrell, R. W., and Winterbourn, C. C.: The unstable hemoglobins. *In* Schneider, R., Charache, S., and Schroeder, W. (eds.): Texas Reports on

Biology and Medicine: Human Hemoglobins and Hemoglobinopathies, 1981, pp. 431–446.
160. White, J. M., and Dacie, J. V.: In vitro synthesis of Hb Hammersmith (CD1 Phe–Ser). Nature 225:860, 1970.
161. White, J. M., and Brain, M. C.: Defective synthesis of an unstable haemoglobin Koln (beta 98 Val–Met). Br. J. Haematol. 18:195, 1970.
162. Zalusky, R., Ross, J., and Katz, J. H.: Dissociation and exchange of alpha chains in an unstable haemoglobin. Proceedings of the XIII Congress of the International Society of Hematology, Munich, 1970.
163. Shaeffer, J. R.: Structure and synthesis of the unstable hemoglobin Sabine (alpha 2 beta 2–91 Leu–Pro). J. Biol. Chem. 248:7473, 1973.
164. Shaeffer, J. R., Schmidt, G. J., Kingston, R. E., and Bunn, H. F.: Synthesis of hemoglobin Cranston, an elongated beta chain variant. J. Mol. Biol. 140:377, 1980.
165. Rieder, R. F., and James, G. W., III: Imbalance in alpha and beta globin synthesis associated with a hemoglobinopathy. J. Clin. Invest. 54:948, 1974.
166. Rieder, R. F. and James, G. W., III: Translation of human globin mRNA: Globin synthesis in cells containing Hb Leiden. Blood 47:489, 1976.
167. Adams, J. G., Steinberg, M. H., Newman, M. V., Morrison, W. T., Benz, E. J., and Iyer, R.: Beta thalassemia present in cis to a new beta chain structural variant, Hb Vicksburg beta75 (E19) Leu–0. Proc. Natl. Acad. Sci. USA 78:469, 1981.
167a. Goosens, M., Lee, K. Y., Liebhaber, S. A., and Kan, Y. W.: Globin structural mutant $\alpha 125$ Leu→Pro is a novel cause of α-thalassemia. Nature 296:864, 1982.
168. Tentori, L., Bruni, E., and Marinucci, M.: Three examples of association between beta thalassemia and rare hemoglobin variants. International Istanbul Symposium on Abnormal Hemoglobins and Thalassemia, 1974, pp. 53–62.
168a. Bunn, H. F., Bradley, T. B., Davis, W. E., Drysdale, J. W., Burke, J. F., Beck, W. S., and Laver, M. B.: Structural and functional studies on hemoglobin Bethesda ($\alpha_2\beta_2^{145\ His}$), a variant associated with compensatory erythrocytosis. J. Clin. Invest. 51:2299, 1972.
168b. Stamatoyannopoulos, G., Nute, P. E., and Miller, M.: De novo mutations producing unstable hemoglobins or hemoglobins M. Hum. Genet. 58:396, 1981.
169. Tatsis, B., Dosik, H., Rieder, R., et al.: Hemoglobin Hasharon: Severe hemolytic anemia and hypersplenism associated with a mildly unstable hemoglobin. Birth Defects 8:25, 1972.
170. Levine, R. L., Lincoln, D. R., Buchholz, W. M., Gribble, J., and Schwartz, H. C.: Hemoglobin Hasharon in a premature infant with hemolytic anemia. Pediatr. Res. 9:7, 1975.
170a. Bender, J. W., Reilly, M. P., and Asakura, T.: Molecular stability and function of hemoglobins Hasharon ($\alpha_2 47(CD5)Asp \rightarrow His\ \beta_2$ and Hasharon ($\alpha_2 47(CD5)Asp \rightarrow His\ \delta_2$). Hemoglobin 8:61, 1984.
171. Zinkham, W. H., Liljestrand, J. D., Dixon, S. M., and Hutchison, J. L.: Observations on the rate and mechanism of hemolysis in individuals with Hb Zürich [His E7(63) beta-Arg]: II. Thermal denaturation of hemoglobin as a cause of anemia during fever. Johns Hopkins Med. J. 144:109, 1979.
172. Frick, P. G., Hitzig, W. H., and Betke, K.: Hemoglobin Zurich. A new hemoglobin anomaly associated with acute hemolytic episodes with inclusion bodies after sulfonamide therapy. Blood 20:261, 1982.
173. Rieder, R. F., Zinkham, W. H., and Holtzman, N. A.: Hemoglobin Zurich: Clinical, chemical and kinetic studies. Am. J. Med. 39:4, 1965.
174. Dickerman, J. D., Holtzman, N. A., and Zinkham, W. H.: Hemoglobin Zurich. A third family presenting with hemolytic reactions to sulfonamides. Am. J. Med. 55:638, 1973.
175. Prato, V., Gallo, E., Ricco, G., et al.: Haemolytic anemia due to haemoglobin Torino. Br. J. Haematol. 19:105, 1970.
176. Sansone, G., Sciarratta, G. V., Lang, A., Lorkin, P. A., and Lehmann, H.: A drug induced haemolytic anaemia due to Hb Torino (alpha 43(CD1) Phe–Val). Second finding in an Italian family. Acta Haematol. 56:225, 1976.
177. Adams, J. G., Heller, P., Abramson, R. K., and Vaithianathan, T.: Sulfonamide-induced hemolytic anemia and hemoglobin Hasharon. Arch. Intern. Med. 137:1449, 1977.
178. Grove, S. S., Jenkins, T., Kamuzora, H. L., and Lehmann, H.: Congenital Heinz body haemolytic anaemia due to haemoglobin Perth in a Nama child seemingly aggravated by the high nitrate content of the water supply. Acta Haematol. 57:57:143, 1977.
179. Schmid, R., Brecher, G., and Clemens, T.: Familial hemolytic anemia with erythrocyte inclusion bodies and a defect in pigment metabolism. Blood 14:991, 1959.
179a. Eisinger, J., Flores, J., Tyson, J. A., and Shohet, S. B.: Fluorescent cytoplasm and Heinz bodies of Köln erythrocytes: Evidence for intracellular heme catabolism. Blood 65:886, 1985.
180. Kreimer-Birnbaum, M., Pinkerton, P. H., Bannerman, R. M., and Hutchison, H. E.: Dipyrrolic urinary pigments in congenital Heinz-body anaemia due to Hb Koln and in thalassaemia. Br. Med. J. 2:396, 1966.
181. Kreimer-Birnbaum, M., Pinkerton, P. H., Bannerman, R. M., and Hutchison, H. E.: Urinary "dipyrroles"; their occurrence and significance in thalassemia and other disorders. Blood 28:993, 1966.
182. Tenhunen, R., Marver, H. S., and Schmid, R.: The enzymatic conversion of heme to bilirubin by microsomal heme oxygenase. Proc. Natl. Acad. Sci. USA 61:748, 1968.
183. Goldstein, G. W., Hammaker, L., and Schmid, R.: The catabolism of Heinz bodies: An experimental model demonstrating conversion to non-bilirubin catabolites. Blood 31:388, 1968.
184. Hutchison, H. E., Pinkerton, P. H., Waters, P., Douglas, A. S., Lehmann, H., and Beale, D.: Hereditary Heinz body anaemia, thrombocytopenia and haemoglobinopathy (Hb Köln) in a Glasgow family. Br. Med. J. 2:1099, 1964.
185. Pederson, P. R., McCurdy, P. R., Wrightstone, R. N., Wilson, J. B., Smith, L. L., and Huisman, T. H. J.: Hemoglobin Köln in a black: Pre- and postsplenectomy red cell survival (DF 32 P and 51 Cr) and the pathogenesis of hemoglobin instability. Blood 42:771, 1973.

186. Tatsis, B., Dosik, H., Rieder, R., et al.: Hemoglobin Hasharon: Severe hemolytic anemia and hypersplenism associated with a mildly unstable hemoglobin. Birth Defects 8:25, 1972.
187. White, J. M.: The unstable haemoglobin disorder. Clin. Haematol. 3:333, 1974.
188. Bentley, S. A., Lewis, S. M., and White, J. M.: Red cell survival studies in patients with unstable hemoglobin disorders. Br. J. Haematol. 26:85, 1974.
189. Schneiderman, L. J., Junga, I. G., and Fawley, D. E.: Effects of phosphate and non-phosphate buffers on thermolability of unstable haemoglobins. Nature 225:1041, 1970.
190. Carrell, R. W., and Kay, R.: A simple method for the detection of unstable hemoglobins. Br. J. Haematol. 23:615, 1972.
191. Brosious, E. M., Morrison, B. Y., and Schmidt, R. M.: Effects of hemoglobin F levels, KCN, and storage on the isopropanol precipitation test for unstable hemoglobins. Am. J. Clin. Pathol. 66:878, 1976.
192. Asakura, T., Adachi, K., Shapiro, M., Friedman, S., and Schwartz, E.: Mechanical precipitation of hemoglobin Köln. Biochim. Biophys. Acta 412:197, 1975.
193. Vella, F.: Mechanical stability of human haemoglobins. Acta Haematol. 54:257, 1975.
194. North, M. L., Thillet, J., and Rosa, J.: Effect of some physical features of and of amino acid substitutions on the mechanical precipitation of hemoglobin. Hemoglobin 5:379, 1981.
195. Carrell, R. W., and Lehmann, H.: Zinc acetate as a precipitant of unstable haemoglobins. J. Clin. Pathol. 34:796, 1981.
196. Fairbanks, V. F., and Pettit, R. M.: Sickledex test in unstable hemoglobin disorders. J.A.M.A. 220:128, 1972.
197. Bellingham, A. J., and Huehns, E. R.: Compensation in haemolytic anaemias caused by abnormal haemoglobins. Nature 218:924, 1968.
198. Egan, E. L., and Fairbanks, V. F.: Postsplenectomy erythrocytosis in hemoglobin Köln disease. N. Engl. J. Med. 288:929, 1973.
199. Desforges, J. F.: Unstable oxygen delivery. N. Engl. J. Med. 288:965, 1973.
200. Woodson, R. D., Heywood, J. D., and Lenfant, C.: Oxygen transport in hemoglobin Köln. Effect of increased oxygen affinity in absence of compensatory erythrocytosis. Arch. Intern. Med. 134:711, 1974.
201. Stamatoyannopoulos, G., Parer, J. T., and Finch, C. A.: Physiologic implications of a hemoglobin with decreased oxygen affinity (hemoglobin Seattle). N. Engl. J. Med. 281:915, 1969.
202. Wajcman, H., Byckova, V., Haidas, S., and Labie, D.: Consequences of heme loss in unstable hemoglobins: A study of hemoglobin Köln. FEBS Lett. 13:145, 1971.
203. Sharma, V. S., Noble, R. W., and Ranney, H. M.: Structure-function relationship in hemoglobin Köln (beta 98 Val–Met). J. Mol. Biol. 82:139, 1974.
204. Smith, L. L., Barton, B. P., and Huisman, T. H. J.: Subunit dissociation of the unstable hemoglobin Bibba ($\alpha_2^{136\,Pro}$ (H19) β_2). J. Biol. Chem. 245:2185, 1970.
205. DeFuria, F. G., and Miller, D. R.: Oxygen affinity in hemoglobin Köln disease. Blood 39:398, 1972.
206. Gacon, G., Krishnamoorthy, R., Wajcman, H., Labie, D., Tabon, J., and Cosson, A.: Hemoglobin Djelfa β98 (FG5) Val→Ala: Isolation and functional properties of the heme saturated form. Biochim. Biophys. Acta 490:156, 1977.
207. Nagel, R. L., Reider, R. F., Bookchin, R. M., and James, G. W.: Some functional properties of hemoglobin Leiden. Biochem. Biophys. Res. Commun. 53:1240, 1973.
208. May, A., and Huehns, E. R.: The control of oxygen affinity of red cells with Hb Shepherds Bush. Br. J. Haematol. 22:599, 1972.
209. Hirsh, J., and Dacie, J. V.: Persistent post-splenectomy thrombocytosis and thrombo-embolism: A consequence of continuing anaemia. Br. J. Haematol. 12:44, 1966.
210. Adams, J. G., III: Hemoglobin Ann Arbor: Disturbance in the coordinated biosynthesis of globin chains? Ann. N.Y. Acad. Sci. 241:232, 1974.

HEMOGLOBINOPATHY DUE TO ABNORMAL OXYGEN BINDING

14

In 1966, an 81-year-old man with erythrocytosis was seen in the hematology clinic at Johns Hopkins Hospital.[1,2] He had mild angina pectoris that developed late in life but no other significant clinical problems. Dr. Samuel Charache discovered that he had a hemoglobin of 19.9 g/dl and an abnormal hemoglobin band on electrophoresis. In an attempt to relate these two findings, he determined an oxygen dissociation curve on the patient's blood and found that it was significantly displaced to the left. This observation suggested the intriguing possibility that the patient's erythrocytosis might be a secondary compensation to a primary defect in oxygen unloading. A thorough family study revealed 15 other members with both erythrocytosis and the electrophoretically abnormal hemoglobin.[1] Charache then purified the hemoglobin variant and confirmed that it had a marked increase in oxygen affinity. Structured analysis established that hemoglobin Chesapeake is an α-chain variant with a substitution of leucine for arginine at position 92.[3] This series of observations opened up a new chapter in the developing story of hemoglobin.

Forty-two other variants with increased oxygen affinity have been encountered thus far in individuals with secondary erythrocytosis (Table 14–1). These variants generally have amino acid substitutions at sites crucial to hemoglobin function. Indeed, the understanding of structure-function relationships of human hemoglobin is sufficiently advanced that, in most cases, the abnormal oxygen binding of the variant can be readily explained by its specific structural alteration (see below). In addition, a number of other variants are known to have increased oxygen affinity, although they are not associated with secondary erythrocytosis. As shown in Figure 14–1 and Table 14–2, these variants generally do not have such marked increases in oxygen affinity as those listed in Table 14–1. Until recently, measurements of oxygen affinity were not generally included in studies on new hemoglobin var-

Table 14–1. VARIANTS WITH HIGH OXYGEN AFFINITY ASSOCIATED WITH ERYTHROCYTOSIS

Variant	Structure	Area Affected	% of Total Hb	Hb Level (g/dl)	WB P_{50} (mm Hg)	$\frac{P_{50}X}{P_{50}A}$	% Bohr Effect	Response to 2,3-DPG	Electrophoresis	Comment	Reference(s)
Milledgeville	α 44 (CE2) Pro→Leu	$α_1β_2$		15.6–18.1	11–15		NI (RBC)	NI (RBC)	IEF:0 CAc:0 CAg:0 CAc:0		4
Chesapeake	α 92 (FG4) Arg→Leu	$α_1β_2$	25–30	15–20	19	$\frac{0.39}{2.38}$	NI	NI	CAg:0 SG IEF		1, 3, 5
J-Cape Town	α 92 (FG4) Arg→Gln	$α_1β_2$	10–100	15–17		$\frac{0.8}{3.1}$	NI	NI	CAc	Associated with α thal homozygote—more severe	6–8a
Tarrant	α 126 (H9) Asp→Asn	$α_1β_1$	23, 46	15–19	15/22	$\frac{0.25}{2}$	NI	NI	CAc CAg:0	Homozygote—more severe	9–10
Legnano	α 141 (HC3) Arg→Leu	$α_1β_2$	33	16–20	21	$\frac{1.8}{5.7}$	50%	↓	CAc		11, 12
Suresnes	α 141 (HC3) Arg→His	$α_1β_2$	39	15–16.5	17.5	$\frac{1.85}{12.2}$ $\frac{0.4}{1.9}$	60%	↓	CAc		13, 14
Olympia	β 20 (B2) Val→Met			18–20	18.6		NI (H)		IEF:0 CAg:0 CAc:0		15
Palmerston-North	β 23 (B5) Val→Phe		28	17.8	19				IEF SG:0 CAg	Mildly unstable	15a
Petie-Salpetriere	β 34 (B16) Val→Phe	$α_1β_2$	37	17.5, 20	17	$\frac{0.6}{6}$	25%	NI	IEF CAc:0		16, 17
Brisbane Great Lakes	β 68 (E12) Leu→His	$α_1β_2$		15–20	16.1		NI (N)		IEF:0 CAg:0 CAc:0	Mildly unstable	18, 19
Rahere	β 82 (EF6) Lys→Thr	DPG		19	18	$\frac{3.7}{4.7}$	NI	↑	IEF CAg CAc:0	↑WBC ↓Plasma volume	20
Helsinki	β 82 (EF6) Lys→Met	DPG		14–16.8	23	$\frac{7.0}{8.0}$	70%	↓↓	CAc		21
Providence*	β 82 (EF6) Lys→Asn→Asp*	DPG	19 Asn 32 Asp	15	20.6	3 (Asn) 4.5 Asp) 2 (A)	65%	↓↓	CAc CAg	Partial deamidation in vivo	22–24
Creteil	β 89 (F5) Ser→Asn	?	50	21	14.5	$\frac{1.3}{14}$	45%	0	IEF CAg:0 CAc:0	Splenomegaly	25

Name	Mutation	Interface						↓ (H)		Comments	Ref
Vanderbilt	β 89 (F5) Ser→Arg	?	40	19–22	14.5				CAc		26
Barcelona	β 94 (FG1) Asp→His		37–40	17.7	21	3.0/6.3	75%	NI		Prevents important intra-subunit salt bond	26a, 26b 27–29
Malmö	β 97 (FG4) His→Gln	α₁β₂		17–21	14.5	2.6/14	70%	NI	IEF CAg CAc:0		
Wood	β 97 (FG4) His→Leu	α₁β₂	50	17–22	12.8				IEF CAg CAc:0		30
Yakima	β 99 (G1) Asp→His	α₁β₂	37	16–18	12	0.36/5.4			SG		31, 32
Kempsey	β 99 (G1) Asp→Asn	α₁β₂	46	17–20	13.5/33	0.23/2.4/0.28/5.4	40%	→	SG		33, 34
Ypsilanti	β 99 (G1) Asp→Tyr	α₁β₂	~34	15–19		0.8/4.6			SG	Forms stable hybrids	35, 36
Radcliffe	β 99 (G1) Asp→Ala	α₁β₂	47	17–19	12		75%	→	SG	Forms stable hybrids	37
Hotel Dieu	β 99 (G1) Asp→Gly	α₁β₂	48	20–24	15	0.6/6	40%	SI↓	IEF CAc	Pulmonary disease	17, 38
Chemilly	β 99 (G1) Asp→Val	α₁β₂	40	19	15	1/4.6	50%		CAc		38a
Brigham	β 100 (G2) Pro→Leu	α₁β₂	?	16–18	19		NI (H)		IEF:0 CAg:0 CAc:0		39
British Columbia	β 101 (G3) Glu→Lys	α₁β₂	54(?)	17	23.2				CAc	Forms stable hybrids	40
Alberta	β 101 (G3) Glu→Gly	α₁β₂	45	20		1.3/7.8	NI		CAc SG	Forms stable hybrids	41–43
Potomac	β 101 (G3) Glu→Asp	α₁β₂	?	17–19	12.5		NI (H)		IEF:0 CAg:0 CAc:0		44, 45
Heathrow	β 103 (G5) Phe→Leu	Heme	?	16–21	9.5				IEF:0 CAc:0	Sulfhydryl separation	46, 47
San Diego	β 109 (G11) Val→Met	α₁β₂	?	16–18	16.4		NI (H)		IEF:0 SG:0		48
Ty Gard	β 124 (H2) Pro→Gln	α₁β₂	40	19.2	20.8	1.5/2.2	NI	NI	IEF CAg:0 CAc:0		49
St. Jacques	β 140 (H18) Ala→Thr		~45	19	14.5		NI		CAc:0 CAg:0 IEF:0		49a

Table continued on following page

Table 14-1. VARIANTS WITH HIGH OXYGEN AFFINITY ASSOCIATED WITH ERYTHROCYTOSIS Continued

Variant	Structure	Area Affected	% of Total Hb	Hb Level (g/dl)	WB P_{50} (mm Hg)	$P_{50}X/P_{50}A$	% Bohr Effect	Response to 2,3-DPG	Electro-phoresis	Comment	Reference(s)
Ohio	β 142 (H20) Ala→Asp		48	19–20	16.8	0.3 / 0.7	60%		CAg CAc		50
Little Rock	β 143 (H21) His→Gln	DPG	~45	20–23		0.93 / 3.1	NI	→	CAg IEF SG:0		51, 52
Syracuse	β 143 (H21) His→Pro	DPG	~40	19–24	11	0.32 / 3.1	40%	→	IEF CAg:0 CAc:0		53
Andrew-Minneapolis	β 144 (HC1) Lys→Asn	ββ		20	~16		60%	NI	CAc		54
Rainier	β 145 (HC2) Tyr→Cys	ββ	30	17–21		0.13 / 1.7			CAc:0 CAg	Alkali-resistant	55–58
Bethesda	β 145 (HC2) Tyr→His	ββ	~50	16–21	12.8	0.18 / 3.9	40%	→	IEF:0 CAg CAc:0		58, 59
Osler Fort Gordon Nancy	β 145 (HC2) Tyr→Asp	ββ	30	13; 17–22	12; 13 29.5	0.27 / 2.2 0.32 / 6.6	50% 60%	→	CAg CAc		60–63
McKees Rocks	β 145–146 (HC2–HC3)→0	ββ	46	18–21	10	0.66 / 10	20%	0	CAg CAc:0		64
Hiroshima	β 146 (HC3) His→Asp	ββ	51	11–17	5 / 10.5	0.32 / 1.8	50%	→	CAg CAc		65–67
York	β 146 (HC3) His→Pro	ββ	50			0.62 / 4.7	50%	NI	CAg CAc:0		68
Cowtown	β 146 (HC3) His→Leu	ββ	45	18–19	19	1.9 / 4.7	50%	→	CAg CAc:0		69

*β 82 asparagine is partially deamidated to aspartic acid during the circulation of red cells *in vivo*.

Note: Data herein compiled from references listed in last column. *% Total Hemoglobin* = proportion of abnormal hemoglobin in hemolysate of heterozygote(s). *WB P_{50}* = oxygen tension at which blood is half-saturated at pH 7.4, 37°C (normal = 26 mm Hg). $P_{50} X/P_{50} A$ = ratio of P_{50} value of purified variant hemoglobin to that of Hb A at pH 7.2. (Most measurements were performed at 20° to 25°C in a phosphate-free buffer, $\mu \cong 0.1$.) *% Bohr Effect* = ratio $\Delta \log P_{50}/\Delta$ pH for purified variant hemoglobin over that of Hb A. (Measurements were sometimes on a hemolysate [H] or in intact red cells [RBC].) *Response to 2,3-DPG* = relative effect of added 2,3-DPG on oxygen affinity of the variant hemoglobin compared with that of Hb A.

Electrophoretic data: CAc = cellulose acetate, pH 8.0 to 9.0; SG = starch gel, pH 8.0 to 9.0; CAg = citrate agar, pH 8.0 to 9.0; IEF = isoelectric focusing. When these abbreviations are included, the method was used for the corresponding variant; unless followed by "0," the method achieved electrophoretic separation (e.g., Hb Chesapeake could be separated from Hb A by starch gel [SG] but not by citrate agar [CAg:0]).

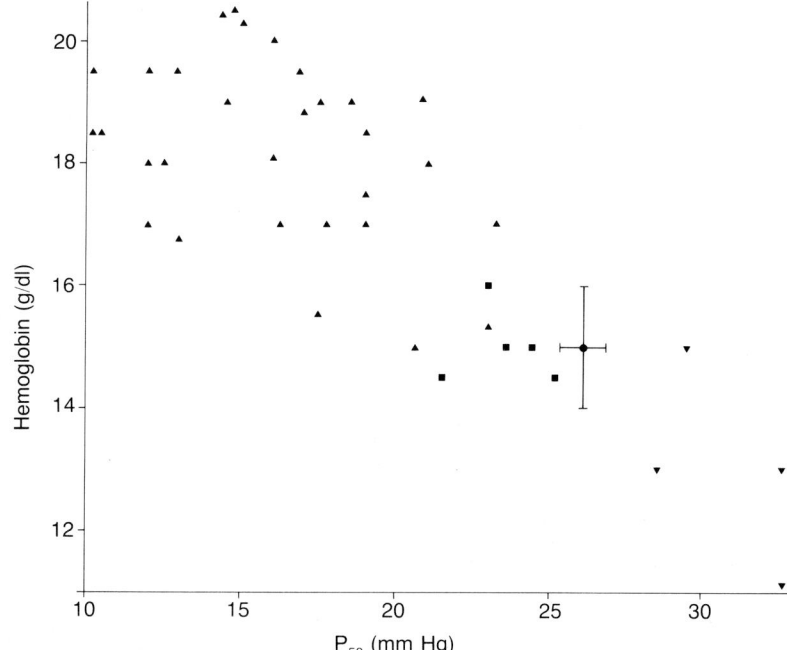

Figure 14–1. Relationship between average hemoglobin level and whole blood oxygen affinity in high-affinity variants associated with familial erythrocytosis (▲) (see Table 14–1), other high-affinity variants (■) (see Table 14–2), and low-affinity variants (▼) (see Table 14–6). (Normal = ●.)

iants. Thus, among the 250-odd variants without clinical manifestations listed in Table 10–1, there are probably additional hemoglobins with increased oxygen affinity as well as other abnormal functional properties.

About 30 per cent of the 90-odd unstable hemoglobin variants have significantly increased oxygen affinity (see Table 13–1). In fact, some of these mutant hemoglobins have higher oxygen affinity than those listed in Table 14–1. However, the predominant clinical manifestations are due to accelerated red cell destruction. The oxygen affinity of unstable hemoglobins appears to be an important determinant of the degree to which the patient's hemolysis is compensated: Those patients with CHBA due to a variant with high affinity tend to have higher hemoglobin levels than those with normal or decreased oxygen affinity[94] (see Chapter 13).

MOLECULAR PATHOGENESIS

The functional behavior of normal hemoglobin depends on a transition in its three-dimensional conformation that accompanies the addition and removal of oxygen. This process is discussed in detail in Chapter 3. As formulated in the allosteric model of Monod, Wyman, and Changeux (MWC),[95] the hemoglobin tetramer exists in equilibrium between two quaternary conformations: R and T. When normal hemoglobin is fully deoxygenated, it is about 99.99 per cent in the T or "tense" structure. In this state, hemoglobin has a relatively low affinity for oxygen and other heme ligands and a relatively high affinity for allosteric effectors such as Bohr protons and 2,3-DPG. Conversely, normal oxyhemoglobin exists almost exclusively in the R or "relaxed" conformation. In this state, it has a relatively high affinity for heme ligands such as oxygen and a low affinity for Bohr protons and 2,3-DPG. The transition between these two conformers involves a considerable free energy change, reflected as cooperativity between subunits or "heme-heme interaction" (see Chapter 3). The change from the T to the R conformation involves a rather well-defined series of structural changes, including the rupture of the salt bonds that stabilize the T conformation and the rotation of the β chains relative to the α chains. A considerable amount of intramolecular "movement" during this conformational isomerization occurs at the $\alpha_1\beta_2$ interface.

A structural alteration that affects the equilibrium between the R and T states would be expected to have a marked effect on hemoglobin function. Thus, if a specific amino acid substitution decreases the stability of the T structure, the transition to the R state will occur at an earlier stage in ligation, and the hemoglobin will have increased oxygen affinity and decreased heme-heme interaction. This

Table 14–2. VARIANTS WITH HIGH OXYGEN AFFINITY UNASSOCIATED WITH ERYTHROCYTOSIS

Variant	Structure	Area Affected	% of Total Hb	Hb Level (g/dl)	WB P_{50} (mm Hg)	$P_{50}X / P_{50}A$	% Bohr Effect	Response to 2,3-DPG	Electrophoresis	Comment	Reference(s)
Sawara	α 6 (A4) Asp→Ala					2 / 4.6	NI	NI	IEF		70
Dunn	α 6 (A4) Asp→Asn		12–17	NI	23.7	5.1 / 7.6	NI	NI	CAg / CAc		71
Kariya	α 40 (C5) Lys→Glu		6	15.8		1 / 5	~80%		CAc	Slightly unstable	71a
Kawachi	α 44 (CE2) Pro→Arg	$α_1β_2$	26	15.4		2.0 / 5.4	20%		IEF		71b
Fort de France	α 45 (CE3) His→Arg		20	NI	27.5 / 29.5		NI	NI	IEF		72
G-Norfolk	α 85 (F6) Asp→Asn		15	14.9	30	14 / 20	NI	NI	CAc		73
G-Georgia	α 95 (G2) Pro→Leu	$α_1β_2$	24	10.8	30	12 / 17.4	→		SG	↑ Subunit dissociation	74, 75
Rampa	α 95 (G2) Pro→Ser	$α_1β_2$	24			↑	→		SG	↑ Subunit dissociation	74, 76
Denmark Hill	α 95 (G2) Pro→Ala	$α_1β_2$	19	12		5 / 10.7	85%		CAc		77
St. Luke's	α 95 (G2) Pro→Arg	$α_1β_2$	14	16.4		2.8 / 6.2	100%	NI	SG		78
Dallas	α 97 (G4) Asn→Lys		23	14.5	18.2	0.7 / 5.0	100%	NI	CAc		78a
Tokoname	α 139 (HC1) Lys→Thr		25	15.6		2.4 / 4.8	40%	NI	IEF		78b
Cubujuqui	α 141 (HC3) Arg→Ser	$α_1β_2$	29	14.7		0.32 / 2.0		NI	CA / CAg:0		78c

Name	Mutation									Notes	Ref
Deer Lodge	β 2 (NA2) His→Arg	DPG	45	12.6		0.68 / 1.1	NI	NI	SG		79, 80
Porto Alegre	β 9 (A6) Ser→Cys			14.9		1.1	NI	NI	SG	Homozygote has normal Hb; polymerizes	81, 82
Strasbourg	β 23 (B5) Val→Asp		40	NI	29/30	2.7 / 6.3	NI	NI			83, 83a
Hirose	β 37 (C3) Trp→Ser	α₁β₂	41	10–14		5.1 / 17.3 / 2.6 / 11.0	→		SG		84, 85
Athens-Ga	β 40 (C6) Arg→Lys	α₁β₂	48	13–16	21.5		NI (H)				86
Austin	β 40 (C6) Arg→Ser	α₁β₂	45	NI		9/10	NI	NI	CAc	↑ Subunit dissociation	87
Willamette	β 51 (D2) Pro→Arg		32–39	14–15	25.2	11.7 / 14.4	80%		CAc		88
Pasadena	β 75 (E19) Leu→Arg					2.9 / 4.9	85%	NI			88a
G-Hsi-Tsou	β 79 (EF3) Asp→Gly					2.8 / 3.6		NI			89
Bunbury	β 94 (FG1) Asp→Asn		38	13	21				CAc		89a
Crete	β 129 (H7) Ala→Pro		38	16	23	3.5 / 9	NI	NI	CAg SG CAc	Slightly unstable; Crete/δβ thal heterozygote has Hb 11 g/dl, P₅₀ 11 mm Hg	90
Abruzzo	β 143 (H21) His→Arg	DPG				0.8 / 1.8	NI	↓	SG CAc	Double heterozygote with β⁰ thalassemia	91, 92
Tak	β 147—Elongated	ββ	26	NI		0.19 / 12.2	18%	↓		May be slightly unstable; double heterozygote with β thal	93, Ch. 10

See *Note* at end of Table 14–1.

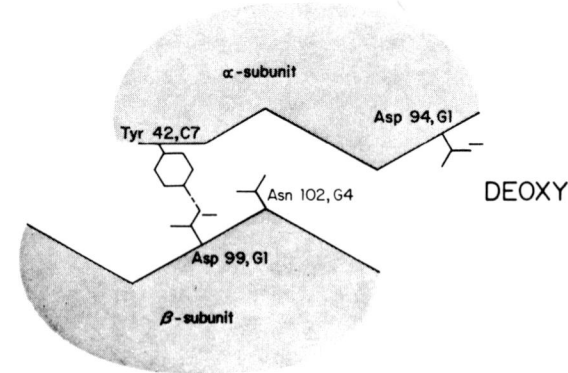

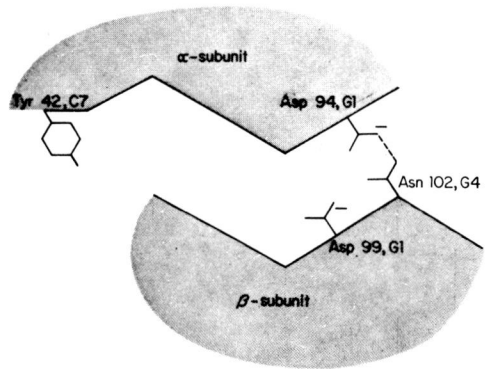

Figure 14–2. Changes at a portion of the $\alpha_1\beta_2$ interface upon oxygenation. The area of contact shifts in a dovetail fashion. Deoxyhemoglobin is stabilized by a hydrogen bond between α 42 Tyr and β 99 Asp. This bond cannot form in Hb Kempsey (β 99 Asp→Asn). Likewise, oxyhemoglobin is stabilized by a bond between α 94 Asp and β 102 Asn. This bond cannot form in Hb Kansas (β 102 Asn→Thr), Hb Beth Israel (β 102 Asn→Thr), and Hb Titusville (α 94 Asp→Asn). (From Perutz, M. F.: New Scient. Sci. J., June, 1971.)

has been demonstrated for a number of chemically modified hemoglobins as well as for many of the high-affinity mutants.[96] Hemoglobin Kempsey is a particularly well studied example.[33, 34, 97-100] It is a β-chain variant in which β 99 aspartic acid has been replaced by asparagine. In deoxyhemoglobin A, this aspartic acid residue normally forms an important hydrogen bond with α 42 tyrosine at the $\alpha_1\beta_2$ interface (Fig. 14–2). Upon oxygenation, the two subunits shift in a dovetail fashion, so that the β 99–α 42 hydrogen bond is broken and another one forms between α 94 aspartic acid and β 102 asparagine.[101] In hemoglobin Kempsey, the substitution at β 99 prevents the formation of the former hydrogen bond and lessens the stability of the "deoxy" or T structure. Thus, when hemoglobin Kempsey is fully deoxygenated, it remains partly in the R state. (The equilibrium constant L in the MWC model is drastically reduced.) This has been verified experimentally in a variety of ways. A number of physical and chemical properties distinguish normal oxy- and deoxyhemoglobin (see Chapter 3). In fact, these can be considered to be properties that distinguish the R and T conformations. In most respects, deoxygenated hemoglobin Kempsey bears more resemblance to oxyhemoglobin A than to deoxyhemoglobin A. These include kinetics of ligand binding, sulfhydryl reactivity, extent of dissociation into αβ dimers, and binding to haptoglobin.[34] In addition, physical probes such as nuclear magnetic resonance spectroscopy[97] and circular dichroism[98, 99] support the conclusion that deoxygenated Hb Kempsey is partially in the R conformation.

Most of the high-affinity variants encountered thus far have substitutions at one of three regions that are crucial to hemoglobin function (see Tables 14–1 and 14–2):

1. The $\alpha_1\beta_2$ interface.
2. The C-terminal end of the β chain.
3. The 2,3-DPG binding site.

Hb Kempsey is one of many high-affinity variants that has an amino acid substitution at the $\alpha_1\beta_2$ interface. As mentioned above, a structural alteration in this important region often affects the relative stability of either the T or the R structure and impairs the orderly transition between the two conformers.

Seventeen high-affinity variants have structural alterations at the C-terminal end of the subunits. As discussed in Chapter 3, the C-terminal portions of the α and β chains contribute greatly to the overall stability of the "deoxy" or T conformation.[102, 103] The penultimate tyrosine of both chains (α 140, β 145) is anchored in a cleft between the F and H helices. In the α chain, the C-terminal arginine is involved in two salt bonds: The guanido group is linked to an aspartate (residue 126) of the same α chain, and the carboxyl group may be linked to the N-terminal amino group of the other α chain. The C-terminal end of the β chain plays an equally important role. The C-terminal histidine (β 146) forms two salt bonds: Its carboxyl group is linked to the ε-amino group of α 40 lysine, and its imidazole group forms an intrasubunit bond with the carboxyl of β 94 aspartate. In addition, β 143 histidine is an important binding site for 2,3-DPG. All these interactions are oxygen-linked. The bonds break upon oxygenation, and the molecule then assumes the relaxed (R) conformation. It is not surprising that variants having substitution at the C-terminal portion of the β chain can have abnormal functional properties, including high oxygen affinity, decreased cooperativity, decreased Bohr effect, and impaired interaction with 2,3-DPG. These will be discussed in more detail in the next section.

Not all variants with substitutions at these strategic sites have abnormal functional properties. For example, Hb Cochin–Port Royal (β 146, His→Arg) has only minor abnormalities in oxygen binding.[104] Even more surprising, Hb J-Altgeld Gardens, β 92 (F8) His→Asp, a substitution at the proximal heme, appears to have normal oxygenation.[105]

PROPERTIES OF THE HIGH-AFFINITY VARIANTS

Oxygen Equilibrium

By definition, this group of hemoglobin variants is associated with a shift to the left of the whole blood oxygen dissociation curve. Under physiologic conditions of pH (7.4) and temperature (37°C), normal red cells in plasma have a P_{50} of 26 mm Hg. That is, at an oxygen tension of 26 mm Hg, hemoglobin in these cells will be half saturated. Increased oxygen affinity is associated with low P_{50}.

In patients with erythrocytosis due to abnormal hemoglobins, whole blood P_{50} values range widely (see Table 14–1). As shown in Figure 14–1, the degree of polycythemia is roughly proportional to the increase in whole blood oxygen affinity. Figure 14–3A shows a whole blood oxygen dissociation curve from a girl with hemoglobin Bethesda. The red cell organic phosphates were within normal limits. Therefore, the marked shift to the left in the

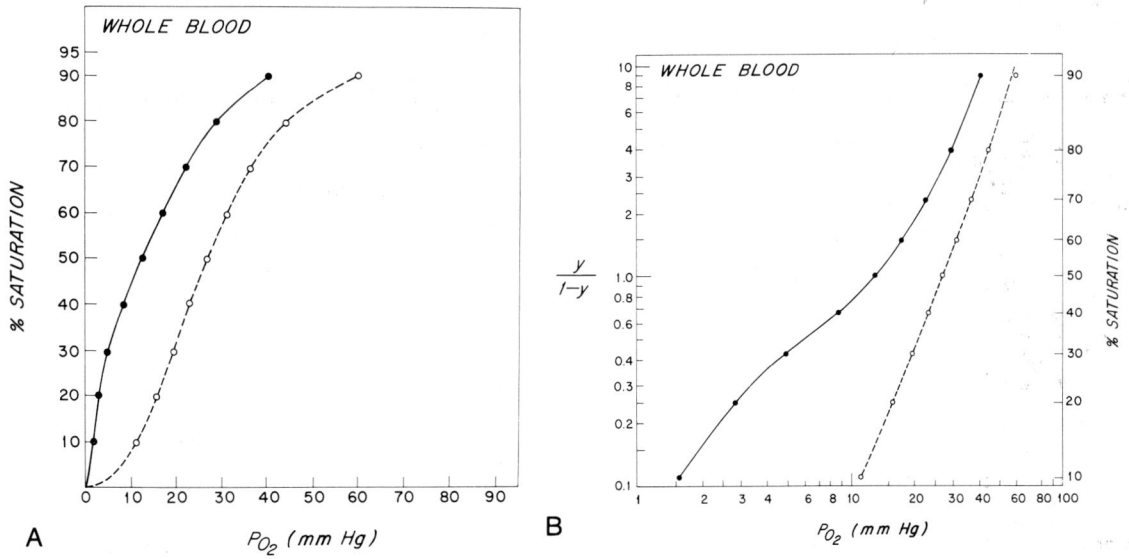

Figure 14–3. A, Oxygen binding curves of a normal individual ○----○ (P_{50} = 26.5 mm Hg) and of a patient with Hb Bethesda ●——● (P_{50} = 12.8 mm Hg). B, Hill plots of data shown in A. Normal (○----○); patient (●——●). Note biphasic curve. (From Bunn, H. F., et al.: J. Clin. Invest. 51:2299, 1972.)

oxygen binding curves indicates the presence of functionally abnormal hemoglobin. From a Hill plot (Fig. 14–3B) of the data shown in Figure 14–3A, it is apparent that the patient has a biphasic curve. The lower portion of the curve is due to the presence of hemoglobin Bethesda. An inflection point is seen at about 50 per cent saturation. The slope of the Hill plot at this point is low, as is the case for a mixture of any two hemoglobins of widely different oxygen affinities. This particular "n" value is *not* a reflection of cooperativity, despite some statements in the literature. The upper portion of the patient's curve in Figure 14–3B approaches the normal curve asymptotically and reflects the oxygenation of normal hemoglobin A that coexists in the red cells with an equal amount of hemoglobin Bethesda.

Although the whole blood oxygen dissociation curve provides information that is physiologically relevant, it does not give precise information on the functional properties of the variant hemoglobin. The whole blood curve is determined by the relative oxygen affinities and proportions of the normal and abnormal hemoglobins as well as by intracellular factors such as organic phosphates, pH, and carbon dioxide tension. These latter variables are eliminated if measurements are made on a phosphate-free hemolysate. A fuller investigation of the variant requires its isolation by some preparative technique such as column chromatography prior to the measurement of its functional properties. It is difficult to compare the 40-odd high-affinity variants because they have been studied in a number of laboratories by a variety of techniques and under different experimental conditions. In Table 14–3, the oxygen equilibria of the variants that have been studied in our laboratory are compared. Some of these mutant hemoglobins have oxygen binding properties approaching those of isolated subunits of hemoglobin A. Generally, those variants having the highest oxygen affinity have the lowest cooperativity. This abnormality reflects a perturbation in the equilibrium between conformational isomers. These hemoglobins flip from T to R at a relatively early stage in ligation. The reduction in the overall energy of interaction between subunits results in a low n value (see Chapter 3). If the R $\rightleftharpoons$ T equilibrium can be shifted back toward T, then the energy of subunit interaction will be enhanced and Hill's n will increase. For example, the cooperativity of several of the high-affinity variants can be significantly increased by the addition of organic phosphates such as 2,3-DPG and inositol hexaphosphate[13, 34, 106-108] (Fig. 14–4).

Bohr Effect

Many of the high-affinity hemoglobins have a decreased alkaline Bohr effect (see Tables 14–1 to 14–3). There are two explanations for this abnormality. In the first place, those variants having substitutions at the C-terminal end of the β chain may have a decreased value because of failure to form the important salt bond (in deoxyhemoglobin) between the im-

Table 14–3. COMPARISON OF FUNCTIONAL PROPERTIES OF HIGH-AFFINITY VARIANTS STUDIED UNDER IDENTICAL CONDITIONS

Hemoglobin Variant	Phosphate-Free Hemolysate		Purified Hemoglobin			
	% Abnormal	P_{50}* (mm Hg)	P_{50}* (mm Hg)	n*	Bohr Effect**	P_{50} DPG/P_{50}†
Chesapeake	30		0.55	1.4		
Kempsey	45	1.2	0.23	1.1	−0.22	1.6
Bethesda	50	1.3	0.18	1.1	−0.21	1.6
Brigham	50	2.7	#			
Hiroshima	50		0.90	2.2		
Syracuse	45	1.5	0.33	1.1	−0.24	1.4
Alberta			0.60	2.3	−0.65	
Cranston	25	3.0	0.20	1.0	−0.20	
A (normal)	0	4.0	3.4	2.8	−0.55	2.4
α^A chains			0.45	1.0		
β^A chains			0.24	1.0		

*0.05 M bis-TRIS buffer (0.1 M Cl⁻), pH 7.2, 20°C; hemoglobin concentration = 0.1 mM tetramer.
**Δ log P_{50}/Δ pH.
†P_{50} (1 mM 2,3-DPG)/P_{50} (no 2,3-DPG).
#Hemoglobin Brigham cannot be separated from Hb A by conventional technqiues.

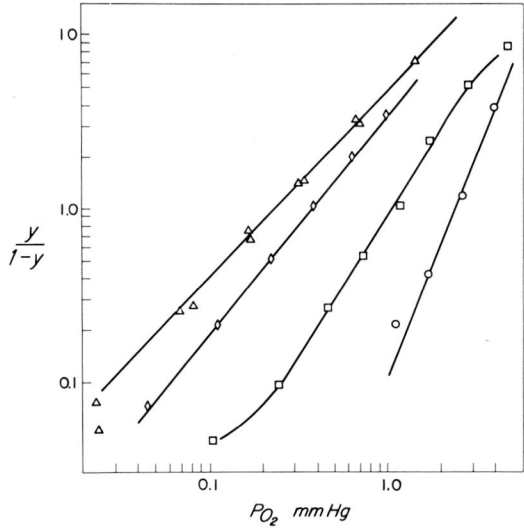

Figure 14–4. Oxygen equilibria of hemoglobin Kempsey and hemoglobin A (isolated from the same column). Hemoglobin (0.4 mM heme) in 0.05 bis-TRIS buffer, pH 7.2, 0.1 M Cl⁻, 20°C.

	P_{50} mm Hg	n
△ Kempsey	0.23	1.1
◇ Kempsey + 1 mM 2,3-DPG	0.37	1.3
□ Kempsey + 1 mM inositol hexaphosphate	1.1	1.7
○ A	2.4	2.6

(From Bunn, H. F., et al.: J. Biol. Chem. 249:7402, 1974.)

idazole of β 146 histidine and the carboxyl group of β 94 aspartic acid. This interaction contributes significantly to the normal alkaline Bohr effect (see Chapter 3). In hemoglobin Hiroshima, the substitution of aspartic acid for histidine at β 146 prevents the formation of this salt bond. The Bohr effect of Hb Hiroshima is half normal. However, certain variants have a reduced Bohr effect, even though their structural alterations are not at or near one of the residues known to contribute Bohr protons. For example, hemoglobin Kempsey (in the absence of organic phosphates) cannot assume a fully T structure upon deoxygenation and thus does not liberate a full complement of Bohr protons upon oxygenation.

Interaction with 2,3-DPG

Red cell 2,3-DPG has been measured in most of these variants and has been consistently normal. However, several of these variants have been shown to have a diminished interaction with 2,3-DPG. Some of these have substitutions at sites normally responsible for binding of 2,3-DPG, specifically β 82 (EF6) Lys and β 143 (H21) His.

Three variants have been encountered with amino acid substitutions at β 82 Lys: Hb Rahere,[20] Hb Providence,[22-24] and Hb Helsinki.[21] All of these are associated with familial erythrocytosis. These hemoglobins have nearly normal oxygen affinity in the absence of organic phosphates but have very little change in P_{50} upon the addition of 2,3-DPG. As a result, heterozygotes have increased whole blood oxygen affinity. The individual with Hb Rahere had a marked increase in hemoglobin (20 g/dl), yet his red cell mass was not significantly elevated.

Hemoglobins Little Rock and Syracuse have amino acid substitutions at β 143 histidine. Hemoglobin Little Rock (β 143 His→Gln) is of particular interest because it has nearly normal heme-heme interaction and Bohr effect.[51] Its high oxygen affinity may be due to *enhanced stability of the R structure*[109] (see below). Bare and associates[52] have done careful and extensive oxygen binding studies on hemoglobin Little Rock in the absence and presence of varying concentrations of 2,3-DPG. They have found that deoxyhemoglobin Little Rock binds 2,3-DPG somewhat more weakly than does deoxyhemoglobin A. However, the binding of oxyhemoglobin Little Rock with 2,3-DPG is even weaker than that of oxyhemoglobin A with 2,3,DPG, so that the overall effect of 2,3-DPG on the oxygenation of hemoglobin Little Rock is normal or even increased.

In contrast, hemoglobin Syracuse (β 143 His→Pro) has decreased 2,3-DPG reactivity, as measured by oxygen affinities.[53] The oxygen binding experiments on hemoglobin Syracuse are difficult to interpret solely in terms of 2,3-DPG interaction with a hemoglobin lacking β 143 histidine because the proline substitution also disrupts the H helix at position 143 and greatly weakens the overall stability of the T structure. This disruption probably explains the impaired heme-heme interaction and decreased Bohr effect in Hb Syracuse.[53]

Kinetics of Ligand Binding

Measurement of the rate of binding of oxygen or other ligands to hemoglobin provides information that cannot be obtained from equilibrium determinations. In particular, kinetic data have provided insights into the conformational transition that occurs on ligand binding and into the differential reactivity of the α and β subunits (see Chapter 3). Gibson and colleagues have developed very sophisticated methods for studying these fast reactions and have applied them not only to normal human hemoglobin A but also to chemically modified hemoglobin and some of the functionally abnormal variants. Those studied in detail at this time include hemoglobins Chesapeake,[5, 110] Rainier,[55, 56] Hiroshima,[65] Bethesda,[106] Kempsey,[34] Syracuse (McDonald and Gibson, unpublished observations), Osler,[60] Suresnes,[13] Providence,[24] and Alberta.[42] In general, when fully liganded, these variants behave like hemoglobin A. The reaction

$$Hb(O_2)_4 \xrightarrow{k_4} Hb(O_2)_3 + O_2$$

is very similar among these hemoglobins. (The value of k_4 is somewhat low for hemoglobins Hiroshima[65] and Syracuse [McDonald and Gibson, unpublished observations] but normal for the others.) Thus, when fully liganded, these variants appear to assume a normal R conformation. When deoxygenated, they tend to have a rapid and monophasic reaction with heme ligands (such as carbon monoxide), indicating that a significant proportion of deoxygenated hemoglobin is in the R state. In contrast, deoxyhemoglobin A has a slow and biphasic reaction with heme ligands, indicating the transition from T to R during heme ligation. In some variants, such as Hiroshima,[65] the abnormal subunit shows particularly fast ligand binding, suggesting that the amino acid substitution has drastically altered the tertiary conformation of the subunit and has exaggerated the asymmetry between α- and β-chain reactivity for heme ligands. Other variants such as hemoglobin Kempsey do not show such asymmetry between subunits.[107]

X-Ray Crystallography

The precise delineation of the high-affinity variants in three-dimensional space should provide the most direct information on structure-function relationships. The structure of normal and variant hemoglobins can be compared by difference Fourier analysis. From such information, electron-density maps can be constructed that indicate specific sites where the two molecules differ. Because the three-dimensional structure of human deoxyhemoglobin A has been solved at high resolution (1.7 Å), difference Fourier analyses can be obtained by examining crystals prepared from deoxygenated variants. Recently, the structures of carboxy[111] and oxy[112] Hb A have been determined. This information will allow difference Fourier analyses of the liganded forms of variants that will complement the existing body of x-ray data on the deoxy derivatives. X-ray studies have been done on the following high-affinity variants: J-Cape Town and Chesapeake,[113] Yakima,[114] Rainier,[115] Hiroshima,[116] Kempsey,[98] San Diego,[117] Nancy,[118] Radcliffe,[37] Creteil,[119] and Cowtown.[119a] In general, difference Fourier analyses of these variants in the deoxy state show marked differences from hemoglobin A that extend beyond the site of amino acid substitution and indicate alterations in both the tertiary structure of the subunit and, in some cases, the quaternary structure of the tetramer. Hemoglobins Chesapeake and Radcliffe appear to be exceptions. Their deoxy structures appear to differ very little from that of hemoglobin A. In contrast, electron-density maps of the oxy form of these two variants at low resolution show marked differences. On occasion, the x-ray studies have provided very specific information. The difference Fourier analysis of deoxyhemoglobin Rainer showed a disulfide bridge between cysteine introduced by mutation at β 145 and the cysteine at β 93.[115] These results indicated that the original structural analysis of hemoglobin Rainier was incorrect. Likewise, x-ray crystallography identified the amino acid substitution of hemoglobin Hiroshima as β 146[116] rather than β 143, as was first reported.

Spectroscopic Studies

Nuclear magnetic resonance (NMR) and electron paramagnetic resonance (EPR) have proved to be useful conformational probes not only of functionally normal hemoglobin but especially of the high-affinity variants.[37, 100, 120–122] Because the primary structural alteration in each of these variants is known, a comparison of its NMR spectrum with that of normal hemoglobin under identical conditions permits assignment of certain peaks to specific structural loci. For example, NMR spectra of hyperfine shifted proton resonance has demonstrated that the environments around the α- and β-chain heme groups are structurally different. From the change in spectra upon partial saturation with ligand, the differential binding to α and β hemes can be demonstrated. This approach was used to show that the β chains of hemoglobin Kempsey have a slightly higher affinity for carbon monoxide than the α chains.[97] From ring current shift resonances of the carboxy derivatives, assignments can be made to certain residues adjacent to the hemes. Specific NMR signals have also been attributed to certain protons involved in hydrogen bonds at the subunit interfaces. These assignments have been largely based on comparisons with certain high-affinity variants that have amino acid substitutions at these sites.[123] Recently, hemoglobin variants, including some with high affinity, have been used by Ho and colleagues[124] to determine which portions of the hyperfine shifted proton resonance spectrum can be assigned to specific histidine residues. These studies have helped to identify the sites on hemoglobin that contribute to the Bohr effect (see Chapter 3).

Synthetic molecules that have paramagnetic resonance (spin labels) have been used to probe the conformation of normal and variant hemoglobins. Spin labels have been employed in several ways: (a) 2,3-DPG analogues[96, 125]; (b) sulfhydryl reagents[126]; and (c) the heme ligand, nitric oxide.[127] Both the binding of organic phosphates to hemoglobin and the environment around the reactive β 93 sulfhydryl group appear to be strongly dependent on quaternary structure. Therefore, these measurements can provide a means of monitoring the transition from the T to R structure during ligation of the hemes. Such information on both normal and high-affinity hemoglobins has been useful in testing models of allosteric behavior.

Subunit Interactions

As discussed in Chapter 3, fully liganded hemoglobin* in solution dissociates readily into dimers:

$$\alpha_2\beta_2 \rightleftharpoons 2\alpha\beta$$

There is ample evidence that the molecule splits at the $\alpha_1\beta_2$ interface. Dissociation at the $\alpha_1\beta_1$ interface is very much slower, except under denaturing solvent conditions. In contrast to liganded hemoglobins, deoxyhemoglobin dissociates much less readily into dimers. This difference is due in part to the inter-subunit salt bonds that stabilize the T structure.[102, 103] As mentioned above and in Table 14-1, many of the high-affinity variants have substitutions at the $\alpha_1\beta_2$ interface. Such structural alterations might be expected to affect the dissociation of the tetramer into dimers. A number of earlier studies showed that certain high-affinity variants, when fully deoxygenated, dissociate into dimers more readily than does deoxyhemoglobin A. These include hemoglobins Bethesda,[106] Kempsey,[34] and Chesapeake.[110] These observations are in accord with other evidence that neither deoxy Bethesda nor deoxy Kempsey can form a stable T quaternary structure. Furthermore, hemoglobin Chesapeake in the liganded state had *decreased* subunit dissociation,[128] indicating that its R structure is relatively more stable than that of hemoglobin A (Fig. 14–5A).

More recently Ackers and colleagues[129] have completed a thorough comparison of a variety of different hemoglobins, including 10 high-affinity variants. By examining both the liganded and unliganded forms, they were able to establish the relationship between subunit dissociation and oxygen affinity. The energy of interaction between hemoglobin subunits in the oxy and deoxy states can be linked thermodynamically to the cooperative binding of ligand to hemes[130-132] (see Chapter 3). As indicated in Figure 14–5B, the oxygen affinity of a mutant or chemically modified hemoglobin will be affected if the relative stabilities of the R and T structures differ significantly from those of native hemoglobin A. Variants having a relatively unstable T structure, such as Hbs Bethesda and Kempsey, will have high oxygen affinity. Similarly, enhanced stability of the R state should also result in high oxygen affinity. Perutz[109] has suggested that the presence of an additional hydrogen bond in oxyhemoglobin Little Rock may be the basis for its high oxygen affinity. If so, this variant in its liganded state should have decreased dissociation into dimers. Perutz's prediction has been confirmed by direct measurement of subunit dissociation of Hb Little Rock.[133] As mentioned above, the liganded form of Hb Chesapeake also has enhanced tetrameric stability.[128, 129] Crystallographic analysis indicates that the conformation of oxyhemoglobin Chesapeake differs markedly from that of oxyhemoglobin A,[113] whereas the deoxygenated hemoglobins have very similar three-dimensional structures. However, there are kinetic[5, 110] and NMR data[122] as well as direct measurements of subunit dissociation[129] indicating that deoxyhemoglobin Chesapeake differs significantly from deoxyhemoglobin A. Thus, both the T form and the R form of this variant have abnormal

---

*Oxyhemoglobin, carboxyhemoglobin, cyanmethemoglobin.

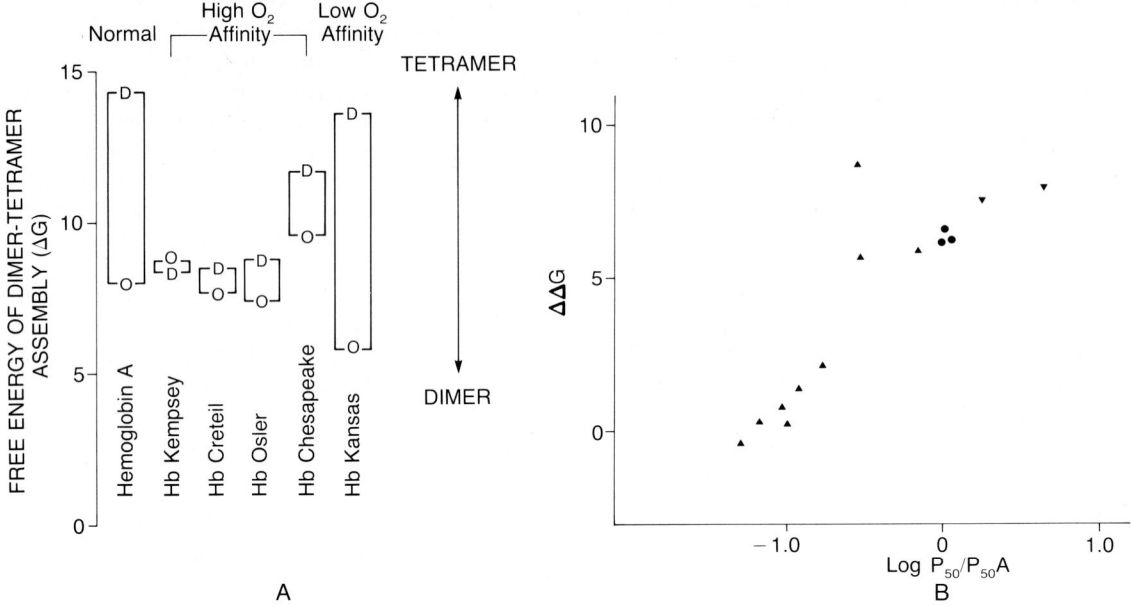

Figure 14–5. *A,* Subunit dissociation of oxygenated and deoxygenated hemoglobins. (Data obtained from Pettigrew, D. W., et al.: Proc. Natl. Acad. Sci. USA 79:1849, 1982.) *B,* Relationship between the oxygen affinity of hemoglobin variants and the difference between the stability of the liganded tetramer versus the deoxygenated tetramer. (▲ = high affinity variants; ● = Hbs A, S, and C; ▼ = low-affinity variants.)

conformations and subunit interaction. This situation is depicted in Figure 14–5A.

A number of "high-affinity" variants, when fully oxygenated, have *increased* dissociation into αβ dimers. These include Hbs Hirose,[84] Richmond,[134] G-Georgia,[74] Rampa,[74] Austin,[87] Malmö,[134a] Osler,[60] and Suresnes.[13] All but the last two have substitutions at the $\alpha_1\beta_2$ interface. The fact that they have increased oxygen affinity must mean that the deoxy form of the hemoglobin is also more "unstable" than normal. Direct measurements of the dissociation of deoxy Hirose,[84, 129] Osler,[60, 129] and Suresnes[13, 139] into dimers support this contention.

A few high-affinity variants with substitutions at the $\alpha_1\beta_2$ interface form stable asymmetrical hybrid molecules. Normally, in an equimolar mixture of two hemoglobins $\alpha_2\beta^A_2$ and $\alpha_2\beta^X_2$, the predominant species is the asymmetrical hybrid tetramer $\alpha_2\beta^A\beta^X$.[135, 136] However, these hybrids are not detected by ordinary electrophoresis because they sort into αβ dimers of different charges when subjected to an electrical field (see Chapter 10). In contrast, some high-affinity variants such as Alberta,[41, 42] British Columbia,[40]* Rush,[137] Yp-silanti,[35] and Radcliffe[37] have substitutions at the $\alpha_1\beta_2$ interface that enhance stability of the oxy or R structures, therefore preserving the asymmetrical hybrids.

Autoxidation

The autoxidation of oxyhemoglobin to methemoglobin involves the dissociation of superoxide anion (see Chapter 16):

$$Hb^{2+}O_2 \rightarrow Hb^{3+} + O_2^-$$

This reaction occurs more readily when the affinity of hemoglobin for oxygen is relatively low. Thus, partially oxygenated hemoglobin autoxidizes more readily than does fully saturated hemoglobin. It follows that high-affinity hemoglobin variants should have a decreased rate of autoxidation, whereas low-affinity mutants should autoxidize more readily than Hb A. Studies on three high-affinity variants, Hb Syracuse,[53] Hb Creteil,[138] and Hb Kempsey,[138a] confirm the predicted low rate of autoxidation, whereas the low-affinity mutant Hb J-Cairo[138] has an increased rate. Once oxidized, the high-affinity mutants appear to have a decreased rate of enzymatic and nonenzymatic reduction from methemoglobin to deoxyhemoglobin.[139]

---

*No direct evidence has been published demonstrating asymmetrical hybrids in mixtures containing Hb British Columbia. However, the unusual electrophoretic behavior of this variant can be explained by the presence of stable $\alpha_2\beta^A\beta^{BC}$ hybrids.

PHYSIOLOGICAL ASPECTS

In normal man, the oxygen dissociation curve is appropriately poised to permit efficient loading and unloading of oxygen during rest and exercise. In Chapter 5 the pathophysiological consequences of significant displacements of the oxygen binding curve are discussed. Most commonly, a "shift to the left" or "shift to the right" can be explained by intracellular factors such as alterations in pH and red cell 2,3-DPG or modification of the heme groups, as in carbon monoxide poisoning or methemoglobinemia. In many instances, the change in oxygen affinity constitutes an adaptation to some form of hypoxia. In contrast, individuals having hemoglobin variants with high oxygen affinity exhibit a *primary* displacement of the whole blood oxygen dissociation curve and respond to this molecular lesion with appropriate physiological adjustments. According to the Fick equation cited in Chapter 5, oxygen delivery to tissues (VO_2) is a function of three independent variables:

$$VO_2 = 0.139 \cdot Q \cdot Hb \cdot (S_aO_2 - S_{\bar{v}}O_2)$$

The primary shift to the left in the oxygen dissociation curve results in a marked decrease in oxygen extraction per gram of hemoglobin ($S_aO_2 - S_{\bar{v}}O_2$). Consequently, tissue oxygenation can be maintained by two adjustments:

Table 14–4. OXYGEN TRANSPORT IN HETEROZYGOTES HAVING HEMOGLOBIN VARIANTS WITH HIGH O_2 AFFINITY*

Variant	Cardiac Index	Mixed Venous PO_2	Reference(s)
A (normal)	3.7 ± 0.3	34–49	
Creteil	5.0	33	147
Heathrow	3.7	41	46
Little Rock	7.2	36	142
Yakima	2.6, 2.3	34, 35	31, 32
McKees Rocks	3.9, 6.4	26, 27	143
Osler	5.2, 6.0	33, 33	143

*Adapted from Charache, S., et al.: Blood 52:1156, 1978.

increase in circulating hemoglobin concentration (Hb) or increase in blood flow (Q). Increased capillary density may be an additional independent way of adapting to hypoxia.

The primary mode of compensation is erythrocytosis (see Figure 14–1). An individual with a stable high-affinity variant (normal red cell life span) will have an increase in red cell mass roughly proportional to the "shift to the left" of the whole bood oxygen dissociation curve. This response appears to be mediated through erythropoietin. Adamson and colleagues[57, 140, 141] have studied individuals with hemoglobins Rainier, Yakima, and Bethesda. The urinary erythropoietin (erythropoietic stimulating factor [ESF]) of these polycythemic subjects was normal. However, when these individuals were bled down to a "normal" red cell mass, urinary ESF increased markedly (Fig. 14–6). Similar results have been reported in patients with hemoglobins Little Rock,[142] McKees Rocks,[143] and Osler.[143] These observations attest to the significant hypoxia that these individuals will develop if they are robbed of an important mode of compensation.

Individuals with high-affinity variants have normal oxygen consumption and normal arterial oxygen tension. The fact that they develop enhanced erythropoietin production indicates that the sensor for this hormonal regulation must be located in the postarterial region of the renal vasculature.[144] As shown in Table 14–4, mixed venous PO_2 is generally normal or somewhat low. Decreased values probably reflect failure of either erythrocytosis or enhancement in blood flow to compensate for the increase in oxygen affinity.

It is difficult to assess alterations in blood flow of individuals with high-affinity variants. Resting cardiac output may be somewhat in-

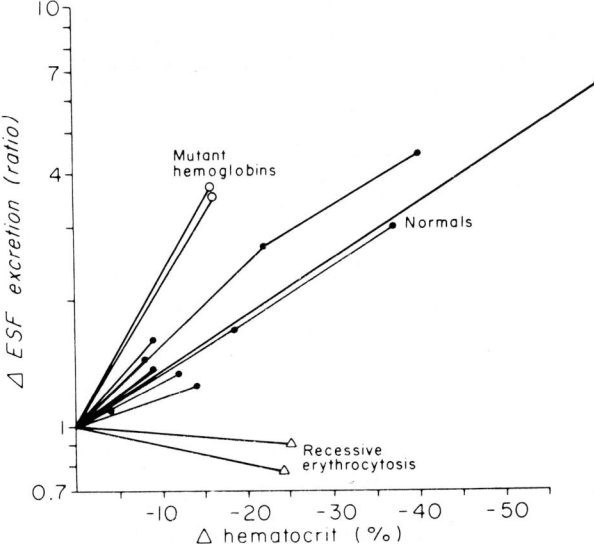

Figure 14–6. Effect of phlebotomy on erythropoietin (ESF) excretion in normal volunteers (●), individuals with high-affinity hemoglobin variants (○), and individuals with autosomal recessive erythrocytosis (△) (see Table 14–5). (From Adamson, J. W., et al.: Blood 41:641, 1973.)

creased. After graded exercise[142, 147]* or phlebotomy to reduce the red cell mass to normal,* cardiac output may increase markedly, accompanied by a fall in mixed venous PO_2. The total cardiac output does not reflect adjustments in blood flow to specific organs. In order to preserve adequate oxygenation of vital tissues, individuals with high-affinity variants probably have appropriate alterations in regional circulation. A patient with hemoglobin Malmö was shown to have greater than normal myocardial blood flow.[148] Cerebral blood flow was also noted to be significantly increased in six individuals with Hb Yakima.[146]†

Individuals with high-affinity variants generally tolerate exercise very well. However, if their red cell mass is lowered, their maximum work capacity falls, and they have a decreased anaerobic threshold.[148a, 148b, 148c]

The physiologic embarrassment that accompanies a "shift to the left" of the oxyhemoglobin dissociation curve does not pertain at reduced ambient oxygen tension. Indeed, if hypoxia is sufficient to cause unsaturation of arterial blood, increased oxygen affinity may be beneficial. Animals adapted to high altitude, such as llamas, alpacas, and vicuñas, have left-shifted curves that enable their arterial blood to be fully saturated (see Chapter 6). Hebbel and colleagues[149] have shown that when individuals with a high-affinity mutant (Hb Andrew-Minneapolis) were taken to high altitude (3100 meters), they tolerated exercise better than their unaffected siblings.

In Chapter 5, the importance of red cell 2,3-DPG in the adaptation to hypoxia is discussed. However, the high-affinity variants represent one type of hypoxia in which this adaptation does not occur. Red cell 2,3-DPG has been measured in most of the different high-affinity variants and has been consistently normal. It is possible that erythrocytosis provides adequate compensation; however, individuals with this disorder should theoretically derive some benefit from increased red cell 2,3-DPG. An extreme example is depicted in Figure 14–7. These red cells contain 50 per cent normal hemoglobin A; the remaining hemoglobin has very high oxygen affinity and, when deoxygenated, the hemolysate fails to form stable mixed hybrid tetramers with normal hemoglobin (e.g., $\alpha_2\beta^A\beta^X$). Such a lack of interaction has been demonstrated for hemoglobins Bethesda[59] and Kempsey[34]—two variants that are unable to form a stable T structure. In red cells containing such a mixture, the two hemoglobins are oxygenated independently. Furthermore, the hemoglobin with high oxygen affinity remains almost fully saturated in all parts of the circulation.[147] Therefore, the abnormal hemoglobin lacks any physiological function and might as well be albumin or some other space-occupying colloid. If so, the individual has a functioning hemoglobin level that is half the total. Such an "anemic" patient should benefit from the interaction of 2,3-DPG on the normal functioning hemoglobin. Actually, in such individuals, red cell 2,3-DPG should be expressed as moles per mole of hemoglobin A, because under physiologic conditions the abnormal hemoglobin remains in the R conformation and therefore fails to bind significantly to 2,3-DPG. Accordingly, many of these variants have impaired interaction with 2,3-DPG, as shown in Table 14–1. Viewed in this way, the individual with a high-affinity variant has elevated red cell 2,3-DPG, similar to other patients with anemia!

---

*Unpublished observations on an individual with Hb Syracuse, courtesy of Dr. Frank Oski.
†J. Wade: Personal communication, 1983.

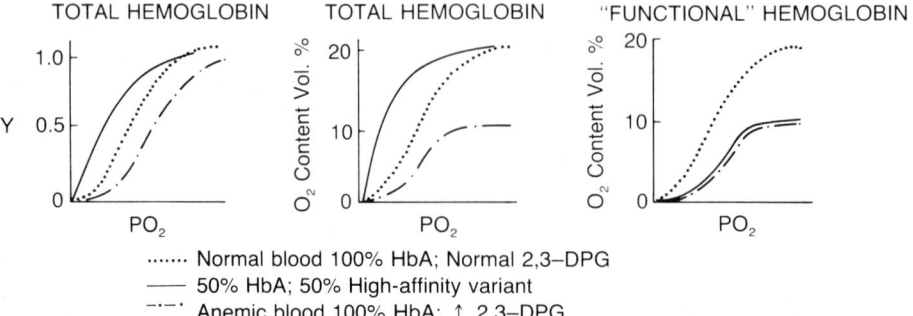

Figure 14–7. Oxygen binding curves of a normal individual (··········), a patient with anemia and increased red cell 2,3-DPG (— • — • —), and a patient with a high-affinity variant (———).

CLINICAL MANIFESTATIONS

Genetics

Like other structurally abnormal hemoglobins, the high-affinity variants follow an autosomal dominant pattern of inheritance. All affected individuals are heterozygotes; their red cells contain at least as much normal hemoglobin A as the abnormal variant.* In most instances, the homozygous state would be incompatible with life. A positive family history is very helpful in evaluating a patient for the presence of a high-affinity hemoglobin. However, spontaneous mutations occasionally occur. We have seen a girl with hemoglobin Bethesda whose parents were both normal.[59]

Clinical Presentation

The great majority of affected individuals are entirely asymptomatic. Physical examination is unremarkable, except for the occasional presence of a ruddy complexion. Most commonly, erythrocytosis is detected on a routine blood count. The increase in packed cell volume and red cell mass is generally not severe. Accordingly, affected individuals do not usually have symptoms due to hyperviscosity of the blood. Some individuals with hemoglobin Malmö may be an exception. One patient reliably reported subjective improvement following phlebotomy and transfusion with normal blood.[148] This patient had severe cardiac dysfunction with a history of myocardial infarction, angina, dyspnea, and decreased exercise tolerance. Interestingly, coronary angiography revealed patent vessels except for an isolated narrow segment in a branch of the right posterior descending artery. As mentioned in the beginning of this chapter, the first patient in whom this disorder was established had mild angina. However, a survey of the 200-odd individuals that have been reported to date does not indicate a high incidence of myocardial ischemia or any other form of tissue hypoxia.

Some have speculated that in a pregnant woman with a high-affinity variant, the transplacental transport of oxygen may be impaired. In both humans and nearly all other mammals that have been tested, the oxygen affinity of fetal blood is significantly higher than that of maternal blood (see Chapter 6). The physiological importance of this phenomenon is not well established. There are several instances in which the oxygen binding curve of the mother was shifted to the left of that of the fetus because of an abnormal hemoglobin; these pregnancies were perfectly uneventful and the babies were healthy. An increased incidence of fetal mortality has been reported in a family with hemoglobin Yakima,[32] but the significance of this is not clear. Charache and colleagues[44, 149a] have reviewed the reproduction histories of affected mothers and offspring and have found no evidence that high-affinity hemoglobins affect the outcome of pregnancy. In contrast, adverse effects have been reported in animal studies.[150, 151]

Diagnosis

Affected individuals usually come to the attention of physicians because of unexplained erythrocytosis. Hemoglobin values vary considerably, with a mean of about 19 g/dl (see Table 14–1). The increase in red cell mass is less marked than that seen in patients with polycythemia vera. The white blood cell count and platelet count are normal, and the peripheral blood smear is unremarkable. However, exceptions have been noted. Occasional individuals with high-affinity variants have had persistent leukocytosis,[20] and three have had splenomegaly.[25, 37] Understandably, these individuals were thought to have polycythemia vera. During the initial evaluation, a number of diagnostic possibilities must be ruled out. Table 14–5 presents one approach to classifying various types of erythrocytosis. If appropriate clinical and laboratory information does not suggest one of the more common etiologies, the possibility remains that the patient's erythrocytosis is due to the presence of a functionally abnormal hemoglobin. The likelihood is considerably strengthened if other blood relatives also have unexplained erythrocytosis. However, not all familial erythrocytosis is due to the presence of a functionally abnormal hemoglobin variant. There is a very rare entity in which familial erythrocytosis is due to a defect in the humoral regulation of red cell mass.[152] Unlike the high-affinity variants, this disorder has an autosomal recessive pattern of inheritance. Moreover, as explained below, familial erythrocytosis may also be

---

*Exceptions include an individual who is doubly heterozygous for Hb Abruzzo and β thalassemia[91] and another who is doubly heterozygous for Hb Crete and β thalassemia.[90] In these individuals, the abnormal hemoglobin comprises 85 to 95 per cent of the total.

• Table 14–5. **DIFFERENTIAL DIAGNOSIS OF ERYTHROCYTOSIS**

I. Autonomous erythroid proliferation (↓ ESF): polycythemia vera
II. Secondary erythroid proliferation
   A. Autonomous or inappropriate increase in ESF
      1. Neoplasm
      2. Renal lesions
      3. Familial erythrocytosis (autosomal recessive inheritance)
   B. Secondary increase in ESF
      1. Hypoxemia (↓ arterial PO_2)
         a. High altitude
         b. Alveolar hypoventilation
         c. Pulmonary disease
         d. Cardiac R→L shunt
      2. Abnormal hemoglobin function (normal arterial (PO_2)
         a. High-affinity variants (autosomal dominant inheritance)
         b. DPG mutase deficiency (autosomal recessive inheritance)
         c. Congenital methemoglobinemia
         d. Carboxyhemoglobinemia (smokers)

caused by defects in red cell metabolism leading to low levels of 2,3-DPG.

If hemoglobin electrophoresis reveals the presence of an abnormal band, the diagnosis is virtually established. However, the failure to demonstrate any electrophoretic abnormality by no means rules out the diagnosis. As shown in Table 14–1, only about half of the high-affinity variants that have been reported to date can be separated from hemoglobin A by routine electrophoresis on cellulose acetate or starch gel at pH 8.6. Some variants can be detected if other types of electrophoresis are employed, such as citrate agar (pH 6.0)[153] or gel electrofocusing (Fig. 14–8). There remains a group that appear to be electrophoretically silent. These include hemoglobins Olympia, Heathrow, Milledgeville, Potomac, San Diego, and Brigham. Certain tricks can be employed to "separate the unseparable," such as taking advantage of the fact that high-affinity mutants may have an altered reactivity to sulfhydryl reagents.[154, 155] This selective chemical modification permits the hemoglobin variant to be separated on the basis of the surface charge.* Variants with reduced Bohr effect will have less of a change in isoelectric point upon deoxygenation than has hemoglobin A.[157] Figure 14–9 shows how deoxygenation was useful in enhancing the electrophoretic separation of hemoglobin Syracuse from hemoglobin A. This approach has been used to prepare purified Hb Potomac by applying a deoxygenated hemolysate to an anaerobic ion-exchange column.[158]

The abnormal subunit of electrophoretically silent high-affinity hemoglobin variants can be identified by isolating the heme-intact α and β chains from hemolysate and making hybrid tetramers with complementary subunits prepared from normal Hb A.[159] Oxygen affinity of these hybrid hemoglobins will establish which subunit is abnormal.

The only way to definitively establish the diagnosis of a variant with high oxygen affinity is to perform some type of oxygen binding measurement. An oxygen dissociation curve done on whole blood will be shifted to the left not only by high-affinity variants but also by conditions causing decreased red cell 2,3-DPG (see Chapter 5) as well as methemoglobinemia (see Chapter 16) and carboxyhemoglobinemia (see Chapter 17). Several oxygen-binding techniques have been proposed to screen for high-affinity hemoglobin variants.[160, 161] An automated system such as that devised by Imai and associates[161] can provide precise data within a relatively short time (~20 minutes). It may be necessary to measure red cell 2,3-DPG to find out if the increase in whole blood oxygen affinity is due to an abnormality in red cell metabolism, leading to deficiency of 2,3-DPG. Rosa and colleagues[162] described an individual with erythrocytosis secondary to DPG mutase deficiency. The oxygen affinity of the patient's red cells was markedly increased (P_{50} = 15 mm Hg) because of a virtual absence of red cell 2,3-DPG. These investigators have also discovered a family in which erythrocytosis was explained by low red cell 2,3-DPG due to enhanced pyruvate kinase activity.[162a] These entities must be very rare. Most red cell enzymopathies are associated with nonspherocytic hemolytic anemia. The distinction between a high-affinity hemoglobin and a defect in 2,3-DPG synthesis can also be made by measuring oxygen affinity on hemolysate stripped of organic phosphates.

The screening procedure used in our laboratory is a four-point spectrophotometric oxygen binding curve on hemolysate thoroughly stripped of all organic phosphates. The visible spectra will reveal the presence of methemoglobin or carboxyhemoglobin. In their absence, a significant alteration in oxygen binding is diagnostic of the presence of a functionally abnormal hemoglobin variant. We restrict this screening test to patients with erythrocytosis

---

*Differential sulfhydryl reactivity has been used to isolate hemoglobin Philly, an unstable variant with a neutral substitution.[156]

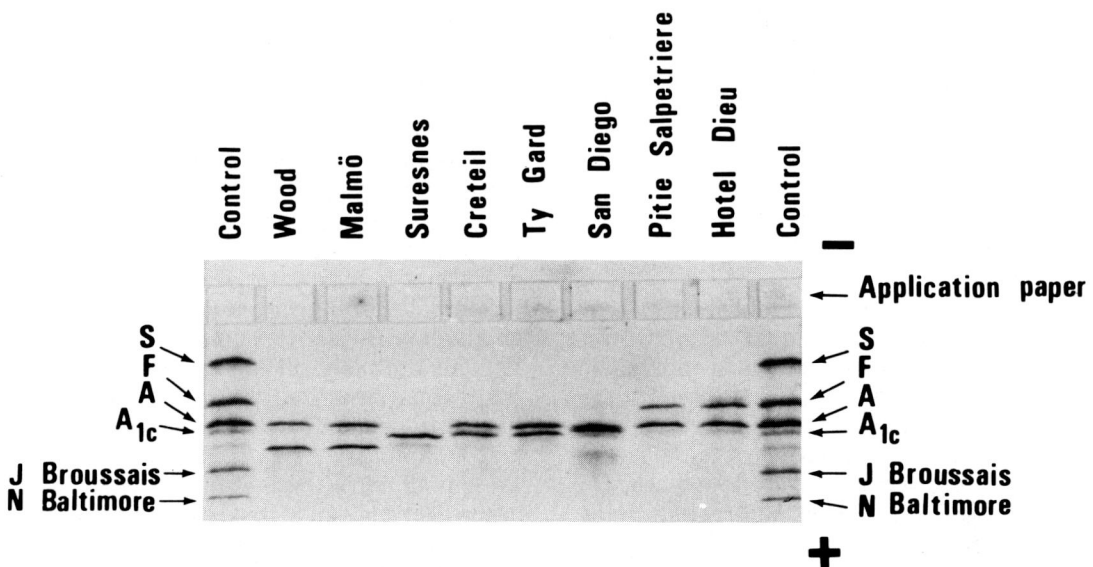

Figure 14–8. Separation of certain hemoglobin variants with high oxygen affinity by isoelectric focusing on a thin polyacrylamide slab. (From Basset, P., et al.: J. Chromatogr. *227*:267, 1982.)

Figure 14–9. Comparison of gel electrofocusing patterns of normal hemolysate and hemolysate of a patient with hemoglobin Syracuse. *Left,* Hemoglobin treated with CO. *Right,* Deoxygenated hemoglobin. The improved separation of Hb Syracuse from Hb A following deoxygenation is a reflection of the fact that Hb Syracuse has a decreased Bohr effect (see text). (From Jensen, M., et al.: J. Clin. Invest. *55*:469, 1975.)

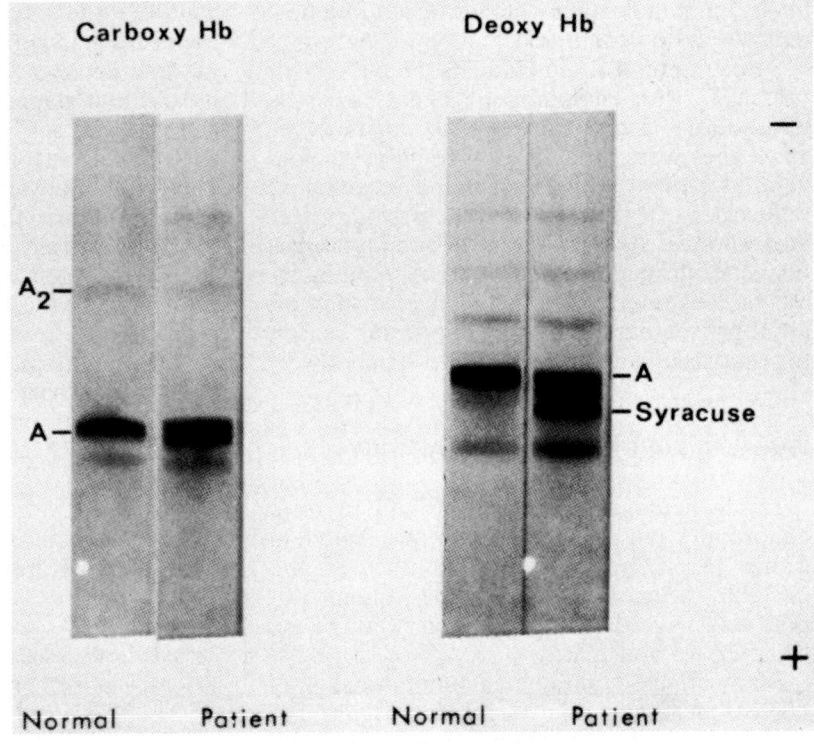

and (1) a positive family history of erythrocytosis; (2) an abnormal hemoglobin electrophoresis and/or isoelectric focusing pattern; or (3) a thorough medical evaluation that has ruled out other recognized causes of polycythemia. Even under these circumstances, the odds that the oxygen binding curve will be abnormal are still very small.

Treatment

Once the diagnosis is established, all affected family members should be reassured that the condition is benign. Most individuals require no treatment at all, although it is prudent to perform follow-up blood counts at regular intervals. In a minority of patients, the hematocrit may become high enough that the viscosity of the blood poses a potential threat. As mentioned earlier, occasional patients have derived subjective benefit from phlebotomy; however, this treatment should be used sparingly, because the increased red cell mass is an important mode of compensation. Charache recommends that if elderly individuals and those with angina pectoris are being considered for phlebotomy, they should undergo electrocardiographic exercise testing before and after treatment. This objective measurement may be useful in indicating whether or not phlebotomy should be continued.

Some affected individuals have been "treated" with radiomimetic agents such as phosphorus-32 or phenylalanine mustard because they were thought to have polycythemia vera. A patient with Hb Yakima received 72 millicuries of ^{32}P over a 10-year period. After an additional 10 years, he developed a preleukemic syndrome followed by frank acute myelocytic leukemia.[163] The avoidance of such inappropriate therapy is one important reason for establishing a diagnosis in these patients.[164]

VARIANTS WITH LOW OXYGEN AFFINITY

Stable hemoglobin variants found to have abnormally low oxygen affinity are listed in Table 14–6. In addition, a number of the unstable variants and some of the M hemoglobins also have decreased oxygen affinity (see Chapters 13 and 15).

Many affected family members have slightly decreased hemoglobin levels (see Figure 14–1). It is likely that this "anemia" is the opposite of the polycythemia found in association with high-affinity variants: The enhanced oxygen release provided by the right-shifted curve reduces the erythropoietin-mediated stimulus to erythropoiesis.* In the evaluation of a mild anemia in an otherwise healthy individual in whom all routine diagnostic tests are negative, hemoglobin electrophoresis coupled with a measurement of oxygen affinity may be a reasonable "last resort." However, considering the high frequency of mild anemia and the rarity of these variants, these diagnostic tests would not be cost-effective.

Several variants listed in Table 14–6 have an alkaline Bohr effect greater than that of Hb A. This probably reflects enhanced stability of the T quaternary structure and therefore an increased value for the allosteric constant L (see Chapter 3).

Hemoglobin Kansas is of particular interest, because it has such strikingly abnormal functional properties and is the most thoroughly studied of the low-affinity variants. In 1961, Reissman, Ruth, and Nomura[173] encountered a mother and son with unexplained cyanosis. The subjects were otherwise asymptomatic and had normal hemoglobin levels without any evidence of hemolysis. The cyanosis was explained by an oxygen saturation of only 60 per cent in samples of arterial blood, despite a PaO_2 of 100 mm Hg. Upon breathing 100 per cent O_2, the oxygen saturation increased by about 35 per cent. These results indicated a marked decrease in whole blood oxygen affinity. At first glance, it is surprising that the red cell mass is "set" at a normal level, in view of such abnormal oxygenation of hemoglobin. However, the amount of oxygen unloaded during the circulation through capillaries is probably within normal limits. Despite the reduced oxygen content of the arterial blood, the shape of the curve permits adequate oxygen release. It seems likely that individuals with hemoglobin Kansas would have a limited tolerance to strenuous muscular exercise, which depends on a marked increase in oxygen unloading. This consideration notwithstanding, the son is reputed to be a fine tennis player.†

The structure-function relationships of hemoglobin Kansas have been studied in con-

---

*Such a mechanism has been offered to explain the anemia in patients with hemoglobin Seattle,[182] an unstable variant. However, this situation is more complex, because the shortened red cell survival in these individuals also contributes to the reduction in red cell mass.

†R. Shulman: Personal communication, 1984.

Table 14–6. STABLE VARIANTS WITH LOW OXYGEN AFFINITY

Variant	Structure	Area Affected	% of Total Hb	Hb Level (g/dl)	WB P_{50} (mm Hg)	$\frac{P_{50}X}{P_{50}A}$	% Bohr Effect	Response to 2,3-DPG	Electro-phoresis	Comment	Reference(s)
Titusville	α 94 (G1) Asp→Asn	$\alpha_1\beta_2$	35	12.5		$\frac{16}{5}$	36%		CAg CAc	↑ Subunit dissociation	165
Raleigh	β 1 (NA1) Val→Acetyl Ala	DPG	45	NI		3.3 1.8	NI	→	CAc	Acetylated at β-NH_2	166
Connecticut	β 21 (B3) Asp→Gly		39	13	28.5	$\frac{4.8}{2.0}$	NI	NI	CAc		167
Rothschild	β 37 (C3) Trp→Arg	$\alpha_1\beta_2$	47			$\frac{3.5}{2}$			IEF CAc	↑ Dissociation of liganded Hb	145, 168
Bologna	β 61 (E5) Lys→Met		48	14.6	31 37.6*	12.3 7.3			CAc	Found with β⁰ Thal	169
J-Cairo	β 65 (E9) Lys→Gln		48	11		$\frac{15}{?}$	NI	NI	CAg:0 CAc		138
Vancouver	β 73 (E17) Asp→Tyr		40	NI	$\frac{41}{31}$ 29.5	9.0	115%		CAc	Found with β⁰ Thal	170
Mobile	β 73 (E17) Asp→Val		42	12		$\frac{6.6}{8.6}$ 6.5	122%		CAg:0 CAc		170
Agenogi	β 90 (F6) Glu→Lys			NI		$\frac{10.5}{0.8}$	NI		CAc		171, 172
Kansas	β 102 (G4) Asn→Thr	$\alpha_1\beta_2$		14	~70	$\frac{20}{4.5}$	60%	→	SG		173–175
Beth Israel	β 102 (G4) Asn→Ser	$\alpha_1\beta_2$	40	13.2	88		NI (H)		CAg:0 SG		176
Saint Mande	β 102 (G4) Asn→Tyr	$\alpha_1\beta_2$	38	12	52	$\frac{16}{6.5}$	70%	NI	IEF		177, 178
Yoshizuka	β 108 (G10) Asn→Asp	$\alpha_1\beta_1$	51	"Slight anemia"		$\frac{14}{10}$	70%		SG		179
Presbyterian	β 108 (G10) Asn→Lys	$\alpha_1\beta_1$	40	10.6–12.4		$\frac{25}{4.2}$	130%	NI	CAc		180
Hope	β 136 (H14) Gly→Asp		40	12–13	$\frac{42}{30}$	$\frac{21}{12}$	NI	→			181

*Bologna/β⁰ Thal—double heterozygote

See Note at end of Table 14–1.

siderable detail. The structural abnormality is a substitution of threonine for asparagine at β 102.[174] Like many of the high-affinity variants, this site is at the $\alpha_1\beta_2$ interface. Indeed, as shown in Figure 14–2, when normal hemoglobin A is oxygenated, β 102 Asn forms a hydrogen bond with α 94 Asp. Such a bond is not possible in oxyhemoglobin Kansas. Therefore, it is interesting to note that oxyhemoglobin Kansas dissociates more readily into αβ dimers than does oxyhemoglobin A.[174] Its low oxygen affinity appears to be due in part to a relatively unstable R structure (see Fig. 14–5A). In hemoglobin Kansas, the transition from the T to the R structure occurs relatively late in heme ligation. Indeed, in the presence of organic phosphates such as 2,3-DPG and inositol hexaphosphate, fully liganded hemoglobin Kansas has the NMR characteristics of the T structure.[183] Difference Fourier analyses of crystals of deoxyhemoglobin Kansas indicate widespread abnormalities in the T structure.[184] Furthermore, isolated β chains of Kansas subunits also have relatively low oxygen affinity.[185] The interpretation of these results is complicated by the fact that these preparations of β subunits showed a considerable amount of kinetic heterogeneity that is unexplained. Shulman and colleagues[186] have done extensive physical-chemical studies in Hb Kansas, taking advantage of the fact that even when fully ligated, it can be frozen in the T structure. These experiments have been valuable in elucidating the localization and extent of energy changes upon sequential ligation of deoxyhemoglobin (see Chapter 3).

Cyanosis has also been encountered in two other low-affinity variants: Hb Beth Israel (β 102 Asn → Ser)[176] and Hb St. Mande (β 102 Asn → Tyr).[177, 178] They have amino acid substitutions at the same site as Hb Kansas. The functional properties of the three variants are very similar. Hb Beth Israel probably arose as a spontaneous mutation, because neither parent is cyanotic.

Hb Titusville (α 94 Asp → Asn)[165] appears to have an oxygen affinity nearly as low as that of Hb Kansas and Hb Beth Israel. The amino acid substitution prevents the formation of the bond between α 94 and β 102 (mentioned above) that normally stabilizes oxyhemoglobin (see Figure 14–2). As a result, Hb Titusville resembles Hb Kansas in having enhanced dissociation of tetramer into dimers. Affected individuals had no apparent clinical or hematological abnormalities.

References

1. Charache, S., Weatherall, D. J., and Clegg, J. B.: Polycythemia associated with a hemoglobinopathy. J. Clin. Invest. 45:813, 1966.
2. Charache, S.: A manifestation of abnormal hemoglobins of man: Altered oxygen affinity. Hemoglobin Chesapeake: From the clinic to the laboratory and back again. Ann. N.Y. Acad. Sci. 241:449, 1974.
3. Clegg, J. B., Naughton, M. A., and Weatherall, D. J.: Abnormal human hemoglobins. Separation and characterization of the α and β chains by chromatography, and the determination of two new variants—Hb Chesapeake and Hb J (Bangkok) J. Molec. Biol. 9:91, 1966.
4. Honig, G. R., Vida, L. N., Shamsuddin, M., Mason, R. G., Schlumpf, H. W., and Luke, R. A.: Hemoglobin Milledgeville (α 44 (CD2) Pro→Leu). A new variant with increased oxygen affinity. Biochim. Biophys. Acta 626:424, 1980.
5. Nagel, R. L., Gibson, Q. H., and Charache, S.: Relation between structure and function in hemoglobin Chesapeake. Biochemistry 6:2395, 1967.
6. Botha, M. C., Beale, D., Isaacs, W. A., and Lehmann, H.: Haemoglobin J Cape Town—$\alpha_2^{92\ Arginine \rightarrow Glutamine}\ \beta_2$. Nature 2:792, 1966.
7. Lines, J. G., and McIntosh, R.: Oxygen binding by haemoglobin J-Cape Town ($\alpha_2^{92\ Arg \rightarrow Gln}$). Nature 215:297, 1967.
8. Charache, S., and Jenkins, T.: Oxygen equilibrium of hemoglobin J Cape Town. J. Clin. Invest. 50:1554, 1971.
8a. Botha, M. C., Stathopoulou, R., Lehmann, H., Rees, J. S., and Plowman, D.: A J-Cape Town homozygote association of Hb J-Cape Town and alpha thalassemia. FEBS Lett. 96:331, 1978.
9. Moo-Penn, W. F., Jue, D. L., Johnson, M. H., Wilson, S. M., Therrell, B., Jr., and Schmidt, R. M.: Hemoglobin Tarrant: α 126(H9) Asp→Asn. A new hemoglobin variant in the $\alpha_1\beta_1$ contact region showing high oxygen affinity and reduced cooperativity. Biochim. Biophys. Acta 490:443, 1977.
10. Ibarra, B., Vaca, G., Cantu, J. M., Wilson, J. B., Lam, H., Stallings, M., Gravely, M. E., and Huisman, T. H. J.: Heterozygosity and homogosity for the high oxygen affinity hemoglobin Tarrant or α 126 (H9) Asp→Asn in two Mexican families. Hemoglobin 5:337, 1981.
11. Mavilio, F., Marinucci, M., Tentori, L., Fontanarosa, P. P., Rossi, U., and Biagiotti, S.: Hemoglobin Legnano (α_2 141 (HC3) Arg→Leu β_2): A new abnormal human hemoglobin with high oxygen affinity. Hemoglobin 2:249, 1978.
12. Giuliani, A., Maffi, D., Cappabianca, M. P., and Tentori, L.: Hemoglobin Legnano (α_2 141 (HC3) Arg→Leu β_2): A new high oxygen affinity variant. J. Biochem. 88:1233, 1980.
13. Poyart, C., Bursaux, E., Arnone, A., Bonaventura, J., and Bonaventura, C.: Structural and functional studies of hemoglobin Suresnes (Arg 141 α_2→His β_2). Consequences of disrupting an oxygen-linked anion-binding site. J. Biol. Chem. 255:9465, 1980.
14. Poyart, C., Krishnamoorthy, R., Bursaux, E., Gacon, G., and Labie, D.: Structural and functional studies of haemoglobin Suresnes or α_2 141 (HC3) Arg→His β_2, a new high oxygen affinity mutant. FEBS Lett. 69:103, 1976.
15. Stamatoyannopoulos, G., Nute, P. E., Adamson, J.

W., Bellingham, A. J., and Funk, D.: Hemoglobin Olympia (β 20 Valine→Methionine): An electrophoretically silent variant associated with high oxygen affinity and erythrocytosis. J. Clin. Invest. 52:342, 1973.

15a. Brennan, S. O., Williamson, D., Whisson, M. E., and Carrell, R. W.: Hemoglobin Palmerston North β23(B5) Val→Phe. A new variant identified in a patient with polycythemia. Hemoglobin 6:569, 1982.

16. Blouquit, Y., Braconnier, F., Cohen-Solal, M., Foldi, J., Arous, N., Ankri, A., Binet, J. L., and Rosa, J.: Hemoglobin Pitie-Salpetriere β 34 (B16) Val→Phe. A new high oxygen affinity variant associated with familial erythrocytosis. Biochim. Biophys. Acta 624:473, 1980.

17. Thillet, J., Arous, N., and Rosa, J.: Functional studies of two new abnormal hemoglobins with their mutation located at intersubunit contacts: Hb Hotel Dieu β 99(G1) Asp→Gly and Hb Pitie Salpetriere β 34(B16) Val→Phe. Biochim. Biophys. Acta 670:260, 1981.

18. Brennan, S. O., Wells, R. M., Smith, H., and Carrell, R. W.: Hemoglobin Brisbane: β 68 Leu→His. A new high oxygen affinity variant. Hemoglobin 5:325, 1981.

19. Rahbar, S., Winkler, K., Louis, J., Rea, C., Blume, K., and Beutler, E.: Hemoglobin Great Lakes (β 68 E12 Leucine→Histidine): A new high affinity hemoglobin. Blood 58:813, 1981.

20. Lorkin, P. A., Stephens, A. D., Beard, M. E. J., Wrigley, P. F. M., Adams, L., and Lehmann, H.: Haemoglobin Rahere (β82 Lys→Thr): A new high affinity haemoglobin associated with decreased 2,3-diphosphoglycerate binding and relative polycythaemia. Br. Med. J. 4:200, 1975.

21. Ikkala, E., Koskela, J., Pikkarainen, P., Rahiala, E.-L., El-Hazmi, M. A. F., Nagai, K., Lang, A., and Lehmann, H.: Hb Helsinki: A variant with a high oxygen affinity and a substitution at a 2,3-DPG binding site (β82 EF6 Lys→Met). Acta Haematol. 56:257, 1976.

22. Charache, S., McCurdy, P., and Fox, J.: Hemoglobin Providence (Hb Prov), a fetal-like hemoglobin. Blood 46:1030, 1975.

23. Moo-Penn, W. F., Jue, D. L., Bechtel, K. C., Johnson, M. H., Schmidt, R. McCurdy, P. R., Fox, J., Bonaventura, J., Sullivan, B., and Bonaventura, C.: Hemoglobin Providence. A human hemoglobin variant occurring in two forms in vivo. J. Biol. Chem. 251:7557, 1976.

24. Bonaventura, J., Bonaventura, C., Sullivan, B., Ferruzzi, G., McCurdy, P. R., Fox, J., and Moo-Penn, W. F.: Hemoglobin Providence. Functional consequences of two alterations of the 2,3-diphosphoglycerate binding site at position β82. J. Biol. Chem. 251:7563, 1976.

25. Thillet, J., Blouquit, Y., Garel, M. C., Dreyfus, B., Reyes, F., Cohen-Solal, M., Beuzard, Y., and Rosa, J.: Hemoglobin Creteil β89 (F5) Ser→Asn: High oxygen affinity variant of hemoglobin frozen in a quaternary R-structure. J. Molec. Med. 1:135, 1976.

26. Paniker, N. V., Lin, K.-T., Krantz, S. B., Flexner, J. M., Wasserman, B. K., and Puett, D.: Haemoglobin Vanderbilt ($\alpha_2\beta_2^{89\ Ser\rightarrow Arg}$): A new haemoglobin with high oxygen affinity and compensatory erythrocytosis. Br. J. Haematol. 39:249, 1978.

26a. Aguilar, i., Bascompte, J. L., Wajcman, H., Poyart, C., and Labie, D.: Hemoglobin Barcelona β94 (FG1) Asp→His: A new hemoglobin variant with increased oxygen affinity. Nouv. Rev. Fr. Hematol. 23:267, 1981.

26b. Wajcman, H., Aguilar, i., Bascompte, J. L., Labie, D., Poyart, C., and Bohn, B.: Structural and functional studies of hemoglobin Barcelona ($\alpha_2\beta_2$ 94 Asp(FG1)→His). J. Molec. Biol. 156:185, 1982.

27. Lorkin, P. A., Lehmann, H., Fairbanks, V. P., Berglund, G., and Leanhardt, T.: Two new pathological haemoglobins: Olmsted β 141 (H19) Leu→Arg and Malmö β 97 (FG4) His→Gln. Biochem. J. 119:68, 1970.

28. Fairbanks, V. F., Maldonado, J. E., Charache, S., and Boyer, S. H.: Familial erythrocytosis due to electrophoretically undetectable hemoglobin with impaired oxygen dissociation (hemoglobin Malmö, $\alpha_2\beta_2^{97Gln}$). Mayo Clin. Proc. 46:721, 1971.

29. Thillet, J., Garel, M. C., Blouquit, Y., Basset, P., Dreyfus, B., Rosa, J., and Arous, N.: Functional studies of Hb Malmö β 97(FG4) His→Gln. FEBS Lett. 84:71, 1977.

30. Taketa, F., Huang, Y., P., Libnoch, J. A., and Dessel, B. H.: Hemoglobin Wood β 97(FG4) His→Leu. A new high-oxygen-affinity hemoglobin associated with familial erythrocytosis. Biochim. Biophys. Acta 400:348, 1975.

31. Novy, M. J., Edwards, M. J., and Metcalfe, J.: Hemoglobin Yakima: II. High blood oxygen affinity associated with compensatory erythrocytosis and normal hemodynamics. J. Clin. Invest. 46:1848, 1967.

32. Jones, R. T., Osgood, E. E., Brimhall, B., and Koler, R. D.: Hemoglobin Yakima. I. Clinical and biochemical studies. J. Clin. Invest. 46:1840, 1967.

33. Reed, C. S., Hampson, R., Gordon, S., Jones, R. T., Novy, M. J., Brimhall, B., Edwards, M. J., and Koler, R. D.: Erythrocytosis secondary to increased oxygen affinity of a mutant hemoglobin, hemoglobin Kempsey. Blood 31:623, 1968.

34. Bunn, H. F., Wohl, R. C., Bradley, T. B., Cooley, M., and Gibson, Q. H.: Functional properties of hemoglobin Kempsey. J. Biol. Chem. 249:7402, 1974.

35. Rucknagel, D. L., Glynn, K. P., and Smith, J. R.: Hemoglobin Ypsi, characterized by increased oxygen affinity, abnormal polymerization and erythremia. Clin. Res. 15:270, 1967.

36. Glynn, K. P., Penner, J. A., Smith, J. R., and Rucknagel, D. L.: Familial erythrocytosis. A description of three families, one with hemoglobin Ypsilanti. Ann. Intern. Med. 69:769, 1968.

37. Weatherall, D. J., Clegg, J. B., Callender, S. T., Wells, R. M. G., Gale, R. E., Huehns, E. R., Perutz, M. F., Viggiano, G., and Ho, C.: Haemoglobin Radcliffe ($\alpha_2\beta_2^{99[G1]Ala}$): A high oxygen-affinity variant causing familial polycythaemia. Br. J. Haematol. 35:177, 1977.

38. Blouquit, Y., Braconnier, F., Galacteros, F., Arous, N., Soria, J., Zittoun, R., and Rosa, J.: Hemoglobin Hôtel-Dieu β 99 Asp→Gly (G1). A new abnormal hemoglobin with high oxygen affinity. Hemoglobin 5:19, 1981.

38a. Rochette, J., Poyart, C., Varet, B., and Wajcman, H.: A new hemoglobin variant altering the $\alpha_1\beta_2$ contact: Hb Chemilly $\alpha_2\beta_2$ 99 (G1) Asp→Val. FEBS Lett. 166:8, 1984.

39. Lokich, J. J., Moloney, W. C., Bunn, H. F., Bruckheimer, S. M., and Ranney, H. M.: Hemoglobin Brigham ($\alpha_2^A\beta_2$ 100 Pro→Leu). Hemoglobin variant associated with familial erythrocytosis. J. Clin. Invest. 52:2060, 1973.

40. Jones, R. T., Brimhall, B., and Gray, G.: Hemoglo-

bin British Columbia ($\alpha_2\beta_2^{101[G3]\ Glu\to Gly}$) A new variant with high oxygen affinity. Hemoglobin 1:171, 1976.
41. Stinson, R. A.: Isolelectric focusing studies of a "stable" asymmetrical hybrid formed with a new hemoglobin variant, hemoglobin Alberta ($\alpha_2\beta_2^{101[G3]Glu\to Gly}$) J. Lab. Clin. Med. 90:623, 1977.
42. McDonald, M. J., Turci, S. M., and Bleichman, M.: Functional properties of hemoglobin Alberta, a variant with abnormal subunit interaction. J. Mol. Biol., in press.
43. Mant, M. J., Salkie, M. L., Cope, N., Appling, F., Bolch, K., Jayalakshmi, M., Gravely, M., Wilson, J. B., and Huisman, T. H. J.: Hb-Alberta or $\alpha_2\beta_2$ (101[G3]Glu→Gly), a new high-oxygen-affinity hemoglobin variant causing erythrocytosis. Hemoglobin 1:183, 1976.
44. Charache, S., Jacobson, R., Brimhall, B., Murphy, E. A., Hathaway, P., Winslow, R., Jones, R., Rath, C., and Simkovich, J.: Hb Potomac (101 Glu→Asp): Speculations on placental oxygen transport in carriers of high-affinity hemoglobins. Blood 51:331, 1978.
45. Rubin, R. N., Ballas, S. K., Atwater, J., Burka, E. R., Adachi, K., Asakura, T., and Schwartz, E.: Hemoglobin Potomac: Clinical picture, biosynthesis and stability. Hemoglobin 2:447, 1978.
46. White, J. M., Szur, L., Gillies, I. D. S., Lorkin, P. A., and Lehmann, H.: Familial polycythaemia caused by a new haemoglobin variant: Hb Heathrow, β103 (G5) phenylalanine-leucine. Br. Med. J. 3:665, 1973.
47. Beard, M. E. J., Hamer, J. W., Brennan, S. O., Jones, J. N., Sheat, J. M., and Maclaurin, J. S.: Familial relative polycythaemia due to haemoglobin Heathrow. Aust. N.Z. J. Med. 9:297, 1979.
48. Nute, P. E., Stamatoyannopoulos, G., Hermodson, M. A., and Roth, D.: Hemoglobinopathic erythrocytosis due to a new electrophoretically silent variant, hemoglobin San Diego (β109 (G11) Val→Met). J. Clin. Invest. 53:320, 1974.
49. Bursaux, E., Blouquit, Y., Poyart, C., and Rosa, J.: Hemoglobin Ty Gard ($\alpha_2^A\beta_2$ 124(H2) Pro→Gln). A stable high O_2 affinity variant at the $\alpha_1\beta_1$ contact. FEBS Lett. 88:155, 1978.
49a. Rochette, J., Varet, B., Boissel, J. P., Clough, K., Labie, D., Wajcman, H., Bohn, B., Magne, P., and Poyart, C.: Structure and function of Hb Saint-Jacques ($\alpha_2\beta_2$ 140 (H18) Ala→Thr): A new high–oxygen-affinity variant with altered bisphosphoglycerate binding. Biochim. Biophys. Acta 785:14, 1984.
50. Moo-Penn, W. F., Schneider, R. G., Shih, T.-B., Jones, R. T., Govindarajan, S., Govindarajan, P. G., and Patchen, L. C.: Hemoglobin Ohio (β142 Ala→Asp): A new abnormal hemoglobin with high oxygen affinity and erythrocytosis. Blood 56:246, 1980.
51. Bromberg, P. A., Alben, J. O., Bare, G. H., et al.: High oxygen affinity variant of haemoglobin Little Rock with unique properties. Nature [New Biol.] 243:177, 1973.
52. Bare, G. H., Alben, J. O., Bromberg, P. A., Jones, R. T., Brimhall, B., and Padilla, F.: Hemoglobin Little Rock (β143 (H21) His→Gln). Effects of an amino acid substitution at the 2,3-diphosphoglycerate binding site. J. Biol. Chem. 249:773, 1974.
53. Jensen, M., Oski, F. A., Nathan, D. G., and Bunn, H. F.: Hemoglobin Syracuse ($\alpha_2\beta_2^{143(H21)\ His\to Pro}$). A new high-affinity variant detected by special electrophoretic methods. J. Clin. Invest. 55:469, 1975.
54. Zak, S. J., Brimhall, B., Jones, R. T., and Kaplan, M. E.: Hemoglobin Andrew-Minneapolis $\alpha_2^A\beta_2^{144\ Lys\to Asn}$: A new high-oxygen-affinity mutant human hemoglobin. Blood 44:543, 1974.
55. Amiconi, G., Winterhalter, K. H., Antonini, E., et al.: Functional properties of hemoglobin Rainier. FEBS Lett. 21:341, 1972.
56. Salhany, J. M.: The deoxygenation kinetics of hemoglobin Rainier ($\alpha_2\beta_2^{145\ Tyr\to Cys}$). Biochem. Biophys. Res. Commun. 47:784, 1972.
57. Adamson, J. W., Parer, J. T., and Stamatoyannopoulos, G.: Erythrocytosis associated with hemoglobin Rainier: Oxygen equilibria and marrow regulation. J. Clin. Invest. 48:1376, 1969.
58. Hayashi, A., and Stamatoyannopoulos, G.: Role of penultimate tyrosine in haemoglobin β subunit. Nature [New Biol.] 235:70, 1972.
59. Bunn, H. F., Bradley, T. B., Davis, W. E., Drysdale, J. W., Burke, J. F., Beck, W. S., and Laver, M. B.: Structural and functional studies on hemoglobin Bethesda ($\alpha_2\beta_2^{145\ His}$), a variant associated with compensatory erythrocytosis. J. Clin. Invest. 51:2299, 1972.
60. Bucci, E., Fronticelli, C., Nicklas, J., and Charache, S.: Conformation in solution of hemoglobin Osler ($\alpha_2^A\beta_2^{145\ Tyr\to Asp}$). J. Biol. Chem. 254:10811, 1979.
61. Charache, S., Brimhall, B., and Jones, R. T.: Polycythemia produced by hemoglobin Osler (β145 (HC2) Ty4→Asp) Johns Hopkins Med. J. 136:132, 1975.
62. Kleckner, H. B., Wilson, J. B., Lindeman, J. G., Stevens, P. D., Niazi, G., Hunter, E., Chen, C. J., and Huisman, T. H. J.: Hemoglobin Fort Gordon or $\alpha_2\beta_2^{145\ Tyr\to Asp}$, a new high-oxygen-affinity hemoglobin variant. Biochim. Biophys. Acta 400:343, 1975.
63. Gacon, G., Wajcman, H., and Labie, D.: Structural and functional study of Hb Nancy, β145 (HC2) Tyr→Asp, a high oxygen affinity hemoglobin. FEBS Lett. 56:39, 1975.
64. Winslow, R. M., Swenberg, M.-L., Gross, E., Chervenick, P. A., Buchman, R. R., and Anderson, W. F.: Hemoglobin McKees Rocks ($\alpha_2\beta_2^{145\ Tyr\to Term}$): A human "nonsense" mutation leading to a shortened β-chain. J. Clin. Invest. 57:772, 1976.
65. Olson, J. S., Gibson, Q. H., Nagel, R. L., and Hamilton, H. B.: The ligand-binding properties of hemoglobin Hiroshima ($\alpha_2\beta_2^{146\ Asp}$). J. Biol. Chem. 247:7485, 1972.
66. Hamilton, H. B., Iuchi, I., Miyaji, T., et al.: Hemoglobin Hiroshima (β143 Histidine-Aspartic acid): A newly identified fast-moving beta chain variant associated with increased oxygen affinity and compensatory erythremia. J. Clin. Invest. 48:525, 1969.
67. Imai, K., Hamilton, H. B., Miyaji, T., and Shibata, S.: Physicochemical studies of the relation between structure and function in hemoglobin Hiroshima (HC3 β, Histidine-Aspartate). Biochemistry 11:114, 1972.
68. Bare, G. H., Bromberg, P. A., Alben, J. O., Brimhall, B., Jones, R. T., Mintz, S., and Rother, I.: Altered C-terminal salt bridges in haemoglobin York cause high oxygen affinity. Nature 259:155, 1976.
69. Schneider, R. G., Bremner, J. E., Brimhall, B., Jones, R. T., and Shih, T.-B.: Hemoglobin Cowtown (β146 HC3 His→Leu): A mutant with high oxygen affinity and erythrocytosis. Am. J. Clin. Pathol. 72:1028, 1979.

70. Sasaki, J., Imamura, T., Sumida, I., Yanase, T., and Ohya, M.: Increased oxygen affinity for hemoglobin Sawara: α A4(6) aspartic acid–alanine. Biochim. Biophys. Acta 495:183, 1977.
71. Charache, S., Brimhall, B., and Zaatari, G.: Oxygen affinity and stability of hemoglobin Dunn (α6 (A4) Asp→Asn): Use of isoelectric focusing in recognition of a new abnormal hemoglobin. Am. J. Hematol. 9:151, 1980.
71a. Harano, T., Harano, K., Shibata, S., Ueda, S., Imai, K., Tsuneshige, A., Yamada, H., and Fukui, H.: Hemoglobin Kariya [α 40 (C5) Lys→Glu]: A new hemoglobin variant with an increased oxygen affinity. FEBS Lett. 153:332, 1983.
71b. Harano, T., Harano, K., Ueda, S., Shibata, S., Imai, K., Ohba, Y., Shinohara, T., Horio, S., Nishioka, K., and Shirotani, H.: Hemoglobin Kawachi [α44 (CE2) Pro→Arg]: A new hemoglobin variant of high oxygen affinity with amino acid substitution at $\alpha_1\beta_2$ contact. Hemoglobin 6:43, 1982.
72. Braconnier, F., Gacon, G., Thillet, J., Wajcman, H., Soria, J., Maigret, P., Labie, D., and Rosa, J.: Hemoglobin Fort de France ($\alpha_2^{45(CD3)His \to Arg} \beta_2$). A new variant with increased oxygen affinity. Biochim. Biophys. Acta 493:228, 1977.
73. Cohen-Solal, M., Manesse, B., Thillet, J., and Rosa, J.: Haemoglobin G Norfolk α 85 (F6) Asp→Asn: Structural characterization by sequenator analysis and functional properties of a new variant with high oxygen affinity. FEBS Lett. 50:163, 1975.
74. Smith, L. L., Plese, C. F., Barton, B. P., Charache, S., Wilson, J. B., and Huisman, T. H. J.: Subunit dissociation of the abnormal hemoglobins G Georgia ($\alpha_2^{95Leu[G2]}\beta_2$) and Rampa ($\alpha_2^{95Ser[G2]}\beta_2$) J. Biol. Chem. 247:1433, 1972.
75. Huisman, T. H. J., Adams, H. R., Wilson, S. B., Efremov, G. D., Reynolds, C. A., and Wrightstone, R. N.: Hemoglobin G Georgia or $\alpha_2^{95 Leu(G2)}\beta_2$. Biochim. Biophys. Acta 200:578, 1970.
76. De Jong, W. W. W., Bernini, L. F., and Khan, P. M.: Haemoglobin Rampa: α 95 Pro→Ser. Biochim. Biophys. Acta 236:197, 1971.
77. Wiltshire, B. G., Clark, K. G. A., Lorkin, P. A., and Lehmann, H.: Haemoglobin Denmark Hill α 95 (G2) Pro→Ala, a variant with unusual electrophoretic and oxygen-binding properties. Biochim. Biophys. Acta 278:459, 1972.
78. Lorkin, P. A., Casey, R., Clark, K. G. A., and Lehmann, H.: The oxygen affinity of haemoglobin St. Luke's. FEBS Lett. 39:111, 1974.
78a. Dysert, P. A., Head, C. G., Shih, T. B., Jones, R. T., and Schneider, R. G.: Hb Dallas α_2 97 (G4) Asn→Lys β_2: A new abnormal hemoglobin with high oxygen affinity. Blood 60(Suppl. 1):53a, 1982.
78b. Harano, T., Harano, K., Shibata, S., Ueda, S., Imai, K., and Seki, M.: Hemoglobin Tokoname (α 139 (HC1) Lys→Thr): A new hemoglobin variant with a slightly increased oxygen affinity. Hemoglobin 7:85, 1983.
78c. Moo-Penn, W. F., Therrell, B. L., Jr., Jue, D. L., and Johnson M. H.: Hemoglobin Cubujuqui (α141 Arg→Ser): Functional consequences of the alteration of the C-terminus of the α chain of hemoglobin. Hemoglobin 5:715, 1981.
79. Labossiere, A., Vella, F., Hiebert, J., and Galbraith, P.: Hemoglobin Deer Lodge: $\alpha_2\beta_2^{2His \to Arg}$. Clin. Biochem. 5:46, 1972.
80. Bonaventura, J., Bonaventura, C., Sullivan, B., and Godette, G.: Hemoglobin Deer Lodge (β 2 His→Arg). Consequences of altering the 2,3-diphosphoglycerate binding site. J. Biol. Chem. 250:9250, 1975.
81. Tondo, C. V., Salzano, F. M., and Rucknagel, D. L.: Hemoglobin Porto Alegre, a possible polymer of normal hemoglobin in a Caucasian Brazilian family. Am. J. Hum. Genet. 15:265, 1963.
82. Tondo, C., Bonaventura, J., Bonaventura, C., Brunori, M., Amiconi, G., and Antonini, E.: Functional properties of hemoglobin Porto Alegre ($\alpha_2^A\beta_2$ 9 Ser→Cys) and the reactivity of its extra cysteinyl residue. Biochim. Biophys. Acta 342:15, 1974.
83. Garel, M. C., Blouquit, Y., Arous, N., and Rosa, J.: Hb Strasbourg $\alpha_2\beta_2$ 20(B2) Val→Asp: A variant at the same locus as Hb Olympia (β 20 Val→Met). FEBS Lett. 72:1, 1976.
83a. Cohen-Solal, M., North, M. L., Albrech-Ellmer, K., Garel, M. C., Blouquit, Y., and Rosa J.: Haemoglobin Strasbourg $\alpha_2\beta_2$ (B5) Val→Asp. FEBS Lett. 90:286, 1978.
84. Sasaki, J., Imamura, T., Yanase, T., Atha, D. H., Riggs, A., Bonaventura, J., and Bonaventura, C.: Hemoglobin Hirose, a human hemoglobin variant with a substitution at the $\alpha_1\beta_2$ interface. Subunit dissociation and the equilibria and kinetics of ligand binding. J. Biol. Chem. 253:87, 1978.
85. Yamaoka, K.: Hemoglobin Hirose: $\alpha_2\beta_2$ 37(C3) tryptophan yielding serine. Blood 38:730, 1971.
86. Brown, W. J., Niazi, G. A., Jayalakshmi, M., Abraham, E. C., and Huisman, T. H. J.: Hemoglobin Athens-Georgia, or $\alpha_2\beta_2$ $^{40(C6) Arg \to Lys}$, a hemoglobin variant with an increased oxygen affinity. Biochim. Biophys. Acta 439:70, 1976.
87. Moo-Penn, W. F., Johnson, M. H., Bechtel, K. C., Jue, D. L., Therrell, B. L., Jr., and Schmidt, R. M.: Hemoglobins Austin and Waco: Two hemoglobins with substitutions in the $\alpha_1\beta_2$ contact region. Arch. Biochem. Biophys. 179:86, 1977.
88. Jones, R. T., Koler, R. D., Duerst, M. L., and Dhindsa, D. S.: Hemoglobin Willamette $\alpha_2\beta_2$ 51 Pro→Arg (D2): A new abnormal human hemoglobin. Hemoglobin 1:45, 1976.
88a. Shih, T. B., Jones, R. T., and Johnson, C. S.: Functional properties of Hb Pasadena, $\alpha_2\beta_2$ 75 (E19) Leu→Arg. Hemoglobin 6:153, 1982.
89. Benesch, R., Edalji, R., and Benesch, R. E.: Oxygenation properties of hemoglobin variants with substitutions near the polyphosphate binding site. Biochim. Biophys. Acta 393:368, 1975.
89a. Como, P. F., Kennett, D., Wilkinson, T., and Kronenberg, H.: A new hemoglobin with high oxygen affinity—hemoglobin Bunbury: $\alpha_2\beta_2$ [94 (FG1) Asp→Asn]. Hemoglobin 7:413, 1983.
90. Maniatis, A., Bousios, T., Nagel, R. L., Balazs, T., Ueda, Y., Bookchin, R. M., and Maniatis, G. M.: Hemoglobin Crete (β 129 Ala→Pro): A new high-affinity variant interacting with β^0- and $\delta\beta^0$-thalassemia. Blood 54:54, 1979.
91. Chiarioni, T., Graziani, B., Nardi, E., Papa, G., Sasso, G. F., and Tentori, L.: Nuova emoglobina anomala (Hb Abruzzo) in sogetto con sindrome emolitica di tipo "Mediterraneo" e spiccata policitemia. Haematologica (Pavia) 58:210, 1973.
92. Tentori, L., Sorcini, M. C., and Buccella, C.: Hemoglobin Abruzzo: beta 143 (H21) His→Arg. Clin. Chim. Acta 38:258, 1972.
93. Imai, K., and Lehmann, H.: The oxygen affinity of haemoglobin Tak, a variant with an elongated beta chain. Biochim. Biophys. Acta 412:288, 1975.
94. Bellingham, A. J., and Huehns, E. R.: Compensa-

tion in haemolytic anaemias caused by abnormal haemoglobins. Nature 218:924, 1968.
95. Monod, J., Wyman, J., and Changeux, J. P.: On the nature of allosteric transitions: A plausible model. J. Molec. Biol. 12:88, 1965.
96. Ogata, R., and McConnell, H. M.: Mechanism of cooperative oxygen binding to hemoglobin. Proc. Natl. Acad. Sci. USA 69:334, 1972.
97. Lindstrom, T. R., Baldassare, J. J., Bunn, H. F., and Ho, C.: Nuclear magnetic resonance and spin-label studies of hemoglobin Kempsey. Biochemistry 12:4212, 1973.
98. Perutz, M. F., Ladner, J. E., Simon, S. R., and Ho, C.: Influence of globin structure on the state of the heme. Biochemistry 13:2163, 1974.
99. Perutz, M. F., Fersht, A. R., Simon, S. R., and Roberts, G. C. K.: Influence of globin structure on the state of the heme. II. Allosteric transitions in methemoglobin. Biochemistry 13:2174, 1974.
100. Nagai, K., La Mar, G. N., Jue, T., and Bunn, H. F.: Proton magnetic resonance investigation of the influence of quaternary structure on the iron-histidine bonding in deoxy hemoglobins. Biochemistry 21:842, 1982.
101. Perutz, M. F.: Nature of haem-haem interaction. Nature [New Biol.] 243:180, 1972.
102. Perutz, M. F.: Stereochemistry of cooperative effects in haemoglobin. Nature 228:726, 1970.
103. Perutz, M. F.: The Bohr effect and combination with organic phosphates. Nature 228:734, 1970.
104. Wajcman, H., Kilmartin, J. V., Najman, A., and Labie, D.: Hemoglobin Cochin–Port Royal—consequences of the replacement of the β chain C-terminal by an arginine. Biochim. Biophys. Acta 400:354, 1975.
105. Adams, J. G., III, Przywara, K. P., Shamsuddin, M., and Heller, P.: Hemoglobin J Altgeld Gardens (β 92(F8) His→Asp): A new hemoglobin variant involving a substitution of the proximal histidine. Am. Soc. Hematol. 18th Annual Meeting, Dallas, Texas, 1975.
106. Olson, J. S., and Gibson, Q. H.: The functional properties of hemoglobin Bethesda ($\alpha_2\beta_2^{145\,His}$). J. Biol. Chem. 247:3662, 1972.
107. Imai, K.: Hemoglobin Chesapeake (92α, Arginine→Leucine)—precise measurements and analyses of oxygen equilibrium. J. Biol. Chem. 249:7607, 1974.
108. Matsukawa, S., Nishibu, M., Nagai, M., Mawatari, K., and Yoneyama, Y.: Analysis of optical properties of hemoglobins in terms of the two state model, especially from studies on abnormal hemoglobins with amino acid substitution in the $\alpha_1\beta_2$ contact region. J. Biol. Chem. 254:2358, 1979.
109. Perutz, M. F.: Sterechemical interpretation of high oxygen affinity of haemoglobin Little Rock ($\alpha_2\beta_2^{143\,His\rightarrow Gln}$). Nature [New Biol.] 243:180, 1973.
110. Gibson, Q. H., and Nagel, R. L.: Allosteric transition and ligand binding in hemoglobin Chesapeake. J. Biol. Chem. 249:7255, 1974.
111. Baldwin, J. M.: The structure of human carbonmonoxy haemoglobin at 2.7 Å resolution. J. Molec. Biol. 136:103, 1980.
112. Shaanan, B.: The structure of human oxyhemoglobin at 2.1 Å resolution. J. Mol. Biol. 171:31, 1983.
113. Greer, J.: Three-dimensional structure of abnormal human haemoglobins Chesapeake and J Cape Town. J. Molec. Biol. 62:241, 1971.
114. Pulsinelli, P. D.: Structure of deoxyhaemoglobin Yakima: A high-affinity mutant form exhibiting oxy-like $\alpha_1\beta_2$ subunit interactions. J. Molec. Biol. 74:57, 1973.
115. Greer, J., and Perutz, M. F.: Three dimensional structure of haemoglobin Rainier. Nature [New Biol.] 230:261, 1971.
116. Perutz, M. F., Pulsinelli, P., Ten Eyck, L., Kilmartin, J. V., Shibata, S., Iuchi, I., Miyagi, T., and Hamilton, H. B.: Haemoglobin Hiroshima and the mechanism of the alkaline Bohr effect. Nature [New Biol.] 232:147, 1971.
117. Anderson, N. L.: Hemoglobin San Diego (β109 [G11] Val→Met): Crystal structure of the deoxy form. J. Clin. Invest. 53:329, 1974.
118. Arnone, A., Gacon, G., and Wajcman, H.: X-ray and functional studies of hemoglobins Nancy and Cochin–Port-Royal. J. Biol. Chem. 251:5875, 1976.
119. Arnone, A., Thillet, J., and Rosa, J.: The structure of hemoglobin Creteil (β89 Ser→Asn) is similar to that of abnormal human hemoglobin having sequence changes at Tyr 145β. J. Biol. Chem. 256:8545, 1981.
119a. Perutz, M. F., Fermi, G., and Shih, T. B.: Structure of deoxyhemoglobin Cowtown (His HC3 (146) beta→Leu), origin of the alkaline Bohr effect and elecrostatic interactions in hemoglobin. Proc. Natl. Acad. Sci. USA 81:4781, 1984.
120. Davis, D. G., Lindstrom, T. R., Mock, N. H., Baldassare, J. J., Charache, S., Jones, R. T., and Ho, C.: Nuclear magnetic resonance studies of hemoglobins. VI. Heme proton spectra of human deoxyhemoglobins and their relevance to the nature of cooperative oxygenation of hemoglobin. J. Molec. Biol. 60:101, 1971.
121. Ho, C., and Lindstrom, T. R.: Functional nonequivalence of α and β hemes in human hemoglobins. Adv. Exp. Med. Biol. 28:65, 1972.
122. Lindstrom, T. R., Noren, I. B. E., Charache, S., Lehmann, H., and Ho, C.: Nuclear magnetic resonance studies of hemoglobins. VII. Tertiary structure around ligand binding site in carbonmonoxy-hemoglobin. Biochemistry 11:1677, 1972.
123. Fung, L. W., and Ho, C.: A proton nuclear magnetic resonance study of the quaternary structure of human hemoglobins in water. Biochemistry 14:2526, 1975.
124. Russu, I., Ho, N. T., and Ho, C.: Role of the β 146 histidine in the alkaline Bohr effect of hemoglobin. Biochemistry 19:1043, 1980.
125. Ogata, R. T., McConnell, H. M., and Jones, R. T.: Binding of triphosphate spin labels to hemoglobin Kempsey. Biochem. Biophys. Res. Commun. 47:157, 1972.
126. Baldassare, J. J., Charache, S., Jones, R. T., and Ho, C.: Electron paramagnetic resonance studies of spin-labeled hemoglobins. II. Roles of subunit interactions and of intermediate structures in the cooperative oxygenation of hemoglobin and the results on hemoglobin Yakima, hemoglobin J Cape Town and carboxypeptidases A- and B-treated hemoglobin A. Biochemistry 9:4707, 1970.
127. Salhany, J. M., Ogawa, S., and Shulman, R. G.: Correlation between quaternary structure and ligand dissociation kinetics for fully liganded hemoglobin. Biochemistry 14:2180, 1975.
128. Bunn, H. F.: Dissociation of haemoglobin Chesapeake into subunits. Nature 227:839, 1970.
129. Pettigrew, D. W., Romeo, P. H., Tsapis, A., Thillet, J., Smith, M. L., Turner B. W., and Ackers, G.

K.: Probing the energetics of proteins through structure perturbation: Localization of the regulatory energy in human hemoglobin. Proc. Natl. Acad. Sci. USA 79:1849, 1982.
130. Briehl, R. W.: Relations between aggregation and oxygen equilibrium in human and lamprey haemoglobin. *In* Goodwin, T. W., Harris, J. I., and Hartley, B. S. (eds.): Structure and Activity of Enzymes. New York, Academic Press, 1964, p. 171.
131. Noble, R. W.: Relation between allosteric effects and changes in the energy of bonding between molecular subunits. J. Molec. Biol. 39:479, 1969.
132. Ackers, G. K., and Halvorson, H. R.: Linkage between oxygenation and subunit dissociation in human hemoglobin. Proc. Natl. Acad. Sci. USA 71:4312, 1974.
133. Perutz, M. F., Kilmartin, J. V., Nishikura, K., Fogg, J. H., Butler, P. J. G., and Rollema, H. S.: Identification of residues contributing to the Bohr effect of human haemoglobin. J. Molec. Biol. 138:649, 1980.
134. Winslow, R. M., and Charache, S.: Hemoglobin Richmond. Subunit dissociation and oxygen equilibrium properties. J. Biol. Chem. 250:6939, 1975.
134a. Adachi, V., Vonk, H., Reilly, M. P., Adachi, H., Schroeder, W. A., Schwartz, E., and Asakura, T.: Relationship between tetramer-dimer assembly and the stability of Hb Malmö ($\alpha_2\beta_2^{97Gln}$). Biochim. Biophys. Acta 790:132, 1984.
135. Park, C. M.: Isoelectric focusing and the study of interacting protein systems: Ligand binding, phosphate binding and subunit exchange in hemoglobin. Ann. N.Y. Acad. Sci. 209:237, 1973.
136. Bunn, H. F., and McDonough, M.: Asymmetrical hemoglobin hybrids. An approach to the study of subunit interactions. Biochemistry 13:988, 1974.
137. Adams, J. G., III, Winter, W. P., Tausk, K., and Heller, P.: Hemoglobin Rush (β101 [G3] Glutamine): A new unstable hemoglobin causing mild hemolytic anemia. Blood 43:261, 1974.
138. Garel, M. C., Hassan, W., Coquelet, M. T., Goossens, M., and Rosa, J.: Hemoglobin J Cairo: 65 (E9) Lys→Gln, a new hemoglobin variant discovered in an Egyptian family. Biochim. Biophys. Acta 420:97, 1976.
138a. Tomoda, A., Takizawa, T., and Yoneyama, Y.: Mechanism of autoxidation of hemoglobin Kempsey (β99 Asp→Asn). Hemoglobin 8:137, 1984.
139. Taketa, F., Matteson, K. J., Chen, J. Y., and Libnoch, J. A.: Methemoglobin reduction in red cells: Effect of a high oxygen affinity hemoglobin. Blood 55:116, 1980.
140. Adamson, J. W., and Finch, C. A.: Erythropoietin and the polycythemias. Ann. N.Y. Acad. Sci. 149:560, 1968.
141. Adamson, J. W., Hayashi, A., Stamatoyannopoulos, G., and Burger, W. F.: Erythrocyte function and marrow regulation in hemoglobin Bethesda (β145 Histidine). J. Clin. Invest. 51:2883, 1972.
142. Bromberg, P. A., Padilla, F., Guy, J. T., and Balcerzak, S. P.: Effect of a new hemoglobin (Hb Little Rock) on the physiology of oxygen delivery. J. Lab. Clin. Med. 78:837, 1971.
143. Charache, S., Achuff, S., Winslow, R., Adamson, J., and Chervenick, P.: Variability of the homeostatic response to altered P_{50}. Blood 52:1156, 1978.
144. Adamson, J. W., and Finch, C. A.: Hemoglobin function, oxygen affinity and erythropoietin. Ann. Rev. Physiol. 37:351, 1975.
145. Sharma, V. S., Newton, G. L., Ranney, H. M., Ahmed, F., Harris, J. W., and Danish, E. H.: Hemoglobin Rothschild (β 37(C3) Trp→Arg): A high/low affinity hemoglobin mutant. J. Molec. Biol. 144:267, 1980.
146. Wade, J. P. H., duBoulay, G. H., Marshall, J., Pearson, T. C., Ross Russell, R. W., Shirley, J. A., Symon, L., Wetherley-Mein, G., and Zilkha, E.: Cerebral blood flow, haematocrit and viscosity in subjects with a high oxygen affinity haemoglobin variant. Acta Neurol. Scand. 61:210, 1980.
147. Poyart, C., Bursaux, E., Teisseire, B., Freminet, A., Duvelleroy, M., and Rosa, J.: Hemoglobin Creteil: Oxygen transport by erythrocytes. In vitro and in vivo studies in a high oxygen-affinity mutant hemoglobin. Ann. Intern. Med. 88:758, 1978.
148. Gau, G. T., Fairbanks, V. F., Maldonado, J. E., Bassingthwaighte, J. B., and Tancredi, R. G.: Cardiac dysfunction in a patient with hemoglobin Malmö treated with repeated transfusions. Clin. Res. 22:276A, 1974.
148a. Butler, W. M., Spratling, L., Kark, J. A., and Schoomaker, E. B.: Hemoglobin Osler: Report of a new family with exercise studies before and after phlebotomy. Am. J. Hematol. 13:293, 1982.
148b. Winslow, R. M., Butler, W. M., Kark, J. A., Klein, H. G., and Moo-Penn, W.: The effect of bloodletting on exercise performance in a subject with a high-affinity hemoglobin variant. Blood 62:1159, 1983.
148c. Wranne, B., Berlin, G., Jorfeldt, L., and Lund, N.: Tissue oxygenation and muscular substrate turnover in two subjects with high hemoglobin oxygen affinity. J. Clin. Invest. 72:1376, 1983.
149. Hebbel, R. P., Eaton, J. W., Kronenberg, R. S., Zanjani, E. D., Moore, L. A., and Berger, E. M.: Human llamas. Adaptation to altitude in subjects with high oxygen affinity. J. Clin. Invest. 62:593, 1978.
149a. Charache, S., Catalano, P., Burns, S., et al.: Pregnancy in carriers of high-affinity hemoglobins. Blood 65:713, 1985.
150. Hebbel, R. P., Berger, E. M., and Eaton, J. W.: Effect of increased maternal hemoglobin oxygen affinity on fetal growth in the rat. Blood 55:969, 1980.
151. Bauer, C., Jelkmann, W., and Moll, W.: High oxygen affinity of maternal blood reduces fetal weight in rats. Respir. Physiol. 43:169, 1981.
152. Adamson, J. W.: Familial polycythemia. Semin. Hematol. 12:383, 1975.
153. Colgan, J. P., Fairbanks, V. F., Libnoch, J. A., Taketa, F., Brimhall, B., Zak, S. J.: Comparison of hemoglobins Wood ($\alpha_2\beta_2^{97\ Leu}$) and Malmö ($\alpha_2\beta_2^{97\ Glu}$). Diagnostic value of citrate agar electrophoresis. Am. J. Clin. Pathol. 71:668, 1978.
154. Garel, M. C., Cohen-Solal, M., Blouquit, Y., et al.: A method for isolation of abnormal haemoglobins with high oxygen affinity due to a frozen quaternary R-structure: Application to Hb Creteil, $\alpha_2^A\beta_2$ (F5) 89 Asn. FEBS Lett. 43:93, 1974.
155. Brennan, S. O., Winterbourn, C. C., and Carrell, R. W.: Isolation of high oxygen affinity hemoglobins. Hemoglobin 1:479, 1977.
156. Rieder, R. F., Oski, F. A., and Clegg, J. B.: Hemoglobin Philly (β35 Tyrosine → Phenylala-

nine): Studies in the molecular pathology of hemoglobin. J. Clin. Invest. 48:1627, 1969.
157. Poyart, C. F., Guesnon, P., and Bohn, B. M.: The measurement of the intrinsic alkaline Bohr effect of various human haemoglobins by isoelectric focusing. Biochem. J. 195:493, 1981.
158. Shih, T.-B., and Jones, R. T.: Application of anaerobic ion-exchange chromatography to the separation of hemoglobins in R from T conformational states. Hemoglobin 4:541, 1980.
159. Harkness, D. R., Yu, C. K., Goldberg, M., and Bradley, T. B.: Novel studies on a "silent" high affinity mutant hemoglobin (San Diego, β109 Val→Met). Hemoglobin 5:33, 1981.
160. Lichtman, M. A., Murphy, M. S., and Adamson, J. W.: Detection of mutant hemoglobins with altered affinity for oxygen. Ann. Intern. Med. 84:517, 1976.
161. Hayashi, A., Kidoguchi, K., Suzuki, T., Yamamura, Y., Miwa, S., and Imai, K.: Application of an automatic oxygenation technique to analysis of oxygen equilibrium curves for hemoglobinopathic red cells and functional screening of clinically important hemoglobinopathies. Hemoglobin 3:429, 1979.
162. Rosa, R., Prehu, M.-O., Beuzard, Y., and Rosa, J.: The first case of a complete deficiency of diphosphoglycerate mutase in human erythrocytes. J. Clin. Invest. 62:907, 1978.
162a. Max-Audit, I., Rosa, I., and Marie, J.: Pyruvate kinase hyperactivity genetically determined: Metabolic consequences and molecular characterization. Blood 56:902, 1980.
163. Bagby, G. C., Jr., Richert-Boe, K., and Koler, R. D.: ^{32}P and acute leukemia: Development of leukemia in a patient with hemoglobin Yakima. Blood 52:350, 1978.
164. Charache, S.: Haemoglobins with altered oxygen affinity. Clin. Haematol. 3:357, 1974.
165. Schneider, R. G., Atkins, R. J., Hosty, T. S., Tomlin, G., Casey, R., Lehmann, H., Lorkin, P. A., and Nagai, K.: Haemoglobin Titusville: α 94 Asp→Asn. A new haemoglobin with a lowered affinity for oxygen. Biochim. Biophys. Acta 400:365, 1975.
166. Moo-Penn, W. F., Bechtel, K. C., Schmidt, R. M., Johnson, M. H., Jue, D. L., Schmidt, D. E., Jr., Dunlap, W. M., Opella, S. J., Bonaventura, J., and Bonaventura, C.: Hemoglobin Raleigh (β 1 Valine→Acetylalanine) structural and functional characterization. Biochemistry 16:4872, 1977.
167. Moo-Penn, W. F., McPhedran, P., Bobrow, S., Johnson, M. H., Jue, D. L., and Olsen, K. W.: Hemoglobin Connecticut (β 21(B3) Asp→Gly): A hemoglobin variant with low oxygen affinity. Am. J. Hematol. 11:137, 1981.
168. Gacon, G., Belkhodja, O., Wajcman, H., and Labie, D.: Structural and functional studies of Hb Rothschild β 37(C3) Trp→Arg. A new variant of the $\alpha_1\beta_2$ contact. FEBS Lett. 82:243, 1977.
169. Marinucci, M., Giuliani, A., Maffi, D., Massa, A., Giampaolo, A., Mavilio, F., Zannotti, M., and Tentori, L.: Hemoglobin Bologna ($\alpha_2\beta_2$ 61(E5) Lys→Met). An abnormal human hemoglobin with low oxygen affinity. Biochim. Biophys. Acta 668:209, 1981.
170. Jones, R. T., Brimhall, B., Pootrakul, S., and Gray, G.: Hemoglobin Vancouver $\alpha_2\beta_2$ 73(E17) Asp→Tyr: Its structure and function. J. Molec. Evol. 9:37, 1976.
171. Miyaji, T., Suzuki, H., Ohba, Y., and Shibata, S.: Hemoglobin Agenogi ($\alpha_2\beta_2^{90Lys}$), a slow-moving hemoglobin of a Japanese family resembling Hb E. Clin. Chim. Acta 14:624, 1966.
172. Imai, K., Morimoto, H., Kotani, M., Shibata, S., Miyaji, T., and Matsutomo, K.: Studies on the function of abnormal hemoglobins. II. Oxygen equilibrium of abnormal hemoglobins: Shimonoseki, Ube II, Hikari, Gifu and Agenogi. Biochim. Biophys. Acta 200:197, 1970.
173. Reissmann, K. R., Ruth, W. E., and Nomura, T.: A human hemoglobin with lowered oxygen affinity and impaired heme-heme interactions. J. Clin. Invest. 40:1826, 1961.
174. Bonaventura, J., and Riggs, A.: Hemoglobin Kansas, a human hemoglobin with a neutral amino acid substitution and an abnormal oxygen equilibrium. J. Biol. Chem. 243:980, 1968.
175. Gibson, Q. H., Riggs, A., and Imamura, T.: Kinetic and equilibrium properties of hemoglobin Kansas. J. Biol. Chem. 248:5976, 1973.
176. Nagel, R. L., Lynfield, J., Johnson, J., Landau, L., Bookchin, R. M., and Harris, M. B.: Hemoglobin Beth Israel. A mutant causing clinically apparent cyanosis. New Engl. J. Med. 295:125, 1976.
177. Arous, N., Braconnier, F., Thillet, J., Blouquit, Y., Galacteros, F., Chevrier, M., Bordahandy, C., and Rosa, J.: Hemoglobin Saint Mande β 102 (G4) Asn→Tyr: A new low oxygen affinity variant. FEBS Lett. 126:114, 1981.
178. Arous, N., Thillet, J., Braconnier, F., and Rosa, J.: Personal communication, 1982.
179. Imamura, T., Fujita, S., Ohta, Y., Hanada, M., and Yanase, T.: Hemoglobin Yoshizuka (G10 [108] β Asparagine→Aspartic acid): A new variant with a reduced oxygen affinity from a Japanese family. J. Clin. Invest. 48:2341, 1969.
180. Moo-Penn, W. F., Wolff, J. A., Simon, G., Vacek, M., Jue, D. L., and Johnson, M. H.: Hemoglobin Presbyterian: β 108(G10) Asparagine→Lysine. A hemoglobin variant with low oxygen affinity. FEBS Lett. 92:53, 1978.
181. Thillet, J., Cabun, J., Brien, B., Cohen-Solal, M., Garel, M. C., Minh, M. N., and Rosa, J.: Abnormal functional properties of Hb Hope: $\alpha_2\beta_2$ (H14) Gly→Asp: A low oxygen affinity hemoglobin with decreased DPG effect. FEBS Lett. 47:47, 1974.
182. Stamatoyannopoulos, G., Parer, J. T., and Finch, C. A.: Physiologic implications of a hemoglobin with decreased oxygen affinity (hemoglobin Seattle). New Engl. J. Med. 281:915, 1969.
183. Ogawa, S., Mayer, A., and Shulman, R. G.: High resolution proton magnetic resonance study of the two quaternary states in fully ligated hemoglobin Kansas. Biochem. Biophys. Res. Commun. 49:1485, 1972.
184. Greer, J.: Three-dimensional structure of abnormal human haemoglobins Kansas and Richmond. J. Molec. Biol. 59:99, 1971.
185. Riggs, A., and Gibson, Q. H.: Oxygen equilibrium and kinetics of isolated subunits from hemoglobin Kansas. Proc. Natl. Acad. Sci. USA 70:1718, 1973.
186. Shulman, R. G., Ogawa, S., and Mayer, A.: The two-state model of hemoglobin, Hb Kansas as a model for the low affinity state. *In* Ho, C. (ed.): Hemoglobin and Oxygen Binding. New York, Elsevier Biomedical, 1982, p. 205.

M HEMOGLOBINS

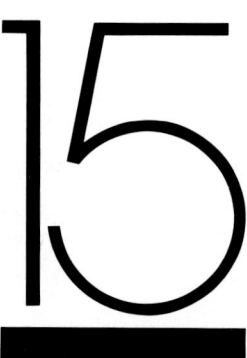

In 1948, a young physician, H. Hörlein, and a medical student, G. Weber, described a family in which certain members had congenital cyanosis.[1] The abnormality was transmitted as an autosomal dominant trait through four generations. The affected individuals had a "lavender-blue" appearance, while their blood appeared brown. Hemolysates had absorption spectra that were similar but not identical to that of methemoglobin. Hörlein and Weber proved that the abnormality lay with the globin and not with the heme by forming hybrids of patient's globin with normal heme and patient's heme with normal globin. Only the former produced the spectral changes present in the native hemolysate. These results provided the first convincing evidence of a familial hemoglobinopathy, antedating by one year Itano and Pauling's discovery of the abnormal electrophoretic behavior of Hb S.[2]

In 1955, Singer[3] designated this type of hemoglobin variant as Hb M. Subsequently other examples of Hb M were discovered[4-6] and were found to have abnormal electrophoretic[7] as well as spectral properties.

The existence of familial cyanosis having an autosomal dominant inheritance pattern has been recognized in Japan since 1800.[8] This disorder, called "Kochikuro" (black mouth) or "Chikuro" (black blood), was restricted to the prefecture of Iwate in the northeast corner of Honshu. In the 1950's, there were about 70 affected individuals residing in this region who had blood "as black as Japanese soy sauce."

The structural analysis of M hemoglobins was first completed by Gerald and Efron.[9] They identified three variants: M-Boston (α 58 His→Tyr), M-Saskatoon (β 63 His→Tyr), and M-Milwaukee-1 (β 67 Val→Glu). Subsequently, the family described by Hörlein and Weber[1] was shown to have Hb M-Saskatoon. The Japanese with "Kochikuro" were found to have a fourth variant. Hb M-Iwate (α 87 His→Tyr).[10] In 1966, Heller and associates[11] described a fifth M hemoglobin: Hyde Park (β 92 His→Tyr). Recently, Hayashi and colleagues

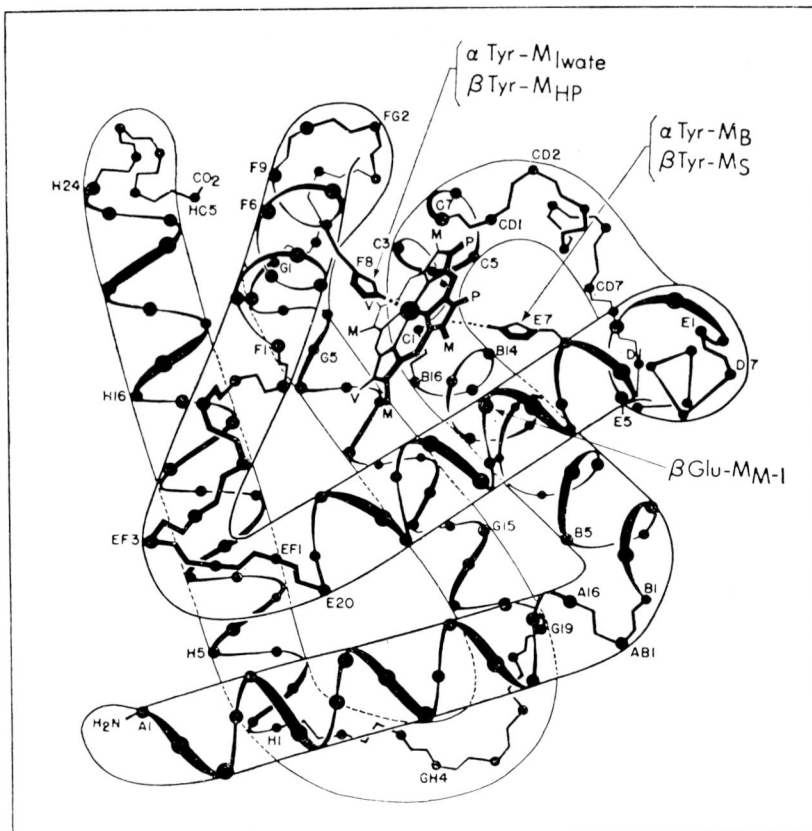

Figure 15–1. Three-dimensional model of hemoglobin subunit modified from Dickerson (1963) showing substituted sites in the M hemoglobins (M_{HP} = M-Hyde Park; M_{M-1} = M-Milwaukee-1; M_B = M-Boston; M_S = M-Saskatoon). (From Ranney, H. M., et al.: Proc. First Inter-Am. Symp. on Hemoglobins, 1971.)

discovered a fetal M hemoglobin. Hb FM-Osaka has the structure γ 63 His→Tyr.[11a] Its properties are very similar to those of Hb M-Saskatoon.*

Because individuals affected with one of the M hemoglobins have a distinctive physical appearance, they have been discovered quite readily in far-flung parts of the globe. For example, Hb M-Saskatoon has been found in Germany, Canada, Britain, the United States, France, Denmark, Norway, Poland, Italy, South Africa, Japan, and the Soviet Union.[14, 15] The various exotic names that have been applied to the M hemoglobins (see Table 10–2*I*) provide further testimony to the worldwide distribution of these variants. Understandably,

---

*The unstable variant Hb St. Louis almost qualifies as an M hemoglobin. The substitution of glutamine for leucine at β 28 causes the heme iron in the abnormal subunits to become completely oxidized to methemoglobin.[12] In addition, other unstable variants such as Hb Freiburg (β 23 Val→0)[13] have an enhanced tendency toward autoxidation. However, these hemoglobins lack the clinical, electrophoretic, and spectral properties shared by the six M hemoglobins.

Hb M has only rarely been recognized in blacks.[11]

As discussed in detail in Chapter 2, the iron atom of the heme group is normally linked to the imidazole group of the proximal (F8) histidine of the α and β chains. Another histidine residue at position E7 is situated on the opposite side, near the sixth coordination position of the heme iron, where oxygen normally binds. Its imidazole group does not form a bond with heme iron unless hemichrome is engendered during hemoglobin denaturation (see Chapter 13). As shown in Figure 15–1, four of the five M hemoglobins involve a substitution of a tyrosine for either the proximal (F8) or distal (E7) histidine in the α or β chain. Gerald and Efron[9] postulated that the phenolic group of the tyrosine residues is able to form a covalent link with the heme iron, thus stabilizing the atom in the oxidized (Fe^{+++}) form.

STRUCTURE-FUNCTION RELATIONSHIPS

Studies on chemically modified hemoglobins have provided important insights into how the protein functions. Among the most thoroughly investigated are the valence hybrids in which the heme iron of either the α or the β chain has been selectively oxidized and then stabilized by the addition of a heme ligand such as cyanide. For example, in $\alpha_2^{CNMet}\beta_2$, the α-chain hemes are frozen in the oxidized state and only the β chains are able to bind oxygen. These valence hybrids, discussed in detail in Chapter 16, may be suitable analogues of partially oxygenated intermediates such as $Hb(O_2)_2$, which have been so difficult to study. Comparable attention has been devoted to the functional properties of the M hemoglobins that are naturally occurring valence hybrids.

Oxygen Equilibria

Because of the close homology between the structure of the α and β chains, one might expect that mutants having a substitution (His→Tyr) at the proximal heme binding site (F8) would have functional properties similar to each other, yet different from those having the substitution at the distal heme binding site (E7). In fact, the experimental results are totally contrary to this expectation. The oxygen equilibria of the M hemoglobins depend primarily on which subunit is affected, rather than whether the substitution is at the proximal or distal histidine. The α-chain M hemoglobins (Boston and Iwate), in which only the β chains react with oxygen, have low oxygen affinity and nearly absent Bohr effect.[16-18] In contrast, the β-chain variants (Saskatoon and Hyde Park), which carry oxygen only on the α chain have nearly normal P_{50} and a substantial Bohr effect.[19-22] Because Hb A binds four oxygen molecules, the total number of protons released upon full oxygenation is $4(\Delta \log P_{50}/\Delta pH)$. Because the M hemoglobins bind only two molecules of oxygen, proton release is only $2(\Delta \log P_{50}/\Delta pH)$. Thus, even though the Bohr coefficients of the β-chain M hemoglobins are substantial and in the case of M-Saskatoon and M-Milwaukee exceed 100 per cent of normal (Table 15–1), the total Bohr effect of these hemoglobins is actually lower than that of Hb A. There is some discrepancy among reported P_{50} and n values. Optimal results are achieved if a methemoglobin-reducing system such as ferredoxin is used, maintaining the normal subunits in the ferrous state but not reducing the variant subunits.[22] Representative oxygen binding curves are shown in Figure 15–2. Hemoglobin M-Milwaukee-1 differs from the other two β variants in having low oxygen affinity (Table 15–1).[23, 24]

Hill plots of oxygen binding curves of the M hemoglobins reveal n values ranging from 1.0 to 1.4. Because only two of the subunits can bind oxygen, the maximal value of n is 2.0 rather than 4.0 as for Hb A. Even so, M hemoglobins have reduced subunit cooperativity compared with Hb A.

When the ferric hemes of the M hemoglobins are converted to the ferrous form by a strong reducing agent, the hemoglobins' functional properties are considerably altered. For example, fully reduced Hb M-Boston acquires nearly full subunit cooperativity ($n = 2.4$) and a normal Bohr effect, whereas fully reduced Hb M-Iwate, which has a substitution at the proximal heme-linked histidine, remains noncooperative.[25] This difference suggests that binding of the ferrous heme iron to the proximal histidine is crucial for normal subunit cooperativity.

Whole blood oxygen binding curves of individuals with M hemoglobin may be right-shifted,[25a] particularly if the variant has low oxygen affinity or if red cell 2,3-DPG is markedly elevated.[26] Because of low subunit cooperativity, the M hemoglobin is less saturated at high oxygen tensions compared with Hb A. These factors increase the amount of deoxyhemoglobin in arterial blood and may contribute to the individual's cyanosis. However, whole blood oxygen affinity is not always decreased.[25a] Individuals with Hb M-Milwaukee and M-Hyde Park have red cells with slightly increased oxygen affinity despite a modest elevation in 2,3-DPG.[27]

X-ray Crystallography

Analysis of the three-dimensional structure of the M hemoglobins by x-ray crystallography has proved useful in explaining their puzzling functional properties. Thus far, four of the variants have been examined: M-Hyde Park,[28] M-Iwate,[28] M-Milwaukee-1,[29] and M-Boston.[30]

When deoxygenated, both Hb M-Hyde Park (β F8 Tyr) and Hb M-Iwate (α F8 Tyr) are isomorphous with deoxy Hb A. This means that the abnormal oxidized subunit assumes the t tertiary conformation. Hb M-Iwate remains in the T quaternary conformation, even after it is fully oxidized. It is likely that the oxygenated form of Hb M-Iwate ($\alpha_2^M \beta_2^{O_2}$) would also remain in the T structure. The stable T structure of Hb M-Iwate and the

Table 15-1. PROPERTIES OF THE M HEMOGLOBINS

	Boston	Iwate	Saskatoon	Hyde Park	Milwaukee
Structure	α 58 His→Tyr	α 87 His→Tyr	β 63 His→Tyr	β 92 His→Tyr	β Val→Glu
Helical residue	E7	F8	E7	F8	E11
% of total Hb		19	35		~50
Hb (g/dl)		17	13–16	10–12.5	14–15
Retic. count			0.8–3.2	4–6	1–2
Whole blood P_{50}	30.8	26.1		21.6 24.7	20.4
P_{50} Hb/P_{50} A (pH 7.2)[16–24]	40/7.1	45/7.1 15/2.9	6.3/6.3	3.0/2.9 1.3/5.0	25/7.1 21/2.9
n value	1.2	1.1, 1.0	1.2	1.4, 1.0	1.5, 1.2
Bohr effect	0%	10%	110%	80%	155%

Quaternary structure[29,30]
  Deoxygenated
  Oxygenated
	
	T*
	T**
		
		T*
		T**
				
				T*
				R**
					
					T*
					R**

Rate of reduction of Fe^{+++} in abnormal chains† by dithionite (T1/2-sec) (Hb A too rapid to be measured)[23]	260		15	55	23
Rate of reduction by NADH-cytochrome b_5 reductase (T 1/2-hr) (Met Hb A = 0.5 hr)[38]	Not reduced	Not reduced	0.5	Not reduced	10
Rate of auto-oxidation of abnormal chains (T 1/2-min) (Hb A = 1440 min)[38]			26		13
Binding of Fe^{+++} in abnormal chains with cyanide (Log K) (Met Hb A = −4.5)[23]	−1.5	−0.6	−3.5	−1.6	−3.2
Rate of heat denaturation[23,54,55]	↓		↑	↑	Sl ↑

*Determined from x-ray data.
**Assumed but unproved (see text).
†With dithionite in presence of CO.

failure to switch to the R structure upon oxygen binding explain the low oxygen affinity and absent Bohr effect of this hemoglobin variant. There was some uncertainty about whether the heme group interacts with the tyrosine at F8 or with histidine at E7, because the analysis of Hb M-Iwate was done at relatively low resolution (5.5 Å). However, recent proton NMR[31,32] and resonance Raman studies* indicate that the heme iron of the abnormal α subunit in Hb M-Iwate is coordinated to F8 tyrosine but when the heme iron is reduced and bound to CO[31] or NO,[33] the iron is then bound to the distal (E7) histidine.

Hb M-Hyde Park differs from Hb M-Iwate in its ability to assume an R conformation when fully oxidized. In view of its Bohr effect, Hb M-Hyde Park probably switches from the T to the R conformation upon full oxygenation. The x-ray data indicated a loss of about 20 to 30 per cent of the β-chain heme groups. This observation helps to explain the relative instability of Hb M-Hyde Park.[21] Because of heme loss, the resolution in the vicinity of the β hemes of Hb M-Hyde Park was reduced,

*K. Nagai and T. Kitagawa: Personal communication, 1982.

M HEMOGLOBINS

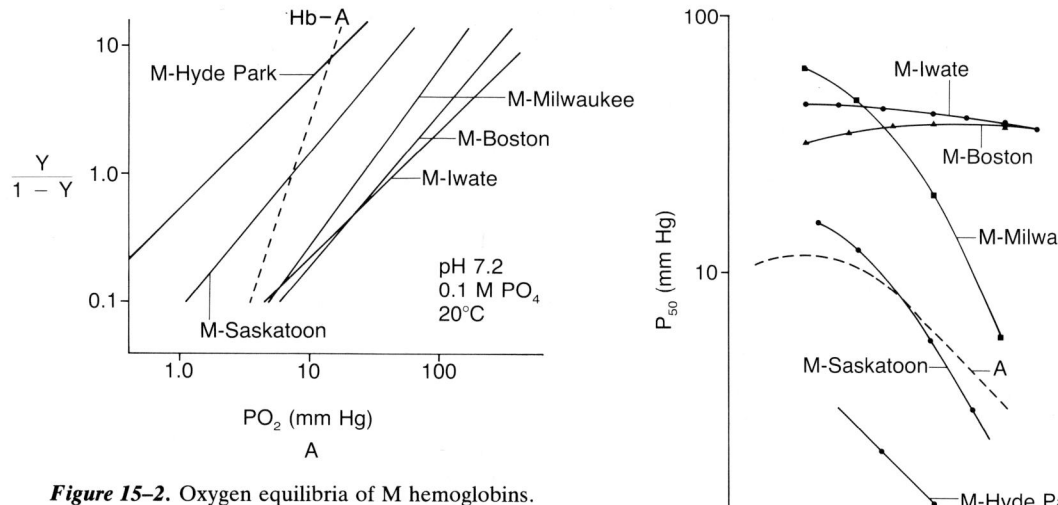

Figure 15–2. Oxygen equilibria of M hemoglobins. *A*, Hill plots. As shown by the slopes of the Hill plots ($n = 1.0$ to 1.3), all the M hemoglobins have decreased subunit cooperativity. In contrast, the n value for hemoglobin A (Hb A) is 3.0 (dotted line). *B*, Bohr effect. (Data from references 17 to 19, 22, and 23; data adjusted to conditions given within graph.)

and therefore, the position of the tyrosine at β F8 remains uncertain. However, from the position of the heme group relative to E7 histidine, F8 tyrosine probably does not act as an internal ligand stabilizing the Fe^{+++} atom. On the other hand, the x-ray data on Hb M-Iwate do indicate that such a linkage occurs as predicted by Gerald and Efron.[9] There are kinetic data that support the structural evidence for a difference between Hb M-Hyde Park and Hb M-Iwate in the stability of the internal ligand at F8. For example, both Hb

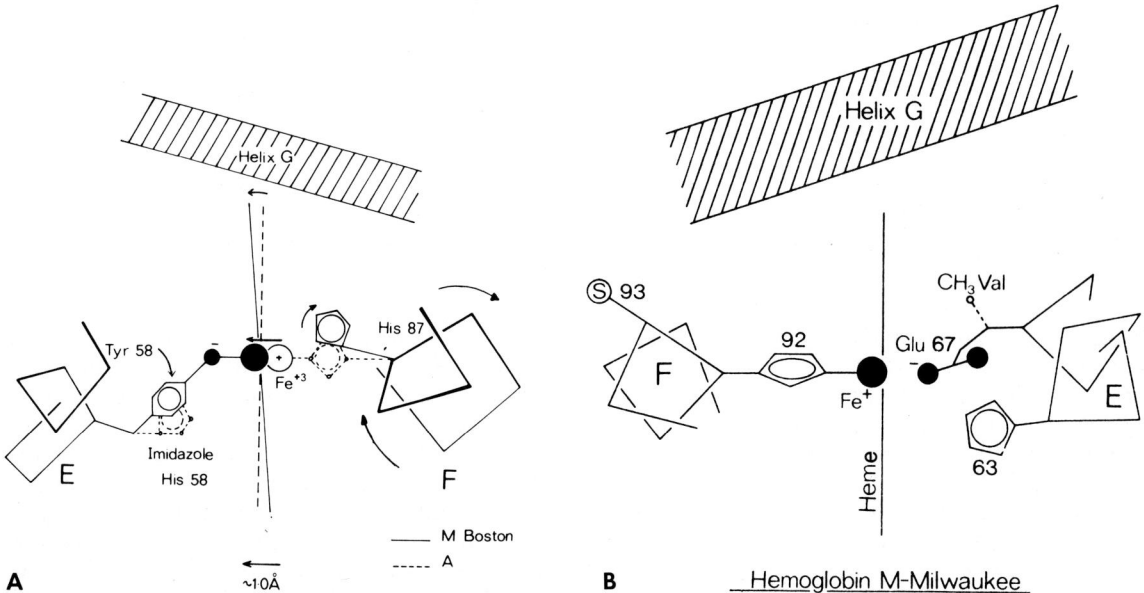

Figure 15–3. *A*, Schematic diagram of the abnormal β chain of Hb M-Boston showing the relationship of the iron atom to the plane of the porphyrin ring (shown as straight and dotted lines) and the substituted tyrosine at α 58 (E7) forming a bond with the iron atom. (From Pulsinelli, P. D., et al.: Proc. Natl. Acad. Sci. USA *70*:3870, 1973.) *B*, Schematic diagram of the abnormal β chain of Hb M-Milwaukee-1 showing the binding of the carboxyl group of the substituted glutamic acid at β 67 with the oxidized iron atom. (From Perutz, M. F., et al.: Nature [New Biol.] *237*:259, 1972.)

M-Iwate and the other α variant, Hb M-Boston, have a much slower rate of reduction of the abnormal subunit's heme Fe^{+++} than have M-Hyde Park and the other two β-chain M hemoglobins[34, 35] (see below). Furthermore, the α-chain M hemoglobins have a very slow rate of reaction with cyanide and weaker binding, in keeping with the presence of a strong internal ligand (see Table 15–1).[36]

The x-ray analysis of Hb M-Boston (α E7 Tyr) produced quite surprising results.[30] Deoxygenated Hb M-Boston is isomorphous with deoxyhemoglobin A. The α heme Fe^{+++} is bonded to the phenolate group of E7 tyrosine. The iron atom is displaced to the distal side of the porphyrin ring and is no longer bonded to the proximal (F8) histidine. Thus, the Fe^{+++} heme of the abnormal subunit is five-coordinated. Proton NMR spectra of Hb M-Boston confirm that the α heme iron is coordinated to E7 tyrosine.[32] These relationships are shown diagrammatically in Figure 15–3A. It is likely that Hb M-Boston remains in the T conformation even after it is oxygenated. Pulsinelli and coworkers[30] found that the x-ray diffraction pattern of the deoxy crystals was preserved even after exposure to air. Failure to undergo a switch to the R conformation would explain the low oxygen affinity and absent Bohr effect of Hb M-Boston. As mentioned above, when Hb M-Boston is chemically reduced to $\alpha_2^{++}\beta_2^{++}$, it has normal heme-heme interaction and near-normal Bohr effect.[25] It is likely that the reduced iron (Fe^{++}) binds to the proximal (F8) histidine, because the phenolate group has a relatively weak affinity for Fe^{++}. This prediction has been verified by EPR measurements.[25] Thus, upon reduction of Hb M-Boston, the iron atom in the α subunit would have to go through the porphyrin ring and come out the other side!

When oxygenated, Hb M-Milwaukee-1 (β E11 Glu) has a quaternary (T) structure like that of deoxyhemoglobin A.[29] The carboxyl group of the substituted glutamic acid at β 67 is coordinated with the heme iron at the sixth position (Fig. 15–3B). In contrast, when fully oxidized, Hb M-Milwaukee-1 assumes an R quaternary structure isomorphous with that of oxyhemoglobin A. Thus, the abnormal β chains of Hb M-Milwaukee-1 can form either the t or the r tertiary structure, depending on the state of the normal α chain. This conclusion gained strong independent support from optical data[29] showing a shift in the red absorption spectrum contributed by the abnormal β chains when the normal α chains reacted with carbon monoxide. In addition, NMR data of Lindstrom and colleagues[37] indicate that such a change in quaternary conformation occurs when deoxyhemoglobin M-Milwaukee is treated with carbon monoxide. The fact that Hb M-Milwaukee-1 has a substantial Bohr effect is also consistent with this conclusion.

Mechanism of Heme Oxidation

The x-ray crystallographic studies described above show how the amino acid substitutions in the M hemoglobins stabilize the heme group in the oxidized form. The redox potentials of the abnormal subunits are abnormally low (see Chapter 16). Compared with normal hemoglobin, the abnormal subunits are much more rapidly oxidized by molecular oxygen.[18, 38] Once oxidized, the abnormal subunit is resistant to reduction both by enzymes[18, 38] and by chemical reducing agents such as dithionite (see Table 15–1).

M. Nagai and colleagues[38] have examined the rate of reduction of the five M hemoglobins by three enzymes: NADH-cytochrome b_5 reductase, NADPH-flavin reductase, and ferredoxin NADP reductase. As discussed in detail in Chapter 16, the first enzyme is responsible for maintaining reduced hemoglobin in normal circulating red blood cells. The M hemoglobins differed markedly in their rates of reduction with these enzymes. As shown in Table 15–1, Hbs M-Iwate, M-Boston, and M-Hyde Park were not reduced at all by cytochrome b_5 reductase. In contrast, Hb M-Milwaukee was reduced slowly (T½ = 10 hr), whereas Hb M-Saskatoon was reduced at the same rate as Met Hb A (T½ = ½ hr). Similar results were obtained with flavin reductase.

These findings pose an enigma: Why are Hbs M-Saskatoon and M-Milwaukee half-oxidized? In fact, individuals with these two variants may have less cyanosis than those with the other M hemoglobins, despite the fact that the proportion of abnormal hemoglobins is higher among these β-chain variants compared with the α-chain variants. Thus, in individuals with Hb M-Saskatoon (and perhaps Hb M-Milwaukee), some of the variant hemoglobin may be fully reduced *in vivo*. That they have cyanosis and that the variant is fully oxidized when examined after *in vitro* isolation can be explained by the fact that the abnormal subunits in these variant hemoglobins autoxidize 50 to 100 times faster than do the subunits of Hb A.[38]

An interesting minor hemoglobin component has been observed in individuals with Hb M-Hyde Park.[39] Cellulose acetate electrophoresis revealed a red hemoglobin band that constituted about 5 per cent of the total and migrated between Hb A_2 and Hbs A and M-Hyde Park. Spectral analysis showed that this minor component was a tetramer containing two normal α chains and two $β^{HP}$ chains, one lacking a heme group but the other having a heme in the reduced form. This species may be an intermediate in the degradation of Hb M-Hyde Park. It would be of interest to determine whether it is present primarily in older red cells.

Physical-Chemical Studies

The M hemoglobins have been used extensively to study subunit cooperativity, because these variants offer several advantages:

1. Since the tetramer binds only two molecules of oxygen (or carbon monoxide) rather than four, formulation of an allosteric model from experimental data is greatly simplified.
2. The cooperativity of ligand binding is sufficiently low that a significant proportion of partially saturated M hemoglobins contains only one ligand per tetramer, permitting their detection and analysis.
3. The electronic or magnetic environment of the oxidized heme on the mutant subunit can be monitored by various physical and chemical probes, such as NMR or EPR.
4. The M hemoglobins are more stable than the valence hybrids prepared from oxidized subunits of normal hemoglobin.

Hemoglobin M-Milwaukee has been investigated exhaustively by means of a broad repertoire of biophysical tools. Both kinetic measurements of ligand binding[40] and proton NMR[41-43] provide strong evidence that the conformation of half-liganded Hb M differs markedly from that of either the unliganded or the fully liganded tetramers. The results pose a stiff challenge to a simple two-state allosteric model. Kinetic studies have also been performed on Hb M-Iwate[44] and Hb M-Saskatoon.[45]

CLINICAL MANIFESTATIONS

Patients have obvious cyanosis but are otherwise totally asymptomatic (see Color Plate IV*A* to *C*). A family history will often elicit a dominant inheritance pattern. However, in a number of affected individuals, the M hemoglobin has apparently arisen as a spontaneous mutation.[14, 46-51] If the individual's cyanosis was apparent at birth, an α-chain M hemoglobin is likely. Alternatively, the newborn could have fetal Hb M.[11a] If so, the cyanosis will disappear when the γ to β switch is complete at about six months of age. The β-chain M hemoglobins do not present clinically until the γ chain has been replaced by β chains at about six months of age.

The blood has a chocolate brown appearance and does not "pink up" when equilibrated with room air. Routine hematological parameters are usually within normal limits. Some but not all individuals with the β-chain M hemoglobins (Hyde Park and Saskatoon) have a mild compensated hemolytic state[34, 46, 49, 52, 53] consistent with the fact that these two hemoglobin variants are slightly unstable when exposed to heat, sodium benzoate,[35] or isopropanol.[54] Heinz bodies have been demonstrated in red cells of individuals with Hb M-Saskatoon.[54] The fact that x-ray crystallography of Hb M-Hyde Park revealed a partial loss of hemes from the β chains also supports this contention and explains the formation of the partially heme-depleted minor hemoglobin component described above. Biosynthetic studies of Hb M-Saskatoon show slightly enhanced turnover of the variant β chain.[54] Another individual with Hb M-Saskatoon had a significant decrease in hematocrit following ingestion of an oxidant drug.[49] Hemichrome has been observed during proteolytic degradation of Hb M-Saskatoon[15] and may be an intermediate in its catabolism. An individual with Hb M-Hyde Park was found to have significant anemia (Hb = 10.7 g/dl) owing to both hemolysis and ineffective erythropoiesis.[27] The basis of the latter finding is unclear. Hb M-Milwaukee also appears to be slightly unstable,[55] but affected individuals do not have significant hemolysis.

Hemoglobin catabolism may be abnormal in individuals with M hemoglobins, even if they have normal red cell survival. Abnormal isomers of biliverdin have been demonstrated when Hb M-Iwate was subjected to nonenzymatic oxidation.[56]

Diagnosis

The presumptive diagnosis of M hemoglobin is made from absorption spectra of hemolysate and hemoglobin electrophoresis.

Spectral abnormalities of the M hemoglobins

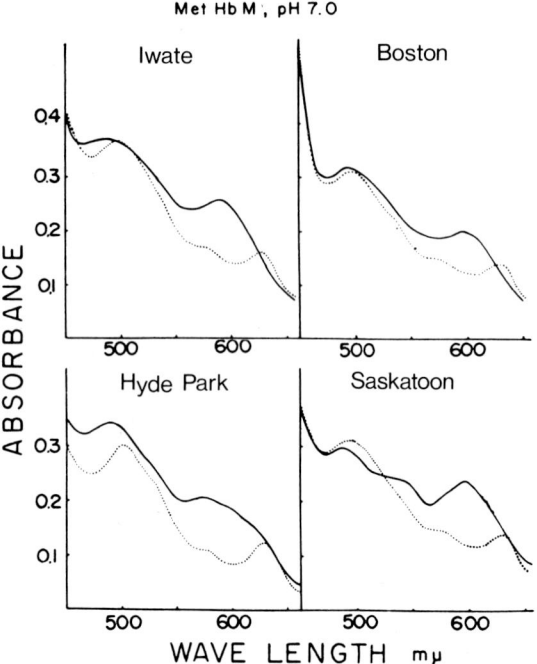

Figure 15–4. Absorption spectra of purified M hemoglobins after they had been fully oxidized with ferricyanide. The absorption spectrum of normal methemoglobin A is shown by the dotted line. (From Shibata, S., et al.: Bull. Yamaguchi Med. Sch. *14*:141, 1967.)

are best seen if all the hemoglobin is oxidized to the Fe^{+++} state with ferricyanide. As Figure 15–4 shows, the absorption spectrum of each of the M hemoglobins differs slightly from the others and can be readily distinguished from that of normal methemoglobin.[8] However, it is not possible to identify any of the M hemoglobins on the basis of absorption spectra, because the results are affected by differences in the composition of the buffer and the purity of the sample. EPR spectroscopy provides a more specific identification of several of the M hemoglobins.[57, 58]

Electrophoresis. The M hemoglobins can also be demonstrated by electrophoresis under appropriate conditions. Routine electrophoresis of the oxygenated hemolysate at pH 8.6 usually fails to separate the normal and abnormal hemoglobins. However, electrophoresis on agar gel at pH 7.1 will generally reveal a brown band (Hb M) running slightly on the anodal side of a red band (Hb A). A much sharper pattern can be obtained with gel electrofocusing (Fig. 15–5). A wider separation of M and A hemoglobins is achieved if the hemolysate is oxidized with ferricyanide.[7] Methemoglobin A has a much higher isoelectric point (more positive surface charge) than methemoglobin M, because the Fe^{+++} atoms of the abnormal subunits are neutralized by an internal ligand.

The *differential diagnosis* rests between hemoglobin M and congenital methemoglobinemia (cytochrome b_5 reductase deficiency). The former has a dominant inheritance pattern, whereas the latter has a recessive pattern. The two disorders can be readily distinguished by a spectral analysis of the hemolysate and hemoglobin electrophoresis. Cytochrome b_5 reductase deficiency is discussed in Chapter 16.

Once the presumptive diagnosis of Hb M is made, the structural abnormality should be identified. The M hemoglobins can be purified by chromatography on Biorex-70. The red Hb A elutes faster than the brown Hbs M, which remain at the top of the column. Once the separation has been achieved, it is convenient to split the column and then elute the purified components. Usually, the α-chain M hemoglobins make up 15 to 30 per cent of the total, and the β-chain variants make up 40 to 50 per cent. The structural abnormality can be identified from peptide maps of tryptic digests of the abnormal subunit. Specific stains for histidine and tyrosine are very useful in interpreting the fingerprints.

Treatment

No specific treatment of these individuals is either indicated or possible. It is important that the patient be thoroughly informed of the benign nature of the disorder. The primary reason for establishing the diagnosis is to provide adequate reassurance and to prevent iatrogenic misadventures that might arise under the mistaken impression that the patient has a cardiac or pulmonary disorder. One member of the original family described by Hörlein and Weber[1] was barred from military service during the Franco-Prussian war. Individuals with M hemoglobins have undergone cardiac catheterization[51, 59] and even exploratory surgery[60] because of presumed heart disease. One woman in labor was refused anesthesia because "she was already cyanotic."[14] A patient believing she had heart disease declined to have abdominal surgery.[61] Another unfortunate subject was confined to a bed-and-chair existence because his solicitous family felt he had a life-threatening illness.[62]

M HEMOGLOBINS 631

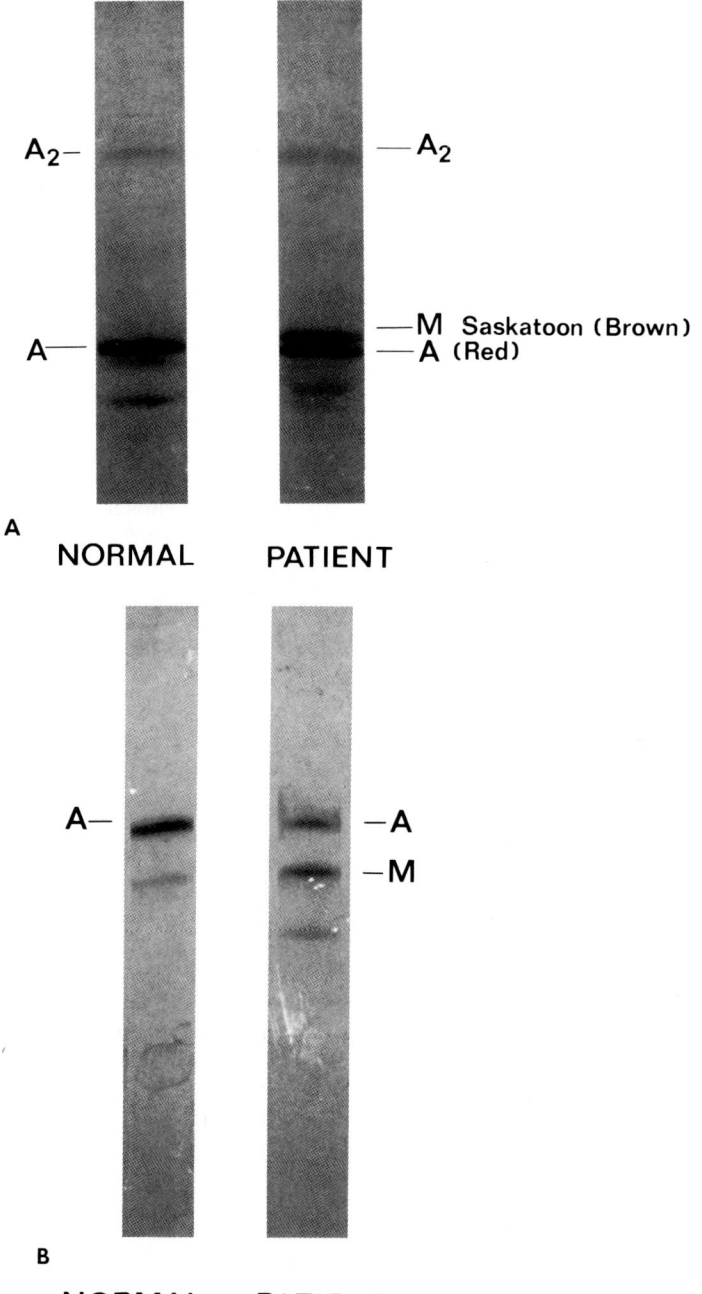

Figure 15-5. Gel electrofocusing patterns obtained on hemolysate of patient with Hb M-Saskatoon. *A*, Pattern obtained on oxygenated specimens showing separation of red Hb A band and brown Hb M-Saskatoon band. *B*, Pattern obtained after ferricyanide, showing wider separation of Hbs A and M-Saskatoon. (The structural analysis of Hb M-Saskatoon was determined by Dr. Thomas Bradley.)

References

1. Hörlein, H., and Weber, G.: Über chronische familiäre Methämoglobinämie und eine neue Modifikation des Methämoglobins. Dtsch. Med. Wochenschr. 73:476, 1948.
2. Pauling, L., Itano, H. A., Singer, S. J., and Wells, I. C.: Sickle cell anemia: A molecular disease. Science 110:543, 1949.
3. Singer, K.: Hereditary hemolytic disorders associated with abnormal hemoglobins. Am. J. Med. 18:633, 1955.
4. Kiese, M., Kurz, H., and Schneider, C.: Chronische Hämoglobinämie durch pathologischen Blutfarbstoff. Klin. Wochenschr. 34:957, 1956.
5. Gerald, P. S., Cook, C. D., and Diamond, L. K.: Hemoglobin M. Science 126:300, 1957.
6. Pisciotta, A. V., Ebbe, S. N., and Hinz, J. E.: Clinical and laboratory features of two variants of methemoglobin M disease. J. Lab. Clin. Med. 54:73, 1959.
7. Gerald, P. S.: The electrophoretic and spectroscopic characterization of Hgb M. Blood 13:936, 1958.
8. Shibata, S., Miyaji, T., Iuchi, I., Ohba, Y., and Yamamoto, K.: Hemoglobins M of the Japanese. Bull. Yamaguchi Med. Sch. 14:141, 1967.
9. Gerald, P. S., and Efron, M. L.: Chemical studies of several varieties of Hb M. Proc. Natl. Acad. Sci. USA 47:1758, 1961.
10. Shibata, S., Miyaji, T., Iuchi, I., and Tamura, A.: Substitution of tyrosine for histidine (87) in the α chain of hemoglobin M_{Iwate}. Acta Haematol. Jpn. 27:13, 1964.
11. Heller, P., Coleman, R. D., and Yakulis, V. J.: Structural studies of haemoglobin M-Hyde Park. Proceedings of the XI Congress of the International Society of Hematology. Sydney, 1966, pp. 427–434.
11a. Hayashi, A., Fujita, T., Fujimura, M., and Titani, K.: A new abnormal fetal hemoglobin, Hb FM-Osaka ($\alpha_2\gamma_2^{63\ His\ Tyr}$). Hemoglobin 4:447, 1981.
12. Cohen-Solal, M., Seligmann, M., Thillet, J., and Rosa, J.: Haemoglobin Saint Louis β28 (B10) leucine→glutamine. A new unstable haemoglobin only present in a ferri form. FEBS Lett. 33:37, 1973.
13. Jones, R. T., Brimhall, B., Huisman, T. H. J., Kleihauer, E., and Betke, K.: Hemoglobin Freiburg: Abnormal hemoglobin due to deletion of a single amino acid residue. Science 154:1024, 1966.
14. Vella, F., Kamuzora, H., Lehmann, H., Duncan, B., and Harold, W.: A second family with hemoglobin M Saskatoon in Saskatchewan. Clin. Biochem. 7:186, 1974.
15. Moldchandva, T. P., Abaturov, L. V., Spivak, V. A., and Ermakov, N. V.: Hemoglobin M Saskatoon alpha 2 beta 2 63 (E7) His→Tyr. Structural identification, hemichrome formation and proteolytic degradation. Mol. Biol. (Mosk.) 14:1253, 1980.
16. Kikochi, G., Hayashi, N., and Tamura, A.: Oxygen equilibrium of hemoglobin M_{Iwate}. Biochim. Biophys. Acta 90:199, 1964.
17. Suzuki, T., Hayashi, A., Yamamura, Y., Enoki, Y., and Tyuma, I.: Functional abnormality of hemoglobin M_{Osaka}. Biochem. Biophys. Res. Commun. 19:691, 1965.
18. Hayashi, N., Motokawa, Y., and Kikuchi, G.: Studies on relationships between structure and function of hemoglobin M_{Iwate}. J. Biol. Chem. 241:79, 1966.
19. Suzuki, T., Hayashi, A., Shimizu, A., and Yamamura, Y.: The oxygen equilibrium of hemoglobin $M_{Saskatoon}$. Biochim. Biophys. Acta 127:280, 1966.
20. Ranney, H. M., Nagel, R. L., Heller, P., and Udem, L.: Oxygen equilibrium of hemoglobin M-Hyde Park. Biochim. Biophys. Acta 160:112, 1968.
21. Hayashi, A., Suzuki, T., Shimizu, A., Imai, K., Morimoto, H., Miyaji, T., and Shibata, S.: Some observations on the physicochemical properties of hemoglobin $M_{Hyde\ Park}$. Arch. Biochem. Biophys. 125:895, 1968.
22. Shih, T.-B., Imai, K., Tyuma, I., Hayashi, A., and Shibata, S.: Further studies on the functional properties of hemoglobin M Hyde Park. Hemoglobin 4:125, 1980.
23. Hayashi, A., Suzuki, T., Imai, K., Morimoto, H., and Watari, H.: Properties of hemoglobin M-Milwaukee-1 variant and its unique characteristics. Biochim. Biophys. Acta 194:6, 1969.
24. Udem, L., Ranney, H. M., Bunn, H. F., and Pisciotta, A.: Some observations on the properties of hemoglobin M-Milwaukee-1. J. Molec. Biol. 48:489, 1970.
25. Nishikura, K., Sugita, Y., Nagai, M., Yoneyama, Y., and Jagenburg, R.: High cooperativity of haemoglobin M Boston in the completely reduced state. Nature 254:727, 1975.
25a. Hayashi, A., Kidoguchi, K., Suzuki, T., Yamamura, Y., Miwa, S., and Imai, K.: Application of an automatic oxygenation technique to analysis of oxygen equilibrium curves for hemoglobinopathic red cells and functional screening of clinically important hemoglobinopathies. Hemoglobin 3:426, 1979.
26. Byckova, V., Wajcman, H., Labie, D., and Travers, F.: Hemoglobin M Saskatoon: Further data on biophysics and oxygen equilibrium. Biochim. Biophys. Acta 243:117, 1971.
27. Shibata, S., Yawata, Y., Yamada, O., Koresawa, S., and Ueda, S.: Altered erythropoiesis and increased hemolysis in hemoglobin M Akita (M Hyde Park β 92 His→Tyr) disease. Hemoglobin 1:111, 1976.
28. Greer, J.: Three-dimensional structure of abnormal human haemoglobins M Hyde Park and M Iwate. J. Molec. Biol. 59:107, 1971.
29. Perutz, M. F., Pulsinelli, P. D., and Ranney, H. M.: Structure and subunit interaction of haemoglobin M Milwaukee. Nature [New Biol.] 237:259, 1972.
30. Pulsinelli, P. D., Perutz, M. F., and Nagel, R. L.: Structure of hemoglobin M Boston, a variant with a five coordinated ferric heme. Proc. Natl. Acad. Sci. USA 70:3870, 1973.
31. Peisach, J., and Gersonde, K.: Binding of CO to mutant α chains of hemoglobin M Iwate; evidence for distal imidazole ligation. Biochemistry 16:2539, 1977.
32. La Mar, G. N., Nagai, K., Jue, T., Budd, D. L., Gersonde, K., Sick, H., Kagimoto, T., Hayashi, A., and Taketa, F.: Assignment of proximal histidyl imidazole exchangeable proton NMR resonances to individual subunits in hemoglobins A, Boston, Iwate and Milwaukee. Biochem. Biophys. Res. Commun. 96:1172, 1980.
33. Nagai, K., Hori, H., Morimoto, H., Hayashi, A., and Taketa, F.: Influence of amino acid replacements in the heme pocket on the electron paramagnetic resonance spectra and absorption spectra of nitrosylhemoglobins M Iwate, M Boston, and M Milwaukee. Biochemistry 18:1304, 1979.
34. Shibata, S., Miyaji, T., Karita, K., et al.: A new type of hereditary nigremia discovered in Akita-hemoglobin M Hyde Park disease. Proc. Jpn. Acad. 43:65, 1967.
35. Hayashi, A., Suzuki, T., Shimizu, A., and Yama-

mura, Y.: Properties of hemoglobin M. Unequivalent nature of the α and β subunits in the hemoglobin molecule. Biochim. Biophys. Acta 168:262, 1968.
36. Hayashi, A., Shimizu, A., Suzuki, T., and Yamamura, Y.: The properties of hemoglobin M. Reactivity of methemoglobin M to cyanide, azide and fluoride. Biochim. Biophys. Acta 140:251, 1967.
37. Lindstrom, T. R., Ho, C., and Pisciotta, A. V.: Nuclear magnetic resonance studies of haemoglobin M Milwaukee. Nature [New Biol.] 237:263, 1972.
38. Nagai, M., Yubisui, T., and Yoneyama, Y.: Enzymatic reduction of hemoglobins M Milwaukee-1 and M Saskatoon by NADH-cytochrome b_5 reductase and NADPH-flavin reductase purified from human erythrocytes. J. Biol. Chem. 255:4599, 1980.
39. Shibata, S., and Iuchi, I.: Characterization of a red minor component of abnormal hemoglobin found in Hb M Hyde Park disease. Hemoglobin 1:829, 1977.
40. Makino, N., Sugita, Y., and Nakamura, T.: Kinetic studies on the cooperative ligand binding by hemoglobin M Milwaukee. J. Biol. Chem. 254:2353, 1979.
41. Fung, L. W.-M., Minton, A. P., and Ho, C.: Nuclear magnetic resonance study of heme-heme interaction in hemoglobin M Milwaukee: Implications concerning the mechanism of cooperative ligand binding in normal hemoglobin. Proc. Natl. Acad. Sci. USA 73:1581, 1976.
42. Fung, L. W.-M., Minton, A. P., Lindstrom, T. R., Pisciotta, A. V., and Ho, C.: Proton nuclear magnetic resonance studies of hemoglobin M Milwaukee and their implications concerning the mechanism of cooperative oxygenation of hemoglobin. Biochemistry 16:1452, 1977.
43. Takahashi, S., Lin, A. K.-L.C., and Ho, C.: Proton nuclear magnetic resonance studies of hemoglobins M Boston (α 58 E7 His→Tyr) and M Milwaukee (β 67 E11 Val→Glu): Spectral assignments of hyperfine-shifted proton resonances and of proximal histidine (E7) NH resonances to the α and β chains of normal human adult hemoglobin. Biochemistry 19:5196, 1980.
44. Salhany, J. M., Castillo, C. L., and Ogawa, S.: Carbon monoxide binding properties of hemoglobin M Iwate. Biochemistry 15:5344, 1976.
45. Makino, N., Sugita, Y., and Nakamura, T.: Kinetic studies on the cooperative ligand binding by valency hybrid hemoglobins. Hemoglobin M Saskatoon and cyanomet hybrids. J. Biol. Chem. 254:10862, 1979.
46. Josephson, A. M., Weinstein, H. G., Yakulis, B. S., Singer, L., and Heller, P.: A new variant of hemoglobin M disease: Hemoglobin $M_{Chicago}$. J. Lab. Clin. Med. 59:918, 1962.
47. Farmer, M. B., Lehmann, H., and Raine, D. N.: Two unrelated patients with congenital cyanosis due to haemoglobinopathy. M. Lancet 2:786, 1964.
48. Becroft, D. M. O., Douglas, R., Carrell, R. W., and Lehmann, H.: Haemoglobin M Hyde Park: A hereditary methaemoglobinaemia in a Caucasian child. N.Z. Med. J. 68:72, 1968.
49. Stavem, P., Strömme, J., Lorkin, P. A., and Lehmann, H.: Haemoglobin M Saskatoon with slight constant haemolysis, markedly increased by sulfonamides. Scand. J. Haematol. 9:566, 1972.
50. Kohne, E., Grosse, H. P., Versmold, K., Kley, H. P., and Kleihauer, E.: Hb M Erlangen: $α_2β_2^{63(E7) Tyr}$: Eine neue Mutation mit Hämolyse und Diaphorasemangel. Z. Kinderheilkd. 120:69, 1975.
51. Stamatoyannopoulos, G., Nute, P. E., Giblett, E., Detter, J., and Chard, R.: Haemoglobin M Hyde Park occurring as a fresh mutation: Diagnostic, structural, and genetic considerations. J. Med. Genet. 13:142, 1976.
52. Hobolth, N.: Haemoglobin $M_{Århus}$. I. Clinical family study. Acta Paediatr. Scand. 54:357, 1965.
53. Heller, P.: Hemoglobin M—an early chapter in the saga of molecular pathology. Ann. Intern. Med. 70:1038, 1969.
54. Baine, R. M., Wright, J. M., Johnson, M. H., and Cadena, C. L.: Biosynthetic evidence for instability of Hb M Saskatoon. Hemoglobin 4:201, 1980.
55. Kohne, E., Wendt, F.-K., and Kleihauer, E.: Hb M Milwaukee in a German family. Hemoglobin 1:759, 1977.
56. Brown, S. B., Docherty, J. C., and Bradley, T. B.: Bile-pigment isomers from degradation of haemoglobin M Iwate. Biochem. Soc. Trans. 5:1020, 1977.
57. Hayashi, A., Shimizu, A., Yamamura, Y., and Watari, H.: Hemoglobins M: Identification of Iwate, Boston and Saskatoon variants. Science 152:207, 1966.
58. Hayashi, A., Suzuki, T., and Fujita, T.: Diagnosis of Hb M disease by electron paramagnetic resonance spectra. Hemoglobin 4:573, 1980.
59. Overly, W. L., Rosenberg, A., and Harris, J. W.: Hemoglobin M Reserve: Studies on identification and characterization. J. Lab. Clin. Med. 69:62, 1967.
60. Nagel, R. L., and Bookchin, R. M.: Human hemoglobin mutants with abnormal oxygen binding. Semin. Hematol. 11:385, 1974.
61. Baltzman, D. M., and Sugarman, H.: Hereditary cyanosis. Can. Med. Assoc. J. 62:348, 1950.
62. Lehmann, H., and Huntsman, R. G.: Man's Haemoglobins. 2nd ed. Philadelphia, J. B. Lippincott Co., 1974.

HEMOGLOBIN OXIDATION: METHEMOGLOBIN, METHEMOGLOBINEMIA, AND SULFHEMOGLOBINEMIA

16

Hemoglobin's color is one of its most appealing properties. Most chemical reactions that involve the heme group cause a detectable change in hemoglobin's visible absorption spectrum. These include not only the reversible binding of ligands such as oxygen and carbon monoxide to heme, but also the oxidation and reduction of the heme iron. When free ferroheme (Fe^{2+}) is exposed to oxygen, it readily autoxidizes to ferriheme (Fe^{3+}). In contrast, when ferroheme is properly inserted into globin subunits, thereby forming hemoglobin, it is able to bind oxygen reversibly without rapid autoxidation. Whatever oxidized hemoglobin (methemoglobin) is formed in red cells is readily reduced back to ferrohemoglobin by an enzyme system.

Investigation of the oxidation and reduction of hemoglobin has provided important insights into its functional behavior. The stepwise transition from fully reduced hemoglobin ($\alpha_2^{2+}\beta_2^{2+}$) to fully oxidized methemoglobin ($\alpha_2^{3+}\beta_2^{3+}$) involves intermediates, called valence hybrids, that are useful models in the study of subunit cooperativity. Indeed, many parallels can be drawn between oxygenation and oxidation of hemoglobin. Furthermore, an understanding of the mechanisms responsible for hemoglobin oxidation is necessary for defining the complex process of hemoglobin degradation. Finally, the oxidation of hemoglobin has clear-cut clinical relevance. The accumulation of significant amounts of methemoglobin in circulating red cells leads to a striking physical finding, cyanosis, as well as impairment of oxygen transport.

In this chapter the physical and chemical properties of methemoglobin will be described, and then the mechanisms, both physiologic and nonphysiologic, that lead to its formation will be considered. The red cell's methemoglobin reducing system, cytochrome b_5 and its reductase, will be described in detail and compared with nonenzymatic means of reducing methemoglobin. This information will be useful in considering clinical disorders: congenital and acquired methemoglobinemia as well as the less common entity, sulfhemoglobinemia.

This colorful topic spans a diverse group of disciplines, including physical biochemistry, enzymology, genetics, toxicology, and pharmacology.

PROPERTIES OF METHEMOGLOBIN

Absorbance and EPR Spectra

When red oxyhemoglobin (or purple deoxyhemoglobin) is treated with an appropriate oxidizing agent such as ferricyanide, the hemoglobin turns a mahogany-brown color. This simple laboratory demonstration appeals equally to Cub Scouts and medical students! The transition from a red to brown color indicates a marked increase in absorbance in the red region of the visible spectrum (600 to 650 nm). As shown in Figure 16–1, methemoglobin has a strong absorbance peak at 630 nm. Note that the absorbance spectrum of methemoglobin is strongly pH-dependent. At low pH, a water molecule occupies the space between the ferric iron and the distal histidine. This species is sometimes called aquomethemoglobin. With increasing pH, there is progressive binding of the negatively charged hydroxyl anion (OH^-) to the positively charged ferric iron (hydroxymethemoglobin). Note that at alkaline pH the absorbance spectrum bears some resemblance to that of methemoglobin bound to other anions such as cyanide, azide, and fluoride.

Methemoglobin and its derivatives have characteristic electron paramagnetic resonance (EPR) spectra reflecting the electronic spin state of the iron atom. In aquomethemoglobin, the iron atom has a fully unpaired electron and therefore has a "high spin" state and is

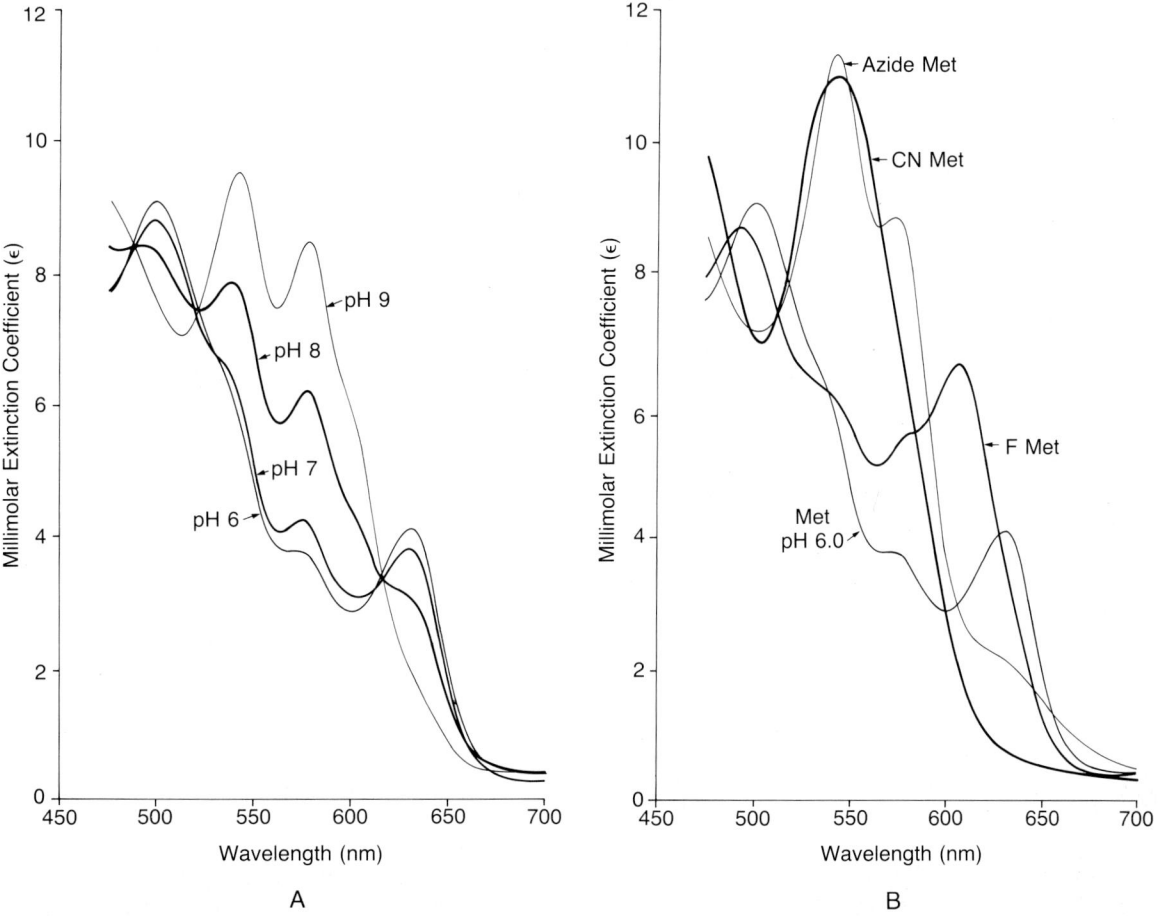

Figure 16–1. Absorption spectra of methemoglobin and its derivatives. *A,* Spectra of normal human hemoglobin A at pH 6.06, 7.01 (in 0.05 M bis-TRIS HCl, 25°C); 7.93, 8.80 (in 0.05 M TRIS HCl, 25°C). *B,* Spectra of methemoglobin, fluoremethemoglobin, azidomethemoglobin, and cyanmethemoglobin (in 0.05 M bis-TRIS HCl, pH 6.0).

strongly paramagnetic. With increasing pH and the formation of hydroxymethemoglobin, the iron atom goes from a high spin state to a low spin state, accompanied by a decrease in atomic radius.

Certain other anions, such as cyanide and azide, can also transform methemoglobin to a low spin state similar to oxyhemoglobin and carboxyhemoglobin. All of these derivatives share a number of physical and chemical properties. In contrast, other anions, such as fluoride, bind weakly to the ferriheme iron and do not lower the spin state.

Three-Dimensional Structure

The earliest studies on the three-dimensional structure of horse hemoglobin in fact pertained to methemoglobin, because the oxyhemoglobin crystals autoxidized to methemoglobin during their prolonged period of analysis. The structure of horse methemoglobin was first solved at 5.5 Å resolution,[1] subsequently at 2.8 Å,[2] and, most recently, at 2.0 Å.[3] Aquomethemoglobin was shown to be isomorphous with carboxyhemoglobin[4] as well as with methemoglobin liganded with cyanide[5] and azide.[6] All of these forms of hemoglobin crystallize in the R conformation. The heme stereochemistry is identical in all of these derivatives, but there are significant differences among them, such as the orientation of the ligand relative to the heme iron.[5,6] Because these derivatives differ in their spin state, as described above, both the displacement of the iron atom from the plane of the porphyrin ring and the distance between the iron atom and the ε-nitrogen of the proximal histidine should also vary correspondingly. However, such small changes in bond length cannot be detected by x-ray crystallography, even at 2 Å resolution. Currently, a powerful spectroscopic probe known as EXAFS* is being used for the assignment of specific bonds involving metal atoms. It will be of interest to see how precise measurements of bond length tally with the electronic state of the heme iron.

As described in detail in Chapter 2, the equilibrium between the R and T quaternary structures is believed to be triggered primarily by the displacement of the ε-nitrogen of the proximal histidine relative to the mean plane of the porphyrin ring. In deoxyhemoglobin, this distance is 2.7 Å, whereas in oxyhemoglobin, the distance is 2.0 Å. In methemoglobin and its liganded derivative fluoromethemoglobin, the N_ϵ-porphyrin distance is intermediate, 2.3 ± 0.1 Å. Thus, the value of the constant $L = [T]/[R]$ from the Monod-Wyman-Changeaux allosteric model should also be intermediate.[7] In this oversimplified but useful view, methemoglobin and fluoromethemoglobin would be expected to undergo a shift from the R to the T quaternary structure more readily than low spin derivatives such as oxyhemoglobin, carboxyhemoglobin, or cyanide methemoglobin. In fact, Fermi and Perutz[7] have analyzed crystals of human fluoromethemoglobin bound to the potent organic phosphate modifier inositol hexaphosphate (IHP) and have found that they were isomorphous with deoxyhemoglobin A.

These structural studies provide solid support for the large body of biochemical evidence that methemoglobin is conformationally metastable and can be pulled to the T quaternary structure under certain solvent conditions such as low pH and the presence of organic phosphates. The demonstration by Perutz and colleagues[8] of a red shift in the visible absorbance spectrum upon addition of IHP to methemoglobin suggests a transition from the R to the T conformation. Their ultraviolet circular dichroism measurements are also consistent with this interpretation.[9] In addition, nuclear magnetic resonance spectra indicate that both fluoromethemoglobin and aquomethemoglobin assume the deoxy T structure in the presence of IHP because they exhibit the same slowly exchanging protons.[10,11] Finally, the change in sulfhydryl reactivity upon addition of IHP also indicates a switch to the T structure.[9]

Chromatographic and Electrophoretic Behavior

Because the oxidation of heme iron involves an increase in positive charge, it might be expected that methemoglobin could be readily separated from oxyhemoglobin by electrophoresis. In fact, routine electrophoresis of partially oxidized hemoglobin fails to achieve a separation because, at the relatively high pH so commonly employed (~ 8.5), the hydroxyl ion binds to the ferriheme group and neutralizes its positive charge. However, when partially oxidized hemoglobin solutions are analyzed at neutral pH, intermediate components can be isolated.[12-15] Gel electrofocusing offers much greater resolution than conventional analytical methods. Following partial oxidation

---

*Extended x-ray absorption fine structure

of hemoglobin either by autoxidation or by ferricyanide, four components can be identified (Fig. 16–2): a red oxyhemoglobin band ($\alpha_2^{2+}\beta_2^{2+}$) with an isoelectric point (pI) of 6.95, a brown methemoglobin band ($\alpha_2^{3+}\beta_2^{3+}$) with a pI of 7.20, and, midway between them, two distinct half-oxidized bands.[15] The intermediate band with the higher pI is $\alpha_2^{3+}\beta_2^{2+}$, and the one with the lower pI is $\alpha_2^{2+}\beta_2^{3+}$.[16–18] The fact that these species have slightly different surface charge testifies further to the subunit inequivalence that is such a dominant feature of hemoglobin chemistry. The separation and quantification of partially oxidized hemoglobins have been very useful in studies of the mechanisms of oxidation and reduction of hemoglobins, which will be described below.

Effect on Oxygen Binding

Hemoglobin subunits that have been oxidized are no longer able to bind oxygen. Thus, the oxygen-carrying capacity of the hemoglobin solution (or blood) is decreased in direct proportion to the amount of methemoglobin. More importantly, the presence of oxidized subunits in a tetramer alters the oxygen binding of the remaining ferrous hemes. Darling and Roughton[19] found that an increase in the amount of methemoglobin in red cells from 0 to 70 per cent was accompanied by a decrease in P_{50} from 27 to 14 mm Hg. Similar observations were made on solutions of partially oxidized hemoglobin (Fig. 16–3). This increase in oxygen affinity can be explained in terms of methemoglobin's tertiary and quaternary structure (described above). Following deoxygenation, the oxidized subunits will remain in the r conformation and the allosteric equilibrium will be shifted toward the R quaternary structure. Therefore, the remaining ferrous hemes will have an increased affinity for oxygen.

The oxygen affinity of partially oxidized hemoglobin depends on the distribution of the oxidized subunits among hemoglobin tetramers. A mixture of fully oxidized and fully reduced tetramers would have normal oxygen affinity but lower capacity. However, this ex-

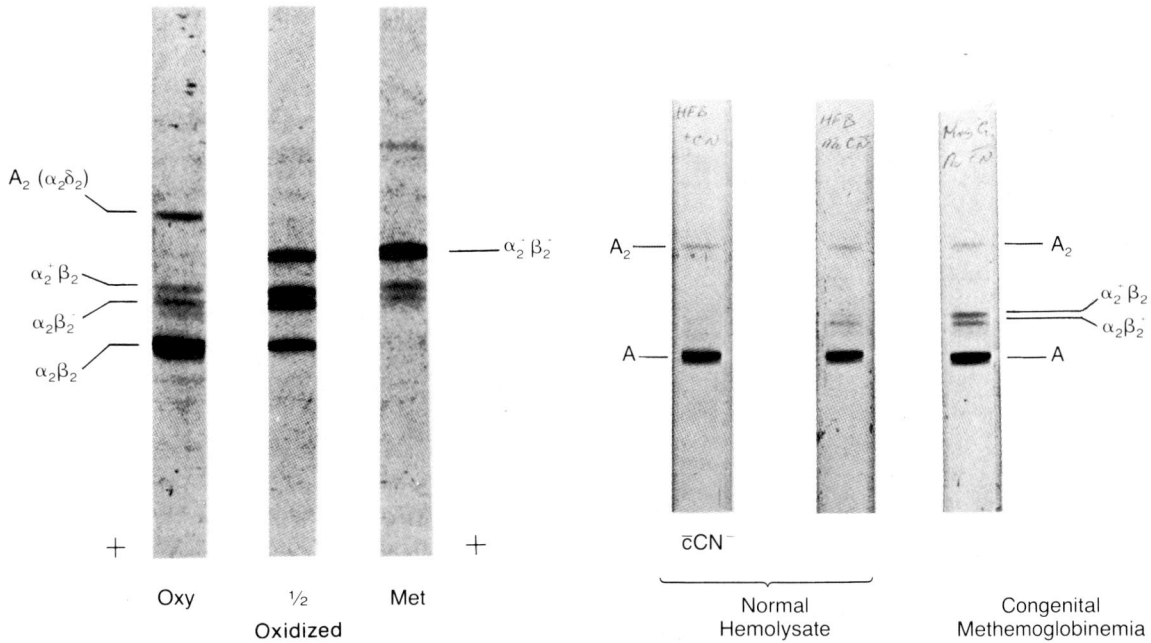

Figure 16–2. Gel electrofocusing patterns of partially oxidized hemoglobin. *A*, Partially oxidized Hb A following the addition of 0.5 equivalents of $K_3Fe(CN)_6$. Note the presence of two bands intermediate between oxyhemoglobin and fully oxidized hemoglobin (methemoglobin): $\alpha_2^{2+}\beta_2^{3+}$ and $\alpha_2^{3+}\beta_2^{2+}$. (From Bunn, H. F.: Methods Enzymol 76:126, 1982.) *B*, Hemolysate of a patient with congenital methemoglobinemia (cytochrome b₅ reductase deficiency). This specimen contained 10 per cent methemoglobin. Note that the intermediate bands are much fainter in the normal hemolysate. If cyanide was added to the hemolysate prior to application (c̄ CN⁻), no intermediate bands were detectable in either the normal hemolysate (left) or the enzyme-deficient hemolysate (not shown). (Cyanmethemoglobin has an isoelectric point identical to that of oxyhemoglobin.) (From Bunn, H. F.: Ann N.Y. Acad. Sci. 209:345, 1973.)

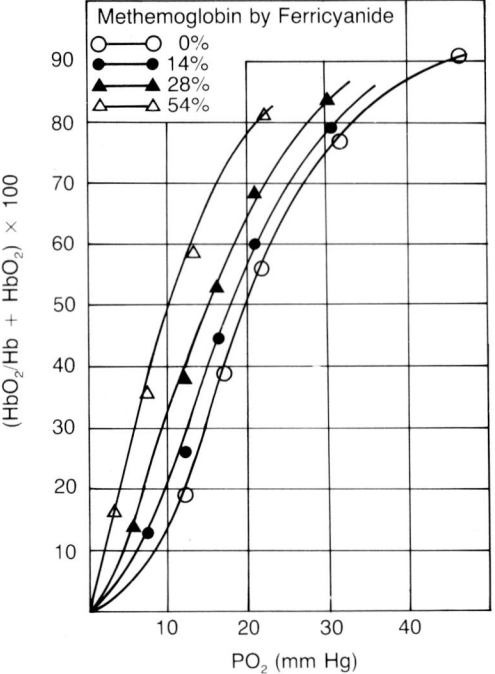

Figure 16–3. Oxygen equilibria of hemoglobin partially oxidized by the addition of increasing amounts of $K_3Fe(CN)_6$. Hemolysate was diluted in 0.6 M phosphate, pH 7.4. Measurements were made at 25°C. (From Darling, R. C., and Roughton, F. J. W.: Am. J. Physiol. *137*:56, 1942.)

periment is easier to conceive than to perform, because both αβ dimer[20] and electron exchange[15, 21, 21a] between the two species soon result in the formation of partially oxidized tetramers. The rate at which electron exchange occurs varies considerably with experimental conditions and is greatly enhanced by the presence of a suitable electron carrier such as methylene blue. In an individual red cell the oxidized subunits are evenly distributed among hemoglobin molecules. In contrast, there is considerable heterogeneity of methemoglobin content among red cells owing to cell aging[22–24] and variation in cytochrome b_5 and cytochrome b_5 reductase[25–27a] (see below). Therefore, the oxygen binding curve of methemoglobinemic blood is less left-shifted than a comparable solution of partially oxidized hemoglobin.

More refined information on the oxygenation of partially oxidized hemoglobin can be obtained from studies of the valence hybrids. These hemoglobins are prepared by mixing oxy α chains and cyanmet β chains and vice versa. Valence hybrid tetramers differ from partially oxidized hemoglobin in two important ways: (1) The former is a homogeneous and symmetrical species in which either the α or β chains are fully oxidized, whereas the latter has a full distribution of partially oxidized species. (2) The former is in the low spin cyanmet form, whereas the methemoglobin in the latter is in a high spin form at low pH. The two valence hybrids differ considerably in their functional properties[28]: $\alpha_2^{3+CN}\beta_2^{2+}$ has markedly increased oxygen affinity and decreased Bohr effect, whereas $\alpha_2^{2+}\beta_2^{3+CN}$ has properties much closer to those of HbA.

THE OXIDATION OF HEMOGLOBIN

Redox Potentials

Oxidation-reduction reactions can be viewed as the coupling of two half-reactions. As one reactant is oxidized, an equivalent amount of the other is reduced. When an atom or compound is oxidized, electrons are released and transferred to the substance undergoing reduction. The relative ease with which a given oxidation or reduction will take place is determined by the electrical potential of the half-reaction. Table 16–1 lists those that are relevant to the oxidation and reduction of hemoglobin both *in vitro* and *in vivo*. The half-reaction

$$HbFe^{3+} + 1e \rightleftharpoons HbFe^{2+} \quad [1]$$

has an electrical potential of 0.14 volt. Those compounds that appear above hemoglobin on the list, when present in the oxidized form, will oxidize hemoglobin to methemoglobin whereas those that appear below hemoglobin, when in the reduced form, will reduce methemoglobin. The electrical potential reflects the relative potency of a given oxidizing or reducing agent. The equilibrium of a coupled redox reaction is determined by the difference between the potentials of the reactants ($\Delta E'_0$). The equilibrium constant K of such a reaction can be determined from the following relationship:

$$K = \exp \frac{nF\Delta E'_0}{RT} \quad [2]$$

where n is the number of electrons transferred, F is the caloric equivalent of the faraday (23.062 kcal), R is the gas constant (1.99 cal/deg/mole), and T is absolute temperature. Application of this equation to the compounds listed in Table 16–1 allows an estimate of the

Table 16–1. OXIDATION-REDUCTION POTENTIALS

Chemical System (Measured at Midpoint; 20° C, pH 7.0)	E'_0 (or E_m) (Volts) (in Decreasing Order of Reduction Potentials)
O_2/H_2O	+ 0.82
Cu^{2+}/Cu^+-hemocyanin	+ 0.54
$S_2O_4^{2-}/S_2O_3^{2-}$	+ 0.48
NO_3^-/NO_2^-	+ 0.42
$Fe(CN)_6^{3-}/Fe(CN)_6^{4-}$	+ 0.36
O_2(gas)/H_2O_2	+ 0.30
Fe^{3+}/Fe^{2+} cytochrome a	+ 0.29
cytochrome oxidase	+ 0.29
Fe^{3+}/Fe^{2+} cytochrome c	+ 0.25
Fe^{3+}/Fe^{2+} cytochrome c_1	+ 0.22
Fe^{3+}/Fe^{2+} β chains in intact Hb†	+ 0.16
Fe^{3+}/Fe^{2+} HEMOGLOBIN	+ 0.14
Fe^{3+}/Fe^{2+} Hb, pH 6.0	+ 0.17
Fe^{3+}/Fe^{2+} α chains in intact Hb†	+ 0.12
Fe^{3+}/Fe^{2+} Isolated β chains of Hb	+ 0.11
Fe^{3+}/Fe^{2+} cytochrome b	+ 0.08 (and + 0.05)
Fe^{3+}/Fe^{2+} Isolated α chains of Hb*	+ 0.05
Fe^{3+}/Fe^{2+} myoglobin	+ 0.05
dehydroascorbic acid/ascorbic acid	+ 0.06 (and + 0.01)
Methylene blue	+ 0.01
Fe^{3+}/Fe^{2+} cytochrome b_5	− 0.002
pyruvate/lactate	− 0.19
FAD/$FADH_2$	− 0.22
glutathione	− 0.23
$NAD^+/NADH$	− 0.32
$NADP^+/NADPH$	− 0.32
cystine/cysteine	− 0.33
xanthine/hypoxanthine	− 0.37
$H^+/(1/2) H_2$	− 0.42
6-P-gluconate/glucose 6-P	− 0.43 (and − 0.47)
$SO_3^{2-}/S_2O_4^{2-}$	− 0.53 (and − 0.47)
pyruvate/acetate (+ CO_2)	− 0.70

*1 M glycine, 5.0° C, pH 7.0[31]
†0.2 M bis-TRIS, room temperature, pH 7.0[32]

extent to which various redox reactions will take place. There is sufficient difference between the potentials of ferricyanide reduction and methemoglobin reduction that when ferricyanide is added to an equimolar amount of hemoglobin, 99.99 per cent of the hemoglobin will be oxidized. In contrast, if an equimolar amount of ferricytochrome c_1 serves as the oxidant, only 95 per cent of the hemoglobin will be oxidized.

Although the redox potentials shown in Table 16–1 indicate which reactions are possible as well as the direction they will take, they are strictly thermodynamic values and therefore provide no information about the rate at which chemical equilibrium is reached. As will be described in detail below, many redox reactions that are of physiologic importance require enzymes to lower the activation energy and allow the reaction to take place.

A second type of oversimplification is apparent in considering the redox potential of hemoglobin. Just as the oxygen affinity depends markedly on hemoglobin's conformation (specifically the equilibrium between the R and T quaternary structures), so does the redox potential. For example, cofactors such as 2,3-DPG and inositol hexaphosphate, which bind preferentially to the T conformation, increase the redox potential,[29] just as they increase P_{50}. Conversely, any chemical modification that shifts the allosteric equilibrium toward R would be expected to lower the redox potential to a level comparable to that of the isolated subunits (Table 16–1). Furthermore, as discussed below, the constituent subunits in the intact tetramer differ in redox potential just as they differ in affinity for heme ligands.

Figure 16–4 shows a plot of the overall redox potential of hemoglobin at different pH values. This redox Bohr effect has clear-cut similarity to the better known oxygenation Bohr effect. However, one striking and puzzling difference between the oxygenation Bohr effect and the redox Bohr effect is apparent. Brunori, Wyman, Antonini, and Rossi-Fanelli[30] have noted that although the shape of the oxygenation curve (conveniently measured by the parameter n in a Hill plot, as in Figure 16–5) is nearly invariant with pH ranging between 6 and 8.5, the shape of the redox equilibrium curve is markedly pH-dependent. At pH 6.0, there is no significant cooperativity ($n = 1.2$), whereas at pH 8.0, there is appreciable cooperativity ($n = 2.0$) (Fig. 16–5). Perutz and colleagues[8, 9, 11] have explained this phenomenon in terms of the equilibrium between the quaternary forms of methemoglobin. At pH 6.0, methemoglobin is primarily in the T conformation, and thus, the reduction to deoxyhemoglobin would involve much less cooperativity than at a higher pH at which hydroxymethemoglobin assumes the R quaternary structure.

An alternative explanation for the shape of the redox equilibrium curves shown in Figure 16–5 involves asymmetry between the α and β subunits. There is considerable experimental evidence that the redox potentials of the α and β chains differ from one another and have different pH dependence. Isolated β chains have a higher redox potential than α chains (see Table 16–1).[31] The β chains exhibit a significant redox Bohr effect, but the α chains do not. The redox potentials of the α and β chains in *intact* hemoglobin show a similar inequivalence[32] (shown in Table 16–1). The β

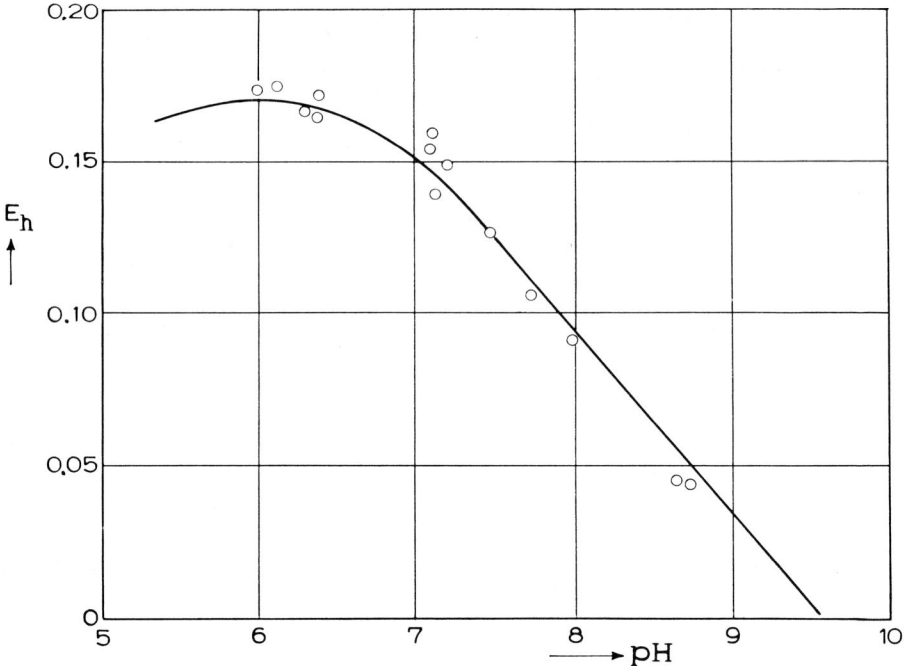

Figure 16–4. Redox Bohr effect of human Hb A. The potential (E_h) at which hemoglobin is half oxidized is plotted against pH. Measurements were performed at 25°C in phosphate or borate buffers. (From Brunori, M., et al.: J. Biol. Chem. *240*:3317, 1965.)

chains have a higher reduction potential and therefore are less likely to be oxidized than are α chains.

Autoxidation of Hemoglobin

When a solution of oxyhemoglobin is incubated for a prolonged period of time, it gradually turns to methemoglobin. The rate at which this oxidation occurs is markedly dependent on solvent conditions; it is favored by increased temperature, hydrogen ion ($\downarrow$pH)[33, 34] organic phosphate,[34, 35] metal ions,[36, 37] and partial oxygenation of the hemoglobin.[33, 38] Under normal circumstances, oxyhemoglobin dissociates into partially deoxygenated hemoglobin and free molecular oxygen:

$$Hb(O_2)_4 \rightarrow Hb(O_2)_3 + O_2 \quad [3]$$

However, occasionally the leaving group is superoxide anion (O_2^-) rather than O_2. As discussed in Chapter 2, it is likely that the oxygenated heme has some portion of iron's d electron transferred to the unoccupied π_2^* orbital of the bound O_2. Thus, O_2^- is bound to low spin ferric heme. The dissociation of O_2^- is accompanied by the removal of an electron from the heme iron; hence, the iron is oxidized to the Fe^{3+} state:

$$HbFe^{2+}O_2 \rightarrow HbFe^{3+}O_2^- \xrightarrow[Cl^-]{H^+} HbFe^{3+} + O_2^- \quad [4]$$

Protons increase the rate of dissociation of superoxide from the iron atom in a catalytic fashion by a relay mechanism involving pro-

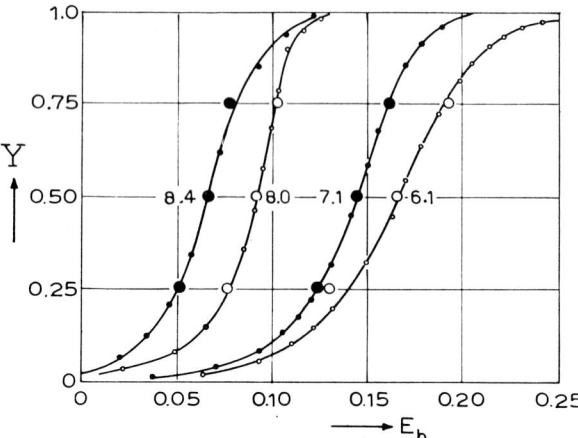

Figure 16–5. Redox equilibrium curves of human Hb A at different pH values. Y is the fraction of oxidized hemoglobin over total hemoglobin. (From Brunori, M. et al.: J. Biol. Chem. *240*:317, 1965.)

tonation of the distal (E7) histidine.[38a] Nucleophiles, including chloride ion, which is weak but abundant in red cells, displace the superoxide anion by nucleophilic attack on the Fe^{3+} iron atom.[38a, 39] In addition, O_2^- can serve as a catalyst to promote further autoxidation[37, 40, 41]:

$$2HbFe^{2+}O_2 + 2O_2^- + 4H^+ \rightarrow \\ 2HbFe^{3+} + 3O_2 + 2H_2O \quad [5]$$

The overall reaction is:

$$4HbFe^{2+}O_2 + 4H^+ \rightarrow 4HbFe^{3+} + 3O_2 + 2H_2O \quad [6]$$

The rate at which autoxidation occurs is markedly dependent on hemoglobin's quaternary conformation. The fact that this reaction is favored by organic phosphates such as 2,3-DPG and IHP[34, 35] suggests that the dissociation of superoxide anion is favored when the molecule assumes the T structure. In support of this conclusion is the fact that the rate is enhanced when hemoglobin is partially deoxygenated[33, 38] or in mutant hemoglobins that have a relatively stable T structure (see Chapter 14).

The autoxidation of hemoglobin can also be enhanced by the presence of trace amounts of certain metal ions.[36, 37] For example, copper ion can serve as a catalyst to promote autoxidation. The reaction is specific for the β-chain hemes and involves the β 93 cysteine sulfhydryl group.[37]

$$Cu^{2+} + HbFe^{2+} \longrightarrow Cu^{1+} + HbFe^{3+} \quad [7]$$

$$Cu^{1+} + O_2 \longrightarrow Cu^{2+} + O_2^- \quad [8]$$

The overall reaction is:

$$HbFe^{2+}O_2 + O_2 \xrightarrow{Cu} HbFe^{3+} + O_2^- \quad [9]$$

The addition of a small amount of a chelating agent will remove the contribution of metal ions that hasten the oxidation of hemoglobin.

During autoxidation of hemoglobin, the α chains are preferentially oxidized[42, 43] (Table 16–2). Flash photolysis experiments indicate that the superoxide anion dissociates from the α-chain heme pocket more readily than from the β-chain heme pocket.[44] In contrast, the direct attack of superoxide anion on hemoglobin (Reaction 5) does not exhibit any subunit preference.

In summary, the autoxidation of hemoglobin is a complex process. There is a reasonable explanation based on chemistry and/or structure-function relationships for all of the factors that are known to influence this process. In the red cell, several of these factors, such as organic phosphates, chloride ion, partial deoxygenation, and body temperature, contribute toward autoxidation of hemoglobin. Fortunately, the red cell is abundantly endowed with superoxide dismutase, catalase, and glutathione peroxidase, enzymes that serve to detoxify the cell of O_2^- and H_2O_2, the unwanted byproducts of autoxidation. For example, the ample amounts of superoxide dismutase in red cells probably prevents reaction 5 from having relevance *in vivo*.[40] These defenses may be necessary to protect both the hemoglobin molecule and the red cell membrane from oxidant damage.

Table 16–2. SUBUNIT SELECTIVITY IN THE OXIDATION AND REDUCTION OF HEMOGLOBINS

Oxidation of $\alpha_2^{2+}\beta_2^{2+}$	
Autoxidation	α > β
Ferricyanide	β > α
Nitrite	β > α
Cupric ion	β
Reduction of $\alpha_2^{3+}\beta_2^{3+}$	
Ascorbic acid	β > α
Cytochrome b_5 reductase	β > α
NADPH-flavin reductase	β > α

Oxidation of Hemoglobin by Chemical Agents

In his comprehensive monograph on methemoglobin, Kiese[45] presents a large body of information on various organic and inorganic compounds that can oxidize hemoglobin both *in vitro* and *in vivo*. These agents can be organized into groups, as shown in Table 16–3. A few substances are able to oxidize hemoglobin directly. Other compounds require the presence of oxygen or need to be chemically modified in order to oxidize hemoglobin. A detailed discussion of the mechanism of action of these agents is beyond the scope of this chapter. Instead, a few compounds of experimental and clinical interest will be discussed.

Direct Oxidation

Hemoglobin can be oxidized directly by compounds that have a higher redox potential. Several of these are listed in Table 16–1. The oxidizing agent most often used in the laboratory is ferricyanide. This compound cannot cause methemoglobinemia because it is unable to penetrate red cells. The addition of ferri-

Table 16-3. AGENTS THAT OXIDIZE HEMOGLOBIN*

I. *Direct Oxidation*
  Ferricyanide
  Copper
  Hydrogen peroxide
  Hydroxylamine
  Others: Chromate, chlorate, nitrogen trifluoride, tetranitromethane, quinones, dyes

II. *Interaction with Oxygen*
  Nitrites†
  Hydrazines
  Thiols
  Others: Arsine, aminophenols, arylhydroxylamines, N-hydroxyurethane, phenylenediamines

III. *Requiring Biochemical Transformation*
  Anilines
  Sulfanilamide
  4,4'-Diaminodiphenylsulfone (dapsone)
  8-Aminoquinolines: primaquine and pamaquine
  N-Acylarylamines: acetanilid, phenacetin

*Adapted from Kiese, M.: Methemoglobinemia: A Comprehensive Treatise. Cleveland, CRC Press, 1974.
†Nitrites can also oxidize hemoglobin directly (see text).

cyanide to a solution of either oxyhemoglobin or deoxyhemoglobin results in the rapid and stoichiometric conversation of the ferrohemes to ferrihemes. Side reactions such as sulfhydryl oxidation are minimal.[46] The oxidation of oxyhemoglobin with ferricyanide appears to involve the bimolecular attack of the oxidizing agent on a deoxygenated heme group:[46]

$$Hb(Fe^{2+}O_2)_4 \rightleftharpoons Hb(Fe^{2+}O_2)_3 Fe^{2+} + O_2 \quad [10]$$

$$Hb(Fe^{2+}O_2)_3 Fe^{2+} + Fe(CN)_6^{3-} \rightarrow Hb(Fe^{2+}O_2)_3 Fe^{3+} + Fe(CN)_6^{4-} \quad [11]$$

Oxidation by ferricyanide is more rapid when hemoglobin is in the T quaternary structure. The lower oxygen affinity of T hemoglobin permits a greater proportion of the deoxygenated heme to be attacked by ferricyanide. Thus, the additon of IHP greatly accelerates the rate of methemoglobin formation by ferricyanide.[47] In contrast to autoxidation (described above), the β-chain hemes are more readily oxidized than the α-chain hemes when hemoglobin is partially reacted with ferricyanide.[48] Thus, the valence hybrid $\alpha_2^{2+}\beta_2^{3+}$ is more abundant than the complementary hybrid $\alpha_2^{3+}\beta_2^{2+}$. As mentioned above, this difference between subunits is even more marked when hemoglobin reacts with cupric ion.[37] This agent oxidizes β-chain heme almost exclusively (see Table 16-2).

Indirect Oxidation

In contrast to ferricyanide, a number of agents oxidize hemoglobin in an indirect and more complex fashion. Most substances that produce toxic methemoglobinemia are reducing agents. Although the precise chemical reactions are not well understood, the overall pathway generally involves the reduction of oxygen to superoxide (O_2^-) and hydrogen peroxide (H_2O_2). These products are oxidizing agents that not only convert hemoglobin to methemoglobin but also engage in a number of side reactions. Compounds that appear to oxidize hemoglobin via the formation of O_2^- and H_2O_2 include nitrite[49] and reduced glutathione.[50]

The mechanism of nitrite-induced hemoglobin oxidation has been studied in considerable detail. This reaction, discovered more than 100 years ago,[51] has assumed considerable importance because nitrites are an important cause of toxic methemoglobinemia (see below). The oxidation of hemoglobin by nitrite has been recognized to be an autocatalytic process.[52, 53] Because nitrite is a univalent reductant of oxygen, it follows that superoxide anion may serve as an intermediate in hemoglobin oxidation. Indeed, the induction of methemoglobin by nitrite is greatly retarded when superoxide dismutase is added to the reaction mixture.[49] Furthermore, the initial lag phase of hemoglobin oxidation can be obliterated by the inclusion of a means for generating superoxide. The following sequence of reactions has been proposed[49]:

$$2HbFe^{2+}O_2 + 2NO_2^- \rightarrow 2HbFe^{3+} + 2NO_3^- + O_2^- + \epsilon \quad [12]$$

$$2NO_2^- + 2O_2^- + 6H^+ + 2\epsilon \rightarrow 2NO + H_2O_2 + 2H_2O + O_2 \quad [13]$$

$$2HbFe^{2+}O_2 + 2NO + \epsilon \rightarrow 2HbFe^{3+} + 2NO_2^- + O_2^- \quad [14]$$

$$H_2O_2 + 2NO_2^- \rightarrow 2H^+ + 2NO_3^- + 2\epsilon \quad [15]$$

The sum of these reactions is:

$$4HbFe^{2+}O_2 + 4NO_2^- + 4H^+ \rightarrow 4HbFe^{3+} + 4NO_3^- + 2H_2O + O_2 \quad [16]$$

This stoichiometry has been confirmed by direct measurements of reaction products.[54] During oxidation by nitrite, the intermediate

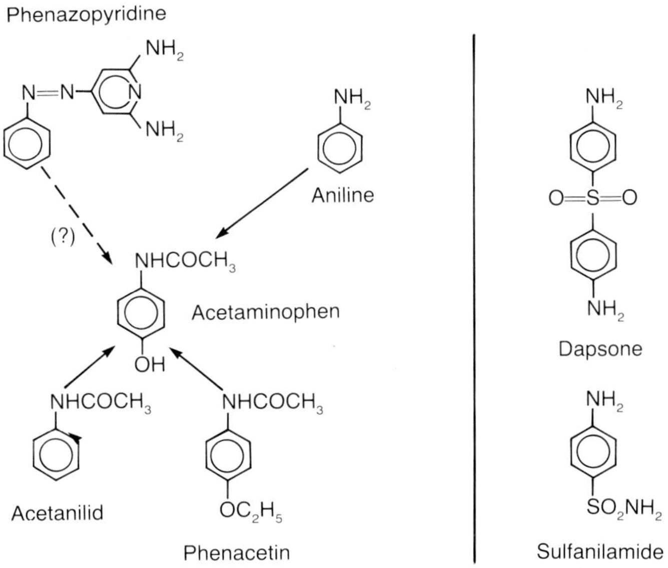

Figure 16-6. Structure of aromatic compounds of the arylamine group that can cause methemoglobinemia. (Courtesy of Dr. V. F. Fairbanks.)

$\alpha_2^{2+}\beta_2^{3+}$ is formed in preference to $\alpha_2^{3+}\beta_2^{2+}$.[49] (See Table 16–2.) Nitrite is also capable of oxidizing deoxyhemoglobin in the total absence of oxygen.[45, 55] This complex process involves the reaction of hemoglobin with nitrous acid; nitric oxide and its dimer serve as intermediates.[55] This anaerobic reaction sequence is of no pathophysiologic importance.

Hydrazine compounds have been used extensively in studies of oxidant-type hemolytic anemia. Deoxyhemoglobin is unaffected by these agents. However, in the presence of oxygen, hydrazines form hydrogen peroxide and can oxidize hemoglobin both *in vitro* and *in vivo*. In addition, further reactions occur, such as the formation of verdoglobin and the oxidation of glutathione. The extent of hemoglobin oxidation and denaturation varies widely among animal species and the various hydrazine derivatives. The primary toxicity of phenylhydrazine and acetylphenylhydrazine is in the induction of Heinz bodies within red cells, resulting in hemolysis. Methemoglobin does not appear to be a necessary intermediate in the formation of Heinz bodies.[56]

Agents Requiring Biochemical Transformation

With the development of the dye industry in Europe during the nineteenth century, a variety of aromatic compounds, particularly the arylamines (Fig. 16–6), emerged as potentially toxic agents. Aniline has probably been responsible for more cases of toxic methemoglobinemia than any other agent (see Toxic Methemoglobinemia, below). Aniline itself is not capable of oxidizing hemoglobin. However, in hepatic microsomes, the drug is converted to phenylhydroxylamine, which serves as a catalyst in mediating hemoglobin oxidation.[57] As shown by the reaction scheme in Figure 16–7, phenylhydroxylamine is stoichiometrically converted to nitrosobenzene as the heme is oxidized. In the red cell, a NADPH-dependent diaphorase (probably NADPH-flavin reductase [see below]) enables NADPH to reduce nitrosobenzene back to phenylhydroxylamine. This cycle keeps operating as the cell regenerates NADPH by shunting glucose into the pentose-phosphate path-

Figure 16-7. Enzymatic cycle that mediates the oxidation of hemoglobin in the presence of an arylamine. (ø-NH-OH = phenylhydroxylamine; ø-NO = nitrosobenzene; G-6-P = glucose-6-phosphate; 6-PGA = 6-phosphogluconic acid).

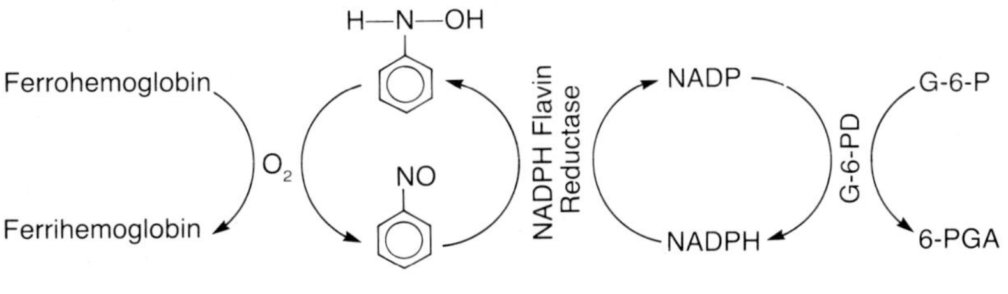

way. Thus, a relatively small amount of phenylhydroxylamine will sustain the oxidation of a large amount of hemoglobin. However, the cycle eventually runs down because the arylamine inside the red cell is eventually disposed of by various side reactions.

A number of other compounds can oxidize hemoglobin after similar *in vitro* transformation. Sulfanilamide is the only "sulfa" drug that induces methemoglobinemia. The increasing use of dapsone in the treatment of malaria and leprosy has been accompanied by sporadic cases of methemoglobinemia. These problems will be considered in more detail in the section below on toxic methemoglobinemia.

THE REDUCTION OF METHEMOGLOBIN

Maintenance of hemoglobin in the reduced (Fe^{++}) state is necessary not only for the red cell but also for investigators who are examining the functional properties of hemoglobin. The reduction of hemoglobin in circulating red cells depends on a well-regulated system of electron carriers and enzymes. Methemoglobin can also be reduced by other enzyme systems and chemical agents. Some of these are useful to the experimentalist in preparing fully deoxygenated hemoglobin and to offset the annoying tendency for partially oxygenated hemoglobin to autoxidize during an experiment.

Nonenzymatic Reduction

A variety of reducing agents will convert methemoglobin to ferrohemoglobin. Examples, listed in order of decreasing potency, include dithionite, metabisulfite, cysteine, reduced glutathione, and ascorbic acid. The redox potentials of these compounds are listed in Table 16–1.

Dithionite is the agent most often used in the laboratory to reduce methemoglobin:

$$S_2O_4^{2-} + 2HbFe^{3+} + 2H_2O \rightarrow \quad [17]$$
$$2SO_3^{2-} + 2HbFe^{2+} + 4H^+$$

In addition, dithionite ($S_2O_4^{2-}$) (as well as metabisulfite [$S_2O_5^{2-}$]) also reduces oxygen to peroxide.

$$S_2O_4^{2-} + O_2 + 2H_2O \rightarrow 2SO_3^{2-} + H_2O_2 + 2H^+ \quad [18]$$

This undesirable side reaction can be minimized if dithionite is used under strictly anaerobic conditions.[58] Furthermore, the time in which dithionite, its by-products, and side products are in contact with hemoglobin should be kept to a minimum. This can be achieved by procedures utilizing gel filtration[59] or a mixed bed ion exchange resin,[60] which effectively separate the reduced hemoglobin from unwanted small charged molecules involved in heme reduction.

A number of molecules encountered in plasma and red cells are weak reducing agents. Ascorbic acid has been used in the treatment of congenital methemoglobinemia, although it is not as effective as methylene blue (see below). The reduction of methemoglobin by ascorbic acid has been thoroughly investigated.[61, 62] The reduction rate is enhanced by the addition of an electron carrier such as methylene blue. Furthermore, the rate is accelerated when inositol hexaphosphate is present.[63] The only intermediate in the reduction is the valence hybrid $\alpha_2^{3+}\beta_2^{2+}$.[63, 64] (See Table 16–2.) The fact that in intact tetramers the β-chain hemes have a somewhat higher redox potential than the α-chain hemes is not a sufficient explanation for this high degree of subunit specificity.

Cysteine reduces methemoglobin more rapidly than does ascorbic acid but is unlikely to have any physiologic significance. In contrast, reduced glutathione reacts more slowly. Even though red cells normally have a high concentraiton of reduced glutathione (1.5 mM), this compound makes a trivial contribution to methemoglobin reduction. Reduced pyridine nucleotides (NADPH and NADH) are also capable of nonenzymatic reduction of methemoglobin but require the presence of an electron carrier.[45, 65]

Nonphysiologic Enzyme Systems

Because strong reducing agents such as dithionite rapidly consume molecular oxygen, they cannot be used in experiments such as oxygen equilibria that depend on the presence of varying amounts of oxyhemoglobin. Methemoglobin that has been generated during such experiments can be reduced by enzyme systems. In a widely used method, methemoglobin is maintained in reduced form by an NADPH-generating system that includes NADP, glucose-6-phosphate, and glucose-6-phosphate dehydrogenase.[66] An alternative system involves the use of pig heart diaphorase, methylene blue, and NADH.[67]

Physiologic Methemoglobin Reduction*

The reduction of methemoglobin in the red cell depends primarily on a linked system consisting of two electron carriers, cytochrome b_5 and NADH, and the enzyme cytochrome b_5 reductase. Only a small proportion of methemoglobin in red cells is reduced by other means.

In the 1940's, while serving as an obstetrician in Ireland, Dr. Quentin Gibson had the opportunity to see two families with congenital methemoglobinemia. His initial investigation of these families led to a classic paper on methemoglobin reduction in red cells[68] and marked the beginning of a distinguished and productive career in research on heme proteins (see also page 54 and Chapters 1 and 3). Gibson showed that when normal red cells, rendered methemoglobinemic by treatment with nitrite, were incubated in the presence of lactate, the accumulation of pyruvate matched the reduction of methemoglobin:

$$\text{Lactate} + 2\text{HbFe}^{3+} \rightarrow \text{Pyruvate} + 2\text{HbFe}^{2+} \quad [19]\dagger$$

This relationship implied that the cofactor NAD^+, which was known to be responsible for the oxidation of lactate, was being converted to NADH, thereby providing reducing equivalents for the reduction of methemoglobin. Thus, reaction 19 is the sum of:

$$\text{Lactate} + NAD^+ \xrightleftharpoons[\text{Dehydrogenase}]{\text{Lactate}} \text{Pyruvate} + NADH \quad [20]\dagger$$

and

$$NADH + 2\text{HbFe}^{3+} \rightarrow NAD^+ + 2\text{HbFe}^{2+} \quad [21]\dagger$$

Furthermore, when nitrite-treated normal red cells were incubated with glucose, the accumulation of pyruvate again matched the reduction of methemoglobin with the same 1:2 stoichiometric ratio. Gibson concluded that the reducing equivalents were provided by the oxidation of triose phosphate because the reduction of methemoglobin was markedly impaired by iodoacetate, which inhibits the enzyme glyceraldehyde-3-phosphate dehydrogenase (G3PD):

$$NAD^+ + G\text{-}3\text{-}P + PO_4^{3-} \xrightleftharpoons{G3PD} NADH + 1,3\text{-}DPG \quad [22]\dagger$$

This observation also suggested that NADH was responsible for reducing methemoglobin. These experiments confirmed and extended prior studies of Kiese,[69] who also demonstrated a relationship between glucose and lactate consumption and methemoglobin reduction. Because of World War II, neither investigator knew of the other's work.

When Gibson performed incubation experiments on red cells of a patient with congenital methemoglobinemia, the rates of methemoglobin reduction and pyruvate accumulation were markedly impaired. (See Figure 16–10 for a later version of this experiment.) From these experiments, Gibson concluded that in normal red cells an NADH-dependent enzyme was responsible for methemoglobin reduction and that this enzyme was deficient in individuals with congenital methemoglobinemia. He went on to identify a second methemoglobin reducing system in the red cells of normal individuals and in those with congenital methemoglobinemia that utilized NADPH for reducing equivalents but required an exogenous electron carrier such as methylene blue for its activity. This NADPH-dependent system will be described in the subsequent section.

Subsequently, Scott and colleagues[70, 71] began to purify and characterize these two methemoglobin-reducing enzymes. They found that the NADH-dependent enzyme was absent in red cells of Eskimos with hereditary methemoglobinemia,[72] in keeping with the earlier conclusion of Gibson.[68] Although the purified enzyme from normal individuals contained very low amounts of flavin, Scott and associates reasoned that this prosthetic group was essential to its function because its reaction kinetics were similar to those of other flavoproteins. Subsequently, higher purification revealed that the enzyme has 1 mole of FAD* per mole of apoenzyme (34,400 M.W.).[73–75] In the presence of the enzyme, the dye 2,6-dichloroindophenol is reduced much more rapidly than is methemoglobin.[70] Therefore, the dye can be used for assaying enzymatic activity.[70] Because of the reduction of exogenous agents such as dyes, the enzyme was called diaphorase-I (Table 16–4). The addition of

---

*This topic has been thoroughly reviewed by Hultquist and colleagues.[67a]

†For the sake of simplicity, reactions 19 to 22 have not been properly balanced.

*Flavin adenine dinucleotide

Table 16–4. NOMENCLATURE OF METHEMOGLOBIN-REDUCING ENZYMES

	Reference(s)
Preferred Term: Cytochrome	
b_5 reductase	77,84
Diaphorase I	70,71
DPNH dehydrogenase I	70,71
NADH dehydrogenase	
NADH methemoglobin reductase	
NADH methemoglobin-ferrocyanide reductase	75
Preferred Term: NADPH-flavin reductase	102,103
Hämiglobinreduktase	99
NADPH methemoglobin reductase	100,101
NADPH dehydrogenase	

ferrocyanide to methemoglobin results in a complex that is rapidly reduced by the NADH-dependent enzyme.[76] This complex can also be used to assay the enzyme.[77] The fact that the reduction of methemoglobin is very slow in the presence of the purified enzyme and NADH suggested that an additional substance is necessary to transport electrons from the enzyme to methemoglobin.

Cytochrome b_5

In 1971, Hultquist and Passon[78] isolated a heme protein from red cells that had visible and EPR spectra characteristic of cytochrome b_5 and, indeed, served as a substrate for hepatic microsomal cytochrome b_5 reductase. This protein greatly accelerated the NADH-dependent enzymatic reduction of methemoglobin, an observation consistent with other studies utilizing hepatic cytochrome b_5.[79, 80] Hultquist and associates then demonstrated that erythrocyte cytochrome b_5 and hepatic cytochrome b_5 have a heme peptide in common[81] and that bovine erythrocyte cytochrome b_5 corresponds to the hydrophilic domain of hepatic cytochrome b_5.[82] The primary structure of the entire bovine hepatic microsomal cytochrome b_5 polypeptide is shown in Figure 16–8. The C-terminal end of the molecule is embedded in the microsomal membrane. Treatment of bovine hepatic cytochrome b_5 with cathepsins D and B removes the hydrophobic tail and yields a species of cytochrome b_5 found in erythrocytes.[82, 83] Accordingly, these investigators proposed that erythrocyte cytochrome b_5 was formed by proteolytic cleavage of a precursor located in the microsomes of erythroid precursors (Fig. 16–9). In support of this scheme, they demonstrated that primitive mouse erythroid cells induced from cells transformed with Friend virus contained microsomal cytochrome b_5 comparable in quantity to the soluble form found in mature red cells.[84]

```
                                  10
(Glx, Glx, Ala)-Ser-Ser-Lys-Ala-Val-Lys-Tyr-Tyr-Thr-Leu-Glu-Gln-Ile-Glu-Lys-

           20                          30
His-Asn-Asn-Ser-Lys-Ser-Thr-Trp-Leu-Ile-Leu-His-Tyr-Lys-Val-Tyr-Asp-Leu-Thr-Lys-

           40                     50
Phe-Leu-Glu-Glu-His-Pro-Gly-Gly-Glu-Glu-Val-Leu-Arg-
                           Fe
                    60                          70
Glu-Gln-Ala-Gly-Gly-Asp-Ala-Thr-Glu-Asp-Phe-Glu-Asp-Val-Gly-His-Ser-Thr-Asp-Ala-Arg-

                   80                      90
Glu-Leu-Ser-Lys-Thr-Phe-Ile-Ile-Gly-Glu-Leu-His-Pro-Asp-Asp-Arg-Ser-Lys-

         95   97   100                107
Ile-Thr-Lys-Pro-Ser-Glu-Ser-Ile-Ile-Thr-Thr-Ile-Asp-Ser-Asn-Pro-Ser-Trp-Trp-

110                  120
Thr-Asn-Trp-Leu-Ile-Pro-Ala-Ile-Ser-Ala-Leu-Phe-Val-Ala-Leu-Ile-Tyr-His-Leu-

130
Tyr-Thr-Ser-Glu-Asn-COO
```

Figure 16–8. Structure of bovine cytochrome b_5 showing heme-binding histidines (residues 43 and 67). The microsomal protein is converted to the cytosolic protein by proteolytic cleavage at 88 Arg and 90 Lys (▼). (The primary sequence data were obtained from Ozols, J., and Strittmatter, P.: J. Biol. Chem. *244*:6617, 1969 and Ozols, J.: Biochemistry *13*:426, 1964.)

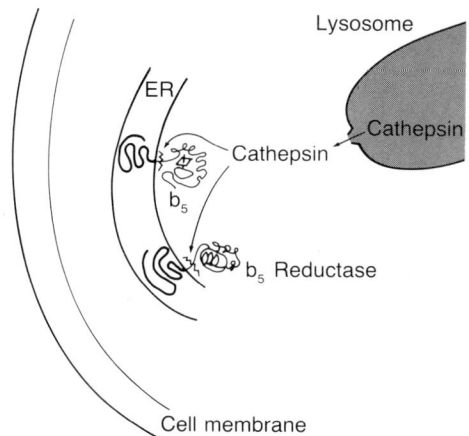

Figure 16–9. Scheme for the solubilization of cytochrome b_5 and cytochrome b_5 reductase from precursor proteins in the endoplasmic reticulum of erythroid progenitor cells. (From Hultquist, D. E., et al.: *In* Brewer, G. (ed.): The Red Cell. New York, Alan R. Liss, Inc., 1978, pp. 199–211.)

Cytochrome b_5 Reductase

The NADH-dependent methemoglobin reductase isolated from human red cells rapidly reduced erythrocyte cytochrome b_5 and had properties similar to those of cytochrome b_5 reductase prepared from hepatic microsomes.[73] Both enzymes contain FAD and show the same substrate specificity, pattern of inhibition, and pH dependency. Furthermore, investigators in three laboratories have shown that the red cell and liver enzymes are immunologically indistinguishable.[85–87] Finally, treatment of these two proteins with cathepsin D yields electrophoretically indistinguishable flavopeptides.[83] Taken together, these studies provide strong evidence that these enzymes have a common structure. Like cytochrome b_5, the soluble erythrocyte cytochrome b_5 reductase is probably cleaved from a microsomal precursor protein. The cleavage of both proteins probably occurs by ATP-dependent proteolysis.[87a] This scheme is depicted in Figure 16–9. In addition, mature red cells also contain an appreciable amount of cytochrome b_5 reductase, which is bound to the plasma membrane and is immunologically indistinguishable from the soluble enzyme.[88] The relationship between the membrane-bound enzyme and the microsomal enzyme has not been established.

In summary, there is compelling evidence that erythrocyte cytochrome b_5 reductase is the NADH-dependent enzyme responsible for methemoglobin reduction and that erythrocyte cytochrome b_5 is the physiologic electron carrier.

In hepatocytes, the microsome-bound cytochrome b_5 and cytochrome b_5 reductase serve to transport electrons for the conversion of saturated to unsaturated fatty acids.[89] Hultquist suggests that these proteins serve the same function in early erythroid cells. However, with the commitment to hemoglobin production, the need for synthesis of membrane lipids diminishes. These electron transport proteins are then released into the cytoplasm, where they are conserved for a different but equally important function: methemoglobin reduction. This is achieved by the following three reactions[83]:

$$NADH + FAD\text{-}Reductase \rightarrow \genfrac{}{}{0pt}{}{NADH}{FAD}\rangle Reductase$$

$$+ H^+ \rightarrow \genfrac{}{}{0pt}{}{NAD^+}{FADH_2}\rangle Reductase \quad [23]$$

$$\genfrac{}{}{0pt}{}{NAD^+}{FADH_2}\rangle Reductase + 2Cytb_5Fe^{3+} \rightarrow$$

$$\genfrac{}{}{0pt}{}{NAD^+}{FAD}\rangle Reductase + 2Cytb_5Fe^{2+} + 2H^+ \quad [24]$$

$$HbFe^{3+} + Cytb_5Fe^{2+} \rightarrow HbFe^{2+} + Cytb_5Fe^{3+} \quad [25]$$

Because cytochrome b_5 has a relatively low redox potential (-0.002 V[90]; see Table 16–1), it is a relatively strong reducing agent. Very small amounts are needed for rapid reduction of methemoglobin. The concentration of cytochrome b_5 in normal human red cells is about 0.5 μM.[80] In view of the relatively high Km of the reductase for cytochrome b_5,[90] only a small proportion of the enzyme is bound to cytochrome b_5, and accordingly, its velocity is far below its maximum.

Interaction of Cytochrome b_5 and Methemoglobin

The reduction of methemoglobin by reduced cytochrome b_5 (see reaction 25) involves the formation of a bimolecular complex. This interaction has been demonstrated by two-dimensional electrophoresis-electrofocusing[91] as well as by direct binding studies.[91a] Kinetic measurements of methemoglobin reduction also provide strong, albeit indirect, evidence for a complex[91b] and indicate that in human red cells the dissociation constant is about 0.5 mM.[83] Accordingly, in the normal red cell, roughly 20 per cent of cytochrome b_5 is expected to be bound to the small amount of methemoglobin that is present. The stability of the cytochrome b_5–methemoglobin complex is much greater, has a lower pH and decreases markedly with increasing ionic strength.[91a] An analysis of the hemoglobin intermediates formed during the reduction of methemoglobin by the cytochrome b_5 enzyme system both in solution[92, 93] and in intact cells[94] indicates that the β chain is reduced preferentially to the α chain (see Table 16–2). This chain heterogeneity is consistent with the redox potential of the individuals subunits in the tetramer (see Table 16–1).

The bimolecular complex involves electrostatic interactions between negatively charged groups around the heme group of the cytochrome and positively charged residues around the heme groups in methemoglobin. A comparable interaction has been proposed[95] and documented[96] for the cytochrome b_5–cytochrome c complex. A comparison of the rates of enzymatic reduction of normal and variant hemoglobins suggests that β 66 Lys and β 95 Lys are among the residues responsible for binding to cytochrome b_5.[97]

Methemoglobin Reduction in Red Cells

A detailed kinetic analysis of the steps in methemoglobin reduction (see reactions [23] to [25]) shows that under conditions simulating those of normal red cells, the first reaction ([23]) proceeds rapidly, whereas the next two reactions ([24] and [25]) are equally slow.[83, 98] This analysis suggests that NADPH may contribute significantly to methemoglobin reduction via the NADH-dependent reductase. Although reaction [23] proceeds 20 to 50 times as rapidly with NADH in comparison with NADPH, this difference is immaterial under physiologic conditions because the reaction is not rate-limiting. Furthermore, red cells normally contain higher levels of NADPH than NADH. However, it is likely that when large amounts of methemoglobin must be reduced through this pathway, NADH is the primary electron donor and is regenerated via glycolysis. There is no evidence that the hexose monophosphate shunt is activated during methemoglobin reduction unless an exogenous electron carrier is present.

The rate of methemoglobin reduction in a mixture of enzymes and cofactors simulating that of the red cell (1.1 to 1.4 μmoles/ml/hr)[74, 90, 98] agrees well with the rate measured in intact red cells (~ 1 μmole/ml/hr).[24, 68] The relative concentrations of cytochrome b_5, cytochrome b_5 reductase, and NADH in normal red cells suggest that both proteins limit the rate of methemoglobin reduction.[83, 98] The level of the enzyme declines with cell aging.[24–27a] Senescent red cells have low levels of enzyme activity. Furthermore, the concentration of cytochrome b_5 decreases to about 20 per cent of its initial value as red cells age *in vivo* ($T_{1/2}$ = 44 days).[27a] Thus, young red cells have a much greater capacity for methemoglobin reduction than older red cells. In view of these considerations, it is not surprising that the content of methemoglobin in normal red cells increases during *in vivo* aging.[27, 27a]

NADPH-Flavin Reductase

As mentioned in the previous section, Gibson[68] observed that methemoglobin reduction in red cells was greatly accelerated by the addition of methylene blue and that the process depended on the presence of NADPH. Kiese and colleagues[99] prepared a flavin-containing enzyme that reduced methemoglobin in the presence of methylene blue. This enzyme utilized NADPH as the electron donor and probably corresponds to the enzyme subsequently isolated by Scott and coworkers[71] and by Huennekens and associates[100, 101] from human erythrocytes. Although all these partially purified preparations required an electron carrier for methemoglobin reduction, there was considerable uncertainty about the nature of the prosthetic group or the specificity for pyridine nucleotide. Recently, a NADPH dehydrogenase from human erythrocytes has been purified to homogeneity.[102, 103] This enzyme can reduce methemoglobin rapidly in the presence of a variety of electron carriers. It is very likely to be the elusive NADPH methemoglobin reductase (see Table 16–3). The protein has a molecular weight of 22,000 and lacks heme or any other chromophore. The enzyme readily reduces not only artificial dyes such as methylene blue and DCIP* but also flavins such as FMN,† FAD, and riboflavin.‡ In contrast, cytochrome b_5 reductase is incapable of reducing flavins. These reduced cofactors can reduce hemoglobin nonenzymatically[104]:

$$H^+ + NADPH + FAD \xrightarrow[\text{Reductase}]{\text{NADPH-Flavin}} NADP^+ + FADH_2 \quad [26]$$

$$FADH_2 + 2HbFe^{3+} \rightarrow FAD + 2HbFe^{2+} + 2H^+ \quad [27]$$

---

*2,6-dichlorophenolindophenol
†FMN = flavin mononucleotide
‡Riboflavin is a precursor of FAD and FMN.

The β heme is reduced more readily than the α heme,[105] as is true for reduction by cytochrome b_5,[92-94]

In the red cell, this process is sustained by the regeneration of NADPH via the hexose monophosphate shunt. However, this pathway is probably not effective in reducing methemoglobin under normal circumstances because the concentration of flavins in the red cell is very low. Nevertheless, the administration of riboflavin, the permeable form of flavin, allows the enzyme to function *in vivo*.[106] This treatment can be considered in lieu of methylene blue in individuals with deficiency of cytochrome b_5 reductase[106-108] (see below).

It is unlikely that NADPH-flavin reductase plays any significant physiologic role. Sass and colleagues[109] described an individual who may be presumed to have deficiency of this enzyme. He had neither methemoglobinemia nor any other apparent clinical or hematologic abnormalities, yet his red cells were unable to reduce methylene blue, even though they contained normal levels of G-6-PD and, therefore, could generate adequate amounts of NADPH. Accordingly, methylene blue was unable to accelerate methemoglobin reduction in the red cells of this individual. Except for methylene blue and brilliant cresyl blue, other oxidant compounds were able to stimulate the hexose monophosphate shunt in these red cells.[110] Thus, this individual appears to be deficient in the enzyme that permits flow of electrons from NADPH to certain redox dyes, including methylene blue.

PATHOPHYSIOLOGIC CONSIDERATIONS

Cyanosis

Cyanosis, or a blue-gray appearance of the skin, can be attributed directly to an alteration in the patient's hemoglobin. As shown in Table 16–5, the most common cause of cyanosis is the presence of relatively high levels of deoxyhemoglobin in the blood, most often due to pulmonary or cardiac dysfunction. Less commonly, cyanosis results from an increase in nonphysiologic forms of hemoglobin: methemoglobin or sulfhemoglobin. A concentration of at least 5 g/dl of deoxyhemoglobin in the blood is required to produce recognizable cyanosis, whereas this sign is observed in individuals with 1.5 g/dl of methemoglobin and as little as 0.5 g/dl of sulfhemoglobin.[111]

Table 16–5. DIFFERENTIAL DIAGNOSIS OF CYANOSIS

I. Inadequate oxygenation of hemoglobin (common)
   A. Pulmonary disorders
   B. Cardiac right-to-left shunt
   C. Congestive heart failure
   D. Cardiovascular collapse (shock)
   E. Low O_2 affinity Hb variant (rare) (see Chapter 14)
II. Methemoglobinemia (rare)
   A. Congenital
     1. Cytochrome b_5 reductase deficiency
     2. M hemoglobins (see Chapter 15)
   B. Acquired
     1. Drugs
     2. Industrial, environmental toxins, etc.
III. Sulfhemoglobinemia (rare)
   A. Congenital (?)
   B. Acquired: drugs, toxins, etc.

Methemoglobin Content in Normal Blood

As normal red cells circulate *in vivo* for 120 days, they are exposed to a variety of endogenous and exogenous agents that are capable of oxidizing hemoglobin (see above). In the absence of an efficient enzymatic reducing system, it is estimated that methemoglobin accumulates at the rate of 2 to 3 per cent per day. However, when the cytochrome b_5 reducing system is operating and there is no unusual exogenous oxidant exposure, red cells contain less than 0.6 per cent methemoglobin. A number of thorough surveys of methemoglobin levels in various normal populations have been published and are summarized in Kiese's monograph.[45] Methemoglobin may be somewhat increased in the red cells of normal infants. The great majority of mammals that have been tested also have less than 1 per cent methemoglobin. In contrast, elevated levels of methemoglobin have often been observed in reptiles and fish. Up to 50 per cent methemoglobin has been reported in turtles (see Chapter 6). In some cases, such high values may be an artifact of sample collection and processing.[111a]

Effect of Methemoglobinemia on Oxygen Transport

As indicated in the previous section on hemoglobin function, the adverse effect of methemoglobinemia is caused by the fact that partial oxidation of hemoglobin results in a marked increase in the oxygen affinity of the remaining hemes in the tetramer. Compare a chronically anemic patient who has a hemoglobin of 7 g/dl with an individual who has a normal hemoglobin concentration (14 g/dl) but a methemoglobin level of 50 per cent. Both patients have a 50 per cent reduction in blood oxygen-carrying capacity. However, the methemoglobinemic individual would be expected to be more symptomatic, because the increased oxygen affinity of his functioning hemoglobin impairs oxygen delivery to tissues (see Chapter 5).

The effect of methemoglobinemia on physiologic function is difficult to establish with accuracy. Animal studies must be interpreted with caution because of species differences and because the oxidizing agents used to induce methemoglobinemia may have additional metabolic and circulatory effects. Furthermore, the pathophysiologic sequelae of induced methemoglobinemia depend on the relative duration of exposure. As in the case of anemia, acutely induced methemoglobinemia is generally tolerated less well than a comparable degree of chronic methemoglobinemia. It is likely that various modes of adaptation to hypoxia are called into play (see Chapter 5).

Individuals with chronic methemoglobinemia due to deficiency of cytochrome b_5 reductase may be asymptomatic even with methemoglobin levels as high as 50 per cent. In contrast, those with acute toxic methemoglobinemia may develop mild fatigue with 20 per cent methemoglobin. Upon exercise, methemoglobinemia of this degree leads to excess lactate production. At 30 per cent, acute induction leads to a significant increase in the heart rate but otherwise causes minimal symptoms. As methemoglobin exceeds 50 per cent, patients generally experience more significant symptoms such as weakness, breathlessness, headache, and confusion. At 70 to 80 per cent, coma and then death may occur. However, newborns exposed to nitrites have been encountered who have survived methemoglobin levels as high as 85 per cent.

CONGENITAL METHEMOGLOBINEMIA: CYTOCHROME b_5 REDUCTASE DEFICIENCY*

Congenital methemoglobinemia is due either to impaired ability to reduce methemoglobin (cytochrome b_5 reductase deficiency) or to the presence of one of the M hemoglobins (see Chapter 15). In acquired methemoglobinemia, the oxidation of hemoglobin results from exposure to an exogenous agent. In this section, cytochrome b_5 reductase deficiency will be considered, and the subsequent section will discuss toxic methemoglobinemia.

Inheritance Pattern

Although sporadic families with congenital methemoglobinemia had been noted since 1932, the inheritance pattern of this disorder was not firmly established until Scott's reports[72, 114] on numerous kindred of Eskimos and Indians. He documented an autosomal recessive inheritance pattern. Furthermore, he proved that the disorder was due to a marked deficiency in the NADH-dependent methemoglobin reductase now known as cytochrome b_5 reductase. By the use of the dye-linked enzyme assay, he showed that heterozygotes had about half normal levels of the enzyme. From the large population that Scott sampled in Alaska, he obtained a gene frequency of 0.07. The distribution of heterozygotes and homozygotes was in excellent agreement with the Hardy-Weinberg equilibrium. Interestingly, a large group of individuals with deficiency of cytochrome b_5 reductase has recently been encountered in northeastern Russia. Perhaps this finding reflects the migration of a population across the Bering Strait. In contrast, the gene frequency is much lower in other parts of the world. Individuals with cytochrome b_5 reductase deficiency are encountered infrequently and sporadically. Because of the autosomal recessive inheritance pattern, often only one member of a family is a clinically recognizable homozygote. In contrast, the M hemoglobins have an autosomal dominant mode of inheritance, and as a result, a larger proportion of family members is affected.

Because a number of variants of cytochrome b_5 reductase have been discovered in deficient individuals (see below), it is likely that in many cases, cyanotic individuals with severe enzyme deficiency are not true homozygotes but actually double (or compound) heterozygotes, inheriting a different mutant enzyme from each parent. Indeed, such a doubly heterozygous state has been documented.[115, 116] There are ample precedents for this phenomenon. Red cell pyruvate kinase deficiency is a well-recognized example. In kindred in whom there is true homozygosity for a cytochrome b_5 reductase variant, either consanguinity[108, 116] or a founder effect is likely.

Heterozygotes generally escape clinical de-

---

*This topic has been thoroughly reviewed by Jaffé.[112, 113]

tection. Even though they have approximately half normal levels of enzyme, they have no significant methemoglobinemia. However, on occasion, they may develop methemoglobinemia and cyanosis when exposed to oxidant compounds such as antimalarials,[117] nitrites, and phenazopyridine.[118a]

Cytochrome b_5 reductase has been assigned to human chromosome 22.[119, 120] It is very likely that a single gene codes for the microsomal enzyme. As explained above, the soluble erythrocyte enzyme is derived from the microsomal protein by proteolytic cleavage.

Clinical Features

Individuals with congenital methemoglobinemia are "more blue than sick."[121] Cyanosis is usually noted at birth. In addition to the skin, the mucous membranes also appear dusky, and when examined by an ophthalmoscope, the fundus has a mauve hue.[122] The extent of cyanosis varies widely, in proportion to the level of methemoglobin. In milder cases or in pigmented individuals, the abnormality may escape notice until the individual encounters an astute observer or his blood specimen is recognized because of its abnormal color. Cyanosis may be more marked during pregnancy[121] or stress such as surgery.[123] The vast majority of individuals have no significant symptoms even with deep cyanosis and levels of methemoglobin as high as 40 per cent. Occasional patients have reported nonspecific symptoms, including fatigue, restlessness, and headache.

Of considerably more concern is a subset of individuals with cytochrome b_5 reductase deficiency who have severe mental retardation. Other neurological abnormalities may also be present, and these patients have a short life expectancy. Kaplan and colleagues[124, 125] have shown that these individuals have a broad deficiency of cytochrome b_5 reductase, including both the cytoplasmic and microsomal forms. Accordingly, the enzyme deficiency is noted not only in the red cells but also in leukocytes, platelets, muscle, liver, brain, and fibroblasts.[124-126] The neurological disorder is probably related to impaired production of unsaturated fatty acids. In fact, the ratio of unsaturated to saturated fatty acids was found to be decreased in myelin, white matter, and gray matter of a patient with generalized enzyme deficiency and mental retardation.[127] In contrast, most individuals with cytochrome b_5 reductase deficiency have a deficiency of only the soluble cytoplasmic enzyme. Thus, enzyme activity in tissues other than the red cells is normal.[119, 126]

Laboratory Features

Individuals whose cyanosis is due to cytochrome b_5 reductase deficiency generally have 10 to 35 per cent methemoglobin. They are either homozygotes or double heterozygotes. Rarely, methemoglobin may reach 50 per cent; such a high level may reflect the superimposition of an oxidant upon severe enzyme deficiency. As mentioned above, methemoglobin levels are normal in heterozygotes unless they are challenged with oxidants.

Although some individuals with cyanosis and cytochrome b_5 reductase deficiency may have mild polycythemia, this finding is often absent. Because the partial oxidation of hemoglobin causes an increase in the affinity of the remaining hemes for oxygen, the resulting impairment in oxygen transport to tissues should result in a compensatory erythrocytosis. The fact that hemoglobin levels are often normal may be explained by the segregation of methemoglobin in the older population of red cells.[24] This phenomenon decreases the interaction between Fe^{3+} subunits and Fe^{2+} subunits, and therefore, the oxygen affinity of the blood is not as increased as it would be if the methemoglobin were evenly distributed among red cells.

The absorption spectrum of hemolysate from an individual with cytochrome b_5 reductase deficiency shows the presence of methemoglobin. The spectrum of methemoglobin from such individuals is indistinguishable from that of methemoglobin prepared by oxidation of normal hemoglobin. As mentioned in the preceding section on the properties of methemoglobin, the decrease in absorption at 630 nm after the addition of cyanide provides a precise measure of methemoglobin. In contrast, when cyanosis is caused by one of the M hemoglobins, the absorption spectrum is abnormal and less affected by the addition of cyanide (see Chapter 15).

The ability of red cells to reduce methemoglobin can be assessed by first pretreating the cells with nitrite in order to oxidize the hemoglobin and then incubating the cells with either glucose or lactate so that NADH can be generated. This approach[68, 69] provides a functional assessment of the cytochrome b_5 system for reducing methemoglobin. The metabolism of purine nucleosides can provide an alternative way of generating NADH.[128] As shown in Figure 16–10, homozygotes for cytochrome b_5 reductase deficiency have marked impairment in the rate of methemoglobin reduction, whereas heterozygotes have an intermediate rate, about half as fast as normal.[68, 112] These observations are consistent with the claim that the enzyme-mediated reduction of cytochrome b_5 is rate-limiting in methemoglobin reduction (see above).

The activity of cytochrome b_5 reductase is usually measured by one of two methods: reduction of DCIP, as developed by Scott and associates,[70, 71] or the assay devised by Hegesh and Avron,[76] which utilizes a ferrocyanide-hemoglobin complex as substrate. If a significant decrease in enzyme activity is noted, the defect can be further characterized by electrophoresis, kinetics, pH optimum, and thermal stability.

Such investigations have revealed considerable heterogeneity in the variant enzymes of deficient individuals. Thus far, at least five cytochrome b_5 reductase variants have been described that appear to function normally but have abnormal electrophoretic behavior.[113] In addition, 10 variants can be distinguished from one another on the basis of low catalytic activity as well as differences in electrophoretic migration[113] (Fig. 16–11). Some of these have

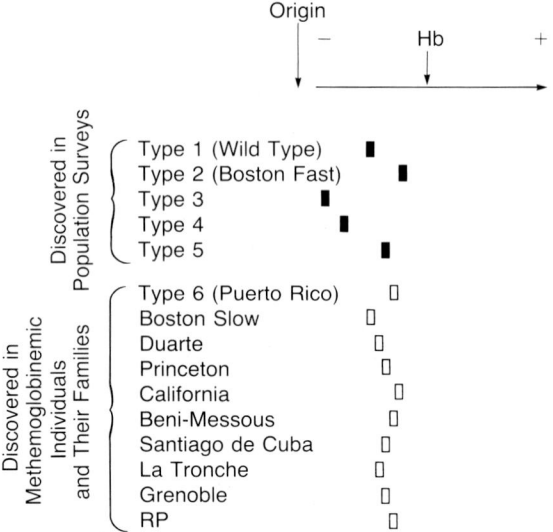

Figure 16–11. Schematic representation of electrophoretic mobilities of variants of cytochrome b_5 reductase. The normal or wild-type enzyme was designated as Type 1 by Hopkinson and associates.[177] In a survey of 3000 normal individuals, they detected an electrophoretic variant in 29 individuals, most commonly Types 2 and 4. These variants (designated as Types 2 to 5) appeared in heterozygotes in amounts approximately equal to the wild type. Thus, it is likely that these variants have normal enzyme activity (■). The other variants shown in this figure were encountered primarily in methemoglobinemic individuals, in whom they often constituted the only enzyme band, suggesting a homozygous state. When present in non-cyanotic relatives (heterozygotes), the variant band was much less prominent than that of the wild type, indicating decreased enzymatic activity (□). (Starch gel electrophoresis pH 8.6 to 9.3.) (This figure was modified from Jaffé[113] and represents data obtained from Hopkinson et al.,[176] Hsieh and Jaffé,[177] Kaplan et al.,[124, 178] Gonzalez et al.,[116] and Bloom and Zarkowsky.[179])

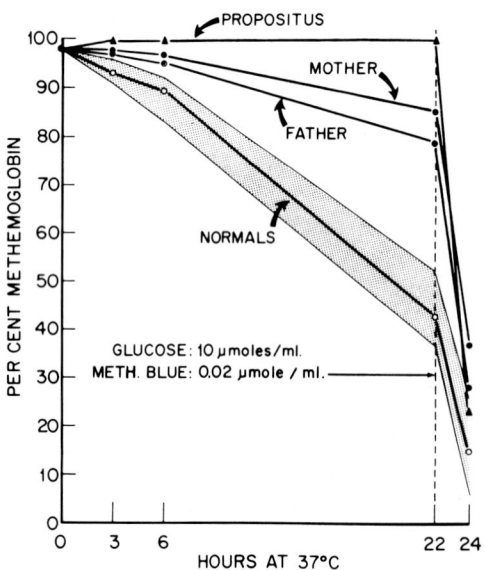

Figure 16–10. Rate of reduction of methemoglobin in nitrite-treated red cells of normal individuals, a homozygote, and obligatory heterozygotes (parents) with cytochrome b_5 reductase deficiency. Note the faster rate of reaction upon addition of methylene blue. (From Jaffe, E. R.: Am. J. Med. *41*:786, 1966.)

been encountered in specific ethnic groups, such as the Puerto Rico variant. Others are designated according to the location in which they were discovered: California, Duarte, Princeton, Boston Fast, Boston Slow, and Santiago de Cuba. As mentioned above, those individuals with associated neurological findings may have no detectable enzyme activity in erythrocytes. Heterogeneity among cytochrome b_5 reductase variants includes differences in the stability of the enzyme. Extreme instability may be responsible for significant deficiency in all tissues; in contrast, those with a less severe degree of instability may be manifested only in erythrocytes, which are long-lived cells incapable of protein synthesis.

In families who have had a child with the generalized deficiency state and severe mental retardation, the diagnosis can be established in fetuses at risk by culturing amniotic cells and measuring cytochrome b_5 reductase.[129]

In summary, the diagnosis of homozygous or doubly heterozygous cytochrome b_5 reductase deficiency can be established by the presence of 10 to 50 per cent methemoglobin and the demonstration of a marked decrease in enzyme activity.

Treatment

Although nearly all enzyme-deficient individuals are asymptomatic, some find their lifelong cyanosis to be a cosmetic handicap. The level of methemoglobin can be reduced to about 5 to 10 per cent by the oral administration of methylene blue (100 to 300 mg/day) or ascorbic acid (200 to 500 mg/day). Thus, these agents effectively reverse the cyanosis. As discussed above, methylene blue serves as an electron carrier and operates via NADPH-flavin reductase. In contrast, ascorbic acid reduces methemoglobin directly. The fact that untreated patients generally have low serum ascorbate levels probably means that the vitamin has been utilized for methemoglobin reduction. As mentioned above, riboflavin has also been found to be effective in lowering the level of methemoglobin in cytochrome b_5 reductase–deficient individuals.[107, 108] Reports of decreased glutathione reductase, a flavin enzyme, in individuals with congenital methemoglobinemia[112, 130] raises the possibility that riboflavin is also utilized for *in vivo* methemoglobin reduction, and therefore, vitamin stores may become depleted. Of these three agents, methylene blue is probably the most efficient. However, this drug should not be used in individuals with glucose-6-phosphate dehydrogenase deficiency because it is ineffective[131-133] and may cause acute oxidant-type hemolysis.[133]

TOXIC METHEMOGLOBINEMIA

Methemoglobinemia can be induced by a wide range of drugs and toxins. These agents are classified in Table 16–3 and discussed in the earlier section entitled "Oxidation of Hemoglobin by Chemical Agents." The extent of methemoglobinemia depends on the agent, its dose, and the duration of exposure. Furthermore, as mentioned above, individuals who are heterozygous for cytochrome b_5 reductase deficiency are more susceptible than normal individuals when exposed to an equivalent dose.[117, 118] There are a large number of anecdotal reports of toxic methemoglobinemia associated with various pharmaceutical and industrial agents. Most cases fall into one of the following groups:

Infants. Newborns and infants appear to be unusually susceptible to the development of toxic methemoglobinemia. This increased risk is due primarily to decreased amounts of cytochrome b_5 reductase in erythrocytes of newborns. The mean level of enzyme is about 60 per cent of that in adult red cells.[134, 135] Furthermore, the more "fetal" population of newborn cells probably has a more marked decreased in enzyme activity. Fetal hemoglobin does not contribute to the susceptibility of newborns to methemoglobinemia. Hb F and Hb A have identical redox potentials[136] and rates of autoxidation *in vitro*.[137]

The most common cause of methemoglobinemia in newborns is the intake of well water containing nitrate.[138] If the surrounding farmland is treated with large amounts of fertilizer, a significant and sometimes toxic amount of nitrate can seep into a well. The ingested nitrate is partially converted to nitrite by intestinal bacteria. Other causes of methemoglobinemia in the newborn include percutaneous absorption of aniline dye used to mark diapers and the administration of menadione (vitamin K_3) to newborns to prevent neonatal hemorrhage. Because of the wide recognition of these toxic effects, the incidence of methemoglobinemia in newborns and infants has decreased markedly in recent years.

Drug Use and Abuse. The incidence of drug-induced methemoglobinemia depends on the availability of drugs and the frequency of use, factors that vary markedly in time and place. Over-the-counter pain medicines have been responsible for the majority of cases of drug-induced methemoglobinemia. In many instances, the drugs have been used inappropriately and in excess. In the 1940's and 1950's, the widespread use of acetanilid and phenacetin for analgesia was associated with a large number of cases of toxic methemoglobinemia.[139] During the past 10 years, this drug has been supplanted by another nitrobenzene derivative, acetaminophen (Tylenol) (see Figure 16–6). Methemoglobinemia generally occurs in those individuals who abuse these agents. Patients often ingest a variety of drugs indiscriminately, so that it may be difficult to establish which were responsible for inducing hemoglobin oxidation. In a recent review of the experience at the Mayo Clinic, Fairbanks[140] has noted that the use of dapsone for dermatologic problems has been the leading cause of drug-induced cyanosis; 35 cases were observed in the interval from 1973 to 1978. During that time, seven cases of drug-induced methemoglobinemia and sulfhemoglobinemia could be attributed to acetaminophen in conjunction with another nitrobenzene, phenacetin, or phenazopyridine (Pyridium). The last drug may also induce hemolytic anemia and impairment of renal function.[141, 142] Furthermore, the drug's oxidant effect is enhanced in the presence of pre-existing renal failure.[143]

Among the antibiotics, the sulfa drugs occasionally cause toxic methemoglobinemia. In the past, sulfanilamide was a common offender. In contrast, the sulfa drugs currently in use rarely, if ever, induce hemoglobin oxidation.

Occasionally, toxic methemoglobinemia is associated with "recreational" use of drugs. Some individuals, particularly homosexuals, sniff or ingest amyl nitrite or isobutyl nitrite in order to achieve a more intense sexual response.[118, 144, 145] Repeated or heavy exposure may oxidize enough hemoglobin to make the individual frankly cyanotic. Occasional deaths have occurred.

The increasing use of nitroprusside for afterload reduction in the treatment of severe congestive heart failure may be associated with sufficient methemoglobinemia to cause cyanosis.[146] This complication can confuse the monitoring and management of these critically ill patients.

A significant proportion of drug-induced methemoglobinemia is caused by the use of local anesthetics.[147-150] Procaine congeners are arylamines and therefore induce methemoglobinemia by the same mechanism as aniline (see above). Recently, a number of cases have been reported following use of topical benzocaine (Cetacaine) prior to intubation or bronchoscopy. In this setting, cyanosis may be mistakenly attributed to the patient's underlying cardiac or pulmonary condition. Cyanosis can also be induced with prilocaine and lidocaine.

Industrial Exposure. As mentioned in the section on hemoglobin oxidation, a large number of cases of toxic methemoglobinemia occurred during the development of the dye industry in Europe in the early part of this century. The arylamines, especially aniline and its derivatives, were the most common offenders. More recently, rigid standards of employee safety have greatly reduced the incidence of significant methemoglobinemia in industry. Occasionally, accidental exposures occur in industry. One of us (H.F.B.) had the opportunity to see a machinist who turned deeply cyanotic within minutes after accidental ingestion of "cutting oil." This material contained a substantial amount of nitrite. The patient was admitted to a local hospital in deep coma with a methemoglobin level of 75 per cent.

Treatment

Patients whose methemoglobin levels exceed 40 per cent or who appear to be symptomatic from methemoglobinemia should be treated promptly with intravenous methylene blue (1 to 2 mg/kg). The level of methemoglobin should fall to normal within an hour after treatment. If not, a second dose of methylene blue can be adminsitered. It is useful but not essential to have spectral documentation of methemoglobinemia either before or soon after treatment is initiated. Failure of the cyanosis to clear promptly may mean that the patient has coexisting G-6-PD deficiency[133] or that he has significant amounts of sulfhemoglobin (> 0.5 g/dl).

If a patient is in extremis, more heroic measures may be indicated. One of us (H.F.B.), in conjunction with Dr. Ernst Jaffé and Dr. Glen Lubash, employed hemodialysis to treat a comatose young woman who had attempted suicide by ingesting a large amount of aniline.[151] A similar case has been treated by exchange transfusion.[152] Both patients recovered.

SULFHEMOGLOBINEMIA

Occasionally, patients who are exposed to oxidant compounds will develop cyanosis that cannot be explained by simple hemoglobin oxidation. The absorbance spectrum differs from that of methemoglobin; as shown in Figure 16–12 and Table 16–6, there is a broad band at 620 nm that is not altered by the addition of cyanide. Because of its high absorbance in the red region of the visible spectrum, sulfhemoglobinemia causes more cyanosis than an equivalent percentage of methemoglobinemia.

Structure and Function

Sulfhemoglobin was discovered in 1863 by Hoppe-Seyler,[153] who observed that when oxyhemoglobin was treated with hydrogen sulfide gas (H_2S), it gradually turned green. Even though it has been investigated with a broad

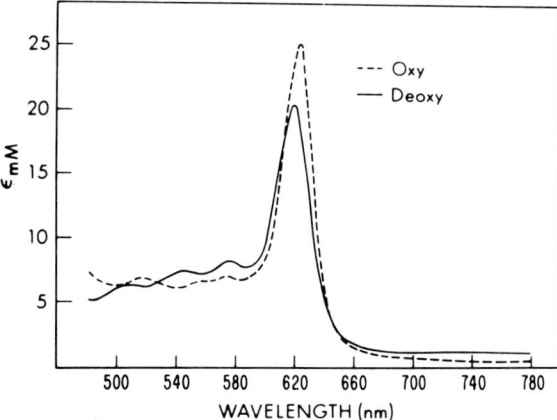

Figure 16–12. Absorbance spectra of deoxy and oxy sulfhemoglobins. (From Carrico, R. J., et al.: J. Biol. Chem. 253:7212, 1978.)

repertoire of analytical techniques, the structure of sulfhemoglobin is not fully established. Indeed, it may not be a single molecular species. The basic problem is that the characteristic sulfhemoglobin spectrum (Fig. 16–12) can be generated by a variety of compounds, but the relevant chemical reactions are complex and not thoroughly understood. The formation of sulfhemoglobin requires the oxidation of the heme iron followed by the interaction of the heme group with a sulfur-containing compound. The highest yield of sulfhemoglobin is obtained if methemoglobin is incubated with a 10-fold excess of hydrogen peroxide followed by the addition of ammonium sulfide or some other sulfide source.[154]

Observations by Morell and colleagues[155, 156] and, more recently, by Berzofsky and Peisach and associates[145, 157–161] on sulfmyoglobin and sulfhemoglobin have gone far toward determining the structure of sulfheme as well as explaining the functional properties of these proteins. It had been known for years that the sulfide does not form a coordination complex with the heme iron. Instead, the sulfur atom is incorporated into heme[155, 160] with a 1:1 stoichiometric ratio.[160] These investigators propose the following scheme for the formation of sulfhemoglobin:

1. In the presence of hydrogen peroxide methemoglobin is converted to ferrylhemoglobin

$$HbFe^{3+} + H_2O_2 \rightarrow HbFe^{4+}O + H_2O + \epsilon \quad [28]$$

2. Upon the addition of hydrogen sulfide, the iron in ferrylhemoglobin is reduced to the ferrous state, and sulfur is incorporated into the porphyrin ring.

$$HbFe^{4+}O + HS^- + 2\epsilon \rightarrow HbSFe^{2+} + OH^- \quad [29]$$

It is likely that this reaction involves the reduction of a β-carbon double bond in one of the pyrroles in protoporphyrin IX to form a chlorin (Fig. 16–13). The higher oxidation state of the heme iron withdraws electrons from the β-β bond, rendering it more susceptible to nucleophilic attack by HS^-.[159, 160] The proposed structure, depicted in Figure 16–13, shows the sulfur in a cyclic thioether. However, other reduction products are possible. Furthermore, it is unclear which, if any, of the four pyrroles in heme is preferentially reduced. Establishing the precise structure of the sulfheme moiety is a formidable challenge. Because of its marked lability, it cannot be analyzed by time-consuming techniques such as nuclear magnetic resonance or mass spectroscopy.

Because the heme iron in sulfhemoglobin is in the reduced (2+) state and not coordinated to sulfur, why does it not bind oxygen? In fact, it does, but with an affinity 100-fold lower than that of unmodified hemoglobin.[158, 161] Although sulfhemoglobin has no significant cooperativity ($n = 1.0$), it has a substantial Bohr effect.[161]

Table 16–6. COMPARISON OF SULFHEMOGLOBIN AND METHEMOGLOBIN

	Methemoglobin	Sulfhemoglobin
Iron valence	Fe^{3+}	Fe^{2+}
Porphyrin	Protoporphyrin	Chlorin
Binds O_2	No	Yes
Absorbance peak (red)	630 nm	620 nm
Absorbance abolished by CN^-	Yes	No
Reversible *in vivo*	Yes	No
Reversible *in vitro*	Yes	No

Figure 16–13. Proposed structure of the modified pyrrole in the porphyrin of sulfhemoglobin. One of the pyrroles (left) in protoporphyrin IX is reduced to a chlorin. (From Berzofsky, J. A., et al.: J. Biol. Chem. 247:3783, 1972.)

Clinical Features

Congenital. Three generations of a family from the United States were found to have congenital cyanosis.[162] The kindred showed an autosomal dominant inheritance pattern. Spectroscopic analysis of the hemoglobin of affected individuals revealed no significant methemoglobinemia but 1.0 to 1.4 g/dl of sulfhemoglobin. No exposure to oxidant agents could be documented. It is possible that these individuals had an unstable hemoglobin variant, a disorder compatible with dominant inheritance (see Chapter 13). Fairbanks* has noted that his patient with Hb Olmstead has significant levels of sulfhemoglobin. Other unstable hemoglobin variants such as Hb Freiburg and Hb St. Louis are associated with methemoglobinemia.

One individual with cyanosis was noted to have sulfhemoglobin and a half normal level of glutathione peroxidase.[163] This patient also ingested an increased amount of sulfur compounds in his diet. It is possible that the combination of impaired defense against peroxide coupled with increased sulfur compounds in the individual's erythrocytes led to the formation of sulfhemoglobin.

Acquired. In the vast majority of cases, sulfhemoglobinemia is associated with exposure to an oxidant compound. The arylamines are the most common offenders. Indeed, when acetanilide and phenacetin were in common use as analgesics, sulfhemoglobinemia was encountered more frequently than it is today.[139, 164, 165] Fairbanks and coworkers[140] noted that in a recent group of patients with cyanosis induced by acetaminophen, the level of sulfhemoglobin exceeded that of methemoglobin. Dapsone can also induce increased levels of both hemoglobin derivatives.[166] It is unclear what factors determine the relative proportions of methemoglobin and sulfhemoglobin in these individuals. Direct exposure to lethal doses of hydrogen sulfide does not usually cause sulfhemoglobinemia.[167] Sometimes the gastrointestinal tract plays a critical role in the development of sulfhemoglobinemia. The association of cyanosis with disturbances of bowel function was recognized by Van den Bergh in 1905 and designated "enterogenous cyanosis."[111, 168, 169] Sulfhemoglobin was often the predominant derivative in patients with constipation, whereas those with diarrhea had predominantly methemoglobin. Van den Bergh[168, 169] described a nine-year-old boy who had a rectal stricture and cyanosis for two years. Following surgical correction of the obstruction, the cyanosis disappeared. Subsequently, several observers noted the association of cyanosis and constipation in individuals who were exposed to aniline derivatives.[164, 170, 171] It is likely that during bowel stasis, the enhanced production of sulfides by bacterial flora converts methemoglobin to sulfhemoglobin. Red cell glutathione (GSH) has been suggested as an alternative source of sulfur that may contribute toward the development of sulhemoglobinemia.[163] Individuals with sulfhemoglobin often have increased GSH in their red cells.[163, 172] The enzyme β-mercaptopyruvate sulfurtransferase, which is abundant in human red cells,[173] may serve in the transfer of HS^- to hemoglobin.

Patients with sulfhemoglobinemia usually have no symptoms other than concern about their skin color. In contrast to methemoglobin, sulfhemoglobin has decreased oxygen affinity and therefore does not impair the unloading of oxygen from the unmodified hemes to tissues.

The diagnosis of sulfhemoglobinemia is established by spectroscopic examination of the patient's hemolysate. As mentioned above, the presence of an absorbance peak at 620 nm after the addition of cyanide indicates the presence of sulfhemoglobin. The percentage of this component can be calculated as follows:

$$\% \text{ SulfHb} \cong \frac{OD_{620} \times \text{Dil (Neutral Buffer} + CN^-)}{1.96 \times OD_{540} \times \text{Dil (Drabkins Solution)}} \quad [30]$$

where Dil is the dilution of the hemolysate. This equation was derived from the molar extinction coefficient:[154] $\epsilon_{\text{DeoSHb}} = 21.4$ (1 mM heme).[154, 174]† It should be noted that this value

---

*V. F. Fairbanks: Personal communication, 1983.

†A reliable spectrophotometric determination of methemoglobin requires that the absorbance measurements be made on hemoglobin solutions that are entirely free of turbidity, owing either to erythrocyte membranes or to precipitated hemoglobin. To minimize turbidity, a detergent such as Sterox SE or Tween 80 should be added to the solution, followed by centrifugation. The use of a scanning spectrophotometer is recommended to document an absorbance peak at 620 nm. Assuming that there is no turbidity, the contributing hemoglobins and their respective millimolar extinction coefficients are: sulfhemoglobin, 21.4; cyanmethemoglobin, 0.82; and oxyhemoglobin, 0.23. If a specimen contains at least 10 per cent sulfhemoglobin, the contribution from oxyhemoglobin to absorbance at 620 nm will be less than 10 per cent. The error in this sulfhemoglobin assay due to absorbance of cyanmethemoglobin at 620 nm will not exceed 10 per cent unless the amount of methemoglobin in the original sample is more than 2.5 times that of sulfhemoglobin.

is about twofold higher than previously published extinction coefficients. Accordingly, earlier formulae for the spectroscopic estimation of sulfhemoglobin are incorrect.

The addition of carbon monoxide causes a characteristic enhancement of the absorbance peak at 620 nm as well as a slight shift to lower wavelength.[174]

When a blood specimen containing sulfhemoglobin is analyzed by isoelectric focusing, a well-defined green band is readily visualized.[175] The fact that its isoelectric point is close to that of deoxyhemoglobin indicates that the sulfhemoglobin is not oxygenated and has the T quaternary structure.

The formation of sulfhemoglobin appears to be irreversible. The red cell lacks the enzymatic and chemical capability for converting it back to functional hemoglobin. Sulfhemoglobinemia is not usually associated with damage to the red cell membrane or hemolysis. In fact, the disappearance of sulfhemoglobin following withdrawal of the inciting agent parallels normal red cell senescence.[111]

Unlike methemoglobinemia, sulfhemoglobinemia cannot be corrected by pharmacologic means. The only treatment is avoidance of oxidant compounds and, when relevant, correction of constipation.

References

1. Perutz, M. F., Rossmann, M. G., Cullis, A. F., Muirhead, H., Will, G., and North, A. C. T.: Structure of haemoglobin: A three-dimensional Fourier synthesis at 5.5 Å resolution obtained by x-ray analysis. Nature 185:416, 1960.
2. Perutz, M. F., Muirhead, H., Cox, J. M., and Goaman, L. C. G.: Three-dimensional Fourier synthesis of horse oxyhaemoglobin at 2.8 Å resolution: The atomic model. Nature 219:131, 1968.
3. Ladner, R. C., Heidner, E. J., and Perutz, M. F.: The structure of horse methemoglobin at 2.0 Å resolution. J. Molec. Biol. 114:385, 1977.
4. Heidner, E. J., Ladner, R. C., and Perutz, M. F.: Structure of horse carbonmonoxyhemoglobin. J. Molec. Biol. 104:707, 1976.
5. Deatherage, J. F., Loe, R. S., and Moffat, K.: Structure of fluoride methemoglobin. J. Molec. Biol. 104:723, 1976.
6. Deatherage, J. F., Obendork, S. K., and Moffat, K.: Structure of azide methemoglobin. J. Molec. Biol. 134:419, 1979.
7. Fermi, G., and Perutz, M. F.: Structure of human fluoromethemoglobin with inositol hexaphosphate. J. Molec. Biol. 114:421, 1977.
8. Perutz, M. F., Heidner, E. J., Ladner, J. E., Beetlestone, J. G., Ho, C., and Slade, E.: Influence of globin structure on the state of heme. III. Changes in heme spectra accompanying allosteric transitions in methemoglobin and their implications for heme-heme interaction. Biochemistry 13:2187, 1974.
9. Perutz, M. F., Fersht, A. R., Simon, S. R., and Roberts, G. C. K.: Influence of globin structure of the state of heme. II. Allosteric transitions in methemoglobin. Biochemistry 13:2174, 1974.
10. Fung, W. M., and Ho, C.: A proton nuclear magnetic resonance study of the quaternary structure of human hemoglobins in water. Biochemistry 14:2526, 1975.
11. Perutz, M. F., Sanders, J. K. M., Chenery, D. H., Noble, R. W., Pennelly, R. R., Fung, L. W.-M., Ho, C., Giannini, I., Pörschke, D., and Winkler, H.: Interactions between the quaternary structure of the globin and the open state of the heme in ferric mixed spin derivatives of hemoglobin. Biochemistry 17:3640, 1978.
12. Itano, H. A., and Robinson, E.: Electrophoretic separation of intermediate compounds in two reactions of ferrihemoglobin. Biochim. Biophys. Acta 29:545, 1958.
13. Chanutin, A., and Curnish, R. R.: Electrophoretic studies of hemoglobin methemoglobin mixtures. Arch. Biochem. Biophys. 113:122, 1966.
14. Huisman, T. H. J.: Studies on the heterogeneity of hemoglobin. XI. Chromatographic studies of intermediate forms of oxy and ferrihemoglobin. Arch. Biochem. Biophys. 113:427, 1966.
15. Bunn, H. F., and Drysdale, J. W.: Separation of partially oxidized hemoglobins. Biochim. Biophys. Acta 229:51, 1971.
16. Park, C. M.: Isoelectric focusing and the study of interacting protein systems: Ligand binding, phosphate binding and subunit exchange in hemoglobin. Ann. N.Y. Acad. Sci. 209:237, 1973.
17. Mast, A., Milo, R., Jurrien, C., Leroux, A., Krishnamoorthy, R., Wajcman, H., Labie, D., and Kaplan, J. C.: Congenital enzymopenic methemoglobinemia. Acta Haematol. 56:174, 1976.
18. Tomoda, A., Takeshita, M., and Yoneyama, Y.: Characterization of intermediate hemoglobin produced during methemoglobin reduction by ascorbic acid. J. Biol. Chem. 253:7415, 1978.
19. Darling, R. C., and Roughton, F. J. W.: Effect of methemoglobin on equilibrium between oxygen and hemoglobin. Am. J. Physiol. 137:56, 1942.
20. Benesch, R. E., Benesch, R., and Macduff, G.: Subunit exchange and ligand binding: A new hypothesis for the mechanism of oxygenation of hemoglobin. Proc. Natl. Acad. Sci. USA 54:535, 1965.
21. Ainsworth, S., and Bingham, W. S. W.: Reactions of partially oxidized hemoglobin solutions. II. A matrix rank analysis of the initial rates of binding carbon monoxide. Biochim. Biophys. Acta 160:10, 1968.
21a. Ainsworth, S., and Ford, W. H.: Reactions of partially oxidized hemoglobin solutions. III. Biochim. Biophys. Acta 160:18, 1958.
22. Jung, F.: Alter, hämolytische Resistenz und Methämoglobingenalt der Erythrocyten. Dtsch. Arch. Klin. Med. 195:454, 1949.
23. Waller, H. D., Schlegel, B., Muller, A. A., and Löhr, G. W.: Der hämiglobingehalt in alternden Erythrocyten. Klin. Wochenschr. 37:898, 1959.
24. Keitt, A. S., Smith, T. W., and Jandl, J. H.: Red cell "pseudomosaicism" in congenital methemoglobinemia. N. Engl. J. Med. 275:397, 1966.
25. Feig, S. A., Nathan, D. G., Gerald, P. S., and Zarkowski, H. S.: Congenital methemoglobine-

mia: The result of age-dependent decay of methemoglobin reductase. Blood 39:407, 1972.
26. Schwartz, J. M., Paress, P. S., Ross, J. M., DiPillo, F., and Rizek, R.: Unstable variant of NADH methemoglobin reductase in Puerto Ricans with hereditary methemoglobinemia. J. Clin. Invest. 51:1594, 1972.
27. Matsuki, T., Tamura, M., Takeshita, M., and Yoneyama, Y.: Age dependent decay of cytochrome b_5 and cytochrome b_5 reductase in human erythrocytes. Biochem. J. 194:327, 1981.
27a. Takeshita, M., Tamura, M., Yubisui, T., and Yoneyama, Y.: Exponential decay of cytochrome b_5 and cytochrome b_5 reductase during senescence of erythrocytes: Relation to the increased methemoglobin content. J. Biochem. 93:931, 1983.
28. Banerjee, R., and Cassoly, R.: Oxygen equilibria of human hemoglobin valency hybrids. Discussion on the intrinsic properties of α and β chains in the native protein. J. Molec. Biol. 42:351, 1969.
29. Desbois, A., and Banerjee, R.: Effects of polyvalent anion binding to hemoglobin on oxidation and oxidation-reduction equilibria and their relevance to allosteric transition. J. Molec. Biol. 92:479, 1975.
30. Brunori, M., Wyman, J., Antonini, E., and Rossi-Fanelli, A.: Studies on the oxidation-reduction potentials of heme proteins. V. The oxidation Bohr effect in normal human hemoglobin and human hemoglobin digested with carboxypeptidase A. J. Biol. Chem. 240:3317, 1965.
31. Banerjee, R., and Cassoly, R.: Preparation and properties of the isolated α and β chains of human hemoglobin in the ferri state. Investigation of oxidation-reduction equilibria. J. Molec. Biol. 42:337, 1969.
32. Banerjee, R., and Lhoste, J.-M.: Nonequivalence of human hemoglobin chains in the oxidation-reduction and heme-transfer reactions. Eur. J. Biochem. 67:349, 1976.
33. Brooks, J.: The oxidation of haemoglobin to methaemoglobin by oxygen. Proc. R. Soc. Lond. [B] 109:35, 1932.
34. Kikugawa, K., Sasahara, T., Sasaki, T., and Kurechi, T.: Factors influencing the autoxidation of hemoglobin A. Chem. Pharm. Bull. 29:1382, 1981.
35. Mansouri, A., and Winterhalter, K. H.: Nonequivalence of chains in hemoglobin oxidation and oxygen binding. Effect of organic phosphates. Biochemistry 13:3311, 1974.
36. Rifkind, J.: Copper and the autoxidation of hemoglobin. Biochemistry 13:2475, 1974.
37. Winterbourn, C. C., and Carrell, R. W.: Oxidation of human hemoglobin by copper. Biochem. J. 165:141, 1977.
38. Brooks, J.: The oxidation of haemoglobin to methaemoglobin by oxygen. II. The relation between the rate of oxidation and the partial pressure of oxygen. Proc. R. Soc. Lond. [B] 118:560, 1935.
38a. Shikama, K.: A controversy on the mechanism of autoxidation of oxymyoglobin and oxyhemoglobin: Oxidation, dissociation, or displacement? Biochem. J. 223:279, 1984.
39. Wallace, W. J., Maxwell, J. C., and Caughey, W. S.: A role for chloride in the autoxidation of hemoglobin under conditions similar to those in erythrocytes. FEBS Lett. 43:33, 1974.
40. Lynch, R. E., Lee, G. R., and Cartwright, G. E.: Inhibition by superoxide dismutase of methemoglobin formation from oxyhemoglobin. J. Biol. Chem. 251:1015, 1976.
41. Demma, L. S., and Salhany, J. M.: Direct generation of superoxide anions by flash photolysis of human oxyhemoglobin. J. Biol. Chem. 252:1226, 1977.
42. Mansouri, A., and Winterhalter, K. H.: Nonequivalence of chains in hemoglobin oxidation. Biochemistry 12:4946, 1973.
43. Tomoda, A., Yoneyama, Y., and Tsuji, A.: Changes in intermediate hemoglobins during autoxidation of haemoglobin. Biochem. J. 195:485, 1981.
44. Demma, L. S., and Salhany, J. M.: Subunit inequivalence in superoxide anion formation during photooxidation of human oxyhemoglobin. J. Biol. Chem. 254:4532, 1979.
45. Kiese, M.: Methemoglobinemia: A Comprehensive Treatise. Cleveland, CRC Press, 1974.
46. Antonini, E., Brunori, M., and Wyman, J.: Studies on the oxidation-reduction potentials of heme proteins. IV. The kinetics of oxidation of hemoglobin and myoglobin by ferricyanide. Biochemistry 4:545, 1965.
47. Tomoda, A., Matsukawa, S., Takeshita, M., and Yoneyama, Y.: Effect of inositol hexaphosphate on hemoglobin oxidation. Biochem. Biophys. Res. Commun. 74:1469, 1977.
48. Tomoda, A., and Yoneyama, Y.: Analysis of intermediate hemoglobins in solutions of hemoglobin partially oxidized with ferricyanide. Biochim. Biophys. Acta 591:128, 1979.
49. Tomoda, A., Tsuji, A., and Yoneyama, Y.: Involvement of superoxide anion in the reaction mechanism of hemoglobin oxidation by nitrite. Biochem. J. 193:169, 1981.
50. Eyer, P., Hertle, H., Kiese, M., and Klein, G.: Kinetics of ferrihemoglobin formation by some reducing agents and the role of hydrogen peroxide. Mol. Pharmacol. 11:326, 1975.
51. Gamgee, A.: On the action of nitrites on blood. Philos. Trans. R. Soc. 158:589, 1869.
52. Martin, H., and Huisman, T. H. J.: Formation of ferrihemoglobin of isolated human hemoglobin types by sodium nitrite. Nature 200:898, 1963.
53. Smith, J. E., and Beutler, E.: Methemoglobin formation and reduction in man and various animal species. Ann. J. Physiol. 210:347, 1966.
54. Kosaka, H., Imaizumi, K., Imai, K., and Tyuma, I.: Stoichiometry of the reaction of oxyhemoglobin with nitrite. Biochim. Biophys. Acta 581:184, 1979.
55. Doyle, M. P., Pickering, R. A., DeWeert, T. M., Hoekstra, J. W., and Pater, D.: Kinetics and mechanism of the oxidation of human deoxyhemoglobin by nitrites. J. Biol. Chem. 256:12,393, 1981.
56. Beutler, E.: Drug induced hemolytic anemia. Pharmacol. Rev. 21:73, 1969.
57. Kiese, M., Reinwein, D., and Waller, H. D.: Die Hämiglobinbildung durch Phenylhydroxylamin und Nitrosobenzol in roten Zellen un vitro. Naunyn-Schmiedebergs Arch. Exp. Pathol. Pharmakol. 210:393, 1950.
58. Dalziel, K., and O'Brien, J. R. P.: Side reactions in the deoxygenation of dilute oxyhaemoglobin solutions by sodium dithionite. Biochem. J. 67:114, 1957.
59. Dixon, H. B. F., and McIntosh, R.: Reduction of methaemoglobin in haemoglobin samples using gel filtration for continuous removal of reaction products. Nature 213:399, 1967.
60. Bauer, C., and Pacyna, B.: The conversion of trivalent to divalent iron in hemoglobin of various species. Anal. Biochem. 65:445, 1975.

61. Vestling, C. S.: The reduction of methemoglobin by ascorbic acid. J. Biol. Chem. *143*:439, 1942.
62. Gibson, Q. H.: The reduction of methaemoglobin by ascorbic acid. Biochem. J. 37:615, 1943.
63. Tomoda, A., Tsuji, A., Matsukawa, S., Takeshita, M., and Yoneyama, Y.: Mechanism of methemoglobin reduction by ascorbic acid under anaerobic conditions. J. Biol. Chem. *253*:7420, 1978.
64. Tomoda, A., Takeshita, M., and Yoneyama, Y.: Characterization of intermediate hemoglobin produced during methemoglobin reduction by ascorbic acid. J. Biol. Chem. *253*:7415, 1978.
65. Kajita, A., Noguchi, K., and Skukuya, R.: A simple non-enzymatic method to regenerate oxyhemoglobin from methemoglobin. Biochem. Biophys. Res. Commun. *39*:1199, 1970.
66. Hayashi, A., Suzuki, T., and Shin, M.: An enzymic reduction system for metmyoglobin and methemoglobin and its application to functional studies of oxygen carriers. Biochim. Biophys. Acta *310*:309, 1973.
67. Suzuki, T., Benesch, R. E., Yung, S., and Benesch, R.: Preparative isoelectric focusing of CO hemoglobins on polyacrylamide gels and conversion to their oxy forms. Anal. Biochem. *55*:249, 1973.
67a. Hultquist, D. E., Sannes, L. J., and Juckett, D. A.: Catalysis of methemoglobin reduction. Curr. Top. Cell. Regul. *24*:287, 1984.
68. Gibson, Q. H.: The reduction of methaemoglobin in red blood cells and studies on the cause of idiopathic methemoglobinemia. Biochem. J. *42*:13, 1948.
69. Kiese, M.: Die Reduktion des Hämiglobins. Biochemische Zeitschrift *316*:264, 1943.
70. Scott, E. M., and McGraw, J. C.: Purification and properties of diphosphopyridine nucleotide diaphorase of human erythrocytes. J. Biol. Chem. *237*:249, 1962.
71. Scott, E. M., Duncan, I. W., and Ekstrand, V.: The reduced pyridine nucleotide dehydrogenases of human erythrocytes. J. Biol. Chem. *240*:481, 1965.
72. Scott, E. M., and Hoskins, D. D.: Hereditary methemoglobinemia in Alaskan Eskimos and Indians. Blood *13*:795, 1958.
73. Passon, P. G., and Hultquist, D. E.: Soluble cytochrome b_5 reductase from human erythrocytes. Biochim. Biophys. Acta *275*:62, 1972.
74. Kuma, F., and Inomata, H.: Studies on methemoglobin reductase. II. The purification and molecular properties of reduced nicotinamide adenine dinucleotide-dependent methemoglobin reductase. J. Biol. Chem. *247*:556, 1972.
75. Yubisui, T., and Takeshita, M.: Characterization of the purified NADH-cytochrome b_5 reductase of human erythrocytes as a FAD-containing enzyme. J. Biol. Chem. *255*:2454, 1980.
76. Hegesh, E., and Avron, M.: The enzymatic reduction of ferrihemoglobin. I. The reduction of ferrihemoglobin in red blood cells and hemolysates. Biochim. Biophys. Acta *146*:91, 1967.
77. Hegesh, E., Calmanovici, N., and Avron, M.: New method for determining ferrihemoglobin reductase (NADH-methemoglobin reductase) in erythrocytes. J. Lab. Clin. Med. *72*:339, 1968.
78. Hultquist, D. E., and Passon, P. G.: Catalysis of methaemoglobin reduction by erythrocyte cytochrome b_5 and cytochrome b_5 reductase. Nature [New Biol.] *229*:252, 1971.
79. Petragnani, N., Nogueria, O. C., and Raw, I.: Methemoglobin reduction through cytochrome b_5. Nature *184*:1651, 1959.
80. Sugita, Y., Nomura, S., and Yoneyama, Y.: Purification of reduced pyridine nucleotide dehydrogenase from human erythrocytes and methemoglobin reduction by the enzyme. J. Biol. Chem. *246*:6072, 1971.
81. Hultquist, D. E., Dean, R. T., and Douglas, R. H.: Homogeneous cytochrome b_5 from human erythrocytes. Biochem. Biophys. Res. Commun. *60*:28, 1974.
82. Slaughter, S. R., Williams, C. H., and Hultquist, D. E.: Demonstration that bovine erythrocyte cytochrome b_5 is the hydrophilic segment of liver microsomal cytochrome b_5. Biochim. Biophys. Acta *705*:228, 1982.
83. Hultquist, D. E., Sannes, L. J., and Schafer, D. A.: The NADH/NADPH-methemoglobin reduction system of erythrocytes from the red cell. In Brewer, G. (ed.): Fifth Ann Arbor Conference on the Red Cell. New York, Alan R. Liss, Inc., 1981, p. 291.
84. Slaughter, S. R., and Hultquist, D. E.: Membrane bound redox proteins of the murine Friend virus-induced erythroleukemia cell. J. Cell Biol. *83*:231, 1979.
85. Kuma, F., Prough, R. A., and Masters, B. S. S.: Studies on methemoglobin reductase: Immunologic similarity of soluble methemoglobin reductase and cytochrome b_5 of human erythrocytes with NADH cytochrome b_5 reductase and cytochrome b_5 of rat liver microsomes. Arch. Biochem. Biophys. *172*:600, 1976.
86. Goto-Tamura, R., Takesue, Y., and Takesue, S.: Immunological similarity between NADH-cytochrome b_5 reductase of erythrocytes and liver microsomes. Biochim. Biophys. Acta *423*:293, 1976.
87. Leroux, A., Torlinski, L., and Kaplan, J. C.: Soluble and microsomal forms of NADH-cytochrome b_5 reductase from human placenta. Similarity with NADH-methemoglobin reductase from human erythrocytes. Biochim. Biophys. Acta *481*:50, 1977.
87a. Raw, I., and Difini, F.: The possible role of ATP-dependent proteolysis on the solubilization of methemoglobin reductase during reticulocyte maturation. Biochem. Biophys. Res. Commun. *116*:357, 1983.
88. Choury, D., Leroux, A., and Kaplan, J. C.: Membrane-bound cytochrome b_5 reductase (methemoglobin reductase) in human erythrocytes. J. Clin. Invest. *67*:149, 1981.
89. Strittmatter, P., Spatz, L., Corcoran, D., Rogers, M. J., Setlow, B., and Redline, R.: Purification and properties of rat liver microsomal stearyl coenzyme A desaturase. Proc. Natl. Acad. Sci. USA *71*:4565, 1974.
90. Abe, K., and Sugita, Y.: Properties of cytochrome b_5 and methemoglobin reduction in human erythrocytes. Eur. J. Biochem. *101*:423, 1979.
91. Righetti, P. G., Gacon, G., Gianazza, E., Lostanleu, D., and Kaplan, J. C.: Titration curves of interacting cytochrome b_5 and hemoglobin by isoelectric focusing. Biochem. Biophys. Res. Commun. *85*:1575, 1978.
91a. Mauk, M. R., and Mauk, A. G.: Interaction between cytochrome b_5 and human methemoglobin. Biochemistry *21*:4730, 1982.
91b. Juckett, D. A., and Hultquist, D. E.: Magnetic

circular dichroism studies of hemoglobin: The reduction of ferrihemoglobin by ferrocytochrome b_5 and characterization of the high-spin hydroxy species of mixed-valence hemoglobin. Biophys. Chem. *19*:321, 1984.
92. Tomoda, A., Yubisui, R., Tsuji, A., and Yoneyama, Y.: Kinetic studies on methemoglobin reduction by human red cell NADH cytochrome b_5 reductase. J. Biol. Chem. *254*:3119, 1979.
93. Mansouri, A.: Non-equivalent behavior of α and β subunits in methemoglobin reduction. Biochim. Biophys. Acta *579*:191, 1979.
94. Tomoda, A., Ida, M., Tsuji, A., and Yoneyama, Y.: Mechanism of methemoglobin reduction by human erythrocytes. Biochem. J. *188*:535, 1980.
95. Salenme, F. R.: A hypothetical structure for an intermolecular electron transfer complex of cytochromes c and b_5. J. Molec. Biol. *102*:563, 1976.
96. Ng, S., Smith, M. B., Smith, H. T., and Millett, F.: Effect of modification of individual cytochrome c lysines on the reaction with cytochrome b_5. Biochemistry *16*:4975, 1977.
97. Gacon, G., Lostanleu, D., Labie, D., and Kaplan, J. C.: Interaction between cytochrome b_5 and hemoglobin: Involvement of β66 (E10) and β95 (FG2) lysyl residues of hemoglobin. Proc. Natl. Acad. Sci. USA *77*:1917, 1980.
98. Sannes, L. J., and Hultquist, D. E.: Effects of hemolysate concentration, ionic strength and cytochrome b_5 concentration on the rate of methemoglobin reduction in hemolysates of human erythrocytes. Biochim. Biophys. Acta *544*:547, 1978.
99. Kiese, M., Schneider, C., and Waller, H. D.: Hämiglobinreduktase. Naunyn-Schmiedeberg's Arch. Exp. Pathol. Pharmakol. *231*:158, 1957.
100. Kajita, A., Kerwar, G. K., and Huennekens, F. M.: Multiple forms of methemoglobin reductase. Arch. Biochem. Biophys. *130*:662, 1969.
101. Niethammer, D., and Huennekins, F. M.: Electrophoretic separation and characterization of the multiple forms of methemoglobin reductase. Arch. Biochem. Biophys. *147*:564, 1971.
102. Yubisui, T., Matsuki, T., Tanishima, K., Takeshita, M., and Yoneyama, Y.: NADPH-flavin reductase in human erythrocytes and the reduction of methemoglobin through flavin by the enzyme. Biochem. Biophys. Res. Commun. *76*:174, 1977.
103. Yubisui, T., Matsuki, T., Takeshita, M., and Yoneyama, Y.: Characterization of the purified NADPH-flavin reductase of human erythrocytes. J. Biochem. *85*:719, 1979.
104. Yubisui, T., Matsukawa, S., and Yoneyama, Y.: Stopped flow studies on the nonenzymatic reduction of methemoglobin by reduced flavin mononucleotide. J. Biol. Chem. *255*:11,694, 1980.
105. Tomoda, A., Yubisui, T., Tsuji, A., and Yoneyama, Y.: Changes in intermediate haemoglobins during methaemoglobin reduction by NADPH-flavin reductase. Biochem. J. *179*:227, 1979.
106. Matsuki, T., Yubisui, T., Tomoda, A., Yoneyama, Y., Takeshita, M., Hirano, M., Kobayashi, K., and Tani, Y.: Acceleration of methemoglobin reduction by riboflavin in human erythrocytes. Br. J. Haematol. *39*:523, 1978.
107. Kaplan, J. C., and Chirouze, M.: Therapy of recessive congenital methemoglobinemia by oral riboflavin. Lancet *2*:1043, 1978.
108. Hirano, M., Matsuki, T., Tanishima, K., Takeshita, M., Shimizu, S., Nagamura, Y., and Yoneyama, Y.: Congenital methaemoglobinemia due to NADH methemoglobin reductase deficiency: Successful treatment with oral riboflavin. Br. J. Haematol. *47*:353, 1981.
109. Sass, M. D., Caruso, C. J., and Farhangi, M.: TPNH-methemoglobin reductase deficiency. A new red cell enzyme defect. J. Lab. Clin. Med. *70*:760, 1967.
110. Sass, M. D.: Observation on the role of TPNH-dehydrogenase in human red cells. Clin. Chim. Acta *21*:101, 1968.
111. Finch, C. A.: Methemoglobinemia and sulfhemoglobinemia. N. Engl. J. Med. *239*:470, 1948.
111a. Board, P. G., Agar, N. S., Gruca, M., and Shine, R.: Methaemoglobin and its reduction in nucleated erythrocytes from reptiles and birds. Comp. Biochem. Physiol. *57B*:265, 1977.
112. Jaffé, E. R.: Hereditary methemoglobinemia associated with abnormalities in the metabolism of erythrocytes. Am. J. Med. *41*:786, 1966.
113. Jaffé, E. R.: Methemoglobinemia. Clin. Haematol. *10*:99, 1981.
114. Scott, E. M.: The relation of diaphorase of human erythrocyte to inheritance of methemoglobinemia. J. Clin. Invest. *39*:1176, 1960.
115. Board, P. G., and Pidcock, M. E.: Methaemoglobinaemia resulting from heterozygosity for two NADH-methaemoglobin reductase variants: Characterization as NADH-ferricyanide reductase. Br. J. Haematol. *47*:361, 1981.
116. Gonzalez, R., Estrada, M., Wade, M., De La Torre, E., Svarch, E., Fernandez, O., Ortiz, R., Guzman, E., and Colombo, B.: Heterogeneity of hereditary methaemoglobinaemia: A study of 4 Cuban families with NADH-methaemoglobin reductase deficiency including a new variant (Santiago de Cuba variant). Scand. J. Haematol. *20*:385, 1978.
117. Cohen, R. J., Sachs, J. R., Wicker, D. J., and Conrad, M.: Methemoglobinemia provoked by malarial chemoprophylaxis in Vietnam. N. Engl. J. Med. *279*:1127, 1968.
118. Horne, M. K., Waterman, M. R., Simon, K. M., Garriott, J. C., and Foerster, E. H.: Methemoglobinemia from sniffing butyl nitrite. Ann. Intern. Med. *91*:417, 1979.
118a. Daly, J. S., Hultquist, D. E., and Rucknagel, D. L.: Phenazopyridine induced methaemoglobinaemia associated with decreased activity of erythrocyte cytochrome b_5 reductase J. Med. Genet. *20*:307, 1983.
119. Fisher, R. A., Povey, S., Bobrow, M., Solomon, E., Boyd, Y., and Carritt, B.: Assignment of the DIA_1 locus to chromosome 22. Ann. Hum. Genet. *41*:151, 1977.
120. Junien, C., Vibert, M., Weil, D., Van-Cong, N., and Kaplan, J. C.: Assignment of NADH-cytochrome b_5 reductase (DIA_1 locus) to human chromosome 22. Hum. Genet. *42*:233, 1978.
121. Jaffé, E. R., and Hsieh, H.-S.: DPNH methemoglobin reductase deficiency and hereditary methemoglobinemia. Semin. Hematol. *8*:417, 1971.
122. Walsh, T. J., and Beehler, W.: Fundus in sulfhemoglobinemia. Arch. Intern. Med. *124*:377, 1969.
123. Gabel, R. A., and Bunn, H. F.: Hereditary methemoglobinemia as a cause of cyanosis during anesthesia. Anesthesiology *40*:516, 1974.

124. Kaplan, J. C., Leroux, A., Bakouri, S., Grangaud, J. P., and Benabadji, M.: La lésion enzymatique dans la méthémoglobinemie congénitale récessive avec encéphalopathie. Nouv. Rev. Fr. Hematol. 14:755, 1974.
125. Leroux, A., Junien, C., Kaplan, J. C., Bamberger, J.: Generalized deficiency of cytochrome b_5 reductase in congenital methaemoglobinaemia with mental retardation. Nature 258:619, 1975.
126. Tanishima, K., Matsuki, T., Fukuda, N., Takeshita, M., and Yoneyama, Y.: NADH-cytochrome b_5 reductase in platelets and leukocytes with special reference to normal levels and to levels in carriers of hereditary methemoglobinemia with or without neurological symptoms. Acta Haematol. (Basel) 63:7, 1980.
127. Mirono, H.: Lipids of myelin, white matter and gray matter in a case of generalized deficiency of cytochrome b_5 reductase in congenital methemoglobinemia with mental retardation. Lipids 15:272, 1980.
128. Jaffé, E. R.: The reduction of methemoglobin in human erythrocytes incubated with purine nucleosides. J. Clin. Invest. 38:1555, 1959.
129. Kaplan, J. C., Junien, C., Leroux, A., Bamberger, J., Bakouri, S., Boue, J., and Boue, A.: Prenatal diagnosis of generalized cytochrome b_5 reductase deficiency (congenital methemoglobinemia with mental retardation, Type II). Ann. Med. Interne (Paris) 132:93, 1981.
130. Das Gupta, A., Vaidya, M. S., Bapat, J. P., Pavri, R. S., Baxi, A. J., and Advani, S. H.: Associated red cell enzyme deficiencies and their significance in a case of congenital enzymopenic methemoglobinemia. Acta Haematol. (Basel) 64:285, 1980.
131. Jaffé, E. R.: The reduction of methemoglobin in erythrocytes of a patient with congenital methemoglobinemia, subjects with glucose-6-phosphate dehydrogenase deficiency and normal individuals. Blood 21:561, 1963.
132. Beutler, E., and Baluda, M.: Methemoglobin reduction. Studies of the interaction between cell populations and the role of methylene blue. Blood 22:323, 1963.
133. Rosen, P. J., Johnson, C., McGehee, W. G., and Beutler, E.: Failure of methylene blue treatment in toxic methemoglobinemia associated with glucose-6-phosphate dehydrogenase deficiency. Ann. Intern. Med. 75:83, 1971.
134. Ross, J. D.: Deficient activity of DPNH dependent methemoglobin diaphorase in cord blood erythrocytes. Blood 21:51, 1963.
135. Bartos, H. R., and DesForges, J. F.: Erythrocyte DPNH-dependent diaphorase levels in infants. Pediatrics 37:991, 1966.
136. Flohé, L., and Uehleke, H.: The oxidation-reduction potential of human hemoglobin F. Life Sci. 5:1041, 1966.
137. Betke, K., Kleihauer, E., and Lipps, M.: Vergleichende Untersuchen Über die Spontanoxydation von Nabelschnur und Erwachenenhämoglobin. Z. Kinderheilkd. 77:549, 1956.
138. Grant, R. S.: Well water nitrate poisoning review: A survey in Nebraska 1973 to 1978. Nebr. Med. J. 66:197, 1981.
139. Brandenburg, R. O., and Smith, H. L.: Sulfhemoglobinemia: A study of 62 clinical cases. Am. Heart J. 42:582, 1951.
140. Fairbanks, V. F.: Personal communication, 1983.
141. Nathan, D. M., Siegel, A. J., and Bunn, H. F.: Acute methemoglobinemia and hemolytic anemia with phenazopyridine: Possible relation to acute renal failure. Arch. Intern. Med. 137:1636, 1977.
142. Zimmerman, R. C., Green, E. D., Ghurabi, W. H., and Colohan, D. P.: Methemoglobinemia from overdose of phenazopyridine hydrochloride. Ann. Emerg. Med. 9:147, 1980.
143. Greenberg, M., and Wong, H.: Methemoglobinemia and Heinz body hemolytic anemia due to phenazopyridine HCl. N. Engl. J. Med. 271:431, 1964.
144. Wason, S., Detsky, A. S., Platt, O. S., and Lovejoy, F. H., Jr.: Isobutyl nitrite toxicity by ingestion. Ann. Intern. Med. 92:637, 1980.
145. Dixon, D. S., Reisch, R. F., and Santinga, P. H.: Fetal methemoglobinemia resulting from ingestion of isobutyl nitrite, a "room odorizer" widely used for recreational purposes. J. Forensic Sci. 26:587, 1981.
146. Bower, P. J., and Peterson, J. N.: Methemoglobinemia after sodium nitroprusside therapy. N. Engl. J. Med. 293:865, 1975.
147. Douglas, W. W., and Fairbanks, V. F.: Methemoglobinemia induced by a topical anesthetic spray (Cetacaine). Chest 71:587, 1977.
148. O'Donohue, W. J., Jr., Moss, L. M., and Angelillo, V. A.: Acute methemoglobinemia induced by topical benzocaine and lidocaine. Arch. Intern. Med. 140:1508, 1980.
149. Sandza, J. G., Jr., Roberts, R. W., Shaw, R. C., and Connors, J. P.: Symptomatic methemoglobinemia with a commonly used topical anesthetic, Cetacaine. Ann. Thorac. Surg. 30:187, 1980.
150. Ludwig, S. C.: Acute toxic methemoglobinemia following dental analgesia. Ann. Emerg. Med. 10:265, 1981.
151. Lubash, G. D., Phillips, R. E., Shields, J. D., and Bonsnes, R. W.: Acute aniline poisoning treated by hemodialysis. Arch. Intern. Med. 114:530, 1964.
152. Harrison, M. R.: Toxic methaemoglobinaemia. A case of acute nitrobenzene and aniline poisoning treated by exchange transfusion. Anaesthesia 32:270, 1977.
153. Hoppe-Seyler, F.: Einwirkung des Schwefelwasserstoffe aus das blut. Zentralbl. Med. Wiss. 1:433, 1863.
154. Carrico, R. J., Peisach, J., and Alben, J. O.: The preparation and some physical properties of sulfhemoglobin. J. Biol. Chem. 253:2386, 1978.
155. Morell, D. B., Chang, Y., and Clezy, P. S.: The structure of the chromophores of sulphmyoglobin. Biochim. Biophys. Acta 136:121, 1967.
156. Nichol. A. W., Hendry, I., Morell, D. B., and Clezy, P. S.: Mechanism of formation of sulphaemoglobin. Biochim. Biophys. Acta 156:97, 1968.
157. Berzofsky, J. A., Peisach, J., and Blumberg, W. E.: Sulfheme proteins. I. Optical and magnetic properties of sulfmyoglobin and its derivatives. J. Biol. Chem. 246:3367, 1971.
158. Berzofsky, J. A., Peisach, J., and Blumberg, W. E.: Sulfheme proteins. II. The reversible oxygenation of ferrous sulfmyoglobin. J. Biol. Chem. 246:7366, 1971.
159. Berzofsky, J. A., Peisach, J., and Alben, J. O.: Sulfheme proteins. III. Carboxysulfmyoglobin: The relation between electron withdrawal from iron and ligand binding. J. Biol. Chem. 247:3774, 1972.

160. Berzofsky, J. A., Peisach, J., and Horecker, B. L.: Sulfheme proteins. IV. The stoichiometry of sulfur incorporation and the isolation of sulfhemin, the prosthetic group of sulfmyoglobin. J. Biol. Chem. 247:3783, 1972.
161. Carrico, R. J., Blumberg, W. E., and Peisach, J.: The reversible binding of oxygen to sulfhemoglobin. J. Biol. Chem. 253:7212, 1978.
162. Miller, A. A.: Congenital sulfhemoglobinemia. J. Pediatr. 51:233, 1957.
163. Tursz, T., Bernard, J. F., Berdier, F., and Boivin, P.: Sulfhemoglobin and glutathione peroxidase deficiency. Nouv. Presse Med. 3:1487, 1974.
164. Kneezel, L. D., and Kitchens, C. S.: Phenacetin-induced sulfhemoglobinemia: Report of a case and review of the literature. Johns Hopkins Med. J. 139:175, 1967.
165. Reynolds, T. B., and Ware, A. G.: Sulfhemoglobinemia following habitual use of acetanilid. J.A.M.A. 149:1538, 1952.
166. Lambert, M., Sonnet, J., Mahien, P., and Hassoun, A.: Delayed sulfhemoglobinemia after acute dapsone intoxication. Clin. Toxicol. 19:45, 1982.
167. Burnett, E., King, E. G., Grace, M., and Hall, W. F.: Hydrogen sulfide poisoning: Review of 5 years' experience. Can. Med. Assoc. J. 117:1277, 1977.
168. van den Bergh, A. A. H.: Enterogene cyanose. Dtsch. Arch. Klin. Med. 83:86, 1905.
169. van den Bergh, A. A. H., and Grutterink, A.: Enterogene cyanose. Berl. Klin. Wochenschr. 43:7, 1906.
170. Lim, T. P., and Lower, D.: "Enterogenous" cyanosis. Am. Rev. Respir. Dis. 101:419, 1970.
171. Basset, P., Bergerat, J. P., Lang, J. M., Oberling, F., and Gillet, B.: Hemolytic anemia and sulfhemoglobinemia due to phenacetin abuse: A case with multivisceral adverse effects. Clin. Toxicol. 18:493, 1981.
172. McCutcheon, A. D.: Sulphaemoglobinaemia and glutathione. Lancet 2:240, 1960.
173. Martensson, J., and Sörbo, B.: Human β-mercaptopyruvate sulfur transferase: Distribution in cellular compartments of the blood and activity in erythrocytes from patients with hematological disorders. Clin. Chim. Acta 87:11, 1978.
174. Nichol, A. W., and Morell, D. B.: Spectrophotometric determination of mixtures of sulphaemoglobin and methaemoglobin in blood. Clin. Chim. Acta 22:157, 1968.
175. Park, C. M., and Nagel, R. L.: Sulfhemoglobinemia: Clinical and molecular aspects. N. Engl. J. Med. 310:1579, 1984.
176. Hopkinson, D. A., Corney, G., Cook, P. J. L., Robson, E. B., and Harris, H.: Genetically determined electrophoretic variants of human red cell NADH diaphorase. Ann. Hum. Genet. 34:1, 1970.
177. Hsieh, H.-S., and Jaffé, E. R.: Electrophoretic and functional variants of NADH-methemoglobin reductase in hereditary methemoglobinemia. J. Clin. Invest. 50:196, 1971.
178. Kaplan, J. C.: Defective molecular variants of glucose-6-phosphate dehydrogenase and methemoglobin reductase. J. Clin. Pathol. 27(Suppl 8):134, 1974.
179. Bloom, G. E., and Zarkowsky, H. S.: Heterogeneity of the enzymatic defect in congenital methemoglobinemia. N. Engl. J. Med. 281:919, 1969.

CARBOXYHEMOGLOBIN AND CARBOXYHEMO-GLOBINEMIA

17

John Burton Sanderson Haldane* was first confronted with the sight of blood just before his fourth birthday. He rushed up to his father and demanded to know whether it was oxyhemoglobin or carboxyhemoglobin.[1] The precocious boy received an authoritative answer. John Scott Haldane,* one of the founding fathers of hemoglobin physiology, was the first to realize that carbon monoxide posed a threat to man and other creatures because it competes so effectively with oxygen in binding to hemoglobin. There was a strong practical bent to the elder Haldane's research. He was elected president of the British Institution of Mining Engineers because of his work on carbon monoxide poisoning in mines. This occupational hazard led him to fundamental studies on the combination of carbon monoxide (CO) with hemoglobin and the relative affinities of CO and oxygen for hemoglobin. According to J. T. Edsall's account[2]:

> Characteristically, after first showing that mice would die when exposed to 0.2 per cent carbon monoxide in air, he experimented on himself, and reached 49 per cent saturation of his hemoglobin with carbon monoxide, at which point he stopped the experiment, recording "vision dim, limbs weak. Had some difficulty in getting up or walking without assistance, movements being very uncertain." These studies led him to recommend the use of small birds in mines, to detect the presence of carbon monoxide, since their very high metabolism made them much more rapidly sensitive than men to the effects of this gas.

In New College, Oxford, there stands a memorial tablet to Haldane; it is worth recording here:

---

*See Chapter 1, pages 4 and 10, and Figure 1–7.

In Memory of
John Scott Haldane
C.H., F.R.S., M.D., LL.D., D.Sc.

Fellow of New College 1901–1936
Honorary Professor and Director of the Mining Research Laboratory in the University of Birmingham

Physiologist and Philosopher
whose researches on respiration on air and in kindred subjects were applied by him to the signal benefit of miners, divers, the crews of submarines and all who work in crowded factories or fly at high altitudes.

a deep thinker
unselfish and single-minded

Born in Edinburgh	Died in Oxford
2nd May 1860	14th March 1936

SOURCES OF CARBON MONOXIDE

Carbon monoxide is a colorless, odorless, and tasteless gas that is generated by incomplete combustion. Its presence in our atmosphere partly reflects man's ever-expanding use of fuels following the Industrial Revolution. At present, oxidation of hydrocarbons, principally gasoline, releases 600 million tons of CO into the atmosphere each year.[3a] Motor vehicles are responsible for more than half of this output. In New York City, automobile traffic produces about 10 million pounds of CO per day.[4] In Los Angeles, more than twice as much CO is released by automobiles. Each car emits about 1/6 pound of CO per mile when traveling at 25 mph. The upward trend in CO production from automobiles abated following the institution of emission controls in 1968. Local concentrations of CO in the air vary enormously, depending on the amount produced, the proximity to the production site, and the degree of ventilation. For example, individuals working in highway toll booths, underground garages, truck loading stations, traffic tunnels, mines, and submarines are exposed to particularly high levels of CO. Various kinds of stationary sources can also increase local levels of CO. Petroleum refineries, iron foundries, and carbon black plants are substantial contributors. In addition, indoor combustion may be a significant source. A number of deaths each year can be attributed to home heating units, particularly gas-fired baseboard heaters, that have faulty ventilation. Open fires and charcoal braziers often produce substantial amounts of CO.[4] Fire fighters and fire victims are also exposed to high levels of CO. Smoking tobacco poses another important type of exposure. Cigarette smoke contains about 2 per cent CO. The effect of smoking on levels of carboxyhemoglobin and on oxygen transport will be discussed in a later section.

National health agencies have attempted to determine the upper limit of CO in the atmosphere that can be regarded as safe.[3] At this time in the United States, the maximal allowable 8-hour concentration is nine parts per million,* not to be exceeded more than once per year. The maximum 1-hour exposure is 35 ppm. In regions of the world free of industry and motor vehicles, the atmospheric CO ranges between 0.01 and <1 part per million.[5,6]

Despite the huge amount of CO that is produced by industrial combustion, it does not appear to contribute significantly to the world's ecosytem. A vast amount of CO is released into the atmosphere by oxidation of methane in the troposphere as well as methane produced in swamps and tropical regions by decomposition of organic matter.[7] In addition, a substantial amount of CO is released by degradation of chlorophyll from dying plants, a process akin to release of CO from heme catabolism, which will be discussed in the following paragraph. Even though the yearly production of CO from industrial combustion is about half the total amount of CO normally present in the atmosphere, the turnover of CO is so rapid that these natural sources of CO production dwarf CO output from automobiles and industrial sources. The major sink of CO is reaction with hydroxyl radicals in the upper atmosphere to produce CO_2. Microorganisms in the soil constitute another important sink. The average residence time of CO in the atmosphere is about 2 to 6 months.[3a] Because of the huge natural sources of CO in the atmosphere and its rapid turnover, man's vigorous production of this gas presents local hazards rather than a global threat.

Endogenous CO Production. In man and other animals, the level of carboxyhemoglobin is determined not only by the partial pressure of CO in the inspired air but also by the endogenous production of CO. As shown in Figure 17–1, about 70 to 80 per cent of endogenous CO production is derived from the degradation of heme in senescent red cells.[4,8] When this cyclic tetrapyrrole is enzymatically

---

*Parts per million (ppm) = moles $CO/10^6$ moles of air ($N_2 + O_2$).

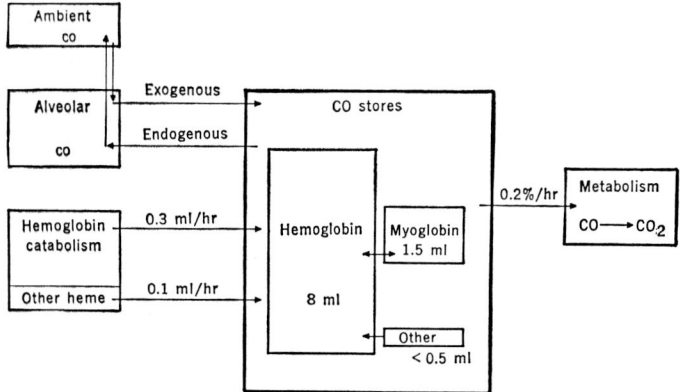

Figure 17–1. Scheme of factors that influence body stores of CO. (From Coburn, R.: Acta Med. Scand. Suppl. 472:269, 1967.)

converted to the linear tetrapyrrole, bilirubin, the α-methene carbon atom, is oxidized to CO. This microsomal enzyme, heme oxygenase, is readily induced in any tissue involved in heme catabolism.[9, 9a] The breakdown of heme from myoglobin and heme-containing enzymes contribute a lesser amount of CO. Finally, oxidation of lipids may also make a small contribution to endogenous CO production.[10] Normal subjects who breathe air free of CO expire approximately 0.4 ml of CO per hour and have a HbCO level of about 0.5 per cent.[11, 14]* This represents the contribution of endogenous CO production to the proportion of HbCO in red cells. Thus, in normal individuals, levels higher than 0.5 per cent represent the inhalation of CO from the atmosphere. The kinetics of CO production *in vivo* have been thoroughly documented by administration of radioactive heme precursors and by montoring recovery of labeled CO. Endogenous production is enhanced in hemolytic anemia and ineffective erythropoiesis. Careful measurement of CO levels in expired air provides an accurate measure of the rate of red cell catabolism.[11] The level of HbCO in blood provides an approximate index of hemolysis.[11–13] A number of variables must be considered in the interpretation of this measurement (as discussed later).

CARBOXYHEMOGLOBIN: STRUCTURE AND FUNCTION

In 1897, J. S. Haldane[15] enunciated a law regarding the relative binding of carbon monoxide and oxygen to hemoglobin. After hemoglobin has been equilibrated with a mixture of the two gases:

$$HbCO/HbO_2 = M\ PCO/PO_2$$

where M is a partition constant. Under physiologic conditions, M for human hemoglobin is approximately 210, which means that CO binds 210 times more strongly than does oxygen. This constant is not altered by pH or organic phosphates but is slightly temperature-dependent ($\Delta H = -3.6$ kcal/mole of heme).[16] Thus, if the partial pressure of CO is 0.5 per cent that of oxygen, the concentration of carboxyhemoglobin at equilibrium will equal that of oxyhemoglobin. The much higher affinity of hemoglobin for carbon monoxide, compared with oxygen, must mean that one or both of the following pertain: (1) the rate of CO binding to hemoglobin is inordinately fast; (2) the rate of dissociation of CO from HbCO is inordinately slow. Precise measurements utilizing stopped-flow kinetics show that CO actually binds to hemoglobin more slowly than does O_2. However, this difference in "on" rates is more than offset by the fact that CO dissociates extremely slowly from HbCO.

As explained in Chapter 2, oxygen binds to the heme iron of hemoglobin as well as of model heme complexes in a bent or off-axis configuration. In contrast, in model heme complexes, CO preferentially binds in an axial configuration.[17] As shown in Figure 17–2, the carbon atom of CO is bonded to the iron atom of heme and the Fe, C, and O atoms form a straight line that, in the model heme complex, is perpendicular to the plane of the heme. A stereoscopic view of the heme pocket of HbCO (Fig. 17–3) shows that steric constraints prevent CO from assuming this perpendicular orientation.[18, 18a] This distortion reduces the strength of the Fe–CO bond. Potential energy

---

*In this chapter, per cent carboxyhemoglobin = % HbCO = (HbCO ÷ total Hb) × 100.

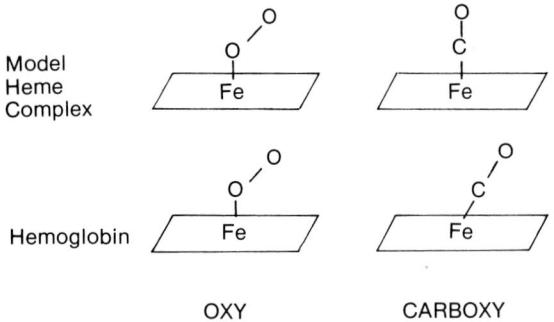

Figure 17-2. Diagram showing orientation of ligands O_2 and CO relative to the plane of the heme. In this figure, the plane is perpendicular to the plane of the page.

calculations indicate that the Fe–C–O unit is linear and displaced from the heme perpendicular by a relatively small strain (< 10 kcal per mole).[19] In the variant Hb Zürich (β 63 (E7) His → Arg), the substitution of the distal histidine allows room for the CO to bind perpendicular to the heme and therefore with considerably higher affinity[20] (see Fig. 13–2A and Chapter 13). A second structural feature distinguishes HbCO from HbO$_2$. In the latter, the distal atom of the oxygen molecule forms a hydrogen bond with the imidazole of the distal histidine (E7 His), pulling this residue further into the heme pocket (see Fig. 17–3).[18a] This hydrogen bond is not formed in carboxyhemoglobin.

Despite the marked difference in affinity between CO and O$_2$, they bind to deoxyhemoglobin with equal cooperativity.[21] The three-dimensional structure of carboxyhemoglobin is identical to that of oxyhemoglobin (except at the site of ligand binding).[18, 18a] Therefore, the same structural transition should take place upon ligand binding, and according to the two-state allosteric model (see Chapter 3), the two ligands would be expected to have equal degrees of cooperativity. Nevertheless, the kinetic basis of cooperativity differs markedly between the two ligands. As explained in Chapter 3, oxygen binds to T and R hemoglobins with approximately equal velocity. Thus, the cooperativity in O$_2$ binding resides almost exclusively in differences in the "off" rates. In contrast, CO binds much more slowly to T hemoglobin than to R hemoglobin. Thus, in carboxyhemoglobin, the "on" rate contributes substantially to the cooperativity. Differences in the kinetic basis of cooperativity have been explained in terms of the transition states formed when the two ligands bind to hemoglobin[22, 23] (see Chapter 3).

Because CO dissociates so slowly from hemoglobin, it is possible to separate deoxyhemoglobin from HbCO by a rapid high-resolution electrophoretic technique. As shown in Figure 17–4,[24] the purple deoxyhemoglobin band has a higher isoelectric point than the red HbCO band, owing to the binding of Bohr protons, which makes the hemoglobin more positively charged. Carboxyhemoglobin and oxyhemoglobin have identical isoelectric points. Recent analyses done at very low temperature have enabled the isolation of partially liganded species of HbCO.[25]

Because of its high affinity, CO readily binds to hemoglobin and triggers the transition from the T to the R quaternary structure. Therefore, hemoglobin partially saturated with CO will have increased affinity for oxygen. Figure 17–5 shows experimental data of the Haldanes[26, 27] on the effect of increasing saturation with CO upon hemoglobin's oxygen affinity. These investigators appreciated the pathophysiologic significance of this phenomenon. A patient or animal with 50 per cent carboxyhemoglobin is much more hypoxic than one with a 50 per cent reduction in total hemoglobin. The pri-

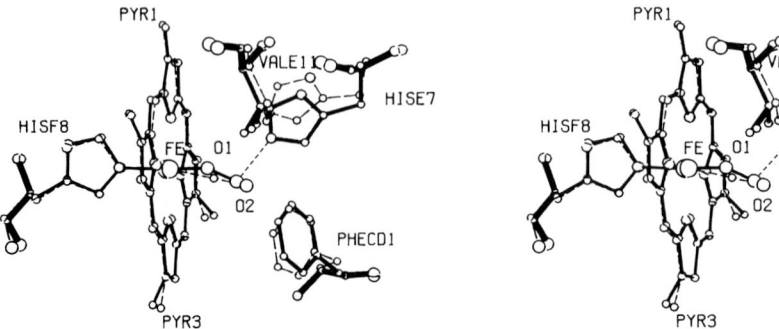

Figure 17-3. Comparison of the structures of the α chain of oxyhemoglobin (solid line) and carboxyhemoglobin (dashed line) in the vicinity of the heme pocket. Note that both O$_2$ and CO are bound in an off-axis configuration. There is a hydrogen bond between the distal atom of the oxygen molecule and the imidazole of E7 His. (From Shaanan, B.: J. Mol. Biol. *171*:31, 1983.)

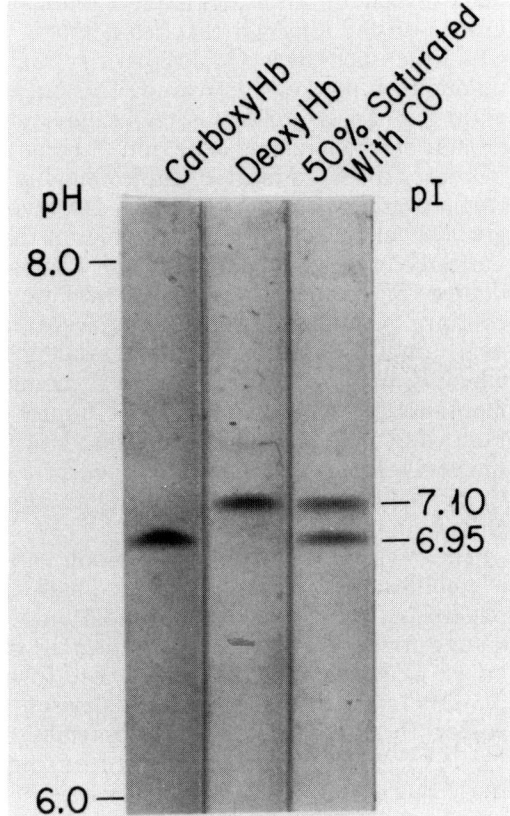

Figure 17–4. Separation of deoxyhemoglobin and carboxyhemoglobin by isoelectric focusing. Carboxyhemoglobin *(left)*, deoxyhemoglobin *(middle)*, and deoxyhemoglobin half saturated with CO *(right)* were applied to cylindrical gels under strict anaerobic conditions. Two bands are seen: purple deoxyhemoglobin and the more negatively charged red carboxyhemoglobin. The binding of CO to deoxyhemoglobin results in a decrease in the isoelectric point (pI) from 7.10 to 6.95 owing to the release of Bohr protons. (*From* Bunn, H. F., and McDonough, M.: Biochemistry *13*:988, 1974.)

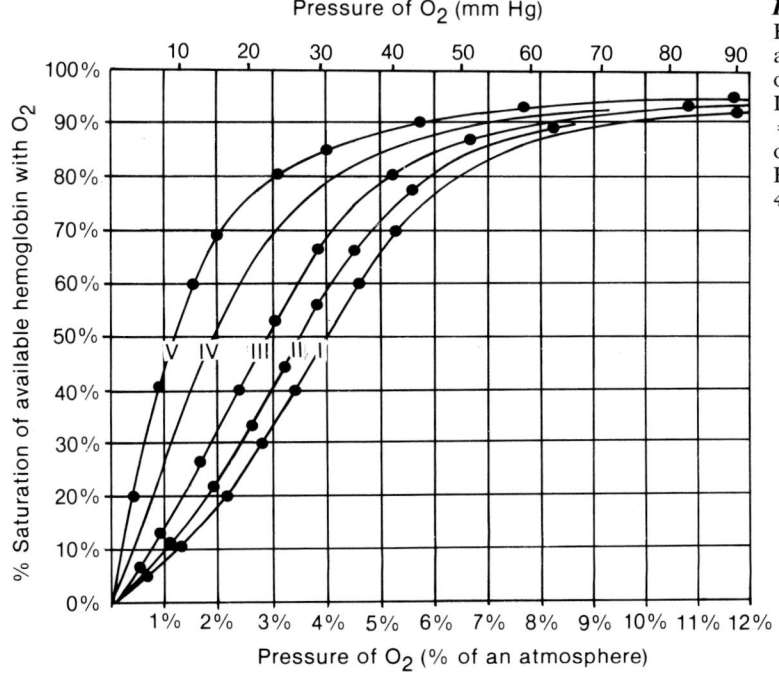

Figure 17–5. Experiment of J. B. S. Haldane showing the effect of increasing amounts of CO in the oxygen equilibrium of normal blood, 38°C (I = 0% HbCO; II = 10% HbCO; III = 25% HbCO; IV = 50% HBCO; V = 75% HbCO). The ordinate shows $HbO_2 \div (HbO_2 + \text{deoxy Hb})$. (From Haldane, J. B. S.: J. Physiol. *45*:xxii, 1912–13.)

mary reason for this is that the remaining heme groups on the tetramer that are not bound to CO have such high O_2 affinity that oxygen unloading is markedly impaired. This phenomenon is entirely analogous to methemoglobinemia, in which partial oxidation of heme iron increases the O_2 affinity of the remaining ferroheme groups on the tetramer. However, a given level of carboxyhemoglobinemia has a more deleterious effect than an equivalent degree of methemoglobinemia because red cells are evenly modified following a sustained exposure to CO, in accord with Haldane's law, whereas methemoglobin tends to be compartmentalized in older red cells (see Chapter 16). Following a brief *in vivo* exposure, HbCO is unevenly distributed among red cells,[28] owing to the slow rate of dissociation of the ligand from hemoglobin.

The oxygen affinity of normal blood samples is significantly increased by even small levels of HbCO. The wide range of whole blood P_{50} values found in normal individuals is influenced by levels of HbCO even more than by 2,3-DPG.[29] Formulas have been devised that correct the P_{50} of blood for the contribution of HbCO.[30, 30a] The slightly increased oxygen affinity due to HbCO persists after lysis of red cells and stripping the hemolysate of organic phosphates.[31] Once the CO is removed by displacement with hyperbaric oxygen, the oxygen affinity of the stripped hemolysates becomes normal.

CARBOXYHEMOGLOBINEMIA

Because hemoglobin has such a high affinity for CO (as discussed previously), the level of HbCO in blood provides an assessment of both exposure to CO in air as well as endogenous CO production. As explained in detail later, the adverse effect of CO in man and other animals depends primarily on its binding to hemoglobin.

Precise measurement of HbCO in blood (as well as CO in air) requires the use of either infrared spectroscopy[32] or gas chromatography.[33, 34] One of these relatively elaborate methods is usually required for studies of endogenous CO production. An indirect but accurate estimate of HbCO can be obtained by measurement of CO in expired air after breath-holding equilibration. The approach obviates the need to obtain blood specimens and therefore is useful in field studies. If the level of HbCO in blood is high ($>$ 10 per cent), it can be measured by an ordinary spectrophotometer utilizing either the visible[35] or the Soret[36, 37, 37a] portion of the hemoglobin spectrum. Blood should be collected in a closed receptacle containing an anticoagulant. A reducing agent such as sodium hydrosulfite is added in order to remove oxygen, converting the hemolysate into a two-component system—HbCO and deoxyhemoglobin. Alternatively, a commercially available instrument (CO-oximeter) utilizes filters to give a rapid estimate of HbCO, HbO_2, and deoxyhemoglobin.[38] Magnetic circular dichroism is an alternative spectroscopic method for measuring HbCO.[39] This method requires no pretreatment of the sample and is reasonably accurate over a HbCO range of 2 to 20 per cent. Its major limitations are the high cost and low availability of the instrument.

Carbon monoxide is absorbed and excreted exclusively by the alveoli of the lungs. There is no transit of CO across the upper respiratory tract, even in a CO-enriched bolus of tobacco smoke.[40] The amount of CO that passes across alveolar membranes per unit time is determined by the tension of CO in the alveolar air and capillaries, the pulmonary diffusing capacity, the rate of ventilation, and the match

$$\frac{d[COHb]}{dt} = \frac{\dot{V}_{CO}}{V_b} - \frac{[COHb]P_{c_{O_2}}}{[O_2Hb]MV_b}\left(\frac{1}{\frac{1}{D_L} + \frac{P_L}{\dot{V}_A}}\right) + \frac{P_{I_{CO}}}{\left(\frac{1}{D_L} + \frac{P_L}{\dot{V}_A}\right) \cdot V_b}$$

COHb	= ml CO/ml blood
O_2Hb	= ml O_2/ml blood
M	= Haldane affinity ratio
V_b	= blood volume (ml)
$\dot{V}_{CO}$	= endogenous CO production (ml/min)
$\dot{V}_A$	= alveolar ventilation rate (ml/min)
D_L	= pulmonary diffusing capacity for CO (ml/min·mm Hg)
$P_{I_{CO}}$	= partial pressure CO in air inhaled (mm Hg)
$P_{c_{O_2}}$	= average partial pressure of O_2 in the lung capillaries (mm Hg)
P_L	= pressure of dry gases in the lungs (mm Hg)

between ventilation and perfusion. The vast proportion of CO that is absorbed is bound to hemoglobin. According to the model developed by Coburn, Forster, and Kane,[11]

Under steady-state conditions, the level of HbCO in man can be roughly predicted from the concentration of CO in the air:

% HbCO ≅ 0.16 (atmospheric CO, ppm)

Following acute CO exposure, the rate of accumulation of HbCO (Fig. 17–6) varies according to an individual's sex, age and level of activity[41] and his body weight and hemoglobin concentration.[42] Likewise, these factors affect the disappearance of HbCO following acute withdrawal. For example, in a 40-year-old man, the HbCO half-life, a measurement of CO disappearance following withdrawal of CO exposure, is 220 minutes at rest and 90 minutes during strenuous exercise.[41] The disappearance time for HbCO has clinical relevance. These data can be used to predict the rate of improvement in patients intoxicated with CO following withdrawal to a CO-free atmosphere. The disappearance time is somewhat reduced if the patient is treated with oxygen (discussed later).

As mentioned, levels of HbCO in normal individuals vary widely according to their geographical location[14] and occupational status. Tobacco smoking is an equally important determinant of HbCO levels in blood. In a given locale, the average smoker has an additional 4 per cent HbCO.[14] This increment in HbCO of smokers is larger at high altitude.[43] Those who inhale tobacco smoke tend to have higher levels of HbCO than those who do not.[44,45] Those who inhale cigar smoke have particularly high HbCO levels. Pipe smoke has a very high CO content but is rarely inhaled. Thus, pipe smokers have only a modest increase in HbCO.[46] Vigorous exercise such as jogging[47] will lower the level of HbCO in smokers owing to increased ventilation. The whole blood dissociation curve of smokers is left-shifted in direct proportion to the level of HbCO.[48] Carboxyhemoglobinemia assumes greater significance if a smoker has an underlying pulmonary disorder that causes arterial hypoxemia (discussed later).

TOXICITY OF CO

How much of the toxicity of CO is due to factors other than carboxyhemoglobinemia? Besides hemoglobin, myoglobin as well as cytochromes, including P-450, can bind CO. The relative affinity constant (M) for myoglobin is approximately 40 (20 per cent that for hemoglobin). Nevertheless, an appreciable amount

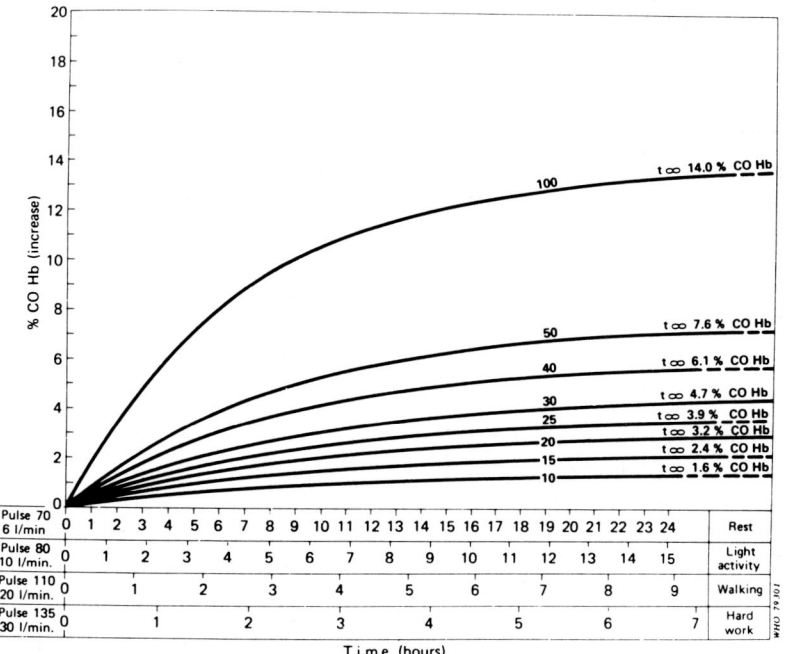

Figure 17–6. Rate of accumulation of HbCO after acute exposure to air containing CO ranging from 10 to 100 ppm. (From Environmental Health Criteria 13, Carbon Monoxide. Geneva, World Health Organization, 1979.)

of carboxymyoglobin is formed during CO exposure. As the tissue PO_2 falls, CO is transferred from hemoglobin to myoglobin. In an individual with 10 per cent HbCO, as much as 30 per cent of cardiac myoglobin may be saturated with CO.[49, 50] It is not at all certain whether such impressive levels of carboxymyoglobin cause impairment of muscle function. In rats, the total amount of myoglobin in heart muscle rises following CO intoxication.[51] This may compensate for high CO saturation. A number of studies on both man and experimental animals indicate that CO exposure lowers exercise tolerance. Clearly, other abnormalities besides carboxymyoglobin could be responsible. Likewise, the significance of CO binding to cytochromes is uncertain. The most likely oxidase to be inhibited *in vivo* is cytochrome P-450. Animal experiments suggest that CO poisoning may impair drug metabolism.[52] However, the M value of cytochrome P-450 is approximately unity, so that it is likely that only a trivial fraction of this protein binds CO, even in individuals or animals with severe CO poisoning.[53] Cytochrome a_3 has a somewhat higher affinity for CO compared with O_2 (M = 5 to 15) but is still unikely to be significantly impaired. Cytochrome oxidase in the brain is unaffected by CO intoxication.[54] At CO tensions compatible with life, there is probably no significant malfunction of the cytochrome system for oxygen consumption.[55] Therefore, in the following discussion of CO toxicity, we make the tacit assumption that the varied clinical manifestations result primarily from the adverse effect of CO on hemoglobin function, decreasing the release of oxygen to tissues.

A Relation of Perſons killed with ſubterraneous Damps.

This Relation was likewiſe made to the *Royal Society*, by that Eminent *Virtuoſo* Sir *R. Moray*, who was pleaſed, upon their deſire, to give it them in writing; as followeth,

In a Coal-pit, belonging to the Lord *Sinclair* in *Scotland*, where the Coal is ſome 18 or 20 foot thick, and antiently waſted to a great depth: The Colliers, ſome Weeks agoe, having wrought as deep as they could, and being to remove into new Rooms (as they call them) did, by taking off, as they retired, part of the Coal that was left as Pillars to ſupport the Roof and Earth over it, ſo much weaken them, that within a ſhort ſpace, after they were gone out of the Pitt, the Pillars falling, the Earth above them filled up the whole Space, where the Colliers had lately wrought, with its ruins. The Colliers being here-by out of work, ſome of them adventured to work upon old remains of Walls, ſo near the old waſtes, that ſtriking through the ſlender partition of the Coal-wall, that ſeperated between them and the place, where they uſed to work, they quickly perceived their Errour, and fearing to be ſtifled by the bad Air, that they knew, poſſeſſed theſe old waſtes, in regard not onely of the Damps, which ſuch waſtes do uſually afford, but becauſe there having for many years been a Fire in thoſe waſtes, that filled them with ſtifling fumes and vapors, retired immediately and ſaved themſelves from the eruptions of the Damp. But next day ſome ſeven or eight of them came no ſooner ſo farr down the ſtaires, that led them to the place, where they had been the day before, as they intended, but upon their ſtepping into the place, where the Air was infected, they fell down dead, as if they had been ſhott: And there being amongſt them one, whoſe Wife was informed he was ſtifled in that place, ſhe went down ſo far without inconvenience, that ſeeing her Husband near her, ventured to go to him, but being choaked by the Damp, as ſoon as ſhe came near him, ſhe fell down dead by him.

This Story of Sir *R. Moray* affirmed to have received from the *Earl* of *Weymes*, Brother in Law to the Lord *Sinclair*. as it was written to him from *Scotland*.

Figure 17–7. The first description of carbon nonoxide poisoning. (*From* Phil. Trans. Roy. Soc. (Lond.) *1*:44, 1665.)

Clinical Manifestations. The first description of carbon monoxide poisoning appeared in 1665[56] (Fig. 17–7). Patients with acute CO poisoning generally begin to develop symptoms when HbCO levels exceed 20 per cent. The diagnosis is usually straightforward. A history of recent exposure is coupled with the development of constitutional symptoms such as weakness, irritability, and breathlessness, often accompanied by headache, nausea, vomiting, and pain in the chest or abdomen. Patients are sometimes confused or dizzy and may appear inebriated. Physical findings are nonspecific. Although clinical lore has stressed a characteristic cherry-red color, this finding is far from obvious in most patients with CO intoxication.[57] Occasionally, flame-shaped retinal hemorrhages are noted. Subacute CO intoxication may be difficult to diagnose. Patients sometimes appear to have flu-like symptoms mimicking gastroenteritis.[57, 58] Uncommon presentations of CO poisoning include aspiration pneumonia, rhabdomyonecrosis, acute renal failure, and peripheral neuropathy.

More severe carboxyhemoglobinemia (40 to 60 per cent) results in stupor, coma and death. Patients who succumb generally have widespread organ dysfunction due to hypoxia. Postmortem examination often reveals acute myocardiopathy and central leukoencephalopathy not encountered in other types of acute hypoxia.

Chronic carboxyhemoglobinemia affects a number of different organ systems, resulting in polycythemia, neuropsychiatric dysfunction, cardiac toxicity, and fetal hypoxia.

Polycythemia. Some heavy smokers have significant polycythemia due to increased oxygen affinity imposed by elevated levels of HbCO.[59] Among reported cases, hematocrits average 55 ± 3 per cent in men and 52 ± 3 per cent in women. The red cell mass is correspondingly increased. These abnormalities revert to normal if these individuals stop smoking. Carboxyhemoglobinemia induced by smoking is probably a relatively common cause of secondary polycythemia. Nevertheless, smoker's polycythemia is infrequently encountered among heavy smokers less than 50 years of age.[60] One of us (H.F.B.) found no difference in hematocrits of 150 military recruits who smoked at least 20 cigarettes per day compared with an equal number who did not smoke. It is likely that other sources of CO, such as the occupational hazards mentioned previously, can cause sufficient sustained carboxyhemoglobinemia to cause secondary polycythemia. Thus, a HbCO level should be determined in any patient with unexplained polycythemia.

Neuropsychiatric Manifestations. In order to maintain normal O_2 consumption, cerebral blood flow must increase in patients with carboxyhemoglobinemia to offset the decrease in the fraction of extracted oxygen.[60a] If this compensation is inadequate, cerebral hypoxia may occur. A vast body of literature has focused on the effects of CO exposure on various neurological and behavioral parameters. Conflicting data abound. These studies are difficult to design and interpret because of a variety of confounding factors, including differences in baseline levels of HbCO in test subjects as well as in the rate and method of CO administration. Moreover, prolonged CO exposure may lead to acclimatization.[61] There is some evidence that relatively low levels of HbCO (3 to 5 per cent) can cause impaired time discrimination and prolonged reaction times as well as disturbances in a number of other perceptual and cognitive processes. However, these reports could not be confirmed by other investigators. Alterations in mood and sleep patterns have been noted in volunteers in whom HbCO has risen to 8 per cent.[62] The threshold for impairment of complex intellectual functions is difficult to assess. At progressively higher levels of HbCO (> 30 per cent), subjects may develop headache, impaired vision, irritability, and confusion.

Cardiovascular Manifestations. The effects of CO intoxication on cardiac function have been thoroughly investigated in dogs. High levels of HbCO (20 to 40 per cent) cause a marked increase in myocardial blood flow but a relative reduction in subendocardial perfusion.[63] Lower levels of HbCO (5 to 10 per cent) can increase the extent and severity of myocardial ischemia caused by coronary artery ligation.[64, 65] However, there is conflicting evidence as to whether comparable levels of HbCO lower the threshold for ventricular arrhythmia[66, 67] or not.[68]

There is little firm evidence in normal man that low levels of HbCO (< 10 per cent) cause significant cardiac toxicity. However, patients with higher HbCO levels (~ 20 per cent) have demonstrated echocardiographic evidence of impaired left ventricular dynamics as well as mitral valve prolapse.[69] More severe carboxyhemoglobinemia can cause serious arrhythmias and progressive myocardial failure.

The hypoxia imposed by carboxyhemoglobinemia can aggravate coronary artery insufficiency. There is convincing evidence that relatively low levels of HbCO (2 to 5 per cent), comparable to that engendered by smoking or even traveling on a crowded freeway, will significantly hasten the onset of angina pectoris and prolong its duration.[70–74] It is likely that this effect is mediated directly via impaired oxygen release to the myocardium. In cholesterol-fed rabbits, CO exposure accelerates the development of atherosclerosis.[75] The relevance of this observation to coronary artery disease in man is unclear. Computer simulation suggests that carboxyhemoglobinemia of ~ 10 per cent induces hypoxia in the midmedial wall of arteries.[76]

Effects on the Fetus. In experimental animals, exposure of the mother to CO has widespread effects on the fetus,[77–79a] including teratogenicity, neurological dysfunction, reduced birth weights, and increased incidence of stillbirths. Babies of women who are heavy smokers weigh less than those born to nonsmoking mothers.[80] Carboxyhemoglobinemia in pregnant women is enhanced by a significant increment in endogenous CO production.[81] It is likely that CO potentiates fetal hypoxia. Because of the higher oxygen affinity of fetal blood, coupled with reduced oxygen content, the PO_2 in arterial blood of the fetus is only 20 to 30 per cent that of the mother.[82] The PO_2 is reduced even further when there is significant carboxyhemoglobinemia.

Interaction with Other Conditions. It is likely that the toxicity encountered with low and moderate levels of HbCO is due to association with other disorders, including coronary artery disease, anemia,[82a] and lung disease. The adverse effect of CO on angina pectoris has already been mentioned. Patients with various types of hypoxic states are more susceptible to the toxic effects of CO. Those with chronic obstructive pulmonary disease are prime examples. In their lungs, ventilation and perfusion are badly mismatched, tantamount

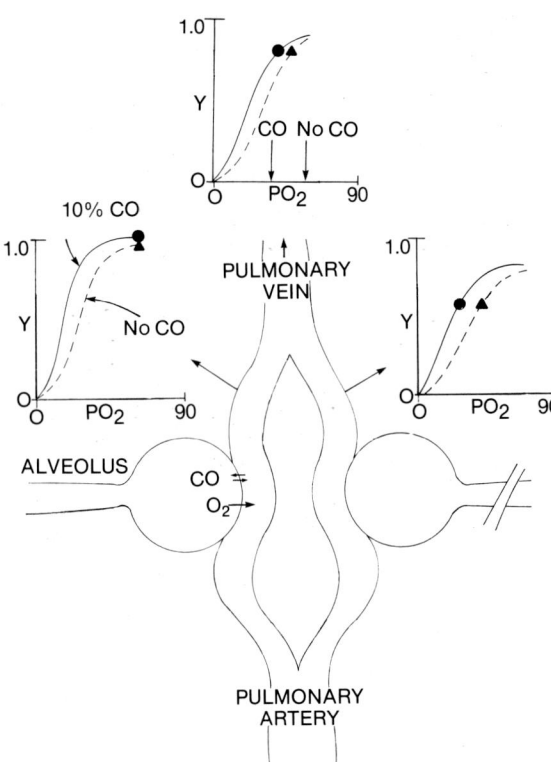

Figure 17–8. Diagram showing the mechanism responsible for the exaggerated reduction in arterial PO_2 in patients with ventilation-perfusion mismatch who have carboxyhemoglobinemia and a left-shifted O_2 binding curve (———). The alveolus on the left is fully ventilated and perfused. The alveolus on the right is perfused but not ventilated. Patients with 10% HbCO (———) will have a significantly lower arterial PO_2 compared to those with minimal HbCO(----).

to pulmonary arteriovenous shunting. When these patients, along with those with cardiovascular right-to-left shunts, have elevated levels of HbCO, the oxygen gradient between the alveoli and the systemic arteries widens significantly.[83] This phenomenon is caused by transfer of O_2 from ventilated blood to partially unsaturated HbCO in shunted blood following their admixture (Fig. 17–8). Because of this enhanced alveolar–arterial gradient, patients with chronic lung disease and elevated levels of HbCO have more severe hypoxemia. Patients with chronic bronchitis and emphysema have a marked reduction in exercise tolerance if their HbCO level rises significantly.[84] This combination of chronic lung disease and CO exposure is further aggravated when the oxygen tension in the inspired air is low. Thus, patients with chronic lung disease who live at high altitude and choose to smoke are under triple jeopardy. A prime example is the copper miner in the Rocky Mountains who eventually develops silicosis and is unaware of the added insult of tobacco smoking.

At a given degree of CO exposure, patients with hypoxemia tend to have more marked carboxyhemoglobinemia than do normal individuals. As mentioned earlier, smokers who live at high altitude have higher levels of HbCO than those at sea level.[43] The highest reported level of HbCO in a smoker (38 per cent) was noted in a patient with chronic obstructive lung disease.[85] Such a patient can ill afford an additional factor that potentiates hypoxia.

Treatment of CO Intoxication. Clearly, the intoxicated patient should be promptly removed from further exposure to CO. The administration of oxygen has a dual benefit: First, the small increment of O_2 dissolved in plasma helps to reverse hypoxia. Second, O_2 therapy hastens the clearance of CO from the body. In a recent epidemic of acute CO poisoning in a public high school, the half-life for HbCO was 137 minutes in patients treated with an oxygen mask, whereas that for untreated patients was 320 minutes.[86] If available, hyperbaric oxygen should be administered to patients with severe intoxication.[87]

References

1. Clark, R. W.: J.B.S. The Life and Work of J.B.S. Haldane. New York, Coward McCann, 1968.
2. Edsall, J. T.: Blood and hemoglobin: The evolution of knowledge of functional adaptation in a biochemical system. J. Hist. Biol. 5:205, 1972.
3. Environmental Health Criteria 13: *Carbon Monoxide.* Geneva, World Health Organization, 1979.

3a. Khalil, M. A. K., and Rasmussen, R. A.: Carbon monoxide in the earth's atmosphere: Increasing trend. Science 224:54, 1984.
4. Goldsmith, J. R., and Landaw, S. A.: Carbon monoxide and human health. Science 162:1352, 1968.
5. Junge, C., Seiler, W., and Warneck, P.: The atmospheric ^{12}CO and ^{14}CO budget. J. Geophys. Res. 76(12):2866, 1971.
6. Cole, P. V.: Comparative effects of atmospheric pollution and cigarette smoking on carboxyhaemoglobin levels in man. Nature 255:699, 1975.
7. Maugh, T. H. II: Carbon monoxide: Natural sources dwarf man's output. Science 177:338, 1972.
8. Landaw, S. A.: Carbon monoxide production as a measurement of heme catabolism. In Goresky, C. A., and Fisher, M. M. (eds.). Jaundice. New York, Plenum Publishing Corporation, 1974, p. 103.
9. Tenhunen, R., Marver, H. S., and Schmidt, R.: Microsomal heme oxygenase: Characterization of the enzyme. J. Biol. Chem. 244:6388, 1969.
9a. Tenhunen, R., Marver, H. S., and Schmidt, R.: Stimulation of microsomal heme oxygenase by hemin. J. Lab. Clin. Med. 75:410, 1970.
10. Wolff, D. G., and Bidlack, W. R.: The formation of carbon monoxide during peroxidation of microsomal lipids. Biochem. Biophys. Res. Commun. 73:850, 1976.
11. Coburn, R. F., Forster, R. D., and Kane, P. B.: Considerations of the physiological variables that determine the blood carboxyhemoglobin concentration in man. J. Clin. Invest. 44:1899, 1965.
12. Coburn, R. F., Williams, W. J., and Kahn, S. B.: Endogenous carbon monoxide production in patients with hemolytic anemia. J. Clin. Invest. 45:460, 1966.
13. Ostrander, C. R., Cohen, R. S., Hopper, A. O., Cowan, B. E., Stevens, G. B., and Stevenson, D. K.: Paired determinations of blood carboxyhemoglobin concentration and carbon monoxide excretion rate in term and preterm infants. J. Lab. Clin. Med. 100:745, 1982.
14. Stewart, R. D., Baretta, E. D., Platte, L. R., Stewart, E. B., Kalbfleisch, J. H., Van Yserloo, B., and Rimm, A. A.: Carboxyhemoglobin concentrations in blood from donors in Chicago, Milwaukee, New York, and Los Angeles. Science 182:1362, 1973.
15. Haldane, J. S., and Smith, J. L.: The absorption of oxygen by the lungs. J. Physiol. (Lond.) 22:231, 1897.
16. Wyman, J., Bishop, G., Richey, B., Spokane, R., and Gill, S.: Examination of Haldane's first law for the partition of CO and O_2 to hemoglobin A_0. Biopolymers 21:1735, 1982.
17. Heidner, E. J., Ladner, R. C., and Perutz, M. F.: Structure of horse carbonmonoxyhemoglobin. J. Mol. Biol. 104:707, 1976.
18. Baldwin, J. M.: The structure of human carbonmonoxyhaemoglobin at 2.7 Å resolution. J. Mol. Biol. 136:103, 1980.
18a. Shaanan, B.: The structure of human oxyhaemoglobin at 2.1 Å resolution. J. Mol. Biol. 171:31, 1983.
19. Case, D. A., and Karplus, M.: Stereochemistry of carbon monoxide binding to myoglobin and hemoglobin. J. Mol. Biol. 123:697, 1978.
20. Tucker, P. W., Phillips, S. E. V., Perutz, M. F., Houtchens, R., and Caughey, W. S.: Structure of hemoglobins Zürich [His E7(63)β → Arg] and Sydney [Val E11(67)β → Ala] and role of the distal residues in ligand binding. Proc. Natl. Acad. Sci. USA 75:1076, 1978.
21. Thomas, J. O., and Edelstein, S. J.: Observation of the dissociation of unliganded hemoglobin. J. Biol. Chem. 247:7870, 1972.
22. Szabo, A.: Kinetics of hemoglobin and transition state theory. Proc. Natl. Acad. Sci. USA 75:2108, 1978.
23. Moffat, K., Deatherage, J. F., and Seybert, D. W.: A structural model for the kinetic behavior of hemoglobin. Science 206:1035, 1979.
24. Bunn, H. F., and McDonough, M.: Asymmetrical hemoglobin hybrids, an approach to the study of hemoglobin interactions. Biochemistry 13:988, 1974.
25. Perrella, M., Benazzi, L., Cremonesi, L., Vesely, S., Viggiano, G., and Rossi-Bernardi, L.: Isolation of intermediate compounds between hemoglobin and carbon monoxide. J. Biol. Chem. 258:4511, 1983.
26. Douglas, C. G., Haldane, J. S., and Haldane, J. B. S.: The laws of combination of haemoglobin with carbon monoxide and oxygen. J. Physiol. 44:275, 1912.
27. Haldane, J. B. S.: The dissociation of oxyhaemoglobin in human blood during partial CO poisoning. J. Physiol. 45:xxii, 1912–13.
28. Blackmore, D. J.: Distribution of HbCO in human erythrocytes following inhalation of CO. Nature 227:386, 1970.
29. Winslow, R. M., Morrissey, J. M., Berger, R. L., Smith, P. D., and Gibson, C. C.: Variability of oxygen affinity of normal blood: An automated method of measurement. J. Appl. Physiol. 45:289, 1978.
30. Ledwith, J. W.: Determining P50 in the presence of carboxyhemoglobin. J. Appl. Physiol. 44:317, 1978.
30a. Rovida, E., Niggeler, M., Carlone, S., and Samaja, M.: Carboxyhemoglobin and oxygen-affinity of human blood. Clin. Chem. 30:1250, 1984.
31. Vanuxem, D., Weiller, P. J., Guillot, C., and Grimaud, Ch.: Action of carbon monoxide on the affinity of hemoglobin for oxygen. Study in whole blood and stripped hemoglobin. Respiration 43:45, 1982.
32. Coburn, R. F., Danielson, G. K., Blakemore, W. S., and Forster, R. E. II: Carbon monoxide in blood: Analytical method and sources of error. J. Appl. Physiol. 19:510, 1964.
33. Collison, H. A., Rodkey, F. L., and O'Neal, J. D.: Determination of carbon monoxide in blood by gas chromatography. Clin. Chem. 14:162, 1968.
34. Dahms, T. E., and Horvath, S. M.: Rapid, accurate technique for determination of carbon monoxide in blood. Clin. Chem. 20:533, 1974.
35. Klendshoj, N. C., Feldstein, M., and Sprague, A. L.: The spectrophotometric determination of carbon monoxide. J. Biol. Chem. 183:297, 1950.
36. Small, K. A., Radford, E. P., Frazier, J. M., Rodkey, F. L., and Collison, H. A.: A rapid method for simultaneous measurement of carboxy- and methemoglobin in blood. J. Appl. Physiol. 31:154, 1971.
37. Rodkey, F. L., Hill, T. A., Pitts, L. L., and Robertson, R. F.: Spectrophotometric measurement of carboxyhemoglobin and methemoglobin in blood. Clin. Chem. 25:1388, 1979.
37a. Beutler, E., and West, C.: Simplified determination of carboxyhemoglobin. Clin. Chem. 30:871, 1984.
38. Malenfant, A. L., Gambino, S. R., Waraska, A. J., and Roe, E. I.: Spectrophotometric determination of hemoglobin concentration and percent oxyhemoglobin and carboxyhemoglobin saturation. Clin. Chem. 14:789, 1968.
39. Wigfield, D. C., Hollebone, B. R., MacKeen, J. E.,

and Selwin, J. C.: Assessment of the methods available for the determination of carbon monoxide in blood. J. Anal. Toxicol. 5:122, 1981.
40. Guyatt, A. R., Holmes, M. A., and Cumming, G.: Can carbon monoxide be absorbed from the upper respiratory tract in man? Eur. J. Respir. Dis. 62:383, 1981.
41. Joumard, R., Chiron, M., Vidon, R., Maurin, M., and Rouzioux, J.-M.: Mathematical models of the uptake of carbon monoxide on hemoglobin at low carbon monoxide levels. Environ. Health Perspect. 41:277, 1981.
42. Tyuma, I., Yoshihiro, U., Imaizumi, K., and Kosaka, H.: Prediction of the carbonmonoxyhemoglobin levels during and after carbon monoxide exposures in various animal species. Jpn. J. Physiol. 31:131, 1981.
43. Brewer, G. J., Eaton, J., Weil, J., and Grover, R.: Studies of red cell glycolysis and interactions with carbon monoxide, smoking and altitude. In Brewer, G. J. (ed.). Red Cell Metabolism and Function. New York, Plenum Press, 1970.
44. Wald, N. J., Idle, M., and Bailey, A.: Carboxyhaemoglobin levels and inhaling habits in cigarette smokers. Thorax 33:201, 1978.
45. Wald, N. J., Idle, M., Boreham, J., and Bailey, A.: Inhaling habits among smokers of different types of cigarettes. Thorax 35:925, 1980.
46. Russell, M. A. H.: Blood carboxyhaemoglobin changes during tobacco smoking. Postgrad. Med. J. 49:684, 1973.
47. Kam, K.-H.: Carboxyhemoglobin levels between jogging and nonjogging smokers. Experientia 36:1397, 1980.
48. Astrup, P., Hellung-Larsen, P., Kjeldsen, K., and Mellemgaard, K.: The effect of tobacco smoking on the dissociation curve of oxyhemoglobin: Investigations in patients with occlusive arterial diseases and in normal subjects. Scand. J. Clin. Lab. Invest. 18:450, 1966.
49. Coburn, R. F.: The carbon monoxide body stores. Ann. N. Y. Acad. Sci. 174:11, 1970.
50. Coburn, R. F., Ploegmakers, F., Gondrie, P., and Abboud, R.: Myocardial myoglobin oxygen tension. Am. J. Physiol. 224:870, 1973.
51. Pankow, D., and Ponsold, W.: Effect of repeated carbon monoxide intoxications on the myoglobin concentration in heart and skeletal muscles of rats. Acta Biol. Med. Ger. 38:1601, 1979.
52. Pankow, D., Schiller, F., and Müller, D.: Effect of repeated carbon monoxide exposure to rats on cytochrome P-450 concentration and activities of monooxygenases in the liver. Acta Biol. Med. Ger. 41:935, 1982.
53. Cooper, D. Y., Levin, S., Narasimhulu, S., Rosenthal, O., and Estabrook, R. W.: Photochemical action spectrum of the terminal oxidase of mixed function oxidase systems. Science 147:400, 1965.
54. Savolainen, H., Kurppa, K., Tenhunen, R., and Kivisto, H.: Biochemical effects of carbon monoxide poisoning in rat brain with special reference to blood carboxyhemoglobin and cerebral cytochrome oxidase activity. Neurosci. Lett. 19:319, 1980.
55. Root, W. S.: Carbon monoxide. In Fenn, W. O., and Rahn, H. (eds.). Handbook of Physiology, Respiration 2. Washington, D. C., American Physiological Society, 1965, p. 1087.
56. Moray, Sir R.: A relation of persons killed with subterraneous damps. Phil. Trans. Roy. Soc. (Lond.) 1:44, 1665.
57. Grace, T. W., and Platt, F. W.: Subacute carbon monoxide poisoning. Another great imitator. JAMA 246:1698, 1981.
58. Hopkinson, J. M., Pearce, P. J., and Oliver, J. S.: Carbon monoxide poisoning mimicking gastroenteritis. Br. Med. J. 281:214, 1980.
59. Smith, J. R., and Landaw, S. A.: Smokers' polycythemia. New Engl. J. Med. 298:6, 1978.
60. Tirlapur, V. G., Gicheru, K., Charlambous, B. M., Evans, P. J., and Mir, M. A.: Packed cell volume, haemoglobin, and oxygen saturation changes in healthy smokers and non-smokers. Thorax 38:785, 1983.
60a. Koehler, R. C., Traystman, R. J., Rosenberg, A. A., Hudak, M. L., and Jones, M. D.: Role of O_2-hemoglobin affinity on cerebrovascular response to carbon monoxide hypoxia. Am. J. Physiol. 245:1019, 1983.
61. Otis, A. B.: The physiology of carbon monoxide poisoning and evidence for acclimatization. Ann. N. Y. Acad. Sci. 174:242, 1970.
62. Groll-Knapp, E., Haider, M., Jenkner, H., Liebich, H., Neuberger, M., and Trimmel, M.: Moderate carbon monoxide exposure during sleep: Neuro- and psychophysiological effects in young and elderly people. Neurobehav. Toxicol. Teratol. 4:709, 1982.
63. Einzig, S., Nicoloff, D. M., and Lucas, R. V., Jr.: Myocardial perfusion abnormalities in carbon monoxide poisoned dogs. Can. J. Physiol. Pharmacol. 58:396, 1980.
64. Becker, L. C., and Haak, E. D., Jr.: Augmentation of myocardial ischemia by low level carbon monoxide exposure in dogs. Arch. Environ. Health 34:274, 1979.
65. Sekiya, S., Sato, S., Yamaguchi, H., and Harumi, K.: Effects of carbon monoxide inhalation on myocardial infarct size following experimental coronary artery ligation. Jpn. Heart J. 24:407, 1983.
66. Aronow, W. S., Stemmer, E. A., Wood, B., Zweig, S., Tsao, K. P., and Raggio, L.: Carbon monoxide and ventricular fibrillation threshold in dogs with acute myocardial injury. Am. Heart J. 95:754, 1978.
67. Aronow, W. S., Stemmer, E. A., and Zweig, S.: Carbon monoxide and ventricular fibrillation threshold in normal dogs. Arch. Environ. Health 34:184, 1979.
68. Foster, J. R.: Arrhythmogenic effects of carbon monoxide in experimental acute myocardial ischemia: Lack of slowed conduction and ventricular tachycardia. Am. Heart J. 102:876, 1981.
69. Corya, B. C., Black, M. J., and McHenry, P. L.: Echocardiographic findings after acute carbon monoxide poisoning. Br. Heart J. 38:712, 1976.
70. Aronow, W. S., Harris, C. N., Isbell, M. W., Rokaw, S. N., and Imparato, B.: Effect of freeway travel on angina pectoris. Ann. Intern. Med. 77:669, 1972.
71. Aronow, W. S., and Isbell, M. W.: Carbon monoxide effect on exercise-induced angina pectoris. Ann. Intern. Med. 79:392, 1973.
72. Anderson, E. W., Andelman, R. J., Stauch, J. M., Fortuin, N. J., and Knelson, J. H.: Effect of low-level carbon monoxide exposure on onset and duration of angina pectoris. Ann. Intern. Med. 79:46, 1973.
73. Aronow, W. S.: Aggravation of angina pectoris by two per cent carboxyhemoglobin. Am. Heart J. 101:154, 1981.
74. Aronow, W. S.: Effect of non-nicotine cigarettes and carbon monoxide on angina. Circulation 61:262, 1980.

75. Astrup, P., Kjeldsen, K., and Wanstrup, J.: Enhancing influence of carbon monoxide on the development of atheromatosis in cholesterol-fed rabbits. J. Atheroscler. Res. 7:343, 1967.
76. Schneiderman, G., and Goldstick, T. K.: Carbon monoxide–induced arterial wall hypoxia and atherosclerosis. Atherosclerosis 30:1, 1978.
77. Penny, D. G., Baylerian, M. S., Thill, J. E., Yedavally, S., and Fanning, C. M.: Cardiac response of the fetal rat to carbon monoxide exposure. Am. J. Physiol. 244:289, 1983.
78. Dominick, M. A., and Carson, T. L.: Effects of carbon monoxide exposure on pregnant sows and their fetuses. Am. J. Vet. Res. 44:35, 1983.
79. Schwetz, B. A., Smith, F. A., Leong, B. K., and Staples, R. E.: Teratogenic potential of inhaled carbon monoxide in mice and rabbits. Teratology 19:385, 1979.
79a. Mactutus, C. F., and Fechter, L. D.: Prenatal exposure to carbon monoxide: Learning and memory deficits. Science, 223:409, 1984.
80. Astrup, P., Olsen, H. M., Trolle, C., and Kjeldsen, K.: Effect of moderate carbon monoxide exposure on fetal development. Lancet 2:1220, 1972.
81. Delivoria-Papadopoulos, M., Coburn, R. F., Longo, L. D., and Forster, R. E.: Endogenous carbon monoxide of mother and fetus. 29th Annual Meeting of the Society of Pediatrics Research, Atlantic City, N. J., 1969, p. 148.
82. Longo, L. D.: Carbon monoxide: Effects on oxygenation of the fetus in utero. Science 194:523, 1976.
82a. Aronow, W. S., Schlueterst, W. J., Williams, M. A., Petratis, M., and Sketch, M. H.: Aggravation of exericse performance in patients with anemia by 3 percent carboxyhemoglobin. Environ. Res. 35:394, 1984.
83. Brody, J. S., and Coburn, R. F.: Carbon monoxide–induced arterial hypoxemia. Science 164:1297, 1969.
84. Calverley, P. M. A., Leggett, R. J., and Flenley, D. C.: Carbon monoxide and exercise tolerance in chronic bronchitis and emphysema. Br. Med. J. 283:878, 1981.
85. Hebbel, R. P., Eaton, J. W., Modler, S., and Jacob, H. S.: Extreme but asymptomatic carboxyhemoglobinemia and chronic lung disease. JAMA 239:2584, 1978.
86. Burney, R. E., Wu, S. C., and Nemiroff, M. J.: Mass carbon monoxide poisoning: Clinical effects and results of treatment in 184 victims. Ann. Emerg. Med. 11:394, 1982.
87. Myers, R. A., Snyder, S. K., Linberg, S., and Cowley, R. A.: Value of hyperbaric oxygen in suspected carbon monoxide poisoning. JAMA 246:2478, 1981.

INDEX

Page numbers in *italics* refer to figures, page numbers followed by t refer to tables

Acidosis, oxygen transport and, 110–111, 110t
Adair, Gilbert S., 5, 7
Adrenalin, 2,3-DPG increase and, 112
Agnatha, hemoglobins of, *141*, 141–142
Aldosterone, oxygen transport and, 112
Alkalosis, oxygen transport in, 110, 110t
Allison, Anthony, 455
Allosteric protein(s), hemoglobin as, 51–57, *52*
Alpha chain(s), carbon dioxide interaction with, 43–44
　E helix of, 19
　G-Philadelphia, 417
　Hb S polymerization and, 463t
　isolation of, 48
　J-Cape Town, 417
　J-Mexico, 417
　J-Tongariki, 417
　oxygen affinity of, 56
　properties of, 48
　Q, 417
　structure of, *16*, 18
　synthesis of, in unstable hemoglobin variants, 577–579, 578t
　variants of, 382–386t
　　CHBA and, 568t
　　globin genotypes and, 261–262, 262t
　　Hb S heterozygosity and, 538
　　high oxygen affinity and, 596t
　　sickle cell disease and, 534t
Alpha helix, disruption of, CHBA and, 572–573
Alpha thalassemia, beta chain variants and, 420, *420*, 420t
　classification of, 327–328, 327t
　codon 125 substitution mutation in, 285–286
　frameshift mutation in, 286–287
　gene deletion in, 242, *243*
　gene mapping of, 256–263, *257*, 261t, 262t
　globin gene DNA in, *244*, 244–245, *245*
　globin gene partial deletion in, 287–288
　globin mRNA studies in, 242–245, *243*, *244*, *245*
　Hb A_2 in, 65t, 66
　Hb G^{Philadelphia} and, 344
　Hb Q and, 343–344
　Hb S and, 344, 419, *419*
　heterozygous, forms of, 244
　　globin chain synthesis in, 226, *226*
　homozygous, 226
　incidence of, 324
　initiation codon mutation in, 287

Alpha thalassemia (*Continued*)
　IVS-1 deletion mutation in, 285, *286*
　molecular variants of, 261, 261t
　mouse model of, 302
　mRNA in, 233
　nondeletion, forms of, 259–261, 285t
　　in blacks, 260–261
　　Mediterranean, 260
　　Saudi Arabian, 260
　　Southeast Asian, 259–260
　　variants of, 260–261
　prenatal diagnosis of, 351
　sequence analysis of, 284–288, 285t, *286*
　sickle cell disease and, 534t, 539–540, *540*
　structural variants and, 299–302
Alpha thalassemia 1, 244
　clinical features of, 328
　globin chain synthesis in, 226, *226*
　globin gene deletion in, 244–245, *245*, 258–259
　homozygous, *332*, 332–333
Alpha thalassemia 2, 244
　clinical features of, 328–329
　cloned genes of, 288
　gene deletion in, 257–259
Alpha^0 thalassemia, gene deletion in, 258–259
Altitude, high, 2,3-DPG levels and, 107, *108*
　oxygen dissociation curve and, 108, *108*
　oxygen transport and, 107–108, *108*
　polycythemia and, 108
Alu I, repetitive DNA sequences of, 186–197, *187*
Ambystoma tigrinum. See *Salamander.*
Amino acids, RNA codons for, 171t
Amphibians, hemoglobins of, *149*, 149–151
Anadara, oxygen affinity in, 139
Anemia, 105–107, *106*, 107t
　2,3-DPG in, 106, 107t
　aplastic, 2,3-DPG in, 107t
　　Hb F in, 74t
　Fanconi's, 74t
　hemolytic, 2,3-DPG in, 107t
　　Hb A_{Ic} in, 78
　　Hb F in, 74
　　Heinz body, 565–593
　　nonspherocytic, 2,3-DPG in, 106–107, 107t
　in sickle cell disease, 542–543
　in thalassemia, 324–326, *325*, *326*
　iron deficiency, 2,3-DPG in, 107t
　megaloblastic, Hb A_2 in, 65t, 66
　O_2 affinity in, 158–159

677

Anemia (*Continued*)
  oxygen dissociation curve in, 106, *106*
  oxygen transport and, 66, 105–107, *106*, 107t
  red cell aging and, 106
  refractory, Hb F in, 74t
  sickle cell. See *Sickle cell anemia.*
  sideroblastic, 65t
    Hb A_2 in, 66
    heme inhibition and, 208
Anesthetics, methemoglobin and, 654
Annelids, chlorocruorins of, 140
  hemoglobin of, 135–139, *136–138*
    functional diversity of, 135, 139
    quaternary structure of, 135, *138*
Aplastic crisis, in sickle cell anemia, 511–512
Apoda, oxygen affinity in, 151
Artarte, hemoglobin of, 139
Arthritis, in sickle cell disease, 519
Arthropods, hemocyanin of, 130, *131*
  hemoglobins of, 139
Arylamines, hemoglobin oxidation and, 643, *643*
  sulfhemoglobinemia and, 656
Asthma, acute, 2,3-DPG and, 109
ATP, hemoglobin oxygen affinity and, 97–98
  in bullfrog hemoglobin, 150
  in fish erythrocytes, 145, *145*, 147
  renal failure and, 111
Autoxidation, 640–641, 641t
  in high-affinity variants, 608
5-Azacytidine, in sickle cell anemia, 548, *549*
  in thalassemia, 358, *359*

Barcroft, Henry, 54
  Sir Joseph, 9, *9*
Benesch, Reinhold, 92, *92*, 95
Benesch, Ruth, 92, *92*, 95
Beta chain(s), amino acid substitutions in, CHBA and, 566–567, *567*, 572, *572*
  carbon dioxide interaction with, 43–44
  Hb S polymerization and, 463t
  homozygous variants of, 404t, 405
  isolation of, 48
  J-Baltimore, *418*
  of Hb A_2, 63–65t
  oxygen affinity of, 56
  properties of, 48
  structure of, *17*, *18*
  synthesis of, in unstable hemoglobin variants, 577–579, 578t
  variants of, 386–391t
    alpha thalassemia and, 420, *420*, 420t
    CHBA and, 568–570t
    oxygen affinity and, 596–598t
    sickle cell disease and, 535t
Beta thalassemia, classification of, 327t, 328
  clinical features of, 333–345
  globin chain synthesis in, 225, *225*
  globin gene analysis in, 271–284, *272*, *273*, 274t, *275*, *277*, *280*, *282*
  Hb A_2 and, 64–66, 65t, 327, *330*, 333–334, 333t
  Hb C and, 343
  Hb E and, 343, 426–427
  Hb F and, 69, 74
  Hb S and, 343, 534t, 536–537
  hemoglobin electrophoresis in, *330*
  heterozygous, bone marrow mRNA in, 232
    clinical features of, 333–335
    hybridization studies in, 240
    types of, 334

Beta thalassemia (*Continued*)
  homozygous, beta globin deficiency in, 236–238, *237*
    bone changes in, *337*
    bone marrow globin chain synthesis in, 226–227
    bone marrow mRNA in, 232
    facial appearance in, *336*
    globin mRNA studies in, 236–238, *237*
    peripheral blood stain in, *338*
    reticulocyte mRNA in, 231–232
    with high Hb A_2, 335–338, *336*, *337*, *338*
      clinical features of, 335–336, *336*, *337*
      laboratory findings in, 336–338, *338*
    with normal Hb A_2, 339–340
    with normal Hb F, 339–340
  incidence of, 324
  inclusion bodies in, 324–326, *325*
  mouse model of, 302–303
  populations affected by, 295–297
  prenatal diagnosis of, 351
  silent carrier state of, 339
  vs. iron deficiency anemia, 333, 333t
  worldwide distribution of, *323*
Beta$^+$ thalassemia, beta mRNA deficiency in, 272, 272–273, *273*
  IVS-1 mutation in, 272, 272–273, *273*
  IVS-2 mutations in, 276, *277*, 278
  mutations causing, 271t
  polyadenylation signal mutation in, 279
  transcription mutations in, 271t, 278–279
Beta^0 thalassemia, base substitution in, 249
  beta chain mRNA in, 232, 238–240, *239*
  Ferrara-type, 232–233
  frameshift mutations in, 281–282, *282*
  gene mapping of, 248
  globin gene DNA in, 240
  homozygous, globin mRNA studies in, 238–240, *239*
  intervening sequence mutations in, 282–284
  IVS-2 mutations in, 276, *277*, 278
  mutations causing, 274, 274t, 276, *280*, 280–284, *282*
  nonsense mutations in, at codon 15, 280
    at codon 17, 280, *280*
    at codon 39, *280*, 280–281
    at codon 121, 281–282
Beta thalassemia intermedia, 339, 340–342, 341t
  types of, 341t
Bicarbonate ion, in crocodilian hemoglobin, 152, *152*
Birds, hemoglobins of, 153–154, *154*
  inositol pentaphosphate regulation of, 153
  ontogenic changes in, 153
Bisphosphoglycerate synthase, 2,3-DPG synthesis and, 100–103, *101*, 101t, *102*
Blood, transfusion of, 113–115, *114*
  in sickle cell disease, 543, 543t
  in thalassemia syndromes, 351–353
Blood flow, 94
  reduction of, oxygen transport and, 117
Bohr, Christian, 8, 39
Bohr effect, 11, 39–42, *40*, *41*
  alkaline, 39, *40*
  contributions to, 41–42
  in fish hemoglobins, 145–146, *146*
  in high affinity variants, 604–605, 604t
  in human hemoglobin, 145–146, *146*
  in tadpole hemoglobin, 150
  in *Xenopus laevis*, 150
Bonaventura, Joseph, 36

Bone, abnormalities of, in sickle cell disease, 518, *518*, 527–529, *528*, *529*
Bone marrow, globin chain synthesis in, in beta thalassemia, 226–228
  transplantation of, in thalassemia, 357–358
Bovine papilloma virus vector system, gene expression analysis by, 270
Boyle, Robert, 1, *2*
Bragg's law, 20
Braunitzer, Gerhard, 7
Brunori, Maurizio, 36, 639
Bullfrog, ontogenic hemoglobin switching in, *149*, 149–151
Busycon, oxygen affinity in, 133

C/D translocation, Hb F and, 72, 196
Calcium, in sickle cells, 489, *489*
Callianassa californiensis, hemocyanin of, oxygen affinity of, 133–134, *134*
Carbamino complex, formation of, 42–44, *43*
Carbamylation, extracorporeal, in sickle cell disease, 547
Carbon dioxide, alpha chain interaction of, 43–44
  beta chain interaction of, 43–44
  hemoglobin binding of, 42–44, *43*
  hemoglobin oxygen affinity and, 97, *97*
Carbon monoxide, 2,3-DPG levels and, 105
  endogenous production of, 664–665
  heme binding of, 666, *666*
  hemoglobin binding of, *55*
  sources of, 664–665, *665*
  toxicity of, 669–672, *670*
    cardiovascular manifestations of, 671
    clinical manifestations of, 670–671
    fetal effects of, 671
    hypoxic states and, 671–672
    neuropsychiatric manifestations of, 671
    polycythemia and, 670–671
    treatment of, 672
Carboxyhemoglobin, 663–675
  chain structures of, *666*
  hemoglobin oxygen affinity and, 98
  isoelectric focusing of, *667*
  structure and function of, 665–668, *666*, *667*
  structure of, three-dimensional, 21, *22*
Carboxyhemoglobinemia, 663–675, 668–669, *669*
Cardiac disorders, oxygen transport and, 109–110
Cardita, hemoglobin of, *138*, 139
Carp, hemoglobins of, 143t, *144*, 145, *145*
  oxygen-binding curve in, hypoxic habitat and, 148, *148*
Castle, William, 454
Cell(s), erythroid, BFU-E–derived, 199
  CFU-E–derived, 199
  development of, 199, *199*
CHBA. See *Congenital Heinz body hemolytic anemia*.
Chironomus, erythrocruorin of, *136*
  globin genes of, 177
  oxygen binding curve in, *137*
Chloride, deoxyhemoglobin binding to, *44*, 44–45
  hemoglobin binding of, *44*, 44–45
  Bohr effect and, 45
Chlorocruorin(s), 127, 129t
  annelid, 140
  color of, 129t
  in animal kingdom, *128*
  molecular weight of, 129t
  subunits of, 129t

Cholestasis, in sickle cell disease, 523
Choriocarcinoma, Hb F in, 74t, 197
Chromatin, structure of, globin gene expression and, 193–194
Circulation, coronary, oxygen affinity and, 109
Cirrhosis, hepatic, 2,3-DPG in, 107t
  oxygen transport and, 111
Clam(s). See *Artarte; Cardita*.
Cloning, gene, *266*, 267–268, *268*
Coagulation, abnormalities in, in sickle cell disease, 515
Codons, globin mRNA usage of, *182–183*, 183–184
  mRNA, for amino acids, 171t
Congenital Heinz body hemolytic anemia (CHBA), 565–593
  alpha helix disruption and, 572–573
  beta chain amino acid substitutions in, 566–567, *567*, 572, *572*
  clinical manifestations of, 579–581
  heme group displacement in, 575–576, *576*, *577*
  hemichrome formation in, *574*, 574–575
  hemoglobin denaturation in, 573–576, *574*
  hemoglobin denaturation tests in, 582–584, 583t, *584*
  hemoglobin instability and, 566–567, *567*, *572*, 572–573
  hemoglobin variants and, 568–571t
  hemolysis in, 576–577
  inheritance of, 579–580
  interior subunit substitutions in, 573
  laboratory diagnosis of, 581–586, *582*, *583*, 583t, *584–586*
  oxygen equilibria in, *585*, 585–586
  pathogenesis of, 566–579, *567*, 568–571t, *572*, *574*, *576*, *577*
  physical findings in, 581
  presentation of, 580–581
  red cell life span in, 581, *582*
  red cell morphology in, 581–582, *583*
  reticulocyte number in, 581, *582*
  splenectomy in, 586–587, *587*
  treatment of, 586–587, *587*
Contrast media, hemoglobin oxygen affinity and, 98
Cooperativity, of hemoglobin subunits, 48–51, *49*
  models of, 51–57
Crocodilians, hemoglobins of, 152, *152*
  bicarbonate ion regulation of, 152, *152*
Crystallography, x-ray, 19–20
Cucumaria minata, hemoglobin of, *137*, 140
Cyanate, hemoglobin oxygen affinity and, 98
Cyanmethemoglobin, absorption spectra of, 4, *5*
Cyanosis, 649, 649t
  differential diagnosis of, 649t
  familial, 623–633
    clinical manifestations of, 629–631, *630*, *631*
Cyclostome(s), hemoglobins of, *141*, 141–142
Cyprinus carpio. See *Carp*.
Cytochrome b_5 reductase, 647, *647*
  electrophoretic mobilities of, 652, *652*
Cytochrome b_5 reductase deficiency. See *Methemoglobinemia, congenital*.

D_1 trisomy, Hb F and, 72, 196
Dactylitis, acute, in sickle cell disease, *517*, 517–518
Davy, Sir Humphrey, 2
Delta beta thalassemia, 339
  Chinese, gene deletion in, 256
  clinical features of, 338
  gamma globin gene control and, 253–256

Delta beta thalassemia (*Continued*)
  gene deletion in, 250–251, *250*
  gene mapping of, 249–251, *250*
  globin mRNA analysis in, 240–242, *241*
  Hb A_2 in, 65t, 66, 327t, 334, 338
  Hb F in, 69, 72, *73*, 327t, 334, 338
  Mediterranean, gene mapping in, 254, *254*
  molecular hybridization results in, 242
  Sardinian, nondeletion, 251
  Sicilian, gene mapping in, 254, *254*
  Spanish, gene deletion in, 256
    gene mapping in, 254, *254*
Delta chain(s), of Hb A_2, 63–65t
  structure of, 18
  variants of, 392t
Delta thalassemia, beta thalassemia and, 339
  clinical features of, 345
  Hb A_2 and, 65t, 339, 345
  Hb F and, 339
  molecular basis of, 288
  primate distribution of, 288
Deoxyhemoglobin, 2,3-DPG binding to, 46, *46*
  site for, *28*, 46–47
  absorption spectra of, 4, *5*
  alpha and beta subunits of, contacts of, 24–25
  alpha chains of, interaction of, 26, *27*
  beta chains of, salt bridges of, 26, *27*
  Bohr proton assignments to, 41–42
  carbon dioxide binding of, 42–44, *43*
  carbon monoxide addition to, 53
  chemical properties of, 47t
  chloride binding to, *44*, 44–45
  dissociation of, 25–26
  electron density map of, *28*
  functional properties of, 47t
  heme group distances of, 23t
  heme-heme interactions of, 32, *33*, 34
  iron atoms of, 31, *31*
  isoelectric focusing of, *667*
  physical properties of, 47t
  structure of, 20
    three-dimensional, *21*, *22*
  vs. oxyhemoglobin, 47–48, 47t
Deoxyhemoglobin S, fiber-crystal transition of, *460*, 460–461
Desferrioxamine, in thalassemia management, 354–356, *355*
Diabetes, glycosylated hemoglobins and, 82
  Hb A_{1c} in, oxygen dissociation curve and, 79, *79*
Diffraction, x-ray, principles of, 20
DiGuglielmo's disease. See *Erythroleukemia.*
2,3-Diphosphoglycerate (2,3-DPG), acid-base balance and, 110, 110t
  acute asthma and, 109
  binding site of, *28*, 46
    sickling inhibition at, 491
  chronic obstructive pulmonary disease and, 108–109
  deoxyhemoglobin binding of, 46, 46–47
  exercise and, 112
  Hb F and, 113, 113t
  Hb F oxygen affinity and, 70–71, *71*
  hemoglobin oxygen affinity and, 44–47, *45*, *46*, *96*, 96–97, *97*
  hepatic cirrhosis and, 111
  high altitude exposure and, 107, *108*
  hyperphosphatemia and, 110–111
  hypophosphatemia and, 110–111
  in anemia, 106, 107t
  in CHBA, 586

2,3-Diphosphoglycerate (2,3-DPG) (*Continued*)
  in diabetes, 78–80, *79*
  in high affinity variants, 605
  in mammalian erythrocytes, 141, *141*
  in stored blood, 113–115, *114*
  mammalian hemoglobin regulation by, 154–158, *155*, *156*, 157t, *158*
  mammalian variation in, *155*, 155–157, *156*, 157t
  metabolic control of, 98–105, *99*, *100*, 101t, *102–104*
  normal levels of, 96
  oxyhemoglobin binding of, *46*, 46–47
  panhypopituitarism and, 112
  pregnancy and, 112
  prematurity and, 113
  regulation of, 99–103, *100–102*, 101t
  renal failure and, 111
  stored blood and, 113–115, *114*
  structure of, 45–46, *46*
  thyroid hormone and, 112
DNA, Alu I family of, 287
  hyperpolymorphic regions of, 190, *190*
  intergene, Alu I family sequences of, 186–187, *187*
    Kpn I family of, 187, *187*
  of globin genes, 185–190, *186*, *187*, *189*, *190*
  sequence variability of, 188–190, *189*, *190*
  simple sequence DNA in, 188
  Kpn I family of, 201
  methylation of, gene expression and, 192–193
cDNA, alpha chain specific, 234, *235*
  beta chain specific, 234, *235*
DNA sequencing, 269
DNase I hypersensitivity, globin gene expression and, 193–194
Douglas, C. G., 6
Down's syndrome, Hb F and, 72, 196
DPG, in bullfrog hemoglobin, 150
2,3-DPG. See *2,3-Diphosphoglycerate.*

Ear(s), abnormality of, in sickle cell disease, 531
Echinoderm, hemoglobins of, 139–140
Elasmobranchs, hemoglobins of, *141*, 142
Electron paramagnetic resonance (EPR), of high affinity variants, 606–607
Electrophoresis, hemoglobin, in CHBA, 584–585
Embiotoca lateralis. See *Sea perch.*
Embryonic hemoglobin(s), 67, 67–68, *68*
  genes for, 172–175, *174*
  Hb F and, 67, *67*, *68*
  in alpha thalassemia, 332–333
  post-translational modifications of, 82–84
Endocrine disorders, oxygen transport and, 111–112
EPR. See *Electron paramagnetic resonance.*
Epsilon chain(s), structure of, 18
Erythrocruorin(s), 134–140, *136–138*
  Chironomus, *136*
  in lower phyla, 135
Erythrocyte(s), oxygen affinity of, 115–117, *117*
Erythrocytosis, differential diagnosis of, 612t
  familial, oxygen affinity in, *599*
  secondary, hemoglobin variants and, 596–597t
  treatment of, 613
Erythroid cell. See *Cell(s), erythroid.*
Erythroleukemia, 74t
  Hb A_2 in, 66
  Hb F in, 74
  Hb H disease in, 262–263, 329–330

Erythropoiesis, fetal-adult hemoglobin switch and, 197
Erythropoietin, hypoxia and, 110
Eudistylia, chlorocruorin of, *137*, *138*, 140
Euzonus, hemoglobin of, *138*
Exercise, 2,3-DPG and, 112
  oxygen transport and, 112
Exon shuffling, 178
Eyes, abnormalities of, in sickle cell disease, 530–531

F thalassemia. See *Delta beta thalassemia*.
Ferroprotoporphyrin IX. See *Heme*.
Fetal hemoglobin. See *Hb F*.
Fetus, oxygen dissociation curve in, 112–113
Fingerprinting, globin peptide analysis by, 15, *15*
Fischer, Hans, 4
Fish, bony. See *Teleosts*.
  catostomid, oxygen transportation of, temperature and, 148
  hemoglobins of, ATP binding site of, *145*
  teleost, oxygen transportation in, temperature and, 148–149
    swim bladder of, 146–147, *147*

G-6-PD deficiency, sickle cell anemia and, 512
Gallstones, in sickle cell disease, 523
Gamma chain(s), structure of, 18
  variants of, 392t
    CHBA and, 568t
Gamma delta beta thalassemia, 339–340
  clinical features in, 344–345
  gene mapping of, *250*, 251–252
Gamma thalassemia, clinical features of, 345
  gene mapping in, 251–252
Gene cloning, *266*, 267–268, *268*
Gene mapping, 246–267
  procedure for, 246–248, *247*
Genes, expression of, 169–171, *170*
  globin. See *Globin genes*.
  replacement of, in sickle cell disease, 548
  in thalassemia, 303–305
Gibbs, Willard, 5, 97
Gibbs-Donnan law, 97
Gibson, Quentin, 53, 54
Gillespie, Elizabeth, 453
Globin, heme linkage of, 29–30, *30*
  polypeptide chains of, *15–17*, 15–18
  synthesis of, heme synthesis and, 205, 207, *207*
Globin chain(s), alpha, heme deficiency and, 208
  inclusion bodies of, 324
  assembly of, in thalassemia, 228–229
  beta, heme deficiency and, 209
    structural variants of, 298–299
  bone marrow synthesis of, 226–228
  synthesis of, initiation of, in thalassemia, 229–230
    thalassemia and, *225*, 225–228, *226*
  termination of, in thalassemia, 230
Globin gene(s), 173–190
  adult expression of, 196–198
  alpha, cloned, 288
    codon 125 substitution mutation in, 285–286
    deletions of, 263–264, *264*, *265*
    initiation codon mutation in, 287
    IVS-1 deletion mutation in, 285, *286*
    organization of, *174*
    sequence analysis of, 284–288, 285t, *286*

Globin gene(s) (*Continued*)
  alpha 1, partial deletion of, 287–288
  ancestral, *204*, 204–205
  beta, intervening sequence mutations in, 282–284
    IVS-1 mutation in, *272*, 272–276, *273*
    IVS-2 mutation in, 276, *277*, 278
    nonsense mutations in, *280*, 280–282, *282*
    polyadenylation signal mutation in, 279
    remote mutations and, 279–280
    transcription mutations in, 271t, 278–279
  chromosomal localization of, 172–173
  chromosomal organization of, 173–175, *174*, 201, *202*
  coding sequences of, 181–185, *182*, *183*
  deletions of, mechanisms of, 263–265, *264*, *265*, 267
    prenatal diagnosis of, 291
  evolution of, 201–209, *202*, *203*, *204*, *207*
    trees for, 202–203, *203*
  evolutionary considerations of, 201–209
  exon-intron junctions of, 177–178
  expression of, 190–200
    chromatin structure and, 193–194
    deletions and, 253–256, *254*
    DNA methylation and, 192–193
    DNase I sensitivity and, 193–194
    HMG 14 and, 193, 195
    HMG 17 and, 193, 195
    nuclear matrix and, 194–195
    regulation of, 192–196
    trans-acting factors and, 195
  expression tests of, *170*, 269–271
  fetal expression of, 196–198
  fine structure of, 175–190
  in beta thalassemia, 271–284, *272*, *273*, 274t, *275*, *277*, *280*, *282*
  intergene distances of, 174
  intergene DNA of, 185–190, *186*, *187*, *189*, *190*
  intervening sequences of, *175*, 175–179, 176t, *177*
    size of, 176t
  manipulation of expression, in thalassemia management, 358–359
  mutations in, in beta$^+$ thalassemia, *272*, 272–273, *273*, 276, 277
    in beta^o thalassemia, 274–276, 274t, *275*
  non-alpha, deletion of, 264–265
    organization of, 174, *174*
  non-alpha globin, origins of, *204*, 204–205
  number of, 172
  organization of, 172, *173*
  preserved sequences in, 179
  psi beta 1, 204–205
  restriction-site polymorphisms of, *188*, 188–189
  RNA of, biogenesis of, 190–192
  tRNA isoacceptor species and, 184
  3' untranslated sequences of, *180*, 181
  5' untranslated sequences of, 180, *180*
  zeta, 174
Globin mRNA. See *RNA*.
Globin pseudogenes, 173–175, *174,* 185, 201, *202*
Glycera, hemoglobin of, *136*
  oxygen binding curve in, *137*
Glycera dibranchiata, hemoglobin of, 135, *136*, *137*
Glycolysis, 2,3-DPG synthesis and, 99, 100
Glycosylated hemoglobin(s), affinity chromatography for, 80, *81*, 81t
  biosynthesis of, 77–78, *78*
  colorimetric analysis of, 81
  electrophoretic analysis of, 81
  functional properties of, 78–79, *79*
  hyperglycemia and, 82

Glycosylated hemoglobins (*Continued*)
  immunologic assays for, 81
  in diabetes, *81*, 81t
  ion-exchange chromatography for, 80
  measurement methods for, 76, 77t, 79t, 80–82, *81*, 81t
  structural studies of, 75–77, *77*, 77t
Graves' disease, oxygen transport and, 111
Growth, impairment of, in sickle cell disease, 513–514, *514*
GTP. See *Guanosine triphosphate.*
Guanosine triphosphate (GTP), in fish erythrocytes, 145, *145*, 147

Hahn, Vernon, 453
Haldane, J. B. S., 6, 507, 663
  John Scott, 4, *6*, 10, 663–665
Ham, Thomas Hale, 454
Hamburger effect, 40, *41*
Haplotype, analysis of, 189, 268, *269*
Harris, John, 455
Harvey, William, 1
Haurowitz, Felix, 8
Hb A, 62t
  A_{Ic} conversion of, 78
  Bohr effect of, 71–72, *72*
  Hb F switch to, 196–197
  Hb S and, 467
  oxygen affinity of, 2,3-DPG and, 70, *71*
    chloride ion and, 70, *71*
  oxygen dissociation of, *55*
  solubility of, 423t
  subunit dissociation of, *608*
  viscosity of, 472, *473*
  vs. Hb F, 70
Hb A_2, 61–67, *62*, 62t, 63t, 64t, 65t, *66*
  acquired disorders and, 65t, 66
  congenital disorders and, 64–66, 65t
  functional properties of, 62, 64
  globin subunit structure of, 63–65t
  Hb S and, 467
  measurement of, 64
  structure of, 61–62, 63t
Hb Abraham-Lincoln, red cell morphology in, 581–582, *583*
Hb AC, 422
Hb A_{Ia}, 62t
Hb A_{Ia1}, oxygen affinity of, 79
  structure of, 76–77, *77*
Hb A_{Ia2}, oxygen affinity of, 79
  structure of, 76–77, *77*
Hb A_{Ib}, 62t
Hb A_{Ic}, 62t
  blood-glucose concentration and, 78
  from Hb A, 78
  in diabetes, 78–79
  oxygen affinity of, 78–79
  structure of, 77
Hb anti-Lepore, 297–298
  genetic basis of, 417
Hb Bart's, 62t
  gene deletion in, *243*, 244, *244*, *245*, 257, 258–259
  hydrops fetalis and, 243–244, *244*
    clinical features of, *332*, 332–333
Hb Bethesda, oxygen binding curve of, *603*
Hb Boyle Heights, genetic basis of, 412t
Hb Bristol, base substitution of, 406, 407t

Hb C, 404t, *421*, 421–425, 422t, 423t
  beta thalassemia with, 343, 422
  detection of, 421–422
  geographical distribution of, *421*
  solubility of, 423t
Hb CC, 422–423, 422t
  cation leak and, 424
  cell dehydration and, 424, *425*
  intracellular crystallization of, 423
  oxygen affinity and, 424–425
Hb Constant Spring, 299–301, *330*
  biosynthetic studies of, 411, 413
  clinical features of, 331–332
  clinical significance of, 414
  genetic basis of, *182*, 242, *243*, 407–408, 408t
  molecular basis of, *182*, 299–301
Hb Coventry, genetic basis of, 412t
Hb Cranston, 301
  biosynthetic studies of, 413
  clinical significance of, 414
  genetic basis of, 410
  oxygen affinity of, 413
Hb D, 425
Hb D–Los Angeles, 404t, 425
Hb D–Punjab, 425
Hb Dakar, genetic basis of, 411
Hb E, 276, 298, 404t, 425–427, *426*
  beta thalassemia and, 343, 426–427
  biosynthesis of, 427
  electrophoresis of, 427
  in Southeast Asia, 426
  mRNA metabolism with, 298–299
  mRNA splicing with, *275*, 276
  properties of, 427
Hb E trait, 426
Hb Edmonton, base substitution of, 406
Hb F, 62t, 68–75, *69*, *71*, *72*, *73*, 74t, 338
  adult production of, 198–200
  and embryonic hemoglobins, 67, *67*, 68
  Bohr effect of, 71–72, *72*
  detection of, 72
  2,3-DPG and, 113, 113t
  genetic heterogeneity of, 69
  Hb S and, 467
  Hb sickling and, 485
  hereditary persistence of. See *Hereditary persistence of Hb F.*
  in mammals, 159–160, 159t, *160*
  measurement of, 72, *72*
  normal levels of, 72–73, *73*, 348
  oxygen affinity of, 70–72, *71*, *72*, 113, 113t
    chloride ion and, 70, *71*
    2,3-DPG and, 70, *71*
  post-translational modifications of, 69
  Saudi sickle cell anemia and, 349–350
  sickle cell disease and, 541
  structure of, 68–70, *69*
    three-dimensional, 70
  switch to Hb A, 196–197
  synthesis of, in sickle cell disease, 548, *549*
  vs. Hb A, 70
Hb F-Poole, 405
Hb F-Sardinia, 69
Hb F_I, 62t, 83
Hb FM–Osaka, 405
Hb Freiburg, absorption spectra of, *574*
  genetic basis of, 412t
Hb G–Coushatta, 404t
Hb G–Galveston, 404t

Hb G–Szuhu, 404t
Hb Gower-1, 62t, 67, *67*
Hb Gower-2, 62t, 67, *67*
Hb G–Philadelphia, alpha thalassemia and, 262t, 344
Hb Grady, biosynthetic studies of, 413
    genetic basis of, 410, 412t, 415
    oxygen affinity of, 413
Hb Gun Hill, genetic basis of, 412t, 414–415, *415*
Hb H, 62t, 427
Hb H disease, acquired, clinical features of, 329–331
    molecular basis of, 262–263
    alpha globin gene deletion in, *243–245*, 244
    beta chain proteolysis in, 227
    clinical features of, 329
    gene deletion in, 259
    globin chain synthesis in, 226, *226*
    hemoglobin electrophoresis in, *330*
    in myeloproliferative disorders, 262–263, 329–331
    inclusion bodies in, 326, *326*
    mental retardation with, 263, 331
    mRNA in, 242
    pathophysiology of, 331
    with beta thalassemia, 342
    with Hb Constant Spring, 331
Hb Hasharon, 461
Hb I, 427–428
    electrophoresis of, *405*
    gene conversion with, 262
Hb Icaria, 299–300
    genetic basis of, 408, 408t
Hb Indianapolis, 299, 342, 419
Hb J–Kurosh, base substitution of, 406
Hb K–Woolwich, 404t
Hb Kansas, 614, 615t, 616
Hb Kempsey, 602, *602*
    oxygen dissociation of, time course of, *55*
    oxygen equilibrium of, *605*
    subunit dissociation of, *608*
Hb Kenya, 172, 254
    genetic basis of, 417
    globin genes in, 255
    HPFH and, 347
Hb Knossos, 276, 298
    silent beta thalassemia and, 339
Hb Köln, 413
    base substitution in, 405, *406*
Hb Korle–Bu, 404t, 427
Hb Koya Dora, 299–300
    genetic basis of, 408, 408t
Hb Leiden, 299
    genetic basis of, 412t
Hb Lepore, 172, 297–298, 340
    beta thalassemia intermedia with, 341, 341t
    clinical features of, 340
    electrophoresis of, *330*
    gene deletion in, *250*, 297
    genetic basis of, 297–298, *416*, 416–417
Hb Lepore trait, 334
Hb Lepore–Boston, 297
    genetic basis of, 416
Hb Lepore–Washington, 297
Hb Lincoln Park, genetic basis of, 412t, 417
Hb Little Rock, oxygen binding of, 605
Hb Lyon, genetic basis of, 412t
Hb M's, 623–633
    absorption spectra of, *630*
    diagnosis of, 629–630, *630*
    electrofocusing patterns of, *631*
    electrophoresis of, 629–630, *630*

Hb M's (*Continued*)
    heme oxidation in, 628
    physical-chemical studies of, 628–629
    structure-function of, 624–629, *626*, *627*
    substituted sites in, 624, *624*
    treatment of, 630
    vs. congenital methemoglobinemia, 630
    x-ray crystallography of, 625–628, *627*
Hb M–Boston, 626t
    x-ray analysis of, *627*
Hb M–Hyde Park, 626t
    heme oxidation in, 628
Hb M–Iwate, 626t
Hb M–Milwaukee, 626t
    base substitution of, 406, 407t
Hb M–Saskatoon, 626t
    electrofocusing pattern of, *631*
Hb McKees Rocks, genetic basis of, 412t, 415–416
Hb Memphis, sickle cell disease and, 538
Hb Miyada, genetic basis of, 417
Hb New York, 302
Hb Niteroi, genetic basis of, 412t
Hb North Shore, 299
Hb O–Arab, 404t
Hb P–Congo, 417
Hb P–Nilotic, genetic basis of, 417
Hb Parchman, genetic basis of, 417
Hb Petah Tikva, 301
Hb Philly, 573
Hb Portland, 62t, 67, 174
Hb Porto Alegre, 404t
    polymerization in, 151
Hb Q, alpha thalassemia with, 343–344
Hb Quong Sze, 285–286, 299, 301, 419, 579
Hb S. See *Sickle hemoglobin*.
Hb S/D–Los Angeles disease, 537–538
Hb S/HPFH disease, 538–539
Hb S/Lepore disease, 538
Hb S/O–Arab disease, 538
Hb Sabine, 413
Hb San Diego, base substitution in, 405, *406*
Hb Saverne, genetic basis of, 410
Hb SC, 422
Hb SC disease, 533, 536, *536*
Hb Seal Rock, 299–300
    genetic basis of, 408, 408t
Hb Siriraj, 404t
Hb St. Antoine, genetic basis of, 412t
Hb Suan-Dok, 301
Hb Sydney, base substitution of, 407t
Hb Syracuse, electrofocusing pattern of, *613*
    oxygen binding of, 605
Hb Tak, 301
    clinical significance of, 414
    genetic basis of, 409–410
    oxygen affinity of, 413
Hb Tampa, 404t
Hb Titusville, 615t, 616
Hb Tochigi, genetic basis of, 412t
Hb Tours, genetic basis of, 412t
Hb Trout–I, *143*, 143–144
    oxygen affinity in, 143, *143*
    Root effect of, *143*
Hb Trout–IV, *143*, 144–145
    oxygen affinity in, *143*, 144
Hb Vicksburg, 299
    genetic basis of, 412t
Hb Wayne, 300–301
    biosynthetic studies of, 413
    clinical significance of, 414

Hb Wayne (*Continued*)
  genetic basis of, 408t, 409
  oxygen affinity of, 413
Hb Zürich, 580
  CHBA and, 567, 572, *572*
HCG. See *Human chorionic gonadotropin.*
Hearing loss, in sickle cell disease, 531
Heart, size of, sickle cell disease and, 520, *521*
Heart disease, congenital, 2,3-DPG in, 109
    oxygen transport and, 109
  sickle cell disease and, 520–522, *521*
Heart failure, congestive, oxygen transport and, 109
Heinz body, 324
Heinz body hemolytic anemia, congenital, 565–593
Helisoma, hemoglobin of, *138*
Helix pomatia, hemocyanin structure in, *131*
Hematin, 29
Hematuria, in sickle cell disease, 524–526, *525*
Heme, 27, *29*, 29–30, *30*, 205–207
  biosynthesis of, globin synthesis and, 205, 207, *207*
  deficiency of, globin chain synthesis and, 208
  dissociation of, in CHBA, 575–576, *576*, *577*
  globin binding of, 29–30, *30*
  iron atom of, *31*, 31–32
  oxygen-iron linkage of, 32
  synthesis of, 29, 205–207, *207*
    disorders of, 207–208
    mitochondrial localization of, 205, *207*
Hemerythrin, 127, *129*, 129–130, 129t, *130*
  color of, 129t, 130
  in animal kingdom, *128*
  molecular weight of, 129t
  myohemerythrin and, 130
  oxygen binding of, 129–130, *130*
  structure of, quaternary, 129, *129*
  subunits of, 129t
    analysis of, 129, *129*
Hemichrome, formation of, in CHBA, 574, *574*–575
Hemin, 29
  in CHBA, 586
  polypeptide chain synthesis and, 209
  protein synthesis and, 209
Hemocyanin, 127, 129t, 130–134
  arthropod, 130, *131*
  Callianassa californiensis, oxygen affinity of, 133–134, *134*
  color of, 129t
  Hill plots of, *134*
  in animal kingdom, *128*
  Limulus, absorption spectra of, 132, *132*
    oxygen affinity of, 133, *133*
    oxygen binding site of, 132, *132*
  molecular weight of, 129t
  mollusc, *131*, 132
  oxygen affinity of, 132–133, *133*
  structure of, quaternary, 130, *131*, 132
  subunits of, 129t
Hemoglobin, acetaldehyde adducts of, 83
  acetylated, 83
  adult, fetal switch to, 196–197
  Agnatha, *141*, 141–142
  allosteric models of, 51–57, *52*
  alpha chains of, carbon dioxide interaction with, 43–44
  alpha helix component of, 18–19, *19*
  arthropod, 139
  as reporter molecule, 83–84
  autoxidation of, 640–641, 641t

Hemoglobin (*Continued*)
  beta chains of, carbon dioxide interaction with, 43–44
  biosynthesis of, 169–222
  bony fish, 142–149, *143*, 143t, *144–148*
  carbamylated, 82
  carbon dioxide binding of, 42–44, *43*
  cysteine content of, 7
  denaturation of, 577, *577*
    cyanide inhibition of, 576, *576*
    heme ligands and, 576, *576*
    in CHBA, 573–576, *574*, *576*
  denaturation rates of, 6
  dimer dissociation of, 48
  2,3-DPG binding to, 44–47, *45*, *46*
    site for, *28*, 46–47
  2,3-DPG regulation of, 154–158, *155*, *156*, 157t, *158*
  echinoderm, 139–140
  elasmobranch, *141*, 142
  electrophoresis of, 584–585
  embryonic. See *Embryonic hemoglobin(s).*
  erythrocruorin, 134–140, *136–138*
  fetal. See *Hb F.*
  fetal-adult switch of, 196–198
  function of, 37–60
  Glycera, *136*
  glycosylated, *75–79*, 75–82, 77t, *81*, 81t. See also *Glycosylated hemoglobin(s).*
  heme-heme interactions of, 32, *33*, 34
  high-affinity variants of, 600–601t. See also *Erythrocytosis.*
    clinical manifestations of, 611–614, 612t, *613*
    diagnosis of, 611–614, 612t, *613*
    electron paramagnetic resonance of, 606–607
    ligand binding of, 605–606
    molecular pathogenesis of, 599–603, *602*
    nuclear magnetic resonance of, 606–607
    physiological aspects of, *609*, 609–610, 609t, *610*
    properties of, 603–614
    structural alterations in, *602*, 602–603
    subunit interactions in, 607–608, *608*
    x-ray crystallography of, 606
  Hill plot of, 49, *49*
  human, electrophoretic comparison of, 400–401, *402*
    variants of, 382–399t. See also *Hemoglobin variants.*
      alphabetized, 395–399t
      clinically important, 403t
  in animal kingdom, *128*
  in lower phyla, 135
  invertebrate, 127–140
    electron micrographs of, *138*
  kinetics of, 53, 55–56
  low affinity variants of, 614–616, 615t
  molecular evolution of, 160–162, *161*, 202–205, *203*
  molecular genetics of, 169–222
  molecular weight of, 6
  molluscan, 138
  noncooperative, 50
  oxygen affinity of. See *Oxygen affinity.*
  phylogenetic tree of, *161*, *203*
  polypeptide chains of, 13–18, *15–17*
  protein structure of, 7–8
  solubilities of, 7
  structure of, 4–8, *5–7*

Hemoglobin (*Continued*)
  structure of, isomorphous replacement method for, 20
    primary, 12–18, *15–17*
    quaternary, 19–34, *21–31, 33, 34*
      relaxed (R), 20
      tense (T), 20
    tertiary, 19–34, *21–31, 33, 34*
    three-dimensional, 8, *21*
  subunit cooperativity of, 48–51, *49*
  subunits of, interaction of, 21–27, *21–27*, 23t
  sulfhydryl groups of, 48
  thermodynamic analyses of, 50–51
  unstable variants of, biosynthesis of, 577–579, 578t
    CHBA and, 565–593
    denaturation tests for, 582–584, 583t, *584*
  viscosity of, 93
Hemoglobin subunits, social behavior of, *419*
Hemoglobin variants, assembly of, *417*, 417–421, *418, 419, 420*, 420t
  chain termination codon mutations and, 407–409, 408t
  CHBA and, 565–593
  distribution of, *418*
  due to chain termination mutation, 407–409, 408t
  due to deletions, 394t
  due to extended chains, 393–394t
  due to fusion subunits, 393t, *416*, 416–417
  due to multiple point mutations, 394t
  due to single base substitutions, 405–407, 406t, 407t
  elongated subunits of, 407–414, 407t, 408t, 413t
  genetic basis of, 403–417
  mendelian inheritance of, *403*, 403–405, 404t, *405*
  shortened subunits of, 414–416, *415*
  spontaneous mutation and, 404
Hemoglobinuria, nocturnal, paroxysmal, Hb F in, 74t
Hemolysis, in CHBA, 576–577
Hendersen, L. J., 11
Hepatoma, Hb F in, 74t
Hereditary persistence of Hb F, 72, *73*, 240–242, *241*
  clinical features of, 345–350
  deletion-type, 252
  gamma globin gene control and, 255
  gene deletion and, 253–254
  gene mapping of, 252–253
  Greek type, 290, *290*
  Hb Kenya and, 347
  Hb S and, 538–539
  heterocellular, 348–350, 539
    Atlanta-type, 349
    British-type, 349
    Georgia-type, 349
    Seattle-type, 349
    Swiss-type, 348–349
  in blacks, 345–347
  in Greeks, 347–348
  Indian-type, gene deletion in, 256
  molecular hybridization in, 242
  nondeletion, molecular basis of, 252–253, 289–290, *290*
  pancellular, 345–346, 538
  sickle cell disease and, 534t, 541
Hexokinase, deficiency of, 2,3-DPG in, 107
  oxygen transport and, 117, *117*
Hibernation, O_2 affinity and, 159
High mobility group. See *HMG*.

Hill, Archibald Vivian, 10, *10*, 48, 49
Hill equation, 10, 49
Hip, avascular necrosis of, in sickle cell disease, 528, *529*
HMG 14, globin gene expression and, 193, 195
HMG 17, globin gene expression and, 193, 195
Hoppe-Seyler, Felix, 2, *4*
Horse, methemoglobin of, *136*
Horseshoe crab. See *Limulus polyphemus*.
HPFH. See *Hereditary persistence of Hb F*.
Human chorionic gonadotropin (HCG), Hb F and, 197
Hybridization assay, for globin mRNA, 234–236, *235, 236*
  procedure for, 234, *235*
Hydatidiform mole, Hb F in, 73, 74t
Hydrops fetalis, Hb Bart's and, 243–244, *244, 332*, 332–333
Hyperbaric environment, hemoglobin oxygen affinity and, 98
Hyperlipemia, oxygen transport and, 111
Hyperlipoproteinemia, familial, oxygen transport and, 111
Hyperphosphatemia, oxygen transport and, 110–111
Hyperthyroidism, Hb A_2 in, 65t, 66
  oxygen transport and, 111
Hypertransfusion, in thalassemia, 352–353
Hyponatremia, in sickle cell disease, 547
Hypophosphatemia, oxygen transport and, 110–111
Hypoxemia, chronic, 2,3-DPG levels and, 105
  in sickle cell disease, 522
  oxygen transport and, 116, *116*
Hypoxia, 2,3-DPG and, *104*, 104–105
  erythropoietin levels and, 110
  O_2 affinity and, in humans, 158
  oxygen transport and, 105–110, *106*, 107t, *108*

IgG, sickle cell anemia and, 512
Immunization, pediatric, in sickle cell disease, 542
Inclusion body, 324–326, *325, 326*
Infarction, bone, in sickle cell disease, 518, *518*
  myocardial, oxygen transport and, 109
Infection, in sickle cell disease, 512–513
Infection(s), *Salmonella*, in sickle cell disease, 528–529
Ingram, Vernon, 452, 455
Inosine, red cell, 2,3-DPG production and, 114, *114*
Inositol pentaphosphate, in avian hemoglobin, 153
Inositol tetraphosphate, in avian hemoglobin, 153
Intervening sequences, *175*, 175–179, *177*
  explanations for, 178
  size of, 176t
  splicing of, 176–178, *177*
Intron. See *Intervening sequences*.
Invertebrates, hemoglobin of, electron micrographs of, *138*
  oxygen binding curves in, *137*
Iron, chelation of, in thalassemia management, 354–356, *355*
  elemental, 31
  ferric, 31
  ferrous, 31
  in heme, *31*, 31–32
Iron deficiency, 2,3-DPG in, 107t
  Hb A_2 in, 65t, 66
  sickle cell anemia and, 512
Iron deficiency anemia, treatment of, Hb F and, 75
  vs. beta thalassemia, 333, 333t

Jaundice, in sickle cell disease, 522–523

Kala-azar, Hb F in, 74t
Kidney, tubular function of, in sickle cell disease, 523–525, *524*
Kidney failure. See *Renal failure.*
Kinetics, hemoglobin, 53, 55–56
Kpn I, repetitive DNA sequences of, 187, *187*
Krogh, August, *8*, 39

Lamprey, hemoglobin of, *136*, *141*, 141–142
    structure of, 142
Lavoisier, Antoine Laurent, 2, *3*
Lehmann, Hermann, 380
Leukemia, 2,3-DPG in, 107t
    acute, Hb F in, 74t
    myeloid, chronic, Hb F in, 74t
Limulus, hemocyanin of, absorption spectra of, 132, *132*
    oxygen affinity of, 133, *133*
    oxygen binding site of, 132, *132*
Limulus polyphemus, hemocyanin structure in, 130, *131*
London, Irving M., 206, *206*
Lower, Richard, 1, *2*
Lumbricus terrestris, hemoglobin of, 135
Lung(s), cancer of, Hb F in, 74t
    damage to, in sickle cell disease, 522

Magnesium, red cell, 2,3-DPG and, 103, *103*
Malaria, falciparum, Hb S and, *507*, 507–508, *508*
    Old World distribution of, *505*
    Hb A_2 in, 66
Malocclusion, dental, in sickle cell disease, 528, *528*
Malpighi, Marcello, 1
Mammal(s), 2,3-DPG variation in, *155*, 155–157, ·*156*, 157t
    Hb F in, 159–160, 159t, *160*
    hemoglobins of, 154–162, *155*, *156*, 157t, *158*, 159t, *160*, *161*
    2,3-DPG regulation of, 154–158, *155*, *156*, 157t, *158*
    high altitude adaptation of, 158, *158*
    phylogenetic tree of, *156*
    red cell O_2 affinity and, 157–158, *158*
Maniatis, Tom, 168, *168*
Maxilla, deformity of, in sickle cell disease, 528, *528*
Mean corpuscular hemoglobin concentration (MCHC), hemoglobin oxygen affinity and, 98
Megaloblastic crisis, sickle cell anemia and, 512
Mental retardation, Hb H disease in, 263
Metabolic disorders, oxygen transport and, 110–111, 110t
Methemoglobin, absorption spectra of, 4, *5*, *635*, 635–636
    chromatographic behavior of, 637–638, *638*
    cytochrome b_5 reductase and, 647–648
    electron paramagnetic resonance spectra of, 635–636
    electrophoretic behavior of, 637–638, *638*
    equine, *136*
    horse, structure of, 20, 21
    normal red cell content of, 649

Methemoglobin (*Continued*)
    oxygen binding and, 637–638, *638*
    properties of, *635*, 635–638, *637*, *638*
    reducing enzymes of, 646, 646t
    reduction of, 644–649, *646*, 646t, *647*, 652, *652*
        enzyme system, 644–648, *646*, 646t, *647*
        nonenzymatic, 644
        steps of, 648
    spin state of, 32
    T quaternary structure of, 467–468
    three-dimensional structure of, 636
    vs. sulfhemoglobin, 655t
Methemoglobinemia, congenital, 650–653, *652*
    2,3-DPG and, 105
    clinical features of, 651
    inheritance pattern of, 650–651
    laboratory features of, 651–653, *652*
    treatment of, 653
    vs. Hb M, 630
    vs. hemoglobin M, 630
    drug-induced, 653–654
    in reptiles, 151
    oxygen transport and, 649–650
    toxic, 653–654
    treatment of, 654
Methylation, DNA, gene expression and, 192–193
Molluscs, hemocyanins of, *131*, 132
    hemoglobins of, 139
Molpodia arenicola, hemoglobin of, 140
mRNA. See *RNA.*
Murex, hemocyanin of, 132
Mutase. See *Phosphoglycerate mutase.*
Myelofibrosis, Hb F in, 74t
Myoglobin, oxygen binding curve of, *38*, 39
    oxygen transport and, 94
    sperm whale, *136*
Myohemerythrin, hemerythrin and, 130

NADPH-flavin reductase, methemoglobin reduction and, 648–649
Nephrotic syndrome, in sickle cell disease, 526
Newborn, oxygen transport in, 113, 113t
Nitrites, hemoglobin oxidation and, 642–643
Nitrogen mustard, sickling inhibition by, 491–492, 491t
Nitroglycerin, oxygen affinity and, 110
Nitroprusside, methemoglobin and, 654
Nuclear magnetic resonance (NMR), in sickle cell disease, 477, *478*
    of high affinity variants, 606–607

Osteomyelitis, in sickle cell disease, 528
Osteopetrosis, Hb F in, 74t
Ostwald, Wolfgang, 4
Oxidation, 634–662, *639–644*, 639t, *640*, 641t, 642t, *643*
    chemical agents and, 641–644, 642t, *643*
    direct, 641–642, 642t
    indirect, 642–643, 642t
    nitrite-induced, 642–643
    redox potentials and, 638–640, 638t, *640*
Oxygen, dissociation curve of. See *Oxygen dissociation curve.*
    hemoglobin affinity for, *95*, 95–98, *96*, *97*
    2,3-DPG and, *95*, *96*, 96–97, *97*
    ATP and, 97–98

Oxygen (*Continued*)
  hemoglobin affinity for, Bohr effect and, *95*, *96*
    carbon dioxide and, 96, 97, *97*
    carboxyhemoglobin and, 98
    in clinical states, 95–96, 105–115, *106*, 107t, *108*, 110t, *113*, *114*
    MCHC and, 98
    pH and, *95*, *96*
    temperature and, *95*, 95–96
  hemoglobin binding curve of, *49*, 49–51
    temperature and, 50
Oxygen affinity, 9, 55, 94–98, *95*, *96*, *97*
  2,3-DPG and, 42–43, *43*, *97*
  abnormal, hemoglobinopathy and, 595–622
  anemia and, 158–159
  ATP and, 42–43, *43*
  carbon dioxide and, 42–43, *43*
  carboxyhemoglobin and, 98
  determinants of, *95*, 95–98, *96*, *97*
  Hb CC and, 424
  hibernation and, 159
  hypoxia and, in humans, 158
  in CHBA, *585*, 585–586
  in clinical states, 95–98, *96*, *97*, 105–115, *106*, 107t, *108*, 110t, *113*, *114*
  in mammals, 157–158, *158*
  in salamanders, 151
  in *Telmatobius culeus*, 151
  in trout hemoglobin, 143, *143*, 144
  MCHC and, 98
  pH and, 39, *40*, 42–43, *43*
  subunit interaction and, in high affinity variants, 607–608, *608*
Oxygen binding, methemoglobin and, 637–638, *638*
  of Hb M, 625, *627*
Oxygen binding curve, 2,3-DPG and, *38*, 39
  in invertebrates, *137*
  ionic strength and, *38*, 39
  pH and, *38*, 39
Oxygen dissociation curve, 37, *38*, 39, *106*
  diabetes and, 79, *79*
  glycosylated hemoglobins and, 78–79
  high altitude exposure and, 108, *108*
  in high affinity variants, 609
  right-shifted, *106*
  temperature and, 50
  time course of, 55
Oxygen equilibrium, carbon dioxide and, *667*
  in high affinity variants, *603*, 603–604, 604t, *605*
  of Hb M, 625, 626t
Oxygen saturation, arterial, in sickle cell disease, 521
Oxygen transport, 50, 91–95, *94*
  acidosis and, 110–111, 110t
  acute myocardial infarction and, 109
  alkalosis and, 110, 110t
  blood flow reduction and, 117
  Bohr effect and, 39, *40*, *41*
  cardiac disorders and, 109–110
  cardiogenic shock and, 109
  compensatory mechanisms for, 115–116
  congestive heart failure and, 109
  coronary circulation and, 109
  endocrine disorders and, 111–112
  exercise and, 112
  Fick equation for, 93–94
  Graves' disease and, 111
  hepatic cirrhosis and, 111
  hexokinase deficiency and, 117
  high altitude and, 107–108, *108*

Oxygen transport (*Continued*)
  hormones and, 112
  hyperlipoproteinemia and, 111
  hyperphosphatemia and, 110–111
  hyperthyroidism and, 111
  hypophosphatemia and, 110–111
  hypoxemia and, 116, *116*
  hypoxia and, 105–110, *106*, 107t, *108*
  in catostomid fish, 148
  in high affinity variants, 609t
  in teleost fish, 148–149
  in tuna, 148–149
  intracellular PO_2, 115
  maternal-fetal, 159–160, 159t, *160*
    in fish, 149
  metabolic disorders and, 110–111, 110t
  methemoglobin and, 649–650
  methemoglobinemia and, 649–650
  myoglobin and, 95
  PO_2 and, 95
  pregnancy and, 112
  pulmonary disease and, 108–109
  pyruvate kinase deficiency and, 117
  renal failure and, 111
  septic shock and, 109
  thyrotoxicosis and, 111–112
Oxyhemoglobin, 2,3-DPG binding to, 46, *46*
  absorption spectra of, 4, *5*
  Bohr proton assignments to, 41–42
  carbon dioxide binding of, 42–44, *43*
  chain structure of, *666*
  chemical properties of, 47t
  dissociation of, 25
  functional properties of, 47t
  heme group distances of, 23t
  heme-heme interactions of, 32, *33*, 34
  iron atoms of, 31, *31*
  oxygen CO_2 replacement in, 31
  oxygen dissociation from, 53
  physical properties of, 47t
  spin state of, 32
  structure of, three-dimensional, *21*
  vs. deoxyhemoglobin, 47–48, 47t

P_{50}, *38*, 39
Pain, crises of, in sickle cell disease, 543–544
Panhypopituitarism, 2,3-DPG and, 112
Panulirus interruptus, hemocyanin structure in, 130
Parkinson's disease, 2,3-DPG and, 112
Pauling, Linus, 7, 11, 51
Pentoxifylline, in sickle cell disease, 548
Perutz, Max, 7–8, 14, 34, 41
pH, carbamino complex formation and, 42–44, *43*
  hemoglobin oxygen affinity and, 39, *40*, *95*, *96*
Phosphoglycerate mutase, 2,3-DPG synthesis and, 100–101, 101t
  deficiency of, 102
Plasmid vector system, gene expression test by, 270
Pneumonia, vs. pulmonary infarction, 516t
PO_2, arterial, oxygen transport and, 116, *116*
  intracellular, 115
  oxygen transport and, 95
Polycythemia, 2,3-DPG levels and, 105
  high altitude exposure and, 108
Polycythemia vera, 2,3-DPG in, 107
  Hb F in, 74t
Polypeptide chains, biosynthesis of, *170*, 170–171
Prednisone, 2,3-DPG increase and, 112

Pregnancy, Hb F during, 73
  in sickle cell disease, 544–545
  oxygen transport and, 112
Prematurity, 2,3-DPG and, 113
  Hb F and, 72
Prenatal diagnosis. See *Thalassemia, prenatal diagnosis of.*
Priapism, in sickle cell disease, 526
Primer extension procedure, mRNA analysis by, 271
Proliferative sickle retinopathy. See *Retinopathy, proliferative.*
Propranolol, hemoglobin oxygen affinity and, 98
Proteins, synthesis of, 169–171, *170*
Pseudogenes, 173, 185, 201
Pulmonary disease, chronic, 2,3–DPG and, 108–109
Pyruvate kinase, deficiency of, 2,3–DPG in, 107
  oxygen transport in, 117

Rana catesbeiana. See *Bullfrog.*
Rapoport-Luebering shunt, 99, *100*
Red cell, 2,3-DPG of, metabolic control of, 98–105, 99, *100*, 101t, *102, 103, 104*
  regulation of, 99–103, *100, 101*, 101t, *102*
  aging of, 105
    anemia and, 106
  contour of, 93
  glycolytic pathway of, 99, *99*
  mass reduction in, oxygen transport and, 117, *117*
  membrane of, 2,3-DPG and, 103
  metabolism of, 99, *99*
Redox potentials, 638–640, 638t, *640*
Reichlin, Morris, 36
Renal failure, in sickle cell disease, 526
  oxygen transport and, 111
Renal tubular acidosis, in sickle cell disease, 525
Reptiles, fetal red cell O_2 affinity in, 151
  hemoglobins of, 151–154, *152*
  methemoglobinemia in, 151
Rete mirabile, of teleost fish, 146, *147*
Retinopathy, nonproliferative, in sickle cell disease, 531
  proliferative, *530*, 530–531
Rhinesmith, H. S., 7
mRNA, globin, atypical transcripts of, 191
  biogenesis of, 190–192
  cap structure of, 180
  codon usage in, *182–183*, 183–184
  electrophoretic analysis of, 245–246, *246*
  encoding sequences of, 179–185, *180, 182, 183, 184*
  functional studies of, *231*, 231–233
  in beta° thalassemia, 238–240, *239*
  nucleotide sequences of, *182–183*
  oligonucleotide fingerprint analysis of, 246, *247*
  post-transcriptional processing of, 191–192
  precursor splicing of, 176–177, *177*
  quantitative studies of, 234–246, *235–237, 239, 241, 243*
  S1 nuclease assay of, *270*, 270–271
  transcription site of, 190–191
  untranslated regions of, 180–181, *180*
tRNA, isoacceptor species of, mRNA codon usage and, 184
Root effect, in trout hemoglobin, *143*, 144
  molecular basis of, *144*, 145
Roughton, F. J. W., 10, 53

S1 nuclease assay, globin mRNA analysis by, *270*, 270–271
Salamander, oxygen affinity in, 151
Salmo gairdneri, hemoglobin of, 143
Salmo irideus, hemoglobin of, 143–144
Salmonella, infections with, in sickle cell disease, 528–529
Schroeder, Walter, 7
Sea perch, maternal-fetal O_2 transport in, 149
Serpula, chlorocruorins of, 140
Servetus, Michael, 1
Sherman, Irving, 454
Shock, cardiogenic, oxygen transport and, 109
  septic, 109
Sickle/beta thalassemia, 343, 534t, 536–537
  inheritance of, *403*
Sickle cell(s), calcium in, 489, *489*
  heterogeneity of, *474*, 474–475, *475*
  in microcirculation, 489–490
  intracellular polymerization of, 475–479, *476*, 477t, *478, 479*
  kinetics of, 479–484, *480–484*
  irreversible type of, 484–486, *485, 486*
  membrane of, 484–490, *485–489*
    Hb S and, 487–488, *488*
    lipids of, 486, *487*
    morphology of, 486–489, *487, 488, 489*
    oxidant damage to, *488*, 488–489
    protein of, 486–487
  oxygenation of, 469–470, *470*
  polymerization of, 474–484, *475, 476*, 477t, *478–484*
    inhibition of, 490–492, 491t, *492*
  sodium-potassium pump and, 489, *489*
  viscosity of, 476, *476*, 477t
Sickle cell anemia, Hb A_2 in, 65t
  Hb F in, 74
  inheritance of, *403*
  Saudi high Hb F determinant and, 349–350
Sickle cell crises, 515–516
Sickle cell disease, 502–564
  abdominal crises in, 519
  alpha chain variants and, 534t
  alpha thalassemia and, 344, 534t, 539–540, *540*
  anemia of, 511–512, 542–543
    G-6-PD deficiency and, 512
    iron deficiency and, 512
    megaloblastic crisis and, 512
    red cell IgG and, 512
    splenic sequestration in, 512
  antenatal diagnosis of, *549*, 550
  antisickling agents in, 545–548, 545t, 546t
  aplastic crisis in, 511–512
  arterial oxygen saturation and, 521
  arthritis in, 519
  5-azacytidine in, 548, *549*
  beta globin gene mutation and, 506, *506, 549*
  bone abnormalities in, 527–529, *528, 529*
  bone infarction in, 518, *518*
  cardiac damage in, 520–522, *521*
  causes of death in, 539, 539t, *540*
  cellular pathogenesis of, 453–501
  chest crises in, 516, 516t
  cholestasis in, 523
  coagulation abonormalities in, 514–515
  dactylitis in, *517*, 517–518
  differential diagnosis of, 531, 532t, 533
  early studies of, 502–503, *503*
  epidemiology of, 504–508, *505, 506, 507, 508*

Sickle cell disease (*Continued*)
  extracorporeal carbamylation in, 547
  gallstones in, 523
  gene replacement in, 548
  genitourinary damage in, 523–526, *524, 525*
  growth impairment in, 513–514, *514*
  Hb F persistence and, 534t
  hearing loss in, 531
  hematuria in, 524–526, *525*
  hemoglobin fiber structure in, 455–464, *456–459, 462,* 463t
  hemoglobin manipulation in, 548, *549*
  hepatobiliary damage in, 522–523
  hip deformity in, 528, *529*
  historical background of, 453–455
  HPFH and, 541
  hyponatremia in, 547
  infection and, 512–513
  inheritance of, 503–504, *504*
  jaundice in, 522–523
  left ventricular function in, 520–521
  lung damage in, 522
  maxillary deformity in, 528, *528*
  molecular pathogenesis of, 453–501
  musculoskeletal crises in, 516–519, *517, 518,* 519t
  nephrotic syndrome in, 526
  neurological crises in, 519–520
  NMR results in, 477, *478*
  nonproliferative retinopathy in, 531
  ocular abnormalities of, *530,* 530–531
  organ damage in, 520–533, *521, 524, 525, 528, 529*
  pain crises in, 515–516
    therapy in, 543–544
  partial exchange transfusion for, 543t
  pathogenesis of, *456*
  pediatric immunization in, 542
  pentoxifylline in, 548
  pregnancy in, 544–545
  prevention of, 550
  priapism in, 526
  prognosis for, 539–541, 539t, *540*
  renal failure in, 526
  renal tubular acidosis in, 524–525
  renal tubular function in, 523–525, *524*
  skin ulcers in, 529–530
  sodium cyanate treatment of, 546t, 547
  spinal deformity in, 528, *529*
  splenectomy in, 544
  splenic sequestration crises in, 519
  stroke in, 526–527
  sudden death in, 520
  supportive therapy for, 542–545, 543t
  surgery in, 544
  treatment of, 541–550, 543t, 545t, 546t, *549*
Sickle cell trait, clinical features of, 508–510, 509t
  diagnosis of, 510
  electrophoresis in, *330*
  NMR results in, 477
  screening for, 510
Sickle hemoglobin, 404t
  alpha thalassemia and, 344, 419, 534t, 539–540, *540*
  beta chain variants and, 535t
  beta thalassemia and, 343, 534t, 536–537
  deoxy, equilibrium of, 464–467, *466*
  Edelstein fiber model of, *462*
  electrophoresis of, *405*
  falciparum malaria and, *507,* 507–508, *508*

Sickle hemoglobin (*Continued*)
  fiber structure of, 456, *456, 457, 458*
  geographic distribution of, 504, *505*
  Hb A and, 467
  Hb A$_2$ and, 467
  Hb D and, 425
  Hb F and, 467
  intermolecular contacts of, 459–462, *461*
  non-S hemoglobins and, 462–464
  oxygen saturation of, polymerization and, 467–470, *468, 470*
  oxygenation of, 468–469
  polymerization of, 464–474, *466, 468, 470, 471*
    kinetics of, 470–472, *471, 472*
  rheology of, 472, *473,* 474
  solubility of, *460, 468,* 468
  viscosity of, 472, *473*
  x-ray diffraction of, 456, *458, 459,* 459
Sickle/beta thalassemia, 536–537, *537*
Sickling, non-SS disorders of, 533–539, 534–535t, *536, 537*
Singer, Karl, 455
Singer, Lily, 455
Skin, ulcers of, in sickle cell disease, 529–530
Snails, planorbid, hemoglobin of, 139
Sodium cyanate, in sickle cell disease treatment, 546t, 547
  sickling inhibition by, 490–491, 491t
Sodium-potassium pump, sickle cells and, 489, *489*
Sperm whale, myoglobin of, *136*
Spherocytosis, hereditary, 2,3-DPG in, 107
Spleen, enlargement of, sickle cell anemia and, 512
Splenectomy, in CHBA, 586–587, *587*
  in sickle cell disease, 544
  in thalassemia, 353–354
Splenomegaly, in sickle cell disease, 519
Splicing, defective, causing alpha thalassemia, 285, *286*
  causing beta thalassemia, 272–278, *273, 275, 277*
  of globin precursor mRNA, 176–177, *177*
Stokes, George G., 2–4, *5*
Stroke, in sickle cell disease, 526–527
Sudden death, in sickle cell disease, 520
Sulfhemoglobin, clinical features of, 656
  structure and function of, 654–657, *655,* 655t
  vs. methemoglobin, 655t
Sulfhemoglobinemia, 654–657, *655,* 655t
  acquired, 656
  arylamines and, 656
Sulfhydryl groups, hemoglobin conformation and, 48
Surgery, in sickle cell disease, 544
SV40 virus vector system, gene expression analysis by, 270
Svedberg, The, 6, *7*
Switching factor, 200
Synthase. See *Bisphosphoglycerate synthase.*

Teleosts, hemoglobins of, 142–149, *143,* 143t, *144–148*
Temperature, hemoglobin oxygen affinity and, *95,* 95–96
  oxygen dissociation curve and, 50–51
Testes, cancer of, Hb F in, 74t
Thalassemia, 223–371
  abnormal hemoglobin and, 342–345

Thalassemia (*Continued*)
  alpha. See *Alpha thalassemia*.
  Belgrade rat model of, 302
  beta. See *Beta thalassemia*.
  classification of, 327–328, 327t
  clinical manifestations of, 322–371
  delta beta. See *Delta beta thalassemia*.
  gamma. See *Gamma thalassemia*.
  gamma delta beta. See *Gamma delta beta thalassemia*.
  gene therapy for, 303–304
  globin chain assembly in, 228–229, 417–421
  globin chain initiation in, 228–230
  globin chain synthesis and, *225*, 225–228, *226*
  globin chain termination in, 230
  globin mRNA in, 234–246, *235–237*, *237*, *241*, *243*
  incidence of, *323*, 323–324
  population genetics of, *323*, 323–324
  population groups affected by, 295–297
  prenatal diagnosis of, 291–295, 293t, *294*
    denaturing gradient gel analysis for, 295
    gene mapping for, 291-292
    oligonucleotide probe analysis for, 293–295, *294*
    restriction endonuclease cleavage site test for, 292–293, 293t
  ribosome function in, 228
  sickle/beta. See *Sickle/beta thalassemia*.
Thalassemia syndromes, management of, 350–259
  bone marrow transplantation for, 357–358
  globin gene manipulation in, 358–359
  hypertransfusion regimen for, 352
  iron-chelating agents for, 354–356, *355*
  splenectomy for, 353–354
  transfusion regimens for, 351–353
  vitamin supplements in, 357
  prevention of, 350–351
Thixotrophy, 472, *473*
Thyroid hormone, 2,3-DPG and, 112
Thyrotoxicosis, Hb F in, 197–198
  oxygen transport and, 111–112
Trans-acting factors, globin gene expression and, 195

Transfusion, in sickle cell disease, 543, 543t
  in thalassemia syndromes, 351–353
Transplantation, bone marrow, in thalassemia, 357–358
Trout, hemoglobins of, *143*, 143–145, 143t, *144*, *145*
Tuna, oxygen transport in, temperature and, 148–149
Typhlonectes, oxygen affinity in, 151

Uremia, 2,3-DPG in, 107t
  carbamylated hemoglobin and, 82
  oxygen transport and, 111

Vertebrae, H-shaped deformity of, in sickle cell disease, 528, *529*
Vertebrates, hemoglobins of, 140–162, *141*, *143–149*, *152*, *154–156*
  amino acid beta chain replacements in, 143t
  mediators of, 140–141, *141*
von Hufner, Gustav, 9

Watson, Janet, 454
Weatherall, David J., 224, *224*
Worms, segmented. See *Annelids*.
Wyman, Jeffries, 36, *36*. 51, 639

Xenopus laevis, hemoglobin of, 150

Zeta chain(s), structure of, 18
Zinc chloride, hemoglobin oxygen affinity and, 98
Zinc deficiency, in sickle cell disease, 514
Zinc sulfate, sickle leg ulcers and, 530